W9-CCJ-913

PROCEDURES

Ch. 1 The Medical Record

1-1 Completion of a Consent to Treatment Form, 20
1-2 Release of Medical Information, 23
1-3 Preparing a Medical Record, 28
1-4 Obtaining and Recording Patient Symptoms, 41

Ch. 2 Medical Asepsis and the OSHA Standard

2-1 Handwashing, 56
2-2 Applying an Alcohol-Based Hand Rub, 58
2-3 Application and Removal of Clean Disposable Gloves, 59

Ch. 3 Sterilization and Disinfection

3-1 Sanitization of Instruments, 93
3-2 Chemical Disinfection of Articles, 100
3-3 Wrapping Instruments Using Paper or Muslin, 107
3-4 Wrapping Instruments Using a Pouch, 109
3-5 Sterilizing Articles in the Autoclave, 114

Ch. 4 Vital Signs

4-1 Measuring Oral Body Temperature—Electronic Thermometer, 133
4-2 Measuring Axillary Body Temperature—Electronic Thermometer, 135
4-3 Measuring Rectal Body Temperature—Electronic Thermometer, 137
4-4 Measuring Aural Body Temperature—Tympanic Membrane Thermometer, 138
4-5 Measuring Pulse and Respiration, 147
4-6 Measuring Apical Pulse, 149
4-7 Measuring Blood Pressure, 157
4-8 Determining Systolic Pressure by Palpation, 160

Ch. 5 The Physical Examination

5-1 Measuring Weight and Height, 178
5-2 Sitting Position, 180
5-3 Supine Position, 181
5-4 Prone Position, 183
5-5 Dorsal Recumbent Position, 184
5-6 Lithotomy Position, 185
5-7 Sims Position, 186
5-8 Knee-Chest Position, 187
5-9 Fowler's Position, 189
5-10 Assisting With the Physical Examination, 196

Ch. 6 Eye and Ear Assessment and Procedures

6-1 Assessing Distance Visual Acuity—Snellen Chart, 213
6-2 Assessing Color Vision—Ishihara Test, 215
6-3 Performing an Eye Irrigation, 217
6-4 Performing an Eye Instillation, 219
6-5 Performing an Ear Irrigation, 227
6-6 Performing an Ear Instillation, 229

Ch. 7 Physical Agents to Promote Tissue Healing

7-1 Applying a Heating Pad, 241
7-2 Applying a Hot Soak, 242
7-3 Applying a Hot Compress, 243
7-4 Applying an Ice Bag, 244
7-5 Applying a Cold Compress, 245
7-6 Applying a Chemical Pack, 246
7-7 Administering an Ultrasound Treatment, 249
7-8 Measuring for Axillary Crutches, 260
7-9 Instructing the Patient in Crutch Gaits, 261
7-10 Instructing the Patient in Use of a Cane, 264
7-11 Instructing the Patient in Use of a Walker, 264

Ch. 8 The Gynecologic Examination and Prenatal Care

8-1 Breast Self-Examination Instructions, 283
8-2 Assisting With a Gynecologic Examination, 286
8-3 Assisting With a Return Prenatal Examination, 313

Ch. 9 The Pediatric Examination

9-1 Measuring the Weight and Length of an Infant, 344
9-2 Measuring the Head and Chest Circumference of an Infant, 346
9-3 Calculating Growth Percentiles, 347
9-4 Applying a Pediatric Urine Collector, 356
9-5 Newborn Screening Test, 367

Ch. 10 Minor Office Surgery

10-1 Applying Sterile Gloves, 387
10-2 Removing Sterile Gloves, 389
10-3 Opening a Sterile Package, 390
10-4 Pouring a Sterile Solution, 391
10-5 Changing a Sterile Dressing, 395
10-6 Removing Sutures and Staples, 401
10-7 Applying and Removing Adhesive Skin Closures, 404
10-8 Assisting With Minor Office Surgery, 411
10-9 Applying a Tubular Gauze Bandage, 426

Ch. 11 Administration of Medication

11-1 Administering Oral Medication, 469
11-2 Preparing the Injection, 480
11-3 Reconstituting Powdered Drugs, 483
11-4 Administering a Subcutaneous Injection, 484
11-5 Administering an Intramuscular Injection, 486
11-6 Z-Track Intramuscular Injection Technique, 488
11-7 Administering an Intradermal Injection, 497
11-8 Administering and Reading a Tine Test, 500

Ch. 12 Cardiopulmonary Procedures

12-1 Running a 12-Lead, Three-Channel Electrocardiogram, 524
12-2 Applying a Holter Monitor, 529
12-3 Spirometry Testing, 539

Ch. 13 Colon Procedures and Male Reproductive Health

13-1 Fecal Occult Blood Testing, 551
13-2 Developing the Hemoccult Slide Test, 554
13-3 Assisting With a Flexible Sigmoidoscopy, 556

Ch. 15 Introduction to the Clinical Laboratory

15-1 Collecting a Specimen for Transport to an Outside Laboratory, 599

Ch. 16 Urinalysis

16-1 Clean-Catch Midstream Specimen Collection Instructions, 618
16-2 Collection of a 24-Hour Urine Specimen, 619
16-3 Measuring Specific Gravity of Urine: Refractometer Method, 622
16-4 Quality Control: Calibration of the Refractometer, 624
16-5 Chemical Testing of Urine With the Multistix 10 SG Reagent Strip, 633
16-6 Microscopic Examination of Urine: Kova Method, 646
16-7 Performing a Rapid Urine Culture Test, 649
16-8 Performing a Urine Pregnancy Test, 652

Ch. 17 Phlebotomy

17-1 Venipuncture—Vacuum Tube Method, 671
17-2 Venipuncture—Butterfly Method, 678
17-3 Venipuncture—Syringe Method, 683
17-4 Separating Serum From Whole Blood, 689
17-5 Skin Puncture—Disposable Lancet, 695
17-6 Skin Puncture—Disposable Semiautomatic Lancet Device, 697
17-7 Skin Puncture—Reusable Semiautomatic Lancet Device, 698

Ch. 18 Hematology

18-1 Hematocrit, 714
18-2 Preparation of a Blood Smear for a Differential Cell Count, 719

Ch. 19 Blood Chemistry and Serology

19-1 Blood Glucose Measurement Using the Accu-Chek Advantage Glucose Monitor, 741

Ch. 20 Medical Microbiology

20-1 Using the Microscope, 762
20-2 Collecting a Specimen for a Throat Culture, 767
20-3 Preparing a Smear, 774

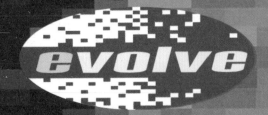

The Latest *Evolution* in Learning.

Evolve provides online access to free learning resources and activities designed specifically for the textbook you are using in your class. The resources will provide you with information that enhances the material covered in the book and much more.

Visit the Web address listed below to start your learning evolution today!

LOGIN: *http://evolve.elsevier.com/Bonewit/*

Evolve Student Learning Resources for Bonewit-West: *Clinical Procedures for Medical Assistants,* 6th edition, offer the following features:

- **WebLinks**
  An exciting resource that lets you link to hundreds of websites carefully chosen to supplement the content of the textbook. The WebLinks are regularly updated, with new ones added as they develop.

- **Content Updates**
  The latest content updates from the author of the textbook to keep you current with recent developments in medical assisting, updated procedures, and more!

- **Chapter Resources**
  Additional materials, including chapter summaries, to enhance each chapter.

Think outside the book... *evolve.*

Clinical Procedures for Medical Assistants

for

Sixth Edition

Clinical Procedures for Medical Assistants

Sixth Edition

Kathy Bonewit-West, BS, MEd, CMA

Coordinator and Instructor
Medical Assistant Technology
Hocking College
Nelsonville, Ohio
Former Member, Curriculum Review Board of the American
Association of Medical Assistants

SAUNDERS
An Imprint of Elsevier

SAUNDERS
An Imprint of Elsevier

11830 Westline Industrial Drive
St. Louis, Missouri 63146

CLINICAL PROCEDURES FOR MEDICAL ASSISTANTS, SIXTH EDITION   0-7216-0286-X
Copyright © 2004, Elsevier. All rights reserved.

Notice

Medical assisting is an ever-changing field. Standard safety precautions must be followed, but as new research and clinical experience broaden our knowledge, changes in treatment and drug therapy may become necessary or appropriate. Readers are advised to check the most current product information provided by the manufacturer of each drug to be administered to verify the recommended dose, the method and duration of administration, and contraindications. It is the responsibility of the licensed health care provider, relying on experience and knowledge of the patient, to determine dosages and the best treatment for each individual patient. Neither the publisher nor the editor assumes any liability for any injury and/or damage to persons or property arising from this publication.

Previous editions copyrighted 2000, 1995, 1990, 1984, 1979

International Standard Book Code Number ISBN 0-7216-0286-X

Publishing Director: Andrew Allen
Executive Editor: Adrianne Cochran
Senior Developmental Editor: Rae L. Robertson
Publishing Services Manager: John Rogers
Project Manager: Mary Turner, Kathleen L. Teal
Senior Designer: Kathi Gosche

Printed in the United States of America

Last digit is the print number: 9   8   7   6   5   4   3   2   1

Sixth Edition Editorial Review Board

For my mom,
Phyllis Rae,
with love

Preface

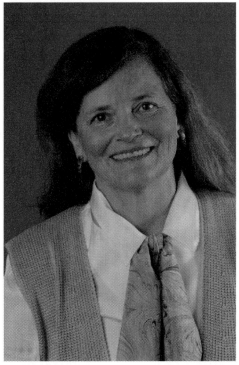

Kathy Bonewit-West

Medical assistants, for many years an integral part of most physicians' staff, now fulfill an ever-expanding and varied role in the medical office, both clinically and administratively. With increased responsibilities has come a greater need for professional knowledge and skills. This text has been designed to meet that need.

The underlying principle of the text is to provide a format for the achievement of professional competency in clinical skills performed in the medical office and the understanding of their application to real-life or on-the-job situations. When professional competency is achieved in the classroom, less of a gap should exist between the academic world and the real world, and thus the transition from student to practicing medical assistant is made more easily.

Although I have emphasized the book's usefulness to students in medical assisting training programs, the practicing medical assistant will also find this text helpful as a learning and reference source. The organization of the text lends itself well to individualized instruction and convenient reference use.

New Features in This Edition

In this sixth edition, the text has been expanded to encompass additional clinical procedures and the theory relating to each. This additional material will help students and instructors meet the demand for the increasing number and variety of clinical skills required of the practicing medical assistant by providing the most current and up-to-date procedures performed in the medical office. The reader will find that nearly every chapter incorporates new information and illustrations to assist in the educational process.

Important Additions Include the Following:

- Current information on the OSHA Bloodborne Pathogens Standard including safer medical devices and alcohol-based hand rubs
- Step-by-step procedure for the breast self-examination
- Liquid-based Pap test procedure
- Guidelines for measuring pediatric blood pressure
- Information on using the PDR

- Comprehensive pharmacology drug table of medications commonly administered and prescribed in the medical office
- Guidelines for writing a prescription.

Other very important features to the sixth edition are the inclusion of some valuable learning aids:

- **Case Studies** are designed to assist the student in responding to "real-life" situations that occur in the medical office. A practitioner's response is given for each case study too, as a means of comparison for the student.

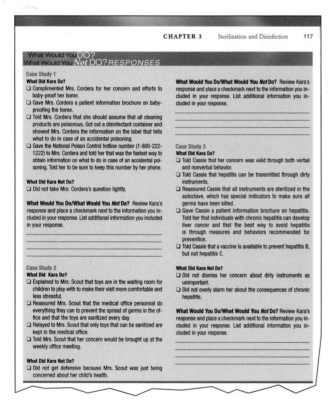

- **Apply Your Knowledge** questions are included at the end of each chapter to give students the opportunity to assess their understanding of the chapter material.

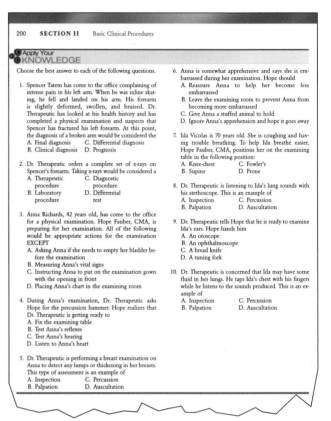

- **Resources on the Web** have been completely updated. These resources allows students to access websites containing additional information relating to the chapter.

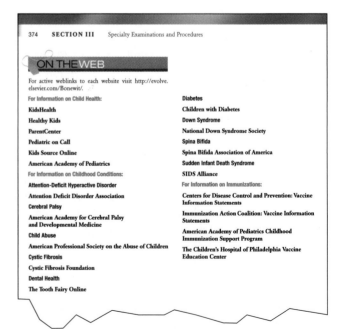

• The organizational format of this edition facilitates the learning process by providing students and educators with detailed objectives and an in-depth study of the most current and up-to-date clinical procedures performed in the medical office. Presented at the beginning of each chapter are **Learning Objectives** and related **Procedures,** a **Chapter Outline, National Competencies,** and **Key Terms.** The learning objectives address the cognitive knowledge required to perform the procedures. Procedures coincide with the objectives to delineate the task or skill to be mastered by the student. (In the student manual, most procedures are expanded into detailed performance objectives, including outcomes, and conditions and standards of acceptable performance.) The chapter outline provides a quick reference of the cognitive knowledge included in that chapter. National competencies indicate the AAMA/CAAHEP competencies met by both the theory and procedures in the chapter. The Key Terms list designates the terms and definitions that should be mastered for each chapter.

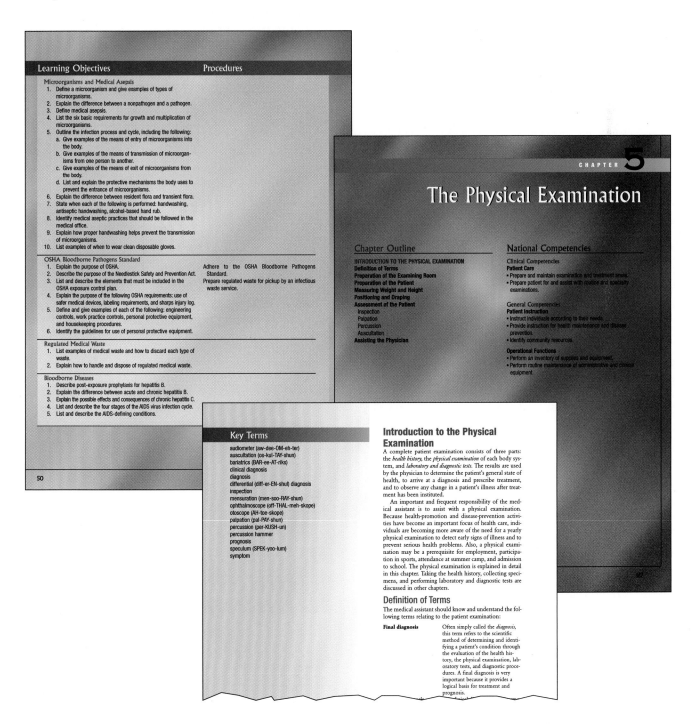

Learning Objectives

Microorganisms and Medical Asepsis
1. Define a microorganism and give examples of types of microorganisms.
2. Explain the difference between a nonpathogen and a pathogen.
3. Define medical asepsis.
4. List the six basic requirements for growth and multiplication of microorganisms.
5. Outline the infection process and cycle, including the following:
   a. Give examples of the means of entry of microorganisms into the body.
   b. Give examples of the means of transmission of microorganisms from one person to another.
   c. Give examples of the means of exit of microorganisms from the body.
   d. List and explain the protective mechanisms the body uses to prevent the entrance of microorganisms.
6. Explain the difference between resident flora and transient flora.
7. State when each of the following is performed: handwashing, antiseptic handwashing, alcohol-based hand rub.
8. Identify medical aseptic practices that should be followed in the medical office.
9. Explain how proper handwashing helps prevent the transmission of microorganisms.
10. List examples of when to wear clean disposable gloves.

OSHA Bloodborne Pathogens Standard
1. Explain the purpose of OSHA.
2. Describe the purpose of the Needlestick Safety and Prevention Act.
3. List and describe the elements that must be included in the OSHA exposure control plan.
4. Explain the purpose of the following OSHA requirements: use of safer medical devices, labeling requirements, and sharps injury log.
5. Define and give examples of each of the following: engineering controls, work practice controls, personal protective equipment, and housekeeping procedures.
6. Identify the guidelines for use of personal protective equipment.

Regulated Medical Waste
1. List examples of medical waste and how to discard each type of waste.
2. Explain how to handle and dispose of regulated medical waste.

Bloodborne Diseases
1. Describe post-exposure prophylaxis for hepatitis B.
2. Explain the difference between acute and chronic hepatitis B.
3. Explain the possible effects and consequences of chronic hepatitis C.
4. List and describe the four stages of the AIDS virus infection cycle.
5. List and describe the AIDS-defining conditions.

Procedures

Adhere to the OSHA Bloodborne Pathogens Standard.
Prepare regulated waste for pickup by an infectious waste service.

50

CHAPTER **5**

The Physical Examination

Chapter Outline

INTRODUCTION TO THE PHYSICAL EXAMINATION
Definition of Terms
Preparation of the Examining Room
Preparation of the Patient
Measuring Weight and Height
Positioning and Draping
Assessment of the Patient
   Inspection
   Palpation
   Percussion
   Auscultation
Assisting the Physician

National Competencies

Clinical Competencies
Patient Care
• Prepare and maintain examination and treatment areas.
• Prepare patient for and assist with routine and specialty examinations.

General Competencies
Patient Instruction
• Instruct individuals according to their needs.
• Provide instruction for health maintenance and disease prevention.
• Identify community resources.

Operational Functions
• Perform an inventory of supplies and equipment.
• Perform routine maintenance of administrative and clinical equipment.

107

Key Terms

audiometer (aw-dee-OM-eh-ter)
auscultation (os-kul-TAY-shun)
bariatrics (BAR-ee-AT-riks)
clinical diagnosis
diagnosis
differential (diff-er-EN-shul) diagnosis
inspection
mensuration (men-soo-RAY-shun)
ophthalmoscope (off-THAL-meh-skope)
otoscope (AH-toe-skope)
palpation (pal-PAY-shun)
percussion (per-KUSH-un)
percussion hammer
prognosis
speculum (SPEK-yoo-lum)
symptom

Introduction to the Physical Examination

A complete patient examination consists of three parts: the *health history,* the *physical examination* of each body system, and *laboratory and diagnostic tests.* The results are used by the physician to determine the patient's general state of health, to arrive at a diagnosis and prescribe treatment, and to observe any change in a patient's illness after treatment has been instituted.

An important and frequent responsibility of the medical assistant is to assist with a physical examination. Because health-promotion and disease-prevention activities have become an important focus of health care, individuals are becoming more aware of the need for a yearly physical examination to detect early signs of illness and to prevent serious health problems. Also, a physical examination may be a prerequisite for employment, participation in sports, attendance at summer camp, and admission to school. The physical examination is explained in detail in this chapter. Taking the health history, collecting specimens, and performing laboratory and diagnostic tests are discussed in other chapters.

Definition of Terms

The medical assistant should know and understand the following terms relating to the patient examination:

Final diagnosis   Often simply called the *diagnosis,* this term refers to the scientific method of determining and identifying a patient's condition through the evaluation of the health history, the physical examination, laboratory tests, and diagnostic procedures. A final diagnosis is very important because it provides a logical basis for treatment and prognosis.

- The **knowledge** or **theory** that the student must acquire to perform each skill is presented in a clear and concise manner. **Numerous illustrations** accompany the theory section to aid the student in acquiring the knowledge relating to each skill.
- **Procedures** for each skill follow the theory section and are designed to help the student perform the skill with the level of competency required on the job. Each procedure is presented in an organized step-by-step format, with underlying principles and illustrations accompanying the techniques. A charting example follows each procedure to provide the student with a guide for charting his or her own procedure. Students should find it much easier to acquire competency in charting with these examples.

- The unique and memorable **Medical Assistant Biographical Profiles (Memories of Externship** and **Putting it All Into Practice)** help students "connect" with their future beyond the classroom. The MAs featured are real people sharing their fears, likes, hopes, and aspirations, providing a "real world" feel to the book and an inspiration for the student.

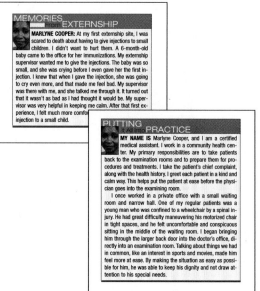

- **Patient Teaching** boxes emphasize this important aspect of the medical assistant's job, and present it in context to make it more relevant, thereby making it more memorable.

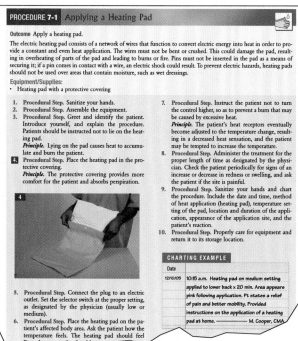

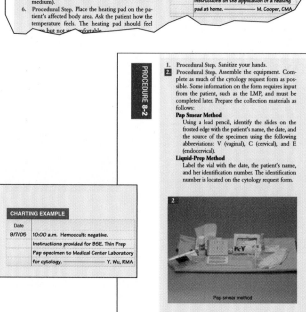

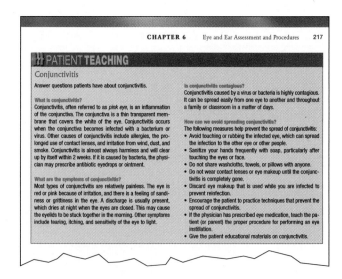

- **Key Terms** identified at the beginning of the chapter are defined at the end of the chapter in the **Terminology Review,** providing students with a valuable terminology overview for each chapter.

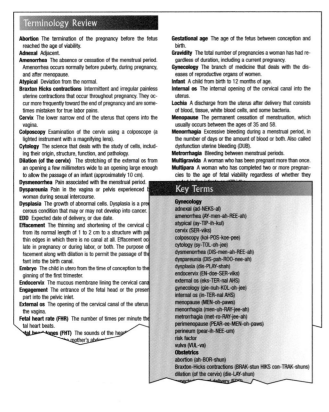

- A **Certification Review** of important points to know after each chapter helps the student to master the important elements covered in the medical assisting certification examination.

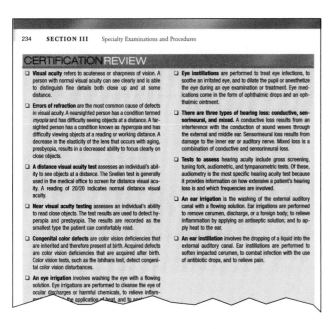

- Legal issues are important for medical assisting students to understand; it is damage control for the medical practice for which they will eventually work. **Medical Practice and the Law** boxes at the end of each chapter provide the student with current legal information pertaining to the chapter.

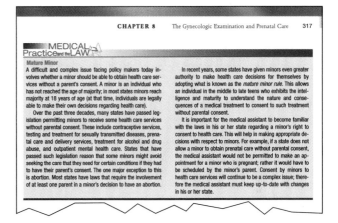

Continuing education is of utmost importance in such a rapidly changing profession. New techniques and developments in the field of medicine have a direct influence on the medical assisting profession. Continuing education helps the medical assistant maintain and improve existing skills and to learn new skills. The AAMA is a professional organization for medical assistants that is dedicated to continuing education. Information on the AAMA can be obtained by writing to:

American Association of Medical Assistants
20 N. Wacker Dr., No.1575
Chicago, IL 60606–2903
312-899-1500
www.aama-ntl.org

It is the author's hope that individuals who use this approach to medical assisting will view this text not as a stopping place but as a means of opening doors to new paths to be explored in the medical assisting profession.

Extensive Supplemental Resources

Student Software Program

The free CD-ROM that comes with the textbook includes two programs designed for students to apply the key content and skills learned throughout the text. *The Virtual Medical Office Challenge* provides realistic scenarios, with students making the decisions and getting feedback on each decision they make, plus a skill-building section that lets students practice clinical competencies. *The Body Spectrum,* an interactive Anatomy and Physiology coloring book, helps strengthen students' knowledge of the body and medical terminology.

Student Mastery Manual

The *Student Mastery Manual* that accompanies the textbook greatly enhances the learning value of the textbook. In addition, its outcome-based approach meets the criteria required for outcome-based program accreditation as stipulated by the Commission on Accreditation of Allied Health Educational Programs (CAAHEP) and the Curriculum Review Board of the American Association of Medical Assistants (AAMA). This edition contains extensive exercises for each chapter and performance checklists. A new color board game is included, providing students with a fun way to refine their knowledge and skills.

Evolve Learning Resources

The Evolve site includes all instructors' materials (for instructors only), content updates, weblinks, a link to Clinical Medical Assisting Online, online research activities, and more.

Clinical Medical Assisting Online

Clinical Medical Assisting Online is a complete online course that can stand alone as a distance education course (when combined with an on-site lab component) or provide additional reinforcement to a traditional classroom course. It covers all key accredited clinical competencies in an exciting, interactive format.

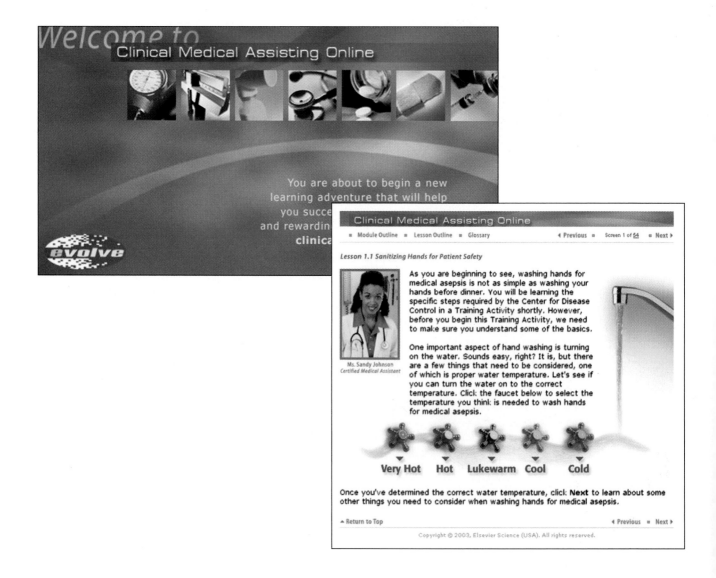

Acknowledgments

The completion of the sixth edition of this text permits the opportunity to relay appreciation to the medical assisting educators who so eagerly and enthusiastically use and enjoy this text. To them I am also indebted for their helpful assistance and suggestions for the sixth edition.

The following professionals served as invaluable consultants and reviewers and deserve special recognition and appreciation:

Sharlene K. Aasen, CMA.-C, Globe College, Oakdale, Minnesota.

Diana Bennett, RN, BSN, MAT, Indiana Vocational Technical College, Indianapolis, Indiana.

Julie A. Benson, AS, RMA, RPhbt, EKG, Medical Program Director, Platt College, Tulsa, Oklahoma.

Cathy Bierly, CMA, Athens Obstetrics and Gynecology, Athens, Ohio.

Lisa Breitbard, AA, LVN, Maric College of Medical Careers, San Diego, California.

Carol S. Champagne, RMA, CMA-C, ICEA, CCE, Clearwater Family Practice Clinic, Clearwater, Kansas; Chairperson, RMA, Continuing Education Committee; Certified Childbirth Education, Private Practice.

Gary A. Clarke, PhD, Assistant Professor of Biology, Roanoke College, Salem, Virginia.

Beverly G. Dugas, TN, Douglas College, New Westminster, British Columbia, Canada.

Amy Fought, CMA, Medical Assistant, Athens, Ohio.

Julie D. Franklin, MT(ASCP), MHE, Former Program Director, Medical Office Assisting, Chattanooga State Technical Community College, Chattanooga, Tennessee.

Cathy Goodwin, CMA-AC, Medical Assistant, San Diego, California

Jeanne Howard, CMA, AAS, Medical Assisting Technology, El Paso Community College, El Paso, Texas.

Tanya L. Howe, Administrative Assistant, School of Health and Nursing, Hocking College, Nelsonville, Ohio.

Susan K. Ipacs, RN, MS, Associate Dean, School of Nursing, Hocking College, Nelsonville, Ohio.

Gail I. Jones, MS, MT(ASCP), Dettman-Connell School of Medical Technology, Fort Worth, Texas.

Jeannette Keiter, CMA, Athens Orthopedic Center, Athens, Ohio.

Richard W. Kocon, PhD, Laboratory Director, Damon Medical Laboratory, Inc., Needham Heights, Massachusetts.

Louis Komarmy, MD, Clinical Pathologist, Children's Hospital, San Francisco, California.

Albert B. Lowenfels, MD, Associate Director of Surgery, Westchester County Medical Center, Valhalla, New York.

Susan J. Matthews, RN, BSN, MEd, Watterson College, Louisville, Kentucky.

Sharon McCaughrin, CMA, Corporate Director of Education, Ross Medical Education Centers, Warren, Michigan.

Tracy Metcalf, CMA, Office Manager, Athens Bone and Joint Surgery, Athens, Ohio.

Deborah Montone, BS, RN, RMA, LLS-P, RCS, Dean of Academics, Hohokus School of Medical Sciences, Ramsey, New Jersey.

Sally A. Murdock, BSN, MS, RN, California Public Health Nursing Certification, Medical Assisting, San Diego Mesa College, San Diego, California.

Kathryn L. Murphy, RN, CMA, Medical Program Director, Department Chair, and Instructor, Springfield College, Springfield, Missouri.

Donna F. Otis, LPN, Medical Instructor, MAA Program, Metro Business College, Rolla, Missouri.

Raymond E. Phillips, MD, FACP, Senior Attending Physician, Phelps Memorial Hospital, North Tarrytown, New York.

Traci Powell, CMA, University Medical Associates, Athens, Ohio.

Vicki Prater, CMA, Concorde Career Institute, San Bernardino, California.

Linda Reed, Indiana Vocational Technical College, Indianapolis, Indiana.

Marjorie J. Reif, PA-C, CMA, Rochester Community College, Rochester, Minnesota.

Alan M. Rosich, Instructor of Radiologic Technology, Lorain County Community College, Elvira, Ohio.

Kimberly Rubesne, MA, Median School of Allied Health Careers, Pittsburgh, Pennsylvania.

Latisha Sharpe, CMA, Athens Orthopedic Center, Athens, Ohio.

Lynn G. Slack, CMA, ICM School of Business and Medical Careers, Pittsburgh, Pennsylvania.

Robin Snider-Flohr, MBA, RN, CMA, Jefferson Community College, Steubenville, Ohio.

Edward R. Stapleton, EMT-P, Assistant Clinical Professor and Director of Prehospital Care and Education, Department of Emergency Medicine, School of Medicine, University Hospital and Medical Center, State University of New York, Stony Brook, New York.

Rachel Stapleton, CMA, Neal J. Nesbitt, MD, Athens, Ohio.

Sandra E. Sterling, MT(ASCP), Boulder Valley Vocational-Technical School, Boulder, Colorado.

Marie Thomas, CLT(NCA), Berdan Institute, Totowa, New Jersey.

Joan K. Werner, PT, PhD, Director, Physical Therapy Program, University of Wisconsin, Madison, Wisconsin.

The photographs in the textbook were taken by Jack Foley and Brian Blauser, professional photographers. I am indebted to them for their careful precision and patience in taking and editing the photographs, thus greatly enhancing the learning value of this text.

A very special thanks to Dawn Bennett for her dedication and hard work, not only on this edition, but for also in the field of medical assisting education as a whole. She has contributed immensely to the recognition of medical assisting students and practitioners as valued members of the health care community.

I would like to gratefully acknowledge the following practicing medical assistants for contributing many hours to be photographed for demonstration of the clinical procedures in the text: Megan Baer, Dawn Bennett, Trudy Browning, Janet Canterbury, Theresa Cline, Marlyne Cooper, Hope Fauber, Dori Glover, Jennifer Hawk, Kevin Hickey, Cammie Lindner, Judy Markins, Korey McGrew, Natalie Morehead, Traci Powell, Linda Proffitt, Latisha Sharpe, Michelle Shockey, Kara Van Dyke, Michelle Villers, and Huang Ying.

I would also like to acknowledge the following individuals who portrayed patients in the text: Brian Adevc, Kim Bingham, Pamela Bitting, Caitlin Brennan, David Brennan, Hollie Bonewit, Phillip Carr, Chloe Cline, Angie Coffin, Chad Cron, Dawn Decaminada, Aja Fox, Markly Georges, Connie Hazlett, Gary Hazlett, Isabella Ipacs, Joey Ipacs, Susan Ipacs, Charles Larimer, Pam Larimer, Christopher Mace, Deborah Murray, Delaney Murray, Michael Nkrumah, Heather Pike, Jan Six, Megan Skidmore, Colton Smith, Sydney Smith, Clinton Swart, Tristen West, and Lynn Witkowski.

I would like to extend my appreciation to the authors, publishers, and equipment companies who have granted me permission to use their illustrations.

The publication of the sixth edition was accomplished through the capable guidance of many talented individuals at Elsevier. Many thanks to Mary Turner and Kathleen Teal for their outstanding production work. This edition could not have attained this level of excellence without the exceptional capabilities of Rae Robertson, Senior Developmental Editor. The sixth edition has been completely redesigned through the capable efforts of Kathi Gosche. I want to relay a very special thank you to Adrianne Cochran, Executive Editor, for her dedication to quality medical assisting education and her encouragement in helping me achieve my very best in this edition.

With warm regard, I would like to recognize those very important individuals—the medical assisting students, graduates, and practicing medical assistants—who continually strive for excellence in meeting the demands and ever-increasing requirements of such a challenging profession. A quote by an unknown author really says it better: "Celebrate your talents, for they are what make you unique."

Kathy Bonewit-West

Clinical Procedure Icons

The OSHA Bloodborne Pathogens Standard must be followed when performing many of the clinical procedures presented in this text. To assist the student in following the OSHA Standard, icons have been incorporated into the procedures. An illustration of each icon along with its description is outlined below.

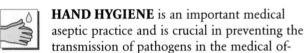 **HAND HYGIENE** is an important medical aseptic practice and is crucial in preventing the transmission of pathogens in the medical office. The medical assistant should sanitize the hands frequently, using proper technique. When performing clinical procedures, the hands should always be sanitized before and after patient contact, before applying gloves and after removing gloves, and after contact with blood or other potentially infectious materials.

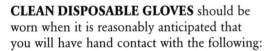 **CLEAN DISPOSABLE GLOVES** should be worn when it is reasonably anticipated that you will have hand contact with the following: blood and other potentially infectious materials, mucous membranes, nonintact skin, and contaminated articles or surfaces.

BIOHAZARD CONTAINERS are closable, leakproof, and suitably constructed to contain the contents during handling, storage, transport, or shipping. The containers must be labeled or color coded and closed before removal to prevent the contents from spilling.

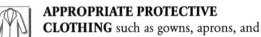 **APPROPRIATE PROTECTIVE CLOTHING** such as gowns, aprons, and laboratory coats should be worn when gross contamination can reasonably be anticipated during performance of a task or procedure.

FACE SHIELDS OR MASKS IN COMBINATION WITH EYE-PROTECTION DEVICES must be worn whenever splashes, spray, spatter, or droplets of blood or other potentially infectious materials may be generated, posing a hazard through contact with your eyes, nose, or mouth.

Contents

SECTION I   INFECTION CONTROL

1   The Medical Record, 3
Introduction to the Medical Record, 4
Components of the Medical Record, 4
Medical Office Administrative Documents, 4
Medical Office Clinical Documents, 6
Laboratory Documents, 10
Diagnostic Procedure Documents, 11
Therapeutic Service Documents, 12
Hospital Documents, 12
Consent Documents, 19
  Procedure 1-1: Completion of a Consent to Treatment Form, 20
  Procedure 1-2: Release of Medical Information, 23
Medical Record Formats, 24
Preparing a Medical Report for a New Patient, 27
  Procedure 1-3: Preparing a Medical Record, 28
Taking a Health History, 29
Charting in the Medical Record, 34
  Procedure 1-4: Obtaining and Recording Patient Symptoms, 41

2   Medical Asepsis and the OSHA Standard, 50
Introduction to Medical Asepsis and the OSHA Standard, 52
Microorganisms and Medical Asepsis, 52
  Procedure 2-1: Handwashing, 56
  Procedure 2-2: Applying an Alcohol-Based Hand Rub, 58
  Procedure 2-3: Application and Removal of Clean Disposable Gloves, 59
OSHA Bloodborne Pathogens Standard, 61
Regulated Medical Waste, 69
Bloodborne Diseases, 71

3   Sterilization and Disinfection, 84
Introduction to Sterilization and Disinfection, 86
Hazard Communication Standard, 87
Sanitization, 91
  Procedure 3-1: Sanitization of Instruments, 93
Disinfection, 97
  Procedure 3-2: Chemical Disinfection of Articles, 100
Sterilization, 102
  Procedure 3-3: Wrapping Instruments Using Paper or Muslin, 107
  Procedure 3-4: Wrapping Instruments Using a Pouch, 109
  Procedure 3-5: Sterilizing Articles in the Autoclave, 114

SECTION II   BASIC CLINICAL PROCEDURES

4   Vital Signs, 122
Introduction to Vital Signs, 124
Temperature, 124
  Procedure 4-1: Measuring Oral Body Temperature—Electronic Thermometer, 133
  Procedure 4-2: Measuring Axillary Body Temperature—Electronic Thermometer, 135
  Procedure 4-3: Measuring Rectal Body Temperature—Electronic Thermometer, 137
  Procedure 4-4: Measuring Aural Body Temperature—Tympanic Membrane Thermometer, 138
Pulse, 141
Respiration, 144
  Procedure 4-5: Measuring Pulse and Respiration, 147
  Procedure 4-6: Measuring Apical Pulse, 149
Blood Pressure, 150
  Procedure 4-7: Measuring Blood Pressure, 157
  Procedure 4-8: Determining Systolic Pressure by Palpation, 160

5 **The Physical Examination, 166**
Introduction to the Physical Examination, 168
Definition of Terms, 168
Preparation of the Examining Room, 170
Preparation of the Patient, 172
Measuring Weight and Height, 173
   Procedure 5-1: Measuring Weight and Height, 178
Positioning and Draping, 180
   Procedure 5-2: Sitting Position, 180
   Procedure 5-3: Supine Position, 181
   Procedure 5-4: Prone Position, 183
   Procedure 5-5: Dorsal Recumbent Position, 184
   Procedure 5-6: Lithotomy Position, 185
   Procedure 5-7: Sims Position: 186
   Procedure 5-8: Knee-Chest Position, 187
   Procedure 5-9: Fowler's Position, 189
Assessment of the Patient, 190
Assisting the Physician, 196
   Procedure 5-10: Assisting With the Physical Examination, 196

SECTION III SPECIALTY EXAMINATIONS AND PROCEDURES

6 **Eye and Ear Assessment and Procedures, 204**
Introduction to Eye and Ear Assessment, 206
The Eye, 206
Structure of the Eye, 206
Visual Acuity, 207
Assessment of Color Vision, 212
   Procedure 6-1: Assessing Distance Visual Acuity—Snellen Chart, 213
   Procedure 6-2: Assessing Color Vision—Ishihara Test, 215
Eye Irrigation, 216
Eye Instillation, 216
   Procedure 6-3: Performing an Eye Irrigation, 217
   Procedure 6-4: Performing an Eye Instillation, 219
The Ear, 221
Structure of the Ear, 221
Assessment of Hearing Acuity, 221
Ear Irrigation, 226
Ear Instillation, 227

   Procedure 6-5: Performing an Ear Irrigation, 227
   Procedure 6-6: Performing an Ear Instillation, 229

7 **Physical Agents to Promote Tissue Healing, 236**
Introduction to Tissue Healing, 238
Local Application of Heat and Cold, 238
   Procedure 7-1: Applying a Heating Pad, 241
   Procedure 7-2: Applying a Hot Soak, 242
   Procedure 7-3: Applying a Hot Compress, 243
   Procedure 7-4: Applying an Ice Bag, 244
   Procedure 7-5: Applying a Cold Compress, 245
   Procedure 7-6: Applying a Chemical Pack, 246
Therapeutic Ultrasound, 247
   Procedure 7-7: Administering an Ultrasound Treatment, 249
Casts, 251
Splints and Braces, 256
Ambulatory Aids, 257
   Procedure 7-8: Measuring for Axillary Crutches, 260
   Procedure 7-9: Instructing the Patient in Crutch Gaits, 261
   Procedure 7-10: Instructing the Patient in Use of a Cane, 264
   Procedure 7-11: Instructing the Patient in Use of a Walker, 264

8 **The Gynecologic Examination and Prenatal Care, 270**
Introduction to the Gynecologic Examination and Prenatal Care, 272
The Gynecologic Examination, 272
Gynecology, 272
The Breast Examination, 274
The Pelvic Examination, 275
   Procedure 8-1: Breast Self-Examination Instructions, 283
   Procedure 8-2: Assisting With a Gynecologic Examination, 286
Vaginal Infections, 289
Prenatal Care, 294
Obstetrics, 294
Prenatal Visits, 295
   Procedure 8-3: Assisting With a Return Prenatal Examination, 313
Six-Weeks-Postpartum Visit, 315

9 The Pediatric Examination, 326
Introduction to the Pediatric Examination, 328
Pediatric Office Visits, 328
Developing a Rapport, 340
Carrying the Infant, 342
Growth Measurements, 342
   Procedure 9-1: Measuring the Weight and Length of an Infant, 344
   Procedure 9-2: Measuring the Head and Chest Circumference of an Infant, 346
   Procedure 9-3: Calculating Growth Percentiles, 347
Pediatric Blood Pressure Measurement, 354
Collection of a Urine Specimen, 355
   Procedure 9-4: Applying a Pediatric Urine Collector, 356
Pediatric Injections, 358
Immunizations, 359
Newborn Screening Test, 362
   Procedure 9-5: Newborn Screening Test, 367

SECTION IV ADVANCED CLINICAL PROCEDURES

10 Minor Office Surgery 376
Introduction to Minor Office Surgery, 378
Surgical Asepsis, 378
Instruments Used in Minor Office Surgery, 380
Commercially Prepared Sterile Packages, 386
   Procedure 10-1: Applying Sterile Gloves, 387
   Procedure 10-2: Removing Sterile Gloves, 389
   Procedure 10-3: Opening a Sterile Package, 390
   Procedure 10-4: Pouring a Sterile Solution, 391
Wounds, 392
Sterile Dressing Change, 394
   Procedure 10-5: Changing a Sterile Dressing, 395
Sutures, 397
   Procedure 10-6: Removing Sutures and Staples, 401
   Procedure 10-7: Applying and Removing Adhesive Skin Closures, 404

Assisting With Minor Office Surgery, 407
   Procedure 10-8: Assisting With Minor Office Surgery, 411
Medical Office Surgical Procedures, 415
Bandaging, 422
   Procedure 10-9: Applying a Tubular Gauze Bandage, 426

11 Administration of Medication, 434
Introduction to Administration of Medication, 436
Food and Drug Administration, 440
Drug Nomenclature, 440
Classification of Drugs Based on Preparation, 440
Classification of Drugs Based on Action, 441
Systems of Measurement for Medication, 455
Converting Units of Measurement, 458
The Prescription, 462
The Medication Record, 465
Factors Affecting Drug Action, 467
Guidelines for Preparation and Administration of Medication, 468
Oral Administration, 468
   Procedure 11-1: Administering Oral Medication, 469
Parenteral Administration, 470
   Procedure 11-2: Preparing the Injection: 480
   Procedure 11-3: Reconstituting Powdered Drugs, 483
   Procedure 11-4: Administering a Subcutaneous Injection, 484
   Procedure 11-5: Administering an Intramuscular Injection, 486
   Procedure 11-6: Z-Track Intramuscular Injection Technique, 488
Tuberculin Testing, 489
Allergy Testing, 493
   Procedure 11-7: Administering an Intradermal Injection, 497
   Procedure 11-8: Administering and Reading a Tine Test, 500

SECTION V   DIAGNOSTIC TESTING

12   Cardiopulmonary Procedures, 510

Introduction to Electrocardiography, 512
Structure of the Heart, 513
Conduction System of the Heart, 514
Cardiac Cycle, 514
Electrocardiograph Paper, 515
Standardization of the Electrocardiograph, 516
Electrocardiograph Leads, 516
Maintenance of the Electrocardiograph, 519
Electrocardiographic Capabilities, 519
Artifacts, 521
Procedure 12-1: Running a 12-Lead, Three-Channel Electrocardiogram, 524
Holter Monitor Electrocardiography, 526
Procedure 12-2: Applying a Holter Monitor, 529
Cardiac Dysrhythmias, 531
Pulmonary Function Tests, 536
Procedure 12-3: Spirometry Testing, 539

13   Colon Procedures and Male Reproductive Health, 546

Introduction to Colon Procedures, 548
Fecal Occult Blood Testing, 548
Procedure 13-1: Fecal Occult Blood Testing, 551
Procedure 13-2: Developing the Hemoccult Slide Test, 554
Flexible Sigmoidoscopy, 555
Procedure 13-3: Assisting With a Flexible Sigmoidoscopy, 556
Introduction to Male Reproductive Health, 558
Prostate Cancer Screening, 558
Testicular Self-Examination, 559

14   Radiology and Diagnostic Imaging, 564

Introduction to Radiology, 566
Radiographs, 566
Contrast Media, 566
Fluoroscopy, 568
Positioning the Patient, 568
Specific Radiographic Examinations, 568
Introduction to Diagnostic Imaging, 573
Ultrasonography, 573
Computed Tomography, 574
Magnetic Resonance Imaging, 575

SECTION VI   PHYSICIAN'S OFFICE LABORATORY

15   Introduction to the Clinical Laboratory, 584

Introduction to the Clinical Laboratory, 586
Laboratory Tests, 586
Purpose of Laboratory Testing, 587
Types of Clinical Laboratories, 588
Laboratory Requests, 589
Laboratory Reports, 593
Patient Preparation and Instructions, 595
Collecting, Handling, and Transporting Specimens, 596
Clinical Laboratory Improvement Amendments, 601
The Physician's Office Laboratory, 602
Quality Control, 605
Laboratory Safety, 605
Procedure 15-1: Collecting a Specimen for Transport to an Outside Laboratory, 599

16   Urinalysis, 612

Structure and Function of the Urinary System, 614
Composition of Urine, 615
Collection of Urine, 616
Procedure 16-1: Clean-Catch Midstream Specimen Collection Instructions, 618
Procedure 16-2: Collection of a 24-Hour Urine Specimen, 619
Analysis of Urine, 620
Procedure 16-3: Measuring Specific Gravity of Urine: Refractometer Method, 622
Procedure 16-4: Quality Control: Calibration of the Refractometer, 624
Procedure 16-5: Chemical Testing of Urine With the Multistix 10 SG Reagent Strip, 633
Procedure 16-6: Microscopic Examination of Urine: Kova Method, 646
Rapid Urine Cultures, 649
Procedure 16-7: Performing a Rapid Urine Culture Test, 649
Urine Pregnancy Testing, 651
Serum Pregnancy Test, 652
Procedure 16-8: Performing a Urine Pregnancy Test, 652

17 Phlebotomy, 658
Introduction to Phlebotomy, 660
Venipuncture, 660
General Guidelines for Venipuncture, 661
Vacuum Tube Method
  of Venipuncture, 667
    Procedure 17-1: Venipuncture–Vacuum
    Tube Method, 671
Butterfly Method of Venipuncture, 676
    Procedure 17-2: Venipuncture–Butterfly
    Method, 678
Syringe Method of Venipuncture, 682
    Procedure 17-3: Venipuncture–Syringe
    Method, 683
Problems Encountered With
  Venipuncture, 686
Obtaining a Serum Specimen, 687
    Procedure 17-4: Separating Serum From
    Whole Blood, 689
Obtaining a Plasma Specimen, 691
Skin Puncture, 692
    Procedure 17-5: Skin Puncture–
    Disposable Lancet, 695
    Procedure 17-6: Skin Puncture–
    Disposable Semiautomatic Lancet
    Device, 697
    Procedure 17-7: Skin Puncture–Reusable
    Semiautomatic Lancet Device, 698

18 Hematology, 706
Introduction to Hematology, 708
Components and Function of Blood, 708
Hemoglobin Determination, 712
Hematocrit, 713
    Procedure 18-1: Hematocrit, 714
White Blood Cell Count, 716
Red Blood Cell Count, 717
White Blood Cell Differential
  Count, 717
    Procedure 18-2: Preparation of a Blood
    Smear for a Differential Cell
    Count, 719

19 Blood Chemistry
and Serology, 726
Introduction to Blood Chemistry
  and Serology, 728
Blood Chemistry, 728
Automated Blood Chemistry
  Analyzers, 728
Quality Control, 733
Cholesterol, 733
Blood Urea Nitrogen, 736
Blood Glucose, 736
Fasting Blood Sugar, 737
Self-Monitoring of Blood Glucose, 740
    Procedure 19-1 Blood Glucose
    Measurement Using the Accu-Chek
    Advantage, Glucose Monitor, 741
Serology, 743
Serologic Tests, 743
Rapid Mononucleosis Testing, 744
Blood Typing, 744
Blood Antigen and Antibody
  Reactions, 747
Agglutination and Blood Typing, 748

20 Medical Microbiology, 754
Introduction to Microbiology, 756
The Normal Flora, 757
Infection, 757
Microorganisms and Disease, 757
Microscope, 759
    Procedure 20-1: Using the
    Microscope, 762
Microbiologic Specimen Collection, 765
    Procedure 20-2: Collecting a Specimen
    for a Throat Culture, 767
Cultures, 768
Streptococcus Testing, 769
Sensitivity Testing, 771
Microscopic Examination
  of Microorganisms, 772
Prevention and Control of Infectious
  Diseases, 773
    Procedure 20-3: Preparing a Smear, 774

*SECTION VII EMERGENCY MEDICAL
              PROCEDURES*

21 **Emergency Medical
    Procedures, 782**
    **Introduction to Emergency Medical
    Procedures, 784**
    The Office Crash Cart, 784
    Emergency Medical Services System, 788
    First Aid Kit, 788
    OSHA Safety Precautions, 788
    Guidelines for Providing Emergency
    Care, 789

APPENDICES

A Medical Abbreviations,
   815
B The Human Body:
   Highlights of Structure
   and Function, 825

GLOSSARY, 845

Clinical Procedures for Medical Assistants

for

Sixth Edition

Infection Control

1 The Medical Record

2 Medical Asepsis and
   the OSHA Standard

3 Sterilization and Disinfection

Components of the Medical Record

1. List and describe the functions served by the medical record.
2. Identify the information contained in each of the following medical office administrative documents: patient registration record and correspondence.
3. Identify the information contained in each of the following medical office clinical documents: health history report, physical examination report, progress notes, medication record, consultation report, and home health care report.
4. List and describe the information included in the following diagnostic procedure documents: electrocardiogram report, Holter monitor report, sigmoidoscopy report, colonoscopy report, spirometry report, radiology report, and diagnostic imaging report.
5. State the purpose of each of the following therapeutic services: physical therapy, occupational therapy, and speech therapy.
6. Identify the information contained in the following hospital documents: history and physical report, operative report, discharge summary report, pathology report, and emergency room report.

Prepare a medical record for a new patient.

Consent Documents

1. Identify the information contained in the following consent documents: consent to treatment form and release of medical information form.

Obtain patient consent for treatment.

Assist a patient in completing a release of medical information form.

Release information according to a completed release of medical information form.

Medical Record Formats

1. Describe the organization of a source-oriented medical record and a problem-oriented medical record.
2. List and define the four subcategories included in the progress notes of a problem-oriented record (POR).
3. Explain the difference between a paper-based patient record (PPR) and an electronic medical record (EMR).

Identify the parts of a source-oriented medical record and a problem-oriented medical record.

Health History

1. List and describe the seven parts of the health history.
2. List the guidelines that should be followed in recording the chief complaint.

Complete or assist the patient in completing a health history form.

Charting

1. List and describe the guidelines to follow to ensure accurate and concise charting.
2. List and describe the types of progress notes that are charted by the medical assistant.
3. List examples of subjective symptoms and objective symptoms.
4. List and describe common symptoms.

Chart the following:
  Procedures
  Administration of medication
  Specimen collection
  Laboratory tests
  Progress notes
  Instructions given to the patient
Obtain and record patient symptoms.

CHAPTER 1

The Medical Record

Chapter Outline

Introduction to the Medical Record
Components of the Medical Record
Medical Office Administrative Documents
  Patient Registration Record
  Correspondence
Medical Office Clinical Documents
  Health History Report
  Physical Examination Report
  Progress Notes
  Medication Record
  Consultation Report
  Home Health Care Report
Laboratory Documents
  Hematology
  Clinical Chemistry
  Serology
  Urinalysis
  Microbiology
  Parasitology
  Cytology
  Histology
Diagnostic Procedure Documents
  Electrocardiogram Report
  Holter Monitor Report
  Sigmoidoscopy Report
  Colonoscopy Report
  Spirometry Report
  Radiology Report
  Diagnostic Imaging Report
Therapeutic Service Documents
  Physical Therapy
  Occupational Therapy
  Speech Therapy
Hospital Documents
  History and Physical Report
  Operative Report
  Discharge Summary Report
  Pathology Report
  Emergency Room Report
Consent Documents
  Consent to Treatment Form
  Release of Medical Information Form

Medical Record Formats
  Source-Oriented Record
  Problem-Oriented Record
Preparing a Medical Record for a New Patient
  Medical Record Supplies
Taking a Health History
  Components of the Health History
Charting in the Medical Record
  Charting Guidelines
  Charting Progress Notes
  Charting Patient Symptoms
  Other Activities That Need to Be Charted

National Competencies

Clinical Competencies
Patient Care
- Perform telephone and in-person screening.
- Obtain and record patient history.
- Maintain medication and immunization records.

General Competencies
Professional Communications
- Respond to and initiate written communications.
- Recognize and respond to verbal communications.
- Recognize and respond to nonverbal communications.
- Demonstrate telephone techniques.

Legal Concepts
- Identify and respond to issues of confidentiality.
- Perform within legal and ethical boundaries.
- Establish and maintain the medical record.
- Document appropriately.
- Demonstrate knowledge of federal and state health care legislation and regulations.

Patient Instruction
- Explain general office policies.

Operational Functions
- Utilize computer software to maintain office systems.

Key Terms

attending physician
charting
consultation report
diagnosis (dye-ag-NOE-sis)
diagnostic procedure
discharge summary report
electronic medical record (EMR)
familial (fah-MIL-yul)
health history report
home health care
informed consent
inpatient
medical impressions
medical record
medical record format
objective symptom
paper-based patient record (PPR)
patient
physical examination
physical examination report
problem
prognosis (prog-NOE-sis)
reverse chronological order
SOAP format
subjective symptom
symptom (SIMP-tum)

Introduction to the Medical Record

A **medical record** is a written record of the important information regarding a patient, including the care of that individual and the progress of the patient's condition. Medical records are a critical part of a medical practice.

The patient's medical record serves a number of important functions. The physician uses the information in the medical record as a basis for decisions regarding the patient's care and treatment. The medical record also serves to document the results of treatment and the patient's progress. The medical record provides an efficient and effective method by which information can be communicated to authorized personnel in the medical office.

The medical record also serves as a legal document. The law requires that a record be maintained to document the care and treatment being received by the patient. If something goes wrong, good documentation works to legally protect the physician and the medical staff. On the other hand, incomplete records could be used as evidence in court to show that the patient did not receive the quality of care that meets generally accepted standards.

The medical assistant must always keep in mind that the information contained in the patient's medical record is strictly confidential and must not be read by or discussed with anyone except the physician or medical staff involved with the care of the patient (Highlight on the HIPAA Privacy Rule).

Components of the Medical Record

A medical record consists of numerous documents. Each document in the medical record has a specific function or purpose. Most of these documents are preprinted forms that contain specific information entered by a physician or other health professional. A large variety of forms are available; the type of form used is based on the specific requirements of each medical office.

Medical record documents can be classified into categories. Each of these categories is outlined in the box presented on p. 6, along with the specific documents included in each.

It is important that the medical assistant be familiar with each type of document in the medical record. A description of the function or purpose of each type of medical record document follows (by category), along with the specific information that each contains.

Medical Office Administrative Documents

Administrative documents contain information necessary for the efficient (record-keeping) management of the medical office. Medical office administrative documents include the patient registration record and patient-related correspondence.

Highlight on the HIPAA Privacy Rule

What Is the HIPAA Privacy Rule?

The acronym HIPAA stands for the Health Insurance Portability and Accountability Act. HIPAA is a federal law consisting of several components, one of which contains provisions to protect a patient's privacy, known as the HIPAA Privacy Rule.

The HIPAA Privacy Rule went into effect on April 14, 2003. The primary purpose of this rule is to provide patients with more control over the use and disclosure of their health information. All health care providers, health plans, and health care clearinghouses (e.g., billing services) that use, store, maintain, or transmit health information must comply with this rule.

What Is Included in the HIPAA Privacy Rule?

The *Highlight on the HIPAA Privacy Rule* is outlined below as it relates to the medical office:

1. The medical office must develop a written document known as a *Notice of Privacy Practices (NPP)*. The NPP must explain to patients how their protected health information (PHI) will be used and protected by the medical office. **Protected health information** includes health information in any form (written, electronic, or oral) that contains patient-identifiable information (e.g., name, social security number, telephone number). The medical office must make a reasonable effort to provide an NPP to each patient and to obtain a signed acknowledgment from the patient that he or she has received an NPP.

2. A patient's written consent is not required for the use or disclosure of PHI for the purpose of medical treatment, payment, and health care operations.

3. Patients have the right to access their medical records and to request changes to the records if they believe them to be inaccurate.

4. To prevent unnecessary or inappropriate access to PHI, the medical office must make an effort to limit the use of, disclosure of, and requests for PHI to the minimum necessary to accomplish the intended purpose (e.g., a request from an insurance company for health information). This requirement, however, does not apply to the use of PHI for the routine practice of medicine within the medical office.

5. Patients have a right to request an accounting of the transfer of their information for purposes other than treatment, payment, or health care operations.

6. Business associates to whom the medical office may disclose PHI must respect the HIPAA Privacy Rule. The medical office must execute a written agreement with each business associate to handle PHI in accordance with HIPAA. Business associates could include the following organizations and firms:
   Medical laboratories
   Transcription services
   Law firms
   Accounting firms
   Software and hardware consultants
   Billing services

7. The medical office must implement a basic training program in privacy and security of PHI for all employees.

8. The medical office is required to put in place appropriate administrative, physical, and technical security safeguards to protect the privacy of PHI from accidental use or disclosure or violation of the above requirements.

What If a Medical Office Does *Not* Comply With the HIPAA Privacy Rule?

There are severe penalties if a medical office fails to comply with the HIPAA Privacy Rule, which can include both civil and criminal penalties.

Where Can More Information on the HIPAA Privacy Rule Be Found?

The following websites contain current information on HIPAA:
www.cms.hhs.gov/hipaa
www.hhs.gov/ocr/hipaa

What Would You DO?
What Would You *Not* DO?

Case Study 1

Moira Celeste, an account executive for a large insurance company, comes to the office complaining of insomnia and depression. Three months ago her husband of 27 years left, and now they are legally separated. Since then Moira has had a lot of trouble sleeping at night. She also feels lethargic during the day and hasn't been eating much. Moira says that she's been having some problems with alcohol. She wants to know of any community agencies that could help her with her problem but who would be sure to keep the information confidential. She has a very responsible job with her firm and doesn't want anyone to know about her alcohol problem. She also doesn't want any information about her problem put in her chart, and she especially doesn't want the physician to know about it because he is friends with many of her colleagues at work.

Categories of Medical Record Documents

Medical Office Administrative Documents
Patient registration record
Correspondence

Medical Office Clinical Documents
Health history report
Physical examination report
Progress notes
Medication record
Consultation report
Home health care report

Laboratory Documents
Hematology report
Clinical chemistry report
Serology report

Laboratory Documents—cont'd
Urinalysis report
Microbiology report
Parasitology report
Cytology report
Histology report

Diagnostic Procedure Documents
Electrocardiogram report
Holter monitor report
Sigmoidoscopy report
Colonoscopy report
Spirometry report
Radiology report
Diagnostic imaging report

Therapeutic Service Documents
Physical therapy report
Occupational therapy report
Speech therapy report

Hospital Documents
History and physical report
Operative report
Discharge summary report
Pathology report
Emergency room report

Consent Documents
Consent to treatment form
Release of medical information form

Patient Registration Record

The patient registration record (Figure 1-1) consists of demographic and billing information. The patient registration form must be completed by all new patients.

In most offices the information on the patient registration record is entered into a computer. This allows the information to be used for a number of functions, such as scheduling appointments, posting patient transactions, and processing patient statements and insurance claims.

Demographic Information

Demographic information required on a patient registration form includes the following:
- Full name
- Address
- Phone (home and work)
- Date of birth
- Gender
- Marital status
- Employer

Billing Information

Billing information is required to bill charges to the patient or an insurance company. Billing information required on a patient registration form includes the following:
- Name of responsible party (person responsible for the account)
- Social security number
- Address of responsible party
- Name of insured (policyholder)
- Insurance company
- Policy number and group number

Correspondence

Correspondence is an important part of the medical record. Correspondence regarding a patient may be received from a number of individuals or facilities. Examples include the patient's insurance company, the patient's attorney, or even the patient himself or herself. Insurance correspondence includes such documents as a precertification authorization for a hospital admission and a request for additional information from the insurance company.

Correspondence also includes copies of letters concerning the patient that are sent out of the office; examples include a copy of a letter referring the patient to a specialist and a copy of a collection letter sent to the patient.

Medical Office Clinical Documents

Medical office clinical documents include a variety of records and reports that assist the physician in the care and treatment of the patient. Common medical office clinical documents are listed and described next.

Health History Report

A **health history report** is a collection of subjective data about the patient. This information may be requested on a preprinted form filled out by the patient, or it may be obtained by the physician or medical assistant during an interview.

Along with the physical examination and laboratory and diagnostic tests, the health history report is used for the following reasons: to determine the patient's general state of health, to arrive at a diagnosis and prescribe treatment, and to observe any change in a patient's illness after treatment has been instituted. The term **diagnosis** refers to the scientific method of determining and identifying a patient's condition.

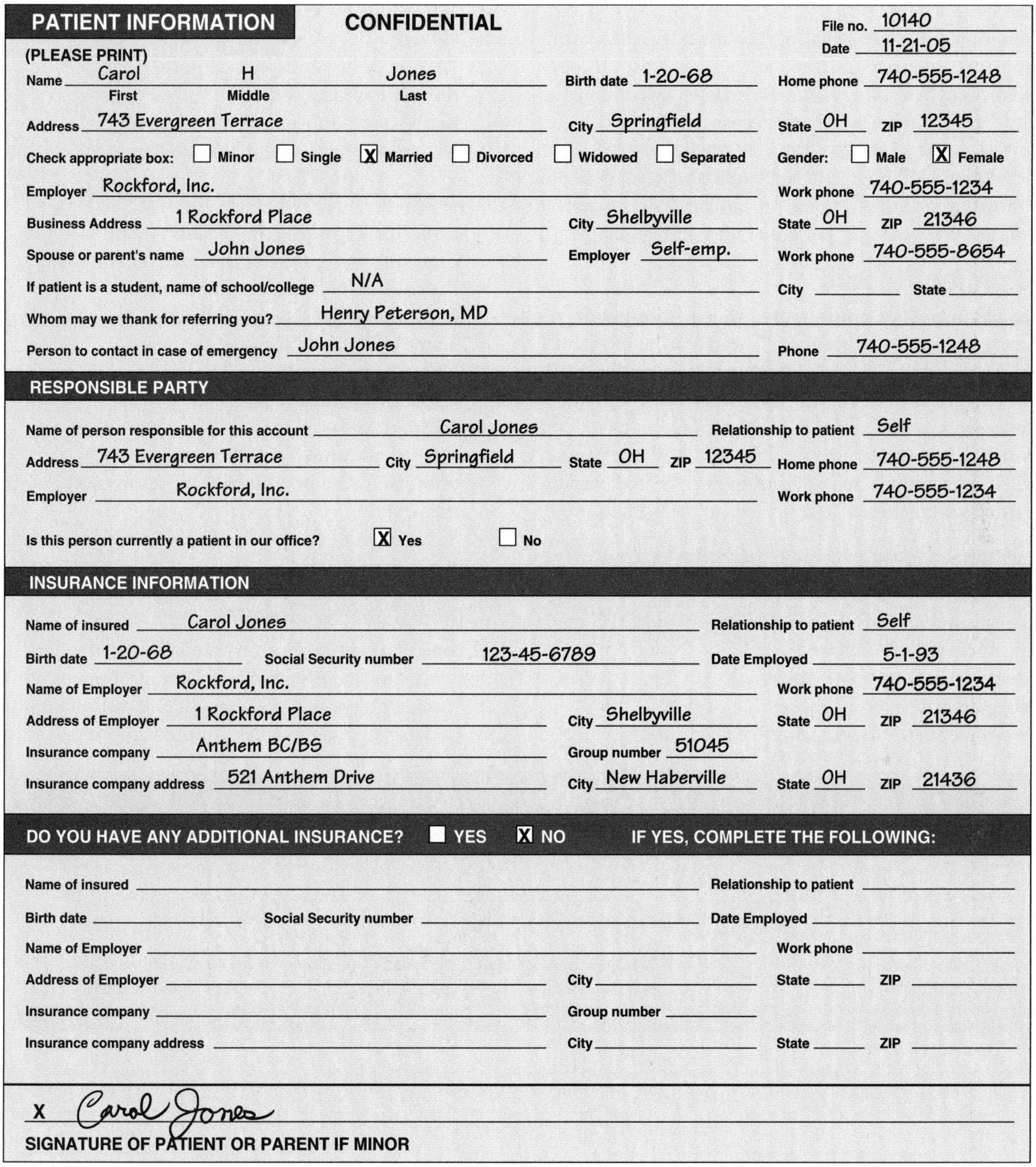

PATIENT INFORMATION **CONFIDENTIAL**

File no. 10140
Date 11-21-05

(PLEASE PRINT)

Name Carol (First) H (Middle) Jones (Last) Birth date 1-20-68 Home phone 740-555-1248

Address 743 Evergreen Terrace City Springfield State OH ZIP 12345

Check appropriate box: ☐ Minor ☐ Single ☒ Married ☐ Divorced ☐ Widowed ☐ Separated Gender: ☐ Male ☒ Female

Employer Rockford, Inc. Work phone 740-555-1234

Business Address 1 Rockford Place City Shelbyville State OH ZIP 21346

Spouse or parent's name John Jones Employer Self-emp. Work phone 740-555-8654

If patient is a student, name of school/college N/A City State

Whom may we thank for referring you? Henry Peterson, MD

Person to contact in case of emergency John Jones Phone 740-555-1248

RESPONSIBLE PARTY

Name of person responsible for this account Carol Jones Relationship to patient Self

Address 743 Evergreen Terrace City Springfield State OH ZIP 12345 Home phone 740-555-1248

Employer Rockford, Inc. Work phone 740-555-1234

Is this person currently a patient in our office? ☒ Yes ☐ No

INSURANCE INFORMATION

Name of insured Carol Jones Relationship to patient Self

Birth date 1-20-68 Social Security number 123-45-6789 Date Employed 5-1-93

Name of Employer Rockford, Inc. Work phone 740-555-1234

Address of Employer 1 Rockford Place City Shelbyville State OH ZIP 21346

Insurance company Anthem BC/BS Group number 51045

Insurance company address 521 Anthem Drive City New Haberville State OH ZIP 21436

DO YOU HAVE ANY ADDITIONAL INSURANCE? ☐ YES ☒ NO **IF YES, COMPLETE THE FOLLOWING:**

Name of insured Relationship to patient

Birth date Social Security number Date Employed

Name of Employer Work phone

Address of Employer City State ZIP

Insurance company Group number

Insurance company address City State ZIP

X Carol Jones

SIGNATURE OF PATIENT OR PARENT IF MINOR

Figure 1-1. Patient registration record. (Courtesy Colwell Systems, Champaign, Ill.)

A thorough history of personal health is obtained for each new patient, and subsequent office visits provide additional information regarding changes in the patient's condition or treatment. A complete discussion of the health history report is presented later in this chapter.

Physical Examination Report

A **physical examination** is an assessment of each part of the patient's body. The purpose of the physical examination is to provide objective data about the patient, which assists the physician in determining the patient's state of health. (The physical examination is described in detail in Chapter 5.)

The **physical examination report** is a summary of the physician's findings from the assessment of each part of the patient's body and includes the following:

- General appearance
- Head and neck
- Eyes
- Ears
- Nose
- Mouth and pharynx
- Arms and hands
- Chest and lungs
- Heart
- Breasts
- Abdomen
- Genitalia and rectum
- Legs and feet

Progress Notes

Progress notes involve updating the medical record with new information each time the patient visits or telephones the medical office. Progress notes serve to document the patient's health status from one visit to the next. It is important that the date and time be included with each progress note, along with the signature and credentials of the individual making the entry. A thorough discussion of charting progress notes is presented later in this chapter.

Medication Record

A medication record consists of detailed information related to a patient's medications. The record may include one or more of the following categories: prescription medications, over-the-counter (OTC) medications, and medications administered at the medical office.

Most medical offices use one form to record prescription and OTC medications and another form to record medications actually administered to the patient at the medical office.

Prescription and Over-the-Counter Medication Record Form

A medication record form for prescription and OTC medications includes the following:
- Patient's name and date of birth
- Drug allergies
- Date the patient began taking the medication
- Name of the medication
- Dosage
- Frequency of administration of the medication
- Route of administration
- Refills (prescription medications only)
- Date the patient stopped taking the medication

Medication Administration Record Form

A form for recording medications administered at the medical office (Figure 1-2) includes the following:
- Patient's name and date of birth
- Drug allergies
- Name of the medication
- Dosage administered
- Route of administration
- Injection site
- Date of administration
- Manufacturer, lot number, and expiration date of the medication
- Signature and credentials of the individual administering the medication

Consultation Report

A **consultation report** is a narrative report of a clinical opinion about a patient's condition by a practitioner other than the primary physician (Figure 1-3). The consultant is usually a specialist in a certain field of medicine (e.g., cardiology,

---

MEDICATION ADMINISTRATION RECORD

PATIENT NAME _Kristen Antle_ BIRTH DATE _1/9/73_

ALLERGIES _∅_

SITE ABBREVIATIONS:

RD: Right deltoid   RDG: Right dorsogluteal   RVL: Right vastus lateralis
LD: Left deltoid   LDG: Left dorsogluteal   LVL: Left vastus lateralis

MEDICATION AND DOSAGE	ROUTE	DATE	MANUFACTURER	LOT#	EXP DATE	SITE	ADMIN BY
Rocephin 500 mg	IM	2/5/05	Roche	1053	10/5/06	RDG	D. Bennett, CMA
Depo-Provera 150 mg	IM	8/14/05	Pharmacia & Upjohn	68FUF	12/5/05	LDG	D. Bennett, CMA
Fluzone 0.5 ml	IM	11/4/05	Aventis Pasteur	OF1120	6/10/06	RD	D. Bennett, CMA
Depo-Provera 150 mg	IM	11/4/05	Pharmacia & Upjohn	87FUF	12/7/06	RDG	D. Bennett, CMA

Figure 1-2. Medication record.

HAROLD B. COOPER, M.D.
6000 MAIN STREET
VENTURA, CA 93003

June 15, 2005

John F. Millstone, M.D.
5302 Main Street
Ventura, CA 93003

Dear Dr. Millstone:

RE: Elaine J. Silverman

This 69-year-old woman was seen at your request. The patient was admitted to the hospital yesterday because of chills, fever, and abdominal and back pain.

REVIEW OF HEALTH HISTORY: The history has been reviewed. A prominent feature of the history is the presence of intermittent, severe, shaking chills for four days with associated left lower back pain, left lower quadrant abdominal pain, and fever to as high as 103 or 104 degrees. The patient has had hypertension for a number of years and has been managed quite well with Aldomet 250 mg twice a day.

PHYSICAL EXAMINATION: On examination her temperature at this time is 100.6 degrees. The pulse is 110 and regular. Blood pressure is 190/100. The patient has partial bilateral iridectomies, the result of previous cataract surgery. Otherwise, the head and neck are not remarkable. Lung fields are clear throughout. The heart reveals a regular tachycardia, heart sounds are of good quality. No murmurs heard and there is no gallop rhythm present. The abdomen is soft. There is no spasm or guarding. A well-healed surgical scar is present in the right flank area. There is considerable tenderness in the left lower quadrant of the left mid abdomen, but as noted, there is no spasm or guarding present. Bowel sounds are present. Peristaltic rushes are noted, and the bowel sounds are slightly high pitched. The extremities are unremarkable.

IMPRESSIONS: I believe the patient has acute diverticulitis. She may have some irritation of the left ureter in view of the findings on the urinalysis. She appears to be responding to therapy at this time in that her temperature is coming down and there has been a slight reduction in the leukocytosis from yesterday.

RECOMMENDATIONS: I agree with the present program of therapy, and the only suggestion would be to possibly increase the dose of gentamicin to 60 mg q8h, rather than the 40 mg q8h that she is now receiving.

Thank you for asking me to see this patient in consultation.

Sincerely,

Harold B. Cooper

Harold B. Cooper, M.D.

mtf

Figure 1-3. Consultation report. (Modified from Diehl MO, Fordney MT: *Medical transcription: techniques and procedures,* ed 5, Philadelphia, 2003, Saunders.)

endocrinology, urology). The consultant's opinion is based on a review of the patient's record and an examination of the patient.

The consultation report must include the following:
- Documentation that the consultant reviewed the patient's health history
- Documentation that the consultant examined the patient
- A report of the consultant's impressions
- Any care or treatment provided by the consultant
- A report of the consultant's recommendations

Home Health Care Report

Home health care is the provision of medical and nonmedical care in a patient's home or place of residence. The purpose of home health care is to minimize the effect of disease or disability by promoting, maintaining, and restoring the patient's health. There is a growing preference for home health care over equivalent health care options. Research shows that familiar surroundings contribute positively to a patient's emotional and physical well-being.

Home health care must be ordered by the patient's physician and is provided by skilled professionals. Home health care professionals include nurses, home health aides, dietitians, physical therapists, occupational therapists, speech therapists, and social workers. Examples of specialized services available through home health care include cardiac home care, infusion therapy, respiratory care, pain management, diabetes management, rehabilitation, and maternal-child care. Home health care providers must periodically provide a summary report (Figure 1-4) to the patient's physician that includes the following:
- Observations and evaluations
- Type of care or service provided
- Instructions given to the patient on medications
- Safety measures recommended for the home
- Diet
- Activities permitted

Laboratory Documents

A laboratory report is a report of the analysis or examination of body specimens. Its purpose is to relay the results of laboratory tests to the physician to assist in diagnosing and treating disease. A thorough discussion of laboratory documents is presented in Chapter 15.

The specific categories of laboratory tests follow.

Hematology. Laboratory analysis in hematology deals with the examination and analysis of blood for the detection of abnormalities and includes areas such as blood cell counts, cellular morphology, clotting ability of the blood, and identification of cell types.

Home Health Agency—Visit Report		Date of visit: 11/21/05		Start: 7	Mileage Finish: 9
		Patient's name: Clarence Castor			
BP:(LA): 160/82 BP:(RA): 160/82 T: 97.7		Financial:	Med. A:		Med. B:
		GH: VA:		Pvt:	Other: Hospice
P:(A): 78 P:(R): 76 R: 18 Wt: 151		Area:		Diagnosis: Lung cancer	
Pt. Instruction: Continue O₂ as needed		Procedures:		Age: 74	
Comments/Observations: (Physical, Mental, Emotional, Activity Level, Environ., S/S, Treatments and Effects, Procedures, Med. Effects, Other)					
Pt complaining of some difficulty breathing and swelling of his feet. Pt was given					
Proventil Atrovent neb tx and started on oxygen at 2 liters per nasal cannula.					
Tx was discussed with Dr. Shay.					
Plan: Monitor vitals every 2 hrs.					
Supplies Used: O₂ @ 2 liters					
Signature: D. Talley, RN		Next visit: 11/22/05	RN ✓ PT	HHA MSN	Other
		Freq of visits: daily	✓		
Supervisory visit:		Travel time:		Service time:	

Figure 1-4. Home health care report. (Courtesy Briggs, Des Moines, Iowa.)

Clinical Chemistry. Laboratory analysis in clinical chemistry involves detecting the presence of chemical substances or determining the amount of substances in body fluids, excreta, and tissues (e.g., blood, urine, cerebrospinal fluid). The largest area in clinical chemistry is blood chemistry.

Serology. Laboratory analysis in serology deals with studying antigen-antibody reactions to assess the presence of a substance or to determine the presence of disease.

Urinalysis. Laboratory analysis in urinalysis involves the physical, chemical, and microscopic analysis of urine.

Microbiology. Laboratory analysis in microbiology deals with the identification of pathogens in specimens taken from the body (e.g., urine, blood, throat, sputum, wound, urethral, vaginal, and cerebrospinal).

Parasitology. Laboratory analysis in parasitology deals with the detection of disease-producing human parasites or eggs in specimens taken from the body (e.g., stool, vagina, blood).

Cytology. Laboratory analysis in cytology deals with the detection of abnormal cells.

Histology. Laboratory analysis in histology deals with the detection of diseased tissues.

MY NAME IS Dawn Bennett, and I work for an orthopedic surgeon. I work in the front area of the office as an administrative supervisor in billing and collections.

Working in billing and collections is very challenging and sometimes stressful. It can even be embarrassing. We are a new practice, and when we opened, there was no collections system. When it came time to review our accounts, we realized that, like every other business, we needed a collections system. We immediately jumped in and took charge.

The primary physician at our office is from New York, and we were unfamiliar with his family members. One day he walked into our office with a very puzzled look. I asked him what was wrong. He replied, "You guys are doing a great job with our collection rate. I asked you to be stern, but thoughtful, when sending our patients collection letters—but did you have to send one to my mother-in-law?!" Needless to say, we fixed the error immediately. This incident prompted us to restructure our collections system, and we added a comment screen to our computer system on all of our patients' accounts. Going into a medical office that already has a system in place may be easier, but you can learn a lot more by setting up an office system yourself.

Diagnostic Procedure Documents

A diagnostic procedure report consists of a narrative description and interpretation of a diagnostic procedure. A **diagnostic procedure** is a type of procedure performed to assist in the diagnosis, management, or treatment of a patient's condition. The procedure may be performed by a physician, the medical assistant, or a technician specially trained in the procedure. The interpretation of the results of the diagnostic procedure is made by a physician.

Examples of diagnostic procedure reports include the following:

Electrocardiogram Report

An electrocardiogram (ECG) report is a narrative description of a cardiologist's interpretation of an ECG, including the implications for the patient. The graphic tracing is usually included with the report.

Holter Monitor Report

A Holter monitor report is a narrative description of the interpretation of an ambulatory electrocardiogram, including the evaluator's impressions. Portions of the graphic tracing are usually included with the report.

Sigmoidoscopy Report

A sigmoidoscopy report is a narrative description of the interpretation of a sigmoidoscopic examination, including the practitioner's impressions.

Colonoscopy Report

A colonoscopy report is a narrative description of a colonoscopic examination, including the practitioner's impressions.

Spirometry Report

A spirometry report is a narrative and graphic description of the interpretation of pulmonary function tests.

Radiology Report

A radiology report is a narrative description of a diagnostic or therapeutic radiologic procedure (Figure 1-5). A radiologist examines the radiograph and provides a written report, which includes a detailed interpretation of the radiograph and his or her impressions. The patient's physician receives a copy of the radiology report; the actual radiograph is kept on file in the hospital's radiology department but is available for review by the patient's physician.

Diagnostic Imaging Report

A diagnostic imaging report is a narrative description of a diagnostic imaging procedure (Figure 1-6, p. 13). The report includes a detailed interpretation of the diagnostic image, along with the practitioner's impressions. Examples of common diagnostic imaging procedures include ultrasonography,

COLLEGE HOSPITAL
4567 BROAD AVENUE
WOODLAND HILLS, MD 21532

RADIOLOGY REPORT

Examination Date:	June 14, 2005	Patient:	Rose Baker
Date Reported:	June 14, 2005	X-ray No.:	43200
Physician:	Harold B. Cooper	Patient:	19
Examination:	PA Chest, Abdomen	Hospital No.:	80-32-11

FINDINGS

PA CHEST: Upright PA view of chest shows the lung fields are clear, without evidence of an active process. Heart size is normal. There is no evidence of pneumoperitoneum.

IMPRESSION: NEGATIVE CHEST

ABDOMEN: Flat and upright views of the abdomen show a normal gas pattern without evidence of obstruction or ileus. There are no calcifications or abnormal masses noted.

IMPRESSION: NEGATIVE STUDY

RADIOLOGIST: *Marian B. Skinner*
Marian B. Skinner, MD

Figure 1-5. Radiology report. (From Diehl MO, Fordney MT: *Medical keyboarding, typing, and transcribing*, ed 4, Philadelphia, 1997, Saunders.)

computed tomography (CT) scan, and magnetic resonance imaging (MRI). The diagnostic computer image is kept on file at the hospital but is available for review by the patient's physician.

Therapeutic Service Documents

A therapeutic service report documents the assessments and treatments designed to restore a patient's ability to function. Examples of therapeutic services that the physician may order follow.

Physical Therapy. Physical therapy involves the use of therapeutic exercise, thermal modalities, cold, hydrotherapy, electrical stimulation, massage, and other physical means. The purpose of physical therapy is to restore function and promote healing following an illness or injury. For example, a physical therapist might help a football player with a knee injury to regain normal functioning of the knee or assist a patient recovering from a stroke to use his or her legs to walk again. Figure 1-7, p. 14 shows an example of a physical therapy report.

Occupational Therapy. Occupational therapy helps the patient learn new skills to adapt to a physical, developmental, emotional, or mentally disabling condition. This enables the patient to perform the activities of daily living and to achieve as much independence as possible. For example, an occupational therapist might help an individual with a physical disability learn how to get dressed and how to prepare meals.

Speech Therapy. Treatment for the correlation of a speech impairment resulting from birth, disease, injury, or prior medical treatment.

Hospital Documents

Hospital documents are prepared by the physician responsible for the care of a patient while at the hospital; this physician is known as the **attending physician.** The attending physician may be the patient's regular physician or a different physician. An example of the latter is a physician attending a patient at an urgent care center or the emergency department of a hospital.

DIAGNOSTIC IMAGING REPORT			
Mt. Carmel Hospital, Columbus, OH 43201			
DATE REQUESTED 6/6/2005	DATE TO BE DONE 6/10/2005	TODAY'S DATE 6/10/2005	DATE OF BIRTH 8/19/1943
☐ WHEELCHAIR	☐ PORTABLE	☐ AMBULATORY	☐ CART

PATIENT: Vera Ruth	INSURANCE: Industrial

SEX F	ROOM NO. OP	RESPONSIBLE PERSON OR EMPLOYER J.B. Warren, Inc.	RADIOLOGIST Richard W. Adams
CLINICAL INFORMATION AND PROVISIONAL DIAGNOSIS Back injury			ATTENDING PHYSICIAN Dr. Robb
			NURSE

EXAMINATION REQUESTED (PINPOINT AREA OF CONCERN IF POSSIBLE)
CT LUMBAR SPINE

TECHNIQUE:

CT of the lumbar spine without contrast was performed from L-3 through S-1.

FINDINGS:

The L3-4 level appears satisfactory without evidence of osseous proliferation or disc protrusion.

At the L4-5 level there is some increased density at the disc level, which may be more prominent on the left. This is partially obscured due to facet artifact crossing obliquely.

There does appear to be some retention, however, of epidural fat plane. This however, may represent left sided disc bulge or protrusion with the appropriate corresponding clinical appearance. Osseous variation at this level is not identified.

At the L5-S1 level, significant variation is not apparent.

IMPRESSION:

Variation at the L4-5 level on the left, which may represent annular disc bulge or perhaps protrusion on the left. However, confirmation with myelography and/or Ampaque enhanced computed tomography of the lumbar spine should be suggested prior to any surgical intervention.

Richard W. Adams, MD

Figure 1-6. Diagnostic imaging (CT scan) report.

Hospital documents are dictated by the attending physician and transcribed at the hospital. The original document is filed in the patient's hospital medical record, and a copy is sent to the patient's physician. Hospital documents assist the patient's physician in reviewing the patient's hospital visit and in providing follow-up care.

History and Physical Report

The term *inpatient* is used to refer to a patient who has been admitted to the hospital for at least one overnight stay. A health history must be obtained and a physical examination performed on all inpatients. There is one exception to this: if a patient history and physical are performed at the medical office within a week before admis-sion, a copy of these documents may be used. In the event that a reliable health history cannot be obtained from the patient, it must be obtained from the person best able to relay the facts.

The history and physical report is a physician's narra-tive report of the patient's history and physical exami-nation, along with the physician's medical impressions (Figure 1-8). The purpose of the history is to document the patient's current complaints and symptoms, whereas the purpose of the physical examination is to assess the patient's current health status. **Medical impressions,** or simply impressions, are conclusions drawn from an in-terpretation of data. In this case the physician interprets the data from the health history and physical examina-tion and draws conclusions as to the patient's state of

PHYSICAL THERAPY EVALUATION AND TX PLAN

INSTRUCTIONS: This form must be completed by a licensed professional physical therapist.

PERTINENT BACKGROUND INFORMATION

Facility __North Side Physical Therapy__

Resident _____ Room no. _____ Admission date __/ /__ D.O.B. __9/23/28__

Medicare No. _____ ☐Part A ☐Part B Other insurance _____

Treatment diagnosis __SIP Ⓛ TKR__ ICD-9 code _____ Onset __/ /__

MD referral and date __Michael Howe__ __9/15/05__ Date plan established __9/23/05__

Prior level of function __Ⓘ__

Prior living situation/support system __Lives c̄ spouse__

Describe pertinent medical/social history and/or previous therapy provided: __Hx Ⓛ knee pain x 5 yrs; little relief c̄ PT__

MUSCLE STRENGTH/FUNCTIONAL ROM EVALUATION

AREA	STRENGTH RIGHT	STRENGTH LEFT	ACTION	ROM RIGHT	ROM LEFT
Shoulder	5	5	Flex/Extend	5	5
	5	5	Abd./Add.	5	5
	5	5	Int.rot./Ext.rot.	5	5
Elbow	5	5	Flex/Extend	5	5
Forearm	5	5	Sup./Pron.	5	5
Wrist	5	5	Flex/Extend	5	5
Fingers (Grip)	5	5	Flex/Extend	5	5
Hip	5	2 (knee pain)	Flex/Extend	5	3 (10% to 70%)
	5	3	Abd./Add.	5	3
	5	3	Int.rot./Ext.rot.	5	4
Hip	5	2+→3⁻	Flex/Extend	5	3
Ankle	5	3	Plant./Dors.	5	4
Foot	5	3	Inver./Ever.	5	4

ADDITIONAL SKIN/MUSCLE FUNCTIONAL EVALUATION CRITERIA

TRUNK/NECK POSTURE __FHP__

MUSCLE TONE __Good__

SPECIFIC DEFICITS _____

PALPATION __Knee bandaged__

SKIN CONDITION _____

EDEMA __Mild distal Ⓛ UE/foot__

REHAB POTENTIAL __Good__

PAIN: ☒Intermittent ☐Variable ☐Constant

intensity scale: 1 __Ranges from 2 to 8__ 10

FUNCTIONAL INDEPENDENCE/BALANCE EVALUATION

	AREA	ASSIST GRADE	ASSISTIVE DEVICES/ COMMENTS
BED MOBILITY	Roll/turn	Not assessed	2° surgery
	Sit/supine	2	Assist to Ⓛ LE
	Scoot/bridge	2	Uses overhead trapeze
TRANSFERS	Sit/stand	2	
	Bed/wheelchair	2	
	Toilet	2	
	Floor	Not assessed	
	Auto	Not assessed	
BALANCE	Sit Static	5	
	Sit Dynamic	5	
	Stand Static	3	
	Stand Dynamic	3	
W/C SKILLS	Propulsion	N/A	
	Weight shift	N/A	
	Foot rests	N/A	
	Brakes	N/A	

ADDITIONAL FUNCTIONAL EVALUATION CRITERIA

ENDURANCE __Fair__

COGNITION:: ☒Alert ☐Oriented x __3__ ☐Confused

☒Good judgment in regards to safety

☐ST Memory ☐LT Memory

☒Follows __full__ step commands

VISION __glasses__ HEARING _____ SPEECH _____

PROPRIOCEPTION __WNL__ COORDINATION __WNL__

GAIT ANALYSIS

ASSIST __Min A +1__ DEVICE __Walker__

ANALYSIS __Pt. able to ambulate normal heel-to-toe pattern, PWB Ⓛ LE__

WEIGHT BEARING STATUS __PWB Ⓛ LE__ LEG LENGTH __N/A__

NAME-Last	First	Middle	Attending Physician	Chart No.
Johnson	Thomas	J.	Michael Howe	

Figure 1-7. Physical therapy report. (Courtesy Briggs, Des Moines, Iowa.)

HISTORY AND PHYSICAL
ST. MERCY HOSPITAL

Patient Name: _Carol Jacobs_   Room #: _215_

Physician: _Charles Thomas, MD_   Hospital #: _5422_

Admission Date: _12/14/05_

CHIEF COMPLAINT: Chest pain

HISTORY OF PRESENT ILLNESS: Patient is an 85-year-old female complaining of chest pain. Patient was found to have abnormal cardiac enzymes in the Emergency Room consistent with acute myocardial infarction. Patient denied any pain radiating; however, she did complain of left-sided chest pain and lower back pain. Patient did not admit to any shortness of breath, nausea, or diaphoresis.

MEDICATIONS: Lasix, Darvocet-N 100, Lisinopril, Lopressor, Glynase, Relafen, Cytotec, and Micro K.

ALLERGIES: No drug allergies known.

PAST MEDICAL HISTORY: Significant for congestive heart failure, chronic obstructive pulmonary disease, diabetes mellitus type 2, coronary atherosclerosis, hypertension, and osteoporosis.

SOCIAL HISTORY: Not a drinker and not a smoker. Patient resides in a nursing home.

PHYSICAL EXAMINATION:

General: Patient is in acute distress. She is obese.
HEENT: She has 2 centimeters jugular venous distention. Pupils are equal and reactive to light and accommodation. No evidence of scleral or conjunctival icterus.
Chest: +2 bibasilar rales.
Heart: Regular rate and rhythm. +2/6 systolic ejection murmur in the left sternal border.
Abdomen: Soft, nontender, no splenomegaly and no hepatomegaly and positive bowel sounds.
Extremities: No evidence of edema or deep venous thrombosis.
Neurological: Cranial nerves II through XII grossly intact.

IMPRESSIONS: Congestive heart failure
                   Rule out myocardial infarction

Charles Thomas

_____

Charles Thomas, MD

Figure 1-8. Hospital history and physical examination report.

health. Other terms for impressions include *provisional diagnosis* and *tentative diagnosis*.

Operative Report

An operative report (Figure 1-9) must be completed for all patients who have had a surgical procedure. This report describes the surgical procedure and must be completed and signed by the surgeon who performed the operation.

The operative report must include the following:
- Patient identification information
- Date of the surgery
- Preoperative diagnosis
- Name of the surgical procedure
- Full description of the findings at surgery (both normal and abnormal)
- Description of the technique and procedures used during surgery

OPERATIVE REPORT
ST. MARY'S HOSPITAL

Name: __Natalie Boyer__

Hospital #: __291734__   Room #: __OP__

Surgeon: __Paul Cain, M.D.__   Date of Surgery: __1/6/05__

Anesthesiologist: __John Adams, M.D.__   Anesthesia: __General__

PRE-OP DIAGNOSIS: Abnormal Pap test with history of cervical carcinoma.

POST-OP DIAGNOSIS: Same and awaiting path report.

OPERATION: D&C, laser cone of the cervix.

PROCEDURE: The patient to the operating room, lithotomy position, perineum and vagina were prepped, and moist sterile drape was used. Laser precautions all in place. Bimanual examination revealed a uterus enlarged with a second-degree uterine prolapse. The cervix was dilated. Uterus sounded to around 9 cm. The endocervical canal was dilated and D&C was performed with tissue recovered and submitted to Pathology. The cervix was stained with iodine, and the nonstaining area was identified. The laser was brought in, 50 watts of current were used to remove laser cone, and we submitted that to Pathology. We then vaporized beyond the margins of the cone, 3-4 mm to a depth of 4-5 mm. Hemostasis was adequate. We placed O Vicryl figure-of-eight sutures at the 3 and the 9 o'clock positions in the cervix, and then we put Monsel solution on the cervix. Hemostasis adequate. Sponge and needle counts correct times two. The patient tolerated the procedure well, and she returned to the recovery room in stable condition. She will be discharged home when awake and stable on Cipro 250 mg twice a day for a week, Darvocet-N 100, #20 as needed for pain. If she continues to have abnormal Pap tests, we will probably want to do a vaginal hysterectomy.

SURGEON: _Paul Cain_____

Paul Cain, MD

Figure 1-9. Operative report.

- Ligatures and sutures used
- Number of packs, drains, and sponges used
- Description of any specimens removed
- Condition of the patient at the completion of the surgery
- Postoperative diagnosis
- Name of the surgeon

Discharge Summary Report

The discharge summary report is a brief (usually one-page) summary of the significant events of the patient's hospitalization (Figure 1-10). The report must be completed and signed by the attending physician. The discharge summary report includes a concise account of the patient's illness, course of treatment, response to treatment and condition of the patient at the time of discharge from the hospital. The purpose of this report is to provide information to the patient's family physician for the continuity of future care. It is also used to respond to authorized requests for information regarding the patient's hospitalization.

The discharge summary report must include the following:
- Patient identification information
- Dates of hospitalization
- Reason for the hospitalization (provisional diagnosis)
- Brief health history
- Significant findings from examinations and tests
- Course of treatment
- Response to treatment
- Condition of the patient at discharge
- Discharge diagnosis (final diagnosis)
- Prognosis
- Discharge instructions
- Recommendations and arrangements for follow-up care

DISCHARGE SUMMARY

Brennan, Susan
97-32-11
June 18, 2005

ADMISSION DATE: June 14, 2005   **DISCHARGE DATE:**   June 16, 2005

HISTORY OF PRESENT ILLNESS:
This 19-year-old female, nulligravida, was admitted to the hospital on June 14, 2005, with fever of 102°, left lower quadrant pain, vaginal discharge, constipation, and a tender left adnexal mass. Her past history and family history were unremarkable. Present pain had started two to three weeks prior to admission. Her periods were irregular, with latest period starting on May 30, 2005, and lasting for six days. She had taken contraceptive pills in the past but had stopped because she was not sexually active.

PHYSICAL EXAMINATION:
She appeared well developed and well nourished, and in mild distress. The only positive physical findings were limited to the abdomen and pelvis. Her abdomen was mildly distended, and it was tender, especially in the left lower quadrant. At pelvic examination, her cervix was tender on motion, and the uterus was of normal size, retroverted, and somewhat fixed. There was a tender cystic mass about 4-5 cm in the left adnexa. Rectal examination was negative.

PROVISIONAL DIAGNOSIS:
1. Probable pelvic inflammatory disease (PID).
2. Rule out ectopic pregnancy.

LABORATORY DATA ON ADMISSION:
Hgb 10.8, Hct 36.5, WBC 8,100 with 80 segs and 18 lymphs. Sedimentation rate 100 mm in one hour. Sickle cell prep+ (turned out to be a trait). Urinalysis normal. Electrolytes normal. SMA-12 normal. Chest x-ray negative, 2-hour UCG negative.

HOSPITAL COURSE AND TREATMENT:
Initially, she was given cephalothin 2 gm IV q6h, and kanamycin 0.5 gm IM bid. Over the next two days the patient's condition improved. Her pain decreased and her temperature came down to normal in the morning and spiked to 101° in the evening. Repeat CBC showed Hgb 9.8, Hct 33.5. The pregnancy test was negative. She was discharged on June 16, 2005 in good condition. She will be seen in the office in one week.

DISCHARGE DIAGNOSIS:
Pelvic inflammatory disease.

Harold B. Cooper
Harold B. Cooper, MD

Figure 1-10. Discharge summary report. (Modified from Diehl MO, Fordney MT: *Medical transcription: techniques and procedures,* ed 5, Philadelphia, 2003, Saunders.)

Pathology Report

A pathology report consists of a macroscopic (gross) and a microscopic description of tissue removed from a patient during surgery or a diagnostic procedure. The report also includes a diagnosis of the patient's condition (Figure 1-11). A pathologist is required to examine the tissue, complete the report, and sign it.

Emergency Room Report

The emergency room report is a record of the significant information obtained during an emergency room visit (Figure 1-12). The report is prepared and signed by the emergency room physician, and a copy is sent to the patient's physician for the purpose of providing follow-up care.

COLLEGE HOSPITAL
4567 BROAD AVENUE
WOODLAND HILLS, MD 21532

PATHOLOGY REPORT

Date:	June 20, 2005	Pathology No.:	430211
Patient:	Molly Ramsdale	Room No.:	1308
Physician:	Harold B. Cooper, M.D.		
Specimen Submitted:	Tumor, right axilla		

FINDINGS

GROSS DESCRIPTION: Specimen A consists of an oval mass of yellow fibroadipose tissue measuring 4 x 3 x 2 cm. On cut section, there are some small, soft, pliable areas of gray apparent lymph node alternating with adipose tissue. A frozen section consultation at time of surgery was delivered as NO EVIDENCE OF MALIGNANCY on frozen section, to await permanent section for final diagnosis. Majority of the specimen will be submitted for microscopic examination.

Specimen B consists of an oval mass of yellow soft tissue measuring 2.5 x 2.5 x 1.5 cm. On cut section, there is a thin rim of pink to tan-brown lymphatic tissue and the mid portion appears to be adipose tissue. A pathological consultation at time of surgery was delivered as no suspicious areas noted and to await permanent sections for final diagnosis. The entire specimen will be submitted for microscopic examination.

MICROSCOPIC DESCRIPTION: Specimen A sections show fibroadipose tissue and nine fragments of lymph nodes. The lymph nodes show areas with prominent germinal centers and moderate sinus histiocytosis. There appears to be some increased vascularity and reactive endothelial cells seen. There is no evidence of malignancy.

Specimen B sections show adipose tissue and 5 lymph node fragments. These 5 portions of lymph nodes show reactive changes including sinus histiocytosis. There is no evidence of malignancy.

DIAGNOSIS: A & B: TUMOR, RIGHT AXILLA: SHOWING 14 LYMPH NODE FRAGMENTS WITH REACTIVE CHANGES AND NO EVIDENCE OF MALIGNANCY.

Stanley T. Nason

Stanley T. Nason, MD

Figure 1-11. Pathology report. (From Diehl MO, Fordney MT: *Medical transcription: techniques and procedures,* ed 5, Philadelphia, 2003, Saunders.)

EMERGENCY ROOM REPORT
CAMDEN CLARK HOSPITAL

Name: John Larimer

DOB: 2/2/65

ER Physician: John Parsons, MD

Date: 7/7/05

ER Number: 07398

Physician: James Woods, MD

NATURE OF ILLNESS/INJURY: This 40-year-old male presents to the Emergency Department complaining of a laceration of the sole of his right foot. Patient cut his foot on a rock 2 days ago and thinks he might have an infection now. Patient also complains of coughing over the past several days.

PHYSICAL EXAMINATION: Temperature 97.4, Pulse 76, Respirations 20, Blood Pressure 120/70. Patient is alert and oriented and is in no acute distress. ENT is normal. Lungs show diffuse rhonchi without crackles or wheezing. Heart has a regular rate and rhythm. Right great toe with marked tenderness with edema and erythema and heat.

DIAGNOSIS: Asthmatic Bronchitis
   Cellulitis, right foot first MTP

TREATMENT: PCMX scrub to right foot. Bacitracin dressing. Tetanus Diphtheria 0.5 cc IM. Biaxin 500 mg bid x 10 days. Guaifenesin with codeine 2 tsp q4h prn. Entex LA,1 bid prn. Debridement of skin flap.

PATIENT INSTRUCTIONS: Patient to follow up with family doctor in 7 days. Discussed bronchospasms with the patient.

James Woods

James Woods, MD

Figure 1-12. Emergency room report.

The emergency room report includes the following:
- Date of service
- Patient identification information
- Nature of the illness or injury
- Any laboratory or diagnostic test results
- Procedures performed
- Treatment rendered
- Diagnosis
- Condition of the patient at discharge
- Instructions regarding follow-up care

Consent Documents

Consent forms are legal documents required in order to perform certain procedures or to release information contained in the patient's medical record.

Consent to Treatment Form

The completion of a consent to treatment form (Procedure 1-1) is required for all surgical operations and nonroutine diagnostic and therapeutic procedures performed in the medical office (e.g., minor office surgery, sigmoidoscopy). The form must be signed by the patient or his or her legally authorized representative and provide written evidence that the patient agrees to the procedure(s) listed on the form (Figure 1-13).

In order for the patient's consent to be valid, it must be informed consent. **Informed consent** means that the patient has received the following information before giving consent:
- The nature of the patient's condition
- The nature and purpose of the recommended procedure
- An explanation of risks involved with the procedure
- Alternative treatments or procedures available
- The likely outcome (prognosis) of the procedure
- The risks of declining or delaying the procedure

The explanation must be in terms the patient can understand, and the patient should be given an opportunity to ask questions regarding the information.

PROCEDURE 1-1   Completion of a Consent to Treatment Form

Outcome Complete a consent to treatment form.

Equipment/Supplies:
- Consent to treatment form

1. **Procedural Step.** Type or print all required information on the consent to treatment form in the spaces provided (e.g., patient's full name, name of the procedure to be performed, and so on).

2. **Procedural Step.** Ensure that the physician has had a discussion to give the patient complete information about the procedure to be performed.
   Principle. In order for the patient's consent to be valid, it must be informed consent.

3. **Procedural Step.** Greet and identify the patient. Introduce yourself, and explain the purpose of the consent form.

4. **Procedural Step.** Give the consent form to the patient and ask him or her to read it. Ask the patient if he or she has any questions.

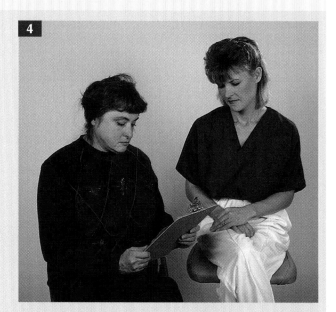

5. **Procedural Step.** Ask the patient to sign the consent form. Witness the patient's signature by signing your name in the appropriate space on the form. Include today's date.
   Principle. Witnessing a signature means only that the medical assistant verified the identify of the patient and watched the patient sign the form; it does not mean that the medical assistant is attesting to the accuracy of the information provided.

6. **Procedural Step.** Provide the patient with a copy of the completed consent form for his or her files.

7. **Procedural Step.** File the original consent to treatment form in the patient's medical record.
   Principle. Maintaining the form provides legal documentation that the patient gave permission for treatment.

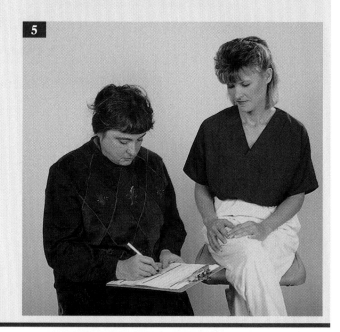

The consent to treatment form should not be signed until the patient has been provided with all necessary information related to the procedure. The patient's signature must be witnessed; this is usually the responsibility of the medical assistant. *Witnessing a signature* means only that the medical assistant verified the patient's identity and watched the patient sign the form; it *does not* mean that the medical assistant is attesting to the accuracy of the information provided.

The consent to treatment form outlines the details of the discussion with the patient and includes the following information:
- Patient's full name
- Name of the procedure to be performed

(Attach label or complete blanks.)

First name: _____   Last name: _____

Date of Birth: _____ Month _____ Day _____ Year

Account Number: _____

Procedure Consent Form

I, _____ , hereby consent to have

Dr. _____ perform _____ .

I have been fully informed of the following by my physician:

1. The nature of my condition
2. The nature and purpose of the procedure
3. An explanation of risks involved with the procedure
4. Alternative treatments or procedures available
5. The likely results of the procedure
6. The risks involved with declining or delaying the procedure

My physician has offered to answer all questions concerning the proposed procedure.

I am aware that the practice of medicine and surgery is not an exact science, and I acknowledge that no guarantees have been made to me about the results of the procedure.

Patient _____   Date _____
        (or guardian and relationship)

Witnessed _____   Date _____

Figure 1-13. Consent to treatment form.

- Name of the surgeon
- A statement indicating the patient agrees to receive the procedure
- Acknowledgment that a disclosure of information has been made
- Acknowledgment that all questions were answered in a satisfactory manner
- A statement that no guarantee as to the outcome has been made
- Signature of the patient or his or her legal representative
- Signature of the witness

Release of Medical Information Form

As previously explained in the box entitled *Highlight on the HIPAA Privacy Rule* (p. 5), a patient's written consent is not required for the use or disclosure of protected health information (PHI) for the purpose of medical treatment, payment, and health care operations (TPO). On the other hand, if a request for PHI is required for purposes that are not part of TPO, a detailed form must be completed, known as a *release of medical information form* (Figure 1-14). For example, if a patient is moving to another state and wants to transfer his or her medical record to a new physician, a release of medical information form must be completed.

The release of medical information form must be signed by the patient authorizing the disclosure of his or her PHI (Procedure 1-2). If the patient is a minor, the form must be signed by the parent or legal guardian of the minor.

The release of medical information form must stipulate the following:
- Patient's full name and address
- Name of the medical practice releasing the information
- Name of the individual or facility to receive the information
- Specific information to be released
- The purpose of or the need for the information
- Method of release of the information
- Signature of the patient or his or her legal representative
- Date that the consent was signed
- The expiration date of the consent form

RELEASE OF MEDICAL INFORMATION

All information contained in the medical record is confidential, and the release of information is closely controlled. A properly completed and signed authorization form is required for the release of the following information.

PATIENT INFORMATION

Patient Name _____

Address _____ Social Security # _____

City _____ State _____ ZIP _____ Birth date _____ / _____ / _____

Phone (Home) _____ Work _____

RELEASE FROM:

Name _____

Address _____

City _____ State _____ ZIP _____

RELEASE TO:

Name _____

Address _____

City _____ State _____ ZIP _____

INFORMATION TO BE RELEASED:

1. GENERAL RELEASE:

____ Entire Medical Record (excluding protected information)

____ Hospital Records only (specify) _____

____ Lab Results only (specify) _____

____ X-ray Reports only (specify) _____

____ Other Records (specify) _____

2. INFORMATION PROTECTED BY STATE/FEDERAL LAW:
If indicated below, I hereby authorize the disclosure and release of information regarding:

____ Drug Abuse Diagnosis/Treatment

____ Alcoholism Diagnosis/Treatment

____ Mental Health Diagnosis/Treatment

____ Sexually Transmitted Disease

PURPOSE/NEED FOR INFORMATION:

____ Taking records to another doctor

____ Moving

____ Legal purposes

____ Insurance purposes

____ Workman's Compensation

____ Other/Explain: _____

METHOD OF RELEASE:

____ US Mail

____ Fax

____ Telephone

____ To Patient

PATIENT AUTHORIZATION TO RELEASE INFORMATION:

Authorization is valid for 60 days only from the date of my signature. I reserve the right to revoke this authorization at any time prior to 60 days (except for action that has already been taken) by notifying the medical office in writing.

I understand that my records are protected under HIPAA (Health Insurance Portability and Accountability Act) Standards for Privacy of Individually Identifiable Information (45 CFR Parts 160 and 164) unless otherwise permitted by federal law. Any information released or received shall not be further relayed to any other facility or person without my written authorization. I also understand that such information will not be given, sold, transferred, or in any way relayed to any other person or party not specified above without my further written authorization.

I hereby grant authorization to release the information listed above. I certify that this request has been made voluntarily and that the information given above is accurate to the best of my knowledge.

_____ _____

Signature of Patient/Legally Responsible Party **Date**

_____ _____

Witness Signature **Date**

OFFICE USE ONLY

Information indicated above released on _____

Date

Explanation of information released: _____

_____

Signature and credentials of individual releasing information: _____

Figure 1-14. Release of medical information form.

PROCEDURE 1-2 Release of Medical Information

Outcome
1. Assist a patient in the completion of a release of medical information form.
2. Release medical information according to a completed release of medical information form.

Equipment/Supplies:
- Release of medical information form

1. **Procedural Step.** Greet and identify the patient. Introduce yourself, and explain the purpose of the release of medical information form. (NOTE: If you do not recognize the patient, ask him or her to provide a picture identification such as a driver's license.)
2. **Procedural Step.** Provide the patient with a release of medical information form and ask the patient to complete the form. Provide assistance if needed.
   Principle. Information from a patient's medical record can be released only upon written authorization of the patient (except when permitted by law).
3. **Procedural Step.** Check to make sure all the requested information on the form has been completed by the patient.
4. **Procedural Step.** Ask the patient to sign the form. Witness the patient's signature by signing your name in the appropriate space on the form. Include today's date. If required by your medical office policy, ask the physician to initial the completed release of medical information form.
   Principle. In order to release information, the form must be signed by the patient authorizing the disclosure of medical information.

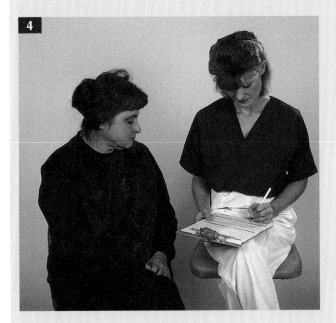

4

5. **Procedural Step.** Provide the patient with a copy of the release of medical information form for his or her files.
6. **Procedural Step.** Copy the information requested on the form. Be sure to release only the information requested. Include a copy of the completed release form with the medical information.
7. **Procedural Step.** Document what information is being released and the date of its release. Sign the document with your name and credentials.
8. **Procedural Step.** File the original document and the release of medical information form in the patient's medical record.
   Principle. Maintaining the release form provides legal documentation that the patient gave permission for the release of his or her medical information.
9. **Procedural Step.** Send the medical information to the appropriate site according to your medical office policy.

Mailed or Faxed Requests for Release of Medical Information
The following steps should be followed when a completed release of medical information form has been mailed or faxed to the medical office:
1. **Procedural Step.** Check the expiration date on the release of medical information form. If the authorization is outdated, a new release form needs to be completed.
2. **Procedural Step.** Verify the authenticity of the signature on the form. This can be accomplished by comparing the patient's signature on the form with the patient's signature in his or her medical record. If you have any doubt as to the authenticity of the signature, do not release the records.
3. **Procedural Step.** Copy the information requested on the form. Be sure to release only the information requested. Include a copy of the completed release form with the medical information.
4. **Procedural Step.** Document what information is being released and the date of its release. Sign the document with your name and credentials.
5. **Procedural Step.** File the original document and the release of medical information form in the patient's medical record.
6. **Procedural Step.** Send the medical information according to your medical office policy.

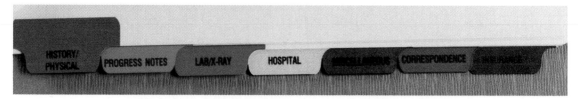

Figure 1-15. Chart dividers in a source-oriented record.

Mailed or Faxed Requests for Release of Medical Information

Most medical offices require that the patient come to the office to sign the release of medical information form; however, this may not always be possible. An example is a patient who has moved away and is requesting the transfer of his or her medical records to a new physician. In this instance a completed and signed release of medical information form may be mailed or faxed to the medical office. The procedure for processing this type of request is outlined at the end of Procedure 1-2.

Medical Record Formats

Most medical offices rely on the use of paper medical records, known as **paper-based patient records (PPRs).** Currently some patient data are maintained on the computer; these include patient registration information and patient charges and payments. As technology advances, more offices may elect to use an **electronic medical record (EMR),** meaning that the entire record is stored in a database on the computer, including the health history report and physical examination report, progress notes, laboratory and diagnostic reports, hospital reports, and so on. Since that is not yet the case, this chapter focuses on the paper-based record.

The way a PPR is organized is known as its *format.* The two main types of medical record formats are the **source-oriented record** and the **problem-oriented record.** Each of these formats is described next.

Source-Oriented Record

The source-oriented format is used most often in the medical office for organizing a medical record. The documents in a source-oriented record are organized into sections based on the department, facility, or other source that generated the information (e.g., laboratory, hospital, consultant). Because documents from each source are filed together, it is easier to compare information from laboratory and diagnostic test results, assessments and treatments, and so on.

Each section in a source-oriented record is separated from the other sections by a chart divider. Attached to each divider is a color-coded tab labeled with the title of its section (Figure 1-15). Within each of these sections, the documents are arranged according to date. Most offices use the reverse chronological order to arrange the documents. **Reverse chronological order** means that the most recent document is placed on top or in front of the others, which means the oldest document is on the bottom or at the end of that section.

The titles that identify each section vary depending on the medical office's preference; however, typical examples include the following:

- History and Physical
- Progress Notes
- Medications
- Laboratory Reports
- ECG
- X-ray Reports
- Consultations
- Rehabilitation Therapy
- Home Health Care
- Hospital Reports
- Insurance
- Consents
- Correspondence
- Miscellaneous

Problem-Oriented Record

The documents in a problem-oriented record (abbreviated POR or POMR for problem-oriented medical record) are organized according to the patient's health problems. The advantage of using the POR is that each of the patient's problems can be defined and followed individually. The POR is developed in four stages:

1. Establishing a *database*
2. Compiling a *problem list*
3. Devising a *plan* of action for each problem
4. Following each problem with *progress notes*

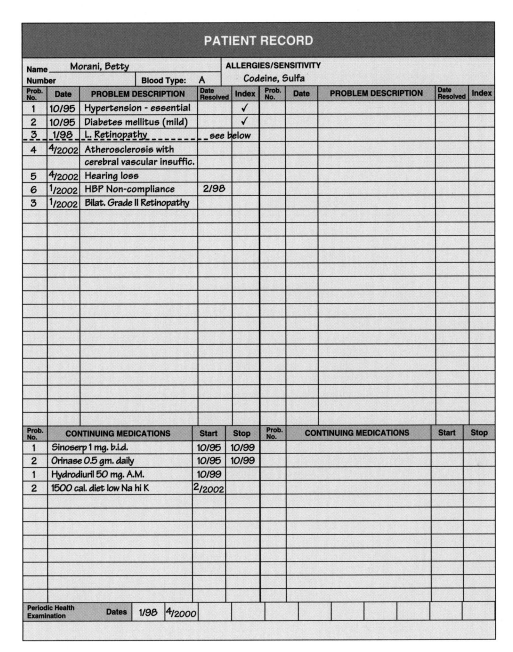

Figure 1-16. POR problem list. (Courtesy Miller Communications, Norwalk, Conn.)

Database

The first step in developing a POR is to establish a database. The database consists of a collection of subjective and objective data. These data include the health history report, physical examination report, and results of baseline laboratory and diagnostic tests. The information in the database is used to identify and compile a problem list.

Problem List

The problem list is developed shortly after the database is completed and consists of a list of all the patient's problems (Figure 1-16). A **problem** is defined as any patient condition that requires observation, diagnosis, management, or patient education. This includes not only medical problems but also psychologic and social problems. The problem list is a crucial part of the POR and is always located in the front of the medical record.

The problem list should be thought of as a table of contents for the record. Each problem in the list is numbered and titled. The problem title is stated as a diagnosis, a physiologic finding, a symptom, or an abnormal test result. All subsequent data (plans and progress notes) added to the medical record are cross-referenced to these numbered problems.

The problem list is modified as needed. If a new problem is identified, it is added to the list and dated accordingly.

PROBLEM-ORIENTED PROGRESS NOTES			
Name Jessica Michaels		**DOB** 9/20/02	**Doctor** Frank Edwards, MD
DATE	**TIME**	**PROBLEM NUMBER**	**FORMAT:** Problem Number and TITLE: S = Subjective O = Objective A = Assessment P = Plan
11/5/05	9:30 AM	1	**S:** Mother states that her child has had a runny nose and the back of her throat has been sore for 2 days.
			O: Vital signs: T 98.8 P 108 R 24
			Weight 27 lb.
			General: alert and active. HEENT: sclera clear.
			TMs negative. Positive clear rhinorrhea. Pharynx benign.
			Heart: regular without murmur. Lungs: clear to
			auscultation and percussion. Abdomen: negative
			tenderness. Positive bowel sounds x4. GU: negative
			Neuro: good tone.
			A: Upper respiratory tract infection.
			P: 1. A prescription for Rondec DM, 1/2 tsp q6h prn
			cough and congestion.
			2. Instructed mother to contact office if child does
			not improve.

Figure 1-17. POR SOAP progress notes. (Courtesy Briggs, Des Moines, Iowa.)

DAWN BENNETT: During my externship as a medical assisting student, I was placed in a family practice clinic. I was very nervous my first day, wondering how in the world I would be able to remember everything I had learned in school. My very first patients were an elderly couple. The wife was there for some test results for cancer. I looked at the results, and they were positive. After the physician relayed the results, the husband broke down. He had just lost his granddaughter to a heart attack and his son-in-law to a stroke. You could tell that he just could not bear losing his wife too.

One week later the elderly man's wife was placed in a nursing home. He came into our office for an appointment. As I was working him up, he was telling me stories about himself and his wife when they were first married. He looked so sad. I sat with him for a few minutes after completing his workup and gave his stories my full attention. As I was leaving the room, a smile came across his face and he thanked me for listening to him. I realized that working in a physician's office is more than just knowing what I learned in school. Compassion and showing the patients you really do care about them is just as important. I felt good about myself that day.

When a problem is resolved, it is marked as such and the date is recorded.

Plan

After examining the problem list, the physician develops the third section of the POR. This involves devising a plan of action for further evaluation and treatment of each problem. Each plan begins with a heading that identifies the number of the problem, followed by the plan of action for the problem. This may include plans for laboratory and diagnostic tests, medical or surgical treatment, therapy, and patient education.

Progress Notes

The last stage in the development of the POR is the follow-up for each problem, or the progress notes (Figure 1-17). The progress notes begin with the number of a problem and include the following four categories:

Subjective data: Subjective data obtained from the patient

Objective data: Objective data obtained by observation, physical examination, diagnostic tests, and so on

Assessment: The physician's interpretation of the current condition based on an analysis of the subjective and objective data

Plan: Proposed treatment for the patient

The acronym for this process is **SOAP,** and the writing of progress notes in this format is called *soaping.* Some physicians who use the source-oriented format have found

What Would You DO? What Would You *Not* DO?

Case Study 3

Brett Oberlin is 21 years old and lives at home. He commutes to a local college and is a junior majoring in art education. His mother and father have come to the medical office and ask to see his medical record. The physician is attending a medical conference and will not return for another 4 days. Mr. and Mrs. Oberlin found some medications in Brett's room and looked them up on the Internet. They found out that they are used to treat HIV infection. Brett would not talk to them about the medications and told them he is an adult and it is none of their business. Mr. and Mrs. Oberlin are very concerned about Brett. They are also worried about other members of the family being exposed to HIV. They say that since they are supporting him, they should be allowed to see his record.

it advantageous to record progress notes in SOAP format. This structured type of note increases the physician's ability to deal with each problem clearly and to analyze data in an orderly, systematic manner.

Preparing a Medical Record for a New Patient

When a patient comes to the medical office for his or her first visit, a medical record must be prepared for that patient (Procedure 1-3). The method used to prepare the record depends on the following criteria: the format used to organize the record, the filing system, and the type of storage equipment. Most medical offices use the source-oriented format to organize their medical records, the alphabetic filing system to arrange the records, and shelf filing units to store the medical records. Methods used to prepare a medical record are described in the following sections and are based on these criteria.

Medical Record Supplies

Certain supplies are required to prepare a medical record. These supplies are categorized and described next.

File Folders. A file folder is a protective cover made of a heavy material such as manila card stock. A file folder is used to hold medical record documents in an organized format. Flexible metal fasteners are typically used to hold documents in the folder. Folders are available with fasteners located on the top or left side of the folder.

Folders are available with tabs. A tab is a projection extending from a folder and is used to identify its contents. The tab is located on either the side or top of the folder. A folder with a tab extending across its entire side or top is called a *full cut tab.*

PROCEDURE 1-3   Preparing a Medical Record

Outcome Prepare a medical record.

The following procedure outlines the method for preparing a medical record for a new patient using the following organization: a source-oriented format stored in shelf files using a color-coded alphabetic filing system.

Equipment/Supplies:
- Patient registration form
- Notice of Privacy Practices (NPP)
- NPP acknowledgment form
- File folder with a full cut side tab
- Metal fasteners
- Name labels
- Color-coded alphabetic bar labels
- Miscellaneous chart labels
- Set of chart dividers
- Blank preprinted forms
- Two-hole punch

1. **Procedural Step.** Greet and identify the patient when he or she arrives at the medical office. Introduce yourself, and verify that the patient is a new patient.
2. **Procedural Step.** Ask the patient to do the following:
   a. Complete a patient registration form.
   b. Read a Notice of Privacy Practices (NPP).
   c. Sign an NPP acknowledgment form.
   Provide the patient with the appropriate forms, a pen, and a hard surface (such as a clipboard) on which to write. Offer to answer any questions.
3. **Procedural Step.** When the patient returns the completed forms, check the patient registration form for accuracy and make sure that you can read the patient's handwriting. If you have any questions regarding the information on the form, ask the patient for clarification. If required by the medical office policy, ask the patient for his or her insurance card and make a copy of it.
   Principle. A copy of the patient's insurance card is used for third-party billing.
4. **Procedural Step.** Enter the data on the completed registration record into the computer.
5. **Procedural Step.** Assemble supplies needed to prepare the medical record. Type the patient's full name on a name label following these guidelines:
   a. Type the patient's name in transposed order as follows: last name, first name, middle name (or initial).
   b. Type the patient's name two or three typewritten spaces from the left edge of the label and one line down from the top of the label.
   c. Make sure the patient's name is spelled correctly.
   Principle. Following these guidelines facilitates the accurate and efficient filing of the patient's medical record.
6. **Procedural Step.** Determine the first two letters of the patient's last name and select the appropriate alphabetic color-coded labels. Attach the color-coded labels to the (full cut) side tab. The labels should be affixed to the folder using the label placement indentations on the tab.
   Principle. Using the label placement indentations ensures that all labels on medical records are affixed at the same place.
7. **Procedural Step.** Affix the name label immediately above the first color-coded alphabetic label.

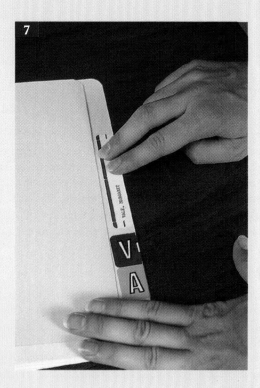

8. **Procedural Step.** Attach any additional chart labels, such as a year label and miscellaneous chart labels (e.g., allergy, insurance), to the folder according to the office policy.

9. **Procedural Step.** Insert the chart dividers onto the metal fasteners of the file folder.

10. **Procedural Step.** Place the original patient registration form in the front of the medical record. Place the signed NPP acknowledgment form and the copy of the patient's insurance card in the appropriate section of the record.

11. **Procedural Step.** Label preprinted forms to be placed in the record with required information such as the patient's name and date. These forms typically include the medical history form, physical examination form, progress note sheets, and a medication record form. If the forms are not prepunched, the medical assistant must use a two-hole punch to insert two holes into the top or side of the form.

12. **Procedural Step.** Insert each form under its proper chart divider. Refer to the box on p. 30 for a list of chart divider subject titles and documents typically filed under each title.

13. **Procedural Step.** Check the medical record to ensure that it has been prepared properly.

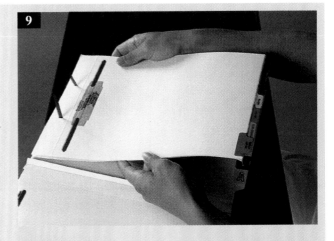

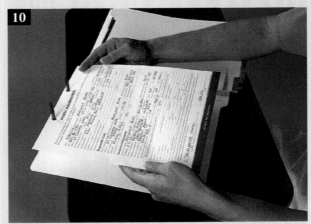

PROCEDURE 1-3

In the medical office, a file folder with a full cut side tab is typically used to prepare a new patient's chart. There are indentations at intervals along the full cut tab to indicate the placement of adhesive labels. This ensures that the labels on all the medical records are affixed at the same place on the file folders.

Folder Labels. Labels to identify the medical record are commercially available in rolls or continuous folded strips for typewriter use. Labels are also available on 8½ × 11-inch sheets for use with a computer and printer. The most common types of labels used in the medical office include name labels, alphabetic color-coded labels, color-coded year labels, and miscellaneous chart labels.

Chart Dividers. Chart dividers are used to identify each section of the medical record by subject (see Figure 1-15). Chart dividers consist of a heavy material such as manila card stock. Attached to each divider is a color-coded tab labeled with a subject title; the most frequently used subject titles are illustrated in the box on the following page, along with the documents typically filed under each title.

Taking a Health History

The health history is a collection of data obtained by interviewing the patient. A thorough history is taken for each new patient, and subsequent office visits (in the form of progress notes) provide information regarding changes in the patient's illness or treatment. A quiet, comfortable room that allows for privacy encourages the patient to communicate honestly and openly. Showing genuine interest in and concern for the patient reduces apprehension and facilitates the collection of data.

Components of the Health History

The health history is taken before the physical examination, providing the physician the opportunity to compare findings. The health history consists of seven parts or sections, which are listed and described next.

Identification Data

The identification data section is included at the beginning of the health history form to obtain basic data on the patient (Figure 1-18, *A*). The identification data section is completed by the patient.

Chart Divider Subject Titles and Documents Typically Filed Under Each Title

History and Physical
Health history
Physical examination report

Progress Notes
Progress notes
Medication record

Lab/X-ray
Hematology report
Clinical chemistry report
Serology report
Urinalysis report
Microbiology report
Parasitology report
Cytology report
Histology report
Electrocardiogram report
Holter monitor report

Lab/X-ray—cont'd
Sigmoidoscopy report
Colonoscopy report
Spirometry report
Radiology report
Diagnostic imaging report

Hospital
History and physical report
Operative report
Pathology report
Discharge summary report
Emergency room report

Correspondence
Consultation report
Letter from patient
Letter from patient's attorney
Referral letter

Insurance
Copy of patient's insurance card
Precertification authorization for hospital admission
Request for additional information from insurance company

Miscellaneous
Consent to treatment form
Release of medical information form
Home health care report
Physical therapy report
Occupational therapy report
Speech therapy report

Chief Complaint

The chief complaint (CC) identifies the patient's reason for seeking care—that is, the symptom causing the patient the most trouble. The chief complaint is used as a foundation for the more detailed information that will be obtained for the present illness and review of systems sections of the health history. The medical assistant is usually responsible for obtaining the chief complaint from the patient and recording it in the patient's chart. In most offices this information is recorded on a preprinted, lined form (Figure 1-18, *G*). Certain guidelines must be followed in obtaining and recording the chief complaint:

- An open-ended question should be used to elicit the chief complaint from the patient. Examples: What seems to be the problem? How can we help you today? What can we do for you today?
- The chief complaint should be limited to one or two symptoms and should refer to a specific, rather than vague, symptom.
- The chief complaint should be recorded concisely and briefly, using the patient's own words as much as possible.
- The duration of the symptom (onset) should be included in the chief complaint.
- The medical assistant should avoid using names of diseases or diagnostic terms to record the chief complaint.

Recording Chief Complaints

The following are correct and incorrect examples of recording chief complaints.

Correct Examples
- Burning during urination that has lasted for 2 days.
- Pain in the shoulder that started 2 weeks ago.
- Shortness of breath for the past month.

Incorrect Examples
- Has not felt well for the past 2 weeks. (This statement refers to a vague, rather than a specific, complaint.)
- Ear pain and fever. (The duration of the symptoms is not listed.)
- Pain upon urination indicative of a urinary tract infection. (Names of diseases should not be used to record the chief complaint; the duration of the symptom is not listed.)

Present Illness

The present illness (PI) is an expansion of the chief complaint and includes a full description of the patient's current illness from the time of its onset. The medical assistant is often responsible for completing this section of the health history, which is recorded on the same form as the chief complaint (see Figure 1-18, *G*). To complete this section of the health history, the medical assistant asks the patient questions to obtain a detailed description of the symptom causing the greatest problem. Much skill and practice in asking the proper questions are required to elicit detailed information. A general guide for

Text continued on p. 34

PATIENT HEALTH HISTORY

A **IDENTIFICATION DATA**   Please print the following information.

Today's date _____

Name _____   ___ Male ___ Female

Address _____   ___ Married ___ Separated ___ Divorced ___ Widowed ___ Single

_____   Date of Birth _____

Telephone _____   _____
         Home number   Work number

B **PAST HISTORY**

Have you ever had the following: (Circle "no" or "yes", leave blank if uncertain)

Measles _____ no yes	Heart Disease _____ no yes	Diabetes _____ no yes	Hemorrhoids _____ no yes
Mumps _____ no yes	Arthritis _____ no yes	Cancer _____ no yes	Asthma _____ no yes
Chickenpox _____ no yes	Sexually Transmitted ___ no yes Disease	Polio _____ no yes	Allergies _____ no yes
Whooping Cough ___ no yes	Anemia _____ no yes	Glaucoma _____ no yes	Eczema _____ no yes
Scarlet Fever _____ no yes	Bladder Infections ___ no yes	Hernia _____ no yes	AIDS or HIV+ _____ no yes
Diphtheria _____ no yes	Epilepsy _____ no yes	Blood or Plasma ___ no yes Transfusions	Infectious Mono ___ no yes
Pneumonia _____ no yes	Migraine Headaches ___ no yes	Back Trouble _____ no yes	Bronchitis _____ no yes
Rheumatic Fever ___ no yes	Tuberculosis _____ no yes	High Blood ___ no yes Pressure	Mitral Valve Prolapse no yes
Stroke _____ no yes	Ulcer _____ no yes	Thyroid Disease ___ no yes	Any other disease ___ no yes Please list: _____
Hepatitis _____ no yes	Kidney Disease _____ no yes	Bleeding Tendency ___ no yes	_____

MAJOR HOSPITALIZATIONS: If you have ever been hospitalized for any major medical illness or operation, write in your most recent hospitalizations below.

Hospitalizations	Year	Operation or illness	Name of hospital	City and state
1st Hospitalization				
2nd Hospitalization				
3rd Hospitalization				
4th Hospitalization				

TESTS AND IMMUNIZATIONS: Mark an X next to those that you have had.

Tests: Immunizations:

☐ TB Test   ☐ Electrocardiogram   ☐ Influenza
☐ Rectal/Hemoccult   ☐ Chest x-ray   ☐ Hepatitis B
☐ Sigmoidoscopy   ☐ Mammogram   ☐ Tetanus
☐ Colonoscopy   ☐ Pap Test   ☐ MMR
                                              ☐ Polio

ALLERGIES: List all allergies (foods, drugs, environment). ☐ None

_____
_____
_____
_____

CURRENT MEDICATIONS: List the following that you are currently taking: Prescription medications, over-the-counter (OTC) medications, vitamin supplements, and herbal supplements. ☐ None

Medication   Frequency
_____
_____
_____
_____

ACCIDENTS/ INJURIES: Describe all serious accidents, severe injuries, head injury, or fractures. Include the date each occurred. ☐ None

Accident/Injury: Date:
_____
_____
_____
_____

Figure 1-18. A health history form.   *Continued*

C   FAMILY HISTORY

For each member of your family, follow the purple or blue line across the page and check boxes for:
1. His or her present state of health
2. Any illnesses he or she has had

	Good Health	Poor Health	Deceased	If deceased, write in age and cause of death.	Allergies or Asthma	Diabetes	Heart Disease	Stroke	Cancer	High Blood Pressure	Glaucoma	Arthritis	Ulcer	Kidney Disease	Mental Health Problems	Alcohol/Drug Abuse	Obesity	High Cholesterol	Thyroid Disease
Father:																			
Mother:																			
Brothers/Sisters:																			

D   SOCIAL HISTORY

EDUCATION _____ High school   _____ College   _____ Postgraduate

Occupation _____ Years _____

Previous occupations _____ Years _____

_____ Years _____

Have you ever been exposed to any of the following in your environment?

☐ Excess dust (coal, lime, rock)   ☐ Cleaning fluids/solvents   ☐ Radiation   ☐ Other toxic materials
☐ Sand   ☐ Hair spray   ☐ Insecticides
☐ Chemicals   ☐ Smoke or auto exhaust fumes   ☐ Paints

Please answer the follwing questions by placing an X in the box in front of the word Yes or No, except where you are asked for specific information. This information is obviously highly confidential and will be released to other healthcare professionals or insurance carriers ONLY with your consent.

DIET:
Do you eat a good breakfast? ☐ Yes ☐ No
Do you snack between meals (soft drinks, chips, candy bars)? ☐ Yes ☐ No
Do you eat fresh fruits and vegetables each day? ☐ Yes ☐ No
Do you eat whole grain breads and cereals? ☐ Yes ☐ No
Is your diet high in fat content? ☐ Yes ☐ No
Is your diet high in cholesterol content? ☐ Yes ☐ No
Is your diet high in salt content? ☐ Yes ☐ No
Are you allergic to any foods? ☐ Yes ☐ No
How many glasses of water do you drink each day? _____
How would you describe your overall eating habits? ☐ Excellent   ☐ Good   ☐ Fair   ☐ Poor

PERSONAL HISTORY:
Do you find it hard to make decisions? ☐ Yes ☐ No
Do you find it hard to concentrate or remember? ☐ Yes ☐ No
Do you feel depressed? ☐ Yes ☐ No
Do you have difficulty relaxing? ☐ Yes ☐ No
Do you have a tendency to worry a lot? ☐ Yes ☐ No
Have you gained or lost much weight recently? ☐ Yes ☐ No
Do you lose your temper often? ☐ Yes ☐ No
Are you disturbed by any work or family problems? ☐ Yes ☐ No
Are you having sexual difficulties? ☐ Yes ☐ No
Have you ever considered committing suicide? ☐ Yes ☐ No
Have you ever desired or sought psychiatric help? ☐ Yes ☐ No

EXERCISE:
Do you exercise on a regular basis? ☐ Yes ☐ No
Does your job require strenuous, sustained physical work? ☐ Yes ☐ No

SLEEP PATTERNS:
Do you seem to feel exhausted or fatigued most of the time? ☐ Yes ☐ No
Do you have difficulty either falling asleep or staying asleep? ☐ Yes ☐ No

USE OF TOBACCO/ALCOHOL/CAFFEINE/DRUGS: Amt:
How much do you smoke per day?   ☐ Cigarettes __
☐ Don't smoke   ☐ Cigars/pipes __

Do you take two or more alcoholic drinks per day? ☐ Yes ☐ No
Do you drink six or more cups of coffee or tea per day? ☐ Yes ☐ No
Are you a regular user of sleeping pills, marijuana, tranquilizers, pain killers, etc? ☐ Yes ☐ No
Have you ever used heroin, cocaine, LSD, PCP, etc? ☐ Yes ☐ No

List any country outside the USA you have visited in the past six months. _____

When did you have your last physical examination? _____

Figure 1-18, cont'd. A health history form.

Patient's Name_____

E | **REVIEW OF SYSTEMS**

HEAD AND NECK
_____ Frequent headaches
_____ Neck pain
_____ Neck lumps or swelling

EYES
_____ Wears glasses
_____ Blurry vision
_____ Eyesight worsening
_____ Sees double
_____ Sees halo
_____ Eye pain or itching
_____ Watery eyes
_____ Eye trouble

EARS
_____ Hearing difficulties
_____ Earaches
_____ Running ears
_____ Buzzing in ears
_____ Motion sickness

MOUTH
_____ Dental problems
_____ Swellings on gums or jaws
_____ Sore tongue
_____ Taste changes

NOSE AND THROAT
_____ Congested nose
_____ Running nose
_____ Sneezing spells
_____ Head colds
_____ Nosebleeds
_____ Sore throat
_____ Enlarged tonsils
_____ Hoarse voice

RESPIRATORY
_____ Wheezes or gasps
_____ Coughing spells
_____ Coughs up phlegm
_____ Coughed up blood
_____ Chest colds
_____ Excessive sweating, night sweats

CARDIOVASCULAR
_____ High blood pressure
_____ Racing heart
_____ Chest pains
_____ Dizzy spells
_____ Shortness of breath
_____ Shortness of breath at night
_____ More pillows to breathe
_____ Swollen feet or ankles
_____ Leg cramps
_____ Heart murmur

DIGESTIVE
_____ Heartburn
_____ Bloated stomach
_____ Belching
_____ Stomach pains
_____ Nausea
_____ Vomited blood
_____ Difficulty swallowing
_____ Constipation
_____ Loose bowels
_____ Black stools
_____ Grey stools
_____ Pain in rectum
_____ Rectal bleeding

URINARY
_____ Night frequency
_____ Day frequency
_____ Wets pants or bed
_____ Burning on urination
_____ Brown, black, or bloody urine
_____ Difficulty starting urine
_____ Urgency

MALE GENITAL
_____ Weak urine stream
_____ Prostate trouble
_____ Burning or discharge
_____ Lumps on testicles
_____ Painful testicles

FEMALE GENITAL
__/__/__ Last menstrual period
__/__/__ Last Pap test
_____ Postmenopausal or hysterectomy
_____ Noticed vaginal bleeding
_____ Abnormal LMP
_____ Heavy bleeding during periods
_____ Bleeding between periods
_____ Bleeding after intercourse
_____ Recent vaginal itching/discharge
_____ No monthly breast exam
_____ Lump or pain in breasts
_____ Complications with birth control

OBSTETRIC HISTORY
_____ Gravida
_____ Para
_____ Preterm
_____ Miscarriages
_____ Stillbirths
_____ Has had an abortion

MUSCULOSKELETAL
_____ Aching muscles
_____ Swollen joints
_____ Back or shoulder pains
_____ Painful feet
_____ Disability

SKIN
_____ Skin problems
_____ Itching or burning skin
_____ Bleeds easily
_____ Bruises easily

NEUROLOGICAL
_____ Faintness
_____ Numbness
_____ Convulsions
_____ Change in handwriting
_____ Trembles

F | **PROGRESS NOTES**

Date	

Figure 1-18, cont'd. A health history form.

obtaining further information on symptoms is presented in Procedure 1-4, and a more thorough study for analyzing a symptom is included in the *Student Mastery Manual* (Chapter 1).

Past History

The past medical history is a review of the patient's past medical status (Figure 1-18, *B*). Obtaining information on past medical care assists the physician in providing optimal care for the current problem. Most medical offices ask the patient to complete this section of the health history through a checklist type of form. The medical assistant should assist the patient with this section as necessary by offering to answer any questions regarding the information required. The past history includes the following areas:

- Major illnesses
- Childhood diseases
- Unusual infections
- Accidents and injuries
- Hospitalizations and operations
- Previous medical tests
- Immunizations
- Allergies
- Current medications

Family History

The family history is a review of the health status of the patient's blood relatives (Figure 1-18, *C*). This section of the health history focuses on diseases that tend to be familial. A **familial** disease is one that occurs in or affects blood relatives more frequently than would be expected by chance. Examples of familial diseases include hypertension, heart disease, allergies, and diabetes mellitus. The patient usually completes this section of the health history and is asked to provide the following information about each blood relative:

- State of health
- Presence of any significant disease
- If deceased, cause of death

Social History

This section of the health history includes information on the patient's lifestyle, such as health habits and living environment (Figure 1-18, *D*). The social history is important because the patient's lifestyle may have an impact on his or her condition and may also influence the course of treatment chosen by the physician. The social history also provides the physician with information regarding the effect that the illness may have on the patient's daily living pattern. If it is necessary for the individual to make a major lifestyle adjustment (e.g., stop smoking, reduce working hours), the physician may recommend support services to assist in this transition. This section of the history is usually completed by the patient and includes the following areas:

- Education
- Occupation (past and present)
- Living environment
- Diet
- Personal history
- Exercise
- Sleep patterns
- Use of tobacco, alcohol, and drugs
- Travel to foreign countries

Review of Systems

A review of systems (ROS) is a systematic review of each body system in order to detect any symptoms that have not yet been revealed. The importance of the review of systems is that it assists in identifying symptoms that might otherwise remain undetected. The physician usually completes the review of systems by asking a series of detailed and direct questions related to each body system; the results of this section of the health history assist the physician in a preliminary assessment of the type and extent of physical examination required. Figure 1-18, *E,* shows an example of a review of systems form.

Charting in the Medical Record

Charting is the process of making written entries about a patient in the medical record and is performed by medical office personnel who are directly involved with the health care of the patient. The medical record is considered a legal document; therefore the information must be charted as completely and accurately as possible. Developing good charting skills requires a thorough knowledge of charting guidelines combined with much repeated practice. To provide guidance in attaining this important skill, charting guidelines are presented in this section followed by examples of proper charting entries.

Charting Guidelines

To ensure accurate and concise charting, specific guidelines must be followed. These are listed and described as follows:

1. *Check the name on the chart before making an entry to be sure you have the correct chart.* If the medical assistant records in the wrong patient's chart by mistake, information such as a procedure that was performed on a patient may be excluded from the correct patient's record. As previously stated, from a legal standpoint, a procedure not documented was not performed.

2. *Use black ink to make entries in the patient's chart.* Black ink must be used to provide a permanent record. In addition, entries made in black ink are easier to reproduce when a record must be duplicated for insurance company purposes, patient referral, and so on.

3. *Write in legible handwriting.* For the medical record to be meaningful to others, the medical assistant must be sure to chart information legibly. If the medical

Highlight on Cultural Diversity

Culture consists of the values, beliefs, and practices of a particular group of people. Culture is deeply rooted and is passed on from one generation to the next through communication. It includes areas such as religion, dietary practices, family lines of authority, family life patterns, beliefs, and health practices.

As the demographics of the United States continue to change, the medical assistant is faced with the challenge of providing care to an increasing number of cultural groups. Therefore it is important for the medical assistant to learn as much as possible about the cultural values of the patients coming to the medical office. This is known as *cultural awareness* and can be accomplished by carefully observing and listening to patients to acquire knowledge of their cultural values.

Cultural sensitivity is the respect and appreciation for cultural diversity, whereas *cultural competence* is understanding and using the cultural background of a patient to assist with the resolution of a problem. Because health practices are part of a patient's culture, changing them may have a negative impact on the patient. Whenever possible, the medical assistant should incorporate factors from a patient's cultural background into his or her health care.

Guidelines for Achieving Cultural Competence
The following guidelines will help the medical assistant in developing cultural awareness and sensitivity and in achieving cultural competence:

1. *Respect the patient's values, beliefs, and practices.* Even if you do not agree with them, it is important to respect the patient's right to hold these values and not dismiss them as strange or odd. Cultural values play an important role in a patient's lifestyle. For example, patients from some cultures believe that losing blood depletes the body's strength and provides a route for the soul to leave the body. If a blood specimen is needed, these patients may become highly distressed or refuse to have their blood drawn. Members of some cultural groups believe that illness results when the body's natural balance or harmony is disturbed. To restore the balance, alternative forms of medicine, such as herbal remedies and aromatherapy, are used.
2. *Refrain from cultural stereotypes.* Realize that not all people of a cultural group have the same beliefs, practices, and values. Assuming that all members of a cultural group are alike is known as *stereotyping* and should be avoided. Just as one would never assume that all people in the United States like hamburgers and baseball, every individ-

ual must be approached according to his or her specific beliefs and practices.
3. *Always address patients by their last names* (and Mr., Mrs., Miss, Ms.) unless they give you permission to use other names. In most cultures, using a first name to address anyone other than family or friends is considered disrespectful. For example, most older people in the United States dislike being called by their first name and feel it shows a lack of respect.
4. *Speak slowly and clearly.* Communicating with a patient may be difficult if the patient has a limited knowledge of English. With these patients, you should speak slowly and clearly in a normal tone and volume of voice. Speaking loudly does not help the patient understand any better and may even be offensive to the patient.
5. *Show respect for cultural lines of authority.* In many cultures, respect is given based on age and gender. For example, in certain cultures, elders are considered the holders of the culture's wisdom and are highly respected. In other cultures, youth is valued over age. In certain cultures, the male dominates and women have very little status. Because of this a female patient from this type of culture may not be permitted to give her own health history or answer questions. In addition, a male patient from this culture may not accept instructions from a female medical assistant.
6. *Use appropriate eye contact.* In most cultures, direct eye contact is important and generally shows that the other is attentive and listening. It conveys self-confidence, openness, interest, and honesty, whereas the lack of eye contact may be interpreted as secretiveness, shyness, guilt, or lack of interest. Other cultures consider eye contact impolite or an invasion of privacy; hence these patients show respect by avoiding direct eye contact.
7. *Be aware of cultural responses to illness.* The conditions under which an individual assumes the role of a (sick) patient and the way he or she performs in that role vary with culture. For example, individuals of some cultures resist the sick role and blame sickness on external forces as a means of punishment. These individuals may deny their illness and fail to provide much information when the medical assistant takes their symptoms. In other cultures, individuals take an optimistic view of the outcome of health care and because of this are more likely to elicit information and to follow the physician's instructions.
8. *Learn to appreciate the richness of diversity* as an asset rather than as a hindrance to communication and effective interaction with patients.

assistant's cursive script is not legible, the information should be printed.
4. *Chart information accurately, using clear and concise phrases.*
   a. The medical assistant should be brief but complete and should avoid vagueness and duplication of information.

b. It is not necessary to include the patient's name in the entry because the entire medical record centers on one patient; it is therefore assumed the information refers to that patient.
c. Each phrase should begin with a capital letter and end with a period.

d. Each new entry should begin on a separate line and be dated with the month, day, year, and time (either AM/PM or military time).

e. Standard abbreviations, medical terms, and symbols can be used to help save time and space. It is *very* important that the medical assistant first check the office policy to determine the abbreviations, medical terms, and symbols that are commonly used in that office. Using commonly accepted terminology will avoid confusing others who will read the chart. A list of abbreviations and symbols commonly used in medical offices is presented in the box on pp. 37-39.

f. *Spell correctly.* Correct spelling is essential for accuracy in charting. If you are in doubt about the spelling of a word, consult a dictionary.

5. *Chart immediately after performing a procedure.* Once a procedure has been performed, it should be charted without delay. If a time lapse occurs between performing the procedure and charting it, the medical assistant may not remember certain aspects of the procedure, such as the results of the treatment or the patient's reaction. Procedures should never be charted in advance. The individual performing the procedure should be the one to chart it; in other words, never chart for someone else.

6. *Each charting entry should be signed by the person making it.* The signature should include the medical assistant's first initial, full last name, and title (e.g., D. Bennett, CMA). The following title abbreviations are often used for medical assistants:

   CMA: certified medical assistant
   RMA: registered medical assistant
   MA: medical assistant
   SMA: student medical assistant

7. *Never erase or obliterate an entry.* If an error is made in charting, the medical assistant must never erase or obliterate it. Should the physician or medical staff be involved in litigation, erased or obliterated entries tend to reduce credibility. If incorrect information is charted, the medical assistant should draw a single line through the incorrect information, thus permitting it to remain legible. The word *error* is then written above the incorrect data, including the date and the medical assistant's first initial, last name, and credentials. Some medical offices may re-

quest that the reason for the change also be recorded. The correct information is then inserted next to the error (Figure 1-19).

The medical assistant should always take the time to chart properly in the patient's medical record. Good charting helps coordinate efforts in the medical office and leads to high-quality health care.

Charting Progress Notes

After completion of the initial health history, a system is needed to update the medical record with new information each time the patient visits the medical office. Most offices use progress notes to fulfill this function. Progress notes document the patient's health status, as well as the care and treatment being received by the patient, in chronological order. Progress notes provide effective communication among medical office personnel and also serve as a legal document.

The medical assistant is frequently responsible for charting progress notes in the medical record. They are usually charted on special preprinted lined sheets known as *progress note sheets.* These sheets have a column for the date and a column for charting information (Figure 1-18, *F*).

Types of progress notes that are often charted by the medical assistant are presented next, along with a charting example of each.

Charting Patient Symptoms

The medical assistant takes patient symptoms during office visits and telephone conversations. Information conveyed during a telephone conversation helps determine whether the patient needs to be seen and the immediacy of the situation.

A **symptom** is any change in the body or its functioning that indicates the presence of disease. Symptoms can be classified as subjective or objective. A **subjective symptom** is one that is felt by the patient and cannot be observed by another person. Pain, pruritus, vertigo, and nausea are examples of subjective symptoms. An **objective symptom** is one that can be observed by another person, as well as by the patient. Rash, coughing, and cyanosis are objective symptoms. The medical assistant should have a thorough knowledge of common symptoms and should be able to recognize them. The box on p. 40 lists and describes common symptoms.

Text continued on p. 40

		error 10/15/05 ——— D. Bennett, CMA
10/15/05	9:30 a.m. Tubersol Mantoux test: 9mm induration. ———	
	12 ——— D. Bennett, CMA	

Figure 1-19. Proper method for correcting an error in the patient's medical record.

Abbreviations and Symbols Commonly Used in the Medical Office

Abbreviations Used to Chart Symptoms and Procedures—cont'd

a͞a	of each	freq	frequent
Ab	abortion	F/U	follow-up
abd	abdomen	Fx	fracture
abs	absent	GYN	gynecology
ac	before meals	h or hr	hour
ad lib	as desired	H/A	headache
admin	administer	HBP	high blood pressure
AM or a.m.	before noon	HC	head circumference
amt	amount	Hep B	hepatitis B vaccine
AP	apical pulse	Hg	mercury
approx	approximately	H_2O	water
appt	appointment	HR	heart rate
ASA	acetylsalicylic acid (aspirin)	HRT	hormone replacement therapy
ASAP	as soon as possible	hs	at bedtime
BA	backache	ht	height
b/c	because	ID	intradermal
BC	birth control	IM	intramuscular
bid	twice a day	IPV	inactivated polio vaccine
BM	bowel movement	IV	intravenous
BP	blood pressure	lab	laboratory
BPM	beats per minute	lac	laceration
BS	blood sugar	lat	lateral
BSE	breast self-examination	lax	laxative
c̄	with	LB	lower back
caps	capsules	LBP	lower back pain
cath	catheter, catheterize	liq	liquid
CC	chief complaint	LMP	last menstrual period
chemo	chemotherapy	med, meds	medication, medications
CMA	certified medical assistant	min	minute
c/o	complains of	MMR	measles, mumps, and rubella
CS	cesarean section	mod	moderate
Cx	cervix	N/A	not applicable
d	day	NB	newborn
/d	per day	N/C	no complaints
d/c	discontinue	neg	negative
D&I	dry and intact	NH	nursing home
dil	dilute	NICU	newborn intensive care unit
disch	discharge	NKA	no known allergies
DNKA	did not keep appointment	NKDA	no known drug allergies
DOB	date of birth	NMP	normal menstrual period
DOI	date of injury	noct	nocturnal
DRE	digital rectal exam	NS	normal saline
DSD	dry, sterile dressing	N&V	nausea and vomiting
DTaP	diphtheria and tetanus toxoids and acellular pertussis vaccine	NVA	near visual acuity
		NVD	nausea, vomiting, and diarrhea
D&V	diarrhea and vomiting	OB	obstetrics
DVA	distance visual acuity	occ	occasionally
ea	each	oint	ointment
EDD	expected date of delivery	op	operation
ER	emergency room	OR	operating room
Fe	iron	OT	occupational therapy
flex sig	flexible simoidoscopy	OTC	over the counter (nonprescription medication)
		OV	office visit

Continued

Abbreviations and Symbols Commonly Used in the Medical Office—cont'd

Abbreviations Used to Chart Symptoms and Procedures—cont'd

P	pulse
Pap	Pap test
path	pathology
pc	after meals
peds	pediatrics
PEN	penicillin
per	by or through
pharm	pharmacy
PM or p.m.	afternoon
PMS	premenstrual syndrome
po or PO	by mouth
pos	positive
postop	postoperative (after surgery)
preop	preoperative (before surgery)
prep	preparation
prn	as needed
PT	physical therapy
Pt or pt	patient
qd	every day
qh	every hour
q(2,3,4)h	every (2,3,4) hours
qid	four times a day
qn	every night
QNS	quantity not sufficient
qod	every other day
QS	quantity sufficient
quad	quadriplegic
R	respiration
RE	rectal examination
reg	regular
rehab	rehabilitation
RMA	registered medical assistant
Rx	prescription
s̄	without
SC or SQ	subcutaneous
S/E	side effects
sec	second
sigmoid	sigmoidoscopy
sl	slight
sm	small
SOB	shortness of breath
sol	solution
spec	specimen
STAT	immediately
surg	surgery
T	temperature
tab(s)	tablet (tablets)
temp	temperature
ther	therapy
tid	three times a day
TLC	total lung capacity, tender loving care

TPR	temperature, pulse, and respiration
tr	trace
TSE	testicular self-examination
vag	vagina, vaginal
VE	vaginal examination
vit	vitamin
VO	verbal order
VS	vital signs
wk	week
WNL	within normal limits
WO	written order
w/o	without
wt	weight
W/U	workup

Abbreviations Used to Chart Body Parts and Locations

abd	abdomen
AD	right ear
AS	left ear
AU	in each ear, both ears
EENT	eye, ear, nose, and throat
GI	gastrointestinal
GU	genitourinary
(L) or lt	left
(LA)	left arm
(LL)	left leg
LLQ	lower left quadrant
LRQ	lower right quadrant
LUQ	left upper quadrant
OD	right eye
OS	left eye
OU	in each eye, both eyes
(R) or rt	right
(RA)	right arm
(RL)	right leg
RLQ	right lower quadrant
RUQ	right upper quadrant

Abbreviations Used to Chart Measurement

C	Celsius
cc	cubic centimeter
cm	centimeter
dL	deciliter
F	Fahrenheit
g	gram
kg	kilogram
L	liter
l	length
lb	pound
m	meter
mcg	microgram
mg	milligram
ml	milliliter
mm	millimeter

Abbreviations and Symbols Commonly Used in the Medical Office—cont'd

Abbreviations Used to Chart Measurement—cont'd

oz	ounce
pt	pint
qt	quart
ss	one half
tbsp	tablespoon
tsp	teaspoon

Miscellaneous Abbreviations
Patient Examination

Dx	diagnosis
H/O	history of
H&P	history and physical
Hx	history
MHx	medical history
PE or Px	physical examination
prog	prognosis
Sx	symptoms
Tx	treatment

Conditions

BPH	benign prostatic hypertrophy
CA	cancer
CAD	coronary artery disease
CHF	congestive heart failure
COPD	chronic obstructive pulmonary disease
CRC	colorectal cancer
CVA	cerebrovascular accident
DM	diabetes mellitus
Fe def	iron deficiency
GC	gonorrhea
GDM	gestational diabetes mellitus
HTN	hypertension
IBS	irritable bowel syndrome
MI	myocardial infarction
MS	multiple sclerosis
OA	osteoarthritis
OM	otitis media
PID	pelvic inflammatory disease
RA	rheumatoid arthritis
RF	rheumatic fever
STD	sexually transmitted disease
TB	tuberculosis
URI	upper respiratory infection
USI	urinary stress incontinence
UTI	urinary tract infection

Diagnostic Procedures

CT, CAT	computed axial tomography
CXR	chest x-ray
ECG	electrocardiogram
Echo	echocardiogram
EEG	electroencephalogram
FOBT	fecal occult blood test

IVP	intravenous pyelogram
LP	lumbar puncture
MRI	magnetic resonance imaging
NST	nonstress test
PFT	pulmonary function test
TRUS	transrectal ultrasound
US	ultrasound

Laboratory Tests

BG	Blood glucose
Bx	biopsy
CBC	complete blood count
C&S	culture and sensitivity
diff	differential
ESR	erythrocyte sedimentation rate
FBS	fasting blood sugar
GCT	glucose challenge test
GTT	glucose tolerance test
Hct	hematocrit
Hgb	hemoglobin
PPBS	postprandial blood sugar
PSA	prostate specific antigen
PT	prothrombin time
RBC	red blood count
RBS	random blood sugar
SG	specific gravity
trig	triglycerides
UA	urinalysis
U/C	urine culture
WBC	white blood count

Symbols

Ø	none, no
✓	check
>	greater than
<	less than
↑	increase
↓	decrease
♀	female
♂	male
°	degree
@	at
×	times
$\bar{x}$	except
$\bar{p}$	after
#	number
1°	primary
2°	secondary
+	positive
−	negative
Ⓡ	rectal temperature
Ⓐ	axillary temperature
"	inches
'	feet

Taking patient symptoms during an office visit consists of:
1. Obtaining a chief complaint (refer to p. 30)
2. Obtaining additional information about the chief complaint

For example, if the patient complains of pain in the abdomen that has lasted for 2 days (chief complaint), additional information is needed to describe the pain, including the type, specific location, onset, intensity, precipitating factors, and duration of the pain. The procedure for taking patient symptoms during an office visit is outlined in Procedure 1-4. Additional skill and practice on taking patient symptoms is included in Chapter 1 of the *Student Mastery Manual.*

Common Symptoms

Integumentary System

Diaphoresis	Excessive perspiration.
Flushing	A red appearance to the skin, which generally affects the face and neck. A flushed appearance is commonly present with a fever.
Jaundice	A yellow appearance to the skin, first evident in the whites of the eyes.
Rash	An eruption on the skin.

Circulatory System

Bradycardia	An abnormally slow pulse rate.
Dehydration	A decrease in the amount of water in the body. The patient will have a flushed appearance, dry skin, and a decreased output of urine.
Edema	The retention of fluid in the tissues, resulting in swelling. The skin over the area is tight. Edema is most easily observed in the extremities.
Tachycardia	An abnormally fast pulse rate.

Gastrointestinal System

Anorexia	A loss of appetite and a lack of interest in food.
Constipation	A condition in which the stool becomes hard and dry, resulting in difficult passage from the rectum. The consistency of the stool, rather than the frequency of defecation, is used as a guide in determining the presence of constipation. (Frequency of bowel movements varies with the individual. Some people have a bowel movement only every 2 to 3 days but are not constipated.) Other symptoms of constipation include headache, nausea, and general malaise.
Diarrhea	The passage of an increased number of loose, watery stools. The fecal material moves rapidly through the intestinal tract, resulting in decreased absorption by the body of water, electrolytes, and nutrients. Other symptoms usually associated with diarrhea are intestinal cramping and general weakness.

Gastrointestinal System—cont'd

Flatulence	The presence of excessive gas in the stomach or intestines.
Nausea and vomiting	Nausea is a sensation of discomfort in the stomach with a feeling that vomiting may occur. Vomiting is the ejection of the stomach contents through the mouth, also known as *emesis.* The ejected content is known as *vomitus.*

Respiratory System

Cough	An involuntary and forceful exhalation of air followed by a deep inhalation. A cough may be productive (meaning a discharge is produced) or nonproductive (no discharge is present).
Cyanosis	A bluish discoloration of the skin due to a lack of oxygen.
Dyspnea	Labored or difficult breathing.
Epistaxis	Hemorrhaging from the nose (nosebleed).

Nervous System

Chills	A feeling of coldness accompanied by shivering. Chills are generally present with a fever.
Convulsions	Involuntary contractions of the muscles.
Fever, or pyrexia	A body temperature that is higher than normal.
Headache	A feeling of pain or aching in the head. It is a common symptom that accompanies many illnesses. Tension, fatigue, and eyestrain can result in a headache.
Malaise	A vague sense of body discomfort, weakness, and fatigue often marking the onset of a disease and continuing through the course of the illness.
Pain	Irritation of pain receptors, resulting in a feeling of distress or suffering. Pain is an important indication that a part of the body is not working properly.
Pruritus	Severe itching.
Vertigo	A feeling of dizziness or lightheadedness.

Other Activities That Need to Be Charted

Procedures. The medical assistant frequently charts procedures performed on the patient; examples include vital signs, weight and height, visual acuity, and ear irrigations. Procedures should be charted immediately after being performed; from a legal standpoint, a procedure that is not documented was not performed. In general, the following information should be included: the date and time, the type of procedure, the outcome, and the patient reaction. The specific information to be charted is included with each procedure presented in this text.

CHARTING EXAMPLE

Date	
6/30/05	9:15 a.m. Irrigated Ⓡ ear c̄ 200 ml of
	normal saline @ 98.6° F. Mod amt of
	cerumen in returned solution. Pt states can
	hear better. ———————— D. Bennett, CMA

Procedure

PROCEDURE 1-4 Obtaining and Recording Patient Symptoms

PROCEDURE 1-4

Outcome

Obtain and record patient symptoms.

Equipment/Supplies:

- Medical record of the patient to be interviewed
- Black ink pen

1. **Procedural Step.** Assemble the equipment. Make sure you have the correct patient's record and a black ink pen for charting patient symptoms.
   Principle. Black ink must be used to provide a permanent record.
2. **Procedural Step.** Go to the waiting room and ask the patient to come back.
3. **Procedural Step.** Escort the patient to a quiet, comfortable room, such as an examination room, that allows for privacy.
   Principle. Patient symptoms should be taken in a room that encourages communication.
4. **Procedural Step.** In a calm and friendly manner, greet and identify the patient and introduce yourself.
   Principle. A warm introduction sets a positive tone for the remainder of the interview.
5. **Procedural Step.** Ask the patient to be seated. You should seat yourself so that you face the patient at a distance of 3 to 4 feet.
   Principle. This type of seating arrangement facilitates open communication.
6. **Procedural Step.** Use good communication skills to interact with the patient. These include the following:
   a. Use the patient's name of choice.
   b. Demonstrate genuine interest and concern for the patient.
   c. Maintain appropriate eye contact.
   d. Use terminology the patient can understand.
   e. Listen carefully and attentively to the patient.
   f. Pay attention to the patient's nonverbal messages.
   g. Avoid judgmental comments.
   h. Avoid rushing the patient.
7. **Procedural Step.** Locate the progress note sheet in the patient's medical record. Chart the date and time and the abbreviation for chief complaint (CC).
8. **Procedural Step.** Use an open-ended question to elicit the chief complaint, such as "What seems to be the problem?"
   Principle. An open-ended question allows the patient to verbalize freely.
9. **Procedural Step.** Chart the chief complaint following the charting guidelines outlined on pp. 34-36. In addition, these guidelines should be followed:
   a. Limit the chief complaint to one or two symptoms and refer to a specific rather than a vague symptom.
   b. Chart the chief complaint concisely and briefly, using the patient's own words as much as possible.
   c. Include the duration of the symptom (onset) in the chief complaint.
   d. Avoid using names of diseases or diagnostic terms to record the chief complaint.
10. **Procedural Step.** Obtain additional information regarding the chief complaint using *what, when,* and *where* questions. Following proper charting guidelines, chart this information after the chief complaint.

Continued

PROCEDURE 1-4   Obtaining and Recording Patient Symptoms—Cont'd

What **Questions:**

What exactly have you been experiencing?

Does the symptom occur suddenly or gradually?

Does anything make it worse?

Where **Question**

Where is the symptom located?

When **Questions**

When did the symptom first occur?

How long does it last?

Does anything cause it to occur?

Principle. This information provides a complete description of the chief complaint.

11. **Procedural Step.** Thank the patient and proceed to the next step in the patient workup. (This usually includes measuring vital signs and height and weight and preparing the patient as needed for the physical examination, as will be presented in Chapters 4 and 5.)

12. **Procedural Step.** Inform the patient the physician will be with him or her soon.

13. **Procedural Step.** Place the patient's medical record where it can be reviewed by the physician (as designated by the medical office policy).

    Principle. The physician will want to review the patient's medical record before examining the patient.

CHARTING EXAMPLE

Date	
6/30/05	3:15 p.m. CC: Intense pain in the (L) ear for the past 2 days. Pt states pain is sharp and continuous. Pt noted sl yellow discharge from (L) ear. Fever of 101° F began last night about 9 p.m. Took Tylenol 2 tabs @ 8 a.m. ———————— D. Bennett, CMA

Administration of Medication. Charting medications administered to the patient is an important responsibility in the medical office. Included in the recording should be the date and time, the name of the medication, the dosage given, the route of administration, the injection site used (for parenteral medication), and any significant observations or patient reactions.

CHARTING EXAMPLE

Date	
6/30/05	10:15 a.m. Bicillin 900,00 units IM, (L) dorsogluteal. ———— D. Bennett, CMA

Administration of medication

Specimen Collection. Each time a specimen is collected from a patient, the medical assistant should chart the date and time of the collection, the type of specimen, and the area of the body from which the specimen was obtained. If the specimen is to be sent to an outside laboratory for testing, this information also should be charted, including the test(s) requested, the date the specimen was sent, and where it was sent. In this way, the physician will know that the specimen was collected and sent to the laboratory when test results are not back yet.

CHARTING EXAMPLE

Date	
6/30/05	1:30 p.m. Venous blood spec collected from (R) arm. Sent to Ross Lab for CBC and diff on 6/30/05 ———————— D. Bennett, CMA
Date	
6/30/05	2:00 p.m. Throat spec collected. Sent to Ross Lab for C&S on 6/30/05 ——————— ———————— D. Bennett, CMA

Specimen collection

Diagnostic Procedures and Laboratory Tests. Diagnostic procedures and laboratory tests ordered for a patient should always be charted in the medical record. If the patient does not undergo the test, documented proof exists that the test was ordered. Charting diagnostic procedures and laboratory tests protects the physician legally and refreshes the physician's memory of the procedures and tests being run on the patient when results are not yet back from the testing facility. Information to include in the charting entry are the date and time, the type of procedure or test(s) ordered, the scheduling date, and where it is being performed.

CHARTING EXAMPLE

Date	
6/30/05	10:15 a.m. Mammography scheduled for 7/5/05 at Grant Hospital. ———
	——— D. Bennett, CMA
Date	
6/30/05	11:30 a.m. Pt given lab request for GTT at Ross Lab. ——— D. Bennett, CMA

Diagnostic/lab tests

Results of Laboratory Tests. It is usually not necessary to chart results from laboratory reports returned from outside laboratories because the report itself is filed in the patient's record. In case of a STAT request or critical findings, however, the test results are often telephoned to the medical office, thus requiring the medical assistant to record the results on a report form. Careful recording is essential to avoid errors, which in turn could affect the patient's diagnosis. Results of laboratory tests performed by the medical assistant in the office should be charted in the medical record and must include the date and time, name of the test, and test results.

CHARTING EXAMPLE

Date	
6/30/05	8:00 a.m. FBS: 82 mg/dL. ———
	——— D. Bennett, CMA
Date	
6/30/05	4:15 p.m. Quick Vue+ Mono Test: neg ———
	——— D. Bennett, CMA

Test results

Patient Instructions. Many times it is necessary to relay instructions to a patient regarding medical care (e.g., wound care, cast care, care of sutures). The medical assistant should chart this information, making sure to include the date and the type of instructions relayed to the patient. Many medical offices have printed instruction sheets that are given to the patient. The patient is asked to sign a form, which is then filed in the patient's record, indicating that he or she has read and understands the instructions (Figure 1-20). The form should also be signed by the medical assistant, who functions as a witness. This protects the physician legally in the event that the patient fails to follow the instructions and causes further harm or damage to a body part.

CHARTING EXAMPLE

Date	
6/30/05	9:30 a.m. Instructions provided for BSE. Pt given a BSE educational brochure. ———
	——— D. Bennett, CMA
Date	
6/30/05	10:00 a.m. Explained wound care. Written instructions provided. Signed copy in chart. To return in 2 days for suture removal. ———
	——— D. Bennett, CMA
Date	
6/30/05	10:25 a.m. Provided instructions for applying a heating pad to the lower back. ———
	——— D. Bennett, CMA

Patient instructions

Other areas in which the medical assistant is responsible for charting in the medical record include missed or canceled appointments, telephone calls from patients, medication refills, and changes in medication or dosage by the physician.

CHARTING EXAMPLE

Date	
6/30/05	11:15 a.m. Phoned office. States that swelling in the Ⓡ ankle is almost gone. ———
	——— D. Bennett, CMA
Date	
6/30/05	1:15 p.m. Missed appointment scheduled for 6/30/05 @ 1:00 p.m. ——— D. Bennett, CMA

Telephone call and missed appointment.

PATIENT INSTRUCTIONS FOR WOUND CARE

Name of patient: _____

Follow the instructions indicated below for care of your wound:

1. Use ice bag and elevate to reduce swelling and pain. Elevate higher than your heart.
2. You may take aspirin/Tylenol for pain.
3. Keep the dressing clean and dry.
4. Replace the dressing within _____ days.
5. Discard the dressing within _____ days.
6. Cleanse the wound daily as instructed.
7. Stitches should be removed in _____ days.
8. Despite the greatest of care, any wound can become infected. If your wound becomes red or swollen, shows pus or red streaks, or feels more sore instead of less sore, contact the physician **immediately.**

I have received and understand the above instructions:

Patient (or representative): _____

Relationship to patient: _____

Witness: _____   Time and date: _____

Figure 1-20. Instruction sheet for patients.

MEDICAL Practice and the LAW

Documentation can be a deciding factor in a legal case. Everything you do for a patient should be documented in a factual manner in the medical record, or "chart." When a legal issue arises, often several years pass before it comes to trial. If you are involved, you will be asked detailed questions as to your actions on a particular day, for a particular patient. Few people have accurate memories for that long. Juries will give more credibility to documentation performed at the time of the action than to a memory of years ago. Ethically, you owe the patient thorough documentation in order to provide optimal continuity of care. Remember that all patient information is confidential.

Proper charting is a critical skill for a medical assistant to master. Although proper documentation will not prevent a lawsuit, it may determine the outcome. Pay particular attention to the rules for consents and charting guidelines outlined in this chapter, and follow them to the letter.

Case Study 1
What Did Dawn Do?
❑ Listened carefully to Mrs. Celeste and relayed concern through both verbal and nonverbal behavior.
❑ Reassured Mrs. Celeste that her information would be kept completely confidential. Explained to Mrs. Celeste that health care professionals are required by law to keep all patient information confidential.
❑ Told Mrs. Celeste how important it is to chart information that relates to her health. Explained that the physician must have accurate data to diagnose and treat her. Stressed that certain medications can be harmful to a patient if consumed with alcohol.
❑ Gave Mrs. Celeste information (including brochures) on community agencies that could help her. Explained that these agencies are required to maintain confidentiality and encouraged her to contact them.

What Did Dawn Not Do?
❑ Did not tell Mrs. Celeste to go to a different physician to make sure her information remained private.
❑ Did not tell Mrs. Celeste that she needed to stop drinking before it affected her health.

What Would You Do/What Would You *Not* Do? Review Dawn's response and place a checkmark next to the information you included in your response. List the additional information you included in your response.

_____

_____

_____

_____

Case Study 2
What Did Dawn Do?
❑ Reassured Tessa that she and her family have been good patients and apologized for the inconvenience.
❑ Told Tessa that it is against the law to transfer medical records without the patient's written authorization. Explained that the reason for the law is to safeguard a patient's privacy.
❑ Asked Tessa if she has a fax machine because the forms could be faxed to her for signing and then back to the office. If not, explained that both she and her husband would need to come to the office to sign release forms.

What Did Dawn Not Do?
❑ Did not get defensive about Tessa being so annoyed.
❑ Did not send their medical records to the new physician without the signed release forms.

What Would You Do/What Would You *Not* Do? Review Dawn's response and place a checkmark next to the information you included in your response. List the additional information you included in your response.

_____

_____

_____

_____

Case Study 3
What Did Dawn Do?
❑ Listened to and empathized with Mr. and Mrs. Oberlin's concerns.
❑ Told Mr. and Mrs. Oberlin that since Brett is of adult age, it would be against the law to let them see his medical record without his written authorization. Explained that the law is there to protect a patient's right to privacy and just as it protects Brett's right, the law also protects their right as well so that no one can obtain information from their medical records without their authorization.
❑ Suggested that they talk with Brett again regarding the situation.

What Did Dawn Not Do?
❑ Did not give them any information from Brett's medical record.

What Would You Do/What Would You *Not* Do? Review Dawn's response and place a checkmark next to the information you included in your response. List the additional information you included in your response.

_____

_____

_____

_____

Apply Your KNOWLEDGE

Choose the best answer to each of the following questions.

1. Marcus Westerfield exhibits a positive test result on a Hemoccult fecal occult blood test. Dr. Diagnosis has decided to perform a flexible sigmoidoscopy on Marcus to assist in determining the cause of his bleeding. Marcus must sign a consent to treatment form before undergoing this procedure. Before he signs this form, Dawn Bennett, CMA, must make sure that
   A. Marcus has washed his hands.
   B. A notary public is available to witness Marcus's signature.
   C. Dr. Diagnosis has discussed all aspects of the procedure with Marcus.
   D. Someone is available to drive Marcus home after the procedure.

2. After performing the flexible sigmoidoscopy on Marcus, Dr. Diagnosis dictates the results of the examination. Dawn transcribes the report and files it in Marcus's medical record under this chart divider:
   A. History and Physical
   B. Lab/X-ray
   C. Hospital
   D. Progress Notes

3. Michael Johnson has obtained a new job and is moving to Michigan. He calls the office and asks Dawn Bennett, CMA, to transfer his medical record to his new physician. Dawn should
   A. Explain to Michael that his medical record belongs to Dr. Diagnosis and cannot leave the office.
   B. Make a copy of the medical record and send it to Michael.
   C. Tell Michael that the information in a medical record is confidential and cannot be released.
   D. Ask Michael to come into the office and sign a release of medical information form.

4. Eva North, a 52-year-old factory worker, comes to the office complaining of difficulty in breathing and persistent coughing. She smokes 2 packs of cigarettes a day and has tried everything to quit smoking. When taking Eva's symptoms, which of the following would be an appropriate way to communicate with Eva?
   A. Offer Eva some breath mints.
   B. Avoid eye contact so that Eva doesn't feel embarrassed about coughing so much.
   C. Tell Eva that heavy smoking can damage her alveoli, which can cause emphysema, a chronic obstructive pulmonary disease, and that eventually she may need oxygen therapy.
   D. Observe that Eva is coughing a lot and offer her a glass of water.

5. Patricia McGhee comes to the office, and Dawn Bennett, CMA, escorts her to an examining room. Dawn obtains Patricia's vital signs and asks her what problem has brought her to the office. Patricia explains her symptoms as coughing, running a temperature for 5 days, and shortness of breath. Of the following, which would be the best example of charting Patricia's chief complaint?
   A. CC: Dyspneic, febrile, with cough.
   B. CC: Patricia is sick.
   C. CC: Cough, fever, shortness of breath for 5 days.
   D. CC: Patricia is running a fever and coughing a lot. She is short of breath, especially in the morning. She has been feeling this way for the past 5 days.

6. Dr. Diagnosis wants Dawn to check to see if Patricia is allergic to penicillin. Dawn would find this information in Patricia's health history under
   A. Present Illness
   B. Past History
   C. Family History
   D. Social History

7. Dr. Diagnosis asks Dawn to administer a breathing treatment to Patricia. Which of the following represents the correct method for charting the breathing treatment?
   A. Chart the breathing treatment immediately after administering it.
   B. Use a No. 2 lead pencil to chart the breathing treatment.
   C. Chart the breathing treatment just before administering it.
   D. Have the office manager chart the breathing treatment.

8. Patricia is prescribed medication for pneumonia. Two days later she calls the office and says she feels sick to her stomach and vomits after taking her medication. Of the following, which would be the best example of charting this information in Patricia's medical record?
   A. 4/2/05 Nausea with medication. D. Bennett, CMA.
   B. 4/2/05 9:00 AM. Called office. N&V p̄ taking med. Reported sym to Dr. Diagnosis. D. Bennett, CMA.
   C. 4/2/05 9:00 AM. N&V probably due to allergic reaction to the medication. Notified Dr. Diagnosis of the problem. D. Bennett, CMA.
   D. 4/2/05 9:00 AM. Patricia called and said she vomits after taking her medication. I reported this information to Dr. Diagnosis right after he got back from lunch at the Red Lobster. D.B.

9. Inoko Lin comes to the medical office complaining of a skin problem. She is from Japan and is attending college in the United States. Which of the following shows that Dawn Bennett, CMA, is practicing cultural awareness?
   A. Bowing upon greeting Inoko Lin
   B. Speaking loudly so Inoko Lin can understand the conversation
   C. Asking Inoko Lin how she prefers to be addressed
   D. Asking Inoko Lin how to make chop suey

10. Amy Grant is describing her symptoms to Dawn Bennett, CMA. She states that her symptoms include a red, blistery rash, intense itching, nausea, and fatigue. Which of the following symptoms that Amy described is an objective symptom?
    A. Blistery, red rash
    B. Intense itching
    C. Nausea
    D. Fatigue

CERTIFICATION REVIEW

❏ **The patient registration record** must be completed by all new patients and consists of demographic and billing information.

❏ **The health history** (along with the physical examination and laboratory and diagnostic tests) is used to determine the patient's general state of health, to arrive at a diagnosis and prescribe treatment, and to observe any change in a patient's illness after treatment has been instituted.

❏ **The physical examination report** is a summary of the findings from the physician's assessment of each part of the patient's body.

❏ **The medication record** consists of detailed information relating to a patient's medications and includes one or more of the following categories: prescription medications; over-the-counter (OTC) medications; and medications administered at the medical office.

❏ **A consultation report** is a narrative report of a specialist's opinion about a patient's condition and is based on a review of the patient's medical record and an examination of the patient.

❏ **Home health care** provides medical and nonmedical care in a patient's home or place of residence to minimize the effect of disease or disability.

❏ **A laboratory report** is a report of the analysis or examination of body specimens. Its purpose is to relay the results of laboratory tests to the physician to assist him or her in diagnosing and treating disease.

❏ **A diagnostic procedure** report consists of a narrative description and interpretation of a diagnostic procedure and includes the following reports: electrocardiogram, Holter monitor, sigmoidoscopy, colonoscopy, spirometry, radiology, and diagnostic imaging.

❏ **A therapeutic service report** documents the assessments and treatment designed to restore a patient's ability to function, such as physical therapy, occupational therapy, and speech therapy.

❏ **Hospital documents** are prepared by the attending physician and include the history and physical examination of a hospitalized patient, operative report, discharge summary report, pathology report, and emergency room report.

❏ **A consent to treatment form** is required for all surgical operations and nonroutine diagnostic or therapeutic procedures performed in the medical office. The form must be signed by the patient and provides written evidence that the patient agreed to the procedure(s) listed on the form.

❏ **A release of medical information form** is required to release information that is not part of medical treatment, payment, and health care operations.

❏ **A source-oriented medical record** is organized into sections based on the department, facility, or other source that generated the information. Each section of a source-oriented record is separated from the others by a chart divider labeled with the title of its respective section.

❏ **The documents in a problem-oriented record (POR)** are organized by the patient's specific health problems and include a database, problem list, plan of action for each problem, and progress notes. Progress notes for a POR include four categories: subjective data, objective data, assessment, and plan (SOAP).

❏ **A health history** consists of the following components: identification data, chief complaint, present illness, past history, family history, social history, and review of systems. A health history is taken for each new patient, and subsequent office visits (in the form of progress notes) provide information regarding changes in the patient's illness or treatment.

❏ **Charting** is the process of making written entries about a patient in the medical record. The medical record is a legal document, and the information must be charted as completely and accurately as possible, following established charting guidelines.

❏ **Progress notes** update the medical record with new information each time the patient visits or telephones the medical office. Types of progress notes often charted by the medical assistant include patient symptoms, medical procedures, administration of medication, specimen collection, diagnostic procedures and laboratory tests ordered on a patient, results of laboratory tests, instructions given to the patient regarding medical care, missed or canceled appointments, telephone calls from patients, medication refills, and changes in medication or dosage by the physician.

Terminology Review

Attending physician The physician responsible for the care of a hospitalized patient.

Charting The process of making written entries about a patient in the medical record.

Consultation report A narrative report of an opinion about a patient's condition by a practitioner other than the attending physician.

Diagnosis The scientific method of determining and identifying a patient's condition.

Diagnostic procedure A procedure performed to assist in the diagnosis, management, or treatment of a patient's condition.

Discharge summary report A brief summary of the significant events of a patient's hospitalization.

Electronic medical record (EMR) A medical record that is stored on a computer.

Familial Occurring or affecting members of a family more frequently than would be expected by chance.

Health history report A collection of subjective data about a patient.

Home health care The provision of medical and nonmedical care in a patient's home or place of residence.

Informed consent Consent given by a patient for a medical procedure after being informed of the nature of his or her condition, the purpose of the procedure, an explanation of risks involved with the procedure, alternative treatments or procedures available, the likely outcome of the procedure, and the risks involved with declining or delaying the procedure.

Inpatient A patient who has been admitted to a hospital for at least one overnight stay.

Medical impressions Conclusions drawn by the physician from an interpretation of data. Other terms for impressions include *provisional diagnosis* and *tentative diagnosis.*

Medical record A written record of the important information regarding a patient, including the care of that individual and the progress of the patient's condition.

Medical record format The way a medical record is organized. The two main types of medical record formats are the source-oriented record and the problem-oriented record.

Objective symptom A symptom that can be observed by an examiner.

Paper-based patient record (PPR) A medical record in paper form.

Patient An individual receiving medical care.

Physical examination An assessment of each part of the patient's body to obtain objective data about the patient that assists in determining the patient's state of health.

Physical examination report A report of the objective findings from the physician's assessment of each body system.

Problem Any condition that requires further observation, diagnosis, management, or patient education.

Prognosis The probable course and outcome of a disease and the prospects for a patient's recovery.

Reverse chronological order Arranging documents with the most recent document on top or in the front, which means that the oldest document is on the bottom or at the back of a section or file.

SOAP format A method of organization for recording progress notes. The SOAP format includes the following categories: subjective data, objective data, assessment, and plan.

Subjective symptom A symptom that is felt by the patient but is not observable by an examiner.

Symptom Any change in the body or its functioning that indicates that a disease is present.

ON THE WEB

For Information on Cultural Diversity:

For active weblinks to each website visit http://evolve.elsevier.com/Bonewit/.

International Channel Networks

National Geographic Society

U.S. Dept. of the Interior: Workforce Diversity

Generations United

For Information on Communication Assistance:

AT&T Toll-Free Directory

U.S. Postal Service Zip Code Access

United Parcel Service

Federal Express

Airborne Express

Microorganisms and Medical Asepsis

1. Define a microorganism and give examples of types of microorganisms.
2. Explain the difference between a nonpathogen and a pathogen.
3. Define medical asepsis.
4. List the six basic requirements for growth and multiplication of microorganisms.
5. Outline the infection process and cycle, including the following:
   a. Give examples of the means of entry of microorganisms into the body.
   b. Give examples of the means of transmission of microorganisms from one person to another.
   c. Give examples of the means of exit of microorganisms from the body.
   d. List and explain the protective mechanisms the body uses to prevent the entrance of microorganisms.
6. Explain the difference between resident flora and transient flora.
7. State when each of the following is performed: handwashing, antiseptic handwashing, alcohol-based hand rub.
8. Identify medical aseptic practices that should be followed in the medical office.
9. Explain how proper handwashing helps prevent the transmission of microorganisms.
10. List examples of when to wear clean disposable gloves.

OSHA Bloodborne Pathogens Standard

1. Explain the purpose of OSHA.
2. Describe the purpose of the Needlestick Safety and Prevention Act.
3. List and describe the elements that must be included in the OSHA exposure control plan.
4. Explain the purpose of the following OSHA requirements: use of safer medical devices, labeling requirements, and sharps injury log.
5. Define and give examples of each of the following: engineering controls, work practice controls, personal protective equipment, and housekeeping procedures.
6. Identify the guidelines for use of personal protective equipment.

Adhere to the OSHA Bloodborne Pathogens Standard.

Prepare regulated waste for pickup by an infectious waste service.

Regulated Medical Waste

1. List examples of medical waste and how to discard each type of waste.
2. Explain how to handle and dispose of regulated medical waste.

Bloodborne Diseases

1. Describe post-exposure prophylaxis for hepatitis B.
2. Explain the difference between acute and chronic hepatitis B.
3. Explain the possible effects and consequences of chronic hepatitis C.
4. List and describe the four stages of the AIDS virus infection cycle.
5. List and describe the AIDS-defining conditions.

CHAPTER 2

Medical Asepsis and the OSHA Standard

Chapter Outline

Introduction to Medical Asepsis and the OSHA Standard
Microorganisms and Medical Asepsis
  Growth Requirements for Microorganisms
  Infection Process Cycle
  Protective Mechanisms of the Body
  Medical Asepsis in the Medical Office
OSHA Bloodborne Pathogens Standard
  Purpose of the Standard
  Needlestick Safety and Prevention Act
  OSHA Terminology
  Components of the OSHA Standard
  Control Measures
Regulated Medical Waste
  Handling Regulated Medical Waste
  Disposal of Regulated Medical Waste
Bloodborne Diseases
  Hepatitis B
  Hepatitis C
  Other Forms of Viral Hepatitis
  Acquired Immunodeficiency Syndrome

National Competencies

Clinical Competencies
Fundamental Procedures
- Perform handwashing.
- Dispose of biohazardous materials.
- Practice standard precautions.

General Competencies
Legal Concepts
- Identify and respond to issues of confidentiality.
- Perform within legal and ethical boundaries.
- Demonstrate knowledge of federal and state health care legislation and regulations.

Patient Instruction
- Identify community resources.

Key Terms

aerobe (AIR-obe)
anaerobe (AN-er-obe)
antiseptic
asepsis (ay-SEP-sis)
cilia (SIL-ee-ya)
contaminate (kon-TAM-in-ate)
decontamination (DEE-kon-tam-in-AY-shun)
hand hygiene
infection
medical asepsis
microorganism (MYE-kroe-OR-gan-iz-um)
nonintact (NON-in-takt) skin
nonpathogen (non-PATH-oh-jen)
opportunistic (OP-pore-tune-IS-tik) infection
optimum (OP-tuh-mum) growth temperature
parenteral (pare-EN-ter-al)
pathogen (PATH-oh-jen)
perinatal (pare-ee-NAY-tul)
pH (PEE-AYCH)
post-exposure prophylaxis (PEP) (proe-fil-ACKS-is)
regulated medical waste (RMW)
reservoir (REZ-er-vwar) host
resident flora (FLOE-ruh)
susceptible (sus-SEP-tih-bul)
transient (TRAN-zee-ent) flora

Introduction to Medical Asepsis and the OSHA Standard

Medical asepsis and infection control are of critical importance in preventing the spread of disease. The medical assistant should always be sure to practice good medical aseptic techniques to provide a safe and healthy environment in the medical office. The OSHA Bloodborne Pathogens Standard is important for infection control. This standard is required by the federal government to reduce the exposure of health care employees to infectious diseases. This chapter presents a thorough discussion of medical asepsis, infection control, and the OSHA Bloodborne Pathogens Standard.

Microorganisms and Medical Asepsis

Microorganisms are tiny living plants or animals that cannot be seen with the naked eye but must be viewed with the aid of a microscope. Common types of microorganisms include bacteria, viruses, protozoa, fungi, and animal parasites. Most microorganisms are harmless and do not cause disease. They are termed **nonpathogens.** Other microorganisms, known as **pathogens,** are harmful to the body and can cause disease.

In the medical office, practices must be employed to reduce the number and hinder the transmission of pathogenic microorganisms. These practices are known as medical asepsis. **Medical asepsis** means that an object or area is clean and free from infection. Nonpathogens will still be present on a clean or medically aseptic substance or surface, but all the pathogens have been eliminated.

Growth Requirements for Microorganisms

In order for microorganisms to survive, certain growth requirements must be present in the environment. These include the following:

Proper nutrition	Microorganisms that use inorganic or nonliving substances as a source of food are known as *autotrophs.* Microorganisms that use organic or living substances for food are known as *heterotrophs.*
Oxygen	Most microorganisms need oxygen to grow and multiply and are termed **aerobes.** Other microorganisms, known as **anaerobes,** grow best in the absence of oxygen.
Temperature	Each microorganism has a temperature at which it grows best, known as the **optimum growth temperature.** Most microorganisms grow best at 98.6° F (37° C), the human body temperature.
Darkness	Microorganisms grow best in darkness.

Moisture   Microorganisms need moisture for cell metabolism and to carry away wastes.

pH   Most microorganisms prefer a neutral pH. If the environment of the microorganisms becomes too acidic or too basic, they die.

If growth requirements are taken away from the environment of microorganisms, they are unable to survive. Eliminating these conditions is one way to reduce the growth and transmission of pathogens in the medical office.

Infection Process Cycle

For a pathogen to survive and produce disease, a continuous cycle must be followed; this is known as the infection process cycle (Figure 2-1). If the cycle is broken at any point, the pathogen dies. The medical assistant has a responsibility to help break this cycle in the medical office by practicing good techniques of medical asepsis. These techniques are discussed in the next section.

Protective Mechanisms of the Body

The body has protective mechanisms to help prevent the entrance of pathogens. These help break the infection process cycle. Protective mechanisms of the body are as follows:

1. The skin is the body's most important defense mechanism; it serves as a protective barrier against the entrance of microorganisms.
2. The mucous membranes of the body, which line the nose and throat and respiratory, gastrointestinal, and genital tracts, help protect the body from invasion by microorganisms.
3. Mucus and cilia in the nose and respiratory tract fight off pathogens. Mucus traps the smaller microorganisms that enter the body, and the hairlike **cilia** constantly beat toward the outside to remove them from the body.
4. Coughing and sneezing help force pathogens from the body.
5. Tears and sweat are secretions that aid in the removal of pathogens from the body.
6. Urine and vaginal secretions are acidic. Pathogens cannot grow in an acidic environment.
7. The stomach secretes hydrochloric acid, which helps in the process of digestion. This acidic environment discourages the growth of pathogens that enter the stomach.

Medical Asepsis in the Medical Office

Hand Hygiene

Hand hygiene refers to the process of cleansing or sanitizing the hands. Hand hygiene is considered the single most

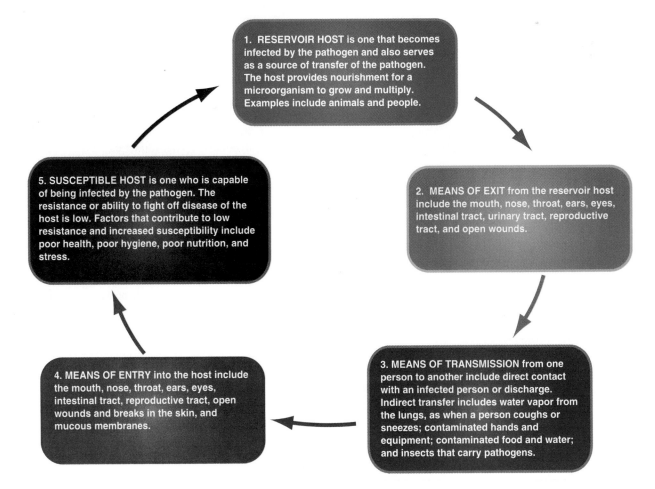

Figure 2-1. The infection process cycle.

important medical aseptic practice in the medical office for preventing the spread of infection. Specific techniques for sanitizing the hands in the medical office include the following:

- Handwashing with a detergent soap and water
- Handwashing with an antimicrobial soap and water
- Using an alcohol-based hand rub

The Centers for Disease Control and Prevention (CDC) recently issued new recommendations for hand hygiene in health care settings. The purpose of these guidelines is to promote improved hand-hygiene practices and to reduce transmission of pathogenic microorganisms to patients and employees in health care settings. The CDC guidelines for hand hygiene are outlined in Table 2-1 as they apply to the medical office. They are also further discussed in this section.

PUTTING It All Into PRACTICE

MY NAME IS Jennifer Hawk, and I work for a large group of physicians in a multispecialty clinic. I work both the front and back areas of the office. I really enjoy experiencing all of these areas of the office, and I definitely never get bored.

The most interesting experience I have had as a practicing medical assistant is seeing the impact that I make in patients' lives. They rely on you and look to you first for help in their health care situation. You are most often the first person they come into contact with in the office, and they look to you for understanding and empathy. Especially patients that must come to your office on a regular basis see you as a kind of family member. They appreciate a familiar face and smile. Most often, you are the individual giving the patient instructions concerning testing they will be having done or medication they will be taking. Patients truly do count on your knowledge and assistance throughout their course of care. I was genuinely surprised at what an impact I could have on others.

Resident and Transient Flora

Microorganisms on the hands are classified into the following categories: resident flora and transient flora. **Resident flora** (also known as normal flora) normally reside and grow in the epidermis and deeper layers of the skin known as the dermis. Resident flora are generally harmless and nonpathogenic. Because resident flora are attached to the deeper skin layers, they are difficult to remove from the skin. Washing the hands with an antimicrobial soap and water will remove some (but not all) resident flora.

Transient flora, on the other hand, live and grow on the superficial skin layers, or epidermis. They are picked up on the hands in the course of daily activities. In the medical office, this may include contact with an infected patient, contaminated equipment, or contaminated surfaces. Transient flora are often pathogenic, but because they are attached loosely to the skin, they can be removed easily with proper handwashing or by applying an alcohol-based hand rub.

Handwashing

Handwashing refers to washing the hands with a detergent soap and water. Detergent soap (commonly known as plain soap) contains agents that help break down and emulsify dirt and oil present on the skin. Soap is used to sanitize the hands through the physical removal of dirt and transient flora. It is important to use adequate friction during handwashing to ensure the removal of all transient flora. Procedure 2-1 outlines the handwashing procedure.

The new CDC hand-hygiene guidelines recommend that handwashing be performed when the hands are visibly soiled with dirt or body fluids, before eating, and after using the restroom (see Table 2-1). If the hands are not visibly soiled, the CDC now recommends that an alcohol-based hand rub be used to sanitize the hands rather than handwashing. This is because repeated handwashing tends to dry out the hands, leading to irritation, chapping, and dermatitis.

TABLE 2-1   CDC Guidelines for Hand Hygiene in Health Care Settings

Wash hands with a detergent soap or an antimicrobial soap at the following times:

- When the hands are visibly soiled with dirt or body fluids (e.g., blood, feces, urine, respiratory secretions)
- Before eating
- After using the restroom

Apply an alcohol-based hand rub in the following clinical situations:

- Before and after patient contact
- Before applying and after removing gloves
- After contact with body fluids or excretions, mucous membranes, nonintact skin, and wound dressings as long as the hands are not visibly soiled
- When moving from a contaminated body site to a clean body site during patient care
- After contact with inanimate objects (e.g., medical equipment) when providing health care

General recommendations:

- Keep natural nail tips less than ¼-inch long.
- Do not add soap to a partially empty liquid soap dispenser. The practice of "topping off" dispensers can lead to bacterial contamination of the soap. The correct procedure is to either (a) dispose of an empty dispenser or (b) rinse an empty dispenser thoroughly and then refill it.
- Disposable paper towels are recommended for drying the hands after handwashing. Multiple-use cloth towels are not recommended.
- Use hand lotions or creams to minimize the occurrence of dermatitis associated with frequent handwashing.
- Change gloves during patient care if moving from a contaminated body site to a clean body site.
- Remove gloves after caring for a patient. Do not wear the same pair of gloves for the care of more than one patient.

Antiseptic Handwashing

Washing the hands with an antimicrobial soap is termed *antiseptic handwashing.* Antimicrobial soaps contains an **antiseptic,** which is an agent that functions to kill or inhibit the growth of microorganisms (Figure 2-2, *A*). Antiseptic handwashing sanitizes the hands through mechanical scrubbing action, as well as through the action of the antiseptic. Proper handwashing with an antimicrobial soap removes all soil and transient flora from the hands. Most antimicrobial soaps also deposit an antibacterial film on the skin that discourages bacterial growth. Examples of antiseptics contained in antimicrobial soaps include triclosan, chlorhexidine, hexachlorophene, iodine, and chloroxylenol (PCMX).

Alcohol-Based Hand Rubs

The new CDC guidelines recommend the use of an alcohol-based hand rub for sanitizing the hands when they are not visibly soiled (see Table 2-1). Alcohol-based hand rubs consist of 60% to 90% alcohol (ethanol or isopropanol) and come in the form of gels, lotions, and foams (see Figure 2-2, *B*). Studies have shown that they are more effective than traditional soap and water handwashing in removing transient flora on the hands.

The advantages alcohol-based hand rubs offer over traditional handwashing are as follows:
- They do not require rinsing; therefore water or hand drying with a towel is not needed.
- Less time is required to perform hand hygiene. It takes between 20 and 30 seconds to sanitize the hands with an alcohol-based hand rub, compared with 1 to 2 minutes to perform proper handwashing.
- Most alcohol-based hand rubs contain emollients, which help prevent the skin of the hands from drying out. As the alcohol dries, protective fats and oils remain on the hands.

Alcohol-based hand rubs have disadvantages. They are more expensive than plain soap. They also cause a brief stinging sensation if they are applied to broken skin, such as a cut or abrasion on the hand. Procedure 2-2 describes the proper steps for performing an alcohol-based hand rub.

Infection Control

In addition to hand hygiene, other good aseptic practices in the medical office include:
1. Follow the OSHA Bloodborne Pathogens Standard (presented in this chapter).
2. Keep the medical office free from dirt and dust, which can collect and carry microorganisms.
3. Make sure that the reception area and examining rooms are well ventilated. Stuffy rooms encourage microorganisms to settle on objects.
4. Keep the reception area and examining rooms bright and airy. Light discourages the growth of microorganisms.
5. Eliminate insects by the use of insecticides or window screens. Insects are a means of transmission of microorganisms.
6. Carefully dispose of wastes, such as urine, feces, and respiratory secretions; all wastes should be handled as if they contained pathogens.
7. Do not let soiled items touch clothing.
8. Avoid coughs and sneezes of patients. The water vapor expelled from the lungs with coughing and sneezing may contain pathogens.
9. Use discretion in the amount of jewelry you wear. Microorganisms can become lodged in the grooves and crevices of jewelry and serve as a means of transmission of pathogens.
10. Teach patients aseptic practices to control the spread of infection at home.

Gloves

The CDC recommends that *clean disposable gloves* be worn when the medical assistant is likely to come in contact with any body substance such as blood, urine, feces, mucous membranes, and nonintact skin. For example, clean disposable gloves should be worn when administering an injection, performing a venipuncture, or performing a urinalysis. *Sterile gloves* are used to perform sterile procedures such as a dressing change or to assist the physician during minor office surgery, which is described in more detail in Chapter 10.

Procedure 2-3 presents the proper method for applying and removing clean disposable gloves.

Text continued on p. 61

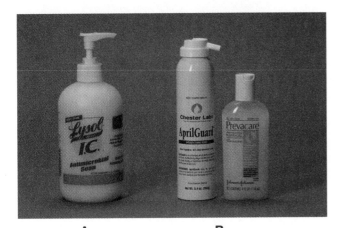

Figure 2-2. A, Antimicrobial soap. **B,** Alcohol-based hand rubs.

What Would You DO?
What Would You *Not* DO?

Case Study 1

Petra Meyer has come in for her annual GYN examination. She notices that alcohol-based hand rubs are being used in the medical office. She says that she has seen them in the grocery store and wants to know if they are as good as regular soap and water for washing hands. Petra wants to know how much to use and how long to rinse the hands after applying them. Petra says she likes to garden and wants to know if hand rubs are effective in removing ground-in soil from the hands. Petra is also curious to know why they are now being used so much in health care settings.

PROCEDURE 2-1 Handwashing

Outcome Perform handwashing.

Equipment/Supplies:
- Liquid or bar soap
- Paper towels

1. **Procedural Step.** Remove your watch or push it up on the forearm so the wrist is clear. Avoid wearing rings. If you wear rings, remove all except a plain wedding band.
   Principle. Microorganisms can lodge in the crevices and grooves of rings.

2. **Procedural Step.** Stand at the sink, making sure clothing does not touch the sink.
   Principle. The sink is considered contaminated, and if the uniform touches the sink, it may pick up microorganisms and transfer them.

3. **Procedural Step.** Turn on the faucets, using a paper towel.
   Principle. The faucets are considered contaminated because they harbor microorganisms.

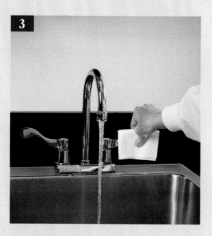

4. **Procedural Step.** Adjust the water temperature. The water should be warm to make the best suds.
   Principle. Water that is too hot or too cold tends to dry the skin, causing chapping and cracking and making it easy for pathogens to enter the body.

5. **Procedural Step.** Discard the paper towel in the trash receptacle.
   Principle. The paper towel is considered contaminated after touching the faucets.

6. **Procedural Step.** Wet hands and forearms thoroughly with water. The hands should be held lower than the elbows at all times. Be careful not to touch the inside of the sink because it is also contaminated.
   Principle. When you hold the hands lower than the elbows, bacteria and debris will be carried away from the arms and body and into the sink.

7. **Procedural Step.** Apply soap to the hands. If you use liquid soap, apply 1 teaspoon of soap (approximately the size of a nickel). If you use bar soap, it must be retained in the hands during sudsing up. Rinse the bar soap before returning it to the soap dish. The soap dish should have drainage holes so that the soap can dry out—moisture encourages the growth of microorganisms.
   Principle. Microorganisms and debris accumulate on the soap during the handwashing procedure. Rinsing the soap helps carry these away.

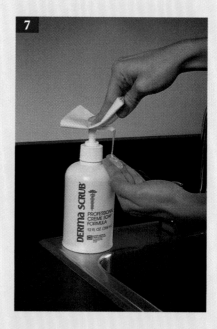

8. **Procedural Step.** Wash the palms and backs of the hands with 10 circular motions. Use friction along with the circular motions to wash the palm and back of each hand.
   Principle. Friction helps dislodge and remove microorganisms from the hands.

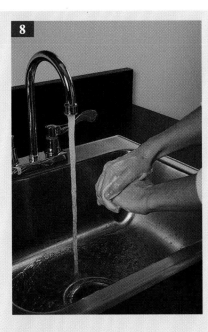

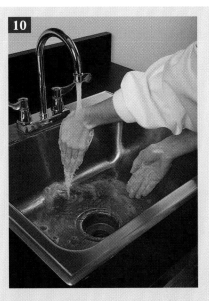

9. **Procedural Step.** Wash the fingers with 10 circular motions. Interlace the fingers and thumbs, and use friction and circular motions while rubbing the fingers back and forth.
Principle. This kind of movement helps remove microorganisms and debris that have accumulated between the fingers.

11. **Procedural Step.** Wash wrists and forearms, using friction along with circular motions. (NOTE: The hands are washed first because they are the most contaminated; thus organisms and dirt are washed away and not spread to the wrists and forearms.)

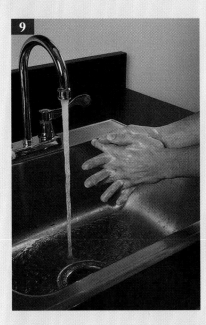

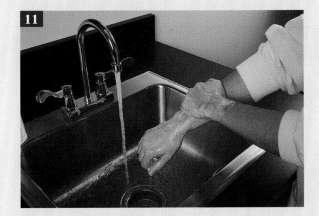

12. **Procedural Step.** Rinse arms and hands.
Principle. The running water rinses away the dirt and microorganisms.
13. **Procedural Step.** Clean the fingernails with a manicure stick. The fingernails should be cleaned at least once daily.
Principle. Dirt and microorganisms collect underneath the fingernails.
14. **Procedural Step.** Repeat the handwashing procedure. For initial handwashing or when the hands come into contact with blood or other potentially infectious materials, the handwashing procedure should be repeated. This is to ensure removal of all pathogens.

10. **Procedural Step.** Rinse well, making sure to hold the hands lower than the elbows.
Principle. Running water helps rinse away dirt and microorganisms.

PROCEDURE 2-1

Continued

PROCEDURE 2-1 Handwashing—Cont'd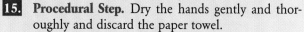

15. **Procedural Step.** Dry the hands gently and thoroughly and discard the paper towel.
Principle. Drying the hands gently prevents them from becoming chapped. Microorganisms can lodge in the crevices of chapped hands. Make sure the hands are dried completely, because wet skin may also cause chapping.

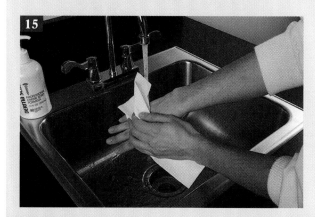

16. **Procedural Step.** Turn off the water, using a paper towel, and discard the paper towel in the trash receptacle.
Principle. The faucet is considered contaminated, whereas the hands are medically aseptic or clean.

17. **Procedural Step.** Do not touch the sink with the bare hands.
Principle. The hands are now medically aseptic, and the sink is considered contaminated.

PROCEDURE 2-2 Applying an Alcohol-Based Hand Rub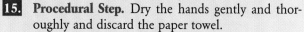

Outcome Apply an alcohol-based hand rub.

Equipment/Supplies:
- Alcohol-based hand rub

1. **Procedural Step.** Inspect the hands to make sure they are not visibly soiled. Hands that are visibly soiled must be washed with soap and water.
Principle. Alcohol-based hand rubs are not intended for the removal of visible soil.

2. **Procedural Step.** Remove your watch or push it up on the forearm. Avoid wearing rings. If you wear rings, remove all except a plain wedding band.
Principle. Microorganisms can lodge in the crevices and grooves of rings.

3. **Procedural Step.** Apply the alcohol-based hand rub to the palm of one hand as follows:
Gel or Lotion. Apply 2 to 3 ml of the gel or lotion, which is an amount approximately equal to the size of a dime.

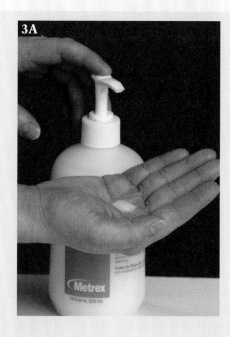

Foam. Apply 3 g of foam, which is an amount approximately equal to the size of a walnut.

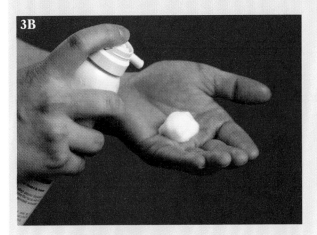

4. **Procedural Step.** Thoroughly spread the hand rub over the surface of both hands up to one-half inch above the wrist.
   Principle. Failure to cover all surfaces can leave areas of the hands contaminated.

5. **Procedural Step.** Rub the hands together until they are dry, which usually takes between 15 and 30 seconds. The hands are now medically aseptic.

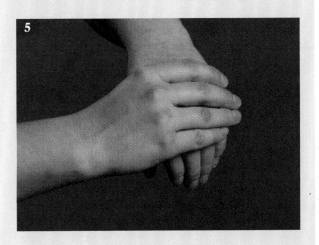

PROCEDURE 2-3 Application and Removal of Clean Disposable Gloves

Outcome Apply and remove clean disposable gloves.

Equipment/Supplies:
- Clean disposable gloves

Applying Clean Disposable Gloves

No special technique is required when clean disposable gloves are applied. This is because the hands are clean and the gloves are clean; therefore the medical assistant can touch any part of the gloves during application without contaminating them.

1. **Procedural Step.** Remove all rings, and sanitize your hands. Handwashing should be performed if the hands are visibly soiled. If this is not the case, use an alcohol-based hand rub to sanitize the hands.
   Principle. Rings may cause the gloves to tear. The warm, moist environment inside gloves provides ideal growing conditions for the multiplication of transient microorganisms present on the hands. Sanitizing the hands removes these microorganisms and prevents the transmission of pathogens.

2. **Procedural Step.** Choose the appropriate size gloves. Apply the gloves and adjust them so that they fit comfortably.

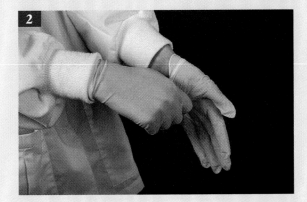

3. **Procedural Step.** Inspect the gloves for tears. If a tear is present, a new pair of gloves must be applied.

Continued

PROCEDURE 2-3 Application and Removal of Clean Disposable Gloves—Cont'd

Removing Clean Disposable Gloves

Gloves must be removed in a manner that protects the medical assistant from contaminating his or her clean hands with pathogens that may be present on the outside of the gloves. This is accomplished by not allowing the bare hands to come in contact with the outside of the gloves.

1. **Procedural Step.** Grasp the outside of the left glove 1 to 2 inches from the top with your gloved right hand. (NOTE: It does not matter which glove is removed first. You may start with the right glove if you prefer.)

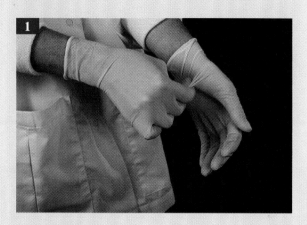

2. **Procedural Step.** Slowly pull the left glove off the hand. It will turn inside out as it is removed from your hand.

3. **Procedural Step.** Pull the left glove free, and scrunch it into a ball with your gloved right hand.

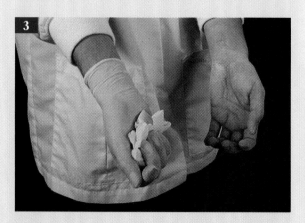

4. **Procedural Step.** Place the index and middle fingers of the left hand on the inside of the right glove. Do not allow your clean hand to touch the outside of the glove.

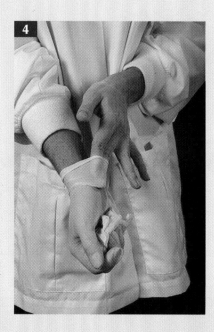

5. **Procedural Step.** Pull the glove off the right hand. It will turn inside out as it is removed from your hand, enclosing the balled-up left glove. Discard both gloves in an appropriate container.

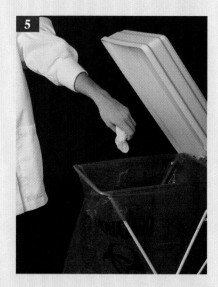

6. **Procedural Step.** Sanitize your hands to remove any microorganisms that may have come in contact with your hands.

OSHA Bloodborne Pathogens Standard

Purpose of the Standard

The Occupational Safety and Health Administration (OSHA) was established by the federal government to assist employers in providing a safe and healthy working environment for their employees. In 1991 OSHA published a comprehensive set of regulations designed to reduce the risk to employees of exposure to infectious diseases. These regulations are known as the *OSHA Occupational Exposure to Bloodborne Pathogens Standard*, which went into effect in March of 1992.

The OSHA Bloodborne Pathogens Standard must be followed by any employee with occupational exposure to pathogens, regardless of the place of employment. In addition to medical assistants, employees with occupational exposure include physicians, nurses, dentists, dental hygienists, medical laboratory personnel, and emergency medical technicians. Employees who may have less obvious occupational exposure are correctional and law enforcement officers, firefighters, hospital laundry workers, morticians, and custodians.

Failure by employers to comply with the OSHA standard could result in a citation carrying a maximum penalty of $7,000 for each violation and a maximum penalty of $70,000 for repeat violations.

Needlestick Safety and Prevention Act

Since the adoption of the OSHA Bloodborne Pathogens Standard in 1992, needlestick injuries among health care workers (HCWs) have continued to be a problem because of their high frequency of occurrence and the severity of the health effects associated with exposure to bloodborne pathogens. To address this problem, on November 6, 2000, Congress passed a law known as the *Needlestick Safety and Prevention Act (NSPA).* The NSPA directed OSHA to revise the Bloodborne Pathogens Standard to incorporate stronger measures to reduce needlesticks and other sharps injuries among HCWs. In response to this mandate, the primary measure instituted by OSHA was to establish detailed requirements that employers identify and make use of safer medical devices. This revised OSHA Bloodborne Pathogens Standard went into effect on April 18, 2001, and is described in detail in this chapter.

OSHA Terminology

The following definitions will help clarify terms relating to the OSHA Bloodborne Pathogens Standard.

Occupational exposure is reasonably anticipated skin, eye, mucous membrane, or parenteral contact with blood or other potentially infectious materials that may result from the performance of an employee's duties.

Parenteral refers to the piercing of the skin barrier or mucous membranes, such as through needlesticks, human bites, cuts, and abrasions.

Blood means human blood, human blood components, and products made from blood. Blood components include plasma, serum, platelets, and serosanguineous fluid (e.g., exudates from wounds). An example of a blood product is a medication derived from blood, such as immune globulins.

Bloodborne pathogens (BBPs) refers to pathogenic microorganisms in human blood that can cause disease in humans. Bloodborne pathogens include, but are not limited to, the hepatitis B virus (HBV), the hepatitis C virus (HCV), and the human immunodeficiency virus (HIV).

Other potentially infectious materials (OPIMs) include:
- Semen and vaginal secretions
- The following body fluids: cerebrospinal, synovial, pleural, pericardial, peritoneal, and amniotic
- Any body fluid that is visibly contaminated with blood
- Any body fluid that has not been identified
- Saliva in dental procedures
- Any unfixed human tissue
- Any tissue culture, cells, or fluid known to be HIV infected

Contaminated is defined as the presence or reasonably anticipated presence of blood or other potentially infected materials on an item or surface.

Decontamination is the use of physical or chemical means to remove, inactivate, or destroy bloodborne pathogens on a surface or item to the point where they are no longer capable of transmitting infectious particles and the surface or item is rendered safe for handling, use, or disposal.

Nonintact skin is skin that has a break in the surface. It includes but is not limited to skin with dermatitis, abrasions, cuts, burns, hangnails, chapping, and acne.

Exposure incident is defined as a specific eye, nose, mouth, other mucous membrane, nonintact skin, or parenteral contact with blood or other potentially infectious materials that results from an employee's duties.

Components of the OSHA Standard

The OSHA Bloodborne Pathogens Standard is presented on the following pages as it pertains to the medical office and includes the following categories:
- Exposure control plan
- Safer medical devices
- Labeling requirements
- Communication of hazards to employees
- Record keeping

Exposure Control Plan

The OSHA standard requires that the medical office develop a written exposure control plan (ECP) (Figure 2-3) designed to eliminate or minimize employee exposure to bloodborne pathogens and other potentially infectious material. The ECP must be made available for review by all medical office staff. The ECP must include the following elements:

1. **An exposure determination:** The purpose of this section of the ECP is to identify employees who must receive training, protective equipment, hepatitis vaccination, and other protections required by the Bloodborne Pathogens Standard. The exposure determination must include (1) a list of all job classifications in which *all* employees are likely to have occupational exposure, such as physicians, medical assistants, and laboratory technicians and (2) a list of job classifications in which only *some* employees have occupational exposure, such as custodians. For the second classification of jobs, the determination must include a list of tasks in which occupational exposure may occur, such as emptying the trash.

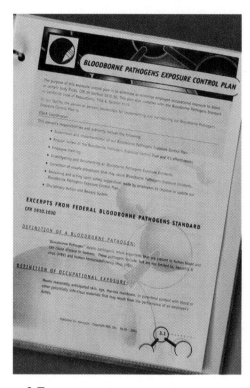

Figure 2-3. An example of an exposure control plan.

2. **The method of compliance:** The method of compliance section of the ECP must document the specific health and safety control measures that are taken in the medical office to eliminate or minimize the risk of occupational exposure. Because these measures must be followed closely by the medical assistant, they are discussed in more detail later (see Control Measures).

3. **Post-exposure evaluation and follow-up procedures:** The post-exposure evaluation and follow-up must specify the procedures to follow in the event of an exposure incident in the medical office, including the method of documenting and investigating an exposure incident, and the post-exposure evaluation, medical treatment, and follow-up that will be made available to the employee. (Refer to the OSHA Post-Exposure Evaluation and Follow-Up Procedures box.)

OSHA requires employers to review and update their ECP at least annually to ensure that the plan remains current with the latest information that eliminates or reduces exposure to bloodborne pathogens. The ECP must also be updated whenever necessary to reflect new or modified tasks and procedures that affect occupational exposure.

OSHA Post-Exposure Evaluation and Follow-Up Procedures

In the event of an exposure incident to bloodborne pathogens or other potentially infectious materials, OSHA requires the following be performed:

1. Perform the initial first aid measures immediately (e.g., wash a needlestick injury thoroughly with soap and water).
2. Document the route of exposure, and the conditions and circumstances of the exposure incident.
3. Identify and document the source individual (unless the employer can establish that identification is not feasible or is prohibited by state or local law). A *source individual* is any person, living or dead, whose blood or OPIMs may be a source of occupational exposure to the health care worker.
4. Obtain consent to test the source individual's blood. Test it as soon as possible to determine HBV, HCV, and HIV infectivity. The following guidelines apply to this requirement:
   a. If consent is not obtained, the employer must document that legally required consent cannot be obtained.
   b. If the source individual's consent is not required by law, the source individual's blood (if available) must be tested and the results documented.
   c. If the source individual is already known to be infected with HBV, HCV, or HIV, testing does not need to be repeated.
5. Provide the exposed employee with the source individual's test results. Inform the employee of applicable laws and regulations concerning disclosure of the identity and infectious status of the source individual.
6. Obtain consent to test the employee's blood. Collect and test the blood of the employee as soon as possible for HBV, HCV, and HIV serological status. If the employee does not give consent for HIV serologic testing, the baseline blood sample must be preserved for at least 90 days. If the employee elects to have the baseline sample tested during the 90-day waiting period, such testing must be done as soon as feasible.
7. When medically indicated, provide the employee with appropriate post-exposure prophylaxis as recommended by the U.S. Public Health Service.

Safer medical devices (described in the next section) must be used to reduce the risk of injuries from sharps. As part of the annual review, the following information must be included: (1) documentation that safer medical devices that reflect changes in technology are being evaluated and implemented in the workplace and (2) documentation that input was obtained from employees in selecting safer medical devices.

Safer Medical Devices

OSHA stipulates specific requirements to reduce needlestick and other sharps injuries among HCWs. These requirements are described as follows. Employers are required to evaluate and implement commercially available safer medical devices and other engineering controls that eliminate occupational exposure to the lowest extent feasible. Input from employees involved in direct patient care must be taken into consideration in making this determination. This helps to ensure that the individuals who are using the devices have the opportunity for input.

A *safer medical device* is a device that, based on reasonable judgment, will make an exposure incident involving a contaminated sharp less likely. Reasonable judgment refers to the judgment of the HCWs who will be using the device. Examples of safer medical devices include sharps with engineered sharps injury protection and needleless systems.

A *sharp with engineered sharps injury protection (SESIP)* is a nonneedle sharp or a needle device with a built-in safety feature that is used for procedures that involve the risk of a sharps injury. Examples of SESIPs include safety engineered syringes and phlebotomy devices (Figure 2-4).

A *needleless system* is a device that does not use a needle for (1) the administration of medication or other fluids, (2) the collection or withdrawal of body fluids after initial access to a vein or artery is established, or (3) any other procedure involving the potential for occupational exposure to bloodborne pathogens as a result of percutaneous injuries from contaminated sharps. An example of a needleless system is a jet injection syringe, which uses compressed air to administer an injection rather than a needle.

Labeling Requirements

The OSHA Bloodborne Pathogens Standard requires that containers and appliances containing biohazardous materials be labeled with a *biohazard warning label.* The biohazard warning label must be fluorescent orange or orange-red and contain the biohazard symbol and the word BIOHAZARD in a contrasting color (Figure 2-5, *A*).

A warning label must be attached to the following: (1) containers of regulated waste, (2) refrigerators and freezers used to store blood and other potentially infectious materials, and (3) containers and bags used to store, transport, or ship blood or other potentially infectious materials (Figure 2-5, *B*). Red bags or red containers may be substituted for biohazard warning labels.

The labeling requirement is designed to alert employees to possible exposure, particularly in situations where the nature of the material or contents is not readily identifiable as blood or other potentially infectious materials.

Communicating Hazards to Employees

According to the OSHA standard, employers must ensure that all medical office employees with risk of occupational exposure participate in a training program. The program must present the ECP for the medical office, focusing on the measures that employees are to take for their safety. Training must be provided at the time an employee is initially assigned to tasks in which occupational exposure may occur and at least annually thereafter.

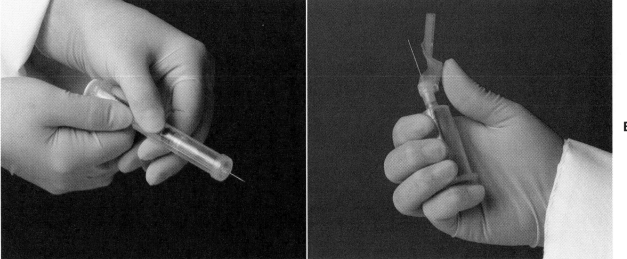

A   **B**

Figure 2-4. A, Safety engineered syringe. **B,** Safety engineered phlebotomy device.

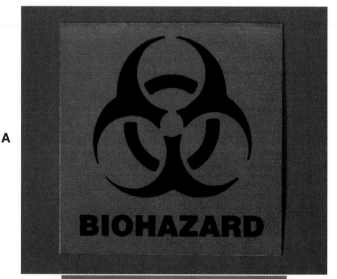

A

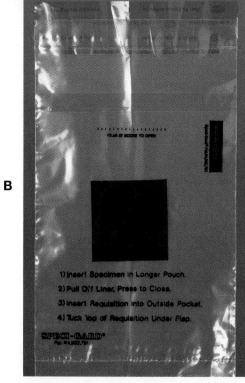

B

Figure 2-5. A, Biohazard warning label. **B,** Biohazard bag used to hold and transport blood or other potentially infectious materials.

Record Keeping

The OSHA Bloodborne Pathogens Standard requires that the following records be maintained:

1. **OSHA Employee Record:** The OSHA standard requires that the employer maintain an accurate OSHA record of every medical office employee at risk for occupational exposure. These records must be kept confidential except for review by OSHA officials and as required by law. The record must include the following: employee's name; social security number; hepatitis B vaccination status, including dates of vaccination; results of any post-exposure examinations, medical testing, and follow-up procedures; a copy of the health care professional's written evaluation following an exposure incident; and a copy of the exposure incident report. The employer is required to maintain records for the duration of employment plus 30 years. The employer must also maintain records of the training sessions, which must include presentation dates, content of the sessions, names and qualifications of the trainers, and names and job titles of employees who attended. These records must be maintained for 3 years from the date of the training session.

2. **Sharps Injury Log:** Employers with more than 10 employees at risk for occupational exposure are required to maintain a log of injuries from contaminated sharps. The sharps injury log must contain the following information:
   - Type and brand of device involved in the injury
   - Location of the incident (i.e., work area)
   - Description of the events that resulted in the injury
   The log must be maintained in a way that protects the privacy of injured employees. The purpose of the log is to help employers and employees keep track of all needlestick injuries. This tracking helps identify problem areas that need attention and ineffective devices that need to be replaced.

Control Measures

There are specific health and safety control measures required by OSHA to eliminate or minimize the risk of occupational exposure in the medical office. These measures are divided into six categories: engineering controls, work practice controls, personal protective equipment, housekeeping, hepatitis B vaccination, and universal precautions. Each of these categories is discussed next.

Engineering Controls

The medical office must use engineering controls to eliminate or minimize the risk of occupational exposure. *Engineering controls* include all control measures that isolate or remove health hazards from the workplace. Engineering controls must be examined and maintained or replaced as required to ensure their effectiveness.

Examples of engineering controls include:
- Readily accessible handwashing facilities
- Safer medical devices
- Biohazard sharps containers and biohazard bags
- Autoclaves

Work Practice Controls

Work practice controls reduce the likelihood of exposure by altering the manner in which the technique is performed.

It is important that the medical assistant consistently adhere to these safety rules, which include the following:

1. Perform all procedures involving blood or other potentially infectious material in a manner to minimize splashing, spraying, spattering, and generation of droplets of these substances.

2. Observe warning labels on biohazard containers and appliances. Bags or containers that bear a biohazard warning label or are color-coded red indicate that they hold blood or other potentially infectious materials. Refrigerators, freezers, and other appliances that contain hazardous materials must also bear a biohazard warning label.

3. Bandage cuts and other lesions on the hands before gloving.

4. Sanitize the hands as soon as possible after removing gloves.

5. If your hands or other skin surfaces come in contact with blood or other potentially infectious material, thoroughly wash the area as soon as possible with soap and water.

6. If your mucous membranes (e.g., eyes, mouth, nose) come in contact with blood or other potentially infectious material, flush them with water as soon as possible.

7. Do not bend, break, or shear contaminated needles.

8. Do not recap a contaminated needle, except in unusual circumstances when no other alternative is possible. Such recapping must be performed through the use of a one-handed technique; using a two-handed technique is strictly prohibited. The one-handed recapping technique involves holding the syringe in the dominant hand and using the needle to pick up the cap, using a scooping motion. The cap is then secured onto the needle by pushing it against a hard surface. (NOTE: Sterile needles may be recapped, such as after the withdrawal of medication from a vial or ampule.)

9. Immediately after use, place contaminated sharps in a puncture-resistant, leakproof container that is appropriately labeled or color coded. *Contaminated sharps* are contaminated objects that can penetrate the skin, including (but not limited to) needles, lancets, scalpels, broken glass, and capillary tubes.

10. Do not eat, drink, smoke, apply cosmetics or lip balm, or handle contact lenses in areas where you may be exposed to blood or other potentially infectious materials.

11. Do not store food or drink in refrigerators, freezers, or cabinets or on shelves or countertops where blood or other potentially infectious materials are present.

12. Place blood specimens or other potentially infectious materials in containers that prevent leakage during collection, handling, processing, storage, transport, or shipping. Make sure the containers are closed before being stored, transported, or shipped and are labeled or color coded for easy identification.

13. Before any equipment that might be contaminated is serviced or shipped for repairing or cleaning, such as a centrifuge, it must be inspected for blood or other potentially infectious material. If such material is present, the equipment must be decontaminated. If it cannot be decontaminated, it must be appropriately labeled to clearly indicate the contamination site, to enable those coming into contact with the equipment to take appropriate precautions.

14. If you are exposed to blood or other potentially infectious materials, perform first-aid measures immediately (e.g., wash a needlestick injury thoroughly with soap and water). After taking these measures, report the incident to your physician-employer as soon as possible so that post-exposure procedures can be instituted. (See the box entitled OSHA Post-Exposure Evaluation and Follow-Up Procedures.) The most obvious exposure incident is a needlestick, but any eye, mouth, or other mucous membrane, nonintact skin, or parenteral contact with blood or other potentially infectious materials constitutes an exposure incident and should be reported.

Personal Protective Equipment

The OSHA standard specifies that personal protective equipment must be used in the medical office whenever occupational exposure remains after instituting engineering and work practice controls. *Personal protective equipment* is clothing or equipment that protects an individual from contact with blood or other potentially infectious materials; examples include gloves, face shields, masks, protective eyewear, laboratory coats, and gowns. The type of protective equipment appropriate for a given task depends on the degree of exposure that is anticipated, as outlined here:

1. Wear gloves when it is reasonably anticipated that your hand(s) will have contact with blood and other potentially infectious materials, mucous membranes, or nonintact skin; when performing vascular access procedures; and when handling or touching contaminated surfaces or items. Gloves will not prevent a puncture, but they could prevent the virus from entering the body through a break in the skin, such as a cut, abrasion, burn, or rash.

2. Face shields or masks in combination with eye-protection devices must be worn whenever splashes, spray, spatter, or droplets of blood or other potentially infectious materials may be generated, posing a hazard through contact with your eyes, nose, or mouth (e.g., removing a stopper from a tube of blood, transferring serum from whole blood) (Figure 2-6).

3. Wear appropriate protective clothing, such as gowns, aprons, and laboratory coats, when gross contamination can reasonably be anticipated during performance of a task or procedure (e.g., laboratory testing procedure). The type of protective clothing will depend on the task and degree of exposure anticipated.

Personal Protective Equipment Guidelines

Certain guidelines must be followed when using protective equipment:

1. Protective equipment must not allow blood or other potentially infectious material to pass through or reach

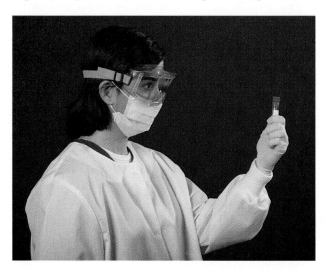

Figure 2-6. Jennifer wears a combination mask and eye-protection device and a laboratory coat to protect against splashes, spray, spatter, and droplets of blood.

your work clothes, street clothes, undergarments, skin, eyes, mouth, or other mucous membranes under normal conditions of use and for the duration of time the protective equipment is used.

2. The employer must provide appropriate personal protective equipment at no cost to you. The employer is responsible for making sure the equipment is available in appropriate sizes, is readily accessible, and is used correctly. In addition, the employer must ensure that the equipment is cleaned, laundered, repaired, replaced, or disposed of as necessary to ensure its effectiveness.

3. If your gloves become contaminated, torn, or punctured, replace them as soon as possible.

4. All eye-protection devices must have solid side shields; therefore face shields, goggles, and glasses with side shields are acceptable (Figure 2-7); standard prescription eyeglasses are unacceptable as eye protection.

5. If a garment is penetrated by blood or other potentially infectious materials, it must be removed as soon as possible and placed in an appropriately designated container for washing.

6. All personal protective equipment must be removed before leaving the medical office.

Highlight on OSHA Bloodborne Pathogens Standard

General Information

The exposure control plan must be made available to OSHA upon request.

OSHA inspectors are responsible for determining whether the medical office meets the Bloodborne Pathogens Standard. This is accomplished through a careful review of the exposure control plan, interviews with the medical office employer and employees, and observation of work activities.

Feces, nasal secretions, saliva, sputum, sweat, tears, urine, and vomitus are not considered by OSHA to be potentially infectious material unless they contain blood.

Control Measures

Employees must be trained in the proper use of the following: engineering controls (including safer medical devices), work practice controls, and personal protective equipment.

General work clothes, such as scrubs, uniforms, pants, shirts, and blouses, are not intended to function as protection against a hazard and are not considered personal protective equipment.

Employees are not permitted to launder contaminated clothing at home; rather, it is the employer's responsibility to have clothing laundered.

If an employee is allergic to the standard latex gloves, the employer must provide a suitable alternative, such as hypoallergenic gloves.

Needlestick Injuries

The CDC estimates that every year between 600,000 and 800,000 health care workers in the United States suffer from needlestick and other sharps injuries and 1,000 of these individuals contract serious infections as a result of these injuries. The CDC estimates that 62% to 88% of sharps injuries can be prevented by the use of safer medical devices.

A wide variety of commercially available safer medical devices have recently been developed to reduce the risk of needlestick and other sharps injuries.

Safer medical devices that eliminate exposure to the lowest extent feasible must be evaluated and implemented in the health care setting. The lack of injuries on the sharps injury log *does not* exempt the employer from this provision.

7. When protective equipment is removed, it must be placed in an appropriately designated area or container for storage, washing, decontamination, or disposal.

8. Utility gloves may be decontaminated and reused unless they are cracked, peeling, torn, or punctured or no longer provide barrier protection.

9. If you believe using protective equipment would prevent proper delivery of health care or would pose an increased hazard to your safety or that of a co-worker, in extenuating circumstances you may temporarily and briefly decline its use. After such an incident, the circumstances must be investigated to determine whether the situation could be prevented in the future.

Housekeeping

The OSHA standard requires that specific housekeeping procedures be followed to ensure that the work site is maintained in a clean and sanitary condition. The medical office must develop and implement a written schedule for cleaning and decontaminating each area where exposure

occurs. The method of decontaminating work surfaces must be specified and should be based on the type of surface to be cleaned, the soil present, and the tasks or procedures that occur in that area. Housekeeping procedures include the following:

1. Clean and decontaminate equipment and work surfaces after completing procedures that involve blood or other potentially infectious materials. Cleaning is accomplished using a detergent soap, and decontamination is performed using an appropriate disinfectant (Figure 2-8).

2. Clean and decontaminate all equipment and work surfaces as soon as possible after exposure to blood or other potentially infectious material.

3. Inspect and decontaminate all reusable receptacles, such as bins, pails, and cans, on a regular basis. If contamination is visible, the item must be cleaned and decontaminated as soon as possible.

4. Do not pick up broken, contaminated glassware with the hands, even if gloves are worn. Use mechanical means, such as a brush and dustpan, tongs, and forceps (Figure 2-9).

5. Protective coverings, such as plastic wrap and aluminum foil, may be used to cover work surfaces or equipment, but they must be removed or replaced if contamination occurs.

6. Handle contaminated laundry as little as possible and with appropriate personal protective equipment. Place all contaminated laundry in leakproof bags that are properly labeled or color coded. Contaminated laundry must not be sorted or rinsed at the medical office.

What Would You DO?
What Would You *Not* DO?

Case Study 2

Tracy Smith is pregnant and is at the medical office to have her blood drawn for a prenatal profile. Tracy says she doesn't understand why gloves have to be worn when her blood is drawn. She says that it makes her feel like a leper and she is absolutely sure that she doesn't have any diseases. Tracy says she has been reading information about the hepatitis B vaccine because she knows her baby will be given this vaccine soon after birth. She wants to know why it is recommended that an infant be immunized for hepatitis B. Tracy says that babies aren't at risk for contracting hepatitis B since the way it is transmitted is mostly through sexual contact and illegal drug use.

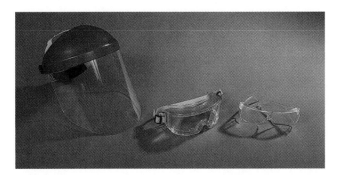

Figure 2-7. Examples of eye-protection devices. *Left,* Face shield; *center,* goggles; *right,* glasses with solid side shields.

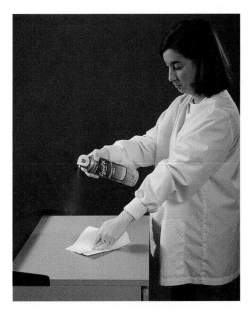

Figure 2-8. Clean and decontaminate work surfaces with an appropriate disinfectant after completing procedures involving blood and other potentially infectious materials.

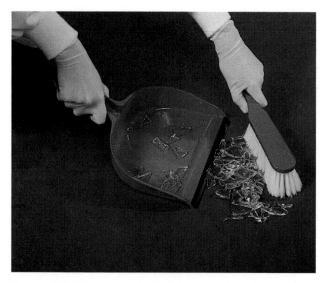

Figure 2-9. Use mechanical means to pick up broken contaminated glass.

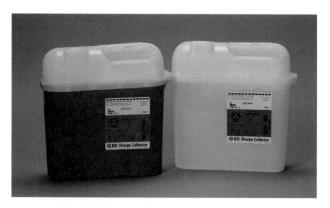

Figure 2-10. Biohazard sharps containers.

7. If the outside of a biohazard container becomes contaminated, it must be placed in a second suitable container.
8. Biohazard sharps containers (Figure 2-10) must be closable, puncture-resistant, and/or leakproof. They must bear a biohazard warning label and be color-coded red to ensure identification of the contents as hazardous. To ensure effectiveness, the following procedures must be observed:
    a. Locate the sharps container as close as possible to the area of use to avoid the hazard of transporting a contaminated needle through the workplace.
    b. Maintain sharps containers in an upright position to keep liquid and sharps inside.
    c. Do not reach into the sharps container with your hand.
    d. Replace sharps containers on a regular basis and do not allow them to overfill. (It is recommended that sharps containers be replaced when they are three-quarters full.)

Highlight on Hepatitis B Vaccine

The hepatitis B vaccine became available in 1982 and is 95% effective in providing immunity.

The hepatitis B vaccine is well tolerated by most patients. The most common side effect is soreness at the injection site, including induration, erythema, and swelling. Occasionally a low-grade fever, headache, and dizziness occur.

It has been determined that the hepatitis B vaccine provides immunity for at least 15 years. At the present time, the CDC does not recommend a routine booster dose.

The hepatitis B vaccine is recommended for all infants, children, and adolescents who are 18 years of age or younger. It also is recommended for adults over the age of 18 who are at increased risk for developing hepatitis B. This population includes employees with occupational exposure (such as health care workers), hemodialysis patients, hemophiliacs, individuals with multiple sex partners, homosexually active men, injection drug users, and household and sexual contacts of individuals with chronic hepatitis B.

The number of health care workers contracting hepatitis B has decreased sharply since the development of the hepatitis B vaccine. As more people become immune to hepatitis B through the immunization of infants, the goal of eliminating hepatitis B in the United States may be realized.

Hepatitis B Vaccination

The OSHA standard requires physicians to offer the hepatitis B vaccination series free of charge to all medical office personnel who have occupational exposure. The vaccination must be offered within 10 days of initial assignment to a position with occupational exposure unless the following factors exists: (a) the individual has previously received the hepatitis B vaccination series, (b) antibody testing has revealed that the individual is immune, or (c) the vaccine is contraindicated for medical reasons.

Medical office personnel who decline vaccination must sign a hepatitis B waiver form documenting refusal. This form must be filed in the employee's OSHA record (Figure 2-11). Employees who decline vaccination may later request the vaccination, which the employer must then provide according to the aforementioned criteria.

Universal Precautions

Before the release of the OSHA standard, the Centers for Disease Control and Prevention issued recommendations for health care workers known as the Universal Precautions. According to the concept of Universal Precautions, all human blood and certain human body fluids are treated as if known to be infectious for HIV,

HEPATITIS B VACCINE REFUSAL

I understand that due to my occupational exposure to blood or other potentially infectious materials, I may be at risk of acquiring hepatitis B virus (HBV) infection. I have been given the opportunity to be vaccinated with hepatitis B vaccine at no charge to myself. However, I decline hepatitis B vaccination at this time. I understand that by declining this vaccine I continue to be at risk of acquiring hepatitis B, a serious disease. If in the future I continue to have occupational exposure to blood or to other potentially infectious materials and I want to be vaccinated with hepatitis B vaccine, I can receive the vaccination series at no charge to me.

_____
Employee Name (printed)

_____   _____
Employee Signature   Date

_____   _____
Witness Signature   Date

Figure 2-11. Hepatitis B vaccine waiver form. This form must be signed by an employee with occupational exposure who declines hepatitis B vaccination.

hepatitis B, hepatitis C, and other bloodborne pathogens. The OSHA standard states that the Universal Precautions must be observed, and in fact, these precautions form the heart of the OSHA standard itself.

Regulated Medical Waste

Medical waste is generated in the medical office through the diagnosis, treatment, and immunization of patients. Some of this waste poses a threat to health and safety and is known as **regulated medical waste (RMW).** The OSHA Bloodborne Pathogens Standard defines regulated waste as follows:

- Any liquid or semiliquid blood or OPIM
- Contaminated items that would release blood or OPIM in a liquid or semiliquid state if compressed
- Items that are caked with dried blood or OPIM and are capable of releasing these materials during handling
- Contaminated sharps
- Pathological and microbiological wastes that contain blood or OPIM

Regulated medical waste must be properly discarded so as not to become a source of transfer of disease. According to the OSHA definition, a dressing saturated with blood is considered regulated medical waste and must be discarded in a biohazard bag. On the other hand, a bandage with a spot of blood on it is not considered regulated medical waste and therefore can be discarded in a regular waste container. Table 2-2 gives the guidelines for discarding medical waste in the medical office.

Handling Regulated Medical Waste

Regulated medical waste must be handled carefully to prevent exposure incidents. The OSHA Bloodborne Pathogens Standard outlines specific actions to take when handling regulated medical waste:

1. Separate regulated waste from the general refuse at its point of origin. This means that disposable items containing regulated medical waste should be placed directly into biohazard containers and not mixed with the regular trash.
2. Make sure that the biohazard containers are closable, leakproof, and suitably constructed to contain the contents during handling, storage, and transport. These containers include biohazard bags and sharps containers.
3. To prevent spillage or protrusion of the contents, close the lid of the sharps container before removal or replacement. Never open, empty, or clean a contaminated sharps container. If there is a chance of leakage from the sharps container, the medical assistant should place it in a second container that is closable, leakproof, and appropriately labeled or color coded.
4. Securely close biohazard bags and tie them before removal. To provide additional protection, some medical offices double-bag by placing the primary bag inside a second biohazard bag.
5. Remove full biohazard containers to a secured area away from the general public, using personal protective equipment (e.g., gloves).

TABLE 2-2	Guidelines for Discarding Medical Waste in the Medical Office

Regular Waste Container

The following items that have been used for health care *are not* considered regulated medical waste and can be discarded in a covered waste container lined with a regular trash bag.

- Disposable drapes
- Disposable patient gowns
- Examining table paper
- Disposable clean or sterile gloves
- Gauze tinged with blood or other body fluids
- Disposable probe covers for thermometers
- Tongue depressors
- Tissues with respiratory secretions
- Disposable ear speculums
- Empty urine containers
- Urine testing strips
- Disposable diapers
- Feminine hygiene products

Biohazard Sharps Container

The following items are sharps. They *are* considered regulated medical waste and must be discarded in a biohazard sharps container:

- Hypodermic syringes and needles
- Venipuncture needles
- Lancets
- Razor blades
- Scalpel blades
- Suture needles
- Blood tubes
- Capillary pipets
- Microscope slides and coverslips
- Broken glassware

Biohazard Bag Waste Container

The following items *are* considered regulated medical waste. They are not sharps and therefore can be discarded in a covered waste container lined with a biohazard bag:

- Any item saturated or dripping with blood or OPIM, such as dressings, gauze, cotton balls, paper towels, and tissues
- Any item caked with dried blood or OPIM, such as dressings and sutures
- Disposable clean or sterile gloves contaminated with blood or OPIM
- Disposable vaginal speculums and collection devices (swabs, spatulas, brushes)
- Tissue or fluid removed during minor office surgery
- Microbiological waste, such as specimen cultures and collection devices
- Discarded live and attenuated vaccines

Sanitary Sewer

Disposal of small quantities of blood and other body fluids to the sanitary sewer is considered a safe method of disposing of these waste materials. The following fluids can be carefully poured down a utility sink, drain, or toilet. (NOTE: State regulations may dictate the maximum volume allowable for discharge of blood or body fluids into the sanitary sewer.)

- Blood
- Body excretions such as urine
- Body secretions such as sputum

Disposal of Regulated Medical Waste

Each state is responsible for developing policies for disposal of regulated medical waste. To avoid noncompliance, it is important for the medical assistant to know and understand the specific regulated waste policies and guidelines set forth in his or her state.

Most medical offices use a commercial medical waste service to dispose of regulated medical waste. The service is responsible for picking up and transporting the regulated waste to a regulated waste treatment facility for incineration or treatment to render it harmless. The waste can then be safely disposed of in a sanitary landfill. Regulated waste treatment facilities must be licensed and hold permits issued by the Environmental Protection Agency (EPA), allowing them to dispose of regulated medical waste.

A series of steps must be followed for packaging and storing regulated medical waste for pickup by the service. Although these steps may vary slightly from state to state, general measures required by most states include the following:

1. Place biohazard bags and sharps containers into a receptacle provided by the medical waste service. The receptacle is usually a cardboard box (Figure 2-12). The box should be securely sealed with packing tape, and a biohazard warning label must appear on two opposite sides of the box.

2. Store the biohazard boxes in a locked room inside the facility or in a locked collection container outside for pickup by the medical waste service. This step is aimed at preventing unauthorized access to such items as needles and syringes. The regulated waste storage area should be labeled with one of the following:
   - An "Authorized Personnel Only" sign
   - The international biohazard symbol

3. Many states require that a tracking record be completed when the waste is picked up by the medical waste service. The form includes such information as the type

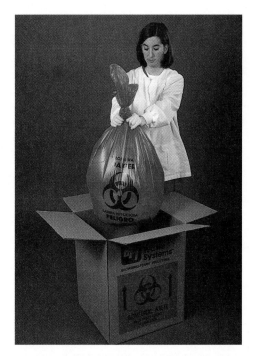

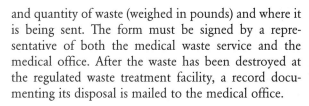

Figure 2-12. Jennifer places a biohazard bag inside a cardboard box in preparation for pickup by the infectious waste service.

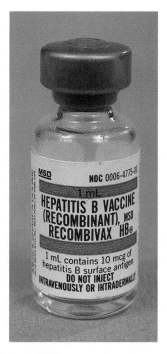

Figure 2-13. Hepatitis B vaccine.

and quantity of waste (weighed in pounds) and where it is being sent. The form must be signed by a representative of both the medical waste service and the medical office. After the waste has been destroyed at the regulated waste treatment facility, a record documenting its disposal is mailed to the medical office.

Bloodborne Diseases

The biggest threats to health care workers from occupational exposure are hepatitis B, hepatitis C, and HIV. Hepatitis is much easier to transmit than is HIV. After a needlestick exposure to blood infected with the hepatitis B virus, health care workers have a 6% to 30% chance of developing hepatitis B. The risk of infection after a needlestick exposure to blood infected with the hepatitis C virus is approximately 2%. After a needlestick exposure to HIV-infected blood, a health care worker has a 0.3% chance of developing AIDS.

These diseases are discussed in detail on the following pages.

Hepatitis B

Hepatitis B is an infection of the liver caused by the hepatitis B virus. The most common means of transmitting hepatitis B in the health care setting are blood and blood products, such as serum and plasma.

Health care workers are most likely to contract hepatitis B through needlesticks and cuts with contaminated sharps. The virus is also spread in the health care setting,

but less effectively, through blood splashes to the eyes, mouth, and nonintact skin and through body fluids such as semen and vaginal secretions.

Every year, approximately 800 health care employees contract hepatitis B in the workplace. Therefore it is important for the medical assistant to carefully follow the OSHA standard to safeguard against exposure to the hepatitis virus and other bloodborne pathogens.

Post-Exposure Prophylaxis

Post-exposure prophylaxis (PEP) refers to treatment administered to an individual after exposure to an infectious disease to prevent the disease. The PEP for individuals exposed to hepatitis B involves the administration of both a passive and an active immunizing agent. The passive immunizing agent provides temporary immunity to hepatitis B, thereby giving the active agent a chance to take effect. The passive agent is hepatitis B immune globulin (HBIG), which contains antibodies that provide immunity to hepatitis B for a period of 1 to 3 months. It is important to administer HBIG as soon as possible after an exposure incident—preferably within 72 hours.

The *active immunizing agent* in the hepatitis B vaccine (Figure 2-13) is produced from genetically altered yeast cells; brand names are Recombivax HB and Engerix-B. The hepatitis B vaccine is administered intramuscularly in a series of three doses. The second dose is given 1 month after the first dose, and the third dose is then administered 6 months after the first dose (i.e., 0, 1 month, and

6 months). Mild side effects, such as soreness at the injection site, may occur, but serious reactions to the vaccine are extremely rare.

As previously discussed, the OSHA standard recommends that all health care workers receive the vaccine as a preventive measure against hepatitis B. Therefore, after an exposure incident, a medical assistant who has previously been vaccinated probably will not require further treatment unless laboratory tests reveal that his or her antibody level is low. In this case, a booster dose of the vaccine is recommended.

Acute Viral Hepatitis B

After a person becomes infected, the acute phase of hepatitis B can last from a few weeks to several months. The symptoms of acute viral hepatitis vary greatly in intensity from mild to severe. Approximately one third of the people who become infected are asymptomatic and unaware that they have the disease. Another third have relatively mild flulike symptoms that often are mistaken for influenza or similar conditions. The remaining one third of infected patients have such severe symptoms that hospitalization may be required.

The initial symptoms, if present, last from 2 to 14 days and include fatigue, headache, loss of appetite, nausea, vomiting, malaise, and muscle and joint pain. In patients with severe acute viral hepatitis, these symptoms progress to abdominal pain, dark urine, and clay-colored stools, followed several days later by jaundice. After the onset of jaundice, the liver enlarges and becomes tender. A very small percentage of patients (0.5% to 2% of those infected) develop fulminant hepatitis, which is almost always fatal. Fulminant hepatitis is characterized by a sudden onset of nausea and vomiting, chills, high fever, severe and early jaundice, convulsions, coma, and death as a result of hepatic failure, usually within 10 days of its onset.

There is no specific treatment or drug to treat acute hepatitis B. Rather, supportive care is prescribed to help the patient's natural defenses overcome the disease; this includes restricted activity, rest, avoidance of alcohol, a well-balanced diet, adequate fluid intake, and precautionary measures to prevent the disease's spread.

Most patients (90%) recover fully after the acute phase, acquire lifelong immunity to hepatitis B, and are not infectious to others.

Chronic Viral Hepatitis B

The remaining 10% of patients who do not recover from the acute phase go on to develop chronic hepatitis. These individuals are unable to remove the virus from their systems and remain infected. Individuals with chronic hepatitis may or may not experience symptoms; nonetheless, they become carriers of hepatitis B and are capable of transmitting the disease to others. In addition, patients with chronic hepatitis face an increased risk of liver damage, which leaves them vulnerable to such diseases as cirrhosis of the liver and liver cancer. A significant number of these patients subsequently die from liver failure.

Hepatitis C

Hepatitis C is an infection of the liver caused by the hepatitis C virus. Currently there is no vaccine available for the prevention of hepatitis C. In the medical office, the most common means of transmission of hepatitis C is through needlesticks and other sharps injuries. The chance of contracting hepatitis C in the health care setting is much lower than that of contracting hepatitis B.

Most individuals with hepatitis C have no symptoms; if symptoms do occur, they are mild and flulike. Approximately 75% to 85% of patients with acute hepatitis C develop chronic hepatitis C. After a period of 10 to 30 years, about 20% of these individuals develop liver disease, including cirrhosis of the liver and cancer of the liver (see the Highlight on Viral Hepatitis).

Highlight on Viral Hepatitis

In the United States there are 500,000 new cases of hepatitis each year. Approximately 43% of these infections are caused by hepatitis B, 32% are caused by hepatitis A, and 23% are caused by hepatitis C.

Symptoms common to all types of hepatitis include fatigue, nausea, loss of appetite, abdominal pain, and jaundice.

In all states, hepatitis A and hepatitis B are reportable diseases. This means that when the physician diagnoses a case of hepatitis A or B, a special form must be completed and filed with the local public health department.

In recent years, antiviral drugs have been developed to treat the chronic forms of hepatitis B and C; however, not all infected individuals are candidates for treatment. These drugs, which must be taken for a prolonged time, are effective in removing the virus from approximately 40% of infected patients.

Hepatitis B

The most common means of transmission of hepatitis B is through sexual contact with an infected person and by sharing needles for illegal drug use with an infected individual.

It is estimated that more than 1 million people in the United States are infected with chronic hepatitis B; therefore they are carriers of hepatitis B and capable of transmitting the disease to others. Many of these individuals do not know that they are carriers.

Every year approximately 6,000 Americans die as a result of the long-term consequences of chronic hepatitis B, such as cirrhosis and liver cancer.

Whether or not an HBV-infected individual develops chronic hepatitis B depends largely on his or her age. Approximately 90% of infected infants born to mothers who are HBV carriers develop chronic hepatitis B, compared with 25% of infected children and 10% of infected adults.

Hepatitis B is capable of surviving for at least a week in a dried state on environmental surfaces, such as contaminated work tables, equipment, and instruments.

Hepatitis C

Chronic hepatitis C is the most common chronic viral infection in the United States. Approximately 2.7 million Americans have been diagnosed with chronic hepatitis C, and each year it causes an estimated 8,000 to 10,000 deaths resulting from cirrhosis and liver cancer.

The most common means of transmission of hepatitis C is by sharing needles for illegal drug use with an infected individual. Hepatitis C is not spread by casual contact, such as sneezing, coughing, hugging, sharing food or water, or sharing eating utensils or drinking glasses. It is rarely transmitted through sexual contact.

Individuals infected with hepatitis C should not share personal items that may have blood on them with other members of the household (e.g., toothbrushes, nail-grooming equipment, and razors).

Chronic hepatitis C is known as "an epidemic that occurred in the past." A large number of individuals became infected with hepatitis C more than 20 years ago and are just now being diagnosed with it. This is because the symptoms of chronic hepatitis C often do not appear until 10 to 30 years after infection, and many times the first symptoms come only with advanced liver disease. In fact, chronic hepatitis C surpasses alcoholism as the leading cause of liver cirrhosis and liver transplantation in the United States.

Before 1992 a blood test to determine the presence of hepatitis C did not exist. Because of this, a significant number of people contracted hepatitis C from HCV-infected blood transfusions. The CDC has begun a campaign to encourage people who received blood transfusions before July 1992 to ask their physicians if they should be tested for hepatitis C.

Post-exposure prophylaxis with immune globulin is not effective in preventing hepatitis C, and no vaccine exists yet to prevent hepatitis C. Vaccines are difficult to develop for hepatitis C because the virus mutates so much.

Other Forms of Viral Hepatitis

In addition to hepatitis B and C, three other strains that cause viral hepatitis have been identified. They include hepatitis A, D, and E. Of these, hepatitis B poses the greatest threat to health care workers and has already been discussed in detail. Hepatitis A has occasionally been transmitted to health care workers but is not considered a major occupational hazard. In all cases of viral hepatitis, the virus invades the liver and causes inflammation, resulting in similar symptoms. The medical assistant should have a general knowledge of each of the forms of viral hepatitis. Table 2-3 outlines the incubation period, means of transmission, characteristics, onset and symptoms, and prognosis for all strains of viral hepatitis.

Acquired Immunodeficiency Syndrome

Acquired immunodeficiency syndrome (AIDS) is a disorder of the immune system that eventually destroys the body's ability to fight off infection. AIDS is caused by a retrovirus known as the human immunodeficiency virus (HIV). When HIV gains entrance into the body, it begins to attack and destroy certain white blood cells known as CD4+ T lymphocytes, which are involved in protecting the body against viral, fungal, and protozoal infections. Over time, more and more CD4+ T lymphocytes are destroyed and the body becomes less able to fight off infection, as well as being more susceptible to opportunistic infections.

AIDS is characterized by the presence of severe and life-threatening opportunistic infections and unusual cancers

TABLE 2-3	Forms of Viral Hepatitis				
	Hepatitis A (HAV)	Hepatitis B (HBV)	Hepatitis C (HCV)	Hepatitis D (HDV)	Hepatitis E (HEV)
Incubation Period	2-6 weeks	2 weeks to 6 months	2 weeks to 6 months	2 weeks to 5 months	3-6 weeks
Means of Transmission	Transmitted almost exclusively by the fecal-oral route through practices of poor hygiene; also transmitted by the consumption of food and water contaminated with human feces	Exposure to contaminated semen and vaginal secretions by personal contact, especially sexual contact; parenteral exposure to contaminated blood and blood products, such as through injecting illegal drugs and accidental needlestick injuries by HCW; perinatally from an infected mother to her neonate	Parenteral exposure to contaminated blood or blood products, primarily from injecting illegal drugs	Same as hepatitis B	Fecal-oral route through practices of poor hygiene; consumption of food and water contaminated with feces
Characteristics	Usually occurs in children and young adults, especially in environments of poor sanitation and overcrowding; often a very mild disease with symptoms similar to the flu and lasting 1 to 2 weeks; there is a vaccine available to prevent hepatitis A	Symptoms usually last 1 to 4 weeks, but it may be as long as 6 months before the patient fully recovers; there is a vaccine available to prevent hepatitis B	At risk are individuals who received a blood transfusion before 1992; currently a vaccine does not exist for hepatitis C	Affects only those already infected with hepatitis B; a person who has received the hepatitis B vaccine is also protected from hepatitis D	Rare in the United States; generally seen in developing countries; usually occurs in epidemics rather than in sporadic cases

Symptoms	Symptoms include fever, malaise, fatigue, anorexia, nausea, vomiting, and abdominal discomfort, followed in some patients by dark urine, clay-colored stools, and mild jaundice	Symptoms include fatigue, headache, loss of appetite, nausea, vomiting, malaise, and muscle and joint pain, followed in some patients by dark urine, clay-colored stools, abdominal pain, and jaundice	Symptoms are similar to those of hepatitis B	Occurs as a coinfection or superinfection with hepatitis B and intensifies the symptoms of hepatitis B	Symptoms are similar to those of hepatitis B
Prognosis	Most people recover fully within 6-10 weeks and become immune to the virus; rarely fatal; chronic hepatitis does not develop; carrier states do not develop	Most people recover fully and become immune to this disease; approximately 0.5%-2% of those infected develop fulminant hepatitis, which is almost always fatal; some patients go on to develop chronic hepatitis and may develop cirrhosis and liver cancer; these patients are also carriers of hepatitis B	Approximately 75% to 85% of patients infected with hepatitis C develop chronic hepatitis, which may lead to liver damage such as cirrhosis and liver cancer	Frequently leads to chronic hepatitis; high fatality rate (as high as 30% of chronic hepatitis patients)	Does not progress to chronic hepatitis; hepatitis E is particularly dangerous if contracted by pregnant women (10% to 20% fatality rate in these individuals)

that rarely afflict individuals with healthy immune systems. An **opportunistic infection** is an infection that results from a defective immune system that cannot defend itself from pathogens normally found in the environment. Opportunistic infections are extremely difficult to treat because the infection tends to recur very quickly once a course of therapy is completed.

Stages of AIDS

The AIDS virus infection cycle has four stages; however, they may not all be experienced by every infected individual. These four stages are described below.

Stage 1: Acute HIV Infection. An individual infected with HIV may first experience a transient mononucleosis-like illness known as acute HIV infection, which occurs 1 to 4 weeks after exposure. On the other hand, many people do not develop any symptoms when they first become infected with HIV. Symptoms of acute HIV infection include fever, sweats, fatigue, loss of appetite, diarrhea, pharyngitis, myalgia, arthralgia, and adenopathy. These symptoms usually disappear within a week to a month and are often mistaken for those of another viral infection.

Stage 2: Asymptomatic Period. After these early symptoms have subsided (if they occur at all), the infected individual normally experiences a long incubation period lasting for years, during which he or she is asymptomatic. At that time, the carrier may not realize the HIV infection is present, because the only evidence of HIV infection during this stage is the production by the body of antibodies to HIV that are detectable by blood tests. These HIV antibodies are unable to destroy the virus; however, they are used as a basis for the test procedure to indicate that the HIV infection is present. Because of the length of time required by the body to develop HIV antibodies, however, these tests may fail to detect HIV for as long as 3 to 6 months after an individual has been infected. Since HIV may be transmitted with or without symptoms, it is during this asymptomatic period that the danger of accidental transmission is greatest.

Stage 3: Symptomatic Period. Before the development of full-blown AIDS, many HIV-infected individuals experience a series of lesser symptoms. One of the first such symptoms experienced by many people infected with HIV is lymph nodes that remain enlarged for more than

Highlight on AIDS

AIDS was first reported in the United States in 1981, but it is most likely that it existed here and in other parts of the world for many years before that. More than 800,000 cases of AIDS have been reported in the United States since 1981, and every year 40,000 people in the U.S. are infected with HIV. The epidemic is growing most rapidly among women between the ages of 25 and 44 and minority populations.

Scientific evidence shows that HIV is not spread through casual, everyday contact. There is no evidence that HIV is spread by sharing facilities or equipment, such as telephones, computers, pencils, cups, doorknobs, and bathrooms. Because HIV is not passed through the air, it is not spread through coughing and sneezing.

The majority of individuals infected with HIV show no symptoms and may not develop full-blown AIDS for many years. Once infected with HIV, the individual is infected for life.

Women can transmit HIV to their fetuses during pregnancy or birth. Approximately one quarter to one third of untreated pregnant women infected with HIV pass the infection to their babies. HIV also can be spread to babies through the breast milk of mothers infected with the virus. If the antiretroviral drug zidovudine (AZT) is taken during pregnancy, the chance of transmitting HIV to the baby is reduced significantly.

The ELISA (enzyme-linked immunosorbent assay) test is widely used as a screening test for the presence of HIV. Because of the possibility of a false-positive result, a second ELISA test is always performed if a blood specimen tests positive. If the second ELISA test is also positive, then a more specific test, such as the Western blot test, is performed to confirm the test results. An individual who tests positive for HIV is *seropositive.*

A negative HIV test is not conclusive for the absence of HIV infection. If an individual has recently been infected with HIV, the antibodies may not have had time to develop. It generally takes 3 to 6 months for the antibodies to show up in the blood.

As scientists learned more about the disease, the CDC's definition of AIDS has changed several times since the beginning of the AIDS epidemic. The current AIDS definition includes the following conditions: HIV positive *and* a CD4+ T cell count below 200 cells/uL or the presence of one or more AIDS-defining conditions. The normal CD4+ T cell count for a healthy individual ranges between 500 cells/uL and 1,500 cells/uL.

There is no cure for AIDS; there is no vaccine to prevent it. Over the past several years, however, drugs have been developed that slow the reproduction of the virus. In many patients, these drugs can delay HIV from progressing to full-blown AIDS. Unfortunately, these drugs do not prevent the spread of the disease and they can have serious side effects.

3 months. Other symptoms often experienced months to years before the onset of AIDS include progressive generalized lymphadenopathy (PGL), lack of energy, unexplained weight loss, recurrent fevers and sweats, diarrhea, persistent or frequent yeast infections (oral or vaginal), and persistent skin rashes or flaky skin. Some people develop frequent and severe herpes infections that cause mouth, genital, or anal sores, or a painful nerve disease known as shingles.

Stage 4: AIDS. AIDS is the last stage of the infection cycle that began with HIV infection. As previously described, full-blown AIDS is characterized by the presence of opportunistic infections and unusual cancers known as AIDS-defining conditions. These conditions do not usually occur, or produce only mild illness, in individuals with healthy immune systems. For example, a severe and rare type of pneumonia caused by the organism *Pneumocystis carinii* is frequently associated with AIDS patients, as is *Kaposi's sarcoma,* a rare type of cancer. Refer to Table 2-4 for a description of these and other AIDS-defining conditions. AIDS is also known to damage the nervous system, which eventually results in varying degrees of dementia and other symptoms. As the HIV infection progresses, the individual becomes overwhelmed by infection and cancer. Because the body is unable to fight back because of a weakened immune system, the patient eventually succumbs to AIDS-defining conditions.

Transmission of AIDS

Research has shown that HIV is not transmitted through casual contact or even extensive contact such as occurs among family members of AIDS patients. In the general population, HIV is spread primarily through sexual contact with an infected person and by sharing drug injection needles with someone who is infected.

Because HIV is not easily transmitted, the risk to health care workers is low; statistics indicate that 35 health care workers across the United States are infected with HIV each year. Despite the low risk of infection, however, the serious nature of HIV infection warrants the use of the OSHA Bloodborne Pathogens Standard by all health care workers. Because most HIV carriers are asymptomatic and may not be aware of their infection, precautions minimizing the risk of exposure to blood and body fluids should be taken with all patients at all times. The precautions are also recommended as a means of protection against other bloodborne pathogens, such as hepatitis B, hepatitis C, and syphilis.

TABLE 2-4 AIDS-Defining Conditions

Neoplasms

Kaposi's Sarcoma

Malignant Neoplasm

Kaposi's sarcoma (KS) is the most common neoplasm occurring in AIDS patients. It is an aggressive tumor that involves multiple body organs but generally occurs initially on the skin. It is characterized by multiple dark red or purplish blotches on the skin. The areas of the body most commonly affected are the trunk, arms, head, and neck. Diagnosis of Kaposi's sarcoma is made by tissue biopsy. Other body sites commonly affected by this neoplasm are the lymph nodes, the lungs, and the gastrointestinal tract. Kaposi's sarcoma is rarely the primary cause of death but does further weaken the AIDS patient, who may succumb eventually to opportunistic infections.

Opportunistic Infections

Pneumocystis carinii **Pneumonia**

Protozoa

Pneumocystis carinii pneumonia (PCP) is the most common opportunistic infection causing death in individuals with AIDS. This protozoan lung infection was at one time considered rare and in most instances not fatal. PCP occurs at least once in more than 65% of AIDS patients, and 25% of those initially infected experience a recurrence. PCP is characterized by moderate-to-severe difficulty in breathing, fever, and a nonproductive cough in the early stages and a productive cough in the later stages of the disease. Death occurs in 30% of PCP-infected patients and is generally caused by acute respiratory failure.

Cytomegalovirus Infection

Virus

Cytomegalovirus (CMV) is a virus that belongs to the herpes virus group, that rarely causes disease in healthy adults. The majority of AIDS patients have active cytomegalovirus infection. The most common symptoms of its presence in AIDS patients are spots on the retina that may lead to blindness. This virus also causes pneumonia, esophagitis, and colitis. Specific symptoms may include fever, profound fatigue, muscle and joint aches, night sweats, impaired vision, cough, dyspnea, abdominal pain, and diarrhea.

Herpes Simplex 1 and 2

Virus

Herpes simplex 1 is spread by contact with oral secretions, and herpes simplex 2 is spread by contact with genital secretions. Herpes simplex causes painful vesicular lesions, usually of the nasopharynx, oral cavity, skin, and genital tract. This virus tends to have periods of latency followed by reactivation of symptoms. In AIDS patients, herpes simplex is apt to cause cervical lymphadenopathy and proctitis.

Continued

TABLE 2-4 AIDS-Defining Conditions—cont'd

Mycobacterial Infections

Bacteria

Mycobacterial infections are one of the most frequent opportunistic infections in AIDS patients. One strain *(Mycobacterium avium complex)* causes fever, fatigue, weight loss, diarrhea, and malabsorption. Another strain *(Mycobacterium tuberculosis)* causes pulmonary tuberculosis, which is not considered an opportunistic infection. In AIDS patients, tuberculosis is characterized by a productive, purulent cough, fever, dyspnea, fatigue, weight loss, and wasting. The AIDS epidemic appears to be causing a resurgence of tuberculosis in the United States. Because tuberculosis is more contagious than most AIDS-defining conditions, it appears to be spreading beyond AIDS patients and into the general population.

Candidiasis

Yeastlike Fungus

Candida albicans is a fungus that inhabits the oropharynx, large intestine, and skin, causing no harm in individuals with healthy immune systems. Infection with *Candida albicans* is often one of the first signs of a weakened immune system in HIV-infected individuals. It is characterized by a white, patchy growth on the mouth, throat, or esophagus (thrush). AIDS patients develop an extremely severe case of candidiasis that makes eating and swallowing both difficult and painful. In female AIDS patients, this organism causes severe vaginitis.

Cryptosporidiosis

Protozoa

In AIDS patients, this condition usually causes profuse, watery diarrhea along with anorexia, vomiting, fatigue, malaise, and fever. This condition may become chronic, resulting in dehydration and electrolyte imbalance, which in turn lead to weight loss and eventual death.

Toxoplasmosis

Protozoa

Toxoplasmosis is one of the most common causes of encephalitis in AIDS patients, resulting in the following symptoms: headache, altered mental state, visual disturbances, cranial nerve palsy, and motor disorders. Toxoplasmosis may also result in infection of the heart, lungs, skin, stomach, abdomen, and testes.

Cryptococcosis

Fungus

Cryptococcosis is a common cause of meningitis in AIDS patients and includes chronic symptoms of low-grade fever, malaise, and headaches. Other symptoms manifested after these initial symptoms include photophobia, stiff neck, nausea, vomiting, and seizures.

⚟ PATIENT TEACHING

Acquired Immunodeficiency Syndrome

Teach patients the ways in which AIDS is transmitted
- Having sex (vaginal, anal, or oral) with someone who is infected with HIV. The virus is most commonly found in semen, blood, and vaginal secretions.
- Sharing needles for illegal injection drug use with someone who is infected with HIV.
- Transmitting in utero: A woman with HIV can pass it on to her unborn child. Babies born with HIV usually develop AIDS by 2 years of age.
- Receiving a blood transfusion or blood products (before 1985) from someone infected with HIV. (In 1985 blood banks began screening blood for AIDS, so this is largely a problem of blood received before then.)

Teach patients how to prevent AIDS
- Know your sexual partner(s) and their sexual history and drug use.
- Use a latex condom during sexual intercourse to minimize the risk of infection. HIV cannot pass through the latex if the condom does not break and is used properly. If a lubricant is used with the condom, it should be water based, such as K-Y Jelly, because an oil-based lubricant, such as petroleum jelly, could break down the latex.

- Avoid sexual practices that involve the exchange of body fluids, such as semen or vaginal secretions.
- If you think that you could have HIV, never let your blood, semen, or vaginal fluid enter another person's body.

Teach patients to recognize the symptoms of AIDS
- Unexplained fatigue.
- Weight loss of 10 to 15 pounds in less than 2 months, but without dieting.
- Unexplained fever, chills, and sweating at night for more than 2 weeks.
- Unexplained swollen glands for more than 1 month.
- Unexplained diarrhea or bloody stools for more than 2 weeks.
- Unexplained persistent dry cough, shortness of breath, or difficulty in breathing.
- White patches on the tongue or mouth that cannot be scraped off.

Explain to patients that these symptoms could also be signs of other diseases. However, if they have any of these symptoms, they should consider having an HIV test. The earlier the infection is detected, the earlier treatment can begin that may delay the onset of other symptoms.

MEDICAL Practice and the LAW

There are three behaviors that are very important in protecting yourself from a lawsuit.
1. Establish a rapport. If patients believe that you truly care about them and have their best interests at heart, they rarely sue, even if you make a mistake.
2. Follow all procedures according to your procedures manual. If you do everything right and the patient has an adverse outcome, you will not likely be found liable.
3. Document everything you do objectively. Lawsuits often come to court years after the incident, and nobody's memory is as good as written documentation. Document only facts, not your opinion. Be sure to document the patient's reaction to treatments.

Ethics and Law
Ethics is the highest standard of behavior and is loosely based on the Golden Rule. No law can force you to behave ethically,

but most major professions have a written code of ethics, including the American Association of Medical Assistants (AAMA). Ethics uses words such as *should* and *may*. If you are angry at someone, ethically, you should not yell at him or her. This is not against the law, but it is unethical.

Law is the lowest standard of behavior and is enforced by federal, state, and local law enforcement personnel. Laws use words such as *must* and *shall*. If you are angry at someone, legally, you must not hit him or her. This behavior is illegal, and you could be charged with assault and battery.

Regarding medical asepsis and infection control, you have a duty and a responsibility to protect yourself, your co-workers, and most important, your patients. Follow specific guidelines established by OSHA and the CDC to prevent the transmission of pathogens.

What Would You DO?
What Would You *Not* DO? RESPONSES

Case Study 1

What Did Jennifer Do?

❑ Told Petra that the hand sanitizers (alcohol-based hand rubs) are as good, if not better, than soap and water for removing germs from the hands.

❑ Explained to Petra that an amount of gel equal to the size of a dime should be rubbed on her hands until the gel dries. Told her that she did not need to rinse her hands afterward.

❑ Stressed to Petra that hand sanitizers are not designed to remove soil from the hands and that she should wash her hands with soap and water when they are visibly soiled.

❑ Explained that the Centers for Disease Control and Prevention now recommends that hand sanitizers be used in health care settings to help prevent the spread of disease.

What Did Jennifer Not Do?

❑ Did not tell Petra that she should switch from soap and water to hand sanitizers.

What Would You Do/What Would You *Not* Do? Review Jennifer's response and place a checkmark next to the information you included in your response. List additional information you included in your response.

_____

_____

_____

_____

Case Study 2

What Did Jennifer Do?

❑ Explained to Tracy that a federal agency known as the Occupational Safety and Health Administration (OSHA) requires gloves be worn when drawing a patient's blood in the office. Told her that the office could be fined if they were not worn.

❑ Told Tracy that having her baby immunized for hepatitis B is an investment in her baby's future. Explained that her child could come into contact with the virus anytime in its life. Stressed that if a young child becomes infected with hepatitis B, the child has a higher risk of developing chronic hepatitis, which can cause serious liver problems later in life.

❑ Gave Tracy a brochure on hepatitis B to take home.

What Did Jennifer Not Do?

❑ Did not ask Tracy if she had been tested to make sure she didn't have any diseases.

What Would You Do/What Would You *Not* Do? Review Jennifer's response and place a checkmark next to the information you included in your response. List additional information you included in your response.

_____

_____

_____

_____

Case Study 3

What Did Jennifer Do?

❑ Explained to Giles that the blood supply was not tested for hepatitis C until 1992, because a test to detect the presence of hepatitis C was not developed until then.

❑ Told Giles that it is possible for someone to have hepatitis C and not exhibit any symptoms.

❑ Told Giles that he should ask the physician his question about giving hepatitis C to others.

What Did Jennifer Not Do?

❑ Did not automatically assume that Giles had hepatitis C since he had not yet been seen by the physician. It would be up to the physician to make a diagnosis of hepatitis C.

❑ Did not tell Giles about the serious complications of hepatitis C. If Giles is diagnosed with hepatitis C, it would be the physician's responsibility to relay this information.

What Would You Do/What Would You *Not* Do? Review Jennifer's response and place a checkmark next to the information you included in your response. List additional information you included in your response.

_____

_____

_____

_____

Apply Your KNOWLEDGE

Choose the best answer to each of the following questions.

1. Jennifer Hawk, CMA, arrives at the medical office and checks to make sure everything is ready to start the day. Jennifer notices that the liquid soap dispenser next to the sink is half empty. Jennifer realizes that she must:
   A. Fill the soap dispenser to the top
   B. Wait until the soap dispenser is empty before taking any action
   C. Dump out the remaining soap and refill the dispenser
   D. Throw away the soap dispenser in the regular trash

2. Jennifer is washing her hands after using the restroom. Jennifer performs all of the following during the handwashing procedure EXCEPT:
   A. Uses hot water to wash her hands
   B. Holds her hands lower than her elbows
   C. Rubs her hands together vigorously as she washes them
   D. Dries her hands thoroughly with paper towels

3. Jennifer notices that the back of her right hand is becoming a little irritated. What would be the best action for Jennifer to take?
   A. Not wash her hands until the irritation has healed
   B. Use only an alcohol-based hand rub until her hand has healed
   C. Apply hand lotion after washing her hands
   D. Wear mittens when performing procedures

4. As Jennifer is pulling on latex gloves, she notices a small tear in the glove of her left hand. Jennifer takes the following action:
   A. Ignores the tear since it's just a small one
   B. Puts on a second pair of gloves over the first pair
   C. Applies an alcohol-based hand rub to the gloves
   D. Takes off the left glove and puts on another one

5. Jennifer has just removed sutures from a patient's lower leg. She removes her gloves and sees that her hands look clean. Jennifer now performs the following:
   A. Applies an alcohol-based hand rub
   B. Washes her hands with an antimicrobial soap
   C. Rinses her hands with a dilute bleach solution
   D. Charts the procedure in the patient's record

6. Jennifer is getting ready to eat lunch in the office break room. Before eating, Jennifer should:
   A. Apply an alcohol-based hand rub
   B. Wash her hands with soap and water
   C. Put on gloves
   D. Call the nearest pizza parlor

7. Clara Mills has come to the office for a hepatitis B vaccine. Jennifer Hawk administers the first dose of the hepatitis B vaccine to Clara. Which of the following statements would NOT be accurate to tell Clara about the hepatitis B vaccine?
   A. You will need a second dose of this vaccine 1 month from now
   B. You will need a third dose of this vaccine 6 months from now
   C. You may experience some soreness at the injection site for a few days
   D. This vaccine will also protect you against hepatitis C

8. Jennifer has just drawn a blood specimen from a patient, and some blood gets on her glove as she is removing the needle from the patient's arm. Jennifer removes her gloves and discards them in:
   A. A waste container lined with a biohazard bag
   B. A biohazard sharps container
   C. A waste container lined with a regular trash bag
   D. The recycling bin

9. The medical office is having a meeting to review and update the OSHA exposure control plan. Which of the following statements indicates that this employee does not fully understand the OSHA Bloodborne Pathogens Standard?
   A. "A new type of safety syringe is available, and I think we should consider using it"
   B. "We need to put a biohazard label on the new refrigerator we just got for storing blood tubes"
   C. "We have never had a sharps injury, so we don't need to use safer medical devices"
   D. "We need to replace our sharps containers when they are three-quarters full"

10. Jennifer is preparing regulated medical waste for disposal. Jennifer performs all of the following **EXCEPT:**
    A. Places biohazard bags and sharps containers in a cardboard box
    B. Makes sure there is a biohazard warning label on two opposite sides of the box
    C. Seals the cardboard box securely with tape
    D. Places the cardboard box outside for pickup with the regular trash

CERTIFICATIONREVIEW

☐ **Microorganisms** are tiny living plants or animals that cannot be seen with the naked eye; examples include bacteria, viruses, protozoa, fungi, and animal parasites. Microorganisms that do not cause disease are nonpathogens. Microorganisms that are harmful to the body and can cause disease are pathogens.

☐ **Medical asepsis** refers to practices that are employed to reduce the number and hinder the transmission of pathogenic microorganisms. Nonpathogens will still be present, but all the pathogens will have been removed.

☐ **Microorganisms** that use inorganic substances as a source of food are autotrophs; those that use organic substances for food are heterotrophs. Aerobes are microorganisms that need oxygen to grow and multiply, and anaerobes are microorganisms that grow best in the absence of oxygen.

☐ **The body has protective mechanisms** to help prevent the invasion of pathogens, which include the following: the skin and mucous membranes, mucus and cilia in the nose and respiratory tract, coughing and sneezing, tears and sweat, urine and vaginal secretions, and hydrochloric acid secreted by the stomach.

☐ **Hand hygiene** refers to the process of cleaning or sanitizing the hands and is the most important medical aseptic practice for preventing the spread of infection. Handwashing refers to washing the hands with a detergent soap; antiseptic handwashing means washing the hands with an antimicrobial soap. The CDC now recommends that an alcohol-based hand rub be used to sanitize the hands when they are not visibly soiled.

☐ **Resident flora,** also known as normal flora, normally reside and grow in the epidermis and dermis. Resident flora are generally harmless and nonpathogenic. Transient flora live and grow on the superficial skin layers and are picked up in the course of daily activities. Transient flora are often pathogenic but can be removed easily by handwashing or applying an alcohol-based hand rub.

☐ **OSHA** was established by the federal government to assist employers in providing a safe and healthy working environment for their employees. The OSHA standard must be followed by any employee with occupational exposure, regardless of the place of employment.

☐ **Occupational exposure** is defined as reasonably anticipated skin, eye, mucous membrane, or parenteral contact with bloodborne pathogens or other potentially infectious materials that may result from the performance of an employee's duties. Bloodborne pathogens are pathogenic microorganisms in human blood that can cause disease in humans. An exposure incident is a specific eye, mouth, other mucous membrane, nonintact skin, or parenteral contact with blood or other potentially infectious materials that results from an employee's duties.

☐ **The OSHA standard** requires that the medical office develop a written exposure control plan designed to eliminate or minimize employees' exposure to bloodborne pathogens and other potentially infectious materials. The ECP must be reviewed and updated annually to ensure that it remains current with the latest information that eliminates or reduces exposure to bloodborne pathogens.

☐ **Engineering controls** include all measures that isolate or remove health hazards from the workplace; examples include safer medical devices and biohazard containers. A safer medical device is a device that, based on reasonable judgment, will make an exposure incident involving a contaminated sharp less likely (e.g., sharps with engineered sharps injury protection and needleless systems).

☐ **Work practice controls** reduce the likelihood of exposure by altering the manner in which a technique is performed and include such practices as bandaging cuts before gloving, sanitizing hands as soon as possible after removing gloves, immediately placing contaminated sharps in a biohazard sharps container, and not eating, drinking, or smoking in areas where you may be exposed to blood or other potentially infectious materials. If exposed to blood or OPIMs, perform first aid measures immediately and then report the incident to the physician so that PEP can be instituted.

☐ **Personal protective equipment** is clothing or equipment that protects an individual from contact with blood or other potentially infectious materials; examples include gloves, face shields, masks, protective eyewear, laboratory coats, and gowns. The type of protective equipment appropriate for a given task depends on the degree of exposure that is anticipated.

☐ **Regulated medical waste (RMW)** is waste that may pose a substantial threat to health and safety if exposed to the public. Regulated medical waste must be properly handled and contained in the medical office so as not to become a source of transfer of disease. Regulated medical waste must be disposed of in accordance with all applicable state laws.

☐ **The biggest threats to health care workers** from occupational exposure are hepatitis B, hepatitis C, and HIV. Hepatitis is an infection of the liver. The most common means of transmission of hepatitis in the health care setting are blood and blood products through needlesticks and cuts with contaminated sharps.

☐ **AIDS** is a disorder of the immune system that eventually destroys the body's ability to fight infection. AIDS is characterized by the presence of severe and life-threatening opportunistic infections and unusual cancers. AIDS is caused by HIV, which is transmitted through contaminated body fluids, particularly blood and semen.

Terminology Review

Aerobe A microorganism that needs oxygen in order to live and grow.

Anaerobe A microorganism that grows best in the absence of oxygen.

Antiseptic An agent that inhibits the growth of or kills microorganisms.

Asepsis Free from infection or pathogens; the actions practiced to make and maintain an area object free from infection or pathogens.

Cilia Slender, hairlike projections.

Contaminate To soil or to make impure. An aseptic object is contaminated when it touches something that is not clean.

Decontamination The use of physical or chemical means to remove, inactivate, or destroy bloodborne pathogens on a surface or item to the point where they are no longer capable of transmitting infectious particles; the surface or item is rendered safe for handling, use, or disposal.

Hand hygiene The process of cleansing or sanitizing the hands.

Infection The condition in which the body, or part of it, is invaded by a pathogen.

Medical asepsis Practices that are employed to reduce the number and hinder the transmission of pathogens.

Microorganism A microscopic plant or animal.

Nonintact skin Skin that has a break in the surface. It includes, but is not limited to, abrasions, cuts, hangnails, paper cuts, and burns.

Nonpathogen A microorganism that does not normally produce disease.

Opportunistic infection An infection that results from a defective immune system that cannot defend the body from pathogens normally found in the environment.

Optimum growth temperature The temperature at which an organism grows best.

Parenteral Taken into the body through the piercing of the skin barrier or mucous membranes, such as through needlesticks, human bites, cuts, and abrasions.

Pathogen A disease-producing microorganism.

Perinatal Relating to the period shortly before and after birth.

pH The degree to which a solution is acidic or basic.

Post-exposure prophylaxis (PEP) Treatment administered to an individual after exposure to an infectious disease to prevent the disease.

Regulated medical waste Medical waste that poses a threat to health and safety.

Reservoir host The organism that becomes infected by a pathogen and also serves as a source of transfer of the pathogen to others.

Resident flora Harmless, nonpathogenic microorganisms that normally reside on the skin and usually do not cause disease. Also known as normal flora.

Susceptible Easily affected; lacking resistance.

Transient flora Microorganisms that reside on the superficial skin layers and are picked up in the course of daily activities. They are often pathogenic but can be removed easily from the skin by sanitizing the hands.

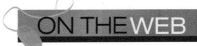

ON THE WEB

For active weblinks to each website visit http://evolve. elsevier.com/Bonewit/.

For Information on Federal Regulations and Recommendations for Infection Control:

Occupational Safety and Health Administration (OSHA)

Centers for Disease Control and Prevention (CDC)

National Institute for Occupational Safety and Health (NIOSH)

Food and Drug Administration (FDA)

Environmental Protection Agency

Association for the Advancement of Medical Instrumentation (AAMI)

Division of Healthcare Quality Promotion (DHQP)

Epidemiology Program Office

Morbidity and Mortality Weekly Report

For Information on Hepatitis:

CDC National Center for Infectious Diseases

Hepatitis Foundation International

HealthTalk

For Information on AIDS:

CDC National Center for HIV, STD, and TB Prevention

AIDS Education Global Information System

AIDS Research Information Center

AIDS Information

The Body—AIDS and HIV Information Resource

Project Inform—HIV Treatment Information

HIV Positive.Com

Learning Objectives	Procedures

Hazard Communication Standard

1. Explain the purpose of the Hazard Communication Standard.
2. List and describe the information that must be included on the label of a hazardous chemical.
3. List and describe the information that must be included in a material safety data sheet (MSDS).

Read and interpret an MSDS.

Sanitization

1. State the purpose of sanitization.
2. State the advantages of using an ultrasonic cleaner to clean instruments.
3. List and describe the guidelines that should be followed when sanitizing instruments.

Sanitize instruments.

Disinfection

1. State the use of the three levels of disinfection: high, intermediate, and low.
2. Explain the differences among the following: critical item, semicritical item, and noncritical item.
3. List and describe the guidelines for disinfecting articles.
4. List and describe the primary use of disinfectants in the medical office.

Chemically disinfect articles.

Sterilization

1. Explain how the autoclave functions to sterilize articles.
2. List the components of a sterilization monitoring program.
3. List and describe types of sterilization indicators.
4. Identify the advantages and disadvantages of the following types of wraps: sterilization paper, sterilization pouches, muslin.
5. List the guidelines that should be followed when the autoclave is loaded.
6. Identify the sterilization times for each of the following categories: unwrapped articles, wrapped articles, liquids, large wrapped packs.
7. Describe the method for storing wrapped articles.
8. Describe the daily, weekly, and monthly maintenance of the autoclave.

Wrap articles to be autoclaved.
Sterilize articles in the autoclave.
Maintain the autoclave.

Other Sterilization Methods

State the primary use of the following types of sterilization methods: dry heat, ethylene oxide gas, chemicals, and radiation.

CHAPTER 3

Sterilization and Disinfection

Chapter Outline

INTRODUCTION TO STERILIZATION AND DISINFECTION
Definition of Terms
Hazard Communication Standard
Hazard Communication Program
Inventory of Hazardous Chemicals
Labeling of Hazardous Chemicals
Material Safety Data Sheets
Employee Information and Training
Sanitization
Sanitizing Instruments
Guidelines for Sanitizing Instruments
Disinfection
Levels of Disinfection
Types of Disinfectants
Guidelines for Disinfection
Sterilization
Sterilization Methods
Autoclave
Other Sterilization Methods

National Competencies

Clinical Competencies
Fundamental Procedures
- Wrap items for autoclaving.
- Perform sterilization techniques.

antiseptic (an-tih-SEP-tik)
autoclave (AU-toe-klave)
contaminate (kon-TAM-in-ate)
critical item
decontamination (DEE-kon-tam-in-AY-shun)
detergent
disinfectant (dis-in-FEK-tant)
incubate (IN-kyoo-bate)
load
material safety data sheet (MSDS)
noncritical item
sanitization (san-ih-tih-ZAY-shun)
semicritical item
spore
sterilization (stare-ill-ih-ZAY-shun)
thermolabile (ther-moe-LAH-bul)

Introduction to Sterilization and Disinfection

The air and all objects around us contain microorganisms. The medical assistant is responsible for helping to reduce and eliminate microorganisms to prevent the spread of disease. This can be accomplished by practicing good techniques of medical and surgical asepsis (refer to Chapters 2 and 10).

Physical and chemical agents are used to destroy microorganisms in the medical office. The agent selected depends on the intended use of the article. For example, articles that penetrate sterile tissue or the vascular system, such as surgical instruments, must be sterilized. Articles that come in contact with the skin should be disinfected, for example, stethoscopes, blood pressure cuffs, and percussion hammers.

Sanitization, disinfection, and sterilization involve hazardous chemicals. Therefore it is essential for the medical assistant to be knowledgeable in the precautions that are required when working with hazardous chemicals.

Definition of Terms

Terms that aid in understanding this chapter are listed and defined here.

Sanitization	Sanitization is a process that removes organic material and lowers the number of microorganisms to a safe level as determined by public health requirements. Sanitization removes all organic material such as blood, body fluids, and tissue from an article. For articles that are used in examinations, treatments, and office surgery to be properly sterilized or disinfected, they must first be sanitized.
Decontamination	The use of physical or chemical means to remove or destroy blood-borne pathogens on an item so that it is no longer capable of transmitting disease; this makes the item safe to handle.
Detergent	A detergent is an agent that cleanses by emulsifying dirt and oil.
Disinfectant	A disinfectant is an agent used to destroy pathogenic microorganisms; however, it does not necessarily kill the resistant bacterial spores. Disinfectants are generally applied to inanimate objects.
Spore	A spore is a hard, thick-walled capsule that some bacteria form by losing moisture and condensing their contents to contain only the essential parts of the protoplasm of the cell. Spores represent a resting and protective stage of the bacterial cell and are more resistant to drying, sunlight, heat, and disinfectants

Sterilization

than is the vegetative form of the bacterium. Favorable conditions cause the spore to germinate into a vegetative bacterium again, capable of reproducing. Two examples of species of bacteria that form spores are *Clostridium botulinum,* which causes botulism, and *Clostridium tetani,* which causes tetanus. Sterilization is the process of destroying all forms of microbial life. An object that is *sterile* is free of all living microorganisms and spores. There can be no relative degrees of sterility—an object is either sterile or not sterile. The device most commonly used to sterilize articles in the medical office is the autoclave.

Hazard Communication Standard

The Hazard Communication Standard (HCS) is a requirement of the Occupational Safety and Health Administration (OSHA). The purpose of the Hazard Communication Standard is to ensure that employees are informed of the hazards associated with chemicals in their workplaces. Chemicals can be in the form of a liquid, solid, or gas. A *hazardous chemical* is any chemical that presents a threat to the health and safety of an individual coming into contact with it. Examples of hazardous chemicals are those that are corrosive, toxic, irritating, carcinogenic, flammable, or reactive.

The Hazard Communication Standard is based on the concept that employees have a right to know about the hazardous chemicals in their workplace, as well as the precautions to take to protect themselves when working with hazardous chemicals. In the medical office, sanitization, disinfection, and sterilization procedures involve the use of hazardous chemicals; therefore the medical assistant must have a thorough knowledge of the Hazard Communication Standard.

The Hazard Communication Standard consists of the following components:
- Development of a hazard communication program
- Inventory of hazardous chemicals
- Labeling requirements
- Material safety data sheet requirements
- Employee information and training

Each of these areas is discussed next.

Hazard Communication Program

As part of the Hazard Communication Standard, employers are required to develop a hazard communication program (HCP). The hazard communication program consists of a written plan that describes what the facility is doing to meet the requirements of the Hazard Communication Standard. The information in the plan must be made available and communicated to all employees who work with hazardous chemicals.

Inventory of Hazardous Chemicals

The employer must develop and maintain a list of hazardous chemicals that are used and stored in the workplace. The list must include the name of the chemical, the name of the manufacturer, the hazardous ingredients, and the health and safety ratings of the chemical. The list must be updated as new chemicals are introduced into the workplace. In the medical office, hazardous chemicals often include the following:
- Chemicals used in the back office (e.g., laboratory reagents)
- Products used for sanitization, disinfection, and sterilization (e.g., chemical disinfectants, autoclave cleaner)
- Pharmaceutical products such as local anesthetics (e.g., Xylocaine)
- Front office products (e.g., toner for copying machine)
- Cleaning products (e.g., drain cleaner)

Labeling of Hazardous Chemicals

The Hazard Communication Standard requires that each container of a hazardous chemical be labeled by the manufacturer with a warning to alert the user that the chemical is dangerous (Figure 3-1). The label must include the possible hazards of the chemical and the steps that can be taken to protect against those risks. The hazard warnings can use words, pictures, or symbols to provide the user with an understanding of the physical and health hazards of the chemical. If a label falls off of a product or is damaged, a replacement label must be applied. If a chemical is transferred to a new container, a label with all the required information must be attached to the new container.

Container Label Requirements

The Hazard Communication Standard requires that manufacturers label the containers of hazardous chemicals they produce with specific information. This information allows the user of the chemical to tell at a glance the hazards of using the chemical and the basic steps to take to protect oneself. The information required by the Hazard Communication Standard includes the following:
1. **Name of the chemical.** The name of the chemical must be clearly indicated on the label.
2. **Manufacturer information.** The name, address, and emergency phone number of the company that manufactures the chemical must be stated on the label.
3. **Physical hazards of the chemical.** Examples of physical hazards that must be stated include the potential of the chemical to catch fire, explode, or react with other chemicals or materials.
4. **Health hazards of the chemical.** Examples of health hazards include the potential of the chemical to produce irritation to tissue, cancer, a sensitivity reaction, or a toxic or corrosive reaction.
5. **Safety precautions.** The protective clothing, equipment, and procedures that are recommended when working with the chemical must be stated on the label.

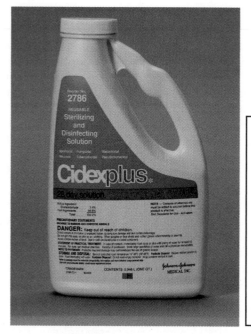

A

B

PRECAUTIONARY STATEMENTS
HAZARDS TO HUMANS AND DOMESTIC ANIMALS
DANGER: Keep out of reach of children.
Direct contact is corrosive to exposed tissue, causing eye damage and skin irritation/damage. Do not get into eyes, on skin or on clothing. Wear goggles or face shield and rubber gloves when handling or pouring. Avoid contamination of food. Use in well ventilated area in closed containers.
STATEMENT OF PRACTICAL TREATMENT: In case of contact, immediately flush eyes or skin with plenty of water for at least 15 minutes. For eyes, get medical attention. Harmful if swallowed. Drink large quantities of water and call a physician immediately.
NOTE TO PHYSICIAN: Probable mucosal damage may contraindicate the use of gastric lavage.
STORAGE AND DISPOSAL: Store at controlled room temperature 15°-30°C (59°-86°F).
Pesticide disposal: Discard residual solution in drain. Flush thoroughly with water.
Container disposal: Do not reuse empty container. Wrap container and put in trash.
Refer to package insert for material compatibility information and more detailed usage/product data.
Use with polycarbonate plastic could cause equipment failure.

*TRADEMARK   CONTENTS: 0.946 L (ONE QT.)
2786 C2-1   830006

Figure 3-1. A, Hazardous chemical container label. **B,** The label must indicate the possible hazards of the chemical.

> **What Would You DO?**
> **What Would You Not DO?**
>
> **Case Study 1**
> Elba Cordera has brought her daughter Maria in for a well-baby visit. Maria is 9 months old and is just starting to crawl. Mrs. Cordera is taking precautions to baby-proof her house to protect Maria from accidents. Mrs. Cordera wants to know how to tell if a cleaning product is poisonous. She also wants to know what she should do if Maria gets into a cleaning product and spills it on herself or swallows it.

6. **Storing and handling the chemical.** Information on how the chemical should be stored and handled must be stated on the label.

Material Safety Data Sheets

A **material safety data sheet (MSDS)** provides more detailed information than the container label regarding the chemical, its hazards, and measures to take to prevent injury and illness when handling the chemical (Figure 3-2). The Hazard Communication Standard requires that a current MSDS be kept on file for each hazardous chemical used or stored in the workplace. MSDSs must be readily accessible to employees and provided to them on request. It is important that the medical assistant review the MSDS before working with a hazardous chemical.

Companies that manufacture and distribute hazardous chemicals must provide an MSDS with every product. A hazardous chemical should never be used unless an MSDS is available. In the event of an accidental exposure, information on the MSDS must be readily available as a reference for emergency treatment. If an MSDS is missing, the supplier or the manufacturer of that chemical should be contacted for a replacement.

An MSDS does not have to be kept on file for a hazardous chemical that is used in the workplace in the same way that a household consumer would use it. For example, correction fluids, such as Wite-Out and Liquid Paper, contain a hazardous chemical. However, if the medical assistant uses it in the same way that a household consumer would use it (i.e., to correct errors on a document), an MSDS does not need to be kept on file. On the other hand, if household bleach (sodium hypochlorite) is used to decontaminate blood spills in the medical office, an MSDS would need to be kept on file because the bleach is not being used in the same way that a household consumer would use it.

Material Safety Data Sheet Requirements

The Hazard Communication Standard requires that manufacturers of hazardous chemicals include the following information on MSDSs (see Figure 3-2):

1. **Identification.** This section provides information used to identify the chemical and must include both the chemical's scientific name and its common name (trade name, brand name, generic name); the name, address, and emergency phone number of the manufacturer; and the date the MSDS was prepared.

2. **Composition of ingredients.** This section provides a list of the ingredients in the hazardous chemical and exposure limits of the chemical.

MATERIAL SAFETY DATA SHEET (MSDS)	
Date of Issue: 4/28/02	Date of Revision: 8/8/03

SECTION 1   IDENTIFICATION

CHEMICAL NAME: Glutaraldehyde	INFORMATION TELEPHONE NUMBER: 1 (800) 733-8690
TRADE NAME: Aldecide	EMERGENCY TELEPHONE NUMBER:
MANUFACTURER'S NAME: Brennan Corporation	1 (800) 331-0766
MFG. ADDRESS: P.O. Box 93	
CITY: Camden STATE: NJ ZIP: 08106	

SECTION 2   COMPOSITION OF INGREDIENTS

CAS NUMBER	CHEMICAL NAME OF INGREDIENTS	PERCENT	PEL	TLV
111-30-8	Glutaraldehyde	2.5	0.2 ppm	0.2 ppm
7732-18-5	Water	97.4	None	None
7632-00-0	Sodium Nitrite	<1	None	None

SECTION 3   PHYSICAL AND CHEMICAL PROPERTIES

BOILING POINT: 212° F	SPECIFIC GRAVITY (H_2O = 1): 1.004
VAPOR PRESSURE (mm Hg): 0.20 at 20° C	VAPOR DENSITY (AIR = 1): 1.1
ODOR: Sharp odor	pH: 7.5-8.5
SOLUBILITY IN WATER: Complete (100%)	MELTING POINT: n/a
APPEARANCE: Bluish-green liquid	FREEZING POINT: 32° F
EVAPORATION RATE: 0.98 (Water = 1)	ODOR THRESHOLD: 0.04 ppm

SECTION 4   FIRE AND EXPLOSION HAZARD DATA

FLASH POINT: Not flammable (aqueous solution)		
FLAMMABILITY LIMITS:	LEL: n/a	UEL: n/a
EXTINGUISHING MEDIA: n/a (aqueous solution)		
SPECIAL FIRE FIGHTING PROCEDURES: n/a		
UNUSUAL FIRE/EXPL HAZARDS: None		

SECTION 5   REACTIVITY DATA

STABILITY: Stable
CONDITIONS TO AVOID: Avoid temperatures above 200° F.
INCOMPATIBILITY (MATERIAL TO AVOID): Acids and alkalines will neutralize active ingredient.
HAZARDOUS DECOMPOSITION BYPRODUCTS: None
HAZARDOUS POLYMERIZATION: Will not occur

Figure 3-2. Material safety data sheet (MSDS).   *Continued*

3. **Physical and chemical properties.** Physical and chemical properties of the chemical must be listed in this section, such as:
   - Appearance and odor
   - Boiling point
   - Vapor pressure
   - Solubility in water
   - Evaporation rate
   - Specific gravity
   - Vapor density
   - pH level
   - Melting point
   - Freezing point
   - Odor threshold

MATERIAL SAFETY DATA SHEET

PAGE 2

SECTION 6 HEALTH HAZARD DATA

ROUTE OF ENTRY: SKIN: yes **EYES:** yes **INHALATION:** yes **INGESTION:** yes

SIGNS AND SYMPTOMS OF OVEREXPOSURE:

SKIN: Moderate irritation. May aggravate existing dermatitis.

EYES: Serious eye irritant. May cause irreversible damage.

INHALATION: Vapors may be irritating and cause stinging sensations in the eyes, nose, and throat.

INGESTION: May cause irritation or chemical burns of the mouth, throat, esophagus, and stomach. May cause vomiting, diarrhea, dizziness, faintness, and general systemic illness.

CARCINOGENICITY DATA: **NTP:** No **AIRC:** No **OSHA:** No

SECTION 7 EMERGENCY FIRST AID PROCEDURES

SKIN: Wash skin with soap and water for 15 minutes. If irritation persists, seek medical attention.

EYES: Immediately flush with water for 15 minutes. Seek medical attention.

INHALATION: Remove to fresh air. If irritation persists, seek medical attention.

INGESTION: Do not induce vomiting. Give large amounts of water. Seek medical attention.

SECTION 8 PRECAUTIONS FOR SAFE HANDLING AND USE

SPILL PROCEDURES: Ventilate area, wear protective gloves and eye gear. Wipe with sponge, mop, or towel. Flush with large quantities of water. Collect liquid and discard it.

WASTE DISPOSAL METHOD: Container must be triple rinsed and disposed of in accordance with federal, state, and/or local regulations. Used solution should be flushed thoroughly with water into sewage disposal system in accordance with federal, state, and/or local regulations.

PRECAUTIONS IN HANDLING AND STORAGE: Store in a cool, dry place (59-86° F) away from direct sunlight or sources of intense heat. Keep container tightly closed when not in use.

SECTION 9 CONTROL MEASURES

VENTILATION: Adequate ventilation to maintain recommended exposed limit.

RESPIRATORY PROTECTION: None normally required for routine use.

SKIN PROTECTION: Wear protective gloves. Butyl rubber, nitrile rubber, polyethylene, or double-gloved latex.

EYE PROTECTION: Safety goggles or safety glasses

WORK/HYGIENE PRACTICES: Prompt rinsing of hands after contact. Handle in accordance with good personal hygiene and safety practices. These practices include avoiding unnecessary exposure.

Figure 3-2, cont'd. Material safety data sheet (MSDS).

4. **Fire and explosion data.** Some hazardous chemicals may cause a fire or explosion if used improperly. This section indicates under what circumstances this may occur and what to do if it does occur.

5. **Reactivity data.** Some chemicals react when combined with other chemicals or materials. The reactivity data list the substances and conditions that the chemical should be kept away from to prevent a dangerous reaction. This information helps in determining where and how to store the chemical.

6. **Health hazard data.** This section is one of the most important areas for health care workers. This section includes the following information:
   - Route of entry (e.g., inhalation, ingestion, skin contact, eye contact)
   - Signs and symptoms of overexposure (e.g., burning eyes, nausea, dizziness, difficulty in breathing)
   - Medical conditions that are aggravated by exposure to the chemical (e.g., asthma, dermatitis).
   - Acute and chronic health hazards that could result from overexposure (e.g., skin irritation, eye damage, lung damage).

This section also indicates if the hazardous chemical has been identified as a potential carcinogen by the National Toxicology Program (NTP), the International Agency for Research on Cancer (IARC), or OSHA

7. **Emergency first aid procedures.** This section identifies the first-aid measures to take if exposed to the chemical (e.g., in case of eye contact, immediately flush eyes with water for 15 minutes).

8. **Precautions for safe handling and use.** This section tells what to do for a spill or leak, the method of disposal of the chemical, and how to handle and store the chemical.

9. **Control measures.** This section lists the engineering controls, work practice controls, and personal protective equipment that should be used to protect oneself from the hazardous chemical. Examples of these measures include using gloves and eye protection and working in a well-ventilated area.

Employee Information and Training

The Hazard Communication Standard requires that employees be provided with information and training regarding hazardous chemicals in the workplace. The training session must be offered at the time of an employee's initial assignment to a work area where hazardous chemicals are present and whenever a new chemical hazard is introduced into the work area. The training program must be an ongoing activity, and each training session must be documented.

The Hazard Communication Standard requires that the following information be relayed to employees who work with hazardous chemicals:

1. The requirements making up the Hazard Communication Standard
2. Physical and health hazards associated with exposure to chemicals in the workplace
3. Measures the employees can take to protect themselves from injury or illness from hazardous chemicals
4. Emergency procedures to take in the event of exposure to a hazardous chemical or a chemical spill
5. The meaning of the information on container labels and how to use that information
6. The meaning of the information on MSDSs and how to use that information
7. The location of the following: hazard communication program plan, list of hazardous chemicals in the workplace, and MSDS for each chemical in the workplace

Sanitization

Sanitization involves a series of steps designed to remove organic material from an article and to lower the number of microorganisms on the article to a safe level (Procedure 3-1). Organic material on an article may result in incomplete sterilization or disinfection. This is because the organic material acts as a physical barrier preventing

the physical or chemical agent from reaching the surface of the article to kill microorganisms.

Sanitizing Instruments

The most frequent items sanitized in the medical office are medical and surgical instruments. Therefore this section focuses on the theory and procedure for sanitizing instruments.

The general steps in the sanitization procedure of instruments are as follows:

1. *Rinse* the instruments to prevent organic material from drying on the instruments.
2. *Decontaminate* the instruments with a chemical disinfectant to remove pathogenic microorganisms.
3. *Clean* the instruments to remove all organic matter.
4. *Thoroughly rinse* the instruments to remove all detergent residue.
5. *Dry* the instruments to prevent stains on the instruments.
6. *Check the instruments* for defects and working condition.
7. *Lubricate* hinged instruments to make the instruments function well and last longer.

Cleaning Instruments

Two methods can be used to perform the cleaning step (step 3 in the preceding list) of the sanitization procedure: the manual method and the ultrasound method.

Manual Method

The manual method is used most often in the medical office. It involves the manual cleaning of instruments using a cleaning solution and a brush. Manual cleaning is recommended for delicate instruments because vibrations that occur with the ultrasound method may damage these instruments.

Ultrasound Method

The ultrasound method uses a machine known as an ultrasonic cleaner (Figure 3-3). The ultrasound method offers a safety advantage in that instruments do not have to be handled during the cleaning process. This decreases the incidence of an accidental puncture or cut from a sharp instrument. An ultrasonic cleaner works by converting sound waves into mechanical energy, which creates small bubbles all over the instruments. When the bubbles burst, vibrations occur that loosen and remove debris from the instruments. Ultrasonic cleaners are especially good at removing debris from hard to reach areas such as box locks of hemostats and screw locks of scissors.

Before the instruments are placed in the ultrasonic cleaner, they should be separated according to the type of metal (e.g., stainless steel, aluminum, brass). Instruments made of dissimilar metals should not be cleaned together in the ultrasonic cleaner. When different metals are in close contact, the ions from one metal can flow to another. This may result in a permanent blue-black stain on an instrument, which can be removed only by having the instrument refinished.

Guidelines for Sanitizing Instruments

The following guidelines should be followed when sanitizing surgical instruments:

1. **Wear gloves during the sanitization process.** Following the OSHA Bloodborne Pathogens Standard, the medical assistant should wear disposable gloves during the entire sanitization procedure. This protects the medical assistant from bloodborne pathogens and other potentially infectious materials. The medical assistant should be especially careful when working with hazardous chemicals and when handling sharp instruments. Heavy-duty utility gloves should be worn over the disposable gloves to provide protection from the irritating effects of chemical agents and accidental punctures or cuts from sharp instruments.

2. **Handle instruments carefully.** Instruments are expensive and delicate, yet durable. They are able to last for many years if handled and maintained properly. Dropping an instrument on the floor or throwing an instrument into a basin may damage it. Instruments should never be piled in a heap, because they will become entangled and may be damaged when separated. Keep sharp instruments separate from the rest of the instruments to prevent damaging or dulling the cutting edge. Also, keep delicate instruments separate to protect them from damage.

3. **Follow instructions on labels of chemical agents.** Before using a chemical agent such as a chemical disinfectant, an instrument cleaner, or an autoclave cleaner, review the product's MSDS and carefully read the label on the container. Check the label to determine the use, mixing, and storage of the chemical agent. Read and observe precautions listed on the label regarding personal safety, such as the use of gloves and eye protection. Also, check the expiration date on the label of the chemical agent. Chemicals have a tendency to lose their potency over time and should not be used past the expiration date.

4. **Use a proper cleaning agent.** A low-sudsing detergent with a neutral pH should be used to clean the instruments. Commercially available instrument cleaners meet these criteria (Figure 3-4). These cleaners usually

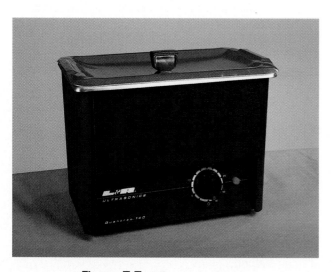

Figure 3-3. Ultrasonic cleaner.

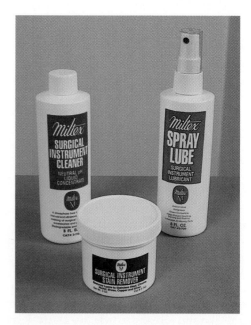

Figure 3-4. Commercially available surgical instrument cleaners. *Left,* Instrument cleaner; *center,* stain remover; *right,* spray lubricant.

come in a concentrated liquid or powder form and must be diluted with water before use. Never substitute any other type of detergent such as dishwasher detergent or laundry detergent; these detergents may not have the proper pH for sanitizing instruments. If a detergent with an alkaline pH is used and not completely rinsed off, it could leave a residue on the instrument. This could result in an orange-brown stain on the instrument that resembles rust. Using an acid detergent can also cause staining and permanent corrosion.

5. **Use proper cleaning devices.** Proper cleaning devices should be used for the manual cleaning of instruments. A stiff nylon brush should be used to clean the surface of the instrument. A stainless-steel wire brush can be used to clean grooves, crevices, or serrations. A stain on an instrument can often be removed using a commercial instrument stain remover (see Figure 3-4). Never use steel wool or other abrasives to remove stains, because damage could occur to the instrument.

6. **Carefully inspect each instrument for defects and proper working condition.** After cleaning and drying the instrument, it is important to check it for defects and proper working condition as follows:
   a. The blades of an instrument should be straight and not bent.

b. The tips of an instrument should approximate tightly and evenly when the instrument is closed.
c. An instrument with a box lock (e.g., hemostatic forceps, needle holders) should move freely but must not be too loose. The pin that holds the box lock together should be flush against the instrument.
d. An instrument with a spring handle (e.g., thumb and tissue forceps) should have sufficient tension to grasp objects tightly.
e. The cutting edge of a sharp instrument should be smooth and devoid of nicks.
f. Scissors should cut cleanly and smoothly. To test for this, the medical assistant should cut into a thin piece of gauze. If they cut all the way to the end of the blade without catching on the gauze, the scissors are in proper working condition.

7. **Lubricate hinged instruments.** Lubricate box locks, screw locks, scissor blades, and any other moving part of each instrument. Use a lubricant that can be penetrated by steam, such as a commercial spray lubricant or a lubricant bath (see Figure 3-4). Be sure to lubricate after performing the final rinse; otherwise the lubricant will be rinsed off the instrument. Never use industrial oils or silicon sprays. These substances are not steam penetrable and can build up on the instrument, affecting its working condition.

Text continued on p. 97

PROCEDURE 3-1

PROCEDURE 3-1   Sanitization of Instruments

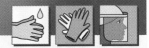

Outcome Sanitize instruments.

Equipment/Supplies:
- Sink
- Disposable gloves
- Heavy-duty utility gloves
- Contaminated instruments
- EPA-approved chemical disinfectant and MSDS
- Disinfectant container
- Cleaning solution and MSDS

- Basin
- Stiff nylon brush
- Stainless-steel wire brush
- Paper towels
- Cloth towel
- Instrument lubricant

1. **Procedural Step.** Review the MSDS for the hazardous chemicals you will be using in the sanitization process.
   Principle. The MSDS provides information regarding the chemical, its hazards, and measures to take to prevent injury and illness when handling the disinfectant.

2. **Procedural Step.** Apply gloves. Transport the contaminated instruments to the cleaning area as soon as possible after use. The instruments should be carried in a covered basin from the examining room to the cleaning area.
   Principle. Disposable gloves act as a barrier to protect the medical assistant from infectious materials. Transporting contaminated instruments in a covered basin promotes infection control.

Continued

PROCEDURE 3-1 Sanitization of Instruments—Cont'd

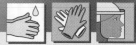

3. **Procedural Step.** Apply heavy-duty utility gloves over the disposable gloves.
   Principle. Utility gloves help protect the hands from the irritating effects of chemical solutions.

4. **Procedural Step.** Separate sharp instruments and delicate instruments from other instruments.
   Principle. Separating sharp instruments from others prevents damage to or dulling of the cutting edge of these instruments. Delicate instruments should be separated to protect them from damage.

5. **Procedural Step.** Immediately rinse the instruments thoroughly under warm, not hot (approximately 110° F [44° C]), running water to remove organic material such as blood, body fluids, tissue, and other debris.
   Principle. Rinsing the instruments as soon as possible prevents organic material from drying on the instruments, making it difficult to remove later. Hot water may cause coagulation of organic material, making it more difficult to remove.

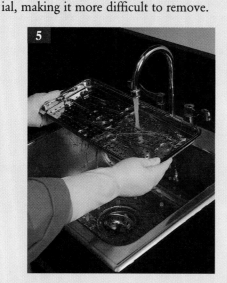

6. **Procedural Step.** Decontaminate the instruments by disinfecting them in an EPA-approved chemical disinfectant as follows:
   a. Select the proper chemical disinfectant and check the expiration date on the container label.
   b. Observe all personal safety precautions listed on the label of the disinfectant (e.g., wearing safety goggles).
   c. Follow the manufacturer's directions on the label for proper mixing and use of the disinfectant.
   d. Immerse the articles in the chemical disinfectant. Make sure the articles are completely submerged in the disinfectant.
   e. Cover the container that holds the chemical disinfectant.
   f. Disinfect the articles for 10 minutes.

Principle. Decontaminating the instruments removes pathogenic microorganisms from them, making them safe to handle. A disinfectant past its expiration date loses its potency and should not be used. An EPA-approved disinfectant has been determined by the EPA (U.S. Environmental Protection Agency) to be effective when used as directed, without causing an unreasonable risk to the public or the environment. The container must be kept covered to prevent the escape of toxic fumes and to prevent evaporation of the disinfectant, which could change its potency.

7. **Procedural Step.** Clean the instruments. The instruments can be cleaned using the manual method or the ultrasound method as follows:

Manual Method for Cleaning Instruments
   a. Obtain the instrument cleaning solution and check its expiration date.
   b. Observe all personal safety precautions listed on the label of the cleaning agent.
   c. Follow the directions on the manufacturer's label for proper mixing and use of the cleaning agent. The detergent may need to be diluted with water.
   d. Remove the articles from the chemical disinfectant and place them in the basin containing the cleaning solution.
   e. Use a stiff nylon brush to clean the surface of each instrument. Be sure to thoroughly scrub all parts of the instrument. Brush delicate instruments carefully to prevent damaging them.

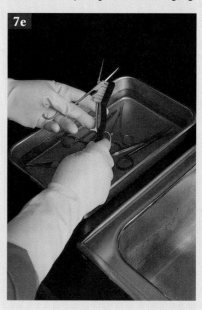

f. Use a stainless-steel wire brush to clean grooves, crevices, or serrations where contaminants such as blood and tissue may collect.

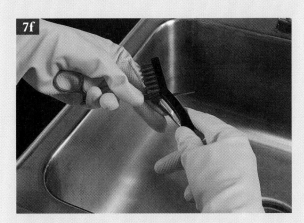

g. If there is a stain on the instrument, attempt to remove it using a damp cloth or sponge to which a commercial stain remover has been applied.

h. Scrub each instrument until it is visibly clean and free from organic material and stains.

i. After cleaning the instruments, dispose of the cleaning solution according to the manufacturer's instructions. It should never be reused.

Principle. A cleaning agent past its expiration date loses its potency and should not be used. Taking appropriate precautions with cleaning agents prevents harm to the medical assistant from hazardous chemicals. All organic material must be removed from the instruments to ensure complete sterilization in the autoclave. Proper disposal of the cleaning solution prevents harm to the environment.

Ultrasound Method for Cleaning Instruments

a. Using a cleaning agent recommended by the manufacturer, prepare the cleaning solution in the ultrasonic cleaner. Make sure to observe all personal safety precautions listed on the label.

b. Remove the articles from the chemical disinfectant and separate instruments made of dissimilar metals such as stainless steel, aluminum, and bronze.

c. Place the instruments in the ultrasonic cleaner with hinged instruments in an open position.

d. Make sure sharp instruments do not touch other instruments.

e. Make sure all instruments are fully submerged in the cleaning solution.

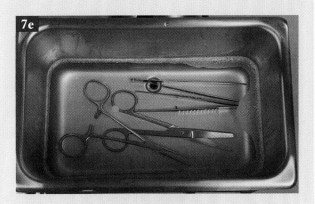

f. Place the lid on the ultrasonic cleaner.

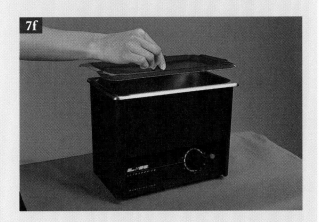

g. Turn on the ultrasonic cleaner and clean the instruments for the length of time recommended by the manufacturer.

h. After completion of the cleaning cycle, remove the instruments from the machine.

i. Change the cleaning solution in the ultrasonic cleaner according to the manufacturer's recommendations.

Principle. Mixing dissimilar metals together could result in permanent stains on the instruments. Instruments must be completely submerged with hinged instruments in an open position so that the solution can reach all parts of the instrument. Taking appropriate precautions with chemical agents prevents harm to the medical assistant from hazardous chemicals.

8. **Procedural Step.** Rinse each instrument thoroughly with warm, not hot (110° F [44° C]), water for at least 20 to 30 seconds to remove all traces of the detergent. Open and close hinged instruments

Continued

PROCEDURE 3-1 Sanitization of Instruments—Cont'd

while rinsing to make sure the solution is completely rinsed out of every part of the instrument.
Principle. Detergent residue left on the instrument could cause stains, which could build up and interfere with the proper functioning of the instrument. Using warm water helps to remove the cleaning solution and facilitates the drying process.

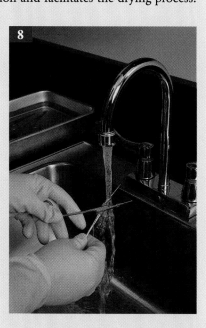

9. **Procedural Step.** Dry each instrument with a paper towel and place the instrument on a cloth towel for additional air drying.
Principle. If the instrument is not completely dry, stains may occur on the instrument.

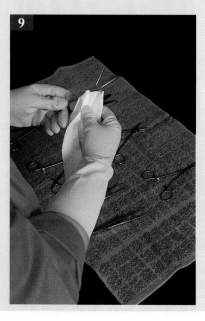

10. **Procedural Step.** Check each instrument for defects and proper working condition. Scissors should cut all the way to the end of a thin piece of gauze without catching. If defects are noted or the instrument is not working properly, it must be discarded or sent to the manufacturer for repair.

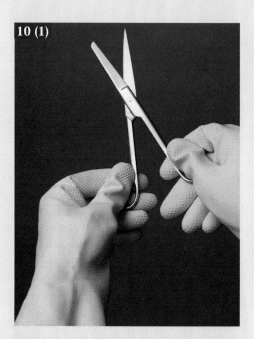

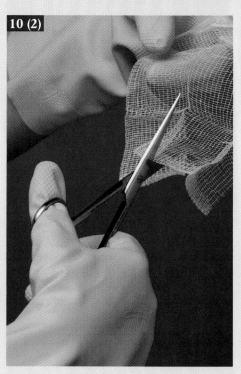

Principle. Instruments that have defects or are not in proper working condition are not safe to use on a patient during a medical or surgical procedure.

11. Procedural Step. Lubricate hinged instruments using a steam-penetrable lubricant as follows:

a. Apply the lubricant to a hinged instrument in its open position.

b. Open and close the instrument after applying the lubricant so that it reaches all parts of the hinged area.

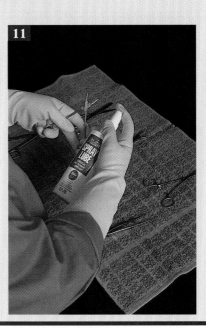

c. Place the instrument back on the towel and allow it to drain. Rinsing and wiping are not necessary.

Principle. Lubricating an instrument makes it function better and last longer.

12. Procedural Step. Remove both sets of gloves and sanitize your hands.

13. Procedural Step. Wrap the instruments and sterilize them in the autoclave according to the medical office policy.

PROCEDURE 3-1

Disinfection

Disinfection is the process of destroying pathogenic microorganisms, but it does not necessarily kill bacterial spores. Disinfection is accomplished in the medical office through the use of liquid chemical agents that are applied to inanimate objects (Procedure 3-2). Chemical disinfection has been discussed with respect to its role in the sanitization process to decontaminate instruments. In this section, chemical disinfection will be discussed in more detail.

Levels of Disinfection

Disinfection can be classified according to three levels of disinfection based on killing action, as follows:

High-Level Disinfection. High-level disinfection is a process that destroys all microorganisms with the exception of bacterial spores. High-level disinfection is used to disinfect semicritical items. A **semicritical item** is an item that comes in contact with nonintact skin or intact mucous membranes such as a flexible fiberoptic sigmoidoscope. A frequently used high-level disinfectant is 2% glutaraldehyde (e.g., Cidex, MetriCide). A newer high-level disinfectant that is growing in popularity is Cidex OPA (ortho-phthalaldehyde). Cidex OPA does not contain glutaraldehyde, which means it is less toxic and safer to handle.

Intermediate-Level Disinfection. Intermediate-level disinfection is a process that inactivates tubercle bacilli (the causative agent of tuberculosis), all vegetative bacteria, most viruses, and most fungi, but does not kill bacterial spores. Intermediate-level disinfection is used to disinfect noncritical items. **Noncritical items** are items that come in contact with intact skin but not mucous membranes; examples include stethoscopes, blood pressure cuffs, tuning

TABLE 3-1	Disinfectants Used in the Medical Office	
Disinfectant	**Common Names**	**Use in the Medical Office**
Glutaraldehyde	Cidex MetriCide ProCide Omnicide Wavicide	Disinfection of flexible fiberoptic sigmoidoscopes
Alcohol	Isopropyl alcohol	Disinfection of stethoscopes, blood pressure cuffs, tuning forks, and percussion hammers; isopropyl alcohol wipes are used to disinfect rubber stoppers of multiple-dose medication vials
Chlorine and chlorine compounds	Sodium hypochlorite (household bleach)	Recommended by OSHA for decontamination of blood spills
Phenolics	Carbolic acid Hydroxybenzene Phenic acid Phenyl hydroxide Phenylic acid	Disinfection of walls, furniture, floors, and laboratory work surfaces
Quaternary ammonium compounds	Benzalkonium chloride	Disinfection of walls, furniture, floors, and laboratory work surfaces

forks, percussion hammers, and crutches. A common intermediate-level disinfectant is isopropyl alcohol.

Low-Level Disinfection. Low-level disinfection is a process that kills most bacteria, some viruses, and some fungi but cannot be relied on to kill resistant microorganisms such as tubercle bacilli nor can it kill bacterial spores. Low-level disinfectants are typically used to disinfect surfaces such as examining tables, laboratory countertops, and walls. Low-level disinfectants used in the medical office include sodium hypochlorite (household bleach) and phenolics.

Types of Disinfectants

The disinfectants used most frequently in the medical office are described next. Table 3-1 provides a list of these disinfectants, along with common names and uses for each.

Glutaraldehyde

Glutaraldehyde is often used as a high-level disinfectant in the medical office. It has a rapid killing action and is not inactivated by the presence of organic material. Because it does not corrode lenses, metal, or rubber, it is the agent of choice for semicritical items that cannot be exposed to heat, such as flexible fiberoptic sigmoidoscopes. Brand names for glutaraldehyde include Cidex and MetriCide.

Glutaraldehyde is highly toxic and can cause harm to the body if not handled properly. When working with glutaraldehyde, the medical assistant must make sure to work in an area that is well-ventilated. Utility gloves and safety goggles must also be worn to protect oneself from the irritating effects of this chemical (Figure 3-5). If the hands or

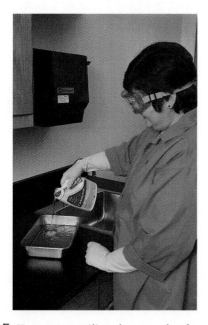

Figure 3-5. Kara wears utility gloves and safety goggles to protect herself from the irritating effects of glutaraldehyde.

any other part of the body comes in contact with glutaraldehyde, the area should be rinsed thoroughly under running water.

Alcohol

Alcohol is frequently used as a disinfectant in the medical office. The two most common types are *ethyl alcohol* and *isopropyl alcohol*. The disinfecting action of alcohol is increased by the presence of water; therefore a 70% solution

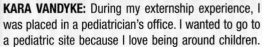

MEMORIES From EXTERNSHIP

KARA VANDYKE: During my externship experience, I was placed in a pediatrician's office. I wanted to go to a pediatric site because I love being around children. One day I was in the examining room with my patient, a 4-year-old boy who was there with his mother. It was standard procedure at this office to take every patient's temperature. I started getting out our electronic thermometer to take his temperature when I noticed he looked a little frightened. He was looking at the thermometer funny, and then he said, "Can you do it in my ear?" I said I was sorry but we didn't have that kind of thermometer. I told him I could do it under his arm or under his tongue. His mom looked at him, and he said, "But I want it in my ear." He finally agreed to let me do it under his arm. When I was finished taking his temperature, he smiled and said, "You're the nicest doctor!"

of alcohol is recommended. Stronger concentrations (95% to 100%) are not as effective. A disadvantage of alcohol is that it tends to dissolve the cement from around the lenses of instruments.

Ethyl alcohol and isopropyl alcohol provide intermediate- to low-level disinfection and can be used to disinfect stethoscopes, blood pressure cuffs, and percussion hammers. Isopropyl alcohol wipes are used to disinfect small surfaces such as the diaphragm of a stethoscope and rubber stoppers on multiple-dose medication vials.

Chlorine and Chlorine Compounds

Chlorine and chlorine compounds are some of the oldest and most used disinfectants. Their most important use is in the chlorination of water.

In the medical office, chlorine is used in the form of hypochlorites, such as liquid sodium hypochlorite (household bleach). A 10% solution of household bleach in water will inactivate tuberculosis bacteria, hepatitis B and C viruses, human immunodeficiency virus, and many bacteria in 10 minutes at room temperature. Because of this, household bleach is recommended by OSHA for the decontamination of blood spills. A disadvantage of this disinfectant is that it can irritate skin and mucous membranes and is highly corrosive to metal.

Phenolics

Phenolics are used mainly to disinfect walls, furniture, floors, and laboratory work surfaces. This disinfectant is a corrosive poison and tends to be irritating to the eyes and skin. Because of this, eye and skin protective devices should be worn when working with phenolics in the pure form. Many derivatives of phenolics are commonly used and are usually nonirritating, including Lysol and hexachlorophene.

Quaternary Ammonium Compounds

The quaternary ammonium compounds are sometimes used in the medical office for the disinfection of noncritical surfaces such as floors, furniture, and walls.

Guidelines for Disinfection

There are certain guidelines that should be followed when disinfecting articles with a chemical agent. They include:

Sanitize the Articles Before Disinfecting Them. The article to be disinfected must first be thoroughly sanitized. As previously described, sanitization includes the following steps: initial rinse, decontamination with a chemical disinfectant, cleaning, rinsing, drying, and checking for working order. It is important to remove all organic matter from the article before it is disinfected. If organic material is still present on the article after it is sanitized, it will prevent the chemical disinfectant from reaching the surface of the article to kill microorganisms. In addition, with some disinfectants, organic material can absorb the chemical disinfectant and inactivate it. The article should be thoroughly rinsed of the detergent after cleaning because detergent residue may interfere with the disinfecting process. The article must be completely dry before placing it in the disinfectant because water dilutes the chemical and decreases its effectiveness.

Observe Safety Precautions. The medical assistant should carefully read the MSDS and the container label before using a chemical disinfectant. All safety precautions should be followed when using the chemical to protect against illness or injury from a hazardous chemical.

Properly Prepare and Use the Disinfectant. Products vary substantially among manufacturers; therefore it is important that the manufacturer's directions on preparation, dilution, and use of the chemical disinfectant be followed very carefully. The disinfectant should be prepared exactly as indicated on the container label. Some disinfectants are used full strength, whereas others require dilution. Some disinfectants (e.g., glutaraldehyde) require the addition of an activator before they can be used. Preparing the disinfectant properly ensures the destruction of microorganisms. A disinfectant must be applied for a certain length of time in order to kill microorganisms. The medical assistant must be sure to disinfect for the length of time indicated on the container label.

Properly Store the Disinfectant. Chemical disinfectants should be closed tightly and stored properly under the storage conditions recommended by the manufacturer. Chemical disinfectants lose their potency over time; therefore the medical assistant should strictly adhere to the manufacturer's recommendations for the disinfectant's shelf life, use life, and reuse life. Each of these terms is defined next as it relates to chemical disinfectants.

Shelf life	Shelf life is the length of time a chemical disinfectant may be stored before use and still retain its effectiveness. The shelf life is indicated by an expiration date on the container.

The expiration date should always be checked before using the chemical. Outdated disinfectants should not be used.

Use life	Some disinfectants must be combined with another chemical, or *activated,* before they are used. Use life is the period of time a disinfecting solution is effective after it has been activated. For example, Cidex Plus (Johnson & Johnson) is effective for 28 days following activation. At the end of this time, any chemical remaining in the container must be discarded. When a chemical disinfectant is activated, the date on which it will expire should be written on the container.
Reuse life	Reuse life is the period of time that a disinfecting solution being used and reused remains active. For example, Cidex Plus can be reused for 28 days. At the end of this time, the disinfectant must be discarded. The date when the disinfectant should be discarded should be written on an adhesive label and affixed to the container holding the disinfectant.

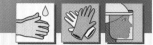

PROCEDURE 3-2   Chemical Disinfection of Articles

Outcome Chemically disinfect articles.

Equipment/Supplies:
- Sink
- Disposable gloves
- Heavy-duty utility gloves
- Contaminated articles

- EPA-approved chemical disinfectant and MSDS
- Disinfectant container
- Paper towels

1. **Procedural Step.** Sanitize the articles by performing procedural steps 1 through 10 in Procedure 3-1.
2. **Procedural Step.** Review the MSDS for the EPA-approved chemical disinfectant that you will be using.
   Principle. The MSDS provides information regarding the chemical disinfectant, its hazards, and measures to take to prevent injury and illness when handling the disinfectant.

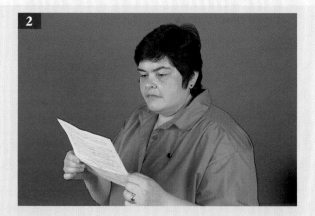

3. **Procedural Step.** Check the expiration date of the chemical disinfectant.
   Principle. A disinfectant past its expiration date loses its potency and should not be used.

(margin tab) PROCEDURE 3-2

4. **Procedural Step.** Observe all personal safety precautions listed on the label. Follow the directions on the manufacturer's label for proper mixing and use of the disinfectant. The disinfectant may need to be diluted with distilled water.
Principle. Taking appropriate precautions with chemical agents prevents harm to the medical assistant from hazardous chemicals.

5. **Procedural Step.** Immerse the articles in the chemical disinfectant. Make sure the articles are completely submerged in the disinfectant.
Principle. The articles must be completely submerged to allow the disinfectant to reach all parts of the instrument.

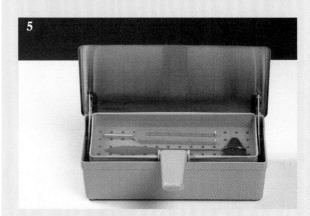

6. **Procedural Step.** Cover the container that holds the chemical disinfectant.
Principle. The container must be kept covered to prevent the escape of toxic fumes and to prevent evaporation of the disinfectant, which could change its potency.

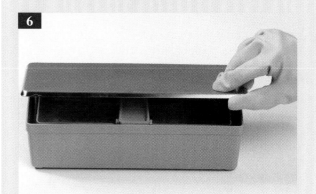

7. **Procedural Step.** Disinfect the articles for the proper length of time as indicated on the label of the container.
Principle. Proper time requirements must be followed to ensure complete destruction of all microorganisms.

8. **Procedural Step.** Remove the articles from the disinfectant and rinse them thoroughly. Dry the articles with paper towels. Dispose of the disinfectant according to the manufacturer's instructions.
Principle. All traces of the chemical disinfectant must be removed to prevent irritation to the patient's tissues. The disinfectant must be disposed of properly to prevent harm to the environment.

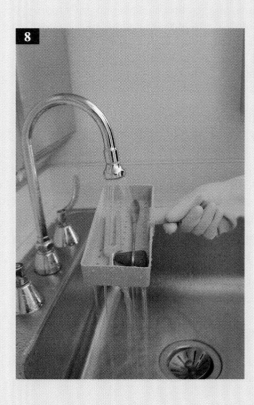

9. **Procedural Step.** Remove both sets of gloves and sanitize your hands.

10. **Procedural Step.** Store the articles according to the medical office policy.

PROCEDURE 3-2

Sterilization

Sterilization is the process of destroying all forms of microbial life, including bacterial spores. An item that is sterile is free of all living microorganisms and spores. Sterilization must be used to process all critical items. A **critical item** is an item that comes in contact with sterile tissue or the vascular system.

As previously described, a semicritical item (one that comes in contact with nonintact skin or with intact mucous membranes) can be chemically disinfected using a high-level disinfectant. However, most offices prefer, instead, to sterilize semicritical items in the autoclave (e.g., nasal specula, vaginal specula). This is because the autoclave provides a convenient, efficient, safe, and inexpensive method for destroying microorganisms. Chemical disinfectants, on the other hand, are not only more expensive to use but are also more hazardous and create problems as to their proper disposal. The exception to this is any semicritical item that is heat-sensitive. For example, flexible fiberoptic sigmoidoscopes would be damaged by the heat of an autoclave and must be chemically disinfected.

Sterilization Methods

Sterilization involves the use of either physical or chemical methods. Each method of sterilization has its advantages and disadvantages. The method used to achieve sterility depends primarily on the nature of the item to be sterilized. The most common physical and chemical sterilization methods include the following:

Physical Methods	**Chemical Methods**
Steam under pressure (autoclave)	Ethylene oxide gas
Hot air (dry heat oven)	Cold sterilization (chemical agents)
Radiation	

The most common method for sterilizing articles in the medical office is steam under pressure using an autoclave. The autoclave is discussed in detail in this chapter, and the other methods of sterilization are briefly described.

Autoclave

The autoclave is dependable, efficient, and economical and can be used to sterilize items that are not harmed by moisture or high temperature. Refer to the box on this page for a list of heat-resistant items that can be sterilized in the autoclave.

An **autoclave** consists of an outer jacket surrounding an inner sterilizing chamber. Under pressure, distilled water is converted to steam, which fills the inner sterilizing chamber. The pressure plays no direct part in killing microorganisms; rather, it functions to attain a higher temperature than could be reached by the steam from boiling water (212° F; 100° C). The cooler, drier air already in the chamber is forced out through the air exhaust valve.

Items Sterilized in the Autoclave	
Surgical instruments	Dressings
Medical instruments	Glassware
Linens	Treatment trays
Liquids	Reusable syringes
Brushes	Utensils

It is important that all the air in the chamber be replaced by steam. When air is present, the temperature in the autoclave is reduced and a temperature that is adequate for sterilization is not reached. When all the air has been removed, the air exhaust valve seals off the inner chamber and the temperature in the autoclave begins to rise.

During the sterilization process, the steam penetrates the materials in the sterilizing chamber. The materials are cooler, so the steam condenses into moisture on them, giving up its heat. This heat serves to kill all microorganisms and their spores.

The autoclave is usually operated at approximately 15 pounds of pressure per square inch (psi) at a temperature of 250° F (121° C). Vegetative forms of most microorganisms are killed in a few minutes at temperatures ranging from 130° to 150° F (54° to 65° C), but certain bacterial spores can withstand a temperature of 240° F (115° C) for more than 3 hours. However, no living organism can survive direct exposure to saturated steam at 250° F (121° C) for 15 minutes or longer.

The sterilization process using the autoclave is discussed in this section (with the exception of sanitization, which was already presented). The sterilization process consists of the following components:

- Monitoring program
- Sanitizing articles
- Wrapping articles
- Operating the autoclave (autoclave cycle)
- Handling and storing packs
- Maintaining the autoclave

Each of these components is discussed next.

Monitoring Program

To ensure that instruments and supplies are sterile when used, the Centers for Disease Control and Prevention (CDC) recommends that the medical office establish and maintain a monitoring program of the sterilization process. The monitoring program should consist of the following:

1. Written policies and procedures for each step of the sterilization process
2. Sterilization indicators to ensure that minimum sterilizing conditions have been achieved

AUTOCLAVE LOG						
Date/Time	Description of the Load	Cycle Time (min)	Temperature (°F)	Indicator (+/−)	Initials	Comments
7/25/05 4:00 PM	Surgical instruments	20	250	—	RR	
7/26/05 3:00 PM	MOS tray setups	30	250	—	RR	

MAINTENANCE: (Indicate date, vendor name, service, etc.)

Figure 3-6. An example of an autoclave log.

3. Records for each cycle maintained in an autoclave log (Figure 3-6)

The information that should be recorded for each autoclave cycle includes the following:

- Date and time of the cycle
- Description of the load
- Exposure time
- Exposure temperature
- Results of the sterilization indicator
- Initials of the operator

Some autoclaves have recorders that automatically print out a portion of this information at the end of the cycle (Figure 3-7).

Sterilization Indicators

Materials that are being sterilized must be exposed to steam at a sufficient temperature and for a proper length of time. Sterilization indicators are available to determine the effectiveness of the procedure and to check against improper wrapping of articles, improper loading of the autoclave, and faulty operation of the autoclave.

An article is not considered sterile unless the steam has penetrated to its center; therefore most sterilization indicators are designed to be placed in the center of the article. The medical assistant should carefully read the instructions that come with the sterilization indicators. The most reliable indicators check for the attainment of

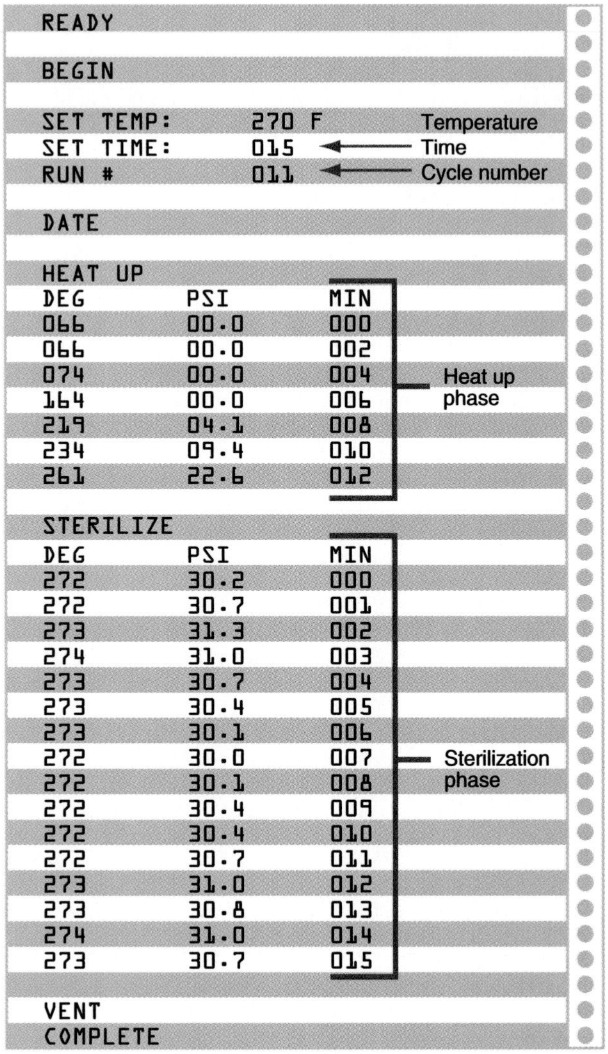

```
READY

BEGIN

SET TEMP:      270 F        Temperature
SET TIME:      015    ←──── Time
RUN #          011    ←──── Cycle number

DATE

HEAT UP
DEG       PSI        MIN
066       00.0       000
066       00.0       002
074       00.0       004       Heat up
164       00.0       006       phase
219       04.1       008
234       09.4       010
261       22.6       012


STERILIZE
DEG       PSI        MIN
272       30.2       000
272       30.7       001
273       31.3       002
274       31.0       003
273       30.7       004
273       30.4       005
273       30.1       006
272       30.0       007  ── Sterilization
272       30.1       008       phase
272       30.4       009
272       30.4       010
272       30.7       011
273       31.0       012
273       30.8       013
274       31.0       014
273       30.7       015


VENT
COMPLETE
```

Figure 3-7. An example of a printout of an autoclave cycle.

the proper temperature and also indicate the duration of the temperature.

If an indicator does not change properly, a defect may be present in the sterilization technique or in the working condition of the autoclave. The manufacturer's guidelines for proper sterilization techniques should be reviewed, and the articles should be resterilized following these guidelines. If the indicator still does not change properly, the autoclave is in need of repair and should not be used until it has been serviced.

Sterilization indicators should be stored in a cool, dry area. Excessive heat or moisture can damage the indicator. The most common sterilization indicators are chemical indicators and biologic indicators, which are described next.

Chemical Indicators

Chemical indicators are impregnated with a **thermolabile** dye that changes color when exposed to the steriliza-

Case Study 3
Cassie Augusta is in the examining room and is being prepared for the removal of a sebaceous cyst. Cassie is very concerned about the instruments that the physician will be using to perform the procedure. She wants to know if they are "safe." Cassie says that her friend Mackenzie got a tattoo several years ago and developed hepatitis 3 weeks later. Mackenzie thinks she got hepatitis from the instruments that were used for her tattoo procedure. Cassie wants to know if it is possible for an instrument to give someone hepatitis. She says she heard that hepatitis can cause liver cancer and wants to know if this is true. Cassie also wants to know if there is a vaccine to prevent hepatitis.

tion process. If the chemical reaction of the indicator does not show the expected results, the item should not be used. Chemical indicators include autoclave tape and sterilization strips.

Autoclave Tape. Autoclave tape contains a chemical that changes color if it has been exposed to steam. The tape is available in a variety of colors, can be written on, and is useful for both closing and identifying the wrapped article (Figure 3-8). Autoclave tape has some limitations as an indicator. Since it is placed on the outside of the pack, it cannot ensure that steam has penetrated to the center of the pack. Nor does it ensure that the item has been sterilized; it merely indicates that an article has been in the autoclave and that a high temperature has been attained.

Sterilization Strips. Sterilization strips are commercially prepared paper or plastic strips that contain a thermolabile dye and that change color when exposed to steam under pressure for a certain length of time (Figure 3-9). Most sterilization strips are designed to change color after being exposed to a temperature of 250° F (121° C) for 15 minutes. The indicator strip should be placed in the center of the wrapped pack with the end containing the dye placed in an area considered to be the hardest for steam to penetrate.

Biologic Indicators

Biologic indicators are the best means available for determining the effectiveness of the sterilization procedure. The CDC recommends that medical office personnel use a biologic indicator to monitor all autoclaves at least once a week.

A biologic indicator is a preparation of living bacterial spores. Biologic indicators are commercially available in the form of dry spore strips in small glassine envelopes. Biologic monitoring of an autoclave requires the use of a

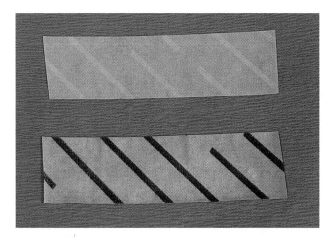

Figure 3-8. Autoclave tape. *Top*, Autoclave tape as it appears before the sterilization process; *bottom:* diagonal lines appear on the tape during autoclaving and indicate that the wrapped article has been autoclaved.

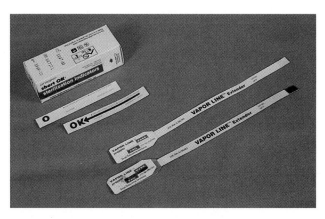

Figure 3-9. Sterilization strips. Sterilization strips contain a thermolabile dye and change color when exposed to steam under pressure for a certain length of time.

preparation of spores of *Bacillus stearothermophilus*, which is a microorganism whose spores are particularly resistant to moist heat.

Each biologic testing unit includes two spore tests that are sterilized and one spore control that is not sterilized (Figure 3-10). The biologic indicator is placed in the center of two wrapped articles. The articles are placed in areas of the autoclave that are the least accessible to steam penetration, such as on the bottom tray of the autoclave, near the front of the autoclave, and in the back of the autoclave.

After the indicators have been exposed to sterilization conditions, they must be processed before the results can be obtained. The two methods for processing results are the in-house method and the mail-in method.

In-house Method. The in-house method involves processing and interpreting the results at the medical office. Following sterilization, the processed spores are incubated for a period of 24 to 48 hours. If sterilization conditions have been met, the color or condition of the processed spores will be different from those of the control. If sterilization conditions have not been met, the processed spores and the unprocessed control will display the same color and condition.

Mail-in Method. With this method, the processed bacterial spores and the (unprocessed) control are mailed to a processing laboratory. The test is performed by the laboratory, and the results are returned to the medical office.

If spores are not killed in routine spore tests, the autoclave should immediately be checked for proper use and function and the spore test repeated. If spore tests

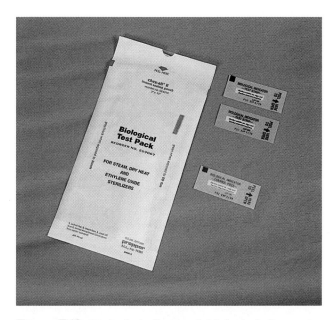

Figure 3-10. Biologic indicator. A biologic indicator includes two spore tests that are sterilized *(top)* and one spore control that is not sterilized *(bottom)*.

remain positive, the autoclave should not be used until it is serviced.

Wrapping Articles

Articles to be sterilized in the autoclave must first be thoroughly sanitized (see Procedure 3-1). Next, the articles are prepared for autoclaving by wrapping them. The purpose of wrapping articles is to protect them from recontamination during handling and storage. Articles that are wrapped and handled correctly will remain sterile after autoclaving until the package seal is broken.

The wrapping material should be made of a substance that is not affected by the sterilization process and should allow steam to penetrate while preventing contaminants such as dust, insects, and microorganisms from entering during handling and storage. It should not tear or puncture easily and should allow the sterilized package to be opened without contamination of the contents. A wrapper should not be used if it is torn or has a hole. Examples of wrapping material used for autoclaving are sterilization paper, sterilization pouches, and muslin.

Sterilization Paper Wrap

Sterilization paper is a disposable and inexpensive wrapping material. It consists of square sheets of paper of different sizes (Figure 3-11). The most common sizes (in inches) are 12×12, 15×15, 18×18, 24×24, 30×30, and 36×36. Articles must be wrapped in such a way that they do not become contaminated when the pack is opened. The proper method for wrapping instruments using sterilization paper is outlined in Procedure 3-3. This method of wrapping can be used for all types of instruments and supplies.

The disadvantage of sterilization paper is that it is difficult to spread open for removal of the contents. It has a "memory" and tends to flip back easily so it may not open flat to provide a sterile field. (*Memory* is the ability of a material to retain a specific shape or configuration.) Because sterilization paper is opaque, it is not possible to view the contents of a pack before opening it.

Sterilization Pouches

Sterilization pouches typically consist of a combination of paper and plastic; paper makes up one side of the pouch, and a plastic film makes up the other side (Figure 3-12). Sterilization pouches are available in different sizes; the most common sizes (in inches) are 3×9, 5×10, and 7×12.

Most pouches have a peel-apart seal on one end that is later used to open the pouch for removal of the sterile item. The other end of the pouch is open and is used to insert the item into the pouch. Once the article has been inserted, this end is sealed with either heat or adhesive tape. The proper method for wrapping an instrument using a pouch is outlined in Procedure 3-4.

Sterilization pouches provide good visibility of the contents on the plastic side. Most manufacturers include a sterilization indicator on the outside of the pouch. After removing a pouch from the autoclave, the medical assistant should check the indicator for proper color change. If the indicator does not change to the appropriate color (specified by the manufacturer), the contents of the pouch must be resterilized.

Muslin

Muslin consists of a reusable woven fabric and is available in different sizes. Muslin is flexible and easy to handle and is considered the most economical sterilization wrap because it can be reused. Because of its durability, muslin is frequently used to wrap large packs such as tray setups for minor office surgery. Muslin is "memory free" so it will lie flat when opened. A pack wrapped in muslin may be opened on a table so that the wrapper becomes a sterile field. The procedure for wrapping an article with muslin is the same as that for sterilization paper (see Procedure 3-3).

Text continued on p. 110

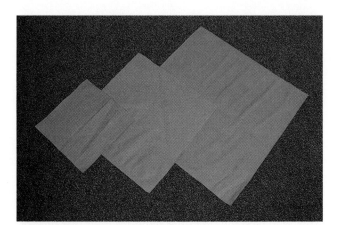

Figure 3-11. Sterilization paper wraps. Sterilization paper consists of square sheets of paper that are available in different sizes.

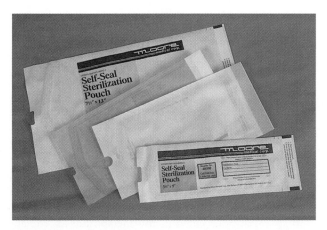

Figure 3-12. Sterilization pouches. Sterilization pouches consist of a combination of paper and plastic and are available in different sizes.

PROCEDURE 3-3   Wrapping Instruments Using Paper or Muslin

Outcome Wrap an instrument for autoclaving.

Equipment/Supplies:
- Sanitized instrument
- Appropriate-sized wrapping material (sterilization paper or muslin)

- Sterilization indicator strip
- Autoclave tape
- Permanent marker

1. **Procedural Step.** Sanitize your hands.
2. **Procedural Step.** Assemble the equipment. Select the appropriate-sized wrapping material for the instrument being wrapped. Check the expiration date on the sterilization indicator box. If the sterilization strips are outdated, do not use them.
   Principle. Instruments are wrapped so that they are protected from recontamination after they have been sterilized. Outdated strip indicators may not provide accurate test results.
3. **Procedural Step.** Place the wrapping material on a clean, flat surface. Turn the wrap in a diagonal position to your body so that it resembles a diamond shape.

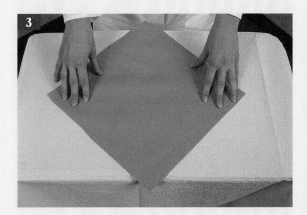

4. **Procedural Step.** Place the instrument in the center of the wrapping material. If the instrument has a movable joint, place it on the wrap in a slightly open position.
   Principle. Instruments with movable joints must be in an open position to allow steam to reach all parts of the instrument. If the instrument is in a closed position, heat exposure could cause the instrument to crack at its weakest part, such as the lock area.

5. **Procedural Step.** Place a sterilization indicator in the center of the pack next to the instrument.
   Principle. Sterilization indicators assess the effectiveness of the sterilization process.

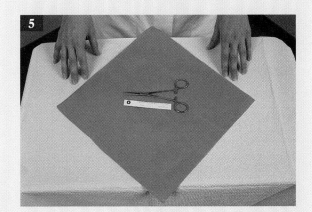

6. **Procedural Step.** Fold the wrapping material up from the bottom and double back a small corner.

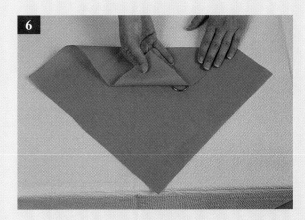

7. **Procedural Step.** Fold over the right edge of the wrapping material and double back the corner.

Continued

PROCEDURE 3-3 Wrapping Instruments Using Paper or Muslin—Cont'd

8. Procedural Step. Fold over the left edge of the wrapping material and double back the corner.

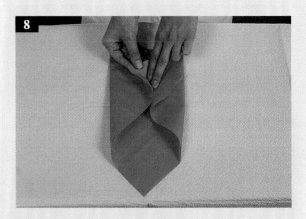

9. Procedural Step. Fold the pack up from the bottom and secure it with autoclave tape. Make sure the pack is firm enough for handling but loose enough to permit proper circulation of steam.
Principle. Instruments must be wrapped properly to permit full penetration of steam and to prevent contaminating them when the wrap is opened. Using autoclave tape will indicate that the pack has been through the autoclave cycle and prevent mixups with packs that have not been processed.

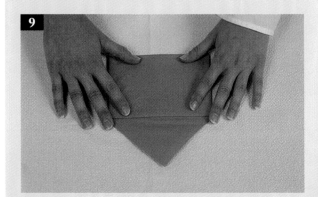

10. Procedural Step. Label the pack according to its contents. Mark the pack with the date of sterilization and your initials.
Principle. Dating the pack ensures that the most recently sterilized packs are stored in back of previously sterilized packs.

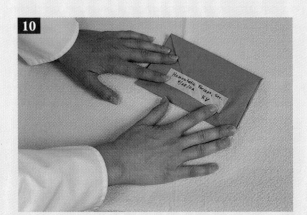

PROCEDURE 3-4   Wrapping Instruments Using a Pouch

Outcome Wrap an instrument for autoclaving.

Equipment/Supplies:
- Sanitized instrument
- Appropriate-sized sterilization pouch
- Permanent marker

1. **Procedural Step.** Sanitize your hands.
2. **Procedural Step.** Assemble the equipment. Select the appropriate-sized sterilization pouch for the instrument being wrapped. For hinged instruments, make sure to use a bag wide enough so the instrument can be placed in a slightly open position inside the bag.
   Principle. Instruments are wrapped so that they are protected from recontamination after they have been sterilized.
3. **Procedural Step.** Place the sterilization pouch on a clean, flat surface.
4. **Procedural Step.** Label the pack according to its contents. Mark the pack with the date of sterilization and your initials.
   Principle. Dating the pack ensures that the most recently sterilized packs are stored in back of previously sterilized packs.

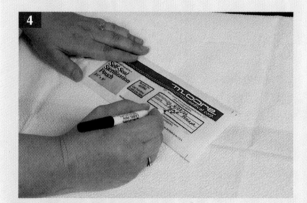

5. **Procedural Step.** Insert the instrument to be sterilized into the unsealed, open end of the pouch.

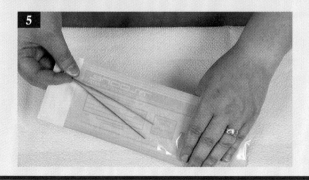

6. **Procedural Step.** Seal the open end of the pouch as follows:
   Adhesive Closure. Peel off the paper strip located above the perforation to expose the adhesive. Fold along the perforation and press firmly to seal the paper to the plastic. Make certain that the seal is secure by running fingers back and forth on both sides of the pouch over the entire sealing area.
   Heat Closure. Seal the pouch using a heat-sealing device.

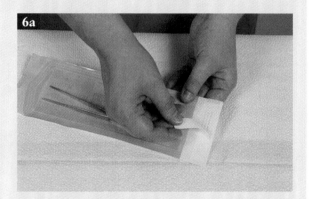

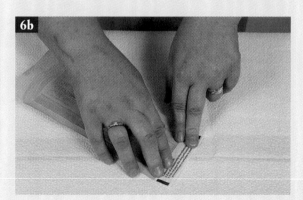

7. **Procedural Step.** Sterilize the pack in the autoclave.

PROCEDURE 3-4

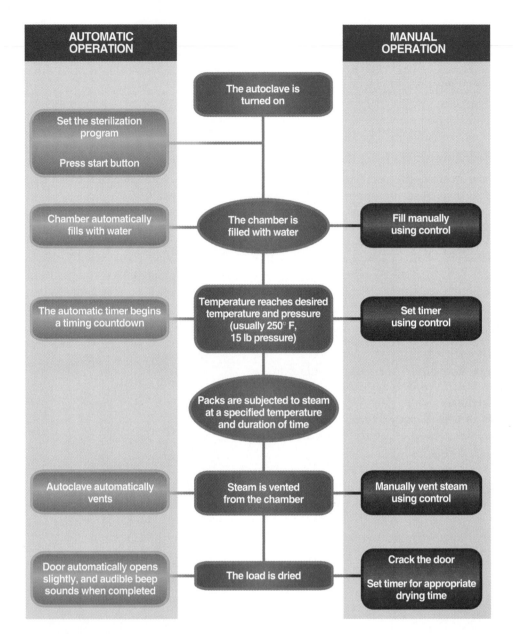

Figure 3-13. The autoclave cycle for manual and automatic operation.

Operating the Autoclave

The autoclave must be operated according to the manufacturer's instructions. The medical assistant should carefully read the operating manual before running the autoclave for the first time. Thereafter, the manual should be kept in an accessible location so that it is available if needed as a reference. Procedure 3-5 outlines a general procedure for sterilizing articles in the autoclave.

The steps involved in achieving sterilization using an autoclave are known as the *autoclave cycle*. Accomplishment of each step varies based on whether the autoclave is operated manually or automatically. Figure 3-13

illustrates the autoclave cycle for both manual and automatic autoclave operation.

Guidelines for Autoclave Operation
General guidelines for operating an autoclave are presented next.

Location of the Autoclave
The autoclave must be placed on a level surface to ensure that the chamber will fill correctly. The front of the autoclave should be near the front of the support surface so water can be easily drained from the drain tube into a container when the autoclave is being flushed out.

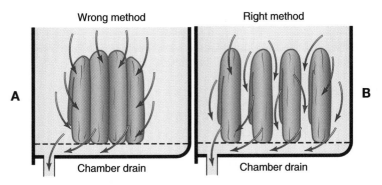

Figure 3-14. Arrangement of packs in the autoclave. **A,** Improper arrangement of packs in the autoclave. A large pack (here consisting of four smaller packs held closely together) prevents adequate penetration of steam, resulting in failure to sterilize the portions in the center of the mass. **B,** The large pack has been broken down into four small packs, and these are slightly separated from each other in the autoclave. Steam will now permeate each pack quickly, and in the much shorter period of exposure needed; there will be no oversterilized outer portions. (Courtesy AMSCO/American Sterilizer Company, Erie, Pa.)

Filling the Water Reservoir

Use distilled water to fill the water reservoir of the autoclave. Normal tap water contains minerals, such as chlorine, which have corrosive effects on the stainless-steel chamber of the autoclave. In addition, using tap water may block the air exhaust valve. This causes air pockets, which prevent the temperature from rising in the autoclave. Fill the water reservoir to the proper level as indicated in the operating manual. An autoclave malfunction may occur if the reservoir is overfilled or if there is not enough water in the reservoir.

Loading the Autoclave

For an item to attain sterility, steam must penetrate every fiber and reach every surface of the item at a required temperature and for a specified period of time. To accomplish this, all packs must be positioned in the chamber to allow free circulation and penetration of steam. These guidelines should be followed when loading the autoclave:

1. Small packs are best, because steam penetrates them more easily; it takes longer for steam to reach the center of a large pack to ensure sterilization. A pack should be no larger than 12×12×20 inches.
2. To allow for proper steam penetration, the packs should be packed as loosely as possible inside the autoclave, with approximately 1 to 3 inches between small packs and 2 to 4 inches between large packs. Packs should not be allowed to touch surrounding walls, and at least 1 inch should separate the autoclave trays. Placing the articles too close together retards the flow of steam (Figure 3-14).
3. Jars and glassware should be placed on their sides in the autoclave with their lids removed. If they are placed upright, air may be trapped in them and they will not be sterilized. Trapped air must flow out and be replaced by steam during the sterilization process (Figure 3-15).

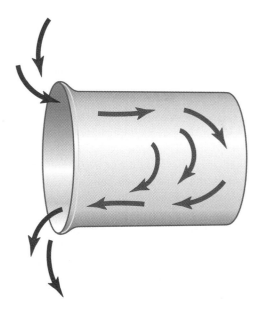

Figure 3-15. Jars and glassware should be placed on their sides in the autoclave with their lids removed. (Courtesy AMSCO/American Sterilizer Company, Erie, Pa.)

4. Packs that contain layers of fabric, such as dressings, should be placed in a vertical position. Because steam flows from top to bottom, this method allows the steam to penetrate the layers of fabric.
5. Sterilization pouches should be positioned on their sides to maximize steam circulation and to facilitate the drying process.

Timing the Load

The autoclave is operated at approximately 15 pounds of pressure per square inch with a temperature of 250° F (121° C). The length of time required for sterilization

TABLE 3-2	Minimum Sterilizing Times	
Items (Manual Operation)*	**Program (Automatic Operation)†**	**Time (min at 250° F or 121° C)**
Unwrapped nonsurgical instruments Open glass or metal canisters Nonsurgical rubber tubing	Unwrapped	15
Wrapped instruments Fabric or muslin Wrapped trays of loose instruments Rubber tubing	Wrapped	20
Minor office surgery tray setup (wrapped)	Packs	30
Liquids or gels	Liquids	30

*Manual operation: The sterilizing time is selected based on the items being sterilized, as indicated in this column. The sterilizing time is set using the manual timing control when the autoclave has reached a temperature of 250° F (121° C).

†Automatic operation: The sterilization program selected from this column is based on the item being autoclaved. The program is selected by pressing the appropriate program button on the front of the autoclave (i.e., unwrapped, wrapped, packs, liquids). The autoclave automatically begins the proper timing countdown when it reaches 250° F (121° C).

varies according to the item that is being sterilized (Table 3-2). For example, steam can easily reach the surfaces of hard, nonporous items such as unwrapped instruments (e.g., vaginal specula) to kill microorganisms; these items require approximately 15 minutes of sterilization time. On the other hand, a large minor office surgery pack requires a longer sterilization time, about 30 minutes, because more time is needed for steam to penetrate to the center of the pack. Rubber goods, however, may be damaged by exposure to excessive heat. To prevent this, the medical assistant should make sure to sterilize rubber items for only the prescribed amount of time.

The sterilizing time should not begin until the desired temperature in the autoclave has been reached. Timing the load is accomplished either automatically or manually. Autoclaves with automatic operation begin timing the load automatically once the desired temperature has been reached. With the manual method of operation, the medical assistant must set the timer by hand using a timing control on the front of the autoclave. The medical assistant should not set the timer until the temperature gauge reaches the desired temperature. The articles in the load are not considered sterile unless they have been subjected to steam for the proper length of time at the proper temperature.

Drying the Load

The sterilized articles are moist and must be allowed to dry before they are removed from the autoclave. This is because microorganisms can move very quickly through the moisture on a wet wrap and onto the sterile article inside, resulting in contamination.

When the load has been subjected to steam for the proper length of time and temperature, the chamber must be vented of steam. Venting the chamber permits the pressure in the autoclave to drop to zero and the chamber to cool, making it safe for the door to be opened. Most autoclaves are designed to vent automatically, which eliminates having to vent them manually.

The door of the autoclave should be opened approximately ½ inch but no more than 1 inch. Opening the door more than 1 inch causes cold air from the outside to rush into the autoclave, resulting in condensation of water on the packs. Cracking the door allows the moisture on the articles to change from a liquid to a vapor and thus to escape through the crack. The residual heat in the inner chamber also helps to dry the articles. The load should be allowed to dry for between 15 and 60 minutes, depending on the type of autoclave and the load. For example, loads that contain large packs require a longer drying time than those with smaller packs. The medical assistant should follow the manufacturer's recommendations for proper drying times of various loads.

Handling and Storing Packs

Sterilized wrapped articles should be handled carefully and as little as possible. If a wrapped article is crushed, compressed, or dropped, the sterility of the contents cannot be assumed and the pack must be resterilized. This is known as *event-related sterility*, meaning that a sterile pack is considered sterile indefinitely unless an event occurs that interferes with the sterility of the article.

Sterilized packs should be stored in clean, dry areas that are free from dust, insects, and other sources of contamination. Wrapped articles should be stored with the most recently sterilized articles placed in the back. The medical assistant should thoroughly check each sterilized pack at least twice: before storing it and before using it. If the pack is torn or opened or if it is wet, it is no longer sterile and must be rewrapped and resterilized.

Maintaining the Autoclave

For the autoclave to work efficiently, it must be maintained properly. The operating manual that accompanies the autoclave provides specific information for the care and maintenance of that type of autoclave.

Safety precautions should be followed when performing maintenance procedures. Before proceeding with preventive maintenance, the autoclave must be cool, the pressure gauge at zero, and the power cord disconnected from the wall socket. Autoclave maintenance is performed on a daily, weekly, and monthly basis as follows:

Daily Maintenance

1. Wipe the outside of the autoclave with a damp cloth and a mild detergent.
2. Wipe the interior of the autoclave and the trays with a damp cloth.
3. Clean the rubber gasket on the door of the autoclave with a damp cloth.
4. Inspect the rubber door gasket for damage that could prevent a good seal.

Weekly Maintenance

1. Wash the inside of the chamber and the trays with a commercial autoclave cleaner according to the manufacturer's instructions, making sure to observe all personal safety precautions. This usually involves the following steps. The water reservoir must first be drained. A soft cloth or a soft brush should be used to clean the chamber, which should be rinsed thoroughly with distilled water. Do not use steel wool or a steel brush or other abrasive agents because they can damage the chamber. The chamber must be dried thoroughly and the door left open overnight.
2. Wash the metal shelves with an autoclave cleaner and rinse them thoroughly with distilled water.

Monthly Maintenance

1. Flush the system to remove any built-up residue, which could cause corrosion of the chamber lines. Carefully follow the manufacturer's directions in the instruction manual to perform this procedure.
2. Check the air trap jet to make sure it is functioning properly. The air trap jet prevents air pockets from occurring in the chamber, to ensure adequate sterilization.
3. Check the safety valve to make sure it is functioning properly. The safety valve releases pressure in the chamber if it gets too high.

Other Sterilization Methods

In addition to the autoclave, other methods can be used to sterilize articles. These methods are not generally used in the medical office and therefore are discussed only briefly in this chapter.

Dry Heat Oven

Dry heat ovens are used to sterilize articles that cannot be penetrated by steam or may be damaged by it. For example, dry heat is less corrosive than moist heat for instruments with sharp edges; it does not dull their sharp edges. Oil, petroleum jelly, and powder cannot be penetrated by steam and must be sterilized in a dry heat oven. Moist heat sterilization tends to erode the ground glass surfaces of reusable syringes, whereas dry heat does not.

Dry heat ovens operate like an ordinary cooking oven. A longer exposure period is needed with dry heat because microorganisms and spores are more resistant to dry heat than to moist heat and also because dry heat penetrates more slowly and unevenly than moist heat. The most commonly used temperature for dry heat sterilization is 320° F (160° C) for a duration of 1 to 2 hours, depending on the article being sterilized. The recommended wrapping material for dry heat sterilization is aluminum foil because it is a good conductor of heat and also protects against recontamination during handling and storage. Dry heat sterilization indicators are available to determine the effectiveness of the sterilization process.

Ethylene Oxide Gas Sterilization

Ethylene oxide is a colorless gas that is both toxic and flammable. It is used to sterilize heat-sensitive items that cannot be sterilized in an autoclave. After items are sterilized with this gas, they must be aerated to remove the toxic residue of the ethylene oxide.

Ethylene oxide sterilization is a more complex and expensive process than steam sterilization. It is frequently used in the medical manufacturing industry for producing prepackaged, presterilized disposable items such as syringes, sutures, catheters, and surgical packs.

Cold Sterilization

Cold sterilization involves the use of a chemical agent for an extended length of time. Only chemicals that are designated *sterilants* by the U.S. Environmental Protection Agency (EPA) can be used for sterilizing articles. If a chemical agent holds this status, the word "sterilant" will be printed on the front of the container.

The item to be sterilized must be completely submerged in the chemical for a long period of time (between 6 and 24 hours depending on the manufacturer's instructions). Prolonged immersion of instruments can damage them. In addition, each time an instrument is added to the instrument container, the clock must be restarted for the entire amount of time. For these reasons, cold sterilization should be used only when steam, gas, or a dry heat oven are not indicated or are unavailable.

Radiation

Radiation uses high-energy ionizing radiation to sterilize articles. Radiation is used by medical manufacturers to sterilize prepackaged surgical equipment and instruments that cannot be sterilized by heat or chemicals.

PROCEDURE 3-5   Sterilizing Articles in the Autoclave

Outcome Sterilize a load of contaminated articles in the autoclave.

Equipment/Supplies:
- Autoclave and instruction manual
- Distilled water
- Wrapped articles
- Heat-resistant gloves

1. **Procedural Step.** Assemble the equipment.
2. **Procedural Step.** Check the level of water in the autoclave and add distilled water, if needed.
   Principle. Water contained in the water reservoir of the autoclave is converted to steam during the sterilization process. Distilled water is used to prevent corrosion of the stainless-steel chamber of the autoclave.

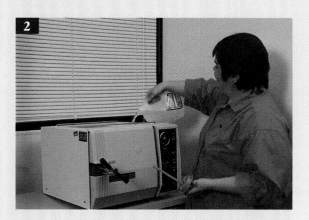

3. **Procedural Step.** Properly load the autoclave following these guidelines:
   a. Do not overload the chamber. Small packs should be placed 1 to 3 inches apart, and large packs should be placed 2 to 4 inches apart. The packs should not touch the chamber walls.
   b. Be sure that at least 1 inch separates the autoclave trays.
   c. Place jars and glassware on their sides.
   d. Place dressings in a vertical position.
   e. When sterilizing dressings and hard goods together, place dressings on the top shelf and hard goods on the lower shelf.
   f. When using sterilization pouches, set the pouches on their sides to maximize steam circulation and to facilitate drying.
   Principle. The autoclave must be loaded properly to ensure adequate steam penetration of all articles.

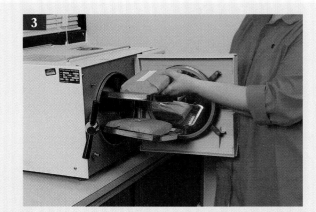

4. **Procedural Step.** Operate the autoclave according to the procedure described in the instruction manual. A general procedure for both the manual and automatic methods of operation follows.

Manually Operated Autoclave
   a. Determine the sterilizing time for the type of articles being autoclaved (see Table 3-2).
   b. Turn on the autoclave.
   c. Fill the chamber with water using the appropriate control.
   d. Securely close and latch the door of the autoclave.
   e. Set the timing control when the temperature gauge reaches the desired temperature (usually 250° F or 121° C). At the end of the steam

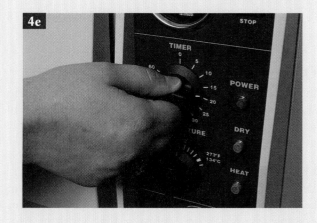

exposure time, an indicator light usually comes on or a beeper sounds.

f. If the autoclave does not vent automatically, use the appropriate control to release steam from the chamber.

g. Dry the load by cracking open the door approximately ½ inch but no more than 1 inch. Set the drying time using the timing control. The drying time will vary between 15 and 60 minutes, depending on the autoclave and the type of load.

Principle. To ensure sterilization, the load should not be timed until the proper temperature has been reached. The sterility of wrapped packs cannot be ensured unless the wrapped articles are allowed to dry fully. Microorganisms can move through the moisture on a wet wrap and contaminate the sterile article inside.

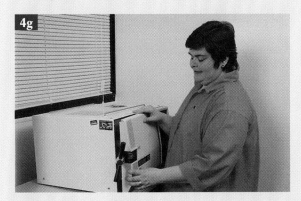

Automatically Operated Autoclave

a. Securely close and latch the door of the autoclave.

b. Turn on the autoclave.

c. Determine the sterilization program according to what is being autoclaved (see Table 3-2). Press the appropriate program button on the front of the autoclave to select the program. Press the start button.

d. Indicators on the front of the autoclave will tell you what is happening (automatically) in the autoclave.

Filling Indicator. Lights up when the chamber is filling with water.

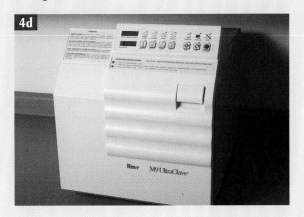

Sterilizing Indicator. Lights up during the heat-up and sterilization phases of the cycle.

Temperature Display. Digital display of the temperature in the autoclave.

Time Display. Digital countdown of the time remaining in the sterilization program.

Drying Indicator. Lights up during the drying phase of the cycle.

Complete or Ready Indicator. Illuminates when the autoclave has completed the cycle and sterilized articles can be removed from the autoclave.

5. Procedural Step. Turn off the autoclave and, wearing heat-resistant gloves, remove the load. Do not touch the inner chamber of the autoclave with your bare hands.

Principle. Heat-resistant gloves protect the medical assistant's hands when the warm packs from the chamber of the autoclave are being removed. The inner chamber of the autoclave is hot and could burn bare skin.

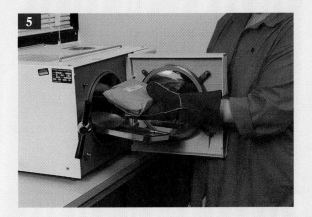

6. Procedural Step. Inspect the packs as you take them out of the autoclave. If the packs show any damage, such as holes or tears, the articles should be rewrapped and resterilized.

Continued

PROCEDURE 3-5

PROCEDURE 3-5   Sterilizing Articles in the Autoclave—Cont'd

7. Procedural Step. Check the sterilization indicators located on the outside of the pack to make sure the proper response has taken place.

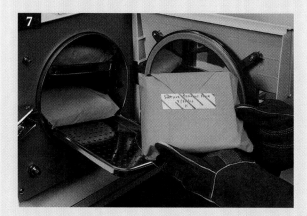

8. Procedural Step. Record monitoring information in the autoclave log. Include the date and time of the cycle, a description of the load, the exposure time and temperature, the results of the sterilization indicator, and your initials.

9. Procedural Step. Store the packs in a clean, dust-proof area with the most recently sterilized packs placed behind previously sterilized packs.

10. Procedural Step. Maintain appropriate daily care of the autoclave, following the manufacturer's recommendations. The daily care of the autoclave includes the following:
  a. Wipe the outside of the autoclave with a damp cloth and a mild detergent.
  b. Wipe the interior of the autoclave and the trays with a damp cloth.
  c. Clean the rubber gasket located on the door of the autoclave with a damp cloth.
  d. Inspect the rubber door gasket for damage that could prevent a good seal.
  Principle. For the autoclave to work efficiently, it must be properly maintained.

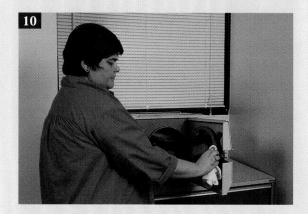

MEDICAL Practice and the LAW

If not performed properly, sterilization and disinfection can adversely affect patients, which can make the medical assistant and other office personnel liable for resultant injuries. Meticulous care must be taken to ensure that all procedures are performed correctly and completely.

Sterilization and disinfection procedures include the use of hazardous chemicals. These chemicals must be stored, used, and disposed of in specific ways mandated by law. The autoclave can be a dangerous machine if it is not used correctly, and it could harm others with hot steam. If you use the autoclave without proper instruction, you could be liable for injuries or accidents resulting from misuse.

Whenever you are dealing with contaminated articles, you have a duty to protect yourself, other employees, patients, and other articles from cross-contamination.

PROCEDURE 3-5

What Would You DO?
What Would You *Not* DO? *RESPONSES*

Case Study 1
What Did Kara Do?
- ❑ Complimented Mrs. Cordera for her concern and efforts to baby-proof her home.
- ❑ Gave Mrs. Cordera a patient information brochure on baby-proofing the home.
- ❑ Told Mrs. Cordera that she should assume that all cleaning products are poisonous. Got out a disinfectant container and showed Mrs. Cordera the information on the label that tells what to do in case of an accidental poisoning.
- ❑ Gave the National Poison Control hotline number (1-800-222-1222) to Mrs. Cordera and told her that was the fastest way to obtain information on what to do in case of an accidental poisoning. Told her to be sure to keep this number by her phone.

What Did Kara Not Do?
- ❑ Did not take Mrs. Cordera's question lightly.

What Would You Do/What Would You *Not* Do? Review Kara's response and place a checkmark next to the information you included in your response. List additional information you included in your response.

_____
_____
_____
_____

Case Study 2
What Did Kara Do?
- ❑ Explained to Mrs. Scout that toys are in the waiting room for children to play with to make their visit more comfortable and less stressful.
- ❑ Reassured Mrs. Scout that the medical office personnal do everything they can to prevent the spread of germs in the office and that the toys are sanitized every day.
- ❑ Relayed to Mrs. Scout that only toys that can be sanitized are kept in the medical office.
- ❑ Told Mrs. Scout that her concern would be brought up at the weekly office meeting.

What Did Kara Not Do?
- ❑ Did not get defensive because Mrs. Scout was just being concerned about her child's health.

What Would You Do/What Would You *Not* Do? Review Kara's response and place a checkmark next to the information you included in your response. List additional information you included in your response.

_____
_____
_____
_____

Case Study 3
What Did Kara Do?
- ❑ Told Cassie that her concern was valid through both verbal and nonverbal behavior.
- ❑ Told Cassie that hepatitis can be transmitted through dirty instruments.
- ❑ Reassured Cassie that all instruments are sterilized in the autoclave, which has special indicators to make sure all germs have been killed.
- ❑ Gave Cassie a patient information brochure on hepatitis. Told her that individuals with chronic hepatitis can develop liver cancer and that the best way to avoid hepatitis is through measures and behaviors recommended for prevention.
- ❑ Told Cassie that a vaccine is available to prevent hepatitis B, but not hepatitis C.

What Did Kara Not Do?
- ❑ Did not dismiss her concern about dirty instruments as unimportant.
- ❑ Did not overly alarm her about the consequences of chronic hepatitis.

What Would You Do/What Would You *Not* Do? Review Kara's response and place a checkmark next to the information you included in your response. List additional information you included in your response.

_____
_____
_____
_____

Apply Your KNOWLEDGE

Choose the best answer to each of the following questions.

1. Kara VanDyke, CMA, is getting ready to sanitize surgical instruments that were used to perform a minor office surgery. Kara performs all of the following steps EXCEPT:
   A. Applies clean disposable gloves
   B. Applies heavy-duty utility gloves
   C. Separates sharp and delicate instruments from other instruments
   D. Rinses the instruments under a stream of hot water

2. Kara next prepares to decontaminate the instruments using Cidex Plus chemical disinfectant. The purpose of decontaminating instruments is to:
   A. Prevent organic material from drying on the instruments
   B. Remove pathogenic microorganisms from the instruments
   C. Remove stains from the instruments
   D. Lubricate the instruments

3. Kara needs to know what personal protective equipment she should use when working with Cidex Plus. Which of the following would provide her with this information?
   A. The MSDS for Cidex Plus
   B. The label on the container of Cidex Plus
   C. Both the MSDS and the container label for Cidex Plus
   D. Her driver's license

4. Kara performs the decontamination process. She performs all of the following steps EXCEPT:
   A. Checks the expiration date on the label of the chemical disinfectant
   B. Completely submerges the instruments in the chemical disinfectant
   C. Scrubs the instruments with a nylon brush
   D. Disinfects the instruments for 10 minutes

5. After the instruments have been decontaminated, Kara prepares to clean them using a commercial instrument cleaner. Kara checks the label of the instrument cleaner to make sure:
   A. It is low sudsing
   B. It has an acidic pH
   C. It destroys bacterial spores
   D. Four out of five dentists recommend this cleaner

6. Kara prepares the cleaning solution and places the instruments in the basin that contains the solution. Which of the following does Kara perform to complete the sanitization procedure?
   A. Cleanses the surface of each instrument with a nylon brush
   B. Rinses each instrument for 20 to 30 seconds
   C. Checks the working order of each instrument
   D. Dries the instruments
   E. All of the above

7. Kara is preparing to autoclave the surgical instruments that she sanitized. She wraps the instruments in sterilization paper before placing them in the autoclave. The purpose of wrapping articles that are to be sterilized is:
   A. To permit better steam penetration during autoclaving
   B. To protect the articles from recontamination after autoclaving
   C. So they can be given as Christmas gifts
   D. To protect the instruments from damage

8. Kara is getting ready to autoclave the wrapped packs of surgical instruments. Which of the following would represent an ERROR in technique during the autoclaving process?
   A. Filling the water reserve with tap water
   B. Loading the autoclave by positioning the packs 1 to 3 inches apart
   C. Setting the timer when the temperature gauge reaches 250° F
   D. Making sure the sterilized packs are dry before removing them from the autoclave

9. When Kara removes a pack from the autoclave, she notices the autoclave tape has changed color. She realizes that this indicates that:
   A. The autoclave is functioning properly
   B. The pack has been exposed to heat
   C. The pack has been exposed to a temperature of 250° F for 15 minutes
   D. The pack needs to be rewrapped and run through the autoclave again

10. Kara properly stores the sterilized packs. Kara performs all of the following steps EXCEPT:
   A. Handles the packs carefully and as little as possible
   B. Rewraps and resterilizes a pack that is torn
   C. Places the packs in a clean, dustproof area
   D. Places the sterilized packs in front of previously sterilized packs

CERTIFICATIONREVIEW

❑ **The Hazard Communication Standard (HCS)** is required by OSHA, and its purpose is to ensure that employees are informed of the hazards associated with chemicals in their workplaces and the precautions to take to protect themselves when working with hazardous chemicals.

❑ **Employers are required** to develop a written hazard communication program describing what their facility is doing to meet the requirements of the Hazard Communication Standard.

❑ **A hazardous chemical** must contain a label that includes the name of the chemical, manufacturer information, physical and health hazards of the chemical, safety precautions, and storing and handling information.

❑ **A material safety data sheet (MSDS)** provides information regarding the chemical, its hazards, and measures to take to prevent injury and illness when handling the chemical. An MSDS must be kept on file for each hazardous chemical used or stored in the workplace.

❑ **The Hazard Communication Standard** requires that employees be provided with information and training regarding hazardous chemicals in the workplace.

❑ **Sanitization** is a process that removes organic material from an article and lowers the number of microorganisms to a safe level. The most frequent items sanitized in the medical office are medical and surgical instruments.

❑ **Instruments can be cleaned** either manually or by using an ultrasonic cleaner. The manual method uses a brush, instrument cleaner, and friction to clean instruments. An ultrasonic cleaner uses a cleaning solution and sound waves to clean the instruments. To prevent the formation of a permanent stain, items made of dissimilar metals should not be cleaned together.

❑ **Disinfection** is the process of destroying pathogenic microorganisms; it does not necessarily kill bacterial spores. Disinfectants consist of chemical agents that are applied to inanimate objects. The disinfectants used most often in the medical office are glutaraldehyde, alcohol, sodium hypochlorite, phenolics, and quaternary ammonium compounds.

❑ **Disinfection can be classified** into the following levels: high, intermediate, and low. High-level disinfection is used to disinfect semicritical items that are heat-sensitive, such as flexible fiberoptic sigmoidoscopes. Intermediate-level disinfection is used for noncritical items such as stethoscopes and blood pressure cuffs. Low-level disinfection is used to disinfect surfaces such as examining tables, countertops, and walls.

❑ **Sterilization** is the process of destroying all forms of microbial life, including bacterial spores. Sterilization must be used for critical items. Critical items are items that come in contact with sterile tissue or the vascular system.

❑ **The autoclave** is used most often in the medical office for sterilization. The autoclave is usually operated at approximately 15 pounds of pressure per square inch at a temperature of 250° F (121° C).

❑ **To ensure that instruments and supplies are sterile** when used, a monitoring program should be established in the medical office. This program should include review of sterilization policies and procedures, checking the use of sterilization indicators, and maintaining records for each autoclave cycle.

❑ **Sterilization indicators** determine the effectiveness of the sterilization process and include chemical indicators and biologic indicators. Chemical indicators use a thermolabile dye that changes color when exposed to the sterilization process. Biologic indicators are the best indicators available and consist of a preparation of heat-resistant bacterial spores.

❑ **The purpose of wrapping articles** for autoclaving is to protect them from recontamination during handling and storage. Examples of wraps commonly used include sterilization paper, sterilization pouches, and muslin.

❑ **The autoclave cycle** refers to the steps involved in achieving sterilization with an autoclave machine. The autoclave must be loaded properly so that steam can easily penetrate the contents of the load. The length of time for sterilization varies according to the item that is being sterilized. The sterilizing time should not begin until the desired temperature in the autoclave has been reached. To prevent recontamination, articles must be completely dry before they are removed from the autoclave. Sterilized wrapped articles should be handled carefully and as little as possible. They should be stored in a clean, dustproof area. A sterile pack is considered sterile indefinitely unless an event occurs that interferes with the sterility of the article. The autoclave should be properly maintained following a daily, weekly, and monthly schedule.

❑ **Other methods that can be used to sterilize articles** include dry heat, ethylene oxide gas, chemical agents, and radiation. Ethylene oxide and radiation are used by the medical manufacturing industry for producing prepackaged and presterilized disposable items.

Terminology Review

Antiseptic A substance that kills disease-producing microorganisms but not their spores. An antiseptic is usually applied to living tissue.

Autoclave An apparatus for the sterilization of materials, using steam under pressure.

Contaminate To soil, stain, or pollute; to make impure.

Critical item An item that comes in contact with sterile tissue or the vascular system.

Decontamination The use of physical or chemical means to remove or destroy bloodborne pathogens on an item so that it is no longer capable of transmitting disease; this makes the item safe to handle.

Detergent An agent that cleanses by emulsifying dirt and oil.

Disinfectant An agent used to destroy pathogenic microorganisms but not necessarily their spores. Disinfectants are usually applied to inanimate objects.

Incubate To provide proper conditions for growth and development.

Load The articles that are being sterilized.

Material safety data sheet (MSDS) A sheet that provides information regarding a chemical, its hazards, and measures to take to prevent injury and illness when handling the chemical.

Noncritical item An item that comes into contact with intact skin but not mucous membranes.

Sanitization A process to remove organic matter from an article and to lower the number of microorganisms to a safe level as determined by public health requirements.

Semicritical item An item that comes into contact with nonintact skin or intact mucous membranes.

Spore A hard, thick-walled capsule formed by some bacteria that contains only the essential parts of the protoplasm of the bacterial cell.

Sterilization The process of destroying all forms of microbial life, including bacterial spores.

Thermolabile Easily affected or changed by heat.

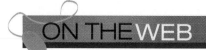

ON THE WEB

For active weblinks to each website visit http://evolve.elsevier.com/Bonewit/.

For Information on Infection Control in the Health Care Setting:

Centers for Disease Control and Prevention

Environmental Protection Agency

National Institute of Environmental Health Sciences

National Institute for Occupational Safety and Health

Office of Public Health and Science

Infection Control Today

Association for Professionals in Infection Control and Epidemiology

To Locate a Material Safety Data Sheet:

MSDS Compliance Solutions

Seton Compliance Resource Center

MSDS-Search

HazCom

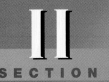

II
SECTION

Basic Clinical Procedures

4 Vital Signs

5 The Physical Examination

Temperature

1. Define a vital sign.
2. Explain the reason for taking vital signs.
3. Explain how body temperature is maintained.
4. List examples of how heat is produced in the body.
5. List examples of how heat is lost from the body.
6. State the normal body temperature range and the average body temperature.
7. List and explain factors that can cause variation in the body temperature.
8. List and describe the three stages of a fever.
9. List the sites for taking body temperature and explain why these sites are used.
10. List and describe the guidelines for using a tympanic membrane thermometer.

Measure oral body temperature.
Measure axillary body temperature.
Measure rectal body temperature.
Measure aural body temperature.

Pulse

1. Explain the mechanism of pulse.
2. List and explain the factors that affect the pulse rate.
3. Identify a specific use of each of the eight pulse sites.
4. State the normal range of pulse rate for each age-group.
5. Explain the difference between pulse rhythm and pulse volume.

Measure radial pulse.
Measure apical pulse.

Respiration

1. Explain the purpose of respiration.
2. State what occurs during inhalation and exhalation.
3. State the normal respiratory rate for each age-group.
4. List and explain the factors that affect the respiratory rate.
5. Explain the difference between the rhythm and depth of respiration.
6. Describe the character of the following abnormal breath sounds: crackles, rhonchi, wheezes, and pleural friction rub.

Measure respiration.

Blood Pressure

1. Define blood pressure.
2. State the normal range of blood pressure for an adult.
3. List and describe factors that affect the blood pressure.
4. Identify the different parts of a stethoscope and a sphygmomanometer.
5. Identify the Korotkoff sounds.
6. Explain how to prevent errors in blood pressure measurement.

Measure blood pressure.
Determine systolic pressure by palpation.

CHAPTER 4

Vital Signs

Chapter Outline

INTRODUCTION TO VITAL SIGNS

Temperature
  Regulation of Body Temperature
  Body Temperature Range
  Assessment of Body Temperature

Pulse
  Mechanism of the Pulse
  Assessment of Pulse

Respiration
  Mechanism of Respiration
  Assessment of Respiration

Blood Pressure
  Mechanism of Blood Pressure
  Assessment of Blood Pressure

National Competencies

Clinical Competencies
Patient Care
- Obtain vital signs.
- Prepare and maintain examination and treatment areas.

General Competencies
Professional Communications
- Recognize and respond to verbal communications.
- Recognize and respond to nonverbal communications.

Patient Instruction
- Provide instruction for health maintenance and disease prevention.

Key Terms

adventitious (ad-ven-TISH-us) sounds
afebrile (uh-FEB-ril)
alveolus (al-VEE-uh-lus)
antecubital (AN-tih-CYOO-bi-tul) space
antipyretic (AN-tih-pye-REH-tik)
aorta (ay-OR-tuh)
apnea (AP-nee-uh)
axilla (aks-ILL-uh)
bounding pulse
bradycardia (BRAY-dee-CAR-dee-uh)
bradypnea (BRAY-dip-NEE-uh)
Celsius (SELL-see-us) scale
conduction (kon-DUK-shun)
convection (kon-VEK-shun)
crisis
cyanosis (sye-an-OH-sus)
diastole (dye-AS-toe-lee)
diastolic (DYE-uh-STOL-ik) pressure
dyspnea (DISP-nee-uh)
dysrhythmia (dis-RITH-mee-uh)
eupnea (YOOP-nee-uh)
exhalation (EKS-hal-AY-shun)
Fahrenheit (FAIR-en-hite) scale
febrile (FEH-bril)
fever
frenulum linguae (FREN-yoo-lum LIN-gway)
hyperpnea (HYE-perp-NEE-uh)
hyperpyrexia (HYE-per-pye-REK-see-uh)
hypertension (HYE-per-TEN-shun)
hyperventilation (HYE-per-ven-til-AY-shun)
hypopnea (hye-POP-nee-uh)
hypotension (HYE-poe-TEN-shun)
hypothermia (HYE-poe-THER-mee-uh)
hypoxia (hye-POKS-ee-uh)
inhalation (IN-hal-AY-shun)
intercostal (IN-ter-KOS-tul)
Korotkoff (kuh-ROT-kof) sounds
malaise (mal-AYZE)
manometer (man-OM-uh-ter)
meniscus (men-IS-kus)
orthopnea (orth-OP-nee-uh)
pulse pressure
pulse rhythm
pulse volume
radiation (RAY-dee-AY-shun)
sphygmomanometer (SFIG-moe-man-OM-uh-ter)
stethoscope (STETH-uh-skope)
systole (SIS-toe-lee)
systolic (sis-TOL-ik) pressure
tachycardia (TAK-ih-KAR-dee-uh)
tachypnea (TAK-ip-NEE-uh)
thready pulse

Introduction to Vital Signs

Vital signs are objective guideposts that provide data to determine a person's state of health. The four vital signs are temperature, pulse, respiration (collectively called TPR), and blood pressure (BP).

The normal ranges of the vital signs are finely adjusted, and any deviation from normal may indicate disease. During the course of an illness, variations in the vital signs may take place. The medical assistant should be alert to any significant changes and report them to the physician because they indicate a change in the patient's condition. When patients visit the medical office, vital signs are routinely checked to establish each patient's usual state of health and establish baseline measurements against which future measurements can be compared. The medical assistant should have a thorough knowledge of the vital signs and attain proficiency in taking them to ensure accurate findings.

General guidelines that the medical assistant should follow when measuring the vital signs are as follows.

1. Be familiar with the normal ranges for all vital signs. Keep in mind that normal ranges vary based on the different age-groups (infant, child, adult, elder).
2. Make sure that all equipment for measuring vital signs is in proper working condition to ensure accurate findings.
3. Eliminate or minimize factors that affect the vital signs, such as exercise, food and beverage consumption, and emotional states.
4. Use an organized approach when measuring the vital signs. The vital signs are usually measured starting with temperature, followed by pulse, respiration, and blood pressure.

Temperature

Regulation of Body Temperature

Body temperature is maintained within a fairly constant range by the hypothalamus, which is located in the brain. The hypothalamus functions as the body's thermostat. It normally allows the body temperature to vary only about 1° to 2° Fahrenheit (F) throughout the day.

Body temperature is maintained through a balance of the heat produced in the body and the heat lost from the body (Figure 4-1). A constant temperature range must be maintained for the body to function properly. When minor changes in the temperature of the body occur, the hypothalamus senses this and makes adjustments as necessary to ensure that the body temperature stays within a normal and safe range. For example, if an individual is playing tennis on a hot day, the body's heat-cooling mechanism is activated to remove excess heat from the body through perspiration.

Heat Production

Most of the heat produced in the body is through voluntary and involuntary muscle contractions. Voluntary muscle contractions involve the muscles over which the person has control, for example, the moving of legs or arms. Involuntary muscle contractions involve the muscles over which the person has no control; examples include physiologic processes such as digestion, the beating of the heart, and shivering.

Body heat is also produced by cell metabolism. Heat is produced when nutrients are broken down in the cells. Fever and strong emotional states can also increase heat production in the body.

Heat Loss

Heat is lost from the body through the urine and feces and in water vapor from the lungs. Perspiration also contributes to heat loss. Perspiration is the excretion of moisture through the pores of the skin. When the moisture evaporates, heat is released and the body is cooled.

Radiation, conduction, and convection all cause loss of heat from the body. **Radiation** is the transfer of heat in the form of waves; body heat is continually radiating into cooler surroundings. **Conduction** is the transfer of heat from one object to another; heat can be transferred by conduction from the body to a cooler object it touches. **Convection** is the transfer of heat through air currents; cool air currents can cause the body to lose heat. These processes are illustrated in Figure 4-2.

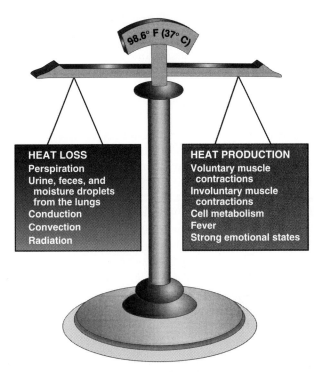

Figure 4-1. Body temperature represents a balance between the heat produced in the body and the heat lost from the body.

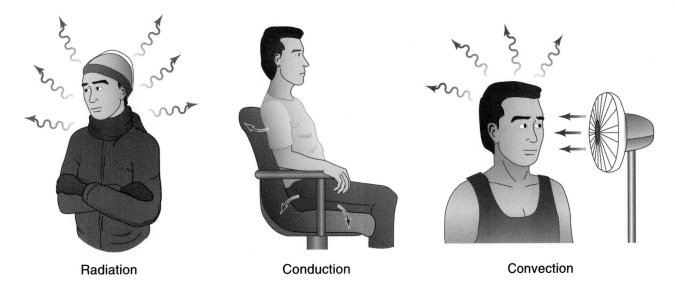

Radiation   Conduction   Convection

Figure 4-2. Heat loss from the body. **Radiation**—the body gives off heat in the form of waves to the cooler outside air. **Conduction**—the chair becomes warm as heat is transferred from the individual to the chair. **Convection**—air currents move heat away from the body.

Body Temperature Range

The purpose of measuring body temperature is to establish the patient's baseline temperature and to monitor an abnormally high or low body temperature. The normal body temperature range is 97° to 99° F (36.1° to 37.2° C), the average temperature being 98.6° F, which is equal to 37° Celsius (C), or centigrade. Body temperature is usually recorded using the Fahrenheit system of measurement. Table 4-1 illustrates comparable Fahrenheit and Celsius temperatures and explains how to convert temperatures from one scale to the other.

Alterations in Body Temperature

A body temperature above 100.4° F (38° C) indicates a **fever,** or *pyrexia.* If the body temperature falls between 99° F (37.2° C) and 100.4° F (38° C), it is termed a *low-grade fever.* When an individual has a fever, the heat that the body is producing is greater than the heat the body is losing. A temperature reading above 105.8° F (41° C) is known as **hyperpyrexia.** Hyperpyrexia is a serious condition, and a temperature above 109.4° F (43° C) is generally fatal.

A body temperature below 97° F (36.1° C) is classified as subnormal, or **hypothermia.** This means that the heat the body is losing is greater than the heat it is producing. A person usually cannot survive with a temperature lower than 93.2° F (34° C). Terms used to describe alterations in body temperature are illustrated in Figure 4-3.

Variations in Body Temperature

During the day-to-day activities of an individual, normal fluctuations occur in the body temperature. Rarely does the body temperature stay the same throughout the course of a day. The medical assistant should take the following points into consideration when evaluating a patient's temperature.

Age. Infants and young children normally have a higher body temperature than adults because their thermoregulatory system is not yet fully established. Elderly people usually have a lower body temperature owing to factors such as loss of subcutaneous fat, lack of exercise, and loss of thermoregulatory control. Table 4-2 shows the normal ranges of body temperature according to age-group.

Diurnal variations. During sleep, body metabolism slows down, as do muscle contractions. The body's temperature is lowest in the morning before metabolism and muscle contractions begin speeding up.

Exercise. Vigorous physical exercise causes an increase in voluntary muscle contractions, which raises the body temperature.

Emotional states. Strong emotions, such as crying and extreme anger, can increase the body temperature. This is important to consider when working with young

TABLE **4-1**	Equivalent Fahrenheit and Celsius Temperatures		
Fahrenheit	**Celsius**	**Fahrenheit**	**Celsius**
93.2	34	101.3	38.5
95	35	102.2	39
96.8	36	104	40
97.7	36.5	105.8	41
98.6	37	107.6	42
99.5	37.5	109.4	43
100.4	38	111.2	44

Temperature Conversion

1. Celsius to Fahrenheit: To convert Celsius to Fahrenheit, multiply by $\frac{9}{5}$ and add 32.

$$°F = (°C \times \tfrac{9}{5}) + 32.$$

2. Fahrenheit to Celsius: To convert Fahrenheit to Celsius, subtract 32 and multiply by $\frac{5}{9}$.

$$°C = (°F - 32) \times \tfrac{5}{9}.$$

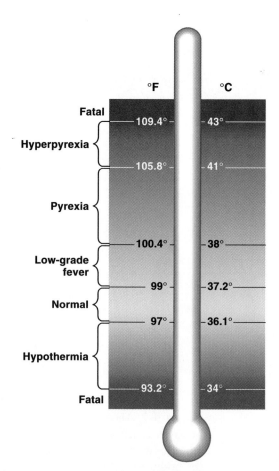

Figure 4-3. Terms that describe alterations in body temperature (adult oral temperature).

children, who frequently cry during examination procedures or when they are ill.

Environment. Cold weather tends to decrease the body temperature, whereas hot weather increases it.

Patient's normal body temperature. Some patients normally run a low or high temperature. The medical assistant should review the patient's past vital sign recordings.

Pregnancy. Cell metabolism increases during pregnancy, which in turn raises body temperature.

PUTTING It All Into PRACTICE

MY NAME IS Sergio Martinez, and I am a registered medical assistant. I work in a large clinic that is associated with a medical school. At present, I work in the family medicine department, but I have also worked in dermatology and internal medicine. Family medicine is the area I enjoy most because of the wide variety of tasks that are performed. There is rarely a dull moment.

I focus primarily on clinical medical assisting. Taking vital signs is a big part of my job responsibilities. It is routine at my clinic to take height, weight, temperature, pulse, respiration, and blood pressure on every patient seen at the clinic, no matter what the reason for his or her visit. I also assist the doctor with various procedures, examinations, and minor office surgery, as well as administering injections, running electrocardiograms, and performing various laboratory tests.

Taking vital signs and length and weight on small children can be very challenging at times. Some children start to cry as soon as they are put on the scale. Taking a temperature on an uncooperative toddler can be very difficult. I try to calm the child as much as possible, and for good behavior, I give a lot of praise. Stickers are also a great reward for cooperative behavior. Usually when small children learn that they can trust you, they are not as frightened by the experience. It is rewarding when a child learns not to be afraid of being evaluated for routine vital signs.

Fever

Fever, or pyrexia, denotes that a patient's temperature has risen above 100.4° F (38° C). An individual who has a fever is said to be **febrile;** one who does not is **afebrile.**

Fever is a common symptom of illness, particularly inflammation and infection. When there is an infection in the body, the invading pathogen functions as a *pyrogen,* which is any substance that produces fever. Pyrogens reset the hypothalamus, causing the body temperature to rise above normal. Fever is not an illness itself but, rather, a sign that the body may have an infection. Most fevers are self-limiting; that is, the body temperature returns to normal after the disease process is completed.

Stages of a Fever

A fever can be divided into the following three stages:
1. The *onset* is when the temperature first begins to rise. The rise may be slow or sudden, the patient experiences coldness and chills, and the pulse and respiratory rate increase.
2. During the *course of a fever,* the temperature rises and falls in one of the following three fever patterns: continuous, intermittent, or remittent. Fever patterns are

Highlight on Fever

Although most fevers indicate an infection, not all do. Noninfectious causes of fever include heatstroke, drug hypersensitivity, neoplasms, and central nervous system damage.

A fever is usually not harmful if it remains below 102° F (38.9° C). In fact, research suggests that fever may serve as a defense mechanism to destroy pathogens that are unable to survive above the normal body temperature range.

The level of the fever is not necessarily related to the seriousness of the infection. A patient with a temperature of 104° F (40° C) may not be any sicker than a patient with a temperature of 102° F (38.9° C).

In children, fever often appears as one of the first signs of illness and has a tendency to become highly elevated. In elderly patients, on the other hand, fever may be elevated only 1 to 2° above normal, even with a severe infection.

During a fever, the body's basal metabolism increases 7% for each degree of temperature elevation. Heart and respiratory rates also increase to meet this metabolic demand.

Chills during a fever result when the hypothalamus has been reset at a higher temperature. In an attempt to reach this temperature, involuntary muscle contractions (chills) occur, which produce heat, causing the temperature of the body to go up. After the higher temperature has been reached, the chills subside and the individual then feels warm.

Increased perspiration during a fever occurs when the hypothalamus has been reset at a lower temperature—for example, after taking an **antipyretic** or after the cause of the fever has been removed. In order to cool the body and reach this lower temperature, the body perspires, often profusely; profuse perspiration is known as *diaphoresis.*

TABLE 4-2	Variations in Body Temperature by Age		
Age	**Site**	**Average Temperature**	
Newborn	Axillary	97-100° F	36.1-37.8° C
1 year	Oral	99.7° F	37.6° C
5 years	Oral	98.6° F	37° C
Adult	Oral	98.6° F	37° C
	Rectal	99.6° F	37.5° C
	Axillary	97.6° F	36.4° C
	Aural	98.6° F	37° C
Elderly (over 70 yr)	Oral	96.8° F	36° C

TABLE 4-3	Fever Patterns	
Pattern	**Description**	**Illustration**
Continuous fever	The body temperature fluctuates minimally but always remains elevated. Occurs with: 　Scarlet fever 　Pneumococcal pneumonia	98.6° F (37° C)
Intermittent fever	The body temperature alternately rises and falls and at times returns to normal or even becomes subnormal. Occurs with: 　Bacterial infections 　Viral infections	98.6° F (37° C)
Remittent fever	A wide range of temperature fluctuations occur, all of which are above normal. Occurs with: 　Influenza 　Pneumonia 　Endocarditis	98.6° F (37° C)

described and illustrated in Table 4-3. During this stage the patient has an increased pulse and respiratory rate and feels warm to the touch. The patient may also experience one or more of the following: flushed appearance, increased thirst, loss of appetite, headache, and malaise. **Malaise** refers to a vague sense of body discomfort, weakness, and fatigue.

3. During the *subsiding stage* the temperature returns to normal. It can return to normal gradually or suddenly (known as a **crisis**). As the body temperature is returning to normal, the patient usually perspires and may become dehydrated.

Assessment of Body Temperature

Assessment Sites

There are four sites for measuring body temperature: mouth, axilla (armpit), rectum, and ear. The locations in which temperatures are taken must be as closed as possible to prevent air currents from interfering with the temperature reading. The body sites should have an abundant blood supply so that the temperature of the entire body is obtained, not the temperature of only a part of the body. The site chosen for measuring a patient's temperature depends on the patient's age, condition, and state of consciousness; the type of thermometer being used; and the medical office policy.

Oral Temperature

The oral method is the most convenient and the most common means for measuring body temperature. When the medical assistant records a temperature, the physician assumes it has been taken through the oral route, unless it is otherwise noted. There is a rich blood supply under the tongue in the area on either side of the **frenulum linguae.**

The thermometer should be placed in this area to receive the most accurate reading. The patient must keep his or her mouth closed during the procedure to provide a closed space for the thermometer.

Axillary Temperature

Axillary temperature is recommended as a site for measuring temperature in toddlers and preschoolers who have trouble holding a thermometer in their mouths. The axillary site should also be used for mouth-breathing patients and for patients with oral inflammation or those who have had oral surgery.

The temperature obtained through the axillary method measures approximately 1° F lower than the same person's temperature taken through the oral route (see Table 4-2). The medical assistant should make a notation to tell the physician that the temperature was taken through the axillary route.

Rectal Temperature

The rectal temperature provides a very accurate measurement of body temperature because few factors can alter the results. The rectum is highly vascular and, of the four sites, provides the most closed cavity. The temperature obtained through the rectal route measures approximately 1° F higher than the same person's temperature taken through the oral route (see Table 4-2). The medical assistant should make a notation on the patient's chart if the temperature has been taken rectally.

The rectal method is generally used for infants and young children, unconscious patients, and mouth-breathing patients and when greater accuracy in body temperature is desired. The rectal site should not be used with newborns because of the danger of rectal trauma.

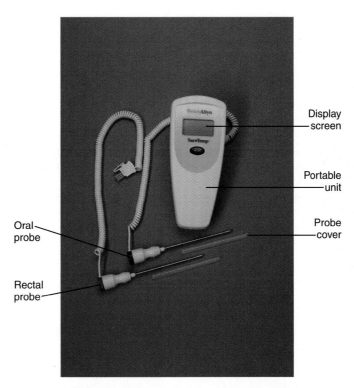

Figure 4-4. Electronic thermometer.

Aural Temperature

The aural (ear) site is used with the tympanic membrane thermometer. The ear provides a closed cavity that is easily accessible. Tympanic membrane thermometers provide instantaneous results, are easy to use, and are more comfortable for the patient. They make is easier to measure the temperature of children younger than 6 years, uncooperative patients, and patients who are unable to have their temperatures taken orally.

Types of Thermometers

The three types of thermometers available for measuring body temperature are electronic thermometers, tympanic membrane thermometers, and chemical thermometers. They are discussed in detail in the following section.

Mercury glass thermometers, once commonly used in medical offices, are no longer used because they break easily and release mercury. Mercury is a chemical that is dangerous to the human body because it can cause damage to the nervous system. In fact, many cities have banned the sale or use of mercury because of its hazards.

Electronic Thermometer

An electronic thermometer is frequently used in the medical office to measure body temperature. Electronic thermometers are portable and measure oral, axillary, and rectal temperatures ranging from 84° F (28.9° C) to 108° F (42.2° C).

An electronic thermometer measures body temperature in a brief time; the time varies between 4 and 60 seconds, depending on the brand of thermometer. The temperature results are then digitally displayed on an LCD screen. An electronic thermometer consists of interchangeable oral and rectal probes attached to a battery-operated portable unit (Figure 4-4). The probes are color-coded for ease in identifying them. The oral probe is color-coded with blue on its collar and is used to take both oral and axillary temperature; the rectal probe is color-coded with red on its collar and is used to take rectal temperatures only.

A disposable plastic cover is placed over the probe to prevent the transmission of microorganisms between patients. Depending on the method of taking temperature, the probe is inserted in the mouth, axilla, or rectum and is left in place until an audible tone is emitted from the thermometer. When the tone sounds, the patient's temperature in degrees Fahrenheit is displayed on the screen. The medical assistant then ejects the plastic probe cover into a regular waste container.

Procedures 4-1, 4-2, and 4-3 outline the methods for measuring oral, axillary, and rectal temperature using an electronic thermometer.

Tympanic Membrane Thermometer

The tympanic membrane thermometer is used at the aural site. The tympanic membrane thermometer functions by detecting thermal energy that is naturally radiated from the body. As with the rest of the body, the tympanic membrane and surrounding ear canal give off heat waves known as infrared waves. The tympanic thermometer functions like a camera by taking a "picture" of these infrared waves, which are considered a documented indicator of body temperature (Figure 4-5). The thermometer then calculates the body temperature from the energy generated by the waves and converts it to an oral or rectal equivalent.

The tympanic membrane thermometer is battery operated and consists of a small handheld device with a sensor probe (Figure 4-6). To operate the thermometer, the probe is covered with a disposable soft plastic cover and placed in the outer third of the external ear canal. An activation button is depressed momentarily, and the results are displayed in 1 to 2 seconds on a digital screen. The probe cover is then ejected into a regular waste container. The procedure for taking aural body temperature using a tympanic membrane thermometer is presented in Procedure 4-4.

Chemical Thermometers

Chemical thermometers contain chemicals that are heat sensitive and include disposable chemical single-use thermometers and temperature-sensitive strips. They are used most often by patients at home to measure body temperature. Although chemical thermometers are less accurate than other types of thermometers, they assist in providing a general assessment of body temperature. Because of their chemical makeup, they should be stored in a cool area,

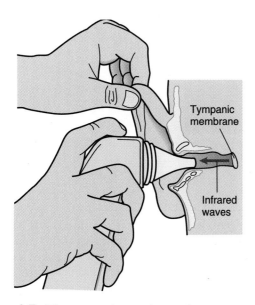

Figure 4-5. The tympanic membrane thermometer functions by detecting thermal energy that is naturally radiated from the tympanic membrane.

What Would You DO?
What Would You *Not* DO?

Case Study 1

Marcela Mason comes in with Olivia, her 5-year-old daughter. Olivia has had a fever and sore throat for the past 2 days. Olivia's aural temperature is taken in her left ear, and it measures 103.3° F. Mrs. Mason says that she has an ear thermometer at home, but when she took Olivia's temperature with it, the readings were always below 97°. She knew that couldn't be right because Olivia felt so warm. Mrs. Mason would like to be able to use her ear thermometer, but she thinks that it might be broken because of the low readings. Mrs. Mason says that she is thinking of switching back to a mercury glass thermometer, but she has heard that it isn't a good idea to use this type of thermometer anymore and wants to know why.

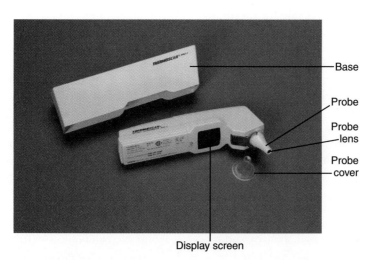

Figure 4-6. Tympanic membrane thermometer.

Guidelines for Using a Tympanic Membrane Thermometer

The following guidelines help ensure accurate aural temperature measurement with a tympanic membrane thermometer.

1. **Determine if a tympanic thermometer can be used to measure the patient's temperature.** The tympanic thermometer should not be used on a patient with inflammation of the external ear canal (e.g., otitis externa) or when the ear contains a discharge such as blood or pus. The presence of otitis media does not significantly affect the temperature reading, nor does a normal amount of cerumen. However, impacted cerumen can result in a falsely low temperature reading.

2. **Select the proper temperature mode.** Tympanic membrane thermometers can be set to oral or rectal equivalent modes. This means that the thermometer translates the tympanic membrane temperature into a more familiar frame of reference for interpretation. The mode selected depends on the age of the patient. To take the temperature of an adult or child older than 3 years, the mode should be set to the oral equivalent (ORAL). To take the temperature of a child younger than 3 years, the mode should be set to the rectal equivalent (RECTAL). The manufacturer's instructions should be followed carefully to change the temperature mode.

3. **Select the temperature measurement system desired.** The temperature of a tympanic membrane thermometer can be displayed in degrees Fahrenheit or degrees Celsius. Follow the manufacturer's instructions to change from one measurement to the other.

4. **Place the probe properly in the patient's ear.** The most important factor in obtaining an accurate temperature is the proper placement of the probe in the patient's ear, as outlined next.

   Straighten the ear canal. The ear canal has an S shape that obstructs the view of the tympanic membrane. To obtain an accurate temperature measurement, the ear canal must be straightened before inserting the probe. This allows the probe sensor to obtain a clear picture of the tympanic membrane.

   Seal the opening of the ear. The probe must be inserted tightly enough to seal the opening of the ear without causing patient discomfort. If the probe does not seal the ear canal, cooler external air can cause the thermometer to register a lower temperature.

   Correctly position the probe. Position the tip of the probe toward the opposite temple (approximately midway between the opposite ear and eyebrow). This allows the sensor to obtain the best possible picture of the tympanic membrane. If the tip is positioned incorrectly, it may be aimed at the ear canal, which results in a falsely low reading.

5. **Verify the accuracy of the temperature reading, if needed.** If you need to take the patient's temperature again, you can use the other ear. There are slight but insignificant differences between the temperature readings in the right ear and the left ear. Before using the same ear, however, you must wait 2 minutes to allow the aural temperature to stabilize.

6. **Check the probe lens before taking the temperature.** The end of the probe is covered with a lens that is transparent to heat waves. To ensure a high level of accuracy, it is very important to keep this lens clean and intact. Before taking a temperature, always check to make sure the lens is shiny and clear. Fingerprints, cerumen, and dust reduce the transparency of the lens, resulting in falsely low temperature readings. If the lens is dirty, it must be cleaned before taking the patient's temperature. If the lens is damaged, the thermometer cannot be used and must be repaired.

7. **Respond appropriately to digital messages.** A message to alert the user is displayed in the digital screen under the following circumstances:

   An attempt is made to take a temperature without changing the cover after the last temperature.

   An attempt is made to take a temperature with no probe cover in place.

   The battery is low.

   The thermometer is in need of repair.

8. **Care for the tympanic thermometer properly.**

   Probe lens. Dust and other minute particles of environmental debris can build up on the probe lens during normal use. The lens should be cleaned as part of routine maintenance or when it becomes dirty. To clean the lens, gently wipe its surface with an alcohol wipe and immediately wipe it dry with a cotton swab. After cleaning, allow at least 5 minutes before taking a temperature.

   Thermometer casing. Clean the casing of the thermometer periodically by wiping it dry with a soft cloth slightly dampened with warm water and a mild detergent or germicidal cleaner. Make sure the cloth is damp but not wet to prevent the cleaning solution from running inside the thermometer, which could damage it.

9. **Store the thermometer properly.** Keep the thermometer away from temperature extremes, which could damage the thermometer. The thermometer should not be exposed to excessive heat (more than 95° F, or 35° C) or excessive cold (less than 60° F, or 15.6° C).

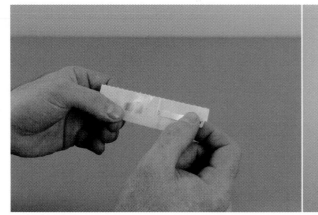
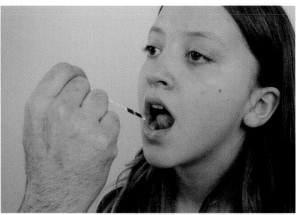

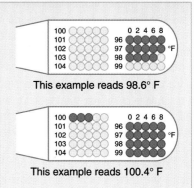

This example reads 98.6° F

This example reads 100.4° F

Figure 4-7. Disposable chemical single-use thermometers. **A,** The thermometer is removed from the wrapper by pulling on the handle. **B,** The thermometer is inserted under the tongue and left in place for 60 seconds. **C,** The thermometer is read by noting the highest reading among the dots that have changed color.

preferably colder than 86° F (30° C), and should not be exposed to direct sunlight because heat may cause the thermometer to register a higher temperature. Each type of chemical thermometer is described here.

Disposable Chemical Single-Use Thermometers. This type of thermometer has small chemical dots at one end that respond to body heat by changing color (Figure 4-7, *A* and *B*). Each thermometer comes in its own wrapper. The protective wrapper must be peeled back to expose the handle of the thermometer. The thermometer is removed from the wrapper by pulling on the handle, being careful not to touch the dotted area. The thermometer is then inserted under the tongue and left in place for the duration of time recommended by the manufacturer (generally 60 seconds). After removal of the thermometer, the dots are observed for a change in color. The thermometer is read by noting the highest reading among the dots that have changed color (Figure 4-7, *C*). The thermometer is then discarded after use.

Temperature-Sensitive Strips. A temperature-sensitive strip consists of a reusable plastic strip that contains heat-sensitive liquid crystals designed to measure body temperature. The plastic strip is pressed onto the forehead and held in place until the colors stop changing, generally 15 seconds. The results are read by observing the color change and noting the corresponding temperature indicated on the strip (Figure 4-8). *Text continued on p. 141*

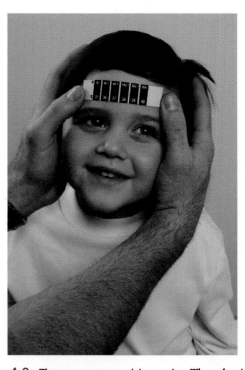

Figure 4-8. Temperature-sensitive strip. The plastic strip is pressed onto the forehead and held in place until the color stops changing (generally 15 seconds). The results are read by observing the color and noting the corresponding temperature indicated on the strip.

PROCEDURE 4-1 Measuring Oral Body Temperature—Electronic Thermometer

Outcome Measure oral body temperature.

Equipment/Supplies:
- Electronic thermometer
- Oral probe (blue collar)
- Plastic probe cover
- Waste container

1. **Procedural Step.** Sanitize your hands and assemble the equipment.

2. **Procedural Step.** Remove the thermometer unit from its base and attach the oral (blue-collar) probe to it. This is accomplished by inserting the latching plug (at the end of the coiled cord of the oral probe) to the plug receptacle on the thermometer unit. Next, insert the probe into the face of the thermometer.

   Principle. The oral probe is color-coded with a blue collar for ease in identifying it.

3. **Procedural Step.** Greet and identify the patient. Introduce yourself and explain the procedure. If the patient has recently ingested hot or cold food or beverages, or has been smoking, you must wait 15 to 30 minutes before taking the temperature.

   Principle. Ingestion of hot or cold food or beverages and smoking could result in an inaccurate reading.

4. **Procedural Step.** Grasp the probe by the collar and remove it from the face of the thermometer. Slide the probe into a disposable plastic probe cover until it locks into place.

   Principle. Removing the probe from the thermometer automatically turns on the thermometer. The probe cover prevents the transfer of microorganisms from one patient to another.

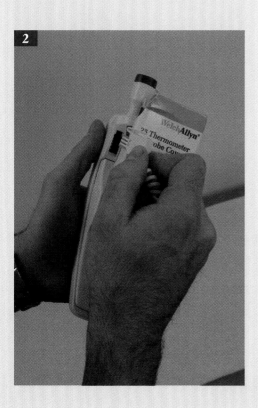

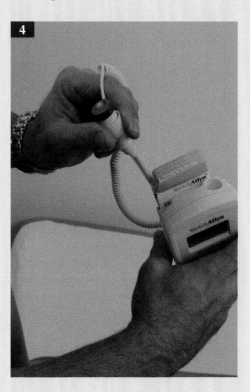

Continued

PROCEDURE 4-1 Measuring Oral Body Temperature—Electronic Thermometer—Cont'd

5. **Procedural Step.** Take the patient's temperature by inserting the probe under the patient's tongue in the pocket located on either side of the frenulum linguae. Instruct the patient to keep his or her mouth closed.

Principle. There is a good blood supply in the tissue under the tongue. The mouth must be kept closed to prevent cooler air from entering and affecting the temperature reading.

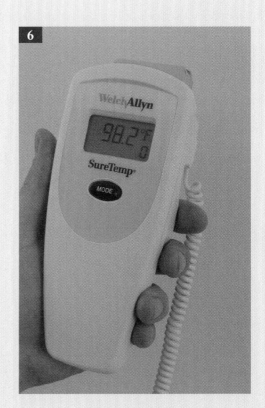

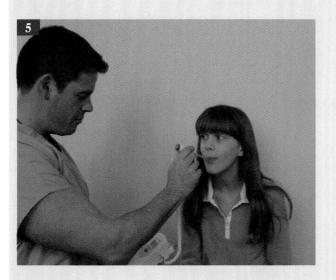

6. **Procedural Step.** Hold the probe in place until you hear the tone. At that time, the patient's temperature appears as a digital display on the screen. (The temperature indicated on this thermometer is 98.2° F [36.8° C]).

7. **Procedural Step.** Remove the probe from the mouth. Discard the probe cover by firmly pressing the ejection button while holding the probe over a regular waste container. Do not allow your fingers to come in contact with the probe cover.

Principle. The probe cover should not be touched to prevent the transfer of microorganisms from the patient to the medical assistant. Saliva is not considered regulated medical waste, and therefore the probe can be discarded in a regular waste container.

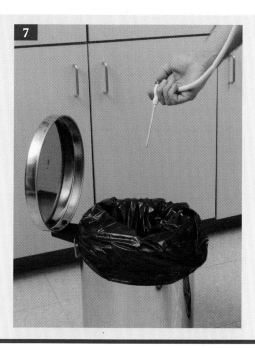

8. **Procedural Step.** Return the probe to its stored position in the thermometer unit. Return the thermometer unit to its base.
   Principle. Returning the probe to the unit automatically turns off and resets the thermometer.

9. **Procedural Step.** Sanitize your hands and chart the results. Include the date, the time, and the temperature reading.
   Principle. Patient data must be recorded properly to aid the physician in the diagnosis and to provide future reference.

CHARTING EXAMPLE

Date	
10/15/05	2:15 p.m. T: 98.2° F.——— S. Martinez, RMA

PROCEDURE 4-2

PROCEDURE 4-2   Measuring Axillary Body Temperature—Electronic Thermometer

Outcome   Measure axillary body temperature.

NOTE: Many of the principles for taking temperature have already been stated and are not included in this procedure.

Equipment/Supplies:
- Electronic thermometer
- Oral probe (blue collar)
- Plastic probe cover
- Waste container

1. **Procedural Step.** Sanitize your hands and assemble the equipment.

2. **Procedural Step.** Remove the thermometer unit from its base and attach the oral (blue-collared) probe to it. This is accomplished by inserting the latching plug (on the end of the coiled cord of the oral probe) to the plug receptacle on the thermometer unit. Next, insert the probe into the face of the thermometer.

3. **Procedural Step.** Greet and identify the patient. Introduce yourself and explain the procedure.

4. **Procedural Step.** Remove clothing from the patient's shoulder and arm. Make sure the axilla is dry. If it is wet, pat it dry with a paper towel or a gauze pad.
   Principle. Clothing removal provides optimal exposure of the axilla for proper placement of the thermometer. Rubbing the axilla causes an increase in the temperature in that area due to friction, resulting in an inaccurate temperature reading.

5. **Procedural Step.** Grasp the probe by the collar and remove it from the face of the thermometer. Slide the probe into a disposable probe cover until it locks into place.

Continued

PROCEDURE 4-2 Measuring Axillary Body Temperature—Electronic Thermometer—Cont'd

6. Procedural Step. Take the patient's temperature by placing the probe in the center of the patient's axilla. Instruct the patient to hold the arm close to the body. Hold the arm in place for small children and other patients who cannot maintain the position themselves.
Principle. Interference from outside air currents is reduced when the arm is held in the proper position.

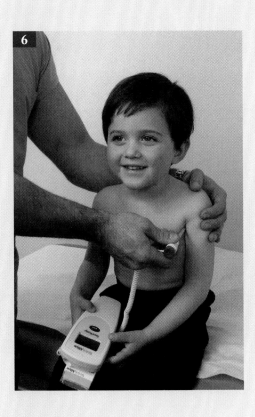

7. Procedural Step. Hold the probe in place until you hear the tone. At that time, the patient's temperature appears as a digital display on the screen.

8. Procedural Step. Remove the probe from the patient's axilla. Discard the probe cover by firmly pressing the ejection button while holding the probe over a regular waste container. Do not allow your fingers to come in contact with the probe cover.

9. Procedural Step. Return the probe to its stored position in the thermometer unit. Return the thermometer unit to its base.

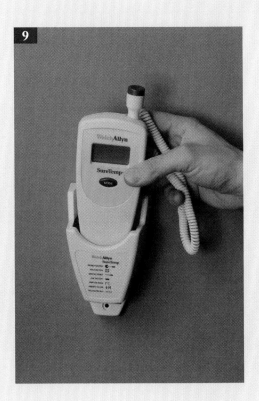

10. Procedural Step. Sanitize your hands and chart the results. Include the date, the time, and the axillary temperature reading. The symbol Ⓐ must be charted next to the temperature reading to tell the physician that an axillary reading was taken.

CHARTING EXAMPLE

Date	
10/15/05	9:30 a.m. T: 97.4° F Ⓐ —S. Martinez, RMA

PROCEDURE 4-3 Measuring Rectal Body Temperature—Electronic Thermometer

Outcome Measure rectal body temperature.

Equipment/Supplies:
- Electronic thermometer
- Rectal probe (red collar)
- Plastic probe cover
- Lubricant
- Disposable gloves
- Tissues
- Waste container

1. **Procedural Step.** Sanitize your hands and assemble the equipment.

2. **Procedural Step.** Remove the thermometer unit from its base. Attach the rectal (red-collar) probe to it. This is accomplished by inserting the latching plug (on the end of the coiled cord of the rectal probe) to the plug receptacle on the thermometer unit. Next, insert the probe into the face of the thermometer.
   Principle. The rectal probe is color-coded with a red collar for ease in identifying it.

3. **Procedural Step.** Greet and identify the patient. Introduce yourself and explain the procedure.
   Principle. It is important to explain what you will be doing because body temperature may be higher in a fearful or apprehensive patient.

4. **Procedural Step.** Apply gloves. Position the patient. *Adults and children:* Position the patient in the Sims position, and drape the patient to expose only the anal area. *Infants:* Position the infant on his or her abdomen.
   Principle. Gloves protect the medical assistant from microorganisms in the anal area and feces. Correct positioning allows clear viewing of the anal opening and provides for proper insertion of the thermometer. Draping reduces patient embarrassment and provides warmth.

5. **Procedural Step.** Grasp the probe by the collar and remove it from the face of the thermometer. Slide the probe into a disposable plastic probe cover until it locks into place. Apply a lubricant to the tip of the probe cover up to a level of 1 inch.
   Principle. A lubricated thermometer can be inserted more easily and does not irritate the delicate rectal mucosa.

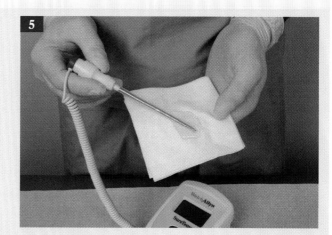

6. **Procedural Step.** Instruct the patient to lie still. Separate the buttocks to expose the anal opening and gently insert the thermometer probe approximately 1 inch into the rectum of an adult, ⅝ inch in children, and ½ inch in infants. Do not force insertion of the probe. Tilt the probe so that it is touching rectal tissue and hold it in place until the temperature registers.
   Principle. The probe must be inserted correctly to prevent injury to the tissue of the anal opening. The probe should be held in place to prevent damage to the rectal mucosa.

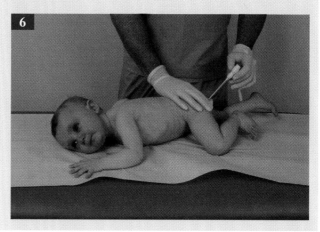

Continued

PROCEDURE 4-3

PROCEDURE 4-3 Measuring Rectal Body Temperature—Electronic Thermometer—Cont'd

7. **Procedural Step.** Hold the probe in place until you hear the tone. At that time, the patient's temperature appears as a digital display on the screen.

8. **Procedural Step.** Gently remove the probe from the rectum in the same direction as it was inserted. Discard the probe cover by firmly pressing the ejection button while holding the probe over a regular waste container. Return the probe to its stored position in the thermometer unit.
Principle. Fecal material is not considered regulated medical waste; therefore the probe can be discarded in a regular waste container.

9. **Procedural Step.** Wipe the patient's anal area with tissues to remove excess lubricant. Dispose of the tissues in a regular waste container. Return the thermometer unit to its base.
Principle. Wiping the anal area makes the patient more comfortable.

10. **Procedural Step.** Remove gloves and sanitize your hands. Chart the results. Include the date, the time, and the rectal temperature reading. The symbol Ⓡ must be charted next to the temperature reading to tell the physician that a rectal reading was taken.

CHARTING EXAMPLE	
Date	
10/15/05	11:15 a.m. T: 99.8° F Ⓡ — S. Martinez, RMA

PROCEDURE 4-4 Measuring Aural Body Temperature—Tympanic Membrane Thermometer

Outcome Measure aural body temperature.

Equipment/Supplies:
• Tympanic membrane thermometer
• Probe cover
• Waste container

1. **Procedural Step.** Sanitize your hands and assemble the equipment.
Principle. Your hands should be clean and free from contamination.

2. **Procedural Step.** Greet and identify the patient. Introduce yourself and explain the procedure.
Principle. It is important to explain what you will be doing because body temperature may be higher in a fearful or apprehensive patient.

3. **Procedural Step.** Remove the thermometer from its base. Check to make sure the probe lens is clean and intact. Check the display screen to make sure the thermometer is set on the proper mode for the patient's age. To take the temperature of an adult or a child older than 3 years, the thermometer should be set on ORAL mode. To take the temperature of children younger than 3 years, the thermometer should be set to RECTAL mode. If the desired mode is not displayed, change the setting according to the manufacturer's instructions.
Principle. A dirty or damaged probe lens could result in a falsely low temperature reading. Tympanic membrane thermometers are set on different modes depending on the age of the patient.

4. **Procedural Step.** Place a cover on the probe by pressing the probe tip straight down into the cover box. You will be able to see and feel the cover snap securely into place on the probe. This procedure automatically turns the thermometer on.
Principle. The probe cover protects the lens and provides infection control. The cover must be seated securely on the probe to activate the thermometer.

PROCEDURE 4-4

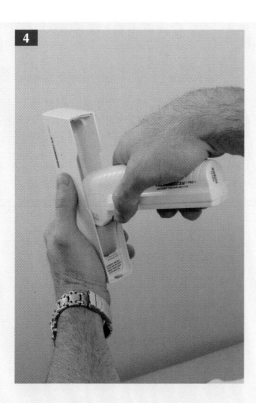

5. Procedural Step. Pull the probe straight up from the cover box. When the thermometer is ready, it will display the word "READY" on the digital screen. Do not take a temperature until the word READY is displayed.

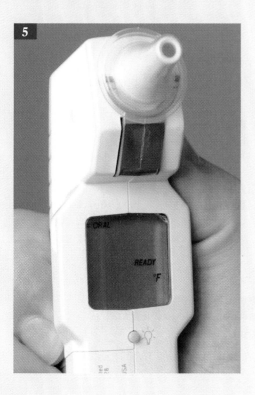

6. Procedural Step. Hold the thermometer in your dominant hand. If you are right handed, you should take the temperature in the patient's right ear. If you are left handed, take the temperature in the patient's left ear.
Principle. Taking the temperature with the dominant hand assists in the proper placement of the probe in the patient's ear.

7. Procedural Step. Straighten the patient's external ear canal with your nondominant hand as follows:
Adults and Children Older Than 3 Years. Gently pull the ear auricle upward and backward.
Children Younger Than 3 Years. Gently pull the ear pinna downward and backward.
Principle. Straightening the ear canal allows the probe sensor to obtain a clear picture of the tympanic membrane, resulting in an accurate temperature measurement.

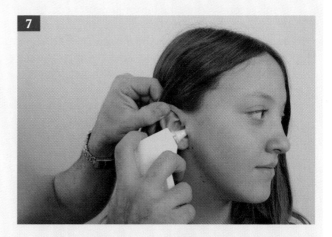

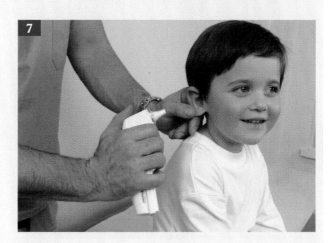

PROCEDURE 4-4

Continued

PROCEDURE 4-4   Measuring Aural Body Temperature—Tympanic Membrane Thermometer—Cont'd

8. **Procedural Step.** Insert the probe into the patient's ear canal tightly enough to seal the opening but without causing patient discomfort. Point the tip of the probe toward the opposite temple (approximately midway between the opposite ear and eyebrow).
   Principle. Sealing the ear canal prevents cooler external air from entering the ear, which could result in a falsely low reading. Correct positioning of the probe optimizes the sensor's view of the tympanic membrane, leading to an accurate temperature reading.

9. **Procedural Step.** Ask the patient to remain still. Hold the thermometer steady and depress the activation button. Hold the button down for 1 full second and then release it.
   Principle. The thermometer cannot take a temperature unless the activation button is depressed for 1 full second. When the button is depressed, the infrared sensor in the probe scans the thermal energy radiated by the tympanic membrane.

10. **Procedural Step.** Turn the digital display of the thermometer toward you and read the temperature. If the temperature appears to be too low, repeat the procedure to ensure that you have used the proper technique. The temperature indicated on this thermometer is 98° F (37° C).

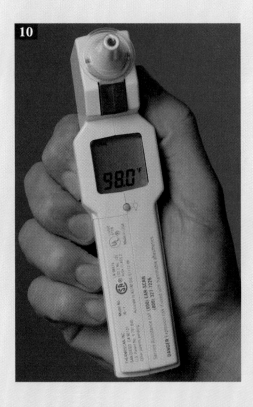

Principle. The temperature remains on the display screen until another cover is inserted on the probe. Improper technique can result in a falsely low temperature reading.

11. **Procedural Step.** Dispose of the probe cover by ejecting it into a regular waste container.

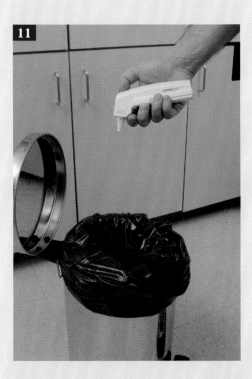

12. **Procedural Step.** Replace the thermometer in its base.
    Principle. The thermometer should be stored in its base to protect the probe lens from damage and dirt.

13. **Procedural Step.** Sanitize your hands.

14. **Procedural Step** Chart the results. Include the date, the time, the aural temperature reading, and which ear was used to take the temperature (AD: right ear; AS: left ear).

CHARTING EXAMPLE

Date	
10/15/05	3:00 p.m. T: 98° F, AD — S. Martinez, RMA

Pulse

Mechanism of the Pulse

When the left ventricle of the heart contracts, blood is forced from the heart into the **aorta,** which is the major trunk of the arterial system of the body. The aorta is already filled with blood and must expand to accept the blood being pushed out of the left ventricle. This creates a pulsating wave that travels from the aorta through the walls of the arterial system. This wave, known as the *pulse,* can be felt as a light tap by an examiner. The pulse rate is measured by counting the number of "taps," or beats per minute. The heart rate can thus be determined by taking the pulse rate.

Factors Affecting Pulse Rate

Pulse rate can vary, depending on a number of factors. The medical assistant should take each of the following into consideration when measuring pulse:

Age. The pulse varies inversely with age. As the age increases, the pulse rate gradually decreases. Table 4-4 gives the pulse rates of the various age-groups.

Gender. Women tend to have a slightly faster pulse rate than men do.

Physical activity. Physical activity, such as jogging and swimming, increases the pulse rate.

Emotional states. Strong emotional states, such as anxiety, fear, excitement, and anger, increase the pulse rate.

Metabolism. Increased body metabolism, such as occurs during pregnancy, increases the pulse rate.

Fever. Fever increases the pulse rate.

Medications. Medications may alter the pulse rate. For example, digitalis decreases the pulse rate and epinephrine increases it.

Pulse Sites

The pulse is felt most strongly when a superficial artery is held against a firm tissue, such as bone. The locations of the sites used for measuring the pulse are shown in Figure 4-9 and are described next.

Radial. The most common site for measuring the pulse is the radial artery, which is located on the inner aspect of the wrist just below the thumb. The radial pulse is easily accessible and can be measured with no discomfort to the patient. This site is also used by individuals at home monitoring their own heart rates, such as athletes, patients taking heart medication, and individuals starting an exercise program. The procedure for measuring radial pulse is outlined in Procedure 4-5.

Apical. The apical pulse has a stronger beat and is easier to measure than the other pulse sites. If the medical assistant is having difficulty feeling the radial pulse or if the radial pulse is irregular or abnormally slow or rapid, the apical pulse should be taken (Procedure 4-6). This pulse site is often used to measure pulse in infants and in children up to 3 years of age because the other sites are difficult to palpate accurately in these age-groups. The apical pulse is measured using a stethoscope. The chestpiece of the stethoscope is placed lightly over the apex of the heart, which is located in the fifth intercostal

TABLE **4-4**	Pulse Rates of Various Age-Groups	
Age-Group	**Pulse Range (beats/minute)**	**Average Pulse (beats/minute)**
Newborn	120-160	140
Toddler	90-140	115
Preschooler	80-110	95
School-age	75-105	90
Adolescent	60-100	80
Adult	60-100	80
After 60th year	67-80	74
Well-trained athletes	40-60	50

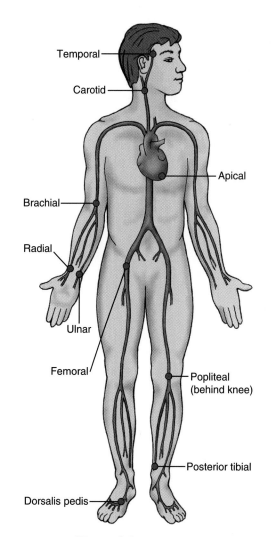

Figure 4-9. Pulse sites.

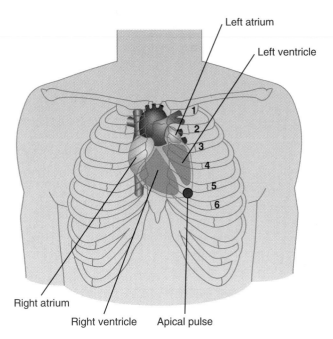

Figure 4-10. The apical pulse is found over the apex of the heart, which is located in the fifth intercostal space at the junction of the left midclavicular line.

(between the ribs) space at the junction of the left mid-clavicular line (Figure 4-10).

Brachial. The brachial pulse is in the antecubital space, which is the space located at the front of the elbow. This site is used to take blood pressure, to measure pulse in infants during cardiac arrest, and to assess the status of the circulation to the lower arm.

Ulnar. The ulnar pulse is located on the ulnar (little finger) side of the wrist. It is used to assess the status of circulation to the hand.

Temporal. The temporal pulse is located in front of the ear and just above eye level. This site is used to measure pulse when the radial pulse is not accessible. It is also an easy access site to assess pulse in children.

Carotid. The carotid pulse is located on the anterior side of the neck, slightly to one side of the midline, and is the best site to find a pulse quickly. This site is used to measure pulse in children and adults during cardiac arrest. The carotid site is also commonly used by individuals to monitor pulse during exercise.

Femoral. The femoral pulse is in the middle of the groin. This site is used to measure pulse in infants and children and in adults during cardiac arrest, as well as to assess the status of the circulation to the lower leg.

Popliteal. The popliteal pulse is at the back of the knee and is detected most easily when the knee is slightly flexed. This site is used to measure blood pressure when the brachial pulse is not accessible and to assess the status of the circulation to the lower leg.

Posterior tibial. The posterior tibial pulse is located on the inner aspect of the ankle just posterior to the ankle bone. This site is used to assess the status of circulation to the foot.

Dorsalis pedis. The dorsalis pedis pulse is located on the upper surface of the foot, between the first and second metatarsal bones. This site is used to assess the status of circulation to the foot.

Assessment of Pulse

The purpose of measuring pulse is to establish the patient's baseline pulse rate and to assess the pulse rate following special procedures, medications, or disease processes that affect heart functioning. Pulse is measured using palpation at all of the pulse sites except the apical site.

A pulse is palpated by applying moderate pressure with the sensitive pads located on the tips of the three middle fingers. The pulse should not be taken with the thumb because the thumb has a pulse of its own. This could result in a measurement of the medical assistant's pulse rather than the patient's pulse. Excessive pressure should not be applied when measuring pulse because it could obliterate, or close off, the pulse. On the other hand, it may not be possible to detect the pulse if too little pressure is applied. An accurate assessment of pulse includes a determination of the pulse rate, the pulse rhythm, and the pulse volume.

Pulse Rate

The pulse rate is the number of heart pulsations or heartbeats that occur in 1 minute; therefore pulse rate is measured in beats per minute. Normal pulse rates vary widely in the various age-groups, as shown in Table 4-4. For the healthy adult, the normal resting pulse rate ranges from 60 to 100 beats per minute, with the average falling between 70 and 80 beats per minute.

An abnormally fast heart rate of more than 100 beats per minute is known as **tachycardia.** Tachycardia may indicate disease states such as hemorrhaging or heart disease. However, an individual's pulse rate may normally exceed 100 beats per minute during vigorous exercise or during strong emotional states.

Bradycardia is an abnormally slow heart rate, fewer than 60 beats per minute. Normally, a pulse rate below 60 may occur during sleep; trained athletes often have low pulse rates. If a patient is exhibiting tachycardia or bradycardia, the apical pulse should also be measured.

Pulse Rhythm and Volume

In addition to measuring the pulse rate, the medical assistant should determine the rhythm and volume of the pulse.

The **pulse rhythm** denotes the time interval between heartbeats; a normal rhythm has the same time interval between beats. Any irregularity in the heart's rhythm is known as a **dysrhythmia** (also termed *arrhythmia*) and is characterized by unequal or irregular intervals between the heartbeats. If a dysrhythmia is detected, the physician often orders diagnostic tests such as an electrocardiogram and Holter monitoring.

The **pulse volume** refers to the strength of the heartbeat. The amount of blood pumped into the aorta by each contraction of the left ventricle should remain constant, making the pulse feel strong and full. If the blood volume decreases, the pulse feels weak and may be difficult to detect. This type of pulse is usually accompanied by a fast heart rate and is described as a **thready pulse.** An increase in the blood volume results in a pulse that feels extremely strong and full, known as a **bounding pulse.**

Any abnormalities in the rhythm or volume of the pulse should be recorded accurately in the patient's chart by the medical assistant. A pulse that has a normal rhythm and volume is recorded as being regular and strong.

PATIENT TEACHING

Aerobic Exercise

- Answer questions patients have about aerobic exercise.

What is aerobic exercise?
Aerobic exercise raises, sustains, and lowers your pulse over time. Aerobic exercise is accomplished through a steady, nonstop activity such as walking, jogging, cycling, or swimming. Each workout should include a warm-up and cool-down period of at least 5 minutes each. This is to prevent muscle or joint injuries.

What are the benefits of an aerobic exercise program?
The benefits of an aerobic exercise program include strengthening of the heart, a slower resting pulse rate, reduction of stress, increased energy, lowering of body fat, a decrease of "bad" (LDL) cholesterol, and an increase of "good" (HDL) cholesterol. The key to a safe and effective aerobic exercise program is your target heart rate (THR).

What is target heart rate?
Your THR is a safe and effective exercise pulse range that indicates you are exercising at the right level for your age and for what you are trying to accomplish with exercise. Exercising at a level below your THR does little to promote fitness; exercising at a level above your THR may not be safe.

How do I determine my target heart rate?
The following formula is used to determine your THR:
1. Subtract your age from 220 to determine your maximum heart rate (MHR), which is the fastest your heart can beat safely for your age. For example, the MHR of a 40-year-old person is calculated as follows:

$$220 - 40 \text{ years old} = 180 \text{ (MHR)}.$$

2. Determine the lower end of your THR range by multiplying your MHR by 0.6. For our example,

$$180 \times 0.60 = 108 \text{ (low end of the THR)}.$$

3. Determine the upper end of your THR range by multiplying your MHR by 0.8. For our example,

$$180 \times 0.80 = 144 \text{ (upper end of the THR)}.$$

Always exercise within your THR range. The 40-year-old person in our example should exercise with a THR between 108 and 144.

How often should aerobic exercise be performed?
A recent report from the Institute of Medicine recommends that adults and children spend at least 60 minutes throughout the day in moderately intense exercise in order to obtain the maximum benefits for heart health. Researchers say that this exercise recommendation is based on studies of the amount of energy burned by people who maintain a healthy weight. However, they stress that there are many ways to accomplish this goal, such as through playing with your children, housework, gardening, mowing the grass, walking the dog, bicycling, golfing, swimming, and other day-to-day activities. In addition, the 60 minutes does not have to be done all at once, but can be interspersed throughout the day; for example, 15 minutes of housework in the morning, 30 minutes of mowing grass later in the day, and 15 minutes of walking the dog in the evening.

Respiration

Mechanism of Respiration

The purpose of respiration is to provide for the exchange of oxygen and carbon dioxide between the atmosphere and the blood. Oxygen is taken into the body to be used for vital body processes, and carbon dioxide is given off as a waste product.

Each respiration is divided into two phases: **inhalation** and **exhalation** (Figure 4-11). During inhalation, or inspiration, the diaphragm descends and the lungs expand, causing air containing oxygen to move from the atmosphere into the lungs. Exhalation, or expiration, involves the removal of carbon dioxide from the body. The diaphragm ascends, and the lungs return to their original state, so that air containing carbon dioxide is expelled. One complete respiration is composed of one inhalation and one exhalation.

Respiration can be classified as either *external* or *internal.* External respiration involves the exchange of oxygen and carbon dioxide between the **alveolus** (thin-walled sacs) of the lungs and the blood (Figure 4-12). The blood, located in small capillaries, comes in contact with the alveoli, picks up oxygen, and carries it to the cells of the body. At this point, the oxygen is given off to the cells and carbon dioxide is picked up by the blood to be transported as a waste product to the lungs. The exchange of oxygen and carbon dioxide between the body cells and the blood is known as internal respiration.

Control of Respiration

The medulla oblongata, located in the brain, is the control center for involuntary respiration. A buildup of carbon dioxide in the blood sends a message to the medulla, which then triggers respiration to occur automatically.

To a certain extent, respiration is also under voluntary control. An individual can control respiration during

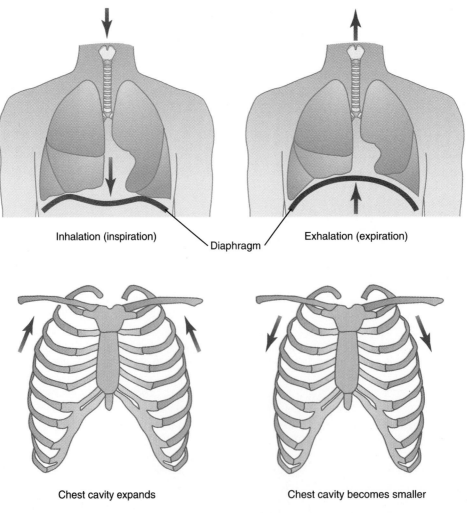

Inhalation (inspiration)   Diaphragm   Exhalation (expiration)

Chest cavity expands   Chest cavity becomes smaller

Figure 4-11. Inhalation and exhalation.

activities such as singing, laughing, talking, eating, and crying. Voluntary respiration is ultimately under the control of the medulla oblongata. The breath can be held for only a certain length of time, after which carbon dioxide begins to build up in the body, resulting in a stimulus to the medulla that causes respiration to occur involuntarily. Small children may voluntarily hold their breath during a temper tantrum. A parent who does not understand the principles of respiration may be concerned that the child will cease breathing. The medical assistant should be able to explain that involuntary respiration will eventually occur and the child will resume breathing.

Assessment of Respiration

Because an individual can control his or her respiration, the medical assistant should measure respirations without the patient's knowledge. Patients may change their respiratory rate unintentionally if they are aware that they are being measured. An ideal time to measure respiration is after the pulse is taken. Procedure 4-5 outlines the procedures for taking both pulse and respiration in one continuous procedure.

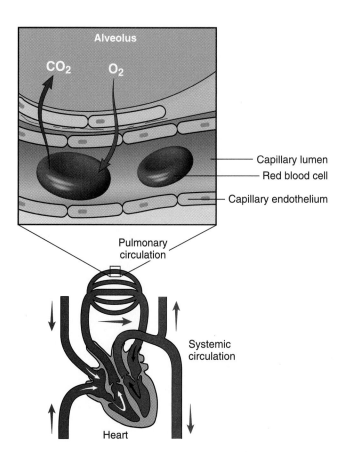

Figure 4-12. Exchange of oxygen and carbon dioxide between the alveoli of the lungs and the blood.

Respiratory Rate

The respiratory rate of a normal healthy adult ranges from 12 to 20 respirations per minute. With most adults, there is a ratio of 1 respiration for every 4 pulse beats. For example, if the respiratory rate is 18, the pulse rate would be approximately 72 beats per minute. An abnormal increase in the respiratory rate of more than 20 respirations per minute is referred to as **tachypnea.** An abnormal decrease in the respiratory rate of fewer than 12 respirations per minute is known as **bradypnea.**

When measuring the respiratory rate, the medical assistant should take into consideration the following factors:

Age. As age increases, the respiratory rate decreases. Therefore we would expect the respiratory rate of a child to be faster than that of an adult. Table 4-5 provides a chart of the respiratory rates for the various age-groups.

Physical activity. Physical activity increases the respiratory rate.

Emotional states. Strong emotional states increase the respiratory rate.

TABLE **4-5**	Respiratory Rates of Various Age-Groups	
Age-Group	**Average Respiratory Range (respirations/minute)**	**Respiratory Average**
Newborn	30-40	35
Toddler	23-35	30
Preschooler	20-30	25
School-age	18-26	22
Adolescent	12-20	16
Adult	12-20	16

What Would You DO? What Would You *Not* DO?

Case Study 2

Alex Jacoby is 18 years old and a senior in high school. He comes to the office complaining of pain in his left shoulder. Alex is an outstanding competitive swimmer and is currently ranked first in the state in the 100-yard butterfly. Alex has a big meet coming up and must do well because he has a chance of getting an athletic scholarship to the University of Florida. He says he thinks he can take 2 seconds off his best time at this meet and he doesn't want anything to interfere with that. Alex wants the physician to do whatever he can to make his shoulder better and thinks that steroids and codeine might be the answer. His vital signs are as follows: Temp: 98.5; Pulse: 48; Resp: 12; and BP: 108/68. Alex asks why his pulse is so slow and wants to know if there is any medication he can take to make it faster.

Fever. A patient with a fever has an increased respiratory rate. One of the ways heat is lost from the body is through the lungs; therefore a fever causes an increased respiratory rate as the body tries to rid itself of the excess heat.

Medications. Certain medications increase the respiratory rate, and others decrease it. The medical assistant who is unsure of what effect a particular drug may have on the respiratory rate should consult a drug reference such as the *Physician's Desk Reference* (PDR).

Rhythm and Depth of Respiration

Both the *rhythm* and *depth* should be noted when measuring respiration. Normally, the rhythm should be even and regular, and the pauses between inhalation and exhalation should be equal.

The depth of respiration indicates the amount of air that is inhaled or exhaled during the process of breathing. Respiratory depth is generally described as normal, deep, or shallow and is determined by observing the amount of movement of the chest. For normal respirations, the depth of each respiration in a resting state is approximately the same. Deep respirations are those in which a large volume of air is inhaled and exhaled, whereas shallow respirations involve the exchange of a small volume of air. Normal respiration is referred to as **eupnea.** The rate is approximately 12 to 20 respirations per minute, the rhythm is even and regular, and the depth is normal.

Hyperpnea is an abnormal increase both in the rate and depth of the respirations. A patient with hyperpnea exhibits a very deep, rapid, and labored respiration. Hyperpnea occurs normally with exercise, and abnormally with pain and fever. It can also occur with any condition in which the supply of oxygen is inadequate, such as heart disease and lung disease.

Hyperventilation is an abnormally fast and deep type of breathing that is usually associated with acute anxiety conditions such as hysteria and panic attacks. An individual who is hyperventilating is "overbreathing," which usually causes dizziness and weakness.

Hypopnea is a condition in which a patient's respiration exhibits an abnormal decrease in the rate and depth. The depth is approximately half that of normal respiration. Hypopnea often occurs in individuals with sleep disorders.

Color of the Patient

The patient's color should also be observed while the respiration is being measured. A lack of oxygen (**hypoxia**) results in a condition known as **cyanosis,** which causes a bluish discoloration of the skin and mucous membranes. Cyanosis is first observed in the nailbeds and lips, because in these areas the blood vessels lie close to the surface of the skin. Cyanosis typically occurs in patients with advanced emphysema and in patients during cardiac arrest.

))) PATIENT **TEACHING**

Chronic Obstructive Pulmonary Disease

- Answer questions that patients have about chronic obstructive pulmonary disease (COPD).

What is COPD?
COPD is a chronic airway obstruction that results from emphysema, chronic bronchitis, or asthma, or any combination of these conditions. COPD is a chronic debilitating, irreversible, and sometimes fatal disease.

How many people are affected with COPD?
COPD affects an estimated 16 million Americans, and its incidence is rising. It is the fourth leading cause of death in the United States behind heart disease, cancer, and strokes. Although COPD is much more common in men than women, the greatest increase of death rates is occurring in females.

What causes COPD?
Cigarette smoking after a period of many years is the leading cause of COPD. Other causes include air pollution and occupational exposure to irritating inhalants, such as noxious dusts, fumes, and vapors.

What types of tests might the physician order?
Respiratory tests to diagnose COPD include various types of pulmonary function tests. Examples of pulmonary function tests are spirometry, lung volumes, diffusion capacity, arterial blood gas studies, pulse oximetry, and cardiopulmonary exercise tests.

What treatment might the physician prescribe?
Treatment is focused on improving breathing difficulties and may include bronchodilator drug therapy, breathing exercises, and oxygen therapy.
- Encourage patients with COPD to comply with the therapy prescribed by the physician.
- Provide the patient with information about smoking, asthma, emphysema, and chronic bronchitis. Educational materials are available from the American Lung Association, American Heart Association, and American Cancer Society.

Apnea is a temporary absence of respirations. Some individuals experience apnea during sleep; this condition is known as *sleep apnea.* Apnea can be a serious condition if the breathing ceases for more than 4 to 6 minutes because the person could suffer brain damage and death.

Respiratory Abnormalities

A patient who is having difficulty in breathing or shortness of breath has a condition known as **dyspnea.**

Dyspnea may occur normally during vigorous physical exertion and abnormally in patients with asthma and emphysema. The patient with dyspnea may find it easier to breathe while in a sitting or standing position. This state is called **orthopnea** and occurs with disorders of the heart and lungs such as asthma, emphysema, pneumonia, and congestive heart failure.

Breath Sounds

Breath sounds are caused by air moving through the respiratory tract. Normal breath sounds are quiet and barely audible. Abnormal breath sounds are referred to as **adventitious sounds** and generally signify the presence of a respiratory disorder. The cause and character of abnormal breath sounds are presented in Table 4-6.

Text continued on p. 150

TABLE 4-6	Abnormal Breath Sounds	
Type	**Cause**	**Character**
Crackles* (rales)	Air moving through airways that contain fluid	Dry or wet intermittent sounds that vary in pitch (this sound can be duplicated by rubbing the hair together next to the ear)
Rhonchi*	Thick secretions, tumors, or spasms that partially obstruct air flow through the large upper airways	Deep, low-pitched, rumbling sound more audible during expiration
Wheezes	Severely narrowed airways caused by partial obstruction in the smaller bronchi and bronchioles; a common symptom of asthma	Continuous, high-pitched, whistling musical sounds heard during inspiration and expiration
Pleural friction rub*	Inflamed pleura rubbing together	High grating sound similar to rubbing leather pieces together, heard on both inspiration and expiration

*Audible only through a stethoscope.

PROCEDURE 4-5 Measuring Pulse and Respiration

Outcome Measure pulse and respiration.

Equipment/Supplies:
- Watch with a second hand

1. **Procedural Step.** Sanitize your hands. Greet and identify the patient. Introduce yourself and explain the procedure. Observe the patient for any signs that might increase or decrease the pulse rate.
   Principle. Pulse rate can vary, according to the factors listed on p. 141.
2. **Procedural Step.** Have the patient sit down. Position the patient's arm alongside the body in a comfortable position. The forearm should be slightly flexed in order to relax the muscles and tendons over the pulse site.
   Principle. Relaxed muscles and tendons over the pulse site make it easier to palpate the pulse.
3. **Procedural Step.** Place your three middle fingertips over the radial pulse site. Never use your thumb to take a pulse.
   Principle. The thumb has a pulse of its own; using the thumb results in a measurement of the medical assistant's pulse and not the patient's pulse.

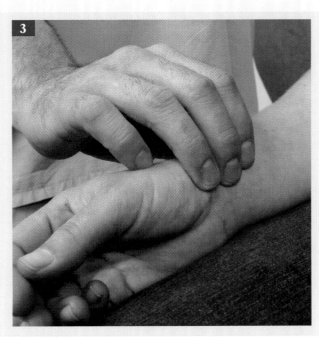

Continued

PROCEDURE 4-5

PROCEDURE 4-5 Measuring Pulse and Respiration—Cont'd

4. **Procedural Step.** Apply moderate, gentle pressure directly over the site until you feel the pulse.
   Principle. A normal pulse can be felt with moderate pressure. Too much pressure applied to the radial artery closes it off, and no pulse is felt.

5. **Procedural Step.** Count the pulse for 30 seconds, and multiply by 2. Note the rhythm and volume of the pulse. If abnormalities occur in the rhythm or volume, count the pulse for 1 full minute.
   Principle. A longer time ensures an accurate assessment of abnormalities.

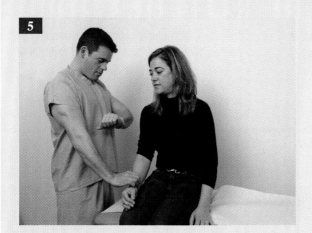

6. **Procedural Step.** After taking the pulse, continue to hold three fingers on the patient's wrist with the same amount of pressure and measure the respirations. This helps to ensure that the patient is unaware that respirations are being monitored.
   Principle. If the patient is aware that respiration is being taken, the breathing may change.

7. **Procedural Step.** Observe the rise and fall of the patient's chest as the patient inhales and exhales.
   Principle. One complete respiration includes one inhalation and one exhalation.

8. **Procedural Step.** Count the number of respirations for 30 seconds and multiply by 2; note the rhythm and depth of the respiration. Also observe the patient's color. If abnormalities occur in the rhythm or depth, count the respiratory rate for 1 full minute.

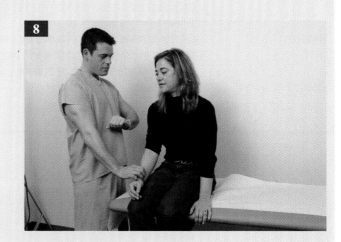

9. **Procedural Step.** Chart the results. Include the date; the time; the pulse rate, rhythm, and volume; and the respiratory rate, rhythm, and depth.

CHARTING EXAMPLE

Date	
10/15/05	2:30 p.m. P: 74. Reg and strong. R: 18. Even and reg. ————— S. Martinez, RMA

PROCEDURE 4-6   Measuring Apical Pulse

Outcome   Measure apical pulse.

Equipment/Supplies:
- Watch with a second hand
- Stethoscope
- Antiseptic wipe

1. **Procedural Step.** Sanitize your hands. Greet and identify the patient. Introduce yourself and explain the procedure.

2. **Procedural Step.** Assemble the equipment. If the stethoscope's chestpiece consists of both a diaphragm and a bell, rotate the chestpiece to the bell position. Clean the earpieces and chestpiece of the stethoscope with an antiseptic wipe.
   Principle. The bell position allows better auscultation of heart sounds. Cleaning the earpieces helps prevent the transmission of microorganisms.

3. **Procedural Step.** Have the patient sit or lie down (supine).
   Principle. A sitting or supine position allows access to the apex of the heart.

4. **Procedural Step.** Warm the chestpiece of the stethoscope with your hand. Insert the earpieces of the stethoscope into your ears, with the earpieces directed slightly forward, and place the chestpiece over the apex of the patient's heart. The apex of the heart is located in the fifth intercostal space at the junction of the left midclavicular line.
   Principle. Warming the chestpiece reduces the discomfort of having a cold object placed on the chest. In addition, a cold chestpiece could startle the patient, resulting in an increase in the pulse rate. The earpieces should be directed forward to follow the direction of the ear canal, which facilitates hearing.

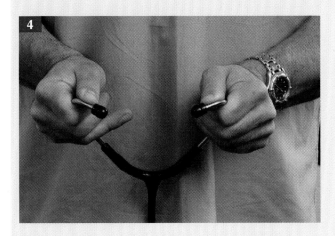

5. **Procedural Step.** Listen for the heartbeat and count the number of beats for 30 seconds (and multiply by 2) if the rhythm and volume are normal or if the apical pulse is being taken on an infant or child. If abnormalities occur in the rhythm or volume, count the pulse for 1 full minute. You will hear a "lubb-dupp" sound through the stethoscope. This sound is the closing of the heart's valves. Each "lubb-dupp" is counted as one beat.

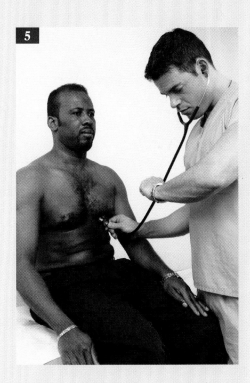

6. **Procedural Step.** Chart the results. Include the date, time, and the apical pulse rate, rhythm, and volume.

7. **Procedural Step.** Clean the earpieces and the chestpiece of the stethoscope with an alcohol wipe.

CHARTING EXAMPLE

Date	
10/15/05	10:15 a.m. AP: 68. Reg and strong.————————————— S. Martinez, CMA

PROCEDURE 4-6

Blood Pressure

Mechanism of Blood Pressure

Blood pressure is a measurement of the pressure or force exerted by the blood on the walls of the arteries in which it is contained. Each time the ventricles contract, blood is pushed out of the heart and into the aorta and pulmonary aorta, exerting pressure on the walls of the arteries. This phase in the cardiac cycle is known as **systole,** and it represents the highest point of blood pressure in the body, or the **systolic pressure.** The phase of the cardiac cycle in which the heart relaxes between contractions is referred to as **diastole.** The **diastolic pressure** (recorded during diastole) is lower because the heart is relaxed. Thus, contraction and relaxation of the heart result in two different pressures, systolic and diastolic.

Interpretation of Blood Pressure

Blood pressure is abbreviated BP, and its measurement is expressed as a fraction. The numerator represents the systolic pressure, and the denominator is the diastolic pressure. Blood pressure is measured in millimeters of mercury, abbreviated mm Hg. A blood pressure reading of 120/80 means that there was enough force to raise a column of mercury 120 mm during systole and 80 mm during diastole.

Based on new guidelines from the National Heart, Lung, and Blood Institute (NHLBI), a blood pressure less than 120/80 mm Hg is classified as normal, whereas a blood pressure between 120/80 and 139/89 is classified as *prehypertension.* These guidelines were issued as a result of scientific studies that showed that the risk of heart disease begins at a blood pressure reading lower than previously thought. The NHLBI guidelines are outlined in Table 4-7.

Blood pressure should be taken during every office visit to allow the physician to compare the patient's readings over time. This is a good preventive measure in guarding against serious illness. A single blood pressure reading taken on one occasion does not characterize an individual's blood pressure accurately. Several readings, taken on different occasions, provide a good index of an individual's baseline blood pressure.

Blood pressure readings always should be interpreted using a patient's baseline blood pressure. A rise or fall of 20 to 30 mm Hg in a patient's baseline blood pressure is significant, even if it is still within the normal accepted blood pressure range.

The most common condition that causes an abnormal blood pressure reading is high blood pressure, or **hypertension.** Hypertension results from excessive pressure on the walls of the arteries. Hypertension is determined by a sustained systolic blood pressure reading of 140 or higher or a sustained diastolic reading of 90 or higher. See Table 4-7 for the NHLBI classifications for hypertension. **Hypotension** results from reduced pressure on the arterial walls. Hypotension is determined by a blood pressure reading below 95/60 mm Hg.

Pulse Pressure

The difference between systolic and diastolic pressure is the **pulse pressure.** It is determined by subtracting the smaller number from the larger. For example, if the blood pressure is 110/70, the pulse pressure would be 40 mm Hg. A pulse pressure between 30 and 50 is considered to be within normal range.

Factors Affecting Blood Pressure

Blood pressure does not remain at a constant value. Numerous factors may affect it throughout the course of the day. An understanding of these factors will help ensure an accurate interpretation of blood pressure readings.

Age. Age is an important consideration when determining whether a patient's blood pressure is normal. As age increases, the blood pressure gradually increases: a 6-year-old child may have a normal reading of 90/60, whereas a young, healthy adult may have a blood pressure reading of 116/76, and it would not be unusual for a 60-year-old man to have a reading of 130/90.

Gender. Following puberty, women usually have a lower blood pressure than men of the same age. After menopause, women usually have a higher blood pressure than men of the same age.

Diurnal variations. Fluctuations in an individual's blood pressure are normal during the course of a day. When one awakens, the blood pressure is lower as a result of the decreased metabolism and physical activity during sleep. As metabolism and activity increase during the day, the blood pressure rises.

Emotional states. Strong emotional states, such as anger, fear, and excitement, increase the blood pressure. If the medical assistant observes such a reaction, an attempt should be made to calm the patient

---

What Would You DO?
What Would You *Not* DO?

Case Study 3

Tyronne Jackson, 45 years old, is at the office to have his blood pressure checked. Three months ago Tyronne started taking a diuretic and an antihypertensive prescribed by the physician to lower his blood pressure. The last recording in his chart indicates that Tyronne's blood pressure fell from 180/112 to 126/84; however, his blood pressure at this visit is 158/98. Tyronne says that he hasn't been very good at taking his medication lately. He says it's really hard to remember to take all those pills every day. He also says that he felt just fine before being put on blood pressure pills, but once he started taking them, he felt awful. He had to urinate more often, when he got up fast, he felt dizzy, and he had some problems with headaches. Tyronne says that he decided to cut back on his pills to see if these problems got better, and sure enough, they went away altogether. Tyronne wants to know if there's anything he can do to lower his blood pressure besides take pills.

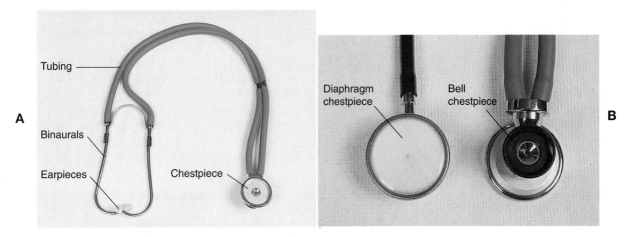

Figure 4-13. A, The parts of a stethoscope. B, Types of chestpieces.

TABLE 4-7	Classification of Blood Pressure for Adults Age 18 and Older		
Blood Pressure Classifications	**Systolic Blood Pressure (mm Hg)**		**Diastolic Blood Pressure (mm Hg)**
Normal	Less than 120	AND	Less than 80
Prehypertension*	120-139	OR	80-89
Hypertension*			
Stage 1	140-159	OR	90-99
Stage 2	160 or higher	OR	100 or higher

From the Seventh Report of The Joint National Committee on Detection, Evaluation, and Treatment of High Blood Pressure. National Heart, Lung, and Blood Institute. U.S. Department of Health and Human Services. NIH Publication, 2003.
*Based on the average of two or more properly measured, seated blood pressure readings taken at each of two or more visits.

before taking blood pressure. Other factors that may increase the blood pressure include pain, a recent meal, smoking, and bladder distention.

Exercise. Physical activity temporarily increases the blood pressure. To ensure an accurate reading, a patient who has been involved in physical activity should be given an opportunity to rest for 20 to 30 minutes before blood pressure is measured.

Body position. In some cases, the blood pressure of a patient who is in a lying or standing position may be different from that measured when the patient is sitting. A notation should be made on the patient's chart if the reading was obtained in any position other than sitting, using the following abbreviations: *L* (lying) and *St* (standing).

Medications. Many medications may either increase or decrease the blood pressure. Because of this factor, it is important to record all prescription and OTC medications that the patient is taking in his or her chart.

Assessment of Blood Pressure

The equipment needed to measure blood pressure includes a stethoscope and a sphygmomanometer. The **stethoscope** amplifies sounds produced by the body and allows the medical assistant to hear them.

Stethoscope

The most common type of stethoscope used in the medical office is the acoustical stethoscope. It consists of four parts: earpieces, sidepieces known as binaurals, plastic or rubber tubing, and a chestpiece (Figure 4-13, *A*).

Stethoscope Chestpiece

There are two types of chestpieces—a *diaphragm,* which is a large, flat disc, and a *bell,* which has a bowl-shaped appearance (Figure 4-13, *B*). The chestpiece of a stethoscope may be a diaphragm, a bell, or both. If a chestpiece consists of both a diaphragm and a bell, the medical assistant must make sure the desired piece is rotated into position before use. Failure to do so will not allow the medical assistant to hear sound through the earpieces.

The diaphragm chestpiece is more useful for hearing high-pitched sounds like lung and bowel sounds, whereas the bell chestpiece is more useful for hearing low-pitched sounds such as those produced by the heart and vascular system. Before using a stethoscope, the medical assistant should make sure that it is in proper working condition.

Sphygmomanometers

The **sphygmomanometer** is an instrument that measures the pressure of blood within an artery. It consists of a

manometer, an inner inflatable bladder surrounded by a covering known as the cuff, and a pressure bulb with a control valve to inflate and deflate the inner bladder. The manometer contains a scale for registering the pressure of the air in the bladder.

The two types of sphygmomanometers are the aneroid and mercury. The *aneroid sphygmomanometer* is lightweight and portable, but the *mercury sphygmomanometer* is more accurate.

Aneroid Sphygmomanometer

The aneroid sphygmomanometer (Figure 4-14) has a gauge with a round scale. The scale is calibrated in millimeters, with a needle that points to the calibrations (Figure 4-15). To ensure an accurate reading, the needle must be positioned initially at zero. The manometer must be placed in the correct position for proper viewing. The medical assistant should be no farther than 3 feet from the scale on the gauge of the manometer, and the manometer should be placed so that it can be viewed directly. At least once a year, an aneroid sphygmomanometer should be recalibrated to ensure its accuracy.

Mercury Sphygmomanometer

The mercury sphygmomanometer (Figure 4-16) has a vertical tube calibrated in millimeters that is filled with mercury. Although more accurate than the aneroid sphygmo-

manometer, the use of the mercury sphygmomanometer is being discouraged because mercury is a hazardous chemical.

If a mercury manometer is used to take blood pressure, it must be placed in the correct position for proper viewing. The medical assistant should be no farther than 3 feet from the scale of the manometer. A portable mercury manometer should be placed on a flat surface so that the mercury column is in a vertical position. The wall model mercury manometer is mounted securely against a wall, thereby placing the mercury column in a vertical position.

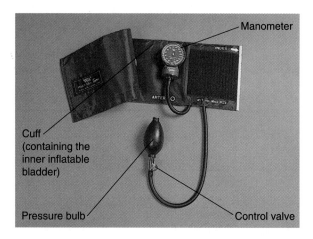

Figure 4-14. The parts of an aneroid sphygmomanometer.

Highlight on Stethoscopes

The stethoscope was first introduced in the 1800s by a French physician named René Laennec. This early stethoscope consisted of a simple wooden tube with a bell-shaped opening at one end.

The selection of a stethoscope is an individual decision. You will hear sounds differently when using different stethoscopes. The primary consideration in choosing a stethoscope should be that it is well made and fits well in your ears. Stethoscopes are available from uniform shops and medical supply companies.

The usual length of tubing on a stethoscope is 12 to 16 inches (30 to 40 cm), but you may prefer the longer 22-inch tubing. An argument against long tubing is that it transmits sound less efficiently. Research has shown, however, that 6 to 8 more inches of tubing does not significantly alter the transmission of most sounds.

The stethoscope should have metal binaurals. The binaurals should allow you to angle the earpieces firmly to follow the direction of your ear canal. Binaurals that are too tight are uncomfortable, and binaurals that are too loose do not allow you to hear as well as you should.

The earpieces should fit comfortably and snugly in the ear canal. If you can understand what someone is saying in the same room, they are too loose, which will interfere with effective auscultation. Some stethoscopes come with removable ear tips in different sizes. This offers the advantage of selecting an

ear tip that fits your ear canal. Flexible ear tips of soft rubber are usually more comfortable than nonflexible tips of hard rubber or plastic.

The chestpiece should be a key factor in the selection of a stethoscope. A stethoscope with both a diaphragm and a bell offers the most versatility for listening to different types of sound. Many stethoscopes have a rubber or plastic nonchill rim around the diaphragm and bell to avoid chilling the patient with a cold chestpiece and to decrease air leaks between the chestpiece and the patient.

The most common problem with use of stethoscopes is air leak. Air leaks interfere with effective sound transmission and also allow environmental noise to enter the stethoscope. Air leaks may result from a cracked earpiece, a cracked or chipped chestpiece, or a break in the tubing.

Stethoscopes must be cared for properly to ensure proper functioning and to prevent the transmission of disease in the medical office. The earpieces should be removed and cleaned regularly with a cotton-tipped applicator moistened with alcohol to remove cerumen. The chestpiece should be cleaned with an alcohol wipe to remove dirt, dust, lint, and oils. The tubing should be cleaned with a paper towel using an antimicrobial soap and water. Alcohol should not be used to clean the tubing because it can dry out the tubing and cause it to crack over time.

The following guidelines must be followed when measuring blood pressure with a mercury sphygmomanometer. Before the blood pressure reading is obtained, the mercury must be even with the zero level at the base of the calibrated tube. Pressure created by inflation of the inner bladder causes the mercury to rise in the tube. The top portion of the mercury column, the **meniscus,** curves slightly upward. The blood pressure should be read at the top of the meniscus, with the eye at the same level as the meniscus of the mercury column.

Cuff Sizes

Blood pressure cuffs come in a variety of sizes and are measured in centimeters (cm) (Figure 4-17). The size of a cuff refers to its inner inflatable bladder rather than its cloth cover. Table 4-8 lists the types of cuffs available and the size of the inner bladder of each cuff.

For accurate blood pressure measurement, the inner bladder of the cuff should encircle at least 80% of the arm circumference and be wide enough to cover two thirds of the distance from the axilla to the antecubital space (Figure 4-18). Child cuffs must often be used for adults with thin arms. The adult cuff is used for the average-sized adult arm, and the thigh cuff is used for taking blood pressure from the thigh or for adults with large arms. If the cuff is too small, the reading may be falsely high, as it would be, for example, when an adult cuff is used on a patient with a large arm. On the other hand, if the cuff is too large, the reading may be falsely low, as it would be when an adult cuff is used with a patient with a thin arm. The cuff should fit snugly and should be applied so that the center of the inflatable bag is directly over the artery to be compressed. The cuff has an interlocking, self-sticking substance (Velcro) that facilitates closing and fastening the cuff in place temporarily.

Korotkoff Sounds

Korotkoff sounds are used to determine the systolic and diastolic blood pressure readings. When the cuff is inflated, the brachial artery is compressed so that no audible sounds are heard through the stethoscope. As the cuff is deflated, at a rate of 2 to 3 mm Hg per second, the sounds become audible until the blood flows freely and they can no longer be heard (Table 4-9). The medical assistant should practice listening to these sounds and be able to identify the various phases.

Procedure 4-7 outlines the procedure for taking blood pressure using an aneroid sphygmomanometer.

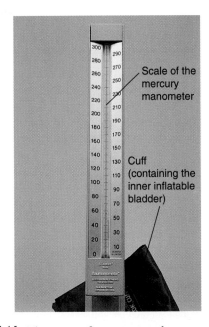

Figure 4-16. The parts of a mercury sphygmomanometer.

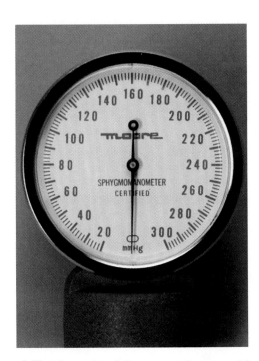

Figure 4-15. The scale of the gauge of an aneroid sphygmomanometer.

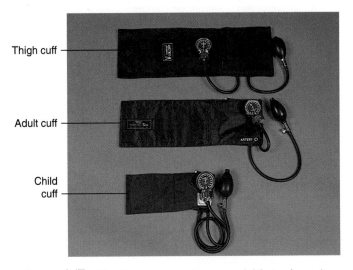

Figure 4-17. Blood pressure cuffs are available in three sizes: child, adult, and thigh.

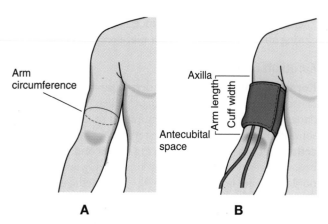

Figure 4-18. Determination of proper cuff size. **A,** The bladder of the cuff should be long enough to encircle 80% of the arm. **B,** The cuff should be wide enough to cover two thirds of the distance from the axilla to the antecubital space.

TABLE 4-8	Types of Blood Pressure Cuffs
Cuff	**Bladder Length (cm)**
Child	21
Small adult	24
Adult	30
Large adult	38
Adult thigh	42

Prevention of Errors in Blood Pressure Measurement

The following guidelines should be followed to prevent errors in blood pressure measurement:

1. **Instruct the patient** not to consume caffeine or use tobacco for 30 minutes before the blood pressure measurement.
2. **The patient should be seated** in a quiet room for at least 5 minutes before blood pressure is taken.
3. **Always use the proper cuff size.** If the cuff is too small, the reading may be falsely high, and if the cuff is too large, the reading may be falsely low. The inner inflatable bladder of the cuff should encircle at least 80% of the patient's arm and cover two thirds of the distance from the axilla to the antecubital space.
4. **Never take blood pressure over clothing.** Roll up the patient's sleeve approximately 5 inches above the elbow. If the sleeve is too tight after being rolled up, remove the arm from the sleeve. A tight sleeve causes partial compression of the brachial artery, resulting in an inaccurate reading.
5. **Position the patient's arm properly.** Position the arm at heart level, and make sure it is well supported with the palm facing upward. If the arm is above heart level, the blood pressure reading may be falsely low.
6. **Avoid extraneous sounds from the cuff.** Position the cuff approximately 1 inch above the bend in the elbow. The cuff should be up far enough to prevent the stethoscope from touching it; otherwise extraneous sounds, which could interfere with an accurate measurement, may be picked up.
7. **Compress the brachial artery completely.** Center the inner bladder of the cuff directly over the artery to be compressed. Most cuffs are labeled with an arrow indicating the center of the bladder. Centering the inner bladder allows for complete compression of the brachial artery.
8. **Apply equal pressure over the brachial artery.** The cuff should be applied so that it fits smoothly and snugly around the patient's arm. This prevents bulging or slipping and permits application of an equal pressure over the brachial artery.
9. **Position the earpieces so you can hear the sounds clearly.** Place the earpieces of the stethoscope in your ears with the earpieces directed slightly forward. This allows the earpieces to follow the direction of the ear canal, which facilitates hearing.
10. **Avoid extraneous sounds.** Make sure the tubing of the stethoscope hangs freely and is not permitted to rub against any object. If the stethoscope tubing rubs against an object, extraneous sounds may be picked up, which could interfere with an accurate measurement.
11. **Position the chestpiece properly.** Palpate the brachial pulse to provide good positioning of the chestpiece over the brachial artery. Place the chestpiece firmly, but gently, over the brachial artery to assist in transmitting clear and audible sounds. Do not allow the chestpiece to touch the cuff to prevent extraneous sounds from being picked up, which could interfere with an accurate measurement.
12. **Release the pressure at a moderate steady rate.** Release the pressure in the cuff at a rate of 2 to 3 mm Hg per second to ensure an accurate blood pressure measurement. Releasing the pressure too quickly or too slowly could cause a falsely low systolic reading and a falsely high diastolic reading.
13. **Avoid venous congestion.** If you need to take the blood pressure in the same arm again, wait 1 to 2 minutes to allow blood trapped in the veins (venous congestion) to be released. Venous congestion can result in a falsely high systolic reading and a falsely low diastolic reading.
14. **Measure and record the blood pressure in both arms during the initial BP assessment of a new patient.** There may normally be a difference of 5 to 10 mm Hg between the two arms. During return visits, the blood pressure should be measured in the arm with the higher initial reading.

TABLE 4-9   Korotkoff Sounds

Phase	Description	Illustration
	Inflation of the cuff compresses and closes off the brachial artery so that no blood flows through the artery.	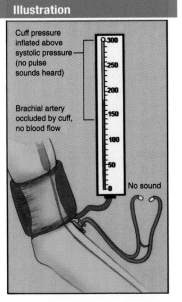
Phase I	The first faint but clear tapping sound is heard, and it gradually increases in intensity. The first tapping sound is the systolic pressure.	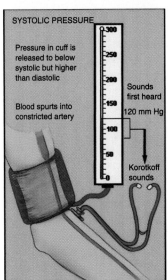
Phase II	As the cuff continues to deflate, the sounds have a murmuring or swishing quality.	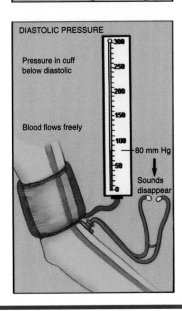
Phase III	With further deflation the sounds become crisper and increase in intensity.	
Phase IV	The sounds become muffled and have a soft, blowing quality. According to the American Heart Association, the onset of muffled sounds is the best index of the diastolic pressure in children. The pressure in the cuff is released at a moderate steady rate of 2 to 3 mm Hg per second.	
Phase V	The sounds disappear. This is typically recorded as the diastolic pressure for an adult. Some authorities believe that the adult diastolic pressure falls midway between phases IV and V; therefore some physicians want the medical assistant to record both phases IV and V as the diastolic pressure (e.g., 120/84/80).	

‖) PATIENT **TEACHING**

Hypertension

- Answer questions patients have about hypertension.

What is high blood pressure?
Blood pressure is the force of blood against the walls of the arteries. High blood pressure, also called **hypertension,** means the pressure in the arteries is consistently above normal (140/90), resulting in excessive pressure on the walls of the arteries.

What are the symptoms of high blood pressure?
Approximately one third of people who have high blood pressure are not aware of it because there are few or no symptoms. Hypertension is the most common life-threatening disease among Americans. It is estimated that 1 in 4 Americans has high blood pressure. The only way to know for sure whether you have high blood pressure is to have it checked regularly.

What causes high blood pressure?
In about 90% of cases, the precise cause of high blood pressure is unknown. This type of hypertension is known as *essential,* or *primary, hypertension.* Certain factors, however, seem to increase the risk of developing essential hypertension. These risk factors include:

- *Heredity.* A family history of high blood pressure increases an individual's risk of developing high blood pressure.
- *Weight.* Individuals who are overweight are two to six times more likely than the general population to develop high blood pressure.
- *Race.* Research has shown that more black than white Americans develop high blood pressure.
- *Age.* Blood pressure normally increases as you grow older.
- *Sodium intake.* Sodium found in salt and processed, canned, and most snack foods does not cause high blood pressure; however, it can aggravate high blood pressure. Most Americans consume more sodium than they need. The current recommendation is to consume less than 2.4 g (2400 mg) of sodium a day. This is equivalent to 6 g (about 1 teaspoon) of salt.

- *Stress.* Research indicates that people who are under continuous stress tend to develop more heart and circulatory problems than those who are not under stress.
- *Smoking.* Smoking tobacco constricts blood vessels, causing an increase in blood pressure.
- *Alcohol consumption.* Heavy alcohol consumption may increase the blood pressure.

What can happen if high blood pressure is not treated?
If high blood pressure is not brought under control, it can cause severe damage to vital organs such as the heart, brain, and kidneys, resulting in a heart attack or heart failure, stroke, or kidney damage. Early detection and treatment of high blood pressure can prevent these complications.

Can high blood pressure be cured?
High blood pressure cannot be cured, but a number of treatments are used to bring it under control. These include lifestyle modifications such as weight reduction, a healthy diet rich in fruits and vegetables and low in saturated fat, limitation of salt intake, regular aerobic exercise, cessation of smoking, limitation or elimination of alcohol consumption, and stress management. If lifestyle modifications alone are not enough, medications are available for lowering blood pressure, allowing the patient to lead a normal, healthy, active life.

How long will I undergo treatment?
Treatment is usually a lifelong process. Even if you feel fine, you'll probably have to continue treatment for the rest of your life to keep your blood pressure down. If you discontinue your diet and lifestyle changes or stop taking your medication, your blood pressure will go up again.

- Encourage patients with hypertension to adhere to the treatment prescribed by the physician. Help patients remember to take their medication by telling them to associate their medication schedule with a daily routine, such as brushing their teeth or having meals.
- Provide the patient with educational materials on high blood pressure available from sources such as the American Heart Association.

PROCEDURE 4-7　Measuring Blood Pressure

Outcome Measure blood pressure.

Equipment/Supplies:
- Stethoscope
- Sphygmomanometer
- Antiseptic wipe

1. **Procedural Step.** Sanitize your hands and assemble the equipment. Be sure to select the proper cuff size. If the chestpiece consists of both a diaphragm and a bell, rotate it to the diaphragm position. Clean the earpieces and chestpiece of the stethoscope with the antiseptic wipe.

Principle. The chestpiece must be rotated to the proper position for sound to be heard through the earpieces.

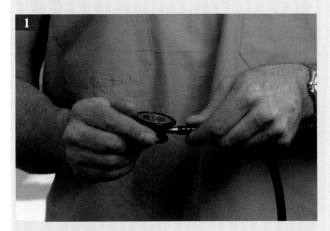

2. **Procedural Step.** Greet and identify the patient. Introduce yourself and explain the procedure. While explaining the procedure, observe the patient for signs that might influence the reading, such as anger, fear, pain, and recent physical activity. If it is not possible to reduce or eliminate these influences, list them in the patient's chart.

3. **Procedural Step.** Have the patient sit in a comfortable position. Roll up the patient's sleeve approximately 5 inches above the elbow. If the sleeve does not roll up or is too tight after being rolled up, remove the arm from the sleeve. The arm should be positioned at heart level and well supported, with the palm facing up. Make a notation in the patient's chart if the lying or standing position was used to take blood pressure. Abbreviations that can be used are L (lying) and St (standing).

Principle. A tight sleeve causes partial compression of the brachial artery, resulting in an inaccurate reading. The position of the arm allows easy access to the brachial artery. Placing the arm above heart level may cause the reading to be falsely low.

4. **Procedural Step.** Select the proper cuff size. The inner inflatable bladder of the cuff should be long enough to encircle at least 80% of the patient's arm and wide enough to cover two thirds of the distance from the axilla to the antecubital space.

Principle. The appropriate size cuff must be used to ensure an accurate measurement.

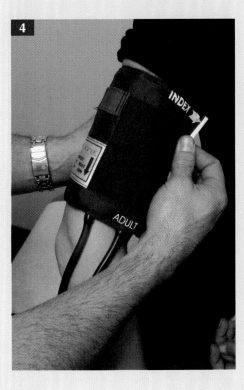

PROCEDURE 4-7

Continued

PROCEDURE 4-7   Measuring Blood Pressure—Cont'd

5. Procedural Step. Locate the brachial pulse with the fingertips. Center the inner bladder over the brachial pulse site. (NOTE: Place the cuff on the patient's arm so that the lower edge of the cuff is approximately 1 inch above the bend in the elbow. Most cuffs are labeled with a right and left arrow indicating the center of the bladder. The right arrow should be placed over the brachial pulse site when you are using the right arm, and the left arrow should be placed over the brachial pulse site when you are using the left arm.)

Principle. The cuff should be placed high enough to prevent the stethoscope from touching it; otherwise, extraneous sounds, which could interfere with an accurate measurement, may be picked up. Centering the inner bladder over the pulse site allows complete compression of the brachial artery.

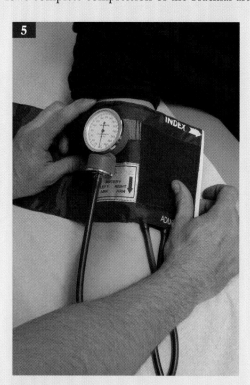

6. Procedural Step. Wrap the cuff smoothly and snugly around the patient's arm, and secure the end of it.

Principle. Applying the cuff properly prevents it from bulging or slipping. This technique permits application of an equal pressure over the brachial artery.

7. Procedural Step. Position the manometer for direct viewing and at a distance of no more than 3 feet.

Principle. The medical assistant may have trouble seeing the scale on the manometer if it is placed more than 3 feet away.

8. Procedural Step. Place the earpieces of the stethoscope in your ears, with the earpieces directed slightly forward. During the blood pressure measurement, the tubing of the stethoscope should hang freely and should not be permitted to rub against any object.

Principle. The earpieces should be directed forward, permitting them to follow the direction of the ear canal, which facilitates hearing. If the stethoscope tubing rubs against an object, extraneous sounds may be picked up, which will interfere with an accurate measurement.

9. Procedural Step. Making sure the arm is well extended, locate the brachial pulse again, and place the diaphragm of the stethoscope over the brachial pulse site. The diaphragm should be positioned to make a tight seal against the patient's skin. Enough pressure should be exerted to leave a temporary ring on the patient's skin when the disk is removed. Do not allow the chestpiece to touch the cuff.

Principle. Locating the brachial pulse is necessary for good positioning of the chestpiece over the brachial artery. A well-extended arm allows easier palpation of the brachial pulse. Good contact of the chestpiece with the skin helps transmit clear and audible Korotkoff sounds through the ear-

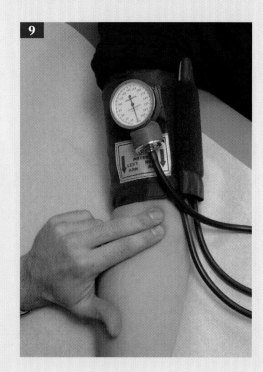

pieces of the stethoscope. If the chestpiece touches the cuff, extraneous sounds may be picked up, which will interfere with an accurate measurement.

10. Procedural Step. Close the valve on the bulb by turning the thumbscrew clockwise until it feels tight. Pump air into the cuff as rapidly as possible, up to a level of 20 to 30 mm Hg above the palpated (see Procedure 4-8) or previously measured systolic pressure. Explain to the patient that this will cause numbing and tingling in the arm.

Principle. Inflation of the cuff compresses and closes off the brachial artery so that no blood flows through the artery. A preliminary determination of the systolic pressure, by palpation, allows the medical assistant to estimate how high to inflate the cuff. Procedure 4-8 explains how to palpate the systolic pressure. If the patient has had the blood pressure measured previously at the medical office, the recorded systolic pressure can be used to determine how high to inflate the cuff.

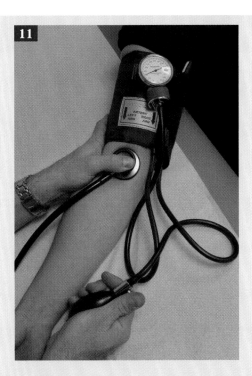

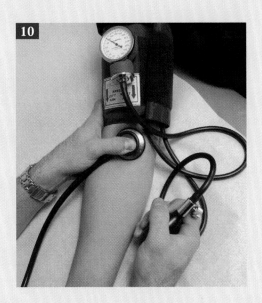

11. Procedural Step. Release the pressure at a moderately steady rate of 2 to 3 mm Hg per second by slowly turning the thumbscrew counterclockwise. This opens the valve and allows the air in the cuff to escape slowly. Listen for the first clear tapping sound (phase I of the Korotkoff sounds). This represents the systolic pressure. Note this point on the scale of the manometer.

Principle. The systolic pressure is the point at which the blood first begins to spurt through the artery as the cuff pressure begins to decrease; it represents the pressure that occurs on the walls of the arteries during systole.

12. Procedural Step. Continue to deflate the cuff while listening to the Korotkoff sounds. Listen for the onset of the muffled sound that occurs during phase IV. Continue to deflate the cuff and note the point on the scale at which the sound ceases (Phase V).

Principle. Phase V marks the diastolic pressure (which represents the pressure that occurs on the walls of the arteries during diastole); the cuff pressure is reduced, and blood is flowing freely through the brachial artery.

13. Procedural Step. Quickly and completely deflate the cuff to zero. If you could not obtain an accurate blood pressure reading, wait 1 to 2 minutes and repeat the blood pressure measurement procedure. Remove the earpieces of the stethoscope from your ears, and carefully remove the cuff from the patient's arm.

Principle. Venous congestion results when blood pressure is taken, which will alter a second reading if it is taken too soon.

14. Procedural Step. Chart the results. Include the date, the time, and the blood pressure reading. Blood pressure is recorded using even numbers.

15. Procedural Step. Clean the earpieces and the chestpiece of the stethoscope with an antiseptic wipe and replace the equipment properly.

CHARTING EXAMPLE

Date	
10/20/05	2:30 p.m. BP: 106/74.— S. Martinez, RMA

PROCEDURE 4-8   Determining Systolic Pressure by Palpation

Outcome Determine systolic pressure by palpation.

Equipment/Supplies:

• Sphygmomanometer

1. **Procedural Step.** Sanitize your hands and assemble equipment.
2. **Procedural Step.** Locate the brachial pulse with the fingertips. Place the cuff on the patient's arm so that the inner bladder is centered over the brachial pulse site.
3. **Procedural Step.** Wrap the cuff smoothly and snugly around the patient's arm and secure the end of it.
4. **Procedural Step.** Position the manometer for direct viewing and at a distance of no more than 3 feet.
5. **Procedural Step.** Locate the radial pulse with your fingertips.
6. **Procedural Step.** Close the valve on the bulb and pump air into the cuff until the pulsation ceases.
7. **Procedural Step.** Release the valve at a moderate rate of 2 to 3 mm Hg per heartbeat while palpating the artery with your fingertips.
8. **Procedural Step.** Record the point at which the pulsation reappears as the palpated systolic pressure.
9. **Procedural Step.** Deflate the cuff completely, and wait 15 to 30 seconds before checking the blood pressure.

MEDICAL Practice and the LAW

Measurement of vital signs is standard procedure for almost every patient in the physician's office. Because vital sign measurements are performed so frequently, the medical assistant may tend to minimize their importance. Changes in vital signs may be the first indicator of disease or illness, so meticulous attention must be paid to the performance and documentation of vital signs, as well as comparing the current measurements with past measurements for each patient.

Most patients want to know their vital signs, especially their blood pressure or temperature if febrile. Although the patient owns the information that you collect, be aware that you may not give this information to family members without the patient's consent. Some offices have a policy that indicates specific information the medical assistant can give the patient; some physicians prefer to disclose this information themselves and discuss it with their patients.

Often the measurement of vital signs is the first contact the patients have with the medical assistant. The most important factor in determining whether a patient will sue is not the skill of the practitioner, but the level of rapport with the patient. In everything you do, convey your caring and concern to every patient.

What Would You DO?
What Would You *Not* DO? *RESPONSES*

Case Study 1

What Did Sergio Do?

❏ Told Mrs. Mason that sometimes ear thermometers can be a little tricky to use.

❏ Showed Mrs. Mason how to use the ear thermometer and let her practice by taking Olivia's temperature.

❏ Explained how to care for and maintain the ear thermometer to prevent inaccurate readings.

❏ Explained to Mrs. Mason that the use of mercury is being discouraged because it can be toxic to both humans and animals.

What Did Sergio Not Do?

❏ Did not ask Mrs. Mason if she had read the directions that came with her ear thermometer.

❏ Did not tell Mrs. Mason that she should switch back to the mercury thermometer.

❏ Did not ask Mrs. Mason why she waited so long to bring Olivia to the office.

What Would You Do/What Would You *Not* Do? Review Sergio's response and place a checkmark next to the information you included in your response. List the additional information you included in your response.

_____

_____

_____

_____

Case Study 2

What Did Sergio Do?

❏ Recognized and congratulated Alex on his swimming achievements.

❏ Told Alex that it is normal for his pulse to be that slow because of his athletic training, and it shows that he is in good shape.

❏ Assured Alex that the physician will do everything he can to help Alex.

❏ Stressed to Alex how important it is to follow the physician's advice so that his shoulder heals as soon as possible.

What Did Sergio Not Do?

❏ Did not comment on Alex's request for steroids or codeine. Made sure to chart the information so that the physician could handle the situation.

❏ Did not criticize Alex for putting a swim meet before his health.

What Would You Do/What Would You *Not* Do? Review Sergio's response and place a checkmark next to the information you included in your response. List the additional information you included in your response.

_____

_____

_____

_____

Case Study 3

What Did Sergio Do?

❏ Empathized with Tyronne about having to take so many pills. Suggested that he get a daily pill container to help him remember.

❏ Stressed to Tyronne the importance of taking his blood pressure medication. Explained to him that high blood pressure is a "silent disease." He may feel just fine, but damage to his body organs can still be taking place if he doesn't take his pills.

❏ Gave Tyronne a brochure about high blood pressure and went over the long-term effects of hypertension and lifestyle changes that could help lower blood pressure.

❏ Encouraged Tyronne to call the office when he experiences side effects from medications because the physician may be able to do something to help.

What Did Sergio Not Do?

❏ Did not tell him it was all right to discontinue his medication.

What Would You Do/What Would You *Not* Do? Review Sergio's response and place a checkmark next to the information you included in your response. List the additional information you included in your response.

_____

_____

_____

_____

Apply Your KNOWLEDGE

Choose the best answer for each of the following questions.

1. Clara Ashworth is a patient who has come to the office for a checkup. She has COPD and is short of breath most of the time. Because of this condition, she always breathes through her mouth. Sergio Martinez, RMA, needs to check her temperature. His office uses electronic thermometers for taking temperature. Which site would Sergio choose to take Clara's temperature?
   A. Mouth   C. Ear
   B. Rectum   D. Axilla

2. Tyler Tompkins is 5 years old. His mother has brought him to the office for his kindergarten physical examination. Sergio Martinez, RMA, needs to take Tyler's vital signs. Before taking Tyler's aural temperature, Sergio checks the lens of the probe to make sure it is clean and shiny because he realizes that a dirty lens can result in
   A. A falsely low temperature reading
   B. A falsely high temperature reading
   C. Otitis media
   D. Beans growing in the ear

3. While taking Tyler's aural temperature, Sergio makes sure to use proper technique. Sergio performs all of the following EXCEPT
   A. Applies a plastic cover to the probe
   B. Pulls Tyler's ear down and back
   C. Seals the opening of Tyler's ear with the probe
   D. Positions the tip of the probe toward Tyler's opposite temple

4. Before putting the ear thermometer away, Sergio cleans the lens of the probe by wiping it with
   A. Hydrogen peroxide   C. Water
   B. Alcohol   D. Bleach

5. Caitlin Perry, age 28, comes to the medical office for an employment physical. Sergio Martinez, RMA, takes Caitlin's pulse for 30 seconds and counts 45 beats. Sergio realizes that Caitlin's pulse rate
   A. Indicates bradycardia
   B. Is normal
   C. Indicates tachycardia
   D. Indicates hyperpnea

6. Sergio is now ready to measure Caitlin's respirations. All of the following would be correct techniques for Sergio to use EXCEPT
   A. Counting the respirations for 30 seconds and multiplying times 2

   B. Continuing to hold his fingers over the wrist area while counting respirations
   C. Instructing Caitlin to remain still so that her respirations can be counted
   D. Noting the rhythm and depth of the respirations

7. Sergio is preparing to take Caitlin's blood pressure using an aneroid sphygmomanometer. To ensure an accurate reading, Sergio makes sure that the
   A. Bladder is centered over the brachial artery
   B. Needle of the gauge is at zero
   C. Chestpiece is not touching the cuff
   D. All of the above

8. Paula Simons has a history of cardiac problems and is on cardiac medication. She has come to the office for a checkup. While taking her radial pulse, Sergio Martinez, RMA, notices that the rhythm is irregular. He recognizes that Paula
   A. Is having a heart attack
   B. Is having side effects from her cardiac medication
   C. Has a dysrhythmia and counts her pulse for 1 full minute
   D. Has a normal pulse

9. Carlos Ramirez has come to the office because he has been sick with an upper respiratory infection. Carlos has suffered from chronic bronchitis for the past 4 years. He is short of breath, and his lips and nailbeds are bluish. Terms that could be used to document his symptoms would be
   A. Dyspnea and cyanosis
   B. Orthopnea and paleness
   C. Tachypnea and flushed
   D. Bradypnea and cyanosis

10. Ivan Peabody, 42 years old, comes to the office for his annual physical examination. Sergio Martinez, RMA, takes his vital signs. His blood pressure is 138/88. Sergio realizes this reading falls into the following category:
   A. Normal
   B. Prehypertension
   C. Hypertension, stage 1
   D. Hypertension, stage 2

11. All of the following statements by Ivan indicate that he may be at risk for hyptertension EXCEPT
   A. "I need to quit smoking."
   B. "I have been overweight since I was a teenager."
   C. "My father and twin brother have high blood pressure."
   D. "I have been having some problems urinating."

CERTIFICATIONREVIEW

Temperature

❑ **Body temperature is maintained** within a fairly constant range by the hypothalamus, which is located in the brain. Body temperature is maintained through a balance of the heat produced in the body and the heat lost from the body. Heat is produced in the body by voluntary and involuntary muscle contractions, cell metabolism, and strong emotional states. Heat is lost from the body through perspiration; in the urine, feces, and moisture droplets from the lungs; and through conduction, convection, and radiation.

❑ **The normal body temperature range** is 97° to 99° F (36.1° to 37.2° C), with the average body temperature being 98.6° F (37° C). Pyrexia describes a temperature above normal, and hypothermia describes a temperature below normal.

❑ **Factors that affect body temperature** include age, diurnal variations, exercise, emotional states, environmental factors, the patient's normal body temperature, and pregnancy. An individual with a fever is said to be febrile, and one without a fever is afebrile. The course of a fever rises and falls in one of the following patterns: continuous, intermittent, or remittent.

❑ **The four sites** for taking body temperature are the mouth, rectum, axilla, and ear. The site chosen for measuring a patient's temperature depends on the patient's age, condition, and state of consciousness; the type of thermometer being used; and the medical office policy. The temperature obtained through the rectal route measures approximately 1° F higher than the same person's temperature taken through the oral route. The axillary temperature measures approximately 1° F lower than the same person's temperature taken through the oral route.

❑ **An electronic thermometer** consists of interchangeable oral (blue) and rectal (red) probes attached to a battery-operated portable unit. A disposable plastic cover is placed over the probe to prevent the transmission of microorganisms between patients.

❑ **The tympanic membrane thermometer** is used at the aural site and provides results within 1 to 2 seconds. The thermometer detects thermal energy given off by the tympanic membrane in the form of infrared waves.

❑ **Chemical thermometers** are less accurate than other types of thermometers and are often used by patients at home to provide a general assessment of body temperature.

Pulse

❑ When the left ventricle of the heart contracts, a pulsating wave travels through the walls of the arterial system; this wave is known as the pulse. Pulse rate can vary due to age, gender, physical activity, emotional states, metabolism, fever, and medications.

❑ **The most common site** for measuring pulse is the radial artery, located on the inner aspect of the wrist just below the thumb. The apical pulse, easier to hear than pulse at other sites, is located in the fifth intercostal space at the junction of the left midclavicular line. Other pulse sites are the brachial, ulnar, temporal, carotid, femoral, popliteal, posterior tibial, and dorsalis pedis.

❑ **The normal resting pulse rate** for an adult ranges from 60 to 100 beats per minute. A pulse rate of more than 100 beats per minute is tachycardia, and a pulse rate below 60 beats per minute is bradycardia.

❑ **The pulse rhythm** is the time interval between heartbeats. An irregularity in the heart's rhythm is known as a dysrhythmia (or arrhythmia). The pulse volume refers to the strength of the heartbeat. A thready pulse feels weak and thin, and a bounding pulse feels very strong and full.

Respiration

❑ **One respiration** consists of one inhalation and one exhalation. During inhalation, the diaphragm descends and the lungs expand; during exhalation, the diaphragm ascends and the lungs return to their original state.

❑ **The respiratory rate** of an adult ranges from 12 to 20 respirations per minute. An abnormal increase in the respiratory rate is known as tachypnea, and an abnormal decrease is known as bradypnea.

❑ **Normally, the rhythm** should be even and regular, and the pauses between inhalation and exhalation should be equal. The depth of each respiration should be the same. Hyperpnea denotes a very deep, rapid, and labored type of respiration. Hyperventilation is an abnormally fast and deep type of breathing usually associated with acute anxiety. Hypopnea is an abnormal decrease in the rate and depth of respiration. Dyspnea, or difficult breathing, can be caused by asthma, emphysema, and vigorous physical exertion. Orthopnea means the patient can breathe easier in a sitting or standing position.

Blood Pressure

❑ **Blood pressure measures** the pressure exerted by the blood on the walls of the arteries. The systolic pressure is the highest pressure, and the diastolic pressure is the point of lesser pressure on the arterial walls.

❑ **A blood pressure** less than 120/80 mm Hg is normal. A single blood pressure reading taken on one occasion does not characterize an individual's blood pressure; several readings must be taken on different occasions.

❑ **Hypertension** is excessive pressure on the walls of the arteries and refers to a sustained systolic pressure of 140 or higher or a sustained diastolic reading of 90 or higher.

❑ **Factors that affect blood pressure** are age, gender, diurnal variations, emotional states, exercise, body position, and medication.

Terminology Review

Adventitious sounds Abnormal breath sounds.

Afebrile Without fever; the body temperature is normal.

Alveolus A thin-walled air sac of the lungs in which the exchange of oxygen and carbon dioxide takes place.

Antecubital space The space located at the front of the elbow.

Antipyretic An agent that reduces fever.

Aorta The major trunk of the arterial system of the body. The aorta arises from the upper surface of the left ventricle.

Apnea The temporary cessation of breathing.

Axilla The armpit.

Bounding pulse A pulse with an increased volume that feels very strong and full.

Bradycardia An abnormally slow heart rate (fewer than 60 beats per minute).

Bradypnea An abnormal decrease in the respiratory rate of fewer than 10 respirations per minute.

Celsius scale A temperature scale on which the freezing point of water is 0° and the boiling point of water is 100°. Also called the centigrade scale.

Conduction The transfer of energy, such as heat, from one object to another.

Convection The transfer of energy, such as heat, through air currents.

Crisis A sudden falling of an elevated body temperature to normal.

Cyanosis A bluish discoloration of the skin and mucous membranes.

Diastole The phase in the cardiac cycle in which the heart relaxes between contractions.

Diastolic pressure The point of lesser pressure on the arterial wall, which is recorded during diastole.

Dyspnea Shortness of breath or difficulty in breathing.

Dysrhythmia An irregular rhythm. Also termed arrhythmia.

Eupnea Normal respiration. The rate is 16 to 20 respirations per minute, the rhythm is even and regular, and the depth is normal.

Exhalation The act of breathing out.

Fahrenheit scale A temperature scale on which the freezing point of water is 32° and the boiling point of water is 212°.

Febrile Pertaining to fever.

Fever A body temperature that is above normal. Synonym for pyrexia.

Frenulum linguae The midline fold that connects the undersurface of the tongue with the floor of the mouth.

Hyperpnea An abnormal increase in the rate and depth of respiration.

Hyperpyrexia An extremely high fever.

Hypertension High blood pressure.

Hyperventilation An abnormally fast and deep type of breathing usually associated with acute anxiety conditions.

Hypopnea An abnormal decrease in the rate and depth of respiration.

Hypotension Low blood pressure.

Hypothermia A body temperature that is below normal.

Hypoxia A reduction in the oxygen supply to the tissues of the body.

Inhalation The act of breathing in.

Intercostal Between the ribs.

Korotkoff sounds Sounds heard during the measurement of blood pressure which are used to determine the systolic and diastolic blood pressure readings.

Malaise A vague sense of body discomfort, weakness, and fatigue that often marks the onset of a disease and continues through the course of the illness.

Manometer An instrument for measuring pressure.

Meniscus The curved surface on a column of liquid in a tube.

Orthopnea The condition in which breathing is easier when an individual is in a standing or sitting position.

Pulse pressure The difference between the systolic and diastolic pressures.

Pulse rhythm The time interval between heartbeats.

Pulse volume The strength of the heartbeat.

Radiation The transfer of energy, such as heat, in the form of waves.

Sphygmomanometer An instrument for measuring arterial blood pressure.

Stethoscope An instrument for amplifying and hearing sounds produced by the body.

Systole The phase in the cardiac cycle in which the ventricles contract, sending blood out of the heart and into the aorta and pulmonary aorta.

Systolic pressure The point of maximum pressure on the arterial walls, which is recorded during systole.

Tachycardia An abnormally fast heart rate (more than 100 beats per minute).

Tachypnea An abnormal increase in the respiratory rate of more than 20 respirations per minute.

Thready pulse A pulse with a decreased volume that feels weak and thin.

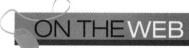

ON THE WEB

For active weblinks to each website visit http://evolve.elsevier.com/Bonewit/.

For Information on Hypertension:

American Heart Association

National Heart, Lung, and Blood Institute

Cardiology Channel

Hypertension Education Foundation

American Society of Hypertension

Novartis Hypertension and Health

For Information on Lung Disease:

American Lung Association

Pulmonology Channel

Lung Cancer Online

Learning Objectives	Procedures

Preparation for the Physical Examination

1. Identify the three components of a complete patient examination.
2. List the guidelines that should be followed in preparing the examining room.
3. Identify equipment and instruments used during the physical examination.

Prepare the examining room.

Operate and care for equipment and instruments used during the physical examination, according to the manufacturer's instructions.

Prepare a patient for a physical examination.

Measuring Weight and Height

1. Explain the purpose of measuring weight and height.
2. List the guidelines that should be followed when measuring weight and height.

Measure weight and height.

Positioning and Draping

1. Explain the purpose of positioning and draping.
2. List one use of each patient position.

Position and drape a patient in the following positions:
Sitting
Supine
Prone
Dorsal recumbent
Lithotomy
Sims
Knee-chest
Fowler's

Assessment of the Patient

1. List and define the four techniques of examining the patient.
2. State an example of the use of each examination technique during the physical examination of a patient.

Assisting the Physician

Describe the responsibilities of the medical assistant during the physical examination.

Assist the physician during the physical examination of a patient.

CHAPTER 5

The Physical Examination

Chapter Outline

INTRODUCTION TO THE PHYSICAL EXAMINATION
Definition of Terms
Preparation of the Examining Room
Preparation of the Patient
Measuring Weight and Height
Positioning and Draping
Assessment of the Patient
  Inspection
  Palpation
  Percussion
  Auscultation
Assisting the Physician

National Competencies

Clinical Competencies
Patient Care
- Prepare and maintain examination and treatment areas.
- Prepare patient for and assist with routine and specialty examinations.

General Competencies
Patient Instruction
- Instruct individuals according to their needs.
- Provide instruction for health maintenance and disease prevention.
- Identify community resources.

Operational Functions
- Perform an inventory of supplies and equipment.
- Perform routine maintenance of administrative and clinical equipment.

Key Terms

audiometer (aw-dee-OM-eh-ter)
auscultation (os-kul-TAY-shun)
bariatrics (BAR-ee-AT-riks)
clinical diagnosis
diagnosis
differential (diff-er-EN-shul) diagnosis
inspection
mensuration (men-soo-RAY-shun)
ophthalmoscope (off-THAL-meh-skope)
otoscope (AH-toe-skope)
palpation (pal-PAY-shun)
percussion (per-KUSH-un)
percussion hammer
prognosis
speculum (SPEK-yoo-lum)
symptom

Introduction to the Physical Examination

A complete patient examination consists of three parts: the *health history,* the *physical examination* of each body system, and *laboratory and diagnostic tests.* The results are used by the physician to determine the patient's general state of health, to arrive at a diagnosis and prescribe treatment, and to observe any change in a patient's illness after treatment has been instituted.

An important and frequent responsibility of the medical assistant is to assist with a physical examination. Because health-promotion and disease-prevention activities have become an important focus of health care, individuals are becoming more aware of the need for a yearly physical examination to detect early signs of illness and to prevent serious health problems. Also, a physical examination may be a prerequisite for employment, participation in sports, attendance at summer camp, and admission to school. The physical examination is explained in detail in this chapter. Taking the health history, collecting specimens, and performing laboratory and diagnostic tests are discussed in other chapters.

Definition of Terms

The medical assistant should know and understand the following terms relating to the patient examination:

Final diagnosis	Often simply called the *diagnosis,* this term refers to the scientific method of determining and identifying a patient's condition through the evaluation of the health history, the physical examination, laboratory tests, and diagnostic procedures. A final diagnosis is very important because it provides a logical basis for treatment and prognosis.
Clinical diagnosis	The clinical diagnosis is an intermediate step in the determination of a final diagnosis. The clinical diagnosis of a patient's condition is obtained through the evaluation of the health history and the physical examination without the benefit of laboratory or diagnostic tests. Outside laboratories provide a space to specify the clinical diagnosis on the laboratory request form; this information assists the laboratory in correlating the clinical laboratory data and the physician's needs. Once the physician has analyzed the test results, a final diagnosis can usually be established.
Differential diagnosis	Two or more diseases may have similar symptoms. The differential diagnosis involves determining

which of these diseases is producing the patient's symptoms so that a final diagnosis can be established. For example, streptococcal sore throat and pharyngitis have similar symptoms. A differential diagnosis is made by obtaining a throat specimen and performing a strep test.

Prognosis   The prognosis is the probable course and outcome of a patient's condition and the patient's prospects for recovery.

Risk factor   A risk factor is a physical or behavioral condition that increases the probability that an individual will develop a particular condition; examples are genetic factors, habits, environmental conditions, and physiologic conditions. The presence of a risk factor for a certain disease does not mean that the disease will develop; it means only that a person's chances of developing that disease are greater than those of a person without the risk factor. For example, cigarette smoking is a risk factor for developing lung cancer and heart disease. A person who smokes has a higher risk of developing lung cancer than one who does not or who has stopped smoking.

Acute illness   An acute illness is characterized by symptoms that have a rapid onset, are usually severe and intense, and subside after a relatively short time. In some cases, the acute episode progresses into a chronic illness. Examples of acute illness include influenza, strep throat, and chickenpox.

Chronic illness   A chronic illness is characterized by symptoms that persist for more than 3 months and show little change over a long time. Examples of chronic illness include diabetes mellitus, hypertension, and emphysema.

Therapeutic procedure   A therapeutic procedure is performed to treat a patient's condition with the goal of eliminating it or promoting as much recovery as possible. Examples of therapeutic procedures include the administration of medication, ear and eye irrigations, and therapeutic ultrasound.

Diagnostic procedure   A procedure performed to assist in the diagnosis of a patient's condition; examples include electrocardiography, x-ray examination, and sigmoidoscopy.

Laboratory testing   The analysis and study of specimens obtained from patients to assist in diagnosing and treating disease.

Highlight on Health Screening

The chance of developing certain diseases is greater at different ages. Periodic health screening is recommended for the detection and early treatment of disease.

Test or Procedure	Gender	Recommended Frequency
Beginning at age 20 years		
Blood pressure	M & F	Every year
Cholesterol level	M & F	Every 5 years
Blood glucose level	M & F	Every 3 to 5 years
Breast self-examination	F	Every month
Beginning at the age specified		
Clinical breast examination (by a physician)	F	Every 3 years beginning at age 29, and every year beginning at age 40
Pap test and pelvic examination	F	Every year starting at the onset of sexual activity or at age 18 years, whichever is earlier
Testicular self-examination	M	Every month beginning at age 15
Rectal examination	M & F	Every year beginning at age 40
Fecal occult blood test	M & F	Every year starting at age 50
Sigmoidoscopy	M & F	Every 5 years beginning at age 50
Prostate cancer screening	M	Every year beginning at age 50
Mammography	F	Every year beginning at age 40
Electrocardiogram	M & F	One baseline recording starting at age 40

Preparation of the Examining Room

Proper preparation of the examining room provides a comfortable and healthy environment for the patient and facilitates the physical examination. The following guidelines should be followed in preparing the examining room:

- Make sure the examining room is free of clutter and well lit.
- Check the examining rooms daily to make sure there are ample supplies. Restock supplies that are getting low.
- Empty waste receptacles frequently.
- Replace biohazard containers as necessary. When removing biohazard containers from the examining room (see Chapter 2), be especially careful to follow the OSHA Bloodborne Pathogens Standard.

- Make sure the room is well ventilated and install an air freshener to eliminate odors.
- Maintain room temperatures that are comfortable not only for a fully clothed person but also for one who has disrobed.
- Clean and disinfect examining tables, countertops, and faucets daily. Remove dust and dirt from furniture and towel dispensers.
- Change the examining table paper after each patient by unrolling a fresh length. Check to make sure there is an ample supply of gowns and drapes ready for use.
- Patients' privacy should be ensured. The medical assistant is responsible for making sure that the door is closed during the examination.

TABLE 5-1	Equipment and Supplies for the Physical Examination
Item	**Description and Purpose**
Patient examination gown	A gown made of disposable paper or cloth that provides patient modesty, comfort, and warmth
Drapes	Lengths of disposable paper or cloth to cover the patient or parts of the patient to reduce exposure
Sphygmomanometer	An instrument used to measure blood pressure
Stethoscope	An instrument used to auscultate body sounds, such as blood pressure and lung and bowel sounds
Thermometer	An instrument used to measure body temperature
Upright balance scale	A device used to measure weight and height
Otoscope	A lighted instrument with a lens, used to examine the external ear canal and tympanic membrane
Tuning fork	A small metal instrument consisting of a stem and two prongs, used to test hearing acuity
Ophthalmoscope	A lighted instrument with a lens, used for examining the interior of the eye
Tongue depressor	A flat wooden blade used to depress the patient's tongue during examination of the mouth and pharynx
Antiseptic wipe	A disposable pad saturated with an antiseptic such as alcohol that is used to cleanse the skin
Tape measure	A flexible device calibrated in inches on one side and centimeters on the other side; it is used to measure the patient (e.g., diameter of a limb, head circumference)
Percussion hammer	An instrument with a rubber head, used for testing neurologic reflexes
Speculum	An instrument for opening a body orifice or cavity for viewing (e.g., an ear speculum, nasal speculum, vaginal speculum)
Disposable gloves	Gloves, usually latex, that are worn only once to provide protection from bloodborne pathogens and other potentially infectious materials
Lubricant	An agent that is applied to the physician's gloved hand or to a speculum that reduces friction between parts to make insertion easier
Specimen container	A container in which a body specimen is placed for transport to the laboratory (after it has been labeled)
Tissues	Tissues are used for wiping body secretions
Cotton-tipped applicator	A small piece of cotton wrapped around the end of a slender wooden stick, for the collection of a specimen from the body
Gooseneck lamp	A light mounted on a flexible movable stand to focus light on an area for good visibility
Basin	A container in which used instruments are deposited
Biohazard container	A specially made container used for receiving items that contain infectious waste
Waste receptacle	A container for used disposable articles that do not contain infectious waste

- Properly clean and prepare equipment, instruments, and supplies that will be used for patient examinations so that they are ready for use by the physician. Table 5-1 lists the equipment and supplies, along with their uses, that may be employed during a physical examination.
- Check equipment and instruments regularly to verify that they are in proper working condition. This protects the patient from harm caused by faulty equipment.

- Have the equipment and supplies ready for the examination. They should be arranged for easy access by the physician. The equipment and supplies needed for the physical examination vary according to the type of examination and the physician's preference (Figure 5-1).
- Know how to operate and care for each piece of equipment and each instrument. The manufacturer includes an operating manual, which should be read carefully and thoroughly and kept available for reference.

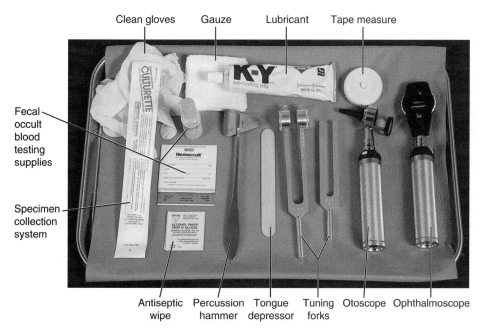

Figure 5-1. Common instruments and supplies used for the physical examination.

Highlight on Patient Teaching

The purpose of patient teaching is to help the patient develop habits, attitudes, and skills that enable the individual to maintain and improve his or her own health.

FACT: Patients who are active, informed participants in their health care are more apt to follow the physician's instructions than those who are passive recipients of medical services.

ACTION: Provide patients with information on health care. Every patient interaction is an opportunity for teaching.

FACT: Adult learners are goal oriented and performance centered. They need and want information that will assist them in managing and improving their health.

ACTION: Review the information that you provide to patients and determine whether it is nice to know or necessary to know. Select subject matter that is practical and useful and relates directly to the patient's needs.

FACT: The more information that is presented, the more the patient is likely to forget. Approximately half the information presented to the patient will be forgotten in the first 5 minutes after giving it.

ACTION: When teaching, use the following pointers to help patients learn and retain information:

- Keep it short and be specific.
- Speak in terms the patient can understand.
- Focus on "how" rather than "why."
- Repeat and reinforce important information.
- Give practical examples and provide ample time for patient practice.
- Ask for feedback from the patient to determine whether he or she understands the information.
- Provide the patient with written information.

Continued

Highlight on Patient Teaching—cont'd

FACT: Each individual has a distinct style of learning and learns best when using his or her preferred learning style. The three main learning styles are reading, listening, and doing. People often use more than one style for learning.

ACTION: Use a variety of teaching strategies to engage the various learning styles of patients. Examples of teaching strategies include explanations, printed handouts, audiovisual aids, demonstrations, and discussions.

FACT: Only two thirds of patients comply with the health care instructions prescribed by the physician. Factors that influence compliance include the patient's adaptation to illness, motivation to change, physical capability, and support systems.

ACTION: The following help increase patient compliance with prescribed treatment:
- Address the patient by name. (Keep in mind that many patients object to being called by their first name by strangers.)
- Encourage the patient to take an active role in personal health care.
- Help the patient set goals and objectives for change.
- Encourage care and support from family members.
- Make the patient aware of outside resources.
- Give positive reinforcement when the patient makes healthful changes.

What Would You DO? What Would You Not DO?

Case Study 1

Abbey Auden, 35 years old, is at the medical office. Her husband got a backyard trampoline for their two school-age children, and she decided to try it out. Abbey landed wrong on the trampoline and hurt her back and neck. For the past 5 days she has been having headaches and back pain. Abbey refuses to have her weight taken because she has gained weight over the past several years and doesn't want to know how much she's gained. She doesn't understand why weight has to be taken at an office visit in the first place. Abbey says that many times when she should go to the doctor, she doesn't, just to avoid being weighed. She says she wouldn't even be here now, except that her husband insisted that she come.

Preparation of the Patient

It is the medical assistant's responsibility to prepare the patient for the physical examination. At this time, the medical assistant takes vital signs and measures weight and height. The results of these procedures are charted in the patient's medical record.

The medical assistant should explain the purpose of the examination and offer to answer any questions. A patient's apprehension and embarrassment can be reduced by addressing the patient by his or her name of choice, by adopting a friendly and supportive attitude, and by speaking clearly, distinctly, and slowly. This also facilitates the physical examination of the patient.

The patient should be asked if he or she needs to empty the bladder before the examination. An empty bladder makes the examination easier and is more comfortable for the patient. If a urine specimen is needed, the patient is requested to void.

PUTTING It All Into PRACTICE

MY NAME IS Hope Fauber, and I am a certified medical assistant. I work in a medical clinic with a family medicine department of 10 physicians and 10 residents and interns. My duties cover a broad spectrum, from pediatrics to geriatrics, and include prenatal care, allergy injections, minor office surgery, electrocardiograms, colposcopies, immunizations, and wound care.

At our clinic many of the patients are elderly. I occasionally come across geriatric patients who are not very cooperative and are "set in their ways." One 90-year-old lady, in particular, had a reputation in the office of being cantankerous and difficult to work with. One day when the physician ordered lab work on her, I prepared to draw blood from her tiny, frail body, praying that everything would go smoothly. As I helped her up after a successful "stick," she, of all people, reached to give me a hug and said to me, "I like you. That didn't even hurt!" She continued to hold my hand and talk to me as I walked her out of the office. This turned out to be the last time I would see her as she moved out of town, but not out of my heart, leaving a lasting impression on my life.

Instructions on disrobing for the examination should be specific, so that the patient understands what items of clothing to remove and where to place the clothing. The disrobing facility should be comfortable and provide privacy. It is helpful to have a place for the patient to sit to make it easier to remove clothing and shoes. The facility should also be equipped with hooks for hanging clothing. Instructions for putting on the examination gown and for locating the gown opening reduce patient confusion. If the medical assistant senses that the patient will have trouble undressing, assistance should be offered. Elderly and disabled patients sometimes have difficulty removing clothing.

PATIENT TEACHING

Health Promotion and Disease Prevention

Teach patients the essentials of health promotion and disease prevention. Help patients become aware of the following patterns of behavior that promote and support health:
- Keeping up to date with immunizations
- Eating nutritiously from the food pyramid
- Exercising regularly
- Maintaining normal weight
- Managing stress
- Maintaining high self-esteem
- Avoiding tobacco and drugs

- Using alcohol wisely
- Understanding how the environment affects health and taking appropriate action to improve it
- Knowing the facts about cardiovascular disease, cancer, infections, sexually transmitted diseases, and accidents and using this knowledge to protect against them
- Understanding the changes that take place through the natural processes of aging
- Developing a sense of responsibility for health by taking an active role in establishing and maintaining a healthy lifestyle

What Would You DO? What Would You Not DO?

Case Study 2

Karen Steiner drops her 17-year-old daughter, Mikayla, off at the office for her sports physical examination. Mikayla is captain of the Varsity Cheerleading squad and getting ready to start her senior year in high school. Mikayla's vital signs are normal, and she measures 5′6″ tall and weighs 105 pounds. With some reluctance, Mikayla admits that she's been having problems with heartburn and she's pretty sure she knows what's causing it. She says that she has to keep her weight down for cheerleading and after eating dinner with her family, she makes herself vomit to get rid of the food in her stomach. Mikayla is not too concerned about doing this because a lot of the popular girls at school are doing the same thing. She says it's the easy way to stay slim and she would like to lose another 10 pounds before football season starts. Mikayla wants some prescription drug samples to help with the heartburn because the OTC pills that she's been taking aren't working anymore. She doesn't want her parents to know about any of this because she's afraid that they wouldn't understand and might make her drop out of cheerleading.

The medical assistant is responsible for making the patient's medical record available for review by the physician. The medical office will have a designated location where the record is placed, such as in a chart holder on the front of the examining room door. Make sure that the medical record is placed so that patient-identifiable information is not visible. This is required by the Health Insurance Portability and Accountability Act (HIPAA) Privacy Rule to protect patient's health information.

The physical examination is performed with the patient positioned on an examining table, which is specially constructed to facilitate the examination. For safety, it is advisable to help the patient on and off the examining table.

Measuring Weight and Height

The medical assistant routinely measures the weight and height of many types of patients. The process of measuring the patient is **mensuration.** A change in weight may be significant in the diagnosis of a patient's condition and in prescribing the course of treatment. Underweight and overweight patients who follow a diet therapy program should be weighed at regular intervals to determine their progress. Prenatal patients are weighed during each prenatal visit to assist in the assessment of fetal development and of the mother's health. Procedure 5-1 describes how to measure height and weight.

An adult's weight is usually measured during each office visit; an adult's height, however, is typically measured only during the first visit or when a complete physical examination of the patient is requested. Children are weighed and measured during each office visit to observe their pattern of growth and to calculate medication dosage.

The patient's height is used to interpret body weight (see the Highlight on Interpreting Body Weight). The weight and height are compared against a standardized chart that serves as a general guide to determine whether the patient's weight falls within normal limits (Figure 5-2).

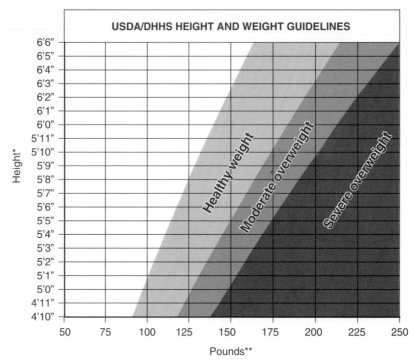

* Without shoes.
**Without clothes. The higher weights apply to people with more muscle and
  bone, such as many men.

Figure 5-2. USDA/DHHS height and weight guidelines. (From *Report of the Dietary Guidelines Advisory Committee on the dietary guidelines for Americans,* Washington, DC, 1995, U.S. Department of Health and Human Services.)

Guidelines for Measuring Weight and Height

When using an upright balance scale to measure weight and height, use the following guidelines.

Weight

1. **Locate the scale to provide privacy for the patient.** Place the scale on a hard, level surface in a private location. Many patients are self-conscious about having their weight measured and prefer that it be done in privacy. Be careful not to make weight-sensitive comments during the procedure. This is especially important for patients with weight control problems such as obesity and eating disorders.
2. **Balance the scale before measuring weight.** If the scale is not balanced, the weight measurement will be inaccurate. The scale is balanced when the upper and lower weights are on zero and the indicator point comes to a rest at the center of the balance area.
3. **Assist the patient.** Make sure to assist the patient on and off the scale platform. The scale platform moves slightly and, therefore, may cause the patient to become unsteady.

4. **Obtain an accurate weight.** Always ask the patient to remove his or her shoes. Measure weight with the patient in normal clothing. Ask the patient to remove heavy outer clothing, such as a sweater or a jacket.
5. **Interpret the calibration markings accurately.** The lower calibration bar is divided into 50-pound increments (Figure 5-3, *A*). The upper calibration bar is divided into pounds and quarter pounds. The longer calibration lines indicate pound increments, and the shorter calibration lines indicate quarter-pound and half-pound increments (Figure 5-3, *B*).
6. **Determine the patient's weight correctly.** Add the measurement on the lower scale to the measurement on the upper scale. The result should be rounded to the nearest quarter pound. Occasionally, the patient's weight may need to be converted to kilograms, which is the metric unit of measurement for weight. This may be required when determining medication dosage. The following formulas are used to convert weight and height measurements from one system to another.

Guidelines for Measuring Weight and Height—cont'd

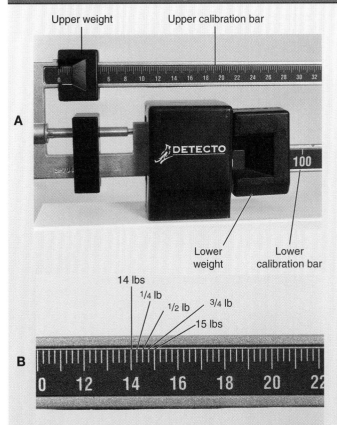

Figure 5-3. Calibration markings for measuring weight on an upright balance scale. **A,** The upper calibration bar is divided into pounds and quarter pounds. **B,** The longer calibration lines indicate pound increments, and the shorter calibration lines indicate quarter-pound and half-pound increments.

Weight Conversion

Pounds to Kilograms. Divide the number of pounds by 2.2; for example,

$$136 \text{ pounds} \div 2.2 = 61.8 \text{ kilograms.}$$

Kilograms to Pounds. Multiply the number of kilograms by 2.2; for example,

$$75 \text{ kilograms} \times 2.2 = 165 \text{ pounds.}$$

Height Conversion

Inches to Centimeters. Multiply the number of inches by 2.5; for example,

$$64 \text{ inches} \times 2.5 = 160 \text{ centimeters.}$$

Centimeters to Inches. Divide the number of centimeters by 2.5; for example,

$$185 \text{ centimeters} \div 2.5 = 74 \text{ inches (or 6 feet 2 inches).}$$

Height

1. **Provide for the patient's safety.** Be very careful to follow the proper procedure when measuring the patient's height. An error in technique could result in injury. For example, if a patient is placed on the scale in a forward position, the measuring bar will open up into the patient's face, causing a facial injury.

2. **Determine the calibration markings accurately.** Depending on the brand of scale, the calibration markings are divided into either inches or feet and inches. (Figure 5-4 is an example of a scale divided into feet and inches.) The calibration rod is also calibrated into centimeters, which is the metric unit of measurement for height. This unit of measurement is not typically used to measure height in the United States.

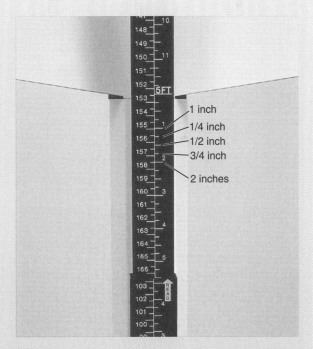

Figure 5-4. Calibration markings for measuring height on an upright balance scale.

3. **Read the measurement correctly.** For most patients, you can read the height measurement at the junction of the stationary calibration rod and the movable calibration rod (Figure 5-5, *A*). However, if the patient's height is less than the top value of the stationary calibration rod, you must read the measurement directly on the stationary rod. For example, (on most scales) the highest calibration on the

Continued

Guidelines for Measuring Weight and Height—cont'd

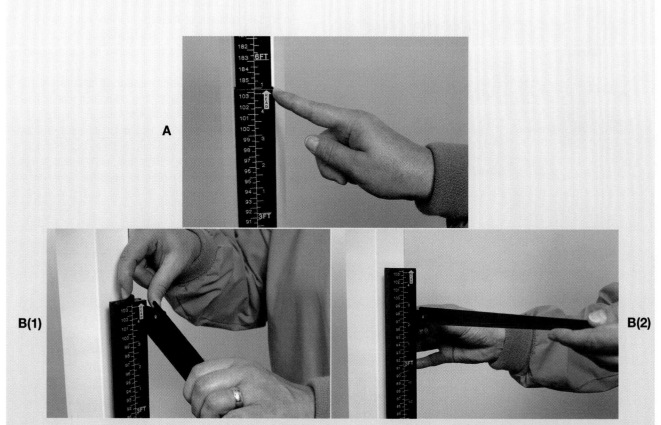

Figure 5-5. **A,** Reading a height measurement at the junction of the stationary calibration rod and the movable calibration rod. The height measurement in this illustration is 6 feet and 1 inch. **B(1),** Reading a height measurement on the stationary calibration rod. NOTE: The measuring bar must first be released and moved down to the stationary bar to measure the patient's height. **B(2),** Reading the height at the junction of the bar and the rod. The height measurement in this illustration is 3 feet and 2 inches.

stationary rod is 50 inches; therefore patients with a height of 50 inches or less will have their height read directly off of the stationary rod (Figure 5-5, *B*).

4. **Record the height measurement correctly.** Record the height measurement in feet and inches. If the scale is calibrated in inches, convert the reading to feet and inches by dividing the number of inches by 12. For example, a height measurement of 60 inches is recorded as 5 feet (60 inches divided by 12 equals 5). If the patient's height measurement is 64 inches, the results would be recorded as 5 feet, 4 inches.

Highlight on Interpreting Body Weight

The two common methods to interpret body weight are (a) weight in relation to standard tables and (b) calculation of the BMI.

Height and Weight Tables

One way to interpret body weight is through the use of standardized height and weight tables. In 1959 the Metropolitan Life Insurance Company (MET) issued a set of tables indicating desirable height and weight ranges for men and women. In 1983 MET issued revised tables for men and women that showed height and weight ranges higher than those in the 1959 table. Many health experts believe that the desirable weight ranges of the revised tables are too high and, therefore, do not represent healthy body weight.

In 1995 the United States Department of Agriculture (USDA) and the Department of Health and Human Services (DHHS) issued a set of weight guidelines (Figure 5-2) that are lower than those of the MET tables. The USDA/DHHS guidelines do not distinguish between weights of men and women, and therefore must be interpreted by each individual as follows. Women usually have smaller bones and less muscle than men, so they should use the lower end of the range. Men and large-boned, muscular women should use the higher end of the weight range to find their healthy body weights.

Body Mass Index

Another method for interpreting body weight is the body mass index, or BMI. The BMI expresses the correlation of an individual's weight to his or her height. Except for trained athletes, the BMI strongly correlates with total body fat content in adults. This, in turn, provides an indication of the risk of developing chronic health conditions associated with obesity. Many health experts believe that the BMI is a more accurate standard for interpreting body weight than height and weight tables.

Method for Calculating BMI

Use the following steps to calculate your BMI:

1. Multiply your weight in pounds (without clothes or shoes) by 703. For example, for an individual who weighs 135 pounds,

$$135 \times 703 = 94{,}905.$$

2. Divide this number by your height in inches. For example, if this person is 66 inches tall,

$$94{,}905 \div 66 = 1438.$$

3. Divide this amount again by your height in inches and round off to the nearest whole number. For our example,

$$1438 \div 66 = 21.79, \text{ or } 22.$$

The BMI of this individual is 22.

Interpretation of the BMI

In June 1998 the National Heart, Lung, and Blood Institute (NHLBI), a federal health agency, issued a set of guidelines for the classification of body weight in adults. One of these guidelines relates to the interpretation of the BMI, as is outlined here.

BMI	Interpretation
Below 18.5	Underweight
18.5 to 24.9	Healthy weight
25 to 29.9	Overweight
30 to 39.9	Obesity
40 or more	Morbid obesity

The NHLBI recommends that the BMI be determined in all adults. People of normal weight should have their BMI reassessed every 2 years.

Adult Obesity

The incidence of obesity in the United States has increased markedly during the past 20 years and is now one of the most common problems encountered by primary care physicians. According to a recent report released by the U.S. Surgeon General's office, more than 61% of Americans are overweight, and 27% of them, or 50 million Americans, are obese. Obesity is associated with premature death and, after smoking, is the second leading cause of preventable death in the United States today.

It has been determined that as the BMI rises above 25, there is an increased risk of developing certain diseases associated with overweight and obesity including:

- Hypertension
- Cardiovascular disease
- Dyslipidemia (high blood cholesterol levels, high blood triglyceride levels, or both)
- Type 2 diabetes
- Colon cancer
- Breast cancer
- Sleep apnea
- Osteoarthritis

Obesity is considered a chronic condition that requires a multiple treatment approach that includes a behavioral therapy program, a low calorie diet, and a suitable aerobic exercise program. Primary care physicians often manage individuals with mild and moderate obesity, but morbidly obese patients are usually referred to a bariatric specialist. **Bariatrics** is the branch of medicine that deals with the treatment and control of obesity and diseases associated with obesity.

PROCEDURE 5-1   Measuring Weight and Height

Outcome Measure weight and height.

Equipment Supplies:
- Upright balance scale

Weight

1. **Procedural Step.** Sanitize your hands.
2. **Procedural Step.** Check the scale to make sure it is balanced as follows:
   a. Make sure the upper and lower weights are on zero. When the weights are on zero, they will be all the way to the left of the calibration bars.

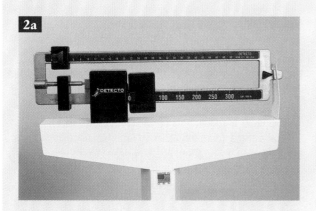

   b. Look at the indicator point. If the scale is balanced, the indicator point is resting in the center of the balance area.
   c. If the indicator point rests below the center, adjust the screw on the balance knob by turning it clockwise (to the right) until the indicator point rests in the center of the balance area.

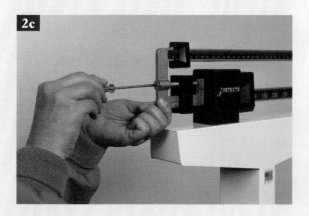

   d. If the indicator point rests above the center, adjust the screw on the balance knob by turning it counterclockwise (to the left) until the indicator point rests in the center of the balance area.

Principle. If the scale is not balanced, the weight measurement will be inaccurate.

3. **Procedural Step.** Greet and identify the patient.
4. **Procedural Step.** Introduce yourself and explain to the patient that you will be measuring his or her height and weight.
5. **Procedural Step.** Instruct the patient to remove his or her shoes and outer clothing such as a jacket or sweater. A good medical aseptic practice is to place a paper towel on the platform of the scale to protect the patient's feet.
   Principle. Removing heavy clothing and shoes allows a more accurate measurement of the patient's weight.
6. **Procedural Step.** Assist the patient onto the scale, and instruct the patient not to move.
   Principle. It is not possible to balance the scale if the patient is moving.
7. **Procedural Step.** Balance the scale as follows:
   a. Move the lower weight to the notched groove that does not cause the indicator point to drop to the bottom of the calibration area. Make sure the lower weight is seated firmly in its groove.
   b. Slide the upper weight slowly along its calibration bar by tapping it gently until the indicator point comes to a rest at the center of the balance area.
   Principle. Not seating the lower weight firmly in its groove results in an inaccurate reading.

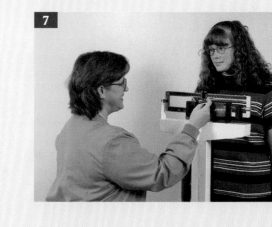

8. **Procedural Step.** Read the results to the nearest quarter pound by adding the measurement on the lower scale to the measurement on the upper scale.
9. **Procedural Step.** Assist the patient off of the scale platform.

Height

1. Procedural Step. Slide the movable calibration rod upward until the measuring bar is well above the patient's apparent height. Open the measuring bar to its horizontal position.

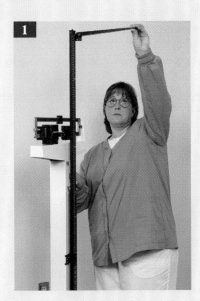

2. Procedural Step. Instruct the patient to step onto the scale platform with his or her back to the scale. Provide assistance if needed. Instruct the patient to stand erect and to look straight ahead.
Principle. Looking straight ahead helps the patient to stand erect and balanced, which ensures an accurate measurement.

3. Procedural Step. Carefully lower the measuring bar (keeping it horizontal) until it rests gently on top of the patient's head. The measuring bar should form a 90-degree angle with the calibration rod.
Principle. The measuring bar must be at a 90-degree angle to ensure an accurate height measurement.

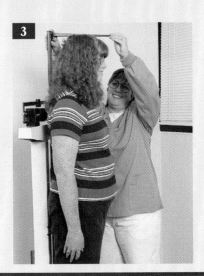

4. Procedural Step. Keeping the measuring bar in a horizontal position, instruct the patient to step down and put on his or her shoes. Be sure to hold the bar in a horizontal position until the patient has stepped off the scale.

5. Procedural Step. Read the height measurement to the nearest quarter inch marking at the junction of the stationary calibration rod and the movable calibration rod. (NOTE: If the patient's height is less than the top value of the stationary rod, read the measurement directly on the stationary calibration rod.)

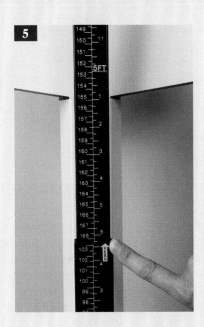

6. Procedural Step. Chart the weight and height measurements. The weight should be charted in pounds to the nearest quarter pound, and the height should be charted in feet and inches to the nearest quarter inch.

7. Procedural Step. Return the weights to zero. Return the measuring bar to its vertical (resting) position, and slide the movable calibration rod to its lowest position.

PROCEDURE 5-1

CHARTING EXAMPLE	
Date	
11/5/05	10:15 a.m. Wt: 155. Ht: 5' 6¼" ————
	———————————— Hope Fauber, CMA

Positioning and Draping

Correct positioning of the patient facilitates the examination by permitting better access to the part being examined or treated. The basic positions used in the medical office are the sitting, supine, prone, dorsal recumbent, lithotomy, Sims, knee-chest, and Fowler's.

The position used depends on the type of examination or procedure to be performed. More than one position may be used to examine the same body part during the physical examination. For example, the sitting and supine positions are both used to examine the chest. It is important to know the correct position for each examination or treatment. When positioning a patient, the medical assistant should explain the position to the patient and assist the patient in attaining it.

It is important to take the patient's endurance and degree of wellness into consideration when positioning a patient. Patients who are weak or ill may not be able to assume a position or may require special assistance in attaining it. Some of the positions, such as the lithotomy and knee-chest, are embarrassing and uncomfortable. Therefore a patient should not be kept in these positions any longer than necessary. Some patients (especially elderly ones) become dizzy after a time in certain positions such as the knee-chest position. These patients should be allowed to rest before they get off the examining table. The medical assistant should also be sure to assist patients off the examining table to prevent falls.

The patient is draped during positioning to provide for modesty, comfort, and warmth. Only the part to be examined should be exposed. Patient gowns and drapes used in the medical office are usually made of paper but may also be made of cloth.

Procedures 2 through 9 present proper positioning and draping of the patient.

Text continued on p. 190

MEMORIES From EXTERNSHIP

HOPE FAUBER: During my externship at a student health center at a four-year college, I was responsible for working up patients for gynecologic examinations. The two-piece drapes had the top opening in the front and the bottom opening in the back. After explaining this to an Asian student who spoke very little English, I noticed that she had the openings opposite of what I had explained. I explained again, with words and gestures, that she needed to reverse the openings. To my surprise, she stood up, turned around in a circle, and sat down!

What Would You DO? What Would You *Not* DO?

Case Study 3

Ben-Yi Sun has brought his father, Chang-Yi Sun, to the medical office. Chang-Yi Sun is 76 years old and lives with Ben-Yi and his family. Because there is a large Asian population in the community, the medical office personnel have learned two things about the Asian culture: (1) They are brought up to respect elders, and elders are always considered first; and (2) Asians have a great respect for harmony. If they do not understand something, they may not admit it to avoid disrupting harmony. Ben-Yi Sun speaks very good English, but his father understands only a few words of English. Chang-Yi Sun has been diagnosed with hypertension, and he needs education about going on a low-sodium diet. He also needs instructions on taking his blood pressure at home and recording the results.

PROCEDURE 5-2   Sitting Position

Outcome Position and drape an individual in the sitting position. The sitting position is used to examine the head, neck, chest, and upper extremities and to measure vital signs.

Equipment/Supplies:
- Examining table
- Patient gown
- Patient drape

1. **Procedural Step.** Sanitize your hands. Greet and identify the patient. Introduce yourself.
2. **Procedural Step.** Explain to the patient the type of examination or procedure that will be performed.

3. **Procedural Step.** Provide the patient with a patient gown. Instruct the patient to remove clothing as appropriate for the type of examination being performed and to put on the patient gown with the opening in front. The disrobing facility should provide privacy, a place to sit, and a place to hang clothing.

4. Procedural Step. Pull out the footrest of the examining table, and assist the patient into a sitting position. The patient's buttocks and thighs should be firmly supported on the edge of the table.

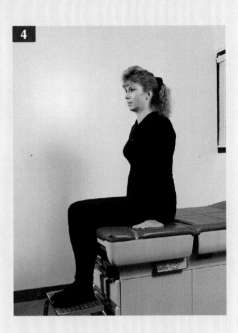

5. Procedural Step. Place a drape over the patient's thighs and legs to provide warmth and modesty.

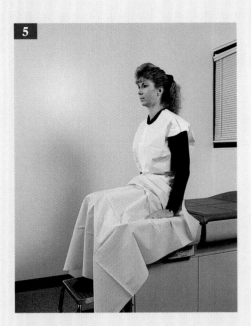

6. Procedural Step. After completion of the examination, assist the patient down from the table. Return the footrest to its normal position. Instruct the patient to get dressed.

PROCEDURE 5-3   Supine Position

Outcome Position and drape an individual in the supine position. The supine position is used to examine the head, chest, abdomen, and extremities.

Equipment/Supplies:
- Examining table
- Patient gown
- Patient drape

1. Procedural Step. Sanitize your hands. Greet and identify the patient. Introduce yourself.

2. Procedural Step. Explain to the patient the type of examination or procedure that will be performed.

3. Procedural Step. Provide the patient with a patient gown. Instruct the patient to remove clothing as appropriate for the type of examination being performed and to put on the patient gown with the opening in front. The disrobing facility should provide privacy, a place to sit, and a place to hang clothing.

4. Procedural Step. Pull out the footrest of the examining table, and assist the patient into a sitting position.

Continued

PROCEDURE 5-3

PROCEDURE 5-3   Supine Position—Cont'd

5. Procedural Step. Ask the patient to move back on the table. As the patient is doing this, pull out the table extension while supporting the patient's lower legs.

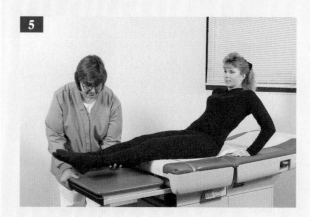

6. Procedural Step. Ask the patient to lie on his or her back with the legs together. Provide assistance if needed. The patient's arms may be placed above the head or alongside the body.

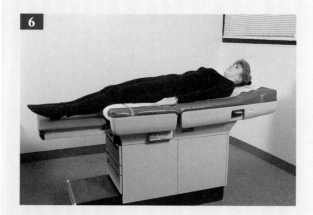

7. Procedural Step. Place a drape over the patient to provide warmth and modesty. As the physician examines the patient, move the drape according to the body parts being examined.

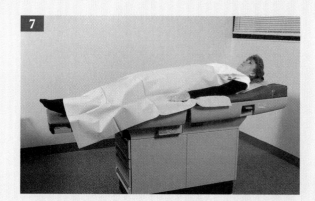

8. Procedural Step. After completion of the examination, assist the patient into a sitting position. Slide the table extension back into place while supporting the patient's lower legs.

9. Procedural Step. Assist the patient down from the table. Instruct the patient to get dressed. Return the footrest to its normal position.

PROCEDURE 5-4 Prone Position

Outcome Position and drape an individual in the prone position. The prone position is used to examine the back and to assess extension of the hip joint.

Equipment/Supplies:
- Examining table
- Patient gown
- Patient drape

1. **Procedural Step.** Sanitize your hands. Greet and identify the patient. Introduce yourself.
2. **Procedural Step.** Explain to the patient the type of examination or procedure that will be performed.
3. **Procedural Step.** Provide the patient with a patient gown. Instruct the patient to remove clothing as appropriate for the type of examination being performed and to put on the patient gown with the opening in back. The disrobing facility should provide privacy, a place to sit, and a place to hang clothing.
4. **Procedural Step.** Pull out the footrest of the examining table, and assist the patient into a sitting position.
5. **Procedural Step.** Ask the patient to move back on the table. As the patient is doing this, pull out the table extension while supporting the patient's lower legs.
6. **Procedural Step.** Ask the patient to lie on his or her back. Provide assistance if needed.
7. **Procedural Step.** Ask the patient to turn onto his or her stomach by rolling toward you. Provide assistance for this step.
   Principle. This step prevents the patient from accidentally rolling off the table.

8. **Procedural Step.** Position the patient with the legs together and the head turned to one side. The arms can be placed above the head or alongside the body.
9. **Procedural Step.** Place a drape over the patient to provide warmth and modesty. As the physician examines the patient, move the drape according to the body parts being examined.

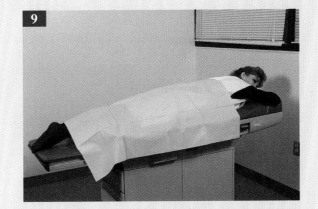

10. **Procedural Step.** After completion of the examination, ask the patient to turn back over by rolling toward you. Assist the patient into a supine position and then into a sitting position. Slide the table extension back into place while supporting the patient's lower legs.
11. **Procedural Step.** Assist the patient down from the table. Return the footrest to its normal position. Instruct the patient to get dressed.

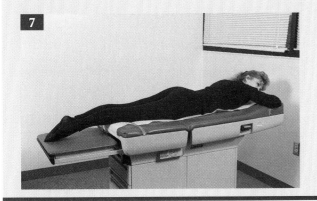

PROCEDURE 5-5   Dorsal Recumbent Position

Outcome Position and drape an individual in the dorsal recumbent position. The dorsal recumbent position is used for vaginal and rectal examinations, for the insertion of a urinary catheter, and to examine the head, neck, chest, and extremities of patients who have difficulty maintaining the supine position. The supine position is not a comfortable position for patients with respiratory problems, a back injury, or low back pain. Bending the legs (rather than lying flat) is more comfortable for these patients and is easier to maintain.

Equipment/Supplies:
- Examining table
- Patient gown
- Patient drape

1. **Procedural Step.** Sanitize your hands. Greet and identify the patient. Introduce yourself.
2. **Procedural Step.** Explain the type of examination or procedure that will be performed.
3. **Procedural Step.** Provide the patient with a patient gown. Instruct the patient to remove clothing as appropriate for the type of examination being performed and to put on the patient gown with the opening in front. The disrobing facility should provide privacy, a place to sit, and a place to hang clothing.
4. **Procedural Step.** Pull out the footrest of the examining table, and assist the patient into a sitting position.
5. **Procedural Step.** Ask the patient to move back on the table. As the patient is doing this, pull out the table extension while supporting the patient's lower legs.
6. **Procedural Step.** Ask the patient to lie on his or her back. Provide assistance if needed. The arms can be placed above the head or alongside the body.
7. **Procedural Step.** Ask the patient to bend the knees and place each foot at the edge of the examining table with the soles of the feet flat on the table. Provide assistance during this step. Push in the table extension and the footrest.

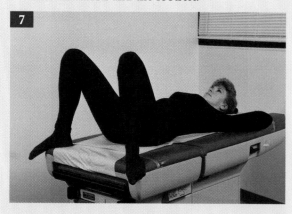

8. **Procedural Step.** Place a drape over the patient to provide warmth and modesty. The drape should be positioned diagonally, with one corner over the patient's chest and the opposite corner over the pubic area.

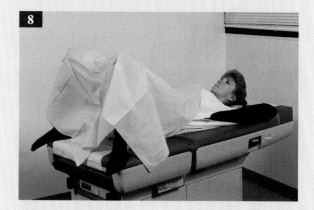

9. **Procedural Step.** When the physician is ready to examine the genital area, the center corner of the drape is folded back over the abdomen.
10. **Procedural Step.** After completion of the examination, pull out the footrest and the table extension. Assist the patient into a supine position and then into a sitting position. Slide the table extension back into place while supporting the patient's lower legs.
11. **Procedural Step.** Assist the patient down from the table. Return the footrest to its normal position. Instruct the patient to get dressed.

PROCEDURE 5-6 Lithotomy Position

Outcome Position and drape an individual in the lithotomy position. The lithotomy position is used for vaginal, pelvic, and rectal examinations. The lithotomy position is the same as the dorsal recumbent position except that the patient's feet are placed in stirrups. The lithotomy position provides maximum exposure to the genital area and facilitates insertion of a vaginal speculum.

Equipment/Supplies:
- Examining table
- Patient gown
- Patient drape

1. **Procedural Step.** Sanitize your hands. Greet and identify the patient. Introduce yourself.
2. **Procedural Step.** Explain the examination or procedure that will be performed.
3. **Procedural Step.** Provide the patient with a patient gown. Instruct the patient to remove clothing as appropriate for the type of examination being performed and to put on the patient gown with the opening in front. The disrobing facility should provide privacy, a place to sit, and a place to hang clothing.
4. **Procedural Step.** Pull out the footrest of the examining table, and assist the patient into a sitting position.
5. **Procedural Step.** Ask the patient to move back on the table. As the patient is doing this, pull out the table extension while supporting the patient's lower legs.
6. **Procedural Step.** Ask the patient to lie on the back. Provide assistance if needed. The arms can be placed above the head or alongside the body.
7. **Procedural Step.** Place a drape over the patient to provide warmth and modesty. The drape should be positioned diagonally with one corner over the patient's chest and the opposite corner over the pubic area.
8. **Procedural Step.** Ask the patient to bend the knees and place each foot at the edge of the examining

table, with the soles of the feet flat on the table. Provide assistance during this step. Push in the table extension and the footrest.

9. **Procedural Step.** Position the stirrups so that they are level with the examining table and pulled out approximately 1 foot from the edge of the table.

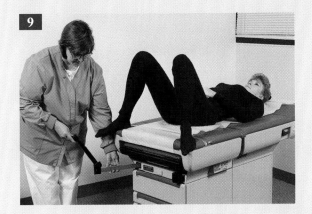

10. **Procedural Step.** Ask the patient to move the feet into the stirrups. Provide assistance during this step.
11. **Procedural Step.** Instruct the patient to slide the buttocks to the edge of the examining table and to rotate the thighs outward as far as is comfortable.

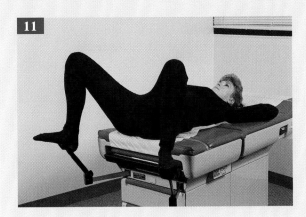

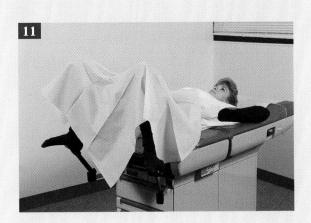

PROCEDURE 5-6

Continued

PROCEDURE 5-6   Lithotomy Position—Cont'd

12. **Procedural Step.** When the physician is ready to examine the genital area, the center corner of the drape is folded back over the abdomen.

13. **Procedural Step.** After completion of the examination, ask the patient to slide the buttocks back from the end of the table. Pull out the footrest and table extension. Lift the patient's legs out of the stirrups at the same time, and place them on the table extension (supine position). Return the stirrups to their normal position. Assist the patient into a sitting position. Slide the table extension back into place while supporting the patient's lower legs. *Principle.* When assisting the patient out of the stirrups, lift both the patient's legs at the same time to avoid strain on the back and abdominal muscles.

14. **Procedural Step.** Assist the patient down from the table. Return the footrest to its normal position. Instruct the patient to get dressed.

PROCEDURE 5-7   Sims Position

Outcome Position and drape an individual in the Sims position. Sims position, also known as the left lateral position, is used to examine the vagina and rectum, to measure rectal temperature, to perform a flexible sigmoidoscopy, and to administer an enema.

Equipment/Supplies:
- Examining table
- Patient gown
- Patient drape

1. **Procedural Step.** Sanitize your hands. Greet and identify the patient. Introduce yourself.

2. **Procedural Step.** Explain the examination or procedure that will be performed.

3. **Procedural Step.** Provide the patient with a patient gown. Instruct the patient to remove clothing from the waist down and to put on the patient gown with the opening in back. The disrobing facility should provide privacy, a place to sit, and a place to hang clothing.

4. **Procedural Step.** Pull out the footrest of the examining table, and assist the patient into a sitting position.

5. **Procedural Step.** Ask the patient to move back on the table. As the patient is doing this, pull out the table extension while supporting the patient's lower legs.

6. **Procedural Step.** Ask the patient to lie on his or her back. Provide assistance if needed.

7. **Procedural Step.** Place a drape over the patient to provide warmth and modesty.

8. **Procedural Step.** Ask the patient to turn onto his or her left side. Provide assistance during this step to prevent the patient from accidentally rolling off the table. The patient's left arm should be positioned behind the body and the right arm forward with the elbow bent. Assist the patient in flexing the legs. The right leg is flexed sharply, and the left leg is flexed slightly.

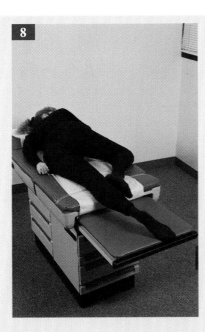

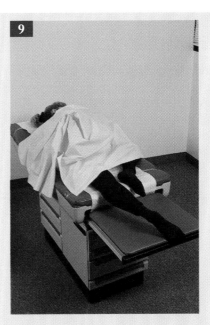

9. **Procedural Step.** Adjust the drape as needed. When the physician is ready to examine the patient, a small portion of the drape is folded back to expose the anal area.

10. **Procedural Step.** After completion of the examination, assist the patient into a supine position and then into a sitting position. Slide the table extension back into place while supporting the patient's lower legs.

11. **Procedural Step.** Assist the patient down from the table. Return the footrest to its normal position. Instruct the patient to get dressed.

PROCEDURE 5-8

PROCEDURE 5-8 Knee-Chest Position

Outcome Position and drape an individual in the knee-chest position. The knee-chest position is used to examine the rectum and to perform a proctoscopic examination because it provides maximal exposure to the rectal area. This is a difficult position to maintain; therefore the patient should not be put into this position until just before the examination.

Equipment/Supplies:
- Examining table
- Patient gown
- Patient drape

1. **Procedural Step.** Sanitize your hands. Greet and identify the patient. Introduce yourself.
2. **Procedural Step.** Explain the examination or procedure that will be performed.
3. **Procedural Step.** Provide the patient with a patient gown. Instruct the patient to remove clothing from the waist down and to put on the gown with the opening in back. The disrobing facility should provide privacy, a place to sit, and a place to hang clothing.
4. **Procedural Step.** Pull out the footrest of the examining table, and assist the patient into a sitting position.
5. **Procedural Step.** Ask the patient to move back on the table. As the patient is doing this, pull out the table extension while supporting the patient's lower legs.

Continued

PROCEDURE 5-8   Knee-Chest Position—Cont'd

6. **Procedural Step.** Assist the patient into the supine position and then into the prone position, making sure to have the patient roll toward you. Place a drape over the patient to provide warmth and modesty.

7. **Procedural Step.** Ask the patient to bend the arms at the elbows and rest them alongside the head. Next ask the patient to elevate the buttocks while keeping the back straight. The patient's head should be turned to one side, and the weight of the body should be supported by the chest. A pillow under the chest can give additional support and aid relaxation. The knees and lower legs are separated approximately 12 inches.

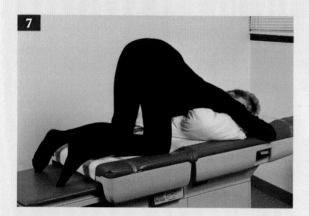

8. **Procedural Step.** Position the drape diagonally with one corner over the patient's back and the opposite corner over the buttocks. When the physician is ready to examine the patient, a small portion of the drape is folded back to expose the anal area.

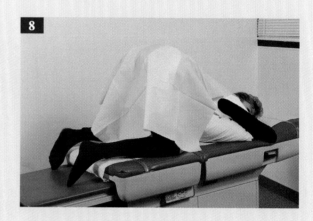

9. **Procedural Step.** After completion of the examination, assist the patient into a prone position and then into a supine position. Allow the patient to rest in the supine position before he or she sits up. *Principle.* Patients (especially elderly ones) frequently become dizzy after being in the knee-chest position and should be allowed to rest before they sit up.

10. **Procedural Step.** Assist the patient into a sitting position. Slide the table extension back into place while supporting the patient's lower legs.

11. **Procedural Step.** Assist the patient down from the table. Return the footrest to its normal position. Instruct the patient to get dressed.

PROCEDURE 5-9 Fowler's Position

Outcome Position and drape an individual in the Fowler's position. Fowler's position is used to examine the upper body of patients with cardiovascular and respiratory problems such as congestive heart failure, emphysema, and asthma. These patients find it easier to breathe in this position than in a sitting or supine position. This position is also used to draw blood from patients who are likely to faint.

Equipment/Supplies:
- Examining table
- Patient gown
- Patient drape

1. **Procedural Step.** Sanitize your hands. Greet and identify the patient. Introduce yourself.
2. **Procedural Step.** Explain the examination or procedure that will be performed.
3. **Procedural Step.** Provide the patient with a patient gown. Instruct the patient to remove clothing as appropriate for the type of examination being performed and to put on the patient gown with the opening in front. The disrobing facility should provide privacy, a place to sit, and a place to hang clothing.
4. **Procedural Step.** Position the head of the table as follows:
    a. For a semi-Fowler's position, the table should be positioned at a 45-degree angle.
    b. For a full Fowler's position, the table should be positioned at a 90-degree angle.
5. **Procedural Step.** Pull out the footrest of the examining table, and assist the patient into a sitting position.
6. **Procedural Step.** Pull out the table extension while supporting the patient's lower legs. Ask the patient to lean back against the table head. Provide assistance during this step.

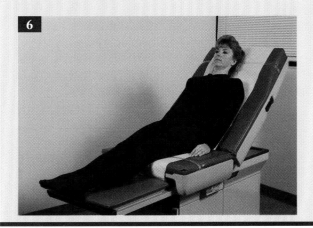

7. **Procedural Step.** Place a drape over the patient to provide warmth and modesty. As the physician examines the patient, move the drape according to the body parts being examined.

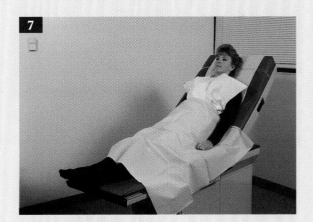

8. **Procedural Step.** After completion of the examination, assist the patient into a sitting position. Slide the table extension back into place while supporting the patient's lower legs.
9. **Procedural Step.** Assist the patient down from the table. Instruct the patient to get dressed. Return the head of the table and the footrest to their normal positions.

PROCEDURE 5-9

Assessment of the Patient

The extent of patient assessment during the physical examination depends on the purpose of the examination and the patient's condition. A complete physical examination involves a thorough assessment of all the body systems. Table 5-2 outlines the specific assessments included in a complete physical examination. In performing a physical examination, the physician uses an organized and systematic approach, starting with the patient's head and proceeding toward the feet. Using this type of approach facilitates the examination process and requires the fewest position changes by the patient.

Text continued on p. 194

TABLE 5-2	Physician Assessment During the Physical Examination		
Body Structure	**Assessment**	**Normal Findings**	**Abnormal Findings**
General Appearance	Observation of body build, posture, and gait	Good posture and balance Steady gait	Poor posture or balance Unsteady, irregular, or staggering gait
	Determination of weight and height	Weight within ideal range	Patient is overweight or underweight
	Observation of hygiene and grooming	Good hygiene and grooming	Poor hygiene and grooming
	Observation for signs of illness	No signs of illness	Obvious signs of illness
	Observation of attitude, emotional state, and mood	Patient speaks clearly and is cooperative	Patient is uncooperative, withdrawn, incoherent, negative, or hostile
Skin	Inspection of the skin for color, vascularity, lesions	Smooth, supple, free of blemishes No unusual color	Blisters, wounds, lesions, rashes, swelling Unusual skin color (e.g., flushing, cyanosis, jaundice, or pallor)
	Palpation of the temperature, moisture, turgor, and texture	Warm to the touch	Rough, dry, flaky skin Poor skin turgor
Arms and Hands	Inspection of the hands and arms for general appearance	Firm, strong muscles Normal range of motion in joints	Muscle weakness, lack of control or coordination Restricted range of motion
	Palpation of arm muscles	Good muscle control and coordination	
	Palpation for tenderness or lumps	No tenderness or lumps	Tenderness or lumps of the hands or arms
	Inspection of the fingernails	Colorless nail plate with a convex curve Smooth nail texture	Indentation, infection, brittleness, thickening, or angulation of the nails Cyanosis or pallor of the nails
Head and Neck	Inspection of the size, shape, and contour of the head	Round head with prominences in the front and back	Head is asymmetric or of unusual size
	Inspection of the hair and scalp	Hair is resilient, evenly distributed, and not excessively dry or oily	Loss of hair Scaliness or dryness of the scalp Presence of lice or other parasites
	Palpation of the head and neck	No lumps, swelling, tenderness, lesions of the head or neck	Lumps, swelling, tenderness, lesions of the head or neck

TABLE 5-2	Physician Assessment During the Physical Examination—cont'd		
Body Structure	**Assessment**	**Normal Findings**	**Abnormal Findings**
Eyes	Evaluation of visual acuity and color vision	Good visual ability with or without glasses or contact lenses Appropriate color perception	Poor visual acuity or blindness Color blindness
	Evaluation of visual field Inspection of the eyelids and eyeballs	No visual field loss Eyes are bright	Gaps in field of vision Dull or glossy eyes
	Inspection of the conjunctiva	Pink mucous membranes	Inflamed mucous membranes Excessive tearing Drainage from the eyes
	Inspection of eye movements	Eyes move equally in all directions	Drooping eyelids Uncoordinated eye movements
	Tests for pupillary reaction using a penlight	Pupils are black, are equal in size, and react appropriately to light	Dilated, constricted, or unequal pupils
	Inspection of the internal eye structures using an ophthalmoscope	Reddish pink retina, even caliber, and intact retinal blood vessels	Cloudy lens or narrowed blood vessels
Ears	Test for hearing using a tuning fork or audiometer	Good hearing ability	Limited hearing or deafness
	Inspection of the size, shape, and symmetry of the ears	Ears are symmetric and proportionate to the head	Ears are asymmetric and not proportionate to the head
	Inspection of the external ear canal and tympanic membrane using an otoscope	Cerumen is soft and easily removed No drainage or discomfort Skin of the ear canal is intact, pink, warm, and slightly moist Tympanic membrane is pearly gray and semitransparent	Lesions, redness, or swelling of the external ear canal Drainage from the ear Pain when the ear is moved Impacted cerumen Tympanic membrane is red, bulging, or perforated
Nose	Inspection of size, shape, and symmetry of the nose	Nose is symmetric, straight, and not tender	Nose is asymmetric, deformed, flaring, or tender
	Inspection of the nostrils using a nasal speculum	Septum is intact and midline Nasal mucosa is moist and pink	Deviation or perforation of septum Redness, swelling, polyps, or discharge Nostrils are obstructed
	Test for the sense of smell	Correct or very few incorrect responses to odors	Absent, decreased, exaggerated, or unequal responses to the test substances
Mouth and Pharynx	Inspection of the lips for contour, color, and texture	Pink, moist, soft, smooth lips	Pallor, cyanosis, blisters, swelling, cracking, excessive dryness of lips
	Inspection of the mucosa	Pink, moist mucous membranes	Pale or dry mucosa with ulcers or abrasions

Continued

TABLE **5-2**	Physician Assessment During the Physical Examination—cont'd		
Body Structure	**Assessment**	**Normal Findings**	**Abnormal Findings**
Mouth and Pharynx—cont'd	Inspection of the gums and palate	Smooth, pink, moist, firm gums Hard palate is firm and white Soft palate is pink and cushiony	Gums are red, bleeding, swollen, tender, spongy, or receding
	Inspection of the teeth	Smooth, white enamel; regularly spaced teeth or well-fitting dentures	Missing or loose teeth, dental caries, poor-fitting dentures
	Inspection of the tongue	Moist, pink, slightly rough-surfaced tongue Pink and smooth pharynx	Tongue is dry, furry, smooth, red, or ulcerated
	Inspection of the pharynx	Tonsils are pink and normal in size Gag reflex is present	Pharynx is red, swollen, or ulcerated Tonsils are red or swollen Absent gag reflex
Chest and Lungs	Inspection of the size and shape of the chest	Chest is symmetric	Abnormal chest contour
	Assessment of respiratory rate, rhythm, and depth	Normal respiratory rate, rhythm, and depth	Labored, slow, rapid, or irregular respirations
	Percussion of the chest		
	Auscultation of breath sounds	Normal breath sounds No cough	Flat or dull lung sounds Noisy breath sounds Productive or nonproductive cough
	Palpation of the ribs	No tenderness of the ribs	Tenderness of the ribs
Heart	Auscultation of heart sounds	Normal heart sounds	Irregular heartbeats or murmur
	Auscultation of apical pulse, rate, rhythm, and volume	Regular, strong heartbeats	Rates slower or more rapid than normal
	Palpation of peripheral pulses	Palpable peripheral pulses	Weak or absent peripheral pulses
	Auscultation of blood pressure	Blood pressure within normal range for age	Low or high blood pressure
	Assessment of peripheral vascular perfusion	Skin is pink, resilient, and moist	Cyanosis, pallor, edema
		Immediate return of color to nailbeds	Poor capillary filling in nailbeds
	Electrocardiogram to assess heart function	Normal heart function	Abnormal electrocardiogram
Breasts	Inspection of size, symmetry, and contour	Breasts are round, smooth, and symmetric	Retraction, dimpling, redness, or swelling of the breasts
	Inspection of the nipple	Nipples are round and equal in size, are similar in color, and appear soft and smooth Areola is round and pink	Bleeding, cracking, discharge, or inversion of the nipples
	Palpation of the breasts Palpation of axillary lymph nodes	No lumps or tenderness of the breasts or axillary lymph nodes	Lumps or tenderness of the breasts or axillary lymph nodes

TABLE 5-2	Physician Assessment During the Physical Examination—cont'd		
Body Structure	**Assessment**	**Normal Findings**	**Abnormal Findings**
Abdomen	Inspection of contour, symmetry, skin condition, and integrity	Symmetric contour Unblemished skin Soft abdomen	Asymmetric contour Rash or other skin lesions Abdominal distention
	Auscultation of bowel sounds	Active bowel sounds	Increased, diminished, or absent bowel sounds
	Percussion to assess underlying organs Palpation of underlying organs, tenderness, and lumps	Normal position and size of the liver and spleen	Tenderness or lumps Enlarged liver or spleen
Genitalia and Rectum	*Male* Inspection of the penis and urethra	Penis is smooth	Ulceration or discharge from the penis
	Inspection of the scrotum and palpation of the testes	Testicles are smooth, firm, and movable within the scrotal sac Scrotum is symmetric	Lumps or tenderness of the scrotum, testes, or prostate gland
	Palpation of the rectum and prostate gland	Increased pigmentation in the anal area Good anal sphincter tone	Enlarged prostate gland Hemorrhoids or relaxed anal sphincter
	Stool specimen to test for occult blood	Absence of occult blood in the stool	Occult blood in the stool
	Female Inspection of the external genitalia	External genitalia are smooth and without lesions	Ulceration or redness or swelling of the external genitalia
	Inspection of the vagina and cervix using a vaginal speculum	Vaginal mucosa is pink and moist Cervix is pink and smooth	Lacerations, tenderness, redness, or discharge from the vagina or cervix
	Specimen collection from the vagina and cervix for the Pap test	Pap test is normal	Pap test is abnormal
	Bimanual pelvic examination	No tenderness or lumps of the uterus and ovaries	Tenderness or lumps of the uterus and ovaries
	Palpation of the rectum Stool specimen to test for occult blood	Good anal sphincter tone Increased pigmentation in the anal area	Hemorrhoids or relaxed anal sphincter Occult blood in the stool
Lower Extremities	Inspection of the legs for general appearance Palpation of the legs	Firm, strong muscles Normal range of motion in joints	Muscle weakness, lack of control or coordination Restricted range of motion Tenderness or lumps Limp or foot dragging during walking
	Inspection of the toenails	Smooth nail texture	Indentation, infection, brittleness, thickening, or angulation of the nails
Neurologic	Determination of mental status and level of consciousness	Alert and responds appropriately Oriented to person, place, and time	Disoriented Responds inappropriately
	Determination of the sense of pain and touch	Normal response to pain and touch	Diminished or absent response to stimuli
	Use of a percussion hammer to test reflexes	Normal reflexes	Abnormal or absent reflexes

The results of the physical examination are charted by the physician in the patient's medical record. Figure 5-6 is an example of a preprinted form for this purpose.

Patients who exhibit symptoms of illness usually require only selected portions of the complete physical examination. For example, a patient who comes to the medical office with the symptoms of bronchitis usually will not require a complete physical examination; rather, the physician examines the body system that is most likely to be associated with the symptoms.

PHYSICAL EXAMINATION

INSTRUCTIONS:
(WNL) Within Normal Limits
(POS) Positive findings (X) Omitted

1. GENERAL
a. Posture
b. Gait
c. Speech
d. Appearance
e. Emotion

2. HEAD
a. Hair
b. Masses
c. Shape
d. Bruits
e. Tenderness
f. Sinus
g. Articulations

3. EYES
a. Lids   R___ L___   f. Pupils   R___ L___
b. Sclera   R___ L___   g. Fundi   R___ L___
c. Conjunctiva   R___ L___   h. Light   R___ L___
d. Muscles   R___ L___   i. Bruits   R___ L___
e. Cornea   R___ L___
j. Accommodation   R___ L___

4. EARS
a. Pinna   R___ L___
b. Canal   R___ L___
c. Drum   R___ L___
d. Weber
e. Rinne

5. NOSE
a. Septum
b. Mucosa   R___ L___
c. Obstruction

6. MOUTH/THROAT
a. Lips   ___   f. Teeth
b. Breath   ___   g. Dentures
c. Tongue   ___   h. Caries
d. Pharynx   ___   i. Larynx
e. Tonsils   ___   j. Floor

7. NECK
a. Thyroid   ___   d. Nodes   R___ L___
b. Trachea   ___   e. Bruits   R___ L___
c. Veins   ___   f. Carotid   R___ L___

8. LUNGS
a. Chest   ___   e. Bruits
b. Symmetry   ___   f. Sounds
c. Diaphragm   ___   g. Fremitus
d. Rubs

9. HEART
a. PMI   ___   e. Rub
b. Rate   ___   f. Murmur
c. Rhythm   ___   g. Palpation
d. Thrill

10. BREASTS
a. Nodes   R___ L___
b. Nipple   R___ L___
c. Areolae   R___ L___
d. Symmetry
e. Discharge

11. ABDOMEN
a. Sounds   ___   e. Hernia   R___ L___
b. Masses   ___   f. Bruits   R___ L___
c. Tenderness   ___   g. Femoral   R___ L___
d. Organs   ___   h. Ing. nodes   R___ L___

12. MUSCULOSKELETAL
a. Cervical
b. Thoracic
c. Lumbar
d. Sacral
e. Pelvic
f. Rib cage

13. FEMALE GENITALS
a. Labia   ___   e. Cervix
b. Bartholin   ___   f. Uterus
   gland   ___   g. Adnexa
c. Urethra   ___   R___ L___
d. Vagina   ___   h. Pap smear
   done   ___

14. MALE GENITALS
a. Penis   ___   e. Scars
b. Scrotum   ___   f. Meatus
c. Testicles   ___   g. Epididymis
d. Discharge

15. RECTAL
a. Masses   ___   f. Fissure
b. Anus   ___   g. Hemorrhoids
c. Sphincter   ___   h. Sigmoid
d. Prostate   ___   ___cm.
e. Pilonidal   ___   i. Mucosa
   j. Other

16. SKIN
a. Scars
b. Marks
c. Texture
d. Sweat
e. Color
f. Ulcers

17. NEUROLOGICAL

	Strength*		Reflex**	
a. Biceps	R___ L___		R___ L___	
b. Triceps	R___ L___		R___ L___	
c. Knee	R___ L___		R___ L___	
d. Ankle	R___ L___		R___ L___	

e. Romberg   ___   i. Coordination
f. Babinsky   ___   j. Tremor
g. Cranial N   ___   k. Vibratory
h. Sensory   ___

*When testing strength use grades:
   Weak (W); Normal (N); Strong (S)

**When testing reflexes use:
   Absent (A); Present (P); Brisk (B)

18. EXTREMITIES

a. Range of Motion
   Shoulder ___   Knee ___
   Elbow ___   Ankle ___
   Wrist ___   Hand ___
   Hip ___   Foot ___
   Phalanges ___

b. General   UR___ UL___ LR___ LL___
c. Muscular   UR___ UL___ LR___ LL___
d. Bruits   UR___ UL___ LR___ LL___
e. Edema   UR___ UL___ LR___ LL___
f. Varicosities   UR___ UL___ LR___ LL___

Signature _____

Figure 5-6. A preprinted form for recording the results of the physical examination.

Four assessment techniques are used to obtain information during the physical examination: inspection, palpation, percussion, and auscultation.

Inspection

Inspection involves observation of the patient for any signs of disease, and of the four assessment techniques, it is the one most frequently used. Good lighting, either natural or artificial, is important for effective observation. The patient's color, speech, deformities, skin condition (e.g., rashes, scars, and warts), body contour and symmetry, orientation to the surroundings, body movements, and anxiety level are assessed through inspection. The medical assistant should develop a high level of detailed observational skills to assist the physician in assessing physical characteristics.

Palpation

Palpation is the examination of the body using the sense of touch (Figure 5-7). The physician uses palpation to determine the placement and size of organs, the presence of lumps, and the existence of pain, swelling, or tenderness. Examining the breasts and taking the pulse are performed by palpation. Palpation often helps verify data obtained by inspection. The patient's verbal and facial expressions are also observed during palpation to assist in the detection of abnormalities.

There are two types of palpation, light and deep, categorized by the amount of pressure applied. *Light palpation* of structures is performed to determine areas of tenderness. The fingertips are placed on the part to be examined and are gently depressed approximately one half inch. *Deep palpation* is used to examine the condition of organs such as those in the abdomen. Two hands are used for deep palpation. One hand is used to support the body from below, and the other hand is used to press over the area to be palpated. For example, deep palpation is used by the physician to perform a bimanual pelvic examination.

Percussion

Percussion involves tapping the patient with the fingers and listening to the sounds produced to determine the size, density, and location of organs. This technique is often used to examine the lungs and abdomen.

The fingertips are used to produce a sound vibration similar to that of tapping a drumstick on a drum. The nondominant hand is placed directly on the area to be assessed, with the fingers slightly separated. The dominant hand is used to strike the joint of the middle finger placed on the patient to produce the sound vibration (Figure 5-8). Structures that are dense, such as the liver, spleen, and heart, produce a dull sound. Empty or air-filled structures, such as the lungs, produce a hollow sound. Any condition

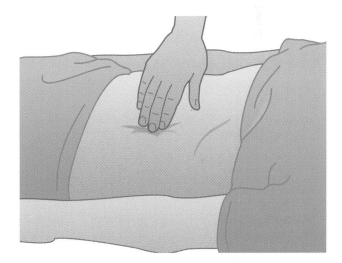

Figure 5-7. Palpation is the examination of the body using the sense of touch.

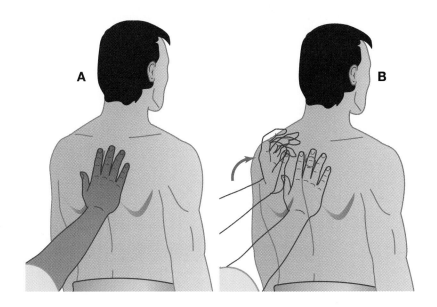

Figure 5-8. Percussion involves tapping the patient with the fingers. **A,** The nondominant hand is placed directly on the area to be assessed, with the fingers slightly separated. **B,** The fingers of the dominant hand are used to strike the joint of the middle finger to produce a sound vibration.

that changes the density of an organ or tissue, such as fluid in the lungs, will change the quality of the sound.

Auscultation

Auscultation is an examination technique that involves listening with a stethoscope to the sounds produced within the body. This technique is used to listen to the heart and lungs or to measure blood pressure. Environmental noise interferes with effective auscultation of body sounds and, therefore, should be minimized. The diaphragm of the stethoscope chestpiece is used to assess high-pitched sounds such as lung and bowel sounds; the bell of the stethoscope chestpiece is used to assess low-pitched sounds such as those produced by the heart and vascular system. The chestpiece should be cleaned with an antiseptic wipe and then warmed with the hand before placing on the patient.

Assisting the Physician

During the patient assessment, the medical assistant should assist the physician as required. This includes helping the patient change positions for the physician's examination of the different parts of the body, handing the physician instruments and supplies, and reassuring the patient to reduce apprehension. Once the examination is completed, the medical assistant should assist the patient off the examining table and provide additional information if needed, such as scheduling a return visit or patient education to promote wellness. Procedure 5-10 describes the procedure for assisting with the physical examination.

PROCEDURE 5-10 **Assisting With the Physical Examination**

Outcome Prepare the patient and assist with a physical examination.

Equipment/Supplies:

- Examining table
- Equipment for the type of examination to be performed

- Patient examination gown
- Drapes

1. **Procedural Step.** Prepare the examining room. Make sure the room is clean, free of clutter, and well lit, and that the room temperature is comfortable for the patient.
2. **Procedural Step.** Sanitize your hands.
3. **Procedural Step.** Assemble the equipment according to the type of examination to be performed and the physician's preference. Arrange the instruments and supplies in a neat and orderly manner on a table or tray. Do not allow one instrument to lay on top of another.

4. **Procedural Step.** Obtain the patient's medical record. Go to the waiting room and ask the patient to come back to the examining room.
5. **Procedural Step.** Escort the patient to the examining room.
6. **Procedural Step.** Ask the patient to be seated. Greet and identify the patient. Introduce yourself to the patient. Use a calm and friendly manner. *Principle.* Using a calm and friendly manner helps to put the patient at ease.

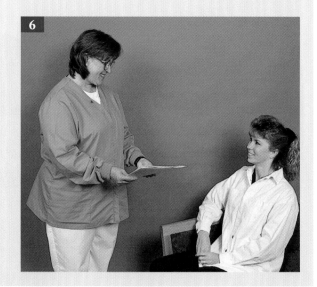

7. **Procedural Step.** Seat yourself so that you face the patient at a distance of 3 to 4 feet.

8. **Procedural Step.** Obtain and record the patient's symptoms following the procedure outlined in Procedure 1-4 in Chapter 1.

9. **Procedural Step.** Measure the patient's vital signs, and chart the results.

10. **Procedural Step.** Measure the weight and height of the patient, and chart the results.

11. **Procedural Step.** Instruct and prepare the patient for the examination as follows:

   a. Ask the patient if he or she needs to empty the bladder before the examination. If a urine specimen is needed, the patient will be required to void into a urine container.

   b. Provide the patient with a patient gown. Instruct the patient to remove all clothing and to put on the patient gown. Offer assistance if you sense the patient may have trouble undressing.

   c. Ask the patient to have a seat and inform the patient that the physician will be with him or her soon.

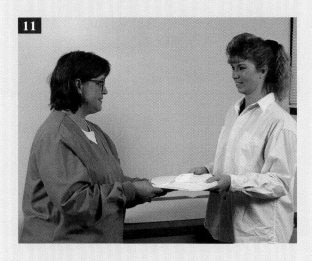

Principle. An empty bladder makes the examination easier and is more comfortable for the patient.

12. **Procedural Step.** Inform the physician that the patient is ready, and make the medical record available to the physician.

13. **Procedural Step.** Assist the physician with the examination of the body systems as follows:

   a. Assist the patient into a sitting position on the examining table so that the physician can examine the patient's head, eyes, ears, nose, mouth and pharynx, neck, chest, lungs, and heart.

   b. Hand the physician the ophthalmoscope, otoscope, and tongue depressor.

   c. Dim the light when the physician is ready to use the ophthalmoscope. The dim light will help dilate the patient's pupils, thus providing the physician better visualization of the interior of the eye.

   d. After use, the tongue depressor should be transferred by holding it at the center to prevent contact with the patient's secretions, which may contain pathogens. Dispose of the tongue depressor in a regular waste container.

   e. Offer reassurance to the patient to reduce apprehension.

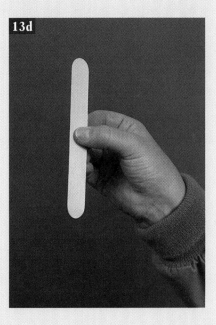

13d

14. **Procedural Step.** Position the patient as required for examination of the remaining body systems. Place and drape the patient in the proper position for examination of a particular part of the body.

PROCEDURE 5-10

Continued

PROCEDURE 5-10   Assisting With the Physical Examination—Cont'd

15. **Procedural Step.** Assist and instruct the patient as follows:
    a. Allow the patient to rest in a sitting position on the examining table before he or she gets off it. Some patients become dizzy after being positioned on the examining table.
    b. Assist the patient off the examining table to prevent falls.
    c. Instruct the patient to get dressed. Provide assistance if needed.
    d. Provide the patient with any necessary instructions, such as patient education and scheduling a return visit. Give instructions involving medical care in terms the patient can understand; do not use medical terms.
    e. Chart any instructions given to the patient in his or her medical record.
    f. Escort the patient to the reception area.
16. **Procedural Step.** Clean the examining room in preparation for the next patient as follows:
    a. Discard the paper on the examining table. If body secretions have gotten on the examining table, apply gloves and clean and disinfect the table. Unroll a fresh length of paper on the table.

    b. Discard all disposable supplies into an appropriate waste container.
    c. Make sure there is an ample number of clean gowns and drapes and other supplies.
    d. Remove reusable equipment to a work area for sanitization, sterilization, or disinfection as required by the medical office policy.

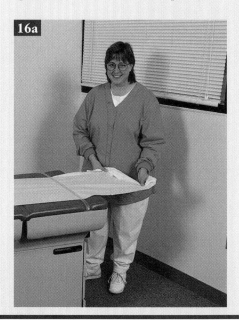

16a

What Would You DO?
What Would You *Not* DO? *RESPONSES*

Case Study 1

What Did Hope Do?

❑ Empathized with Abbey and told her that a lot of patients feel just like she does about having their weight taken.

❑ Told Abbey that weight is important so the doctor can properly diagnose and treat her condition and that medication dosage is often based on a person's weight.

❑ Told Abbey that she could stand on the scale backward while her weight is being measured so she won't see the reading on the scale.

❑ Made sure to return the weights to zero before Abbey got off the scale.

❑ Recorded Abbey's weight in her chart without telling her the results.

❑ Encouraged Abbey to see the physician when she needs to so that she stays as healthy as possible.

What Did Hope Not Do?

❑ Did not make any comments about Abbey's body or weight after weighing her.

❑ Did not criticize Abbey for letting her weight stand in the way of coming in when she needed health care.

What Would You Do/What Would You *Not* Do? Review Hope's response and place a checkmark next to the information you included in your response. List the additional information you included in your response.

_____

_____

_____

_____

Case Study 2

What Did Hope Do?

❑ Listened carefully to Mikayla and showed concern both verbally and nonverbally.

❑ Carefully charted the information relayed by Mikayla so that the physician would be aware of all aspects of Mikayla's problem.

❑ Told Mikayla that she needs to talk to the physician about wanting some medicine for heartburn.

❑ Encouraged Mikayla to talk to her parents about what's been going on with her.

What Did Hope Not Do?

❑ Did not agree with Mikayla that she needs to lose more weight.

❑ Did not make comments about Mikayla's being too thin.

What Would You Do/What Would You *Not* Do? Review Hope's response and place a checkmark next to the information you included in your response. List the additional information you included in your response.

_____

_____

_____

_____

Case Study 3

What Did Hope Do?

❑ Greeted Chang-Yi first before greeting his son.

❑ Spoke clearly and slowly to Ben-Yi in a normal tone of voice.

❑ Gave them a brochure on low-sodium diets and went over the foods that are low in sodium.

❑ Asked Chang-Yi (via Ben-Yi's translating) to indicate the foods he likes that he thinks would be low in sodium. Determined if these foods are low in sodium.

❑ Showed Ben-Yi how to take his father's blood pressure. Had Ben-Yi practice taking his father's blood pressure.

❑ Checked to make sure Chang-Yi and Ben-Yi understood all of the information before they left the office.

What Did Hope Not Do?

❑ Was careful not to ignore Chang-Yi.

What Would You Do/What Would You *Not* Do? Review Hope's response and place a checkmark next to the information you included in your response. List the additional information you included in your response.

_____

_____

_____

_____

Apply Your KNOWLEDGE

Choose the best answer to each of the following questions.

1. Spencer Tatem has come to the office complaining of intense pain in his left arm. When he was inline skating, he fell and landed on his arm. His forearm is slightly deformed, swollen, and bruised. Dr. Therapeutic has looked at his health history and has completed a physical examination and suspects that Spencer has fractured his left forearm. At this point, the diagnosis of a broken arm would be considered the
   A. Final diagnosis
   B. Clinical diagnosis
   C. Differential diagnosis
   D. Prognosis

2. Dr. Therapeutic orders a complete set of x-rays on Spencer's forearm. Taking x-rays would be considered a
   A. Therapeutic procedure
   B. Laboratory procedure
   C. Diagnostic procedure
   D. Differential test

3. Anna Richards, 42 years old, has come to the office for a physical examination. Hope Fauber, CMA, is preparing for her examination. All of the following would be appropriate actions for the examination EXCEPT
   A. Asking Anna if she needs to empty her bladder before the examination
   B. Measuring Anna's vital signs
   C. Instructing Anna to put on the examination gown with the opening in front
   D. Placing Anna's chart in the examining room

4. During Anna's examination, Dr. Therapeutic asks Hope for the percussion hammer. Hope realizes that Dr. Therapeutic is getting ready to
   A. Fix the examining table
   B. Test Anna's reflexes
   C. Test Anna's hearing
   D. Listen to Anna's heart

5. Dr. Therapeutic is performing a breast examination on Anna to detect any lumps or thickening in her breasts. This type of assessment is an example of
   A. Inspection
   B. Palpation
   C. Percussion
   D. Auscultation

6. Anna is somewhat apprehensive and says she is embarrassed during her examination. Hope should
   A. Reassure Anna to help her become less embarrassed
   B. Leave the examining room to prevent Anna from becoming more embarrassed
   C. Give Anna a stuffed animal to hold
   D. Ignore Anna's apprehension and hope it goes away

7. Ida Vicolas is 70 years old. She is coughing and having trouble breathing. To help Ida breathe easier, Hope Fauber, CMA, positions her on the examining table in the following position:
   A. Knee-chest
   B. Supine
   C. Fowler's
   D. Prone

8. Dr. Therapeutic is listening to Ida's lung sounds with his stethoscope. This is an example of
   A. Inspection
   B. Palpation
   C. Percussion
   D. Auscultation

9. Dr. Therapeutic tells Hope that he is ready to examine Ida's ears. Hope hands him
   A. An otoscope
   B. An ophthalmoscope
   C. A bread knife
   D. A tuning fork

10. Dr. Therapeutic is concerned that Ida may have some fluid in her lungs. He taps Ida's chest with his fingers while he listens to the sounds produced. This is an example of
    A. Inspection
    B. Palpation
    C. Percussion
    D. Auscultation

CERTIFICATIONREVIEW

❑ **A patient examination consists of three parts:** the health history, the physical examination, and laboratory and diagnostic tests. The physician uses the results to determine the patient's general state of health, to arrive at a diagnosis and prescribe treatment, and to observe any change in a patient's illness after treatment has been instituted.

❑ **Diagnosis** refers to the scientific method of determining and identifying a patient's condition through the evaluation of the health history, the physical examination, and the results of laboratory tests and diagnostic procedures.

❑ **The clinical diagnosis** is obtained through the evaluation of the health history and the physical examination without the benefit of laboratory or diagnostic tests. The prognosis is the probable course and outcome of a patient's condition.

❑ **The equipment and supplies** needed for the physical examination vary according to the type of examination and the physician's preference. The medical assistant should have the equipment and supplies ready for the examination. They should be arranged for easy access by the physician.

❑ **An adult patient's weight** is usually measured during every office visit, whereas an adult's height is typically measured only during the first visit or when a complete physical examination of the patient is requested. Children are weighed and measured during every office visit to observe their pattern of growth and to calculate medication dosage.

❑ **The scale** must be balanced before measuring a patient's weight to ensure an accurate weight measurement. The weight measurement should be recorded in pounds to the nearest quarter of a pound. The height measurement should be recorded in feet and inches to the nearest quarter of an inch.

❑ **Correct patient positioning** facilitates the examination by permitting better access to the part being examined or treated. The positions used in the medical office are the sitting, supine, prone, dorsal recumbent, lithotomy, Sims, knee-chest, and Fowler's. The position used depends on the type of examination or procedure to be performed.

❑ **The patient is draped** during positioning to provide modesty, comfort, and warmth. The part to be examined is the only part that should be exposed.

❑ **A physical examination** is performed using an organized and systematic approach starting with an examination of the patient's head and proceeding toward the feet.

❑ **Assessment techniques** to obtain information during the physical examination include inspection, palpation, percussion, and auscultation. Inspection involves observation of the patient for signs of disease. Palpation is the examination of the body using the sense of touch. Percussion involves tapping the patient with the fingers and listening to the sounds produced to determine the size, density, and location of underlying organs. Auscultation involves listening with a stethoscope to the sounds produced within the body.

Terminology Review

Audiometer An instrument used to measure hearing.

Auscultation The process of listening to the sounds produced within the body to detect signs of disease.

Bariatrics The branch of medicine that deals with the treatment and control of obesity and diseases associated with obesity.

Clinical diagnosis A tentative diagnosis of a patient's condition obtained through the evaluation of the health history and the physical examination, without the benefit of laboratory or diagnostic tests.

Diagnosis The scientific method of determining and identifying a patient's condition.

Differential diagnosis A determination of which of two or more diseases with similar symptoms is producing the patient's symptoms.

Inspection The process of observing a patient to detect signs of disease.

Mensuration The process of measuring the patient.

Ophthalmoscope An instrument for examining the interior of the eye.

Otoscope An instrument for examining the external ear canal and tympanic membrane.

Palpation The process of feeling with the hands to detect signs of disease.

Percussion The process of tapping the body to detect signs of disease.

Percussion hammer An instrument with a rubber head, used for testing reflexes.

Prognosis The probable course and outcome of a patient's condition and the patient's prospects for recovery.

Speculum An instrument for opening a body orifice or cavity for viewing.

Symptom Any change in the body or its functioning that indicates that a disease might be present.

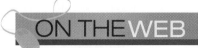

ON THE WEB

For active weblinks to each website visit http://evolve.elsevier.com/Bonewit/.

For Information on Nutrition:

American Dietetic Association

Ask the Dietitian

Healthy Food

For Information on Weight Control and Fitness:

Weight Watchers

Calorie Control Council

Cyber Diet

For Information on Accessing Health Information:

Aetna InteliHealth

Virtual Hospital

Mayo Clinic

U.S. Department of Health and Human Services

American Academy of Family Physicians: Family Doctor

Healthfinder

WebMD

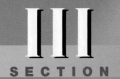

III
SECTION

Specialty Examinations and Procedures

6 Eye and Ear Assessment and Procedures

7 Physical Agents to Promote Tissue Healing

8 The Gynecological Examination and Prenatal Care

9 The Pediatric Examination

Learning Objectives	Procedures

The Eye

1. Identify the structures that constitute the eye, and explain the function of each.
2. Define visual acuity.
3. State the cause and visual difficulty of the following:
   Myopia
   Hyperopia
   Presbyopia
4. Explain the differences among an ophthalmologist, an optometrist, and an optician.
5. Explain the significance of the top and bottom numbers next to each line of letters on the Snellen eye chart.
6. Explain the difference between congenital and acquired color vision defects.
7. List the reasons to perform an eye irrigation and an eye instillation.

Assess distance visual acuity.
Assess near visual acuity.
Assess color vision.
Perform an eye irrigation.
Perform an eye instillation.

The Ear

1. Identify the structures of the external, middle, and inner ear, and explain the function of each.
2. Identify conditions that may cause conductive and sensorineural hearing loss.
3. List and describe the ways in which hearing acuity can be tested.
4. List the reasons to perform an ear irrigation and an ear instillation.

Perform an ear irrigation.
Perform an ear instillation.

CHAPTER 6

Eye and Ear Assessment and Procedures

Chapter Outline

Introduction to Eye and Ear Assessment
THE EYE
Structure of the Eye
Visual Acuity
  Assessment of Distance Visual Acuity
  Assessment of Near Visual Acuity
Assessment of Color Vision
  The Ishihara Test
Eye Irrigation
Eye Instillation
THE EAR
Structure of the Ear
Assessment of Hearing Acuity
  Types of Hearing Loss
  Hearing Acuity Tests
Ear Irrigation
Ear Instillation

National Competencies

Clinical Competencies
Patient Care
- Prepare patient for and assist with routine and specialty examinations.
- Prepare patient for and assist with procedures, treatments, and minor office surgery.

General Competencies
Patient Instruction
- Instruct individuals according to their needs.
- Provide instruction for health maintenance and disease prevention.

Key Terms

audiometer (aw-dee-OM-eh-ter)
canthus (KAN-thus)
cerumen
hyperopia (HYE-per-OP-ee-uh)
instillation (IN-still-AY-shun)
irrigation (EAR-ih-GAY-shun)
myopia (mye-OH-pee-uh)
otoscope (AH-toe-skope)
presbyopia (PRESS-bee-OH-pee-uh)
refraction (ree-FRAK-shun)
tympanic membrane (tim-PAN-ik MEM-brane)

Introduction to Eye and Ear Assessment

The medical assistant is responsible for performing a variety of assessments and procedures that involve the eye and the ear. An understanding of the structure and function of the eye and the ear is essential to mastering skill in these areas.

A visual acuity test is usually part of the routine physical examination. This test is a screening test to detect deficiencies in vision.

The medical assistant may be responsible for assessing color vision with the use of specially prepared colored plates. As a result of this testing, color blindness can be detected. Color blindness is an inability to distinguish certain colors; the most common problem is with the colors red and green. This is particularly significant if the patient is involved in an activity that relies on the ability to distinguish colors, such as electronics and interior decorating.

Hearing tests may also be part of the routine physical examination. During contact with the patient, the medical assistant should be alert to signs that indicate the patient might be having difficulty hearing what is being said. A whispered voice or a ticking watch held next to the patient's ear can be a screening test for hearing acuity. The use of tuning forks or an audiometer provides a more accurate determination of hearing acuity. An **audiometer** is an instrument that emits sound waves at various frequencies. The patient is instructed to indicate when a sound at a given frequency can be heard.

The medical assistant is responsible for performing or teaching the patient to perform eye and ear irrigations and instillations. **Irrigation** is washing a body canal with a flowing solution. **Instillation** is dropping a liquid into a body cavity. Eye and ear irrigations and instillations should be performed using the important principles of medical asepsis outlined in Chapter 2.

THE EYE

Structure of the Eye

The eye has three layers (Figure 6-1). The outer layer is the *sclera,* which is composed of tough, white fibrous connective tissue. The front part of the sclera is modified to form a transparent covering over the colored part of the eye; this covering is the *cornea.*

The middle layer of the eye is the *choroid,* which is composed of many blood vessels and is highly pigmented. The blood vessels nourish the other layers of the eye, and the pigment works to absorb stray light rays. The front part of the choroid is specialized into the ciliary body, the suspensory ligaments, and the iris. The *ciliary body* contains muscles that control the shape of the lens. The function of the *suspensory ligaments* is to suspend the lens in place. The

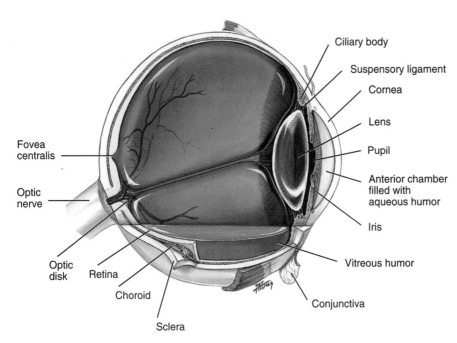

Figure 6-1. The internal structure of the eye. (From Applegate EJ: *The anatomy and physiology learning system*, ed 2, Philadelphia, 2000, Saunders.)

lens is responsible for focusing the light rays on the retina. The colored part of the eye is the *iris,* which controls the size of the pupil. The *pupil* is the opening in the eye that permits the entrance of light rays.

The third and innermost layer of the eye is the *retina.* Light rays come to a focus on the retina and are subsequently transmitted to the brain, by way of the optic nerve, to be interpreted.

The *anterior chamber* is the area between the cornea and the iris, and the *posterior chamber* is the area between the iris and the lens. Both chambers are filled with a substance known as the *aqueous humor.* A transparent jellylike material, known as *vitreous humor,* fills the eyeball between the lens and the retina. Its function is to help maintain the shape of the eyeball.

The *conjunctiva* is a membrane that lines the eyelids and covers the front of the eye, except the cornea. The conjunctiva covering the sclera is transparent except for some capillaries, which allows the white sclera to show through.

Visual Acuity

Visual acuity refers to acuteness or sharpness of vision. A person with normal visual acuity can see clearly and is able to distinguish fine details both close up and at some distance.

Errors of refraction are the most common causes of defects in visual acuity (Figure 6-2). **Refraction** refers to the ability of the eye to bend the parallel light rays coming into it so they can be focused on the retina. An error of refraction means that the light rays are not being refracted or bent properly and therefore are not adequately focused on the retina. A defect in the shape of the eyeball can cause a refractive error. Errors of refraction can be improved with corrective lenses.

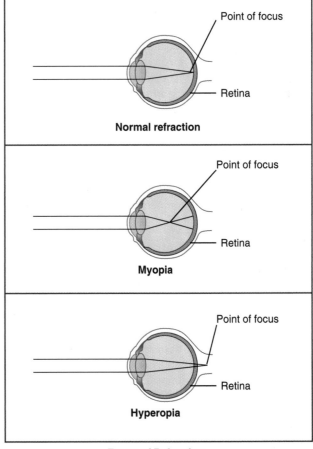

Errors of Refraction

Figure 6-2. Diagram of normal refraction compared with myopia (nearsightedness) and hyperopia (farsightedness), which are errors of refraction that cause visual defects.

A person who is nearsighted has a condition termed **myopia.** The eyeball is too long from front to back, causing the light rays to be brought to a focus in front of the retina. The myopic person has difficulty seeing objects at a distance and may squint and have headaches as a result of eyestrain. A corrective lens (e.g., eyeglasses, contact lenses) can correct this condition by causing the light rays to come to a focus on the retina.

A person who is farsighted has a condition known as **hyperopia.** The eyeball is too short from front to back, resulting in a different type of refractive error, in which the light rays are brought to a focus behind the retina. This person has difficulty viewing objects at a reading or working distance. An individual with hyperopia may experience blurring, headaches, and eyestrain while performing up-close tasks. A corrective lens can correct this condition by causing the light rays to come to a focus on the retina.

In most people, a decrease in the elasticity of the lens of the eye begins to occur after age 40 years. This condition, **presbyopia,** results in a decreased ability to focus clearly on close objects.

If a defect in visual acuity is detected, the patient is referred to an eye specialist for further evaluation. Several types of specialist are involved in the care of the eyes. An *ophthalmologist* is a medical doctor who specializes in diagnosing and treating diseases and disorders of the eye. An ophthalmologist is qualified to prescribe both ophthalmic and systemic medications and to perform eye surgery. An *optometrist* is a licensed primary health care provider who has expertise in measuring visual acuity and prescribing corrective lenses for the treatment of refractive errors. An optometrist is also qualified to diagnose and treat disorders and diseases of the eye and to prescribe ophthalmic medications. An optometrist is not a physician and therefore is not permitted to prescribe systemic medications or to perform eye surgery. An **optician** is a professional who interprets and fills prescriptions for eyeglasses and contact lenses.

Assessment of Distance Visual Acuity

Myopia can be diagnosed (in combination with other tests) by a distance visual acuity (DVA) test. In the medical office, the Snellen eye chart is most often used. Two types of charts are commonly used in the medical office. One type is used for school-age children and adults and consists of a chart of letters in decreasing sizes (Figure 6-3). The other type is used for preschool children, non–English-speaking people, and nonreaders; it is composed of the capital letter E in decreasing sizes and arranged in different directions (Figure 6-4). Visual acuity charts with pictures of common objects are also available for use with preschoolers. Testing with these charts tends to be less accurate than with the Snellen charts. Some children are unable to identify the objects because of lack of recognition, not because of a defect in visual acuity. It is suggested that the Snellen Big E chart be used with preschoolers.

Conducting a Snellen Test

The visual acuity test should be performed in a well-lit room that is free of distractions. The test is usually performed at a distance of 20 feet; this can be conveniently marked off in the medical office with paint or a piece of tape so that it does not have to be remeasured every time the test is given.

At the side of each row of letters on the chart are two numbers, separated by a line. The number above the line

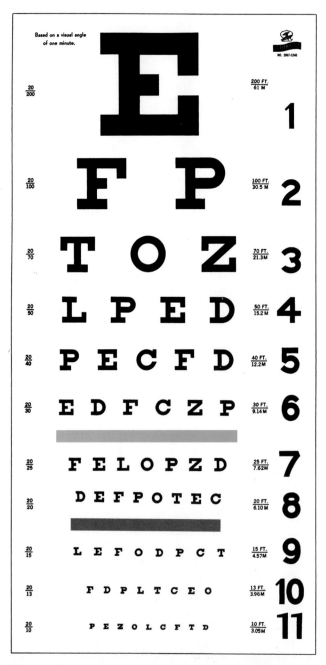

Figure 6-3. A Snellen eye chart consisting of letters in decreasing sizes, which is used to measure distance visual acuity.

represents the distance (in feet) at which the test is conducted. It is usually 20 because most eye tests are conducted at this distance. The number below the line represents the distance from which a person with normal visual acuity can read the row of letters. The line marked 20/20 indicates normal distance visual acuity, or 20/20 vision. This means a person could read what he or she was supposed to read at a distance of 20 feet.

A visual acuity reading of 20/30 means this was the smallest line that the individual could read at a distance of 20 feet. People with normal acuity would be able to read this line at a distance of 30 feet.

A visual acuity reading of 20/15 means this was the smallest line that the individual could read at a distance of 20 feet. It indicates above-average acuity for distance vision. People with normal acuity would be able to read this line at 15 feet.

The acuity of each eye should be measured separately, traditionally beginning with the right eye. Most physicians prefer that the patient wear his or her contact lenses or glasses, except reading glasses, during the test; the medical assistant should record in the patient's chart that corrective lenses were worn by the patient during the test. An eye occluder should be held over the eye not being tested. The patient's hands should not be used to cover the eye because this may encourage peeking through the fingers,

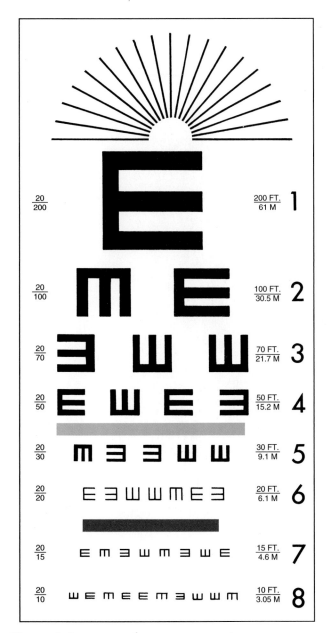

Figure 6-4. A Snellen Big E eye chart consisting of the capital letter E in decreasing sizes and arranged in different directions, which is used to measure distance visual acuity.

Highlight on Eye Assessment

Vision disorders are the fourth most common disability in the United States. Studies show that vision disorders are the most prevalent handicapping condition in children. Because of this, it is recommended that children have a complete eye examination starting at age 3. Both children and adults should have an eye examination every 2 to 3 years up to 60 years of age. Individuals older than 60 years should have yearly eye examinations.

Individuals who have risk factors for eye disorders should have an eye examination every year. Examples of risk factors are diabetes and hypertension.

Visual acuity is considered normal for the various age-groups if it falls within the following values:

Newborn	20/500
Child 1 month to 6 months	20/200 to 20/90
Child 6 to 12 months	20/60
Child 12 to 18 months	20/40
Child 2 to 3 years	20/30
Child 3 to 18 years	20/20
Adult 18 years or older	20/20

Legal blindness is defined as a visual acuity measurement of 20/200 or less in both eyes with the use of corrective lenses.

The term *color blind* is not an accurate term to describe an individual with abnormal color vision because the inability to distinguish any colors at all is extremely rare. Most individuals with a color vision abnormality are unable to distinguish certain hues of color, such as red and green. Therefore a better term is "color vision defect."

Defective color vision is usually congenital. It is found in 8% of men and 5% of women.

Studies show that there is no significant correlation between defective color vision and increased automobile accidents. The majority of drivers who have a color vision defect are able to distinguish traffic lights by the different light intensities and by the position of the light on the traffic signal.

especially in the case of children. The patient should be instructed to leave open the eye not being tested because closing it causes squinting of the eye that is being tested. The procedure for measuring distance visual acuity is outlined in Procedure 6-1.

Assessing Distance Visual Acuity in Preschoolers

With minor variations, Procedure 6-1 can be used to test distance visual acuity in preschoolers. The Snellen Big E chart is used for this purpose.

A child needs a complete and thorough explanation of what is expected of him or her before beginning the test. Tell the child you will be playing a pointing game. Do not force the child to play the game because the results would then tend to be inaccurate. Draw the capital letter E on an index card, and teach the child to point in the direction of the open part of the E by turning the card in different directions (up, down, to the right, and to the left). Using such phrases as the "fingers" or the "legs of the table" to describe the open part of the E helps the child understand what is expected (Figure 6-5). Allow the child to practice the pointing game with the index card until you are sure this level of skill has been mastered. Be sure to praise the child when the correct response is given.

The child might need help holding the eye occluder in place. The aid of another person such as the parent would then be required.

Assessment of Near Visual Acuity

Near visual acuity (NVA) testing assesses the patient's ability to read close objects (i.e., at a reading or working distance); the test results are used to detect hyperopia and presbyopia.

The test is conducted with a card similar to the Snellen eye chart; however, the size of the type ranges from the size of newspaper headlines down to considerably smaller print such as would be found in a telephone directory

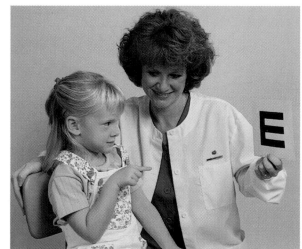

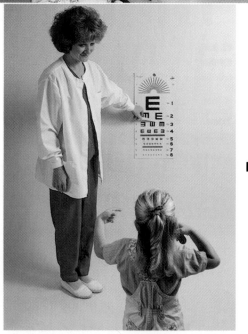

Figure 6-5. **A,** Cammie teaches a preschooler to point in the direction of the open part of the capital letter E. **B,** Cammie performs the Snellen Big E visual acuity test.

(Figure 6-6). The test card is available in a variety of forms such as printed paragraphs, printed words, and pictures.

The test should be performed in a well-lit room free of distractions. It is conducted with the patient holding the test card at a distance between 14 and 16 inches. If the patient wears reading glasses, they should be worn during the test. The acuity should be measured in each eye separately, traditionally beginning with the right eye. An eye occluder should be held over the eye not being tested. The patient should be instructed to keep the covered eye open because closing it may cause squinting of the eye that is being tested. The patient is asked to identify orally each line or paragraph of type. During the test, the patient should be observed for unusual symptoms such as squinting, tilting the head, or watering of the eyes, which may indicate that

What Would You DO? What Would You Not DO?

Case Study 1

Nicole Neason brings her daughter, Haley, to the office for a camp physical. Haley just completed the fourth grade and is going to summer camp for 2 weeks with Tess, her best friend. Tess wears glasses, and Haley thinks they are really cool. She often asks to try on Tess's glasses and wishes she could wear glasses just like her best friend. When Haley is measured for visual acuity, she misses a few letters on the 20/70 line, the 20/50 line, the 20/40 line, and the 20/20 line. She is unable to read any of the letters on the 20/15 line. After the examination, Haley wants to know if she's missed enough letters to be able to get glasses.

No. 1.
.37M

In the second century of the Christian era, the empire of Rome comprehended the fairest part of the earth, and the most civilized portion of mankind. The frontiers of that extensive monarchy were guarded by ancient renown and disciplined valor. The gentle but powerful influence of laws and manners had gradually cemented the union of the provinces. Their peaceful inhabitants enjoyed and abused the advantages of wealth.

No. 2.
.50M

fourscore years, the public administration was conducted by the virtue and abilities of Nerva, Trajan, Hadrian, and the two Antonines. It is the design of this, and of the two succeeding chapters, to describe the prosperous condition of their empire; and afterwards, from the death of Marcus Antoninus, to deduce the most important circumstances of its decline and fall; a revolution which will ever be remembered, and is still felt by

No. 3.
.62M

the nations of the earth. The principal conquests of the Romans were achieved under the republic; and the emperors, for the most part, were satisfied with preserving those dominions which had been acquired by the policy of the senate, the active emulations of the consuls, and the martial enthusiasm of the people. The seven first centuries were filled with a rapid succession of triumphs; but it was

No. 4.
.75M

reserved for Augustus to relinquish the ambitious design of subduing the whole earth, and to introduce a spirit of moderation into the public councils. Inclined to peace by his temper and situation, it was very easy for him to discover that Rome, in her present exalted situation, had much less to hope than to fear from the chance of arms; and that, in the prosecution of

No. 5.
1.00M

the undertaking became every day more difficult, the event more doubtful, and the possession more precarious, and less beneficial. The experience of Augustus added weight to these salutary reflections, and effectually convinced him that, by the prudent vigor of

No. 6.
1.25M

his counsels, it would be easy to secure every concession which the safety or the dignity of Rome might require from the most formidable barbarians. Instead of exposing his person or his legions to the arrows of the Parthians, he obtained, by an honor-

No. 7.
1.50M

able treaty, the restitution of the standards and prisoners which had been taken in the defeat of Crassus. His generals, in the early part of his reign, attempted the reduction of Ethiopia and Arabia Felix. They marched near a thou-

No. 8.
1.75M

sand miles to the south of the tropic; but the heat of the climate soon repelled the invaders, and protected the unwarlike natives of those sequestered regions

No. 9.
2.00M

The northern countries of Europe scarcely deserved the expense and labor of conquest. The forests and morasses of Germany were

No. 10.
2.25M

filled with a hardy race of barbarians who despised life when it was separated from freedom; and though, on the first

No. 11.
2.50M

attack, they seemed to yield to the weight of the Roman power, they soon, by a signal

Figure 6-6. Example of a near visual acuity card.

the patient is having difficulty reading the card. The patient continues until reaching the smallest type that can be read.

The results are recorded as the smallest type that the patient could comfortably read with each eye at the distance at which the card is held (i.e., 14 to 16 inches). The recording will be based on the type of test card used to conduct the test. For example, one type of card uses a recording method similar to that used with the Snellen eye test. For this type of NVA card, the results would be recorded as 14/14 for a patient with normal near visual acuity. This means the patient read what was supposed to be read at a distance of 14 inches. Also included in the recording should be the date and time, corrective lenses worn, and any unusual symptoms exhibited by the patient.

Assessment of Color Vision

Defects in color vision may be classified as congenital or acquired. *Congenital defects* are more common and refer to a color vision deficiency that is inherited and therefore is present at birth. Congenital color vision deficiencies most often affect males. *Acquired defects* refer to a color vision deficiency that is acquired after birth, resulting from such factors as an eye injury, disease, and certain drugs. Color vision tests, such as the Ishihara test

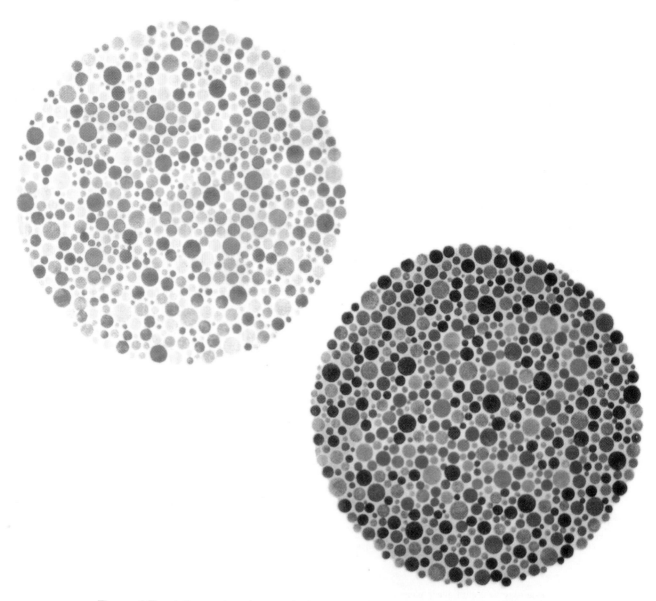

Figure 6-7. Ishihara color plates. Polychromatic plates. In the upper figure the normal person reads 74, but the red-green color-blind person reads 21. In the lower figure the red-blind person (protanope) reads 2, but the green-blind person (deuteranope) reads 4. The normal-vision person reads 42. Note that reproduced plates are not good to test for color deficiency. (From Ishihara J: *Tests for color blindness,* Tokyo, 1920, Kanehara.)

(Figure 6-7), detect congenital color vision disturbances and are commonly performed in the medical office. A basic screening for color vision can be performed by asking the patient to identify the red and green lines on the Snellen eye chart.

The Ishihara Test

The Ishihara test for color blindness is a convenient and accurate method to detect total congenital color blindness and red-green blindness by assessing an individual's ability to perceive primary colors and shades of color.

The Ishihara book contains a series of polychromatic plates of primary colored dots arranged to form a numeral against a background of similar dots of contrasting colors (see Figure 6-7). Patients with normal color vision are able to read the appropriate numeral; however, patients with color vision defects read the dots either as not forming a number at all or as forming a number different from the one identified by the individual with normal color vision. The first plate in the Ishihara book is designed to be read correctly by all individuals (those with normal vision and those exhibiting color vision deficiencies) and should be used to explain the procedure to the patient.

The book includes plates with winding colored lines for patients who are unable to read numbers, such as preschoolers and non–English-speaking people. The patient should be asked to trace the line formed by the colored dots using a cotton swab or the eraser end of a pencil. Soiled fingers can, over time, degrade the polychromatic plates and therefore the patient's finger should not be used to do the tracing.

The Ishihara test should be conducted in a quiet room illuminated by natural daylight. If this is not possible, a room lit with electric light may be used; however, the light should be adjusted to resemble the effect of natural daylight as much as possible. Using light other than just described, such as bright sunlight, may change the appearance of shades of color on the plates, leading to inaccurate test results.

The medical assistant is responsible for performing the color vision test and recording results in the patient's chart. The physician will assess the results to determine whether the patient has a deficiency in color vision.

The Ishihara test consists of 14 color plates. Plates 1 through 11 are used to conduct the basic test, and plates 12, 13, and 14 are used to further assess patients who exhibit a red-green color deficiency. Therefore it is not necessary to include these plates (12, 13, and 14) in the test of patients who exhibit normal color vision. In interpreting the results, if 10 or more plates are read correctly, the patient's color vision is considered normal. If 7 or fewer of the 11 Ishihara plates are read correctly, the patient is identified as having a color vision deficiency. It would be unusual for the medical assistant to obtain results in which the patient read 8 or 9 plates correctly. The test is structured so that a patient with a color vision defect generally does not read 8 or 9 plates correctly and the rest incorrectly.

If a defect in color vision is detected, the patient is referred for additional assessment of color vision to an ophthalmologist or optometrist, who will use more precise color vision tests. The procedure for assessing color vision using the Ishihara color plates is outlined in Procedure 6-2.

PROCEDURE 6-1

PROCEDURE 6-1   Assessing Distance Visual Acuity—Snellen Chart

Outcome Assess distance visual acuity.

Equipment/Supplies:
- Snellen eye chart
- Eye occluder
- Antiseptic wipe

1. **Procedural Step.** Sanitize your hands.
2. **Procedural Step.** Assemble the equipment. Perform the test in a well-lit room that is free of distractions. Wipe the eye occluder with an antiseptic wipe and allow it to dry completely.
   Principle. The eye occluder should be disinfected before use.
3. **Procedural Step.** Greet and identify the patient. Introduce yourself and explain the procedure. Tell the patient that he or she will be asked to read several lines of letters. The patient should not have an opportunity to study or memorize the letters before beginning the test. Instruct the patient not to squint during the test because squinting temporarily improves vision.
4. **Procedural Step.** Determine whether the patient wears contact lenses or glasses (other than reading glasses). If the patient wears such aids, he or she should be told to keep them on during the test.
5. **Procedural Step.** Ask the patient to stand on the marked line located 20 feet from the chart.

Continued

PROCEDURE 6-1 Assessing Distance Visual Acuity—
Snellen Chart—Cont'd

6. **Procedural Step.** Position the center of the Snellen chart at the patient's eye level. Stand next to the chart during the test to indicate to the patient the line to be identified.
   Principle. Make sure the chart is at the patient's eye level rather than your eye level, to provide the most accurate results.

7. **Procedural Step.** Ask the patient to cover the left eye with the eye occluder. If the patient wears eyeglasses, tell him or her to place the occluder in front of the glasses very gently to prevent the glasses from being moved out of their normal position. Instruct the patient to keep the left eye open. During the test, the medical assistant should check to make sure the patient is keeping the left eye open.
   Principle. Eyeglasses moved out of normal position may lead to inaccurate test results. Keeping the left eye open prevents squinting of the right eye.

8. **Procedural Step.** Measure the visual acuity of the right eye first. Ask the patient to identify orally one line at a time on the Snellen chart, starting with the 20/70 line (or a line that is several lines above the 20/20 line).
   Principle. It is best to start at a line above the 20/20 line to give the patient a chance to gain confidence and to become familiar with the test procedure. The medical assistant should establish a pattern of beginning with the same eye (traditionally the right eye) every time the test is performed. This helps to reduce errors during the recording of results.

9. **Procedural Step.** If the patient is able to read the 20/70 line, proceed down the chart until reaching the smallest line of letters the patient can read. If the patient is unable to read the 20/70 line, proceed up the chart until the smallest line of letters the patient can read is reached.

10. **Procedural Step.** While the patient is reading the letters, observe him or her for unusual symptoms such as squinting, tilting of the head, or watering of the eyes.
    Principle. These symptoms may indicate that the patient is having difficulty identifying the letters.

11. **Procedural Step.** Ask the patient to cover the right eye with the eye occluder and to keep the right eye open. Measure the visual acuity in the left eye as described in steps 8 through 10. During the test, check to make sure the patient is keeping the right eye open.
    Principle. Keeping the right eye open prevents squinting of the left eye.

12. **Procedural Step.** Chart the procedure. Include the date and time, the name of the test (Snellen test), the visual acuity results, and any unusual symptoms the patient exhibited during the test. Also chart whether the patient was wearing corrective lenses during the test. Use the following abbreviations:

    s̄c without correction
    c̄c with correction

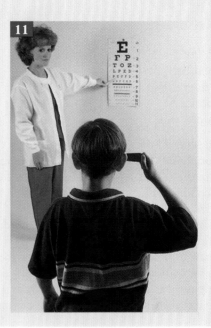

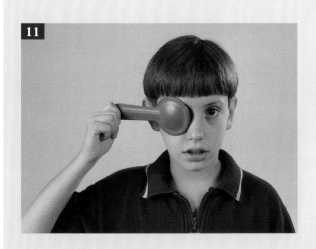

PROCEDURE 6-1

To chart the visual acuity results, observe the numbers to the side of the smallest line of letters that the patient was able to read. If one or two letters were missed, record the visual acuity with a minus sign next to the bottom number, along with the number of letters missed. (If more than two letters were missed, record the previous line.) Latin abbreviations are used to record visual acuity. The abbreviation for the right eye is OD (for *oculus dexter*), the abbreviation for the left eye is OS (for *oculus sinister*), and the abbreviation for both eyes is OU (for *oculus uterque*).

13. **Procedural Step.** Disinfect the eye occluder with an antiseptic wipe and sanitize your hands

CHARTING EXAMPLE	
Date	
11/5/05	3:30 p.m. Snellen test, s̄c: OD 20/20-1.
	OS 20/25. Exhibited squinting, OD. ————
	—————————— C. Lindner, CMA

PROCEDURE 6-2 Assessing Color Vision—Ishihara Test

Outcome Assess color vision.

Equipment/Supplies:
- Ishihara book
- Cotton swab

1. **Procedural Step.** Sanitize your hands. Assemble the equipment.
2. **Procedural Step.** Conduct the test in a quiet room illuminated by natural daylight.
   Principle. Using unnatural light may change the appearance of the shades of color on the plates, leading to inaccurate test results.
3. **Procedural Step.** Greet and identify the patient. Introduce yourself and explain the procedure. Using the first (practice) plate as an example, instruct the patient to orally identify numbers formed by colored dots. Tell the patient that 3 seconds will be given to identify each plate.
   Principle. The first plate is designed to be read correctly by all individuals and is used to explain the procedure to the patient.
4. **Procedural Step.** Hold the first color plate 30 inches (75 cm) from the patient, at a right angle to the patient's line of vision. The patient should keep both eyes open during the test.

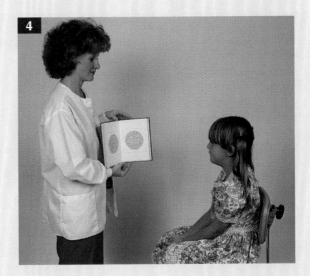

Continued

PROCEDURE 6-2   Assessing Color Vision—Ishihara Test—Cont'd

5. **Procedural Step.** Ask the patient to identify the number on the plate. If the plate consists of a traceable winding colored line, ask the patient to trace the line using a cotton swab or the eraser end of a pencil. The patient's finger should not be used to make the tracing. Record results after each plate. Continue until the patient has viewed all the plates.

To record the color vision results, use the plate identification number and the number given by the patient. If the patient is unable to identify a number, the mark X should be recorded to indicate that the plate could not be read by the patient. Examples:

Plate 5: 21 This means the patient read the number 21 on plate 5.

Plate 6: X This means the patient could not identify a number on plate 6.

Plate 11: Traceable This means that the patient correctly traced a winding line on plate 11.

Principle. The patient's finger should not be used to trace the line because soiled fingers can degrade the plate over time.

6. **Procedural Step.** Chart the results. Include the date and time, the name of the test (Ishihara test), the color vision results, and any unusual symptoms the patient exhibited during the test, such as squinting or rubbing the eyes.

7. **Procedural Step.** Return the Ishihara book to its proper place. The book of color plates must be stored in a closed position to protect it from light. *Principle.* Exposing the plates to excessive and unnecessary light results in fading of the color.

CHARTING EXAMPLE

Plate No.	Normal Person	Results
1	12	12
2	8	8
3	5	5
4	29	29
5	74	74
6	7	7
7	45	45
8	2	2
9	X	X
10	16	16
11	Traceable	Traceable
11/6/05	10:00 a.m.	
	C. Lindner, CMA	

What Would You DO? What Would You *Not* DO?

Case Study 2

Peter Mitchell comes in with his 5-year-old son, Clive. Clive is diagnosed with conjunctivitis, and the physician prescribes Polytrim ophthalmic suspension. Mr. Mitchell says that Clive does not cooperate very well when having drops put in his eyes and asks for any ideas that might make it less of an ordeal. Mr. Mitchell has 7-year-old twin girls at home and wants to know what can be done so they don't get pink eye. He asks if it would be all right to instill the drops in the twins' eyes as a preventive measure.

Eye Irrigation

An eye irrigation involves washing the eye with a flowing solution. Eye irrigations are performed for the following purposes: to cleanse the eye by washing away foreign particles, ocular discharges, or harmful chemicals; to relieve inflammation through the application of heat; and to apply an antiseptic solution. Procedure 6-3 demonstrates how to perform an eye irrigation.

Eye Instillation

Eye instillations are performed to treat eye infections (with medication), to soothe an irritated eye, to dilate the pupil, and to anesthetize the eye during an eye examination or treatment. Medication to be instilled in the eye may come in the form of a liquid, as ophthalmic drops, or as an ophthalmic ointment. The eyedrops may be dispensed in a bottle with an eyedropper or in a flexible plastic container with an attached tip. Eye ointment is dispensed in a small metal tube with a small tip for applying the medication. Procedure 6-4 demonstrates how to perform an eye instillation.

⫘ PATIENT TEACHING

Conjunctivitis

Answer questions patients have about conjunctivitis.

What is conjunctivitis?

Conjunctivitis, often referred to as *pink eye,* is an inflammation of the conjunctiva. The conjunctiva is a thin transparent membrane that covers the white of the eye. Conjunctivitis occurs when the conjunctiva becomes infected with a bacterium or virus. Other causes of conjunctivitis include allergies, the prolonged use of contact lenses, and irritation from wind, dust, and smoke. Conjunctivitis is almost always harmless and will clear up by itself within 2 weeks. If it is caused by bacteria, the physician may prescribe antibiotic eyedrops or ointment.

What are the symptoms of conjunctivitis?

Most types of conjunctivitis are relatively painless. The eye is red or pink because of irritation, and there is a feeling of sandiness or grittiness in the eye. A discharge is usually present, which dries at night when the eyes are closed. This may cause the eyelids to be stuck together in the morning. Other symptoms include tearing, itching, and sensitivity of the eye to light.

Is conjunctivitis contagious?

Conjunctivitis caused by a virus or bacteria is highly contagious. It can be spread easily from one eye to another and throughout a family or classroom in a matter of days.

How can we avoid spreading conjunctivitis?

The following measures help prevent the spread of conjunctivitis:
- Avoid touching or rubbing the infected eye, which can spread the infection to the other eye or other people.
- Sanitize your hands frequently with soap, particularly after touching the eyes or face.
- Do not share washcloths, towels, or pillows with anyone.
- Do not wear contact lenses or eye makeup until the conjunctivitis is completely gone.
- Discard eye makeup that is used while you are infected to prevent reinfection.
- Encourage the patient to practice techniques that prevent the spread of conjunctivitis.
- If the physician has prescribed eye medication, teach the patient (or parent) the proper procedure for performing an eye instillation.
- Give the patient educational materials on conjunctivitis.

PROCEDURE 6-3

PROCEDURE 6-3 Performing an Eye Irrigation

Outcome Perform an eye irrigation.

Equipment/Supplies:
- Disposable gloves (nonpowdered)
- Irrigating solution
- Solution container
- Disposable rubber bulb syringe
- Basin
- Moisture-resistant towel
- Gauze pads

1. **Procedural Step.** Sanitize your hands.
2. **Procedural Step.** Assemble the equipment. Normal saline is generally used to irrigate the eye. Check the irrigating solution carefully with the physician's instructions to make sure you have obtained the correct solution. Check the expiration date of the solution. Check the solution label three times: while removing the solution from the shelf, while pouring the solution, and before returning it to its proper place. Warm the irrigating solution to body temperature (98.6° F, or 37° C).

   Principle. The solution should be carefully compared with the physician's instructions to prevent an error. Outdated solutions may produce undesirable effects. If the solution is too cold or too warm, it will be uncomfortable for the patient.

3. **Procedural Step.** Greet and identify the patient. Introduce yourself and explain the procedure.

   Principle. Explain the purpose of the irrigation to the patient.

Continued

PROCEDURE 6-3 Performing an Eye Irrigation—Cont'd

4. **Procedural Step.** Apply nonpowdered gloves. Position the patient. The patient may be placed in a sitting or lying position with the head tilted in the direction of the affected eye. Position a basin tightly against the patient's cheek under the affected eye to catch the irrigating solution. Place a moisture-resistant towel on the patient's shoulder to protect the patient's clothing. If both eyes are to be irrigated, two sets of equipment must be used to prevent cross-infection from one eye to the other.
Principle. Nonpowdered gloves avoid irritation of the patient's eye with powder that may have gotten on the outside of the glove. The patient is positioned so the solution will flow away from the unaffected eye to prevent cross-infection.

5. **Procedural Step.** Cleanse the eyelids from inner to outer **canthus** with a moistened gauze pad to remove any discharge or debris on the lids. The inner canthus is the inner junction of the eyelids next to the nose. The outer canthus is the junction of the eyelids farthest from the nose. Normal saline or the solution ordered for the irrigation may be used. Discard the gauze pad after each wipe.

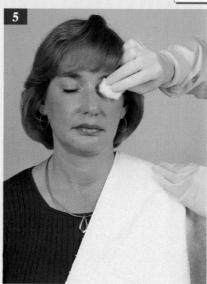

6. **Procedural Step.** Fill the irrigating syringe with the solution by squeezing the bulb and slowly releasing it until the desired amount of solution enters the bulb. Instruct the patient to keep both eyes open and to find a focal point in the room and focus on it.
Principle. Looking at a focal point helps the patient keep the irrigated eye open during the procedure.

7. **Procedural Step.** Separate the eyelids with the index finger and thumb to expose the lower conjunctiva and to hold the upper eyelid open.
Principle. The medical assistant must hold the eye open during the procedure because the patient will have a tendency to close it.

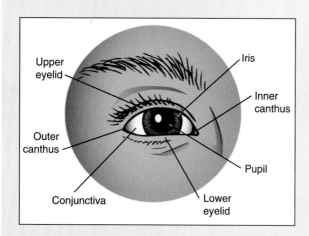

Principle. The eyelids should be clean to prevent foreign particles from entering the eye during the irrigation. Cleansing from inner to outer canthus prevents cross-infection.

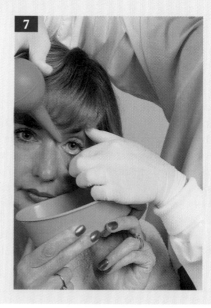

8. **Procedural Step.** Hold the tip of the syringe approximately 1 inch above the eye. Gently release the solution onto the eye at the inner canthus. This allows the solution to flow over the eye at a moderate rate from the inner to the outer canthus. Direct the solution to the lower conjunctiva. To prevent injury, do not allow the syringe to touch the eye.

   Principle. The solution flows away from the unaffected eye to prevent cross-infection. The cornea is sensitive and can be harmed easily. Therefore the irrigating solution must be directed to the lower conjunctiva to prevent injury to the cornea.

9. **Procedural Step.** Refill the syringe and continue irrigating until the desired results have been obtained or all the solution is used, depending on the purpose of the irrigation.

10. **Procedural Step.** Dry the eyelids from inner to outer canthus with a gauze pad.

11. **Procedural Step.** Remove the gloves and sanitize your hands.

12. **Procedural Step.** Chart the procedure. Include the following: the date and time; which eye was irrigated; the type, strength, and amount of solution used; and any significant observations and patient reactions. Use one of these abbreviations to indicate which eye was irrigated:

   OU   Both eyes
   OD   Right eye
   OS   Left eye

CHARTING EXAMPLE	
Date	
11/5/05	10:30 a.m. Irrigated OS c̄ sterile saline @
	98.6° F. No complaints of discomfort.
	———————————— C. Lindner, CMA

PROCEDURE 6-4   Performing an Eye Instillation

Outcome Perform an eye instillation.

Equipment/Supplies:
- Disposable gloves (nonpowdered)
- Ophthalmic drops with a sterile eyedropper or ophthalmic ointment as ordered by the physician
- Tissues
- Gauze pads

1. **Procedural Step.** Sanitize your hands.
2. **Procedural Step.** Assemble the equipment. Check the medication carefully against the physician's instructions to make sure you have obtained the correct medication. The medication label must bear the word *ophthalmic.* Check the expiration date. Check the drug label three times: while removing the medication from the shelf, before removing the cap or withdrawing the medication into the dropper, and before instilling the medication.

   Principle. The medication should be carefully compared with the physician's instructions to prevent a drug error. Medication not bearing the word *ophthalmic* must never be placed in the eye because it could injure the eye. Outdated medications may produce undesirable effects.

3. **Procedural Step.** Greet and identify the patient. Introduce yourself and explain the procedure.

   Principle. Explain the purpose of the instillation to the patient.

4. **Procedural Step.** Help the patient into a sitting or supine position.

5. **Procedural Step.** Apply nonpowdered gloves. Prepare the medication. *Eyedrops:* Withdraw the medication into the dropper. *Eye ointment:* Remove the cap from the tip of the tube.

Continued

PROCEDURE 6-4 Performing an Eye Instillation—Cont'd

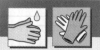

6. **Procedural Step.** Ask the patient to look up at the ceiling, and expose the lower conjunctival sac by using the fingers of the nondominant hand placed over a tissue. The fingers should be placed on the patient's cheekbone just below the eye, and the skin of the cheek should be drawn downward gently.
Principle. Looking up helps keep the dropper from touching the cornea. It also helps keep the patient from blinking when the drops are instilled.

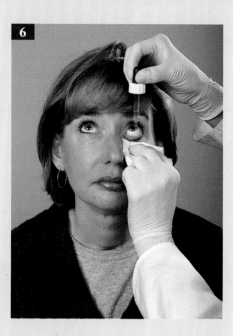

7. **Procedural Step.** Insert the medication. *Eyedrops:* Place the correct number of eyedrops in the center of the lower conjunctival sac. Hold the tip of the dropper approximately $1/2$ inch above the eye sac. Do not allow the dropper to touch the eye. *Eye ointment:* Place a thin ribbon of ointment along the length of the lower conjunctival sac from inner to outer canthus. Be careful not to touch the tip of the ointment tube to the eye. Discontinue the ribbon by twisting the tube.
Principle. Placing the medication in the conjunctival sac, rather than directly on the eyeball, is more comfortable for the patient. Touching the dropper or tube to the eye results in contamination of these items.

8. **Procedural Step.** Discard unused solution from the eyedropper. Do not touch the dropper to the outside of the bottle when returning it to the bottle.
Principle. Touching the dropper to the outside of the bottle contaminates the dropper. Do not return unused solution to the bottle because it will contaminate the medication that is still in the bottle.

9. **Procedural Step.** Ask the patient to close his or her eyes gently and move the eyeballs. Tell the patient that the instillation may blur the vision temporarily.
Principle. Moving the eyeballs helps distribute the medication over the entire eye. If the eyes are shut tightly, the drops or ointment will be pushed out.

10. **Procedural Step.** Dry the eyelid from inner to outer canthus with a gauze pad to remove excess medication.

11. **Procedural Step.** Remove the gloves, and sanitize your hands.

12. **Procedural Step.** Chart the procedure. Include the date and time, the name and strength of the medication, the number of drops or amount of ointment, which eye received the instillation, your observations, and the patient's reaction.

CHARTING EXAMPLE	
Date	
11/5/05	2:30 p.m. Atropine sulfate, 1% gtts ii OU.
	Pt states a temporary blurring of vision. ——
	———————————— C. Lindner, CMA

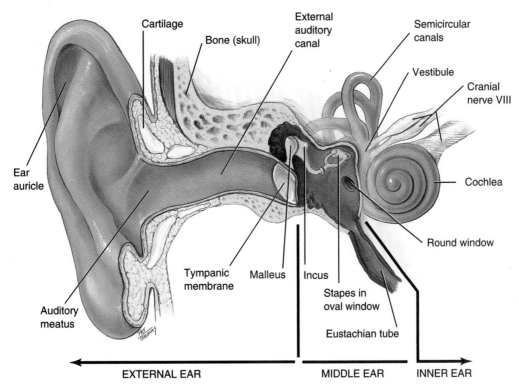

Figure 6-8.   Structure of the ear. (From Applegate EJ: *The anatomy and physiology learning system,* ed 2, Philadelphia, 2000, Saunders.)

THE EAR
Structure of the Ear

The ear has functions in hearing and in maintaining equilibrium. It consists of three divisions: the *external ear,* the *middle ear,* and the *inner ear.* The structures in the ear are illustrated in Figure 6-8 and described next.

The external ear is composed of the auricle (or pinna) and the external auditory canal, also known as the external ear canal. The opening into this canal is the *external auditory meatus.*

The *auricle* is a flap of cartilage covered with skin that projects from the side of the head. Its function is to receive and collect sound waves and to direct them toward the external auditory canal.

The *external auditory canal* is approximately 1 inch long in an adult and extends from the auricle to the tympanic membrane. It is lined with skin that contains fine hairs, nerve endings, and glands. The glands secrete ear wax, or **cerumen,** which lubricates and protects the ear canal. The canal has an S-shaped curve as it leads inward. During an examination with the otoscope or an ear instillation or irrigation, the canal must be straightened.

The **tympanic membrane** is at the end of the external auditory canal. It is a pearly gray semitransparent membrane that receives sound waves.

The middle ear is an air-filled cavity that contains three small bones, or *ossicles:* the malleus, the incus, and the stapes. The *eustachian tube* connects the middle ear to the nasopharynx. Air pressure between the external atmosphere and the middle ear is stabilized through the eustachian tube.

The inner ear contains the *cochlea,* which is the essential organ of hearing. The *semicircular canals* are also located in the inner ear and help to maintain equilibrium.

Assessment of Hearing Acuity

The assessment of hearing acuity is an integral part of a complete physical examination. It is quite possible for an individual to have a hearing loss and not be aware of it. Early detection and treatment of hearing problems help prevent permanent hearing loss.

An individual with normal hearing should be able to hear the frequencies of normal speech, which range from 300 to 4000 Hz (hertz, or cycles per second) at a normal sound intensity. Patients who exhibit hearing loss are referred to an otolaryngologist or an audiologist for further evaluation.

))PATIENT TEACHING

Acute Otitis Media

Answer questions patients have about otitis media.

What is a middle ear infection?

An infection of the middle ear is medically referred to as acute otitis media. It is an inflammation of the middle ear caused by an infection and can occur in one or both ears. It is very common in young children between the ages of 3 months and 3 years but unusual in adults. A middle ear infection is not serious if treated promptly and effectively. If not treated, however, middle ear infections can lead to serious complications such as acute mastoiditis, meningitis, and permanent hearing loss.

What causes a middle ear infection?

It is believed that a middle ear infection as a result of a blocked eustachian tube may be caused by an upper respiratory infection (URI) or allergy. The blockage causes fluid to build up in the middle ear. This fluid is an ideal place for bacteria to grow. If this occurs, the result is acute otitis media.

What are the symptoms of a middle ear infection?

The most common symptoms are intense pain, fever, and temporary hearing loss. Other symptoms may include dizziness, nausea and vomiting, and (if the ear drum ruptures) drainage from the ear.

How does the physician know whether a middle ear infection is present?

The physician examines the ears with an otoscope. If a middle ear infection is present, the eardrum is red and swollen, caused by irritation from the infection, and there is pus and mucus behind the eardrum.

How is it treated?

A middle ear infection is usually treated with an oral antibiotic for 10 to 14 days. It is important to take all the antibiotic prescribed; otherwise the ear infection may recur. The physician may also recommend a decongestant to help open the blocked eustachian tube. After the acute infection is over, fluid may remain trapped in the middle ear. This condition is known as serous otitis media and, if not treated, may last for days, weeks, months, or even a year. Although fluid in the middle ear is painless, it may result in a feeling of fullness or pressure in the ears and temporary hearing loss.

Why are middle ear infections so common in children?

In children, the eustachian tube is positioned horizontally and is shorter and narrower than in adults. Hence, when a child has an upper respiratory infection, bacteria can travel easily to the middle ear. In addition, swelling from the respiratory infection can block this narrow tube, which causes fluid to build up in the middle ear.

- Encourage the patient to complete the entire prescribed course of antibiotics.
- If the physician has prescribed eardrops, teach the patient (or parent) the proper procedure for performing an ear instillation.
- Encourage early treatment of upper respiratory infections.
- Give the patient educational materials on otitis media.

Types of Hearing Loss

There are three types of hearing loss: conductive, sensorineural, and mixed. *Conductive hearing loss* is the most common and results when there is a physical interference with the normal conduction of sound waves through the external and middle ear. Because of the interference, the amount of sound reaching the inner ear is less than normal, resulting in hearing impairment. Conductive loss in the external ear may be caused by an obstruction in the external ear canal, such as impacted cerumen, swelling from external otitis (swimmer's ear), foreign bodies, and benign growths such as polyps. Conductive loss in the middle ear may be caused by serous otitis media (fluid in the middle ear) or acute otitis media (infection in the middle ear), a perforated tympanic membrane, or otosclerosis. The cause of conductive hearing loss often can be detected by examining the external ear canal with an otoscope. Hearing is frequently restored by removing the obstruction (e.g., impacted cerumen) or treating the disorder (e.g., serous otitis media).

Sensorineural hearing loss results from damage to the inner ear or auditory nerve. With this type of hearing loss, the sound is conducted normally through the outer and middle ear structures but, because of a problem with the perception of sound waves, a hearing deficit occurs. Specific causes of sensorineural loss include hereditary factors; intense noise exposure over a period of time; tumors; degenerative changes from the normal aging process; ototoxicity caused by certain medications; and infectious diseases such as measles, mumps, and meningitis. *Mixed hearing loss* is a combination of both conductive and sensorineural loss.

Case Study 3

Willow Basil brings in her 6-year-old daughter, Jade. For the past 3 days, Jade has been running a fever and has had persistent pain and hearing loss in her left ear. Mrs. Basil practices alternative medicine and uses prescription medications as little as possible. She says that she has been trying herbal therapy and aromatherapy to make Jade better, but it doesn't seem to be helping. Jade is diagnosed with acute otitis media, and the physician prescribes amoxicillin for 10 days. Mrs. Basil wants to know if she has to give Jade the amoxicillin for the entire 10 days. She asks if she can stop using it when Jade starts feeling better. Mrs. Basil also wants to know if the ear infection will cause a permanent problem with Jade's hearing.

MEMORIES From EXTERNSHIP

CAMMIE LINDNER: There is one characteristic that is shared by all patients. I first noticed this during my externships, and it does not seem to matter what type of practice it is. Patients like to feel special and to be treated that way. They like consistency in their doctor and in the office staff, in seeing familiar faces. This is especially hard during externship. The time spent is too short to truly get to know the patients, but it is a great learning experience.

It is important to observe the staff and patient communication and interaction skills. By doing this, you can decide which ones you admire and those that you do not wish to copy. The following are just a few of the guidelines that have helped me. (1) Call patients by name, and be sure that they know your name. (2) Follow through with what you have told a patient you will do, and keep them updated if circumstances change. (3) Smile and do not let one patient's negative attitude interfere with your care of others. (4) Take time to listen.

When you do begin your career, it does not take long to get into a routine and to start knowing your patients. When patients see a familiar face, they are more willing to share information that can contribute to improved communication and good health care.

Hearing Acuity Tests

A number of tests can be used to assess hearing acuity. They range from the very simple gross screening test to qualitative tests using a tuning fork to highly specific quantitative tests using an audiometer. It is important to test only one ear at a time because a hearing deficit can exist in one ear only. The ear not being tested should be blocked by an earplug or masked. *Masking* involves the presentation of sound (usually noise) to the ear not being tested so that the patient's response is based only on hearing in the ear being tested.

Gross Screening Test

The gross hearing test is a simple and quick screening test used to identify a very large hearing impairment. It is performed by the physician during the physical examination. Hearing is assessed by asking the patient to repeat a simple word or series of numbers whispered from a distance of 1 to 2 feet from the ear. A gross hearing test may also be conducted by determining whether the patient can hear a watch ticking at 4 to 6 inches from the ear. When a hearing loss is discovered, a tuning fork or audiometer is used for a more precise assessment of hearing.

Tuning Fork Tests

Tuning fork tests provide a general assessment of hearing acuity and may be part of the physical examination. A tuning fork with a frequency of 512 or 1024 Hz is generally used because these frequencies fall within the range of normal speech. The Weber and Rinne tests are the tuning fork tests most commonly performed by the physician; they are used to identify conductive and sensorineural hearing loss.

The Weber test is a useful assessment of hearing loss when one ear hears better than the other. The tuning fork is set in vibration, and the base of the fork is placed on the center of the patient's head. The patient is then asked to indicate where the sound is heard best. A patient with normal hearing will hear the sound equally in both ears or in the center of the head. Figure 6-9 illustrates the Weber test and describes the interpretation of results.

The Rinne test compares the duration of sound perception by air conduction with that of bone conduction. The tuning fork is set in vibration, and the base of the fork is placed against the bone of the mastoid process. The patient is instructed to indicate when the sound is no longer heard. The prongs of the fork (still vibrating) are then placed in the air about 1 inch from the opening of the

Highlight on Hearing Impairment

The number of individuals with a hearing impairment has gradually increased over the past 20 years. Factors that contribute to this increase include an aging population and a noisier environment.

It is estimated that approximately 28 million people in the United States suffer from a hearing loss severe enough to interfere with their daily activities, while another 2 million individuals are profoundly deaf.

Precise screening of preschoolers for hearing loss is difficult. This is because tuning fork tests and audiometry require the ability to signal in response to sound, and children up to the age of 4 or 5 years have trouble mastering this skill.

Most state, county, and local school systems require hearing screening as a prerequisite for entrance to school and again at periodic intervals, usually during the first, third, fifth, and seventh grades.

Risk factors for hearing impairment in children include family history of deafness, premature birth, low birth weight, measles, mumps, high fevers, meningitis, recurrent or chronic ear infections, and the mother's having had rubella during pregnancy.

Signs of hearing impairment in children are poor attentiveness, delayed speech development, and persistent problems with articulation. Signs of hearing impairment in adults include frequent requests for words or statements to be repeated, leaning toward the speaker, turning the head, cupping the ears, and speaking in a loud or unvaried tone of voice.

The most common cause of conductive hearing loss in children is fluid in the middle ear, which prevents the tympanic membrane from vibrating freely. In adults, the most common cause of conductive loss is otosclerosis, a condition in which the stapes becomes fixed because of calcium deposits and less able to pass on vibrations when sound enters the ear.

The loudness of sound is measured in units called *decibels* (dB). Sounds of less than 75 decibels, even after long exposure, are unlikely to cause hearing loss. Normal conversation is approximately 60 decibels and a whisper in a quiet library is 30 to 40 decibels.

Permanent sensorineural hearing loss can result when the ear is repeatedly bombarded with loud sound over a period of time. Standards set by OSHA indicate that continued exposure to noise louder than 85 decibels will eventually harm an individual's hearing by damaging the tiny hair cells in the organ of Corti. The organ of Corti is a structure in the cochlea (inner ear) that converts sound waves into nerve impulses for transmission to the brain. This type of sensorineural hearing loss is known as *noise-induced hearing loss (NIHL)*. It is most often seen in individuals who frequently listen to loud music, fire guns without wearing ear protection, or are exposed to loud noise as part of their jobs. The following are examples of common noises and the decibel level of each:

Noise	Decibels
Normal breathing	10
Humming of a refrigerator	40
Television	70
Vacuum cleaner	60 to 85
Motorcycle	95 to 100
Personal stereo system with earphones (on high)	115
Rock concert	120
Chain saw	120
Auto stereo on high	125
Jet taking off	140
Firecracker	150
Firearms	140 to 170

Many hearing impairments can be helped with the use of a hearing aid. The individual who benefits most from a hearing aid is one with a mild-to-moderate conductive hearing loss. An individual with a sensorineural or mixed loss has more trouble finding a suitable hearing aid and often gets less satisfactory results.

---

patient's ear canal, and the patient indicates when the sound is no longer heard. An individual with normal hearing is able to hear the sound at least twice as long through air conduction as through bone conduction. Figure 6-10 illustrates the Rinne test and describes the interpretation of results.

Audiometry

Audiometry is the measurement of hearing acuity using a special instrument known as an audiometer. An **audiometer** quantitatively measures hearing for the various frequencies of sound waves. Audiometry is a more specific hearing acuity test because it provides information on how extensive a hearing loss is and which frequencies are involved. It is important that the test be conducted in a quiet room because outside noise may affect the results, especially in the lower frequencies. The patient wears headphones placed snugly over the ears (Figure 6-11). The audiometer delivers a single frequency at a time at specific intensities, starting with low-frequency tones of 250 to 500 Hz and going to very high frequencies of 6000 to 8000 Hz. The patient is asked to signal when he or she hears a sound so that the patient's hearing threshold for each frequency can be determined. The hearing acuity in each ear is assessed separately, and the results are plotted on a graph known as an *audiogram*. The medical assistant may be

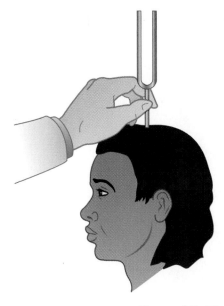

Normal Hearing
The patient hears the sound equally in both ears or in the center of the head.

Conductive Hearing Loss
The patient hears the sound better in the problem ear.

Sensorineural Hearing Loss
The patient does not hear the sound as well in the problem ear.

Figure 6-9. The Weber test.

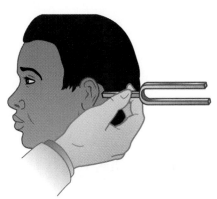

Bone conduction

Normal Hearing
The patient hears the sound at least twice as long through air conduction as through bone conduction.

Conductive Hearing Loss
The patient hears the sound longer by bone conduction than by air conduction.

Sensorineural Hearing Loss
The sound is reduced. The patient will also hear the sound longer through air conduction than through bone conduction but not twice as long.

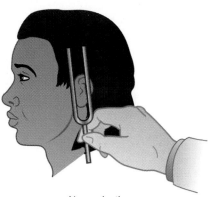

Air conduction

Figure 6-10. The Rinne test.

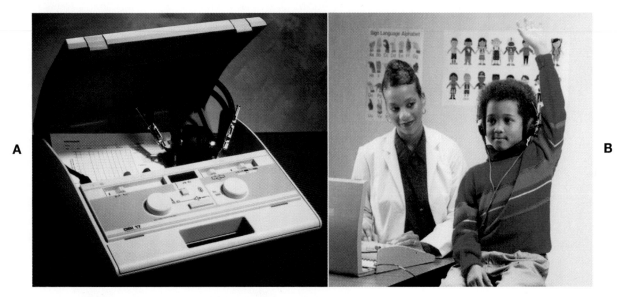

Figure 6-11. A, Audiometer. **B,** The patient signals when he hears a sound. (Courtesy GSI [Grayson-Stadler], Milford, NH.)

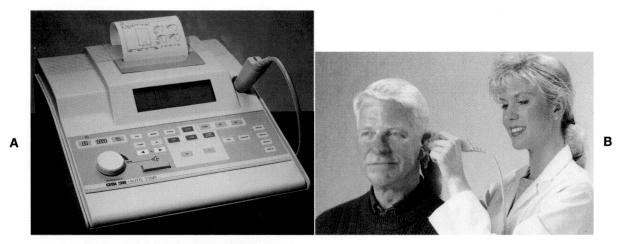

Figure 6-12. A, Tympanometer. **B,** The earpiece is placed snugly in the patient's ear. (Courtesy GSI [Grayson-Stadler], Milford, NH.)

responsible for performing audiometry in the medical office. Before operating an audiometer, however, the medical assistant must receive extensive on-site training by an audiologist to ensure that proper technique is used to conduct the test.

Tympanometry

Tympanometry is not a hearing test, but it does help determine the cause of hearing loss, so it is presented in this section. The tympanometer consists of an earpiece attached to an electronic device (Figure 6-12). The earpiece is placed snugly in the patient's ear, and low-frequency sound waves are directed against the eardrum while pressure is applied in the ear canal. With a normal ear, the eardrum will exhibit mobility in response to the pressure, as indicated on a graphic readout known as a *tympanogram*. If there is fluid in the middle ear, the eardrum will not move but remain stiff, as indicated on the tympanogram. Hence tympanometry is useful in diagnosing serous otitis media (fluid in the middle ear), which is a common cause of hearing loss in children.

Ear Irrigation

An ear irrigation is the washing of the external auditory canal with a flowing solution. Ear irrigations are performed for the following purposes: to cleanse the external auditory canal to remove cerumen, discharge, or a foreign body; to relieve inflammation by applying an antiseptic solution;

and to apply heat to the ear. Before irrigating, impacted cerumen must be softened by instilling warm mineral oil or hydrogen peroxide for 10 to 15 minutes. Procedure 6-5 demonstrates how to perform an ear irrigation.

An ear irrigation should not be performed if the tympanic membrane is perforated because it could result in a severe irritation or infection of the middle ear.

Ear Instillation

An ear instillation involves the dropping of a liquid into the external auditory canal. Ear instillations are performed to soften impacted cerumen, to combat infection with the use of antibiotic eardrops, and to relieve pain. Procedure 6-6 demonstrates how to perform an ear instillation.

PROCEDURE 6-5 Performing an Ear Irrigation

Outcome Perform an ear irrigation.

Equipment/Supplies:
- Disposable gloves
- Irrigating solution
- Solution container
- Irrigating syringe
- Ear basin
- Moisture-resistant towel
- Gauze pads
- Ear wick

1. **Procedural Step.** Sanitize your hands.
2. **Procedural Step.** Assemble the equipment. Check the irrigating solution carefully against the physician's instructions to make sure you have obtained the correct solution. Check the expiration date of the solution. Check the label of the irrigating solution three times: while removing the solution from the shelf, while pouring the solution, and before returning it to its proper place. Warm the irrigating solution to body temperature (98.6° F, or 37° C).
   Principle. Carefully compare the solution with the physician's instructions to prevent an error. Outdated solutions may produce undesirable effects. If the solution is too cold or too warm, it will stimulate the inner ear and the patient will become dizzy.

3. **Procedural Step.** Greet and identify the patient. Introduce yourself and explain the procedure. Explain the purpose of performing the irrigation—for example, to remove cerumen. Tell the patient the procedure is not painful; however, he or she may feel a minimal amount of discomfort and occasional dizziness, fullness, and warmth as the ear solution comes in contact with the tympanic membrane.

4. **Procedural Step.** Help the patient into a sitting position with the head tilted toward the affected ear. Place a moisture-resistant towel on the patient's shoulder under the ear to be irrigated to protect clothing and to prevent water from running down the neck. Instruct the patient to hold the ear basin against the head under the affected ear to catch the irrigating solution.
   Principle. The patient is positioned so gravity aids the flow of the solution out of the ear and into the basin.

5. **Procedural Step.** Apply gloves. Cleanse the outer ear with a moistened gauze pad to remove any discharge or debris present. Normal saline or the solution ordered for the irrigation may be used.
   Principle. The outer ear should be clean to prevent foreign particles from entering the ear canal during the irrigation.

6. **Procedural Step.** Fill the syringe with the irrigating solution (approximately 50 ml). Expel air from the syringe.
   Principle. Air forced into the ear is uncomfortable for the patient.

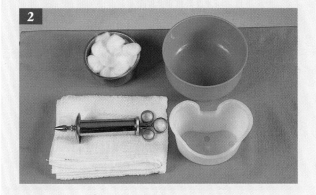

PROCEDURE 6-5

Continued

PROCEDURE 6-5 Performing an Ear Irrigation—Cont'd

7. **Procedural Step.** Straighten the external ear canal. The canal is straightened by gently pulling the ear upward and backward for adults and children over 3 years old and downward and backward for children 3 years of age and younger.
Principle. Straightening the canal permits the irrigating solution to reach all areas of the canal.

8. **Procedural Step.** Insert the syringe tip into the ear and inject the irrigating solution toward the roof of the ear canal. It is important that the solution be injected toward the roof of the canal to prevent it from being injected directly onto the tympanic membrane. Do not insert the tip of the syringe too deeply.
Principle. The tip of the syringe should be directed at the roof of the canal to prevent injury to the tympanic membrane and to aid in the removal of foreign particles by allowing the solution to flow down the length of the canal and out the bottom. In addition, severe patient discomfort and dizziness may occur if the solution is injected directly onto the tympanic membrane. Inserting the tip of the syringe too deeply causes discomfort for the patient.

9. **Procedural Step.** Refill the syringe and continue irrigating until the desired results have been obtained or all the solution is used, depending on the purpose of the irrigation. Make sure the tip of the syringe does not obstruct the canal opening so that the solution can flow freely out of the canal. Observe the returning solution to note the material present (e.g., cerumen, discharge, or a foreign object) and the amount (small, moderate, or large).
Principle. Obstruction of the canal opening causes pressure that results in patient discomfort and possible injury to the tympanic membrane.

10. **Procedural Step.** Dry the outside of the ear with a gauze pad. Have the patient lie on the affected side on the treatment table. Tell the patient that the ear will feel sensitive for a short time. Place a cotton wick loosely in the ear canal for 15 minutes if instructed to do so by the physician.
Principle. Any solution remaining in the ear canal should be allowed to drain out. A cotton wick will make the patient's ear feel less sensitive after the irrigation.

11. **Procedural Step.** Remove the gloves and sanitize your hands.

12. **Procedural Step.** Chart the procedure. Include the following: the date and time; which ear was irrigated; the type, strength, and amount of solution used; the amount and type of material returned in the irrigating solution; any significant observations; and patient reactions. Use one of these abbreviations to indicate which ear was irrigated:

AU	Both ears
AD	Right ear
AS	Left ear

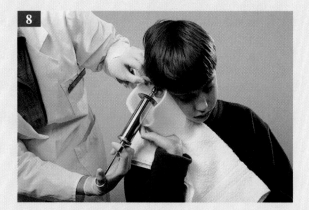

CHARTING EXAMPLE

Date	
11/15/05	2:15 p.m. Irrigated AD c̄ saline, 200 ml @ 98.6° F. Mod amt of cerumen present in returned solution. Cotton wick placed in ear canal × 15 min. No complaints of discomfort.
	———————— C. Lindner, CMA

PROCEDURE 6-6 Performing an Ear Instillation

Outcome Perform an ear instillation.

Equipment/Supplies:
- Disposable gloves
- Otic drops with a sterile dropper
- Gauze pad

1. **Procedural Step.** Sanitize your hands.
2. **Procedural Step.** Assemble the equipment. Check the medication carefully against the physician's instructions to make sure you have obtained the correct medication. The medication label must bear the word *otic*. Check the expiration date. Check the drug label three times: while removing the medication from the shelf, before withdrawing the medication into the dropper, and before instilling the medication.
   Principle. The medication should be carefully compared with the physician's instructions to prevent a drug error. Medication not bearing the word *otic* must not be placed in the ear because it could injure the ear. Outdated medications may produce undesirable effects.
3. **Procedural Step.** Greet and identify the patient. Introduce yourself and explain the procedure.
   Principle. Explain the purpose of the instillation to the patient.
4. **Procedural Step.** Help the patient into a sitting position with the head tilted in the direction of the unaffected ear.
   Principle. Gravity aids in the flow of the medication into the ear canal.
5. **Procedural Step.** Apply gloves. Withdraw the medication into the dropper.

6. **Procedural Step.** Straighten the external auditory canal. The canal is straightened by pulling the ear upward and backward for adults and children over 3 years old and downward and backward for children 3 years of age and younger.
   Principle. Straightening the canal permits the medication to reach all areas of the canal.
7. **Procedural Step.** Place the tip of the dropper at the opening of the ear canal, and insert the proper amount of medication by squeezing the rubber bulb and instilling the correct number of drops along the side of the canal.

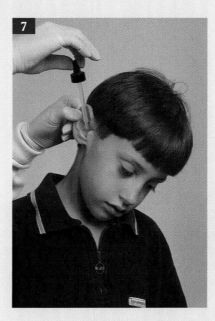

8. **Procedural Step.** Instruct the patient to lie on the unaffected side for 2 to 3 minutes.
   Principle. Lying on the unaffected side prevents the medication from running out and allows complete distribution of the medication.

Continued

PROCEDURE 6-6

PROCEDURE 6-6 Performing an Ear Instillation—Cont'd

9. **Procedural Step.** Place a moistened cotton wick loosely in the ear canal for 15 minutes if instructed to do so by the physician.
   Principle. The cotton wick prevents the medication from running out when the patient is up. Moistening the wick will prevent the medication from being absorbed by the cotton.
10. **Procedural Step.** Remove the gloves and sanitize your hands.
11. **Procedural Step.** Chart the procedure. Include the date and time, the name and strength of the medication, number of drops, which ear(s) received the instillation, any significant observations, and the patient's reaction

CHARTING EXAMPLE

Date	
11/20/05	9:30 a.m. Auralgan gtts ii, AD. No discharge present. Pt states a relief of pain.
	——————————— C. Lindner, CMA

MEDICAL Practice and the LAW

Legal issues concerning eye and ear assessment are similar to those that concern any assessment. Accurate assessments done properly are necessary for accurate diagnoses and treatment and to prevent injuries to these structures.

Patient Rights

Patients entering the office have six major rights, which are enforceable by law. These include:

1. The right to have the physician and medical assistant *do good* for them. Failure results in malpractice.

2. The right to *be treated fairly.* This is enforced by discrimination and employment laws.
3. The right to *be free.* This is exercised by giving informed consent and advance directives.
4. The right *not to be harmed.* Licensure protects patients by ensuring a minimal level of skill.
5. The right of fidelity, or *being true.* This includes confidentiality, telling the truth, and loyalty to the patient.
6. The right to *life.* This appears with cases of abortion, assisted suicide, and euthanasia.
   If any of these rights is violated, the patient has the right to sue.

What Would You DO?
What Would You *Not* DO? *RESPONSES*

Case Study 1
What Did Cammie Do?
- ❑ Talked with Haley (on her level) about why someone needs to wear glasses.
- ❑ Retested Haley with the Snellen chart to see if she missed the same letters.
- ❑ Tested Haley with the Big E chart to give the physician an additional measurement to make an interpretation of Haley's visual acuity.

What Did Cammie Not Do?
- ❑ Did not tell Haley that she needs glasses.
- ❑ Did not scold Haley for trying to miss letters on the text.

What Would You Do/What Would You *Not* Do? Review Cammie's response and place a checkmark next to the information you included in your response. List the additional information you included in your response.

_____

_____

_____

_____

Case Study 2
What Did Cammie Do?
- ❑ Gave Mr. Mitchell some suggestions on how to put drops in Clive's eyes so it is less scary. One idea is to have Clive lie down flat and close his eyes. Place the drops in the inner corner of his eye next to the bridge of his nose, letting them make a little lake there. Then when Clive relaxes and opens his eye, the drops will gently flow into his eye.
- ❑ Talked with Clive (on his level) about why he needs eyedrops.
- ❑ Told Mr. Mitchell that the eyedrops were prescribed for Clive and they should be used only for Clive. Told him that if the twins developed conjunctivitis, he should call the office.
- ❑ Gave Mr. Mitchell suggestions for preventing the twins from getting conjunctivitis (not touching the infected eye, frequent handwashing, not sharing toys or towels.)

What Did Cammie Not Do?
- ❑ Did not tell Mr. Mitchell to hold Clive down or force drops in his eyes.
- ❑ Did not tell Mr. Mitchell that he should know better than to think about giving the twins a medication they don't need.

What Would You Do/What Would You *Not* Do? Review Cammie's response and place a checkmark next to the information you included in your response. List the additional information you included in your response.

_____

_____

_____

_____

Case Study 3
What Did Cammie Do?
- ❑ Explained to Mrs. Basil that Jade may begin to feel better after several days of antibiotics but not all of the germs causing her ear infection will have been killed by then. If she doesn't give Jade the full course of antibiotics, the infection could come back.
- ❑ Documented all the medications that Mrs. Basil has administered to Jade.
- ❑ Gave Mrs. Basil a patient information brochure on acute otitis media.
- ❑ Told Mrs. Basil that she needs to talk to the doctor about her concern regarding hearing loss because he is most qualified to answer that question.
- ❑ Encouraged Mrs. Basil to bring Jade in sooner when she develops fever and ear pain.

What Did Cammie Not Do?
- ❑ Did not criticize Mrs. Basil for waiting so long to bring Jade in.
- ❑ Did not offer a personal opinion about alternative medicine.

What Would You Do/What Would You *Not* Do? Review Cammie's response and place a checkmark next to the information you included in your response. List the additional information you included in your response.

_____

_____

_____

_____

Apply Your KNOWLEDGE

Choose the best answer to each of the following questions.

1. Teresa Lopez has come to the office for a physical examination. She is wearing contact lenses because she has myopia. This type of error of refraction is commonly known as
   A. Nearsightedness
   B. Farsightedness
   C. Hyperopia
   D. Hindsight

2. Cammie Lindner, CMA, is getting ready to check Teresa's visual acuity with the Snellen eye chart. All of the following are appropriate steps in checking Teresa's vision EXCEPT
   A. Having Teresa stand 20 feet away from the chart
   B. Checking to make sure the chart is at Teresa's eye level
   C. Asking Teresa to cover her left eye with an occluder while testing her right eye
   D. Instructing Teresa to keep her covered eye closed

3. Teresa's vision in her right eye is 20/40 with no errors on the Snellen test. The correct interpretation of this reading is that
   A. Teresa did not pass her test and must take it again
   B. Teresa can see at 20 feet from the chart what a person with normal vision can see standing 40 feet from the chart
   C. Teresa can see at 40 feet from the chart what a person with normal vision can see standing 20 feet from the chart
   D. Teresa can see what a normal individual can see 40% of the time

4. Teresa's vision in her left eye is 20/30 with one letter missed. Teresa is wearing contact lenses, and Cammie noticed some squinting while testing her left eye. Cammie would chart her visual acuity as
   A. 4/12/05 9:00 AM Snellen test, c̄c: Ⓡ 20/40. Ⓛ 20/30 −1. C. Lindner, CMA
   B. 4/12/05 9:00 AM Snellen test, s̄c: OD 20/30−1 OS 20/40. C. Lindner, CMA
   C. 4/12/05 9:00 AM Snellen test, s̄c: OD 20/40. OS 20/30−1. Squinting noted. C. Lindner, CMA
   D. 4/12/05 9:00 AM Snellen test, c̄c: OD 20/40. OS 20/30−1. Squinting noted, OS. C. Lindner, CMA

5. Teresa also needs to have her near visual acuity assessed. All of the following are appropriate steps for performing a near visual acuity test EXCEPT
   A. Asking Teresa to hold the NVA card 14 to 16 inches in front of her
   B. Instructing Teresa to remove her reading glasses
   C. Measuring Teresa's NVA beginning with the right eye first
   D. Making sure the room is well lit

6. Quinton Donovan, a 14-year-old boy, is at the office because he has an infection of the external ear canal. His left ear canal is inflamed, red, and swollen. Quinton complains that he is not able to hear as well with that ear. Dr. Canthus performs a Rinne test. During testing of the infected ear, Quinton indicates that he can hear the sound longer through bone conduction than through air conduction. The results of the test indicate that
   A. Quinton has a conductive hearing loss in the left ear
   B. Quinton has a swimmer in his ear
   C. Quinton needs a hearing aid
   D. Quinton has a sensorineural hearing loss in the left ear

7. Dr. Canthus asks Cammie Lindner, CMA, to administer medication to Quinton for external otitis. He directs Cammie to instill 5 drops of ofloxacin into Quinton's left ear. All of the following are appropriate steps for performing an ear instillation EXCEPT
   A. Checking the expiration date of the medication
   B. Having Quinton tilt his head toward the left
   C. Straightening the ear canal by pulling Quinton's ear upward and backward
   D. Instilling the correct number of drops along the side of the canal

8. After instilling the ear medication, Cammie documents the procedure in Quinton's progress notes. She would chart this procedure as
   A. 4/20/05 10:00 AM 5 drops of ofloxacin otic solution instilled in the Ⓛ ear. C. Lindner, CMA
   B. 4/20/05 10:00 AM Ofloxacin otic solution, gtts v̄, AS. C. Lindner, CMA
   C. 4/20/05 10:00 AM Ofloxacin ophthalmic solution, gtts v̄, AS. C. Lindner, CMA
   D. 4/20/05 10:00 AM Ofloxacin drops instilled as directed. C. Lindner, CMA

9. Carrie Engles comes to the office for an employment physical and complains that her right ear has been itching. Dr. Canthus examines her ears and asks Cammie Lindner, CMA, to perform an irrigation on Carrie's right ear to remove cerumen. All of the following are appropriate steps for performing an ear irrigation EXCEPT
   A. Placing Carrie so that her head is tilted toward her right ear
   B. Expelling air from the syringe
   C. Directing the solution toward the roof of the ear canal
   D. Making sure the tip of the syringe seals the opening of the ear canal

10. After performing the ear irrigation, Cammie should relay the following information to Carrie:
    A. "Your ears will feel sensitive for a little while"
    B. "You need to lie on your left side"
    C. "You may have a blood-tinged drainage for a few days"
    D. "You may not be able to hear well for a while"

CERTIFICATIONREVIEW

❑ **Visual acuity** refers to acuteness or sharpness of vision. A person with normal visual acuity can see clearly and is able to distinguish fine details both close up and at some distance.

❑ **Errors of refraction** are the most common cause of defects in visual acuity. A nearsighted person has a condition termed *myopia* and has difficulty seeing objects at a distance. A farsighted person has a condition known as *hyperopia* and has difficulty viewing objects at a reading or working distance. A decrease in the elasticity of the lens that occurs with aging, presbyopia, results in a decreased ability to focus clearly on close objects.

❑ **A distance visual acuity test** assesses an individual's ability to see objects at a distance. The Snellen test is generally used in the medical office to screen for distance visual acuity. A reading of 20/20 indicates normal distance visual acuity.

❑ **Near visual acuity testing** assesses an individual's ability to read close objects. The test results are used to detect hyperopia and presbyopia. The results are recorded as the smallest type the patient can comfortably read.

❑ **Congenital color defects** are color vision deficiencies that are inherited and therefore present at birth. Acquired defects are color vision deficiencies that are acquired after birth. Color vision tests, such as the Ishihara test, detect congenital color vision disturbances.

❑ **An eye irrigation** involves washing the eye with a flowing solution. Eye irrigations are performed to cleanse the eye of ocular discharges or harmful chemicals, to relieve inflammation through the application of heat, and to apply an antiseptic solution.

❑ **Eye instillations** are performed to treat eye infections, to soothe an irritated eye, and to dilate the pupil or anesthetize the eye during an eye examination or treatment. Eye medications come in the form of ophthalmic drops and an ophthalmic ointment.

❑ **There are three types of hearing loss: conductive, sensorineural, and mixed.** A conductive loss results from an interference with the conduction of sound waves through the external and middle ear. Sensorineural loss results from damage to the inner ear or auditory nerve. Mixed loss is a combination of conductive and sensorineural loss.

❑ **Tests to assess** hearing acuity include gross screening, tuning fork, audiometric, and tympanometric tests. Of these, audiometry is the most specific hearing acuity test because it provides information on how extensive a patient's hearing loss is and which frequencies are involved.

❑ **An ear irrigation** is the washing of the external auditory canal with a flowing solution. Ear irrigations are performed to remove cerumen, discharge, or a foreign body; to relieve inflammation by applying an antiseptic solution; and to apply heat to the ear.

❑ **An ear instillation** involves the dropping of a liquid into the external auditory canal. Ear instillations are performed to soften impacted cerumen, to combat infection with the use of antibiotic drops, and to relieve pain.

Terminology Review

Audiometer An instrument used to measure hearing acuity quantitatively for the various frequencies of sound waves.

Canthus The junction of the eyelids at either corner of the eye.

Cerumen Ear wax.

Hyperopia Farsightedness.

Impacted Wedged firmly together so as to be immovable.

Instillation The dropping of a liquid into a body cavity.

Irrigation The washing of a body canal with a flowing solution.

Myopia Nearsightedness.

Otoscope An instrument used to examine the external ear canal and tympanic membrane.

Presbyopia A decrease in the elasticity of the lens that occurs with aging, resulting in a decreased ability to focus on close objects.

Refraction The deflection or bending of light rays by a lens.

Tympanic membrane A thin, semitransparent membrane between the external ear canal and the middle ear that receives and transmits sound waves. Also known as the eardrum.

ON THE WEB

For active weblinks to each website visit http://evolve.elsevier.com/Bonewit/.

For Information on the Eye:

American Optometric Association

American Academy of Ophthalmology

National Eye Institute

All About Vision

Sight and Hearing Association

For Information on the Ear:

American Academy of Audiology

National Institute on Deafness and Other Communication Disorders

Healthy Hearing

Hear It

League for the Hard of Hearing

Learning Objectives

Procedures

Local Application of Heat and Cold

1. Give examples of moist and dry applications of heat and cold.
2. State the factors to consider when applying heat and cold.
3. List the effects of local application of heat, and state reasons for applying heat.
4. List the effects of local application of cold, and state reasons for applying cold.

Apply the following heat treatments:
 Heating pad
 Hot soak
 Hot compress
 Chemical hot pack
Apply the following cold treatments:
 Ice bag
 Cold compress
 Chemical cold pack

Therapeutic Ultrasound

1. Describe the general use of therapeutic ultrasound.
2. Explain the purpose of the ultrasound coupling agent.

Administer an ultrasound treatment.

Casts

1. List reasons for applying a cast.
2. Identify the advantages and disadvantages of synthetic casts.
3. Explain the purpose of each step in the cast application procedure.

Assist with the application of a cast.
Assist with the removal of a cast.
Instruct an individual in proper cast care.

Splints and Braces

1. Describe a splint and explain its use.
2. Explain the purpose of a brace.

Apply a splint following the manufacturer's instructions.
Apply a brace following the manufacturer's instructions.

Ambulatory Aids

1. List factors that are taken into consideration when ambulatory aids are prescribed.
2. Explain the difference between an axillary crutch and a forearm crutch.
3. State conditions that may result when axillary crutches are not fitted properly.
4. List the guidelines that should be followed by the patient to ensure safe use of crutches.
5. State the use of each of the following crutch gaits: four-point gait, two-point gait, three-point gait, swing-to gait, and swing-through gait.
6. List and describe the three types of canes.
7. Identify the patient conditions that warrant the use of a cane or walker.

Measure an individual for axillary crutches.
Instruct an individual in the proper use of crutches.
Instruct an individual in the proper procedure for each of the following crutch gaits:
 Four-point
 Two-point
 Three-point
 Swing-to
 Swing-through
Instruct an individual in the use of a cane.
Instruct an individual in the proper use of a walker.

CHAPTER 7

Physical Agents to Promote Tissue Healing

Chapter Outline

Introduction to Tissue Healing
Local Application of Heat and Cold
  Factors Affecting the Application of Heat and Cold
  Heat
  Cold
Therapeutic Ultrasound
  Parts of the Ultrasound Machine
  Administering Ultrasound Therapy
Casts
  Plaster Casts
  Synthetic Casts
  Cast Application
  Precautions
  Guidelines for Cast Care
  Symptoms to Report
  Cast Removal
Splints and Braces
Ambulatory Aids
  Crutches
  Canes
  Walkers

National Competencies

Clinical Competencies
Patient Care
- Prepare and maintain examination and treatment areas.
- Prepare patient for and assist with procedures, treatments, and minor office surgery.

General Competencies
Patient Instructions
- Instruct individuals according to their needs.
- Provide instruction for health maintenance and disease prevention.

Key Terms

ambulation (AM-byoo-LAY-shun)
ambulatory
brace
compress (KOM-press)
edema (uh-DEE-muh)
erythema (err-uh-THEE-muh)
exudate (EKS-oo-date)
long arm cast
long leg cast
maceration (mass-er-AY-shun)
orthopedist (OR-thoe-PEE-dist)
short arm cast
short leg cast
soak
splint
sprain
strain
suppuration (SUP-er-AY-shun)

Introduction to Tissue Healing

Physical agents are often employed in the medical office to promote tissue healing for individuals who experience a disability as a result of injury, disease, or loss of a body part. Physical agents are used therapeutically to improve circulation, provide support, and promote the return of motion so that the individual can perform the activities of daily living. Physical agents frequently used in the medical office include heat and cold applied locally, therapeutic ultrasound, casts, and ambulatory aids such as crutches, canes, and walkers.

Local Application of Heat and Cold

The application of heat and cold is used therapeutically to treat conditions such as infection and trauma. The medical assistant may be responsible for applying various forms of heat and cold at the medical office or for instructing patients in the proper procedure for applying heat or cold at home. Therefore the medical assistant should have a basic understanding of the physiologic effects of heat and cold on the body and possible adverse reactions if they are not administered correctly.

Heat and cold can be applied in either moist or dry forms. The common applications of dry and moist heat and cold are:

1. Dry heat: heating pad, chemical hot pack
2. Moist heat: hot soak, hot compress
3. Dry cold: ice bag, chemical cold pack
4. Moist cold: cold compress

Heat and cold are applied for short periods (generally 15 to 30 minutes) to produce the desired therapeutic results. The application may be repeated at time intervals specified by the physician. Prolonged application of heat or cold is not recommended because it can result in adverse secondary effects. The type of heat or cold application used for a particular condition depends on the purpose of the application, the location and condition of the affected area, and the age and general health of the patient. The physician will instruct the medical assistant to apply a heat or cold treatment based on these factors.

Heat and cold receptors in the skin readily adapt to changes in temperature, eventually resulting in diminished heat or cold sensations. The temperature actually remains the same and is providing the intended therapeutic effects. However, the patient, not perceiving the same degree of temperature, may want to increase the intensity of the application without realizing the inherent dangers. Excessive heat or cold could result in tissue damage. The medical assistant should fully explain to the patient the necessity of maintaining a safe temperature range during the application.

Factors Affecting the Application of Heat and Cold

Before applying heat or cold, certain factors must be taken into consideration to prevent unfavorable reactions such as tissue necrosis. The temperature may need to be adjusted based on the following conditions:

1. **The age of the patient.** Young children and elderly patients tend to be more sensitive to the application of heat or cold.

2. **Location of the application.** Certain areas of the body are more sensitive to the application of heat or cold, especially thin areas of the skin and areas that are usually covered by clothing, such as the chest, back, and abdomen. The skin on the hands and face is not as sensitive and is able to tolerate temperature change better. Broken skin, such as is found with an open wound, is more sensitive to heat and cold, as well as being more prone to tissue damage.

3. **Impaired circulation.** Patients with impaired circulation tend to be more sensitive to heat and cold. This impairment may be at the site of the application or may be a systemic problem involving the entire body that is a result of conditions such as peripheral vascular disease, diabetes mellitus, or congestive heart failure.

4. **Impaired sensation.** Individuals with impaired sensation, such as diabetic patients, must be watched very carefully because tissue damage may occur from the application of heat or cold without the patient's awareness.

5. **Individual tolerance to change in temperature.** Some individuals cannot tolerate temperature change as easily as others. The medical assistant should observe the area to which the heat or cold has been applied before, during, and after the treatment for signs indicating that a modification of temperature is needed. Prolonged erythema or paleness, pain, swelling, and blisters should be reported to the physician. The medical assistant should also ask the patient if the application feels comfortable or if it is too hot or too cold.

Heat

Local Effects of Heat

The application of moderate heat to a localized area of the body for a short time (approximately 15 to 30 minutes) produces dilatation, or an increase in diameter, of the blood vessels in the area as the body tries to rid itself of excess heat (Figure 7-1). This results in an increased blood supply to the area, and tissue metabolism increases. Nutrients and oxygen are provided to the cells at a faster rate, and wastes and toxins are carried away faster. The skin in the area becomes warm and exhibits erythema. **Erythema** is the reddening of the skin caused by dilation of superficial blood vessels in the skin.

These physiologic effects of moderate heat applied to a localized area promote healing. However, prolonged application of heat (longer than 1 hour) produces secondary

effects that reverse this healing process. Blood vessels constrict, and blood supply to the area decreases. The medical assistant must be careful to apply heat for the length of time specified by the physician.

Purpose of Applying Heat

Heat functions in relieving pain, congestion, muscle spasms, and inflammation. Heat promotes muscle relaxation and, therefore, is often used for the relief of pain caused by excessive contraction of muscle fibers. **Edema,** or swelling, in the tissues can be reduced through the application of heat because the increased blood supply functions to increase the absorption of fluid from the tissues through the lymphatic system.

Heat, usually in the form of a **hot compress,** can be used to soften exudates. An **exudate** is a discharge produced by the body's tissues. At times exudates form a hard crust over an area and require removal. Heat also increases **suppuration,** or the process of pus formation, to HELP IN THE RELIEF OF inflammation by breaking down infected tissues. However, heat is not recommended for the initial treatment of acute inflammation or trauma.

Conditions for which the local application of heat is often prescribed are low back pain, arthritis, menstrual cramping, and localized abscesses. Procedures 7-1, 7-2, 7-3, and 7-6 present proper application of heat with a heating pad, a hot soak, a hot compress, and a chemical hot pack, respectively.

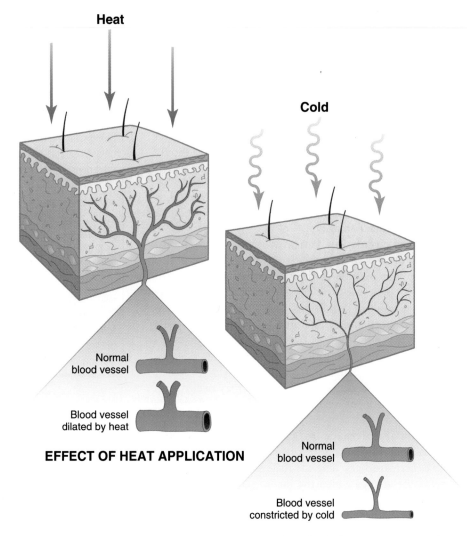

Figure 7-1. Effects of the local application of heat and cold. (From Wood LA, Rambo BJ: *Nursing skills for allied health services,* vol 2, Philadelphia, 1980, Saunders.)

Heat

Cold

Normal
blood vessel

Blood vessel
dilated by heat

EFFECT OF HEAT APPLICATION

Normal
blood vessel

Blood vessel
constricted by cold

EFFECT OF COLD APPLICATION

What Would You DO?
What Would You *Not* DO?

Case Study 1

Aaron Collins is at the office. Aaron recently helped a friend move, and the next day he developed intense pain in his lower back. To alleviate the pain, he slept on a heating pad, but when he woke up, his back was red and blistered. Aaron says he turned the setting on the heating pad to high because he thought that it would help his back feel better sooner. Aaron wants to know the best way to apply heat using a heating pad. He also wants to know what he can do to prevent low back pain in the future.

Cold

Local Effects of Cold

The application of moderate cold to a localized area produces constriction, or a decrease in diameter, of blood vessels in the area as the body attempts to prevent heat loss.

(see Figure 7-1). This constriction leads to decreased blood supply to the area. Tissue metabolism decreases, less oxygen is used, and fewer wastes accumulate. The skin becomes cool and pale. Prolonged application of cold (longer than 1 hour) has a reverse secondary effect. Blood vessels dilate, and there is an increase in tissue metabolism. To prevent secondary effects, the medical assistant must apply cold for the recommended length of time only.

Purpose of Applying Cold

The application of moderate cold for a short time is used to prevent edema. Cold may be applied immediately after an individual has suffered direct trauma such as a bruise, minor burn, **sprain, strain,** joint injury, or fracture. The cold limits the accumulation of fluid in the body tissues by constricting blood vessels and reducing the leakage of fluid into the tissues. Through the constriction of peripheral blood vessels, cold can be used to control bleeding. Cold temporarily relieves pain because of its anesthetic, or numbing, effect, which reduces stimulation of the nerve receptors. Cold also slows the movement of blood and tissue fluids in the affected area, resulting in less pressure against nerve receptors and, therefore, less pain. In the early stages of an infection, the local application of cold will inhibit the activity of microorganisms. In this way suppuration is decreased and inflammation is reduced.

Cold applications should always be placed in a protective covering because applying cold directly to the skin could result in a skin burn.

Procedures 7-4, 7-5, and 7-6 present proper application of cold with an ice bag, a cold compress, and a chemical cold pack, respectively.

Text continued on p. 247

PROCEDURE 7-1   Applying a Heating Pad

Outcome Apply a heating pad.

The electric heating pad consists of a network of wires that function to convert electric energy into heat in order to provide a constant and even heat application. The wires must not be bent or crushed. This could damage the pad, resulting in overheating of parts of the pad and leading to burns or fire. Pins must not be inserted in the pad as a means of securing it; if a pin comes in contact with a wire, an electric shock could result. To prevent electric hazards, heating pads should not be used over areas that contain moisture, such as wet dressings.

Equipment/Supplies:
• Heating pad with a protective covering

1. **Procedural Step.** Sanitize your hands.
2. **Procedural Step.** Assemble the equipment.
3. **Procedural Step.** Greet and identify the patient. Introduce yourself, and explain the procedure. Patients should be instructed not to lie on the heating pad.
   Principle. Lying on the pad causes heat to accumulate and burn the patient.
4. **Procedural Step.** Place the heating pad in the protective covering.
   Principle. The protective covering provides more comfort for the patient and absorbs perspiration.

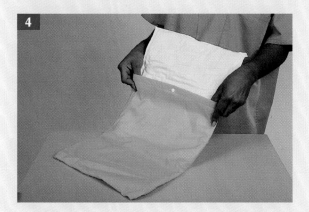

5. **Procedural Step.** Connect the plug to an electric outlet. Set the selector switch at the proper setting, as designated by the physician (usually low or medium).
6. **Procedural Step.** Place the heating pad on the patient's affected body area. Ask the patient how the temperature feels. The heating pad should feel warm but not uncomfortable.

7. **Procedural Step.** Instruct the patient not to turn the control higher, so as to prevent a burn that may be caused by excessive heat.
   Principle. The patient's heat receptors eventually become adjusted to the temperature change, resulting in a decreased heat sensation, and the patient may be tempted to increase the temperature.
8. **Procedural Step.** Administer the treatment for the proper length of time as designated by the physician. Check the patient periodically for signs of an increase or decrease in redness or swelling, and ask the patient if the site is painful.
9. **Procedural Step.** Sanitize your hands and chart the procedure. Include the date and time, method of heat application (heating pad), temperature setting of the pad, location and duration of the application, appearance of the application site, and the patient's reaction.
10. **Procedural Step.** Properly care for equipment and return it to its storage location.

CHARTING EXAMPLE

Date	
12/10/05	10:15 a.m. Heating pad on medium setting applied to lower back x 20 min. Area appears pink following application. Pt states a relief of pain and better mobility. Provided instructions on the application of a heating pad at home. ———————— M. Cooper, CMA

PROCEDURE 7-2 Applying a Hot Soak

Outcome Apply a hot soak.

A **soak** is the direct immersion of a body part in water or a medicated solution. A soak can be applied to an extremity or a part of the torso. Hot soaks are used to cleanse open wounds, increase suppuration, increase the blood supply to an area to hasten the healing process, and apply a medicated solution to an area.

Equipment/Supplies:
- Soaking solution ordered by the physician
- Bath thermometer
- Basin
- Bath towels

1. **Procedural Step.** Sanitize your hands.
2. **Procedural Step.** Assemble the equipment.
3. **Procedural Step.** Greet and identify the patient. Introduce yourself, and explain the procedure.
4. **Procedural Step.** Fill the basin half full with the warmed soaking solution.
5. **Procedural Step.** Check the temperature of the solution with a bath thermometer. The temperature for an adult should range between 105 and 110° F (41 and 44° C).
6. **Procedural Step.** Assist the patient into a comfortable position to avoid fatigue and muscle strain. Pad the side of the basin with a towel for the patient's comfort.
7. **Procedural Step.** Slowly and gradually immerse the patient's affected body part in the solution. Ask the patient how the temperature feels.
   Principle. The affected body part should become accustomed to the change in temperature gradually.
8. **Procedural Step.** Test the temperature of the solution frequently. To keep the solution at a constant temperature, remove cooler fluid every 5 minutes and replace it with hot solution. Pour the hot solution in near the edge of the basin by placing your hand between the patient and solution. Stir the solution as you pour.
   Principle. The solution should be added away from the patient's body part to prevent splashing hot fluid on the patient. Stirring in the solution helps distribute the heat and keep the temperature constant.

9. **Procedural Step.** Apply the hot soak for the proper length of time as designated by the physician (usually 15 to 20 minutes). Check the patient's skin periodically for signs of an increase or decrease in redness or swelling, and ask the patient whether the site is painful.
10. **Procedural Step.** Completely and gently dry the affected part.
11. **Procedural Step.** Sanitize your hands and chart the procedure. Include the date and time, method of heat application (hot soak), name and strength of the solution, the temperature of the soak, location and duration of the application, the appearance of the application site, and the patient's reaction.
12. **Procedural Step.** Properly care for equipment and return it to its storage location.

CHARTING EXAMPLE

Date	
12/12/05	1:15 p.m. Normal saline hot soak @ 105° F applied to (R) ankle x 20 min. Area appears pink following application. Pt states less stiffness in ankle. ———— M. Cooper, CMA

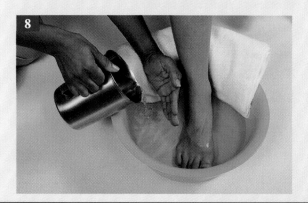

PROCEDURE 7-3   Applying a Hot Compress

Outcome Apply a hot compress.

A **compress** is a soft, moist, absorbent cloth, such as a washcloth, applied to a body part. Hot compresses are used to increase suppuration, to improve circulation to a body part to aid in healing, and to promote drainage from infection. Applying a hot compress to an open wound requires the use of sterile technique.

Equipment/Supplies:
- Solution ordered by the physician
- Bath thermometer
- Basin
- Washcloths

1. **Procedural Step.** Sanitize your hands.
2. **Procedural Step.** Assemble the equipment.
3. **Procedural Step.** Greet and identify the patient. Introduce yourself, and explain the procedure.
4. **Procedural Step.** Fill the basin half full with warmed solution. Check the temperature of the solution with the bath thermometer. The temperature for an adult should range between 105° and 110° F (41° and 44° C).
5. **Procedural Step.** Completely immerse the compress in the solution. Wring the compress to rid it of excess moisture. The compress should be wet but not dripping. Apply it lightly at first to the affected site to allow the patient gradually to become used to the heat. You may want to cover the compress with a waterproof cover to help hold the heat in. Ask the patient how the temperature feels. The compress should be as hot as the patient can comfortably tolerate.

   Principle. The waterproof cover prevents cool air currents from coming in contact with the compress and reduces the number of times the compress needs to be changed.

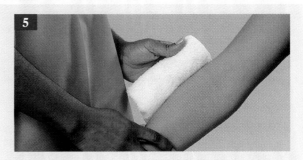

6. **Procedural Step.** Place additional compresses in the solution so they are ready for use.
7. **Procedural Step.** Repeat the application of the compress every 2 to 3 minutes for the duration of time specified by the physician (usually 15 to 20 minutes). Check the patient's skin periodically for signs of an increase or decrease in redness or swelling, and ask the patient whether the site is painful.
8. **Procedural Step.** Check the temperature of the solution periodically. Remove cooler fluid and replace it with hot solution if needed.
9. **Procedural Step.** Thoroughly and gently dry the affected part.
10. **Procedural Step.** Sanitize your hands and chart the procedure. Include the date and time, method of heat application (hot compress), name and strength of the solution, temperature of the solution, location and duration of the application, appearance of the application site, and the patient's reaction.
11. **Procedural Step.** Properly care for equipment and return it to its storage location.

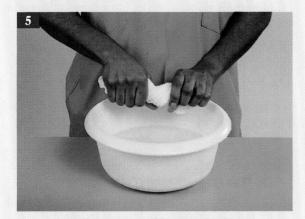

CHARTING EXAMPLE

Date	
12/20/05	10:30 a.m. Normal saline hot compress @ 110° F applied to (R) forearm x 20 min. No complaints of discomfort. — M. Cooper, CMA

PROCEDURE 7-3

PROCEDURE 7-4 Applying an Ice Bag

Outcome Apply an ice bag.

Equipment/Supplies:
- Ice bag with a protective covering
- Small pieces of ice (ice chips or crushed ice)

1. **Procedural Step.** Sanitize your hands.
2. **Procedural Step.** Assemble the equipment.
3. **Procedural Step.** Greet and identify the patient. Introduce yourself, and explain the procedure. Explain the purpose of applying the ice bag, for example, to prevent swelling.
4. **Procedural Step.** Check the ice bag for leakage.
   Principle. A leaking bag will get the patient wet and cause chilling.
5. **Procedural Step.** Fill the bag one-half to two-thirds full with small pieces of ice.
   Principle. Small pieces of ice work better than large pieces because they reduce the air spaces in the bag, resulting in better conduction of cold. In addition, small pieces of ice allow the bag to mold better to the body area.
6. **Procedural Step.** Expel air from the bag by squeezing the empty top half of the bag together and screwing on the stopper.
   Principle. Air is a poor conductor of cold and also makes it difficult to mold the ice bag to the body area.

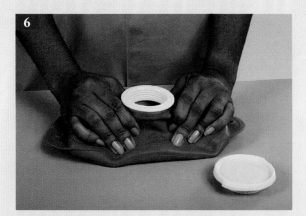

7. **Procedural Step.** Thoroughly dry the bag and place it in the protective covering.
   Principle. The protective covering provides for patient comfort and absorbs the moisture that condenses on the outside of the bag.

8. **Procedural Step.** Place the bag on the patient's affected body area. Ask the patient how the temperature feels. The application of ice is usually uncomfortable, but most patients tolerate it if they know how much benefit may be derived from it.
   Principle. Individuals vary in their ability to tolerate cold.
9. **Procedural Step.** Administer the treatment for the proper length of time, as designated by the physician (*usually until the area feels numb*, approximately 15 to 30 minutes). Check the patient's skin periodically for signs of an increase or decrease in redness or swelling, and ask the patient whether the site is painful. If extreme paleness and numbness or a mottled blue appearance occurs at the application site, remove the bag and notify the physician.
10. **Procedural Step.** Refill the bag with ice as necessary, and change the protective covering if needed.
11. **Procedural Step.** Sanitize your hands, and chart the procedure. Include the date and time, method of cold application (ice bag), location and duration of the application, appearance of the application site, and the patient's reaction.
12. **Procedural Step.** Properly care for the ice bag. Dispose of or launder the protective covering as required. Cleanse the ice bag with a warm detergent, solution, rinse thoroughly, and dry by hanging the bag upside down with the top removed. Store the bag by screwing on the stopper, leaving air inside to prevent the sides from sticking together.

CHARTING EXAMPLE

Date	
12/22/05	11:30 a.m. Ice bag applied to Ⓡ knee x 20 min. Pt complained of slight discomfort during the application. Area appears less swollen following application. Provided instructions on the application of an ice bag at home. ———————— M. Cooper, CMA

PROCEDURE 7-5   Applying a Cold Compress

Outcome Apply a cold compress.

Cold compresses are used to relieve pain and inflammation and to treat conditions such as headaches, injury to the eyes, and pain after tooth extraction.

Equipment/Supplies:

- Ice cubes
- Basin
- Washcloths

1. **Procedural Step.** Sanitize your hands.
2. **Procedural Step.** Assemble the equipment.
3. **Procedural Step.** Greet and identify the patient. Introduce yourself, and explain the procedure.
4. **Procedural Step.** Place large ice cubes in the basin and add a small amount of water.
   Principle. Using larger pieces of ice prevents them from sticking to the compress and slows the rate at which they melt in the water.

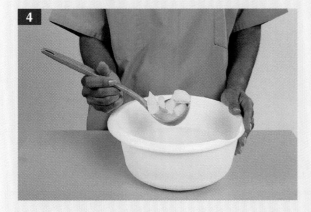

5. **Procedural Step.** Completely immerse the compress in the solution. Wring the compress to rid it of excess moisture. The compress should be wet but not dripping. Apply it lightly at first to the affected site to allow the patient gradually to become used to the cold. You want to cover the compress with an ice bag to help keep it cold and to reduce the number of times it needs to be changed. Ask the patient how the temperature feels.

6. **Procedural Step.** Place additional compresses in the solution to be ready for use.
7. **Procedural Step.** Repeat the application of the compress every 2 to 3 minutes for the duration of time specified by the physician (usually 15 to 20 minutes). Check the patient's skin periodically for signs of an increase or decrease in redness or swelling and ask the patient whether the site is painful.
8. **Procedural Step.** Add ice if needed to keep the water cold.
9. **Procedural Step.** Thoroughly dry the affected part.
10. **Procedural Step.** Sanitize your hands and chart the procedure. Include the date and time, method of cold application (cold compress), location and duration of the application, appearance of the application site, and the patient's reaction.
11. **Procedural Step.** Properly care for equipment and return it to its storage location.

PROCEDURE 7-5

CHARTING EXAMPLE

Date	
12/27/05	9:15 a.m. Cold compress applied to bridge of nose x 15 min. Nose appears less swollen following application. Tolerated application well. ————————— M. Cooper, CMA

PROCEDURE 7-6   Applying a Chemical Pack

Outcome Apply a chemical cold pack and a chemical hot pack.

Chemical Cold Pack

Chemical cold packs are available in a variety of sizes and shapes. Once activated, they provide a specific degree of coldness for a specific period of time (usually 30 to 60 minutes), as indicated on the package label. Most cold packs consist of a vinyl bag of ammonium nitrate crystals. Enclosed in this bag is a smaller vinyl bag of water. The cold pack is activated by applying pressure until the inner bag ruptures. This releases the water into the larger bag, and a chemical reaction occurs between the crystals and water, producing coldness. These packs are disposable, and once the coldness diminishes, they should be discarded in an appropriate receptacle. Chemical cold packs should be stored at room temperature and are used as an alternative to ice bags for the local application of cold.

Chemical Hot Pack

A chemical hot pack is similar to a chemical cold pack except that heat is generated once the bag is activated. The vinyl bag contains calcium chloride crystals, and the smaller bag (encased in the vinyl bag) contains water. Pressure is applied to break the inner bag. The water in the inner bag combines with the calcium chloride crystals to produce heat. After using the pack, it should be discarded in an appropriate receptacle.

The procedure for applying a chemical cold or hot pack is as follows:

1. **Procedural Step.** Shake the crystals to the bottom of the bag.
2. **Procedural Step.** Squeeze the bag firmly to break the inner water bag.
3. **Procedural Step.** Shake the bag vigorously to mix the contents.
4. **Procedural Step.** Cover the bag with a protective covering.
5. **Procedural Step.** Apply the bag to the affected area.
6. **Procedural Step.** Administer the treatment for the proper length of time.
7. **Procedural Step.** Discard the bag in an appropriate receptacle.

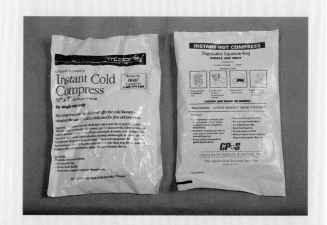

⫸ PATIENT TEACHING

Low Back Pain

Answer questions patients have about low back pain.

What causes low back pain?

Low back pain is one of the most common health problems in the United States. Approximately 80% of Americans are affected by low back pain at some time during their life. The most frequent cause of low back pain is poor posture and poor body mechanics, which strain the muscles and ligaments that support the back. Other causes include physical inactivity, excessive body weight, disc damage, osteoarthritis, and congenital deformities.

How might the physician treat low back pain?

To treat low back pain caused by strain, the physician might prescribe bed rest, local application of heat or cold, massage, medications, back manipulation, the use of back-supporting devices, deep-heating treatments such as ultrasound, and exercises to strengthen the supporting structures of the back and prevent the back pain from recurring or becoming chronic.

What can be done to prevent low back pain?

Most cases of low back pain can be prevented by practicing good posture and body mechanics.

- Encourage patients to follow practices that prevent strain to the lower back.
- Teach the patient the procedure for the local application of heat or cold as prescribed by the physician.
- Provide the patient with a sheet that describes and illustrates the correct way to perform back exercises prescribed by the physician.
- Provide the patient with educational materials on low back pain.

PATIENT TEACHING—Cont'd

Body Mechanics

Teach patients the essentials of good posture and body mechanics as follows:

Standing and Walking

Stand and walk with the chin tucked in, head up, back flattened, and the pelvis held straight. Wear comfortable low-heeled shoes that offer good support.

Lifting

To lift an object, always bend the body at the knees and hips. Never bend from the waist. Lift the object with the leg muscles and hold it close to the body at waist level. Never lift anything heavier than you can easily manage or higher than waist level.

Sitting

Sit in a chair with a firm back. The feet should be flat on the floor, and knees should be level with the hips. Sit firmly against the back of the chair; avoid slumping. Using a pillow in the small of the back or a footstool to raise the knees also reduces strain on the back.

Driving

Make sure the car seat is not too far back. Stretching for the pedals strains the back. The car seat should be positioned so that the driver's back is straight and the knees are raised.

Sleeping

Sleep on a firm, comfortable mattress that supports the back and does not allow it to sag. Sleep on your side with knees bent or on your back with a pillow under the knees. Do not sleep on your stomach because this causes the body to sag into the mattress, which results in strain to the back, neck, and shoulders.

Therapeutic Ultrasound

Therapeutic ultrasound uses high-frequency sound waves as a penetrating, deep-heating agent for the soft tissues of the body, such as tendons and muscles. Many physicians use ultrasound in the medical office for the local application of heat to treat musculoskeletal disorders.

The beneficial physiologic effects of ultrasound result primarily from the deep heat produced in the tissues and include reduction of edema, breakup of exudates increased cellular metabolism, relief of pain, and micromassage. The physician may order ultrasound to treat such musculoskeletal conditions as sprains, joint contractures, neuritis, arthritis, edema, synovitis, scar tissue, bursitis, fibrositis, strains, and dislocations. Therapeutic ultrasound must *not* be used over the eyeball, over malignant tumors, directly over the spinal cord, over the heart or brain, over reproductive organs including a pregnant uterus, or over areas of impaired sensation or inadequate circulation.

The medical assistant is responsible for performing the ultrasound treatment, which includes preparing the patient, operating the machine, and administering the treatment.

Parts of the Ultrasound Machine

The ultrasound machine consists of two main parts: the generator and the transducer. The *generator* is located in the main unit of the machine, which also contains the controls to operate the machine. The *transducer* is a crystal inserted between two electrodes; it is located in a device called the applicator head or sound head. The *applicator head* is a lightweight, handheld device attached to the ultrasound machine by a connector cord (Figure 7-2). The generator produces a high-frequency electric current that causes the crystal in the transducer to vibrate and generate sound

waves. The frequency of the sound waves produced by the transducer is above the frequency of sound waves audible to the human ear; therefore no sound is heard when the machine is in operation.

The controls on the ultrasound machine include a timing control and an intensity control; additional controls may be present, depending on the type of machine. The *timing control* measures time in minutes; the time limit of most machines ranges from 0 to 15 minutes, which is sufficient because the majority of treatments rarely exceed 10 minutes. The *intensity control* governs the intensity of the sound waves, which are measured in watts; therapeutic ultrasound intensity usually ranges from 1 to 4 watts. A digital display screen indicates the intensity at which the machine has been set.

The medical assistant must be able to operate both controls (timing control and intensity control). As an example, if the physician orders an ultrasound treatment at 4 watts for a duration of 5 minutes, the medical assistant must first set the timing control to 5 (minutes) and then set the intensity control until the display screen indicates that the intensity is at 4 watts.

Coupling Agents

Air is a poor conductor of sound; therefore a coupling agent must be used with ultrasound treatments to increase conductivity, thereby providing a good transmission of the sound waves to the patient's tissues. The coupling agent produces an air-free contact between the applicator head and the patient's skin and is available in the form of a gel or lotion.

The coupling agent must be at room temperature and must be applied liberally to the treatment area of the patient's skin. Water may also be used as a coupling agent because it is a good conductor of sound. In this method,

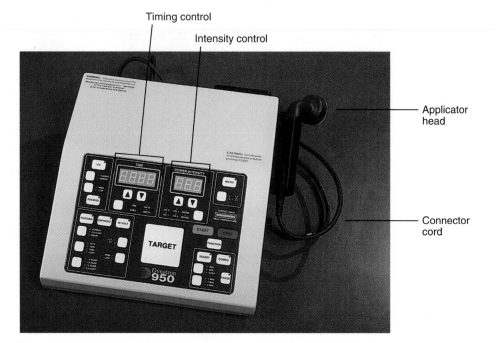

Timing control

Intensity control

Applicator head

Connector cord

Figure 7-2. The parts of an ultrasound machine.

both the patient's skin surface to be treated and the applicator head are completely submerged under water. The applicator head is held ½ to 1 inch away from the patient's skin and is slowly and steadily moved in a circular motion. The underwater method is advocated when the patient's skin is sensitive and cannot tolerate the direct pressure of the applicator head or when the body surface to be treated is uneven, as are the hands and feet, where it would be difficult to obtain a good contact between the patient's skin and the applicator head.

Administering Ultrasound Therapy

The applicator head is placed firmly on the patient's skin and is slowly and steadily moved over the treatment area, which allows the sound waves to penetrate the patient's soft tissues. As the sound waves travel through the tissues, part of the waves are absorbed by the tissues and transformed into heat. This produces a vigorous deep heating in the soft tissues of the body. A micromassage effect is also produced owing to the mechanical vibration of the sound waves as they pass through the tissues, massaging them.

The applicator head must be moved continuously during the treatment in either a back-and-forth stroking motion or in a circular motion at a rate of 1 to 2 inches per second. The method used depends in large part on the area of the body to which the treatment is being applied. It is usually easier to use the stroking motion over larger body areas such as the back and the circular motion over smaller areas such as the ankle. Moving the applicator head ensures a uniform distribution of heat in the tissues

and prevents hot spots. A hot spot is a very small area in which the temperature rises rapidly if the applicator head is allowed to remain stationary. This could burn the patient's tissues.

Ultrasound dosage is expressed in watt-minutes. *Watt* refers to the intensity of the sound waves ordered by the physician, and *minutes* refers to the duration of the treatment. The dosage ordered by the physician depends on the area of the body that is receiving the treatment and the patient's condition. An acute condition requires a lower intensity treatment, whereas a chronic condition warrants a higher intensity treatment. The underwater method also requires a higher intensity because some of the sound waves are absorbed and reflected by the water.

Ultrasound therapy is generally administered in a series of 6 to 12 treatments; the frequency of the treatment varies from once daily to three times per week. The duration of the treatment usually progresses from 5 minutes at the beginning of the series to 8 to 10 minutes near the end of the treatments. An ultrasound treatment should never exceed 20 minutes.

During the treatment, the patient should not feel the ultrasound waves. If the patient indicates a feeling of burning or pain, the medical assistant should stop the treatment immediately and inform the physician. Any pain or discomfort usually indicates that the treatment dosage is too intense. Other causes of pain or discomfort include application of an insufficient amount of coupling medium to the treatment area and keeping the applicator head on one area too long. Procedure 7-7 outlines the procedure for administering an ultrasound treatment to a patient.

Text continued on p. 251

PROCEDURE 7-7 Administering an Ultrasound Treatment

Outcome Administer an ultrasound treatment.

Equipment/Supplies:
- Ultrasound machine
- Coupling agent
- Paper towels

1. **Procedural Step.** Sanitize your hands.
2. **Procedural Step.** Assemble the equipment.
3. **Procedural Step.** Greet and identify the patient. Introduce yourself, and explain the procedure. Tell the patient that the treatment will not take long and that any pain or discomfort experienced during the treatment should be reported immediately.
   Principle. Pain or discomfort during the treatment indicates that the intensity of the treatment dosage might be too high.
4. **Procedural Step.** Ask the patient to remove appropriate clothing to expose the treatment area. Position the patient and prepare the skin. Make sure the coupling agent is at room temperature, and apply it liberally to the treatment area. Tell the patient that the coupling agent will feel cold. Use the applicator head to spread the coupling agent evenly over the treatment area. The coupling agent should completely cover, but should not flood, the area. Do not place the coupling agent on the ultrasound machine.
   Principle. The coupling agent permits a good transmission of the sound waves to the patient's tissues. The coupling agent should be applied at room temperature so as not to be too uncomfortable for the patient.

5. **Procedural Step.** Set the intensity control at the minimum position, and set the timer to the amount of time for the ultrasound treatment specified by the physician. Once the timer has activated the machine, check to make sure the intensity is at 0 watts.
6. **Procedural Step.** Advance the intensity control to the treatment level (measured in watts) specified by the physician. Tell the patient that the applicator head will feel cold. Hold the applicator at a right angle to the patient's skin, and using a firm pressure, place the application head into the coupling agent in the treatment area.

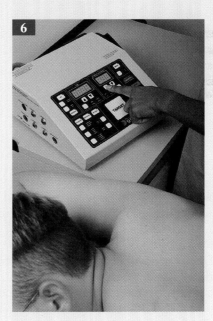

7. **Procedural Step.** Move the applicator head in a back-and-forth stroking motion or in a circular motion. If the stroking method is employed, use short strokes (approximately 1 inch in length), and gradually move the applicator head so that each stroke

Continued

PROCEDURE 7-7

PROCEDURE 7-7   Administering an Ultrasound Treatment—Cont'd

overlaps the previous stroke by one half. Move the applicator head continually at a rate of 1 to 2 inches per second.

Principle. Moving the applicator head continually ensures a uniform distribution of heat in the tissues and prevents overheating of the tissue in a small area (hot spot).

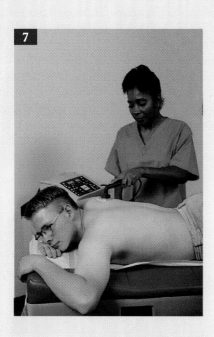

8. **Procedural Step.** Continue the ultrasound treatment until the timer goes off. During the treatment, perform the following:
   a. Move the applicator head continually.
   b. Do not remove the applicator head from the patient's skin and hold it up in the air.
   c. Stop the treatment immediately and notify the physician if the patient complains of pain or discomfort.

   Principle. Holding the applicator head in the air causes it to become hot, and it may burn the patient when it is placed back on the skin. The excessive heat may also damage the crystal in the applicator head.

9. **Procedural Step.** When the treatment time is completed, the timer automatically shuts off the machine. Remove the applicator head from the patient's skin.

10. **Procedural Step.** Wipe the excess coupling medium from the patient's skin and applicator head with a paper towel. Instruct the patient to get dressed.

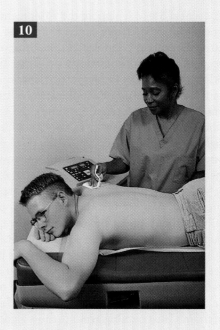

11. **Procedural Step.** Sanitize your hands, and chart the procedure. Include the date and time, the location of the treatment, the duration (in minutes) and the intensity (in watts), and the patient's reaction.

CHARTING EXAMPLE	
Date	
12/10/05	10:45 a.m. Ultrasound applied to Ⓡ upper back @ 2 watts x 5 min. No complaints of discomfort. Pt states a relief of pain and feeling of relaxed muscles. — M. Cooper, CMA

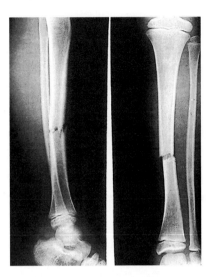

Figure 7-3. A fracture of the tibia in the left lower leg. (From McRae R, Esser M: *Practical fracture treatment,* ed 4, Philadelphia, 2002, Churchill Livingstone.)

Casts

A cast is a stiff cylindrical synthetic or plaster casing that is used to immobilize a body part. Casts are applied most often when an individual sustains a fracture (Figure 7-3). The cast keeps the fractured bones aligned until proper healing takes place. Casts are also used to support and stabilize weak or dislocated joints, to promote healing after a surgical correction such as knee surgery, and to aid in the nonsurgical correction of deformities such as congenital dislocation of the hip.

Casts are applied by an orthopedist, also known as an orthopedic surgeon. An **orthopedist** is a physician who specializes in the diagnosis and treatment of disorders of the musculoskeletal system. An orthopedist treats patients with deformities, injuries, and diseases of the bones, joints, ligaments, tendons, muscles, nerves, and skin.

The role of the medical assistant in cast application is to assemble the equipment and supplies, prepare the patient for the procedure, assist the physician during the application, provide or reinforce cast care instructions, and clean the examining room following the application.

One of the most important goals of cast management is the prevention of pressure areas, which are most apt to occur over bony prominences. A *pressure area* occurs when the cast presses or rubs against the patient's skin and prevents adequate circulation to the area. When this occurs, the patient usually feels a painful rubbing, burning, or stinging sensation under the cast. If permitted to continue, the pressure can cause the skin to break down, leading to the development of a *pressure ulcer.* If not treated, a pressure ulcer progresses from a simple red patch of skin to erosion into the subcutaneous tissue, and then eventually into the muscle and bone. Deep pressure ulcers often become infected by invading organisms and develop gangrene. Therefore it is important to detect the occurrence of a pressure area early so that prompt treatment can be instituted to prevent serious complications.

Plaster Casts

Since the development of synthetic casts, plaster casts are not used as much as they once were. The traditional plaster cast consists of powdered calcium sulfate crystals formed into a bandage that must be soaked in tepid water to activate the crystals. When wet, the plaster bandage becomes pliable and self-adhering, allowing it to be molded to the body part. Plaster bandages are available in individual rolls of widths ranging from 2 to 6 inches. The width used depends on the body part to be casted. Bandages with a smaller width are used for the arms, and bandages with a larger width are used for the legs and trunk.

Some orthopedists initially apply a plaster cast after a patient sustains a fracture. This is because a plaster cast can be easily molded to allow for swelling of the extremity beneath the cast. After the swelling has gone down (several days to a week), the orthopedist removes the plaster cast and applies a synthetic cast, which weighs less and is more durable than a plaster cast.

Synthetic Casts

Synthetic casts consist of a knitted fabric tape made of fiberglass, polyester and cotton, or plastic. The tape is impregnated with polyurethane resin that is activated when soaked in water. Of the three kinds of synthetic material, fiberglass is used most. Synthetic tape comes in different colors and is packaged as an individual roll in an airtight pouch (Figure 7-4). Synthetic tape is available in widths ranging from 2 to 8 inches.

Advantages of Synthetic Casts

The advantages of synthetic casts compared with plaster casts are as follows:

- Synthetic casts dry and set much more quickly than plaster casts. Because of this, they are able to bear weight soon after application.
- Synthetic casts are less likely to become indented because of their fast drying time. Indentations can result in pressure areas.
- Synthetic casts weigh less than plaster casts and, therefore, are less restrictive, which allows the patient greater mobility.
- Synthetic casts are less bulky than plaster casts; therefore patients usually can wear regular clothing over them.
- A synthetic cast is moisture resistant and does not break down when it gets wet, but a plaster cast may break down when wet.

Disadvantages of Synthetic Casts

Disadvantages of synthetic casts compared with plaster casts are as follows:

- Synthetic casts cannot be molded to the body part as easily as plaster casts, so they are less effective for immobilizing severely displaced bones or unstable fractures.
- Because of the cost of the synthetic materials, they are more expensive than plaster casts.

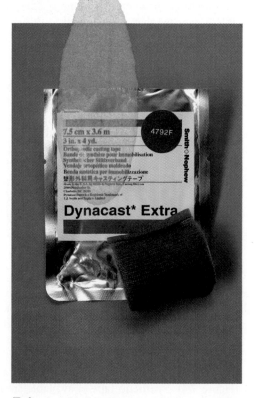

Figure 7-4. A roll of synthetic tape comes packaged in an airtight pouch.

- The surface of a synthetic cast is rougher than that of a plaster cast; therefore there is an increased chance of snagging clothes, scratching furniture, and causing abrasions on other parts of the body with the cast. A newer type of synthetic casting material now available is tightly woven and provides a smoother cast surface, which helps to alleviate this problem.

Cast Application

The physician applies the cast so that it fits snugly but still allows adequate circulation necessary for proper healing. A period of 4 to 6 weeks is usually required for the complete healing of a fracture.

Casts are classified according to the body part they cover. The types of casts most frequently applied in the medical office and common uses of each are illustrated and described in Figure 7-5. The type of cast applied

Short arm cast	
	Extends from below the elbow to the fingers. Use: • Fracture of the hand or wrist • Postoperative immobilization

Long arm cast	
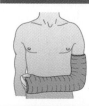	Extends from the upper arm to the fingers, usually with a bend in the elbow. Use: • Fracture of the humerus, forearm, or elbow • Postoperative immobilization

Short leg cast	
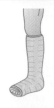	Begins just below the knee and extends to the toes. Use: • Fracture of the foot, ankle, or distal tibia or fibula • Severe sprain or strain • Postoperative immobilization • Correction of a deformity

Long leg cast	
	Extends from the midthigh to the toes. Use: • Fracture of the distal femur, knee, or lower leg • Soft tissue injury to the knee or knee dislocation • Postoperative immobilization

Figure 7-5. Types of casts.

depends on the nature of the patient's injury or condition. For example, a **short arm cast** is used for a dislocated wrist, and a **long arm cast** is used for a fracture of the humerus.

Regardless of the casting material (plaster or synthetic), the following steps are performed in applying a cast:

1. **Inspect the skin.** The area to which the cast will be applied must be clean and dry. The patient's skin should be inspected for redness, bruises, and open areas. This information should be recorded in the patient's chart, which may assist in evaluating patient complaints after the cast has been applied.

2. **Apply the stockinette.** Before applying the cast, the physician covers the body part with a stockinette (Figure 7-6). Stockinette consists of a soft, tubular, knitted cotton material that stretches up to three times its original width to accommodate the diameter of the body part. It is put on like a stocking. The purpose of the stockinette is to provide patient comfort and to cover the rough edges at the ends of the cast.

   Stockinette comes in widths ranging from 2 to 12 inches; the width used depends on the diameter of the part to be covered. Typically a 3-inch width is used for arm casts, a 4-inch width is used for leg casts, and a 10- to 12-inch width is used for body casts.

3. **Apply the cast padding.** Cast padding consists of a soft cotton material that comes in a roll in widths ranging from 2 to 4 inches. The purpose of cast padding is to prevent pressure areas and to shield the patient's skin when the cast is removed. Two or three layers are applied directly over the stockinette, using a spiral turn. Each turn overlaps the preceding one by one-half the width of the roll. Extra layers of padding are applied over bony prominences (Figure 7-7).

4. **Apply the cast bandage or tape.** The plaster cast bandage or synthetic tape is applied over the cast padding. The number of rolls depends on the desired strength of the finished cast. Usually from 4 to 6 layers are applied for a plaster cast and 3 to 5 layers are applied for a synthetic cast.

The physician wears rubber gloves during the procedure to protect the hands from the casting material. Following application, the cast must be allowed to dry. The drying time varies based on the type of casting material. Because of their porous nature, plaster casts require a longer drying period than synthetic casts. Only when a cast is completely dry does it become hard and inflexible and able to bear weight. The physician usually prescribes a supportive device, such as a sling or crutches, to prevent unnecessary strain and to minimize swelling during the healing process. Specific information on applying plaster casts and synthetic casts is presented next.

Plaster Cast

To activate the plaster, the bandage roll must be completely immersed in tepid water (70° to 95° F; 21 to 35° C) until bubbles no longer rise from the roll. The edges of the roll are then gently squeezed (but not wrung) toward the center to remove excess water. A properly squeezed roll should be saturated with water, but not dripping.

The physician wraps the body part with the plaster bandage, using a spiral turn, until the desired number of layers have been applied. The stockinette is folded over the edges of the cast and anchored with the cast bandage to produce a smooth, comfortable edge on the cast. The physician molds and smoothes the plaster to conform to the contours of the body part until the cast is firmly set.

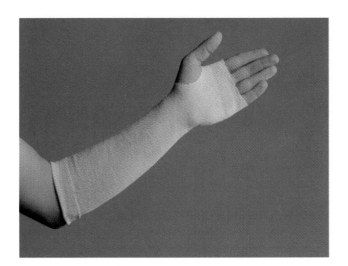

Figure 7-6. Application of stockinette.

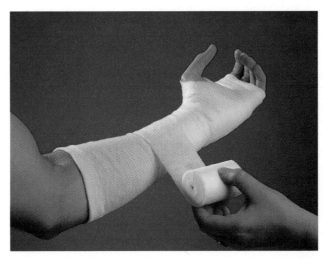

Figure 7-7. Application of cast padding. (Courtesy 3M Health Care, St. Paul, Minn.)

Finally, the physician trims the ends of the cast with a cast knife to remove rough edges and to provide freedom of movement for the uninvolved part of the extremity, such as the thumb, fingers, or toes.

As the plaster begins to harden, a chemical reaction occurs that releases heat. Because of this, the patient may feel warmth during and after the application. The patient should be told that this is normal; in fact, most patients find that the warmth has a soothing effect. The patient should not put weight on the cast until it is completely dry; otherwise the cast may break down. It takes approximately 24 to 48 hours for the standard plaster cast to dry completely.

Synthetic Cast

A synthetic cast is applied in a similar manner to that for a plaster cast. The airtight pouch containing a roll of synthetic tape should remain sealed until just before it is time to immerse the roll in water. This is because air causes the resin in the tape to begin to harden and become rigid. The roll of synthetic tape is fully immersed in cool, room-temperature water (68 to 75° F; 20 to 24° C) for a period of time recommended by the manufacturer. For example, fiberglass tape is immersed for 10 to 15 seconds. The tape is then wrapped over the body part, using a spiral turn, until the desired number of layers have been applied (Figure 7-8). The cast is then allowed to dry for a period of time specified by the manufacturer; for example, a fiberglass cast dries in 30 minutes.

Precautions

The following precautions should be observed during and after cast application:

*   Make sure the temperature of the water used to activate a plaster bandage roll does not exceed 95° F. If a thick cast is being applied, water that is too warm can result in a serious burn to the patient's skin.
*   Do not cover a wet cast with a towel, plastic, or other material. Covers prevent heat from escaping, which could burn the patient's skin.
*   Take precautions to prevent indentations, particularly with a plaster cast, which could lead to pressure areas. This is accomplished by not allowing the cast to come in contact with a hard surface while it is drying and by handling a wet cast with the palms of the hands rather than the fingertips.
*   Remove any crumbs of plaster from the patient's skin, using a cloth dampened with warm water. Remove synthetic casting material with a swab moistened with alcohol or acetone. If cast particles are not removed, they may work their way under the cast and result in irritation and infection.
*   Before the patient leaves the medical office, the physician will check the circulation, sensation, and movement of the extremity to make sure the cast is not too tight. The physician will also make sure that all joints excluded from the cast are free to move.

Guidelines for Cast Care

The medical assistant is often responsible for explaining or reinforcing the guidelines that should be followed by a patient with a cast. These guidelines are often presented on an instruction sheet that is signed by the patient, with a copy filed in the patient's chart. Guidelines for cast care include the following:

*   Wait at least 24 hours before putting any pressure or weight on a plaster cast. This allows the plaster to dry completely and prevents the cast from breaking down. Synthetic casts can bear weight approximately 30 minutes to 1 hour following application.
*   Elevate the cast above heart level for the first 24 to 48 hours to decrease swelling and pain. This can be accomplished by propping the casted extremity up on pillows or some other type of support.
*   Gently move the toes or fingers frequently to prevent swelling and joint stiffness.
*   Ice can be applied to the casted extremity to reduce swelling. Place small pieces of ice in an ice bag and loosely wrap it around the cast at the level of the injury.
*   Take precautions to prevent dirt, sand, powder, and other foreign particles from becoming trapped under the cast. They can cause irritation to the skin and lead to infection.
*   Do not use any object to scratch the skin under the cast. Inserting anything into the cast, such as a pencil, coat hanger, or knitting needle, may cause a break in the skin, which could then become infected. Also, the object may become lost in the cast.
*   Do not engage in activities that could cause injury due to impairment of your physical abilities (e.g., driving a car).

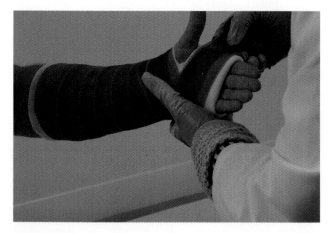

Figure 7-8. Wrapping the tape over the body part, using a spiral turn.

- Keep the cast dry. When taking a bath or shower, cover the cast with a plastic bag and secure the bag to the skin with waterproof tape. If possible, hang the casted limb over the side of the tub or outside of the shower. If a plaster cast becomes wet, it loses its shape and may break down. Although the material making up a synthetic cast is moisture resistant, the cast padding is not. If a synthetic cast becomes wet, it must be dried as soon as possible to prevent maceration. **Maceration** is the softening and breaking down of the skin, which can lead to infection.
- To dry a wet cast, the outside of the cast should first be blotted with an absorbent towel. This should be followed by the application of a blow dryer on a low setting using a sweeping motion over the entire cast until it is completely dry. The patient should be instructed not to use the high setting on the blow dryer because this amount of heat could burn the skin.
- Inspect the skin around the cast at regular intervals to check for redness, sores, or swelling.
- Do not trim the cast or break off any rough edges because this may weaken or break the cast. If the surface of the cast has a rough edge, a metal nail file or emery board can be used to smooth it. Notify the physician if the cast becomes loose, broken, or cracked because the cast may need to be replaced.
- Synthetic casts cannot be signed with a ball-point pen; only permanent markers will write on them.

Symptoms to Report

Report the following symptoms *immediately* to the physician; they may indicate that the cast is too tight or an infection is developing:

- Increased pain or swelling that does not go away with medication, elevation, or rest
- Tingling or numbness of the fingers or toes
- Coldness, paleness, or blueness of the fingers or toes
- Painful rubbing, burning, or stinging under the cast
- Foul odor or drainage coming from the cast
- Sore areas around the edge of the cast
- Chills, fever, nausea, or vomiting

Cast Removal

The easiest and safest way to remove a cast is to bivalve it—this means cutting the cast into two halves, resulting in an anterior shell and a posterior shell. To bivalve a cast, the physician cuts the entire length of the cast on two opposite sides down to the level of the cast padding. The cuts are made with a cast cutter, which is a handheld electric saw with a circular blade that oscillates, which means that the saw vibrates but does not rotate (Figure 7-9, *A*). The medical assistant should reassure the patient that, although the saw is noisy, only a tickling sensation and some heat will be felt from the saw's vibration. After cutting the cast, the physician pries it apart with a cast spreader (Figure 7-9, *B*). Next the physician uses bandage scissors to cut through the cast padding and stockinette (Figure 7-9, *C*). The cast is then carefully removed from the patient's extremity.

The skin of the affected extremity will appear yellow and scaly. The extremity will also appear thinner, and the muscles will be flabby. The medical assistant should explain to the patient that this is normal and results from lack of use of the extremity. The physician may recommend exercises or physical therapy or both to help the patient regain strength and function of the body part.

What Would You DO?
What Would You *Not* DO?

Case Study 2
Christina Themes calls the office. Two days ago Christina fell while she was inline skating and broke the radius and ulna of her right arm. The physician applied a long arm fiberglass cast. While at the medical office Christina had received both oral and written instructions on how to care for her cast. Christina says that in all the confusion she somehow misplaced the instructions. She said she didn't want to bother anyone at the office, so she did what she could to make her arm feel better. She says that it didn't work because now her arm is swollen and hurts. She took a bath, and the cast got wet, so she wants to know how to dry it. Christina asks if it would be possible to have one of those removable casts so she can take it off when she takes a bath.

PATIENT TEACHING

Cast Care

- Teach the patient the important guidelines of cast care.
- Emphasize the importance of contacting the physician immediately if any signs of circulatory impairment or infection occur.
- If the physician has prescribed cold to reduce swelling, teach the patient the procedure for applying an ice bag to the casted extremity.
- Emphasize the importance of returning to have the cast checked by the physician.
- If the physician prescribes isometric exercises to maintain the muscle tone of the affected extremity, provide the patient with a sheet that illustrates the exercises.
- Provide the patient with printed materials on cast care.

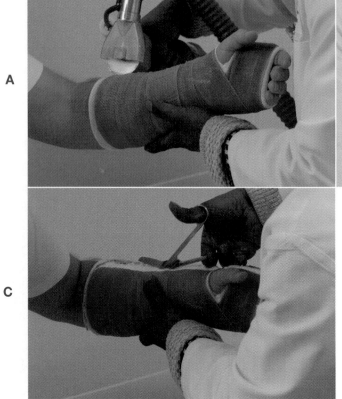

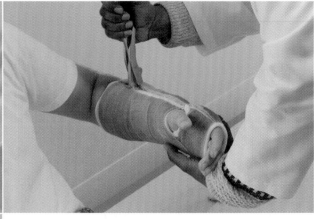

Figure 7-9. Cast removal. **A,** A cast cutter is used to cut the entire length of the cast. **B,** The cast is pried open with a cast spreader. **C,** Bandage scissors are used to cut through the cast padding and stockinette.

Splints and Braces

Along with casts, splints and braces are used to assist in the treatment of fractures. A **splint** is a rigid removable device used to support and immobilize a displaced or fractured part of the body. Splints are also commonly used to protect areas that are sprained or strained. Splints are molded to fit specific parts of the body and are well padded to provide patient comfort and to prevent pressure areas. A splint can be custom made by an orthopedist using plaster or fiberglass casting materials. Splints are also commercially available and consist of two parts: a rigid material such as plastic or fiberglass and straps with Velcro that hold the splint in place (Figure 7-10).

A splint may be applied initially to a fractured limb because it can be adjusted to accommodate swelling from injuries easier than a cast. After the swelling subsides, a cast may be applied. As the fracture heals, another splint may be applied to allow for bathing of the extremity and easy removal for therapy.

A **brace** is designed to support a part of the body and hold it in its correct position to allow for functioning of the body part while healing takes place. An example of a brace is a *short leg walker,* which consists of a rigid lightweight frame with a removable padded liner (Figure 7-11). A short leg walker is often used, instead of a cast, to heal a

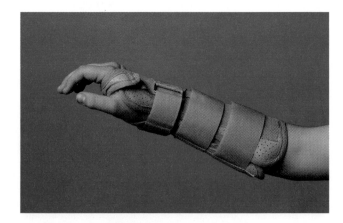

Figure 7-10. Arm splint.

stable fracture of the lower leg. A short leg walker is available in different sizes so that it can be properly fitted to extend from just below the patient's knee to his or her toes. Special fasteners or straps with Velcro are used to hold the walker in place and allow for adjustment of it (see Figure 7-11). A short leg walker permits walking and standing, which encourages healing. It can also be removed to permit bathing of the leg.

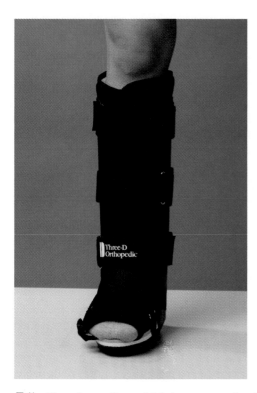

Figure 7-II. Short leg walker, which is an example of a leg brace.

Ambulatory Aids

Mechanical assistive devices are used by individuals who require aid in ambulation. The word **ambulation** means walking; patients who are **ambulatory** are able to walk as opposed to being confined to a wheelchair or a bed. Ambulatory aids include crutches, canes, and walkers. The device used depends on factors such as the type and severity of the disability, the amount of support required, and the patient's age and degree of muscular coordination. The ambulatory aid may be prescribed for a temporary condition, such as a fracture, a sprain to a lower extremity, and disability following orthopedic surgery. It may also be prescribed for a long-term condition such as paralysis, deformity, and permanent weakness of the lower extremities.

Crutches

Crutches are artificial supports that consist of wood or tubular aluminum. They are used for patients who require assistance in walking as a result of disease, injury, or birth defects of the lower extremities. Crutches function by removing weight from the legs and transferring it to the arms. The two main crutch types are the axillary crutch and the forearm crutch (Figure 7-12). Both the axillary and forearm crutch require rubber tips, which increase the surface tension to prevent the crutches from slipping on the floor.

The *axillary crutch* is used most frequently and is made of wood or tubular aluminum. This type of crutch has a shoulder rest and handgrips and extends from the ground almost to the patient's axilla.

Highlight on Ambulatory Aids

Many people who could benefit from ambulatory aids are not using them. The primary reason is that they do not know how to use them correctly, become discouraged, and then quit using them.

Other types of aid available to assist individuals with physical disabilities include raised toilet seats, handle bars carrying devices, tub seats, overbed tables, and swivel cushions for assistance in getting into and out of cars.

If an individual with a physical disability needs help driving, the local bureau of vocational rehabilitation or the state motor vehicle department can provide information on qualified instruction available in the community.

Walking with an ambulatory aid is a physiologic stressor to the body because it requires more energy than normal walking does. Because of this, individuals need to rest frequently when using an ambulatory aid.

Many people need to have their crutches lengthened after they have had them for a while. This is because their posture improves as they gain confidence in walking with them. Children and teenagers who use crutches for a long time also need frequent adjustments as they grow.

A cane can provide security to the individual using it; however, it can be more trouble than it is worth if it is the incorrect size. It is estimated that two thirds of people who buy canes select one that is too long.

Some walkers are designed to fit over chairs and toilets, allowing the user additional support when rising or sitting. Folding walkers are available, and they are easy to store and transport.

The *forearm crutch,* also known as a Lofstrand crutch, consists of a single adjustable tube of aluminum that extends to the forearm. A metal cuff attached to the crutch fits securely around the patient's forearm, and a handgrip covered with rubber extends from the crutch for weight bearing. The metal cuff and the handgrip stabilize the patient's wrists to make walking safer and easier. One advantage of the forearm crutch is that the individual can release the handgrip, enabling use of the hand, while the metal cuff holds the crutch in place. The forearm crutch is most often used by individuals who are paraplegic or have cerebral palsy.

Axillary Crutch Measurement

The patient must be measured for axillary crutches to ensure the correct crutch length and the proper placement of the handgrip. Incorrectly fitted crutches increase the patient's risk of developing back pain, nerve damage, and injuries to the axilla and palms of the hands. Procedure 7-8 presents the correct way to measure a patient for axillary crutches.

If the crutch is too long, the shoulder rest exerts pressure on the patient's axilla. This can injure the radial nerve in the brachial plexus, which eventually may lead to *crutch palsy,* a condition of muscular weakness in the forearm, wrist, and hand. In addition, crutches that are too long force the patient's shoulders forward, preventing the patient from pushing his or her body off the ground. Crutches that are too short force the patient to be bent over and uncomfortable, also making them awkward to use. If the handgrips are too low, pressure is put on the patient's axilla, whereas handgrips that are too high are awkward.

Wooden crutches are made with bolts and wing nuts, which allow proper adjustment of both the length and handgrip level. Aluminum crutches consist of aluminum tubes. Spring-loaded push-buttons on an inner tube "pop out" into holes on an outer tube to allow proper adjustment of the crutch length.

Crutch Guidelines

It is important that the patient receive specific guidelines to ensure safety while using crutches, to prevent injuries and falls. The medical assistant is responsible for instructing the patient in these guidelines:

1. Wear well-fitting flat shoes with firm, nonskid soles to provide good traction and stability.
2. Use correct posture to prevent strain on muscles and joints and to maintain proper body balance.
3. Support your weight with your hands on the handgrips and the axillary pads pressing against the sides of the rib cage. The body weight should not be supported by the axilla because pressure on the axilla may cause crutch palsy.
4. Look ahead when walking rather than down at your feet.
5. Be aware of the surface you are walking on. It should be clean, flat, dry, and well lighted. Throw rugs and objects serving as obstacles should temporarily be removed from your environment to prevent falls.
6. Keep the crutches about 4 to 6 inches out from the side of your feet when walking to prevent obstruction of the pathway for the feet.
7. Take steps by moving the crutches forward a safe and comfortable distance, preferably 6 inches. When first learning to use the crutches, take small steps rather than large ones. Do not move forward more than 12 to 15 inches with each step. A greater distance might cause the crutches to slide forward and you to lose your balance.
8. Report tingling or numbness in the upper body to the physician. You might be using the crutches incorrectly, or they might be the wrong size for you.
9. Extra padding can be added to the shoulder rests of your crutches to make them more comfortable. If you do this, make sure that the extra padding does not press against your axilla, but rather against your lateral rib cage. The handgrips can also be padded for increased comfort.
10. To prevent slipping, keep the crutch tips dry to maintain their surface friction. If they become wet, dry them completely before use.
11. Inspect the crutch tips regularly. They should be securely attached. If the crutch tips are worn down, they should be replaced with tips of the proper size.
12. For wooden crutches, periodically check the wing nuts holding the central strut and handgrips in place to be sure they are tight.

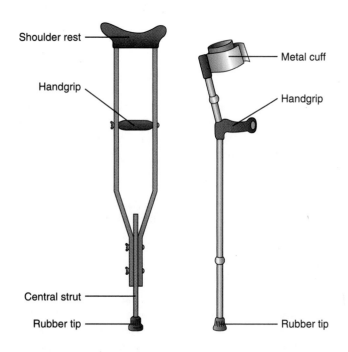

Shoulder rest

Handgrip

Metal cuff

Handgrip

Central strut

Rubber tip

Rubber tip

AXILLARY CRUTCH   **FOREARM CRUTCH**

Figure 7-12. Two kinds of crutches.

> ## ›› PATIENT **TEACHING**
>
> ### Crutches
>
> - Teach patients the guidelines for the proper use of crutches.
> - Provide the patient with an exercise sheet that illustrates exercises to strengthen arm muscles before beginning crutch walking.
> - Teach the patient the crutch gait or gaits prescribed by the physician and have the patient demonstrate the gait(s) before leaving the office.
> - Provide the patient with a list of local vendors who provide crutch services such as repairs and supplies (rubber tips, crutch pads, and so on).
> - Provide the patient with printed educational materials on the use of crutches and crutch gaits.

Crutch Gaits

The type of crutch gait used depends on the amount of weight the patient is able to support with one or both legs and the patient's physical condition and muscular coordination. The patient should learn both a fast and a slow gait. The faster gait is used for making speed in open areas, and the slower one is used in crowded places. In addition, learning more than one gait reduces patient fatigue because a different combination of muscles is used for each gait. Procedure 7-9 provides guidelines and charts for use in instructing the patient on how to walk with crutches.

Canes

A cane is a lightweight, easily movable device made of wood or aluminum with a rubber tip(s) that is used to help provide balance and support. Canes are generally used by patients who have weakness on one side of the body, such as those with hemiparesis, joint disabilities, or defects of the neuromuscular system. The three main types of canes are the *standard cane*, the *tripod cane*, and the *quad cane* (Figure 7-13). The standard cane provides the least amount of support and is used by patients who require only slight assistance in walking. The tripod and quad canes have three and four legs, respectively, a bent shaft, and a T-shaped handle with grips. They are easier to hold and provide greater stability than the standard cane because of the wider base of support. In addition, multilegged canes are able to stand alone, which frees the arms when the patient is getting up from a chair. The disadvantage of the multilegged cane is that it is bulkier and therefore more difficult to move.

A cane is held on the side of the body that is opposite to the side that needs support. The cane length must be properly adjusted to ensure optimum stability. The cane handle should be approximately level with the greater trochanter, and the elbow should be flexed at a 25- to 30-degree angle. The patient should be instructed to stand erect and not lean on the cane to ensure good balance. Procedure 7-10 presents guidelines on instructing the patient on how to walk with a cane.

Walkers

A walker is an ambulatory aid consisting of an aluminum frame with handgrips and four widely placed legs with rubber suction tips and one open side (Figure 7-14). A walker is light and, therefore, easily movable. For proper ambulation, the walker should extend from the ground to approximately the level of the patient's hip joint. Procedure 7-11 presents guidelines on instructing the patient on how to walk with a walker.

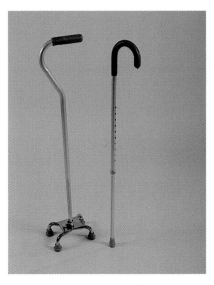

Figure 7-13. Examples of a standard cane *(right)* and a quad cane *(left)*. (Courtesy 3M Health Care, St. Paul, Minn.)

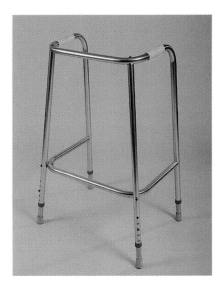

Figure 7-14 A walker.

What Would You DO?
What Would You *Not* DO?

Case Study 3

Thadeus Bernard calls the office. Thadeus fractured the femur of his left leg in a skiing accident 2 weeks ago. The physician applied a long leg fiberglass cast, and Thadeus was properly fitted with aluminum crutches. Thadeus says that he is having some problems with his crutches. He is complaining of weakness in his forearm and hands and some tingling and numbness in his fingers. He also says that he has bruises under his arms. Thadeus says that after he got home, his crutches didn't seem to fit right, so he readjusted them. Thadeus is getting ready to return to college and wants to know the best way to carry his books while using crutches.

Walkers are most often used by geriatric patients with weakness or balance problems. Walkers are also used during the healing process for patients who have had knee or hip joint replacement surgery. These patients need more help with balance and walking than can be provided by crutches or a cane. Because of its wide base, a walker provides the patient with a great amount of stability and security. Disadvantages of a walker include a slow pace and difficulty in maneuvering the walker in a small room.

PROCEDURE 7-8 Measuring for Axillary Crutches

Outcome Measure an individual for axillary crutches.

Determining Crutch Length

In order for you to determine crutch length correctly, the patient must wear shoes while being measured. The measurement can be taken while the patient is standing.

1. **Procedural Step.** Ask the patient to stand erect.
2. **Procedural Step.** Position the crutches with the crutch tips at a distance of 2 inches (5 cm) in front of and 4 to 6 inches (15 cm) to the side of each foot. (The large dots in the figure represent crutch tips.)

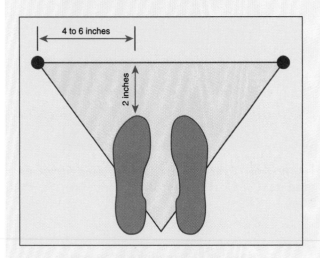

Handgrip Positioning

Once the crutch length has been adjusted, the correct placement of the handgrips must be determined.

1. **Procedural Step.** Ask the patient to stand erect with a crutch under each arm and to support his or her weight by the handgrips.
2. **Procedural Step.** Adjust the handgrips on the crutches so that the patient's elbow is flexed to an angle of approximately 30 degrees. The handgrip level is adjusted by removing the bolt and wing nut and sliding the handgrip upward or downward, as required. The handgrip is then secured by replacing the bolt and tightly fastening the wing nut. The angle of elbow flexion can be verified using a measuring device known as a *goniometer*.
3. **Procedural Step.** Check the fit of the crutches. If the crutches are measured correctly, the medical assistant should be able to insert two fingers between the top of the crutch and the axilla when the patient is standing erect with the crutches under the arms.

3. **Procedural Step.** Adjust the crutch length so that the shoulder rests are approximately 1½ to 2 inches (about 2 finger-widths) below the axilla.
   Wooden Crutches. The length of the crutch is adjusted by removing the bolt and wing nut and sliding the central strut (support piece) at the bottom upward or downward as necessary to attain the proper length. The strut is then secured by replacing the bolt and securely fastening the wing nut.
   Tubular Aluminum Crutches. The length of the crutch is adjusted by pressing the spring-loaded push-button with your thumb and sliding the outer tube upward or downward as necessary to attain the proper length. The spring-loaded button on the inner tube should then be allowed to "pop out" into the appropriate hole on the outer tube.

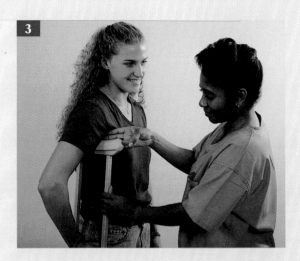

PROCEDURE 7-9 Instructing the Patient in Crutch Gaits

Outcome Instruct an individual in the following crutch gaits: four-point, two-point, three-point, swing-to, and swing-through.

Tripod Position
The tripod position is the basic crutch stance used before crutch walking. It provides a wide base of support and enhances stability and balance.

Instruct the patient in the tripod position as follows:
1. **Procedural Step.** Stand erect, and face straight ahead.
2. **Procedural Step.** Place the tips of the crutches 4 to 6 inches (15 cm) in front of the feet and 4 to 6 inches (10 to 15 cm) to the side of each foot. (The large dots in the figure represent crutch tips.)

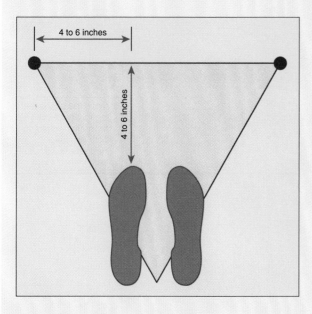

Four-Point Gait
The four-point gait is a very basic and slow gait. In order to use this gait, the patient must be able to bear considerable weight on both legs. The four-point gait is the most stable and safest of the crutch gaits because it provides at least three points of support at all times. It is most often used by patients who have leg muscle weakness or spasticity, poor muscular coordination or balance, or degenerative leg joint disease. Instruct the patient in the procedure for the four-point gait following the steps in the accompanying figure.

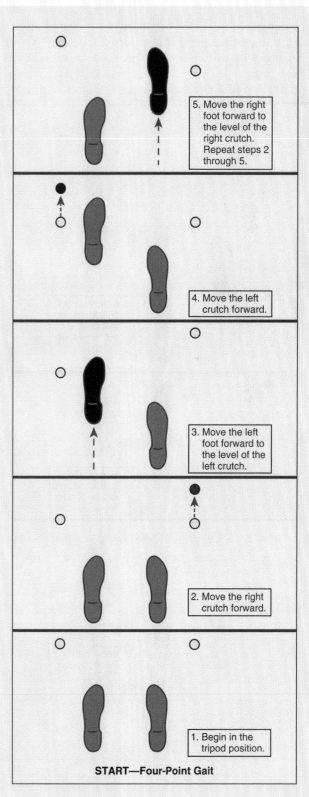

5. Move the right foot forward to the level of the right crutch. Repeat steps 2 through 5.

4. Move the left crutch forward.

3. Move the left foot forward to the level of the left crutch.

2. Move the right crutch forward.

1. Begin in the tripod position.

START—Four-Point Gait

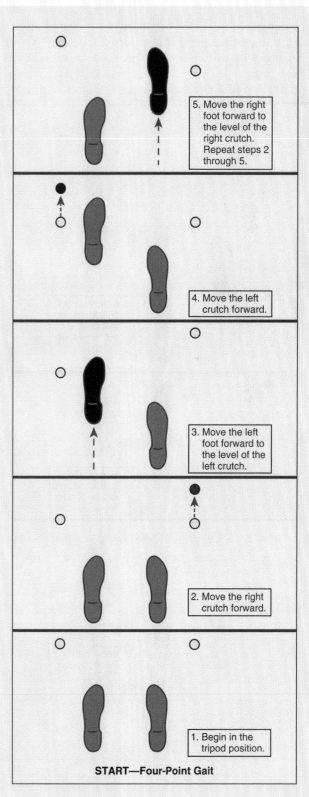
PROCEDURE 7-9

Continued

Two-Point Gait

The two-point gait is similar to, but faster than, the four-point gait. This gait requires more balance because only two points support the body at one time. The two-point gait is used when the patient is capable of partial weight bearing on each foot and has good muscular coordination. Instruct the patient in the procedure for the two-point gait following the steps in the accompanying figure.

Three-Point Gait

The three-point gait is used by patients who cannot bear weight on one leg. The patient must be able to support his or her full weight on the unaffected leg. With this gait, the crutches and the unaffected leg alternatively bear the patient's weight. This gait is used most often by amputees without a prosthesis, patients with musculoskeletal or soft tissue trauma to a lower extremity (e.g., fracture, sprain), patients with acute leg inflammation, and patients who have had recent leg surgery. To use this gait, the patient must have good muscular coordination and arm strength. Instruct the patient in the procedure for the three-point gait, following the steps in the accompanying figure.

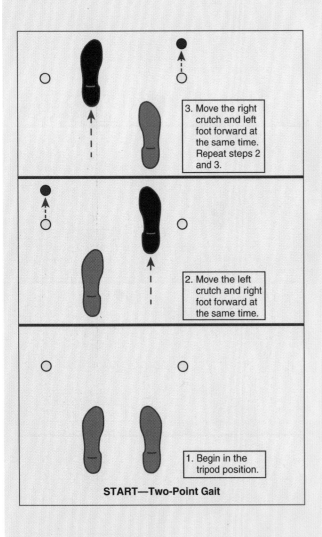

3. Move the right crutch and left foot forward at the same time. Repeat steps 2 and 3.

2. Move the left crutch and right foot forward at the same time.

1. Begin in the tripod position.

START—Two-Point Gait

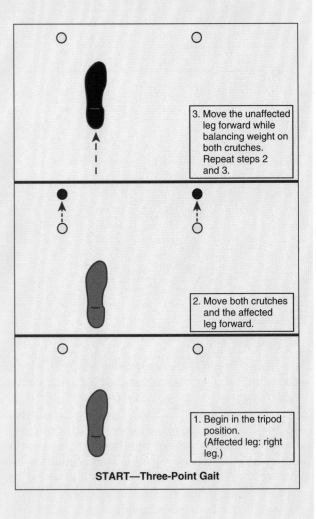

3. Move the unaffected leg forward while balancing weight on both crutches. Repeat steps 2 and 3.

2. Move both crutches and the affected leg forward.

1. Begin in the tripod position. (Affected leg: right leg.)

START—Three-Point Gait

Swing Gaits

The swing gaits include the swing-to gait and the swing-through gait and are used by patients with severe lower extremity disabilities such as paralysis and by patients who wear supporting braces on their legs.

Instruct the patient in the procedure for the swing-to and the swing-through crutch gaits, following the steps in the accompanying figures.

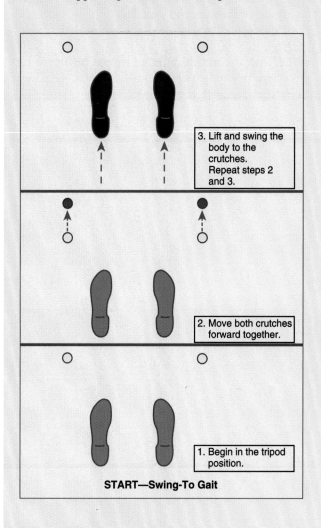

3. Lift and swing the body to the crutches. Repeat steps 2 and 3.

2. Move both crutches forward together.

1. Begin in the tripod position.

START—Swing-To Gait

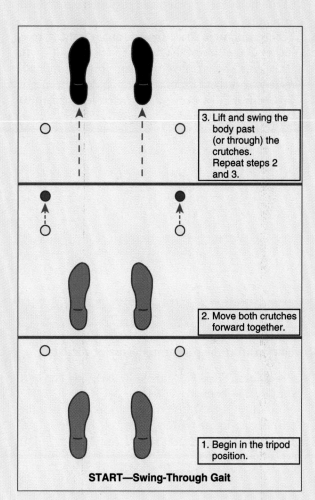

3. Lift and swing the body past (or through) the crutches. Repeat steps 2 and 3.

2. Move both crutches forward together.

1. Begin in the tripod position.

START—Swing-Through Gait

PROCEDURE 7-9

PROCEDURE **7-10** Instructing the Patient in Use of a Cane

Outcome Instruct the patient in the use of a cane.

1. **Procedural Step.** Hold the cane on the strong side of the body (i.e., in the hand opposite the affected extremity).
2. **Procedural Step.** Place the tip of the cane 4 to 6 inches to the side of the foot.
3. **Procedural Step.** Move the cane forward approximately 12 inches (1 foot).
4. **Procedural Step.** Move the affected leg forward to the level of the cane.
5. **Procedural Step.** Move the strong leg forward and ahead of the cane and weak leg.
6. **Procedural Step.** Repeat steps 3 through 5.

NOTE: The cane and the affected leg can be moved forward simultaneously (steps 3 and 4); however, the patient has less support with this method.

PROCEDURE **7-11** Instructing the Patient in Use of a Walker

Outcome Instruct the patient in the use of a walker.

1. **Procedural Step.** Pick up the walker, and move it forward approximately 6 inches.
2. **Procedural Step.** Move the right foot and then the left foot up to the walker.
3. **Procedural Step.** Repeat steps 1 and 2.

PROCEDURE 7-10

MEDICAL Practice and the LAW

The activities described in this chapter deal with the goal of returning full function to an injured area. Sometimes, despite correct treatment, full function does not return. This problem can become a legal issue if the patient believes he or she should have healed fully or cannot return to work. To protect yourself, follow each procedure to the letter, and record the patient's progress (or lack of progress) carefully in the medical record. Sometimes the patient is involved in insurance fraud and falsely complains of pain or impaired function to continue receiving disability benefits. If you suspect this is the case, objectively document the functions you have seen the patient perform.

The application of heat and cold must be performed precisely in order to maximize effectiveness of the treatment without injury to the patient. Failure to follow procedures correctly or to obtain the correct temperature could leave you legally liable.

The ultrasound machine, if used incorrectly, can burn the patient. To protect yourself and benefit the patient, keep the applicator head moving at all times and keep adequate coupling agent on the skin at all times.

Ambulatory aids used correctly can help the patient regain mobility. If crutches are used improperly, the patient could fall or develop nerve or other injuries. When instructing about ambulation aid use, be sure to allow enough time for the patient to give a return demonstration, and send home written instructions to consult in case he or she forgets what was taught.

What Would You DO?
What Would You *Not* DO? *RESPONSES*

Case Study 1
What Did Marlyne Do?
- ❑ Empathized with Aaron for being in so much pain.
- ❑ Explained to Aaron that he should never sleep on a heating pad because the heat builds up and causes the type of burn he experienced.
- ❑ Explained to Aaron that it is best to apply heat for 15 to 30 minutes at a time with the pad set no higher than the medium setting. Told him the pad may not feel warm after his body gets used to it, but that it is still helping him. Told Aaron that the high setting could burn his skin.
- ❑ Told Aaron how to prevent low back pain by using good body mechanics, especially during lifting.

What Did Marlyne Not Do?
- ❑ Did not critcize Aaron for sleeping on the heating pad or turning the pad to the high setting.

What Would You Do?/What Would You *Not* Do? Review Marlyne's response and place a checkmark next to the information you included in your response. List the additional information you included in your response.

_____

_____

_____

_____

Case Study 2
What Did Marlyne Do?
- ❑ Reassured Christina that the medical staff are there to help her and she should never hesitate to call when she needs information or is having a problem
- ❑ Asked Christina what she did to try to make her arm feel better and recorded this information in her chart. Checked with the doctor to determine if he wanted to see Christina.
- ❑ Reeducated Christina in proper cast care instructions over the phone and mailed her another cast care instruction sheet.
- ❑ Explained to Christina how to properly dry her cast by first blotting it and then using a hair dryer. Told her that if she is unable to dry her cast completely, she will need to come in to have it replaced.
- ❑ Explained to Christina that the physician applied the type of cast that would best treat her injury and help her to heal.

What Did Marlyne Not Do?
- ❑ Did not critcize Christina for waiting so long to call the office.
- ❑ Did not tell Christina it would be a good idea for her to have a "removable cast".

What Would You Do?/What Would You *Not* Do? Review Marlyne's response and place a checkmark next to the information you included in your response. List the additional information you included in your response.

_____

_____

_____

_____

Case Study 3
What Did Marlyne Do?
- ❑ Listened carefully and emphathetically to Thadeus's problems and concerns with his crutches.
- ❑ Explained to Thadeus that the crutches were adjusted to fit him properly at the office and that he may have caused some problems by readjusting them.
- ❑ Scheduled an appointment for Thadeus to come in that day so the physician can examine him, and also so that his crutches can be checked for proper length.
- ❑ Went over crutch guidelines and crutch gaits with Thadeus again when he came to the office for his appointment.
- ❑ Told Thadeus that he should use a backpack to carry his books to keep his hands free to move on his crutches. Stressed that he should keep his backpack as light as possible and keep the weight evenly distributed on his back (i.e., use both straps).

What Did Marlyne Not Do?
- ❑ Did not tell Thadeus to readjust the crutches himself.
- ❑ Did not tell Thadeus that he should have paid more attention when he was being instructed in crutch guidelines.

What Would You Do?/What Would You *Not* Do? Review Marlyne's response and place a checkmark next to the information you included in your response. List the additional information you included in your response.

_____

_____

_____

_____

Apply Your KNOWLEDGE

Choose the best answer to each of the following questions.

1. Savannah Uriz recently played in a golf tournament; since then she has been having low back pain. Dr. Walker recommended that she use a heating pad for 30 minutes every 2 hours for the next 3 days. Marlyne Cooper, CMA, is explaining the use of a heating pad to Savannah. Marlyne instructs Savannah to
   A. Place a protective covering over the heating pad before using it
   B. Place a wet towel between her back and the heating pad
   C. Lie down flat with her back on the pad
   D. Turn the setting higher if the pad no longer feels warm enough

2. Brody Adams fell on the playground and has a large "goose egg" on his forehead. Dr. Walker directs Marlyne Cooper, CMA, to apply an ice bag. Marlyne uses small pieces of ice to fill the ice bag. The reason for this is
   A. To prevent Brody's forehead from becoming too cold
   B. So the ice bag will mold better to Brody's forehead
   C. To prevent the goose egg from hatching
   D. To prevent irritation to the affected skin

3. Eunice Faye has osteoarthritis and for the past 3 days has been experiencing intense pain in the joints of the fingers of her right hand. Dr. Walker would be most likely to order which of the following ultrasound treatments for her condition?
   A. Prenatal ultrasound
   B. Direct ultrasound
   C. Underwater ultrasound
   D. Hot wax ultrasound

4. Michael Kasey broke his left wrist while playing football. He had a short arm fiberglass cast applied 3 hours after the accident. Marlyne Cooper, CMA, is instructing Michael on what to do to minimize swelling. Marlyne's explanation would include all of the following EXCEPT
   A. Elevate the cast above heart level for the first 24 to 48 hours
   B. Cover the cast with a plastic bag
   C. Apply an ice bag at the level of the injury
   D. Gently move your fingers as often as possible

5. Marlyne continues to instruct Michael on how to care for his cast. All of the following would be included in Marlyne's discussion EXCEPT
   A. Do not insert anything down into the cast
   B. If the cast gets wet, dry it with a blow dryer on the high setting
   C. Do not trim the cast or break off rough edges
   D. Inspect the skin around the cast periodically

6. Michael calls the office complaining of a problem with his cast. Which of the following would indicate that Michael should be seen immediately?
   A. His friends are unable to sign his cast with a ballpoint pen
   B. He accidentally got his cast wet
   C. There is a foul odor and drainage coming out of his cast
   D. He decided he would rather have a purple cast instead of an orange one

7. Katie Avery severely strained her left ankle. Dr. Walker asks Marlyne Cooper, CMA, to fit her for axillary crutches. If Katie's axillary crutches have been properly fitted,
   A. Her shoulders will be bent over the crutches
   B. Two fingers can be inserted between the top of the crutch and her axilla
   C. Her elbows will be flexed at a 45-degree angle
   D. The axillary pads will fit snugly against her axilla

8. Dr. Walker told Katie not to put weight on her left foot for the next 5 days. The most appropriate crutch gait for Katie to use would be the
   A. Two-point gait
   B. Three-point gait
   C. Four-point gait
   D. Swing-through gait

9. Marlyne instructs Katie in the proper use of her crutches. Which of the following guidelines would be included in Marlyne's explanation?
   A. Support your body weight on your hands
   B. Look straight ahead when walking
   C. Keep the crutch tips dry
   D. Report any tingling or numbness of the upper body
   E. All of the above

10. Marlyne fitted Katie's crutches correctly. However, Katie gets home and adjusts the crutches to a longer length. Katie is putting herself at risk for
    A. Carpal tunnel syndrome
    B. Sciatic nerve damage
    C. Crutch palsy
    D. Chickenpox

CERTIFICATION REVIEW

❑ **The application of heat or cold** is used to treat pathologic conditions such as infection and trauma. Heat and cold are applied for short periods, usually ranging from 15 to 30 minutes. The type of heat or cold application depends on the purpose of the application, the location and condition of the affected area, and the age and general health of the patient.

❑ **The local effects of applying heat** to the body include dilation of the blood vessels in the area. Nutrients and oxygen are provided to the cells at a faster rate, and wastes are carried away faster. Erythema is the redness of the skin caused by congestion of capillaries in the lower layers of the skin. Heat functions in relieving pain, congestion, muscle spasms, and inflammation.

❑ **The local application of cold** constricts the blood vessels. As a result, tissue metabolism decreases, less oxygen is used, and fewer wastes accumulate. The local application of cold is used to prevent edema and may be applied immediately after an individual has suffered direct trauma such as a bruise, sprain, muscle strain, joint injury, or fracture.

❑ **Factors that affect the local application of heat and cold** include the age of the patient, the location of the application, impaired circulation and sensation, and individual tolerance to change in temperature.

❑ **Therapeutic ultrasound** uses high-frequency sound waves as a deep-heating agent for the soft tissues of the body. Ultrasound may be ordered to treat the following conditions: sprains, joint contractures, neuritis, arthritis, edema, synovitis, scar tissue, bursitis, fibrositis, strains, and dislocations. Ultrasound must not be used over the eyeball, over malignant tumors, directly over the spinal cord, over the heart or brain, over reproductive organs including a pregnant uterus, or over areas of impaired sensation or inadequate circulation.

❑ **A cast is a stiff cylindrical casing** that is used to immobilize a body part. Casts are applied most often when an individual sustains a fracture. Other uses of a cast are to support and stabilize weak or dislocated joints, to promote healing after a surgical correction, and to aid in the nonsurgical correction of deformities.

❑ **Casts are classified** according to the body part they cover. The types of cast most frequently applied are short arm cast, long arm cast, short leg cast, and long leg cast. The type of cast applied depends on the nature of the patient's injury or condition.

❑ **Splints and braces** are used to assist in the treatment of fractures. A splint is a rigid removable device used to support and immobilize a displaced or fractured part of the body. A brace is designed to support a part of the body and hold it in its correct position to allow functioning of the body part while healing takes place.

❑ **Mechanical assistive devices** are used by individuals who require help to walk. Ambulatory aids include crutches, canes, and walkers. The device used depends on factors such as the type and severity of the disability, the amount of support required, and the patient's age and degree of muscular coordination.

❑ **Crutches are artificial supports** consisting of wood or tubular aluminum. They are used for patients who require assistance in walking as a result of disease, injury, or birth defects of the lower extremities. Crutches function by removing weight from the legs and transferring it to the arms.

❑ **The type of crutch gait** used depends on the amount of weight the patient is able to support with one or both legs, the patient's physical condition, and muscular coordination. Crutch gaits include the four-point gait, the two-point gait, the three-point gait, and the swing gaits.

❑ **A cane** is a lightweight, easily movable device used to provide balance and support. Canes are generally used by patients who have weakness on one side of the body.

❑ **A walker** is an ambulatory aid that is most often used by geriatric patients with weakness or balance problems.

Terminology Review

Ambulation Walking or moving from one place to another.

Ambulatory Able to walk as opposed to being confined to bed.

Brace An orthopedic device used to support and hold a part of the body in the correct position to allow functioning and healing.

Compress A soft, moist, absorbent cloth that is folded in several layers and applied to a part of the body in the local application of heat or cold.

Edema The retention of fluid in the tissues, resulting in swelling.

Erythema Reddening of the skin caused by dilation of superficial blood vessels in the skin.

Exudate A discharge produced by the body's tissues.

Long arm cast A cast that extends from the axilla to the fingers of the hand, usually with a bend in the elbow.

Long leg cast A cast that extends from the midthigh to the toes.

Maceration The softening and breaking down of the skin as a result of prolonged exposure to moisture.

Orthopedist A physician who specializes in the diagnosis and treatment of disorders of the musculoskeletal system, which includes the bones, joints, ligaments, tendons, muscles, and nerves.

Short arm cast A cast that extends from below the elbow to the fingers.

Short leg cast A cast that begins just below the knee and extends to the toes.

Soak The direct immersion of a body part in water or a medicated solution.

Splint An orthopedic device used to immobilize, restrain, or support a part of the body.

Sprain Trauma to a joint that causes injury to the ligaments.

Strain An overstretching of a muscle caused by trauma.

Suppuration The process of pus formation.

ON THE WEB

For active weblinks to each website visit http://evolve.elsevier.com/Bonewit/.

For Information on Rehabilitation and Disability:

National Rehabilitation Information Center (NARIC)

American Academy of Orthopaedic Surgeons

About.Com: Orthopedics

American Physical Therapy Association

American Chiropractic Association

American Occupational Therapy Association

Cure Paralysis Now (CPN)

National Stroke Association (NSA)

Arthritis Foundation

National Institute of Arthritis and Musculoskeletal and Skin Diseases

Learning Objectives

Procedures

The Gynecologic Examination
1. State the purpose of the gynecologic examination.
2. Identify the components of the gynecologic examination.

The Breast Examination
Explain the purpose of a breast examination.

Instruct a woman in the procedure for a BSE.

The Pelvic Examination
1. Explain the purpose of a pelvic examination.
2. List and describe the four parts of the pelvic examination.
3. State the purpose of a Pap test.
4. List advantages and disadvantages of the liquid-based Pap test.
5. List and describe each category on a cytology request for a Pap test.

Prepare a woman for a gynecologic examination.
Assist the physician with a gynecologic examination.
Complete a cytology requisition.

Vaginal Infections
1. Identify the symptoms of the following:
   - Trichomoniasis
   - Candidiasis
   - Chlamydia
   - Gonorrhea
2. Explain how each of the above is diagnosed and treated.

Assist in the collection of a microbiologic specimen.

Prenatal Visits
1. Explain the purpose of each part of the prenatal record.
2. List and explain the purpose of each procedure included in the initial prenatal examination.
3. List and explain the purpose of each prenatal laboratory test.
4. Explain the purpose of return prenatal visits.
5. Explain the purpose of each of the following:
   - Triple screen test
   - Ultrasound scan
   - Amniocentesis
   - Fetal heart rate monitoring

Record the patient's pregnancy in terms of gravidity and parity.
Calculate the EDD.
Complete a prenatal health history.
Assist with an initial prenatal examination.
Assist with a return prenatal examination.

Six-Weeks Postpartum Visit
1. Explain the purpose of the 6-weeks-postpartum visit.
2. List and explain the purpose of each of the procedures included in the postpartum examination.

Assist with a 6-weeks-postpartum examination.

CHAPTER 8

The Gynecologic Examination and Prenatal Care

Chapter Outline

Introduction to the Gynecologic Examination and Prenatal Care
THE GYNECOLOGIC EXAMINATION
Gynecology
  Terms Related to Gynecology
The Breast Examination
The Pelvic Examination
  Inspection of the External Genitalia, Vagina, and Cervix
  The Pap Test
  Bimanual Pelvic Examination
  Rectal-Vaginal Examination
Vaginal Infections
PRENATAL CARE
Obstetrics
  Obstetric Terminology
Prenatal Visits
  The First Prenatal Visit
  The Prenatal Record
  Initial Prenatal Examination
  Return Prenatal Visits
  Special Tests and Procedures
  Medical Assisting Responsibilities
Six-Weeks-Postpartum Visit

National Competencies

Clinical Competencies
Patient Care
- Obtain and record patient history.
- Prepare and maintain examination and treatment areas.
- Prepare patient for and assist with routine and specialty examinations.

General Competencies
Professional Communications
- Respond to and initiate written communications.
- Recognize and respond to verbal communications.
- Recognize and respond to nonverbal communications.

Patient Instruction
- Instruct individuals according to their needs.
- Provide instruction for health maintenance and disease prevention.

Gynecology

adnexal (ad-NEKS-al)
amenorrhea (AY-men-ah-REE-ah)
atypical (ay-TIP-ih-kul)
cervix (SER-viks)
colposcopy (kol-POS-koe-pee)
cytology (sy-TOL-oh-jee)
dysmenorrhea (DIS-men-ah-REE-ah)
dyspareunia (DIS-pah-ROO-nee-ah)
dysplasia (dis-PLAY-shah)
endocervix (EN-doe-SER-viks)
external os (eks-TER-nal AHS)
gynecology (gie-nuh-KOL-oh-jee)
internal os (in-TER-nal AHS)
menopause (MEN-oh-paws)
menorrhagia (men-uh-RAY-jee-ah)
metrorrhagia (met-ro-RAY-jee-ah)
perimenopause (PEAR-ee-MEN-oh-paws)
perineum (pear-ih-NEE-um)
risk factor
vulva (VUL-va)

Obstetrics

abortion (ah-BOR-shun)
Braxton-Hicks contractions (BRAK-stun HIKS con-TRAK-shuns)
dilation (of the cervix) (die-LAY-shun)
expected date of delivery (EDD)
effacement (eh-FAYS-ment)
embryo (EM-bree-oh)
engagement
fetal heart rate (FHR)
fetal heart tones (FHT)
fetus (FEE-tus)
fundus (FUN-dus)
gestation (jess-TAY-shun)
gestational age (jess-TAY-shun-al)
gravidity (gra-VID-ih-tee)
infant
lochia (LOE-kee-uh)
multigravida (MUL-tee-GRAV-ih-duh)
multipara (mul-TIH-pear-uh)
nullipara (nul-IH-pear-uh)
obstetrics (ob-STEH-triks)
parity (PEAR-ih-tee)
position
postpartum (poest-PAR-tum)
preeclampsia (PREE-ih-KLAMP-see-ah)
prenatal (pree-NAY-tul)
presentation
preterm birth
primigravida (PRIH-mih-GRAV-ih-duh)
primipara (prih-MIH-pear-uh)
puerperium (PYOO-ur-PEER-ee-um)
quickening

term birth
toxemia (tok-SEE-mee-uh)
trimester (try-MES-ter)

Introduction to the Gynecologic Examination and Prenatal Care

The medical assistant should have a knowledge of gynecology and obstetrics to assist in examinations and treatments in these specialties. Gynecologic examinations are frequently and routinely performed in the medical office. Prenatal care consists of a series of scheduled medical office visits for the promotion of the health of both mother and fetus during the pregnancy. Obtaining the patient's cooperation makes the gynecologic or prenatal examination proceed more smoothly and, as a result, makes the patient more comfortable. The medical assistant can help by explaining the purpose of the procedure to the patient. If the individual understands the beneficial results to be derived from the examination, she is more likely to participate as required. This chapter presents a discussion of both the gynecologic examination and prenatal care, as well as the procedures involved with both.

THE GYNECOLOGIC EXAMINATION

Gynecology

Gynecology is the branch of medicine that deals with diseases of the reproductive organs of women. The gynecologic examinations is frequently and routinely performed in the medical office and generally includes a *breast examination* and a *pelvic examination*.

The purpose of the gynecologic examination is to assess the health of the female reproductive organs in order to detect early signs of disease, leading to early diagnosis and treatment. This examination may be part of a general physical examination or it may be performed by itself. Although assisting with the gynecologic examination is a routine procedure for the medical assistant, the patient may not consider it a routine examination. To reduce apprehension or embarrassment, the medical assistant should fully explain the procedure to the patient and offer to answer any questions.

Terms Related to Gynecology

The medical assistant should have a thorough knowledge of the female reproductive system (Figure 8-1), as well as the following terms associated with the female reproductive system:

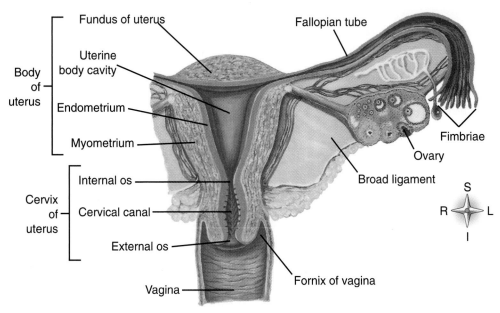

Figure 8-1. Female reproductive system. (Modified from Thibodeau GA, Patton KT: *Anatomy and physiology,* ed 4, St. Louis, 1999, Mosby.)

Amenorrhea	The absence or cessation of the menstrual period. Amenorrhea occurs normally before puberty, during pregnancy, and after menopause.
Cervix	The lower narrow end of the uterus that opens into the vagina.
Colposcopy	Examination of the cervix using a colposcope (a lighted instrument with a magnifying lens).
Dysmenorrhea	Pain associated with the menstrual period.
Dyspareunia	Pain in the vagina or pelvis experienced by a woman during sexual intercourse
Dysplasia	The growth of abnormal cells. Dysplasia is a precancerous condition that may or may not develop into cancer.
Menopause	The permanent cessation of menstruation, which usually occurs between the ages of 35 and 58.
Menorrhagia	Excessive bleeding during a menstrual period, in the number of days or the amount of blood or both. Also called dysfunctional uterine bleeding (DUB).
Metrorrhagia	Bleeding between menstrual periods.
Perimenopause	Before the onset of menopause, the phase during which the woman with regular periods changes to irregular cycles and increased periods of amenorrhea.
Perineum	The external region between the vaginal orifice and the anus in a female and between the scrotum and the anus in a male.

PUTTING It All Into PRACTICE

MY NAME IS Yin-Ling Wu, and I am a Registered Medical Assistant. I work with ten physicians in a large clinic. My primary job responsibilities include documenting patient histories and complaints, taking vital signs, and assisting physicians with patient examinations and procedures.

One experience that has probably affected me more than any other was while I was working in obstetrics and gynecology. A full-term prenatal patient came in for a routine weekly appointment late one afternoon. By this stage of the pregnancy, you have seen them often enough to develop a more personal relationship. I was obtaining her vital signs and asking the routine questions when she said: "I haven't felt the baby move for two days." This immediately sent up a red flag, but I was careful to hide my concern until I was out of her room. The physician was unable to pick up any fetal heart tones, so she immediately did an ultrasound. It showed that the fetus had died. The patient was alone and extremely upset. I stayed with her until her family came.

Although there was little medical treatment given during this time, I do believe that my medical assisting training and experience made a difference in knowing what to do and say to help comfort the patient through this crisis.

Risk factor	Anything that increases an individual's chance of developing a disease. Some risk factors (e.g., smoking) can be avoided, but others cannot (e.g., age and family history).

Highlight on Breast Cancer

Breast cancer is one of the most common types of cancer among American women. The American Cancer Society estimates that one of every nine women in the United States will develop breast cancer at some point in her lifetime. Every year more than 200,000 women learn they have breast cancer and about 40,000 of them die from the disease. Most women (82%) diagnosed with breast cancer are over 50 years old, but breast cancer does occur in younger women.

The 5-year survival rate for breast cancer that has spread to a distant site in the body (metastasized) is only 21%. However, the 5-year survival rate for small, localized tumors is 94%. If the cancer has spread to lymph nodes in the region of the breast, the 5-year survival rate is 73%. These encouraging statistics are the result of advances in early detection of breast cancer, as well as better treatment including improved surgical procedures, radiation therapy, chemotherapy, hormonal therapy, and biological therapy.

The American Cancer Society and the National Cancer Institute recommend a three-point program for the early detection of breast cancer: a monthly breast self-examination, a periodic clinical breast examination by a physician, and screening mammography.

Breast cancer results from the abnormal growth of cells in breast tissue. It occurs more often in the left breast than in the right, and more often in the upper outer quadrant of the breast. The cause of this abnormal growth is unknown; therefore every woman should consider herself at risk for breast cancer.

Certain factors, however, appear to place a woman at higher than normal risk for breast cancer. These risk factors include the following:

Age. The risk of breast cancer increases as women get older. Most women diagnosed with breast cancer are over the age of 50.

Personal history. Women with cancer in one breast have a greater chance of developing a new cancer in the other breast or in another part of the same breast.

Family history. A woman's risk of developing breast cancer increases if her mother, sister, or daughter had breast cancer, especially at a young age.

Breast biopsy. Women who have had a breast biopsy that indicated certain types of benign breast disease (characterized by atypical hyperplasia) have an increased risk of developing breast cancer.

Breast cancer genes. A woman who has inherited mutations in breast cancer genes (mutations of the BRCA1 and BRCA2 genes) from either parent is more likely to develop breast cancer.

Reproductive history. Women who began menstruating at an early age (before age 12) or who went through menopause at a late age (after age 55) have a slightly increased risk of breast cancer.

Childbearing. Women who have never had a child or women who had their first child late (after age 30) have a slightly increased risk of developing breast cancer.

Hormone replacement therapy (HRT). Studies indicate that long-term use of hormone replacement therapy for relief of menopausal symptoms increases the risk of breast cancer.

Radiation treatment. Women who have had radiation of the chest before the age of 30 as a treatment for another type of cancer (e.g., Hodgkin's disease) have a significantly increased risk of developing breast cancer.

Lifestyle factors. Studies suggest that the use of alcohol (more than 2 drinks per day) increases the risk of breast cancer. Obesity, especially for women after menopause, may also increase the risk of breast cancer.

The warning signs of possible breast cancer include a lump, hard knot, or thickening in the breast or armpit, a change in breast color or texture, dimpling or puckering, nipple discharge, changes in the size or shape of the breast, and an enlargement of the lymph nodes.

A biopsy is the only conclusive method of determining whether a breast lump or suspicious area seen on a mammogram is benign or malignant. A biopsy involves the surgical removal and analysis of all or part of the lump. There are several biopsy methods, including needle biopsy, incisional biopsy (removal of a portion of the lump), excisional biopsy (removal of the entire lump), and mammographic localization with biopsy. The physician may recommend one or more of these procedures to evaluate a lump or other change in the breast.

Fortunately, 80% of breast lumps are benign; hence a lump or suspicious area is often the result of a benign breast condition such as normal hormonal changes, fibrocystic breast disease, or a fibroadenoma.

The Breast Examination

The physician usually begins the gynecologic examination with the breast examination. The medical assistant is responsible for the assisting the patient into the supine position. The physician inspects the breasts and nipples for swelling, dimpling, puckering, and change in skin texture.

The nipples are checked for abnormalities such as bleeding and discharge. The breasts and axillary lymph nodes are palpated for lumps, hard knots, and thickening.

The patient should know how to examine her breasts at home for the presence of lumps and other changes by learning to perform a breast self-examination (BSE). Most

⚡ PATIENT TEACHING

Breast Self-Examination

Answer questions patients have about breast self-examination.

When should I examine my breasts?

Beginning at age 20, you should examine your breasts once each month according to your reproductive status as follows:

Regular periods: Approximately 2 to 3 days after your menstrual period has ended. At this time, your breasts are least likely to be tender or swollen, and it will be easier to perform the exam.

No periods (because of menopause or hysterectomy): Any day of the month is fine; however it helps to choose a particular day such as the first day of the month or an easy-to-remember date such as your birthday.

Hormone therapy: If you are taking hormones, talk to the physician about when to examine your breasts.

Why is it important to examine my breasts every month?

The purpose of a breast self-examination is not just to find lumps, but also to notice when there are changes in your breasts. The best way to do this is to become as familiar as possible with your breasts. By examining your breasts once every month, you will learn what is normal for you, and it will be easier to notice changes.

What is considered normal?

Breast tissue normally feels a little lumpy and uneven. The left and right breast may not be the same size; in fact, most women's breasts are slightly different in size. Many women have a normal thickening or ridge of firm tissue under the lower curve of the breast where it attaches to the chest wall. Throughout your life, changes can also occur in the size, shape, and feel of your breasts because of aging, weight changes, the menstrual cycle, pregnancy, breastfeeding, and taking birth control pills or other hormones.

What should be reported to the physician?

Early breast cancer does not usually cause pain. In fact, when breast cancer first develops, there may be no symptoms at all. As the cancer grows, it can cause changes that should be reported to the physician. Contact your physician immediately if any of the following changes takes place:

- Any new lump, hard knot, or thickening in the breast or underarm area
- A change in the size or shape of the breast
- A puckering or dimpling of the skin of the breast or nipple
- A change in skin texture of the breast or nipple
- A nipple that becomes retracted (pulled in)
- A discharge or bleeding from the nipple

---

breast cancers are first discovered by women themselves. The American Cancer Society recommends that women 20 years and older examine their breasts once every month. The medical assistant may be responsible for instructing the patient in this procedure at the medical office. (See Procedure 8-1.) If a lump or other change is discovered, the woman should schedule an appointment with her physician as soon as possible. Most breast lumps are not cancerous, but the physician is the one to make that diagnosis.

The Pelvic Examination

The purpose of the pelvic examination is to assess the size, shape, and location of the reproductive organs and to detect the presence of disease. The pelvic examination consists of the following components:

1. Inspection of the external genitalia, vagina, and cervix
2. Collection of a specimen for a Pap test
3. Bimanual pelvic examination
4. Rectal-vaginal examination

For the pelvic examination the patient is positioned in the lithotomy position. The patient lies on the table on her back, with her feet in the stirrups and her buttocks at the bottom edge of the table. The stirrups should be level with the examining table and pulled out approximately 1 foot from the edge of the table. The patient's knees should be bent and relaxed, and her thighs should be rotated outward as far as is comfortable. This position helps relax the vulva and perineum and facilitates insertion of the vaginal speculum. The patient should be properly draped to reduce exposure and to provide warmth. The lithotomy position is difficult to maintain, and the patient should not be placed in this position until the physician is ready to begin the examination.

The medical assistant can help the patient relax during the examination by telling her to breathe deeply, slowly, and evenly through the mouth. If the patient is relaxed, it is easier for the physician to insert the vaginal speculum and to perform the bimanual pelvic examination; it is also more comfortable for the patient. It is recommended that the medical assistant remain in the room during the pelvic examination to provide legal protection for the physician, to reassure the patient, and to assist the physician. Procedure 8-2 outlines the medical assistant's role in assisting the physician with a gynecologic examination.

Inspection of the External Genitalia, Vagina, and Cervix

The physician begins the pelvic examination with inspection of the external genitalia. The vulva is inspected for swelling, ulceration, and redness.

Next the physician inserts a vaginal speculum into the vagina. Specula are available in two forms—metal and plastic. Metal specula are reusable and therefore must be sanitized and sterilized after each use. Plastic specula are disposable and are designed to be used only once. Vaginal specula come in three sizes: small, medium, and large. The physician determines the size required based on the physical and sexual maturity of the patient. The function of the speculum is to hold the walls of the vagina apart to allow visual inspection of the vagina and cervix (Figure 8-2).

A metal vaginal speculum is cold and should be warmed before use by placing it on a heating pad or by storing it in a warming drawer. A disposable plastic speculum does not hold the cold, and, therefore, does not need to be warmed.

If a specimen needs to be obtained for a Pap smear or a microbiologic test, the speculum should not be lubricated because this would interfere with the test results. In these situations, the speculum can be moistened with warm water, which helps to lubricate it and facilitates insertion.

The physician inspects the vagina and cervix for color, lacerations, ulcerations, tenderness, nodules, and discharge. If an abnormal discharge is present, the physician obtains a specimen for microbiologic examination. Examples of pathologic conditions that produce a discharge include vaginal infections such as *trichomoniasis, candidiasis, chlamydia,* and *gonorrhea,* which are discussed in detail later in this chapter.

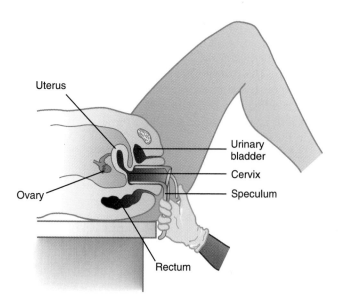

Figure 8-2. Insertion of the vaginal speculum for visualization of the vagina and cervix.

The Pap Test

A Pap test is usually part of the pelvic examination. It is a simple and painless **cytology** evaluation named after its developer, Dr. George Papanicolaou (1883–1962). It is used for the early detection of cervical cancer. Almost all cancers of the cervix can be cured if detected early enough. The Pap test is also used to detect abnormal **(atypical)** cells of the cervix that might develop into cancer if not treated. In some cases, the Pap test can detect cancer of the endometrium; however, it is less reliable in doing so.

Currently the American Cancer Society recommends an annual Pap test and pelvic examination for all women starting at the onset of sexual activity or at age 18 years, whichever is earlier. The guidelines further state that after a woman has tested negative for three or more consecutive examinations, the Pap test may be performed less frequently at the discretion of the physician. Women who are at high risk for cervical cancer or who have had abnormal Pap test results should have a Pap test more often.

Patient Instructions

A Pap specimen must not be collected from a woman during her menstrual period because the red blood cells obscure the specimen and interfere with an accurate evaluation. Therefore the patient should be instructed to schedule her Pap test between 10 and 20 days after the first day of her last menstrual period. The patient should be told not to douche or insert vaginal medications or contraceptive spermicides for 2 days before having a Pap test. Douching reduces the number of cells available for analysis, and vaginal medications and spermicides change the pH of the vagina, making the specimen nonrepresentative or invalid. The patient should also be told to abstain from sexual intercourse for 2 days before the Pap test. Recent sexual intercourse can produce inflammatory changes that can obscure visualization of abnormal cells.

What Would You DO?
What Would You *Not* DO?

Case Study 1

Carol Wooster, 42 years old, has come to the office for a GYN exam. She has not had a GYN examination in 10 years. Mrs. Wooster picked up a BSE brochure at a local health fair and performed a breast examination at home. She is now concerned because she found some unusual things. Her right breast is slightly larger than her left breast, her left nipple is pulled in, and she found some freckles on her right breast. Mrs. Wooster explains that she hasn't had a GYN examination in such a long time because her periods have been normal and regular. She also knows that the doctor will probably want her to have a mammogram, and she has heard that it hurts to have one. Mrs. Wooster is somewhat afraid that the doctor will be annoyed with her for not having had a GYN examination sooner.

Specimen Collection

The outermost layer of the cervix consists of a thin, flat layer of cells, approximately ten layers thick, known as squamous epithelial cells. With the speculum in place, the physician collects a sampling of these cells for evaluation by the laboratory. A scraping of epithelial cells is taken from both the cervix and the endocervical canal. A scraping of cells can also be collected from the vagina; however, this is not usually done unless the physician has observed a lesion on the vaginal wall or the maturation index is to be determined. The technique used by the physician to collect the epithelial cells is described as follows:

Vaginal Specimen.

If a vaginal specimen is needed, it is collected first; in other words before the cervical and endocervical specimens. The rounded end of the plastic spatula is used to collect the specimen. If a routine vaginal specimen is being obtained, it is collected from the vaginal pool in the posterior fornix of the vagina, which is located just below the cervix (Figure 8-3, *A*). If the physician is collecting a specimen from a lesion on the vaginal wall, a scraping of cells is taken from the area of the lesion. To obtain a specimen for a determination of the maturation index (discussed later in this chapter), the physician obtains the vaginal specimen from the upper third of the lateral vaginal wall.

Cervical Specimen.

The physician obtains the cervical specimen by placing the S-shaped end of the plastic spatula just inside the cervical canal at the **external os** and then rotating the blade 360 degrees over the surface of the cervix at the squamocolumnar junction, where cervical cancer is most often found (Figure 8-3, *B*).

Endocervical Specimen.

The physician collects this specimen from the endocervical canal. This is accomplished by inserting an endocervical brush into the endocervical canal and then rotating the brush (Figure 8-3, *C*).

Vaginal Specimen

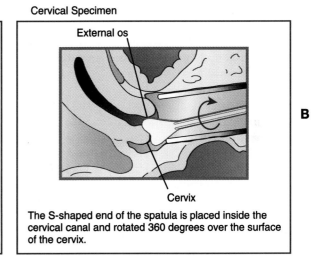

A

The rounded end of the spatula is used to obtain the vaginal specimen from the posterior fornix of the vagina.

The S-shaped end of the spatula is placed inside the cervical canal and rotated 360 degrees over the surface of the cervix.

B

Endocervical Specimen

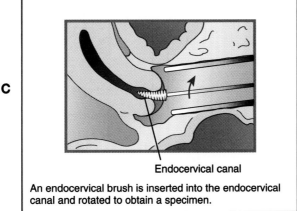

C

An endocervical brush is inserted into the endocervical canal and rotated to obtain a specimen.

Figure 8-3. Obtaining the Pap specimen.

Preparation Methods

There are two methods used to prepare a specimen for a Pap test. The traditional method is the *direct smear* (Pap smear) and the newer method is the *liquid-based preparation*. These methods described next.

Direct Smear

With the direct smear method, the specimen is spread on a glass slide that has a frosted edge. The medical assistant must label each slide on its frosted edge with a lead pencil according to the source of the specimen as follows: V (vaginal), C (cervical), or E (endocervical). Slides are also available on which all three specimens can be placed. Those slides are divided into thirds and prelabeled with V, C, and E.

The smears must be fixed immediately by flooding the slides with 95% ethyl alcohol or by lightly spraying the slides with a commercial cytology spray fixative. The slides must be fixed before they dry to avoid inaccurate results. The purpose of the fixative is to maintain the normal appearance of the cells, to protect the slides from contaminants in the air such as dust and bacteria, and to firmly attach the smear to the slide. The cytology fixative must be allowed to dry thoroughly; the slides are then ready for transport to a laboratory for evaluation. To protect the slides during transport, they must be placed in a slide container designed especially for this purpose.

Liquid-Based Preparation

A newer method to prepare the specimen for evaluation is the liquid-based preparation. Brand names include ThinPrep Pap Test and AutoCyte Pap Test. Although more expensive than the direct smear method, the liquid-based method is growing in popularity. Using this method improves the quality of the specimen, resulting in fewer slides that are unsatisfactory for evaluation. A better

quality specimen also reduces the occurrence of false-negative test results.

The specimen for a liquid-based preparation is usually obtained using the specimen collection technique described earlier. In other words, a plastic spatula is used to collect the cervical specimen and an endocervical brush is used to collect the endocervical specimen. If a vaginal specimen is needed, it is collected using the method previously described.

The Pap specimen can also be collected using a *broom*, a newer collection device made of flexible plastic. The physician inserts the central bristles of the broom into the endocervical canal deep enough to allow the shorter bristles to fully contact the outside of the cervix. The broom is then gently pushed and rotated clockwise five times (Figure 8-4). In this way, a specimen from both the cervix and the endocervical canal can be collected at the same time.

Once the Pap specimen has been collected, the medical assistant is responsible for rinsing the collection device in a vial of liquid preservative. The preservative maintains the specimen and prevents it from drying out during transport to the laboratory. After being received by the laboratory, the vial is placed in an automated slide preparation processor. The automated processor performs several important functions. First it separates the cells from debris present in the specimen, and then it disperses a representative cell sample onto a slide in a thin uniform layer. The slide is next immersed in a fixative to maintain the normal appearance of the cells.

The ways in which the liquid-based method provides a better quality specimen than the direct smear method are as follows:

- With the direct smear method, only a small portion of the specimen is smeared on the slide; most of it is thrown away with the collection device. With the

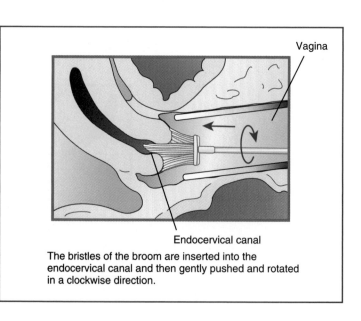

Figure 8-4. Collecting a Pap specimen using a broom.

Vagina

Endocervical canal

The bristles of the broom are inserted into the endocervical canal and then gently pushed and rotated in a clockwise direction.

liquid-based method, the collection device is rinsed in a vial of liquid that preserves almost all of the specimen. Having more of the specimen available allows the laboratory to evaluate it better.

- When a Pap specimen is collected, it includes unnecessary debris such as blood, mucus, and inflammatory cells. With the direct smear method, the debris is smeared on the slide along with the cells. This debris may obscure the cells in the specimen, making it difficult to evaluate them. With the liquid-based method, the automated processor removes debris from the specimen and transfers the cells to a glass slide. This provides the cytotechnologist with a clear, unobstructed view of the epithelial cells.

- With the direct smear method, the cells have a tendency to clump together when they are smeared on the slide, making them more difficult to evaluate. With the liquid-based method, the automated processor disperses the cells onto the slide in a thin even layer. In this way, the cells are spread out, making it easier for the cytotechnologist to evaluate them.

Cytology Request

A cytology request must accompany all Pap specimens. See Figure 8-5 for an example of a cytology request form. The medical assistant is responsible for completing the request, which includes the following categories:

General Information. This information includes the physician's name, address and phone number and the patient's name, address, identification number, date of birth, and LMP (date of last menstrual period). Insurance information is also required in this section for third-party billing.

Date and Time of Collection. The date and time of collection indicates to the laboratory the number of days that have passed since the collection, thus providing the laboratory with information regarding the freshness of the specimen.

Collection Method. Under this category the medical assistant must indicate whether the specimen is a direct smear (Pap smear) or a liquid-based preparation.

Source of the Specimen. The purpose of this category is to identify the origin of the specimen because it is not possible for the laboratory to obtain this information by looking at the specimen. The medical assistant checks one or more of the following boxes on the form: cervical, endocervical, or vaginal.

Collection Technique. The collection device(s) used to obtain the specimen must be indicated in this category. The medical assistant checks one or more of the following boxes on the form: spatula, brush, or broom.

Patient History. Information on the present and past health status of the patient is specified in this category. The medical assistant must check the following boxes that apply to the patient: pregnant, lactating, oral contraceptives, postmenopausal, hormone replacement therapy, postmenopausal bleeding, postpartum, IUD, postcoital bleeding, DES (diethylstilbestrol) exposure, and previous abnormal smear. This information assists the laboratory in evaluating the specimen.

Previous Treatment. Any previous treatment for a precancerous or cancerous condition of the cervix is indicated in this category. The medical assistant checks the appropriate box on the form if any of the following procedures have been performed on the patient: colposcopy and biopsy, cryosurgery, LEEP (loop electrocautery excision procedure), laser vaporization, conization, hysterectomy, radiation, and chemotherapy.

Evaluation of the Pap Specimen

Before a Pap slide can be evaluated, it must be stained. Staining is performed on slides prepared by both the direct smear method and the liquid-based method. The purpose of staining is to allow better viewing of the morphology of the epithelial cells. The slide is then studied under a microscope for evidence of abnormalities by a specially trained technician, known as a *cytotechnologist.* When an abnormality is detected, it is reviewed by a *cytopathologist* (a physician specializing in pathology) who makes a final evaluation. The findings are recorded on a cytology report and returned to the medical office.

A recent development in the evaluation of Pap slides is the use of automated computer-imaging devices. An abnormal slide may contain only a few abnormal cells among thousands of normal cells. Because of this, these abnormal cells may be missed during the evaluation by the cytotechnologist. A computer-imaging device is able to examine every cell on the slide and select and display cells that appear "most abnormal." The cytotechnologist can then further evaluate these cells under a microscope. In this way, the cytotechnologist is able to focus his or her expertise and decision making on preselected areas of the slide.

Maturation Index

The maturation index (MI) must be performed on a sampling of cells taken from the upper third of the lateral vaginal wall. The maturation index refers to the percentage of parabasal, intermediate, and superficial cells present in the specimen. The MI provides the physician with an endocrine evaluation of the patient, which can assist in evaluating the cause of infertility, menopausal or postmenopausal bleeding, or amenorrhea and can help assess the results of treatment with hormones. If the physician orders a maturation index along with the Pap test, the medical assistant must be sure to indicate this on the

GYN CYTOLOGY REQUISITION

THOMAS WOODSIDE, MD
501 MAIN ST
ST. LOUIS, MO 63146
(314) 555–0093

PATIENT INFO

| Patient's Name (Last) | (First) | (MI) | Date of Birth MO | DAY | YR | Collection Time : AM PM | Collection Date MO | DAY | YR | Patient's ID # |

Patient's Address   Phone

City   State   ZIP

RESP. PARTY

Name of Responsible Party (if different from patient)

Address of Responsible Party   APT #

City   State   ZIP

INSURANCE

Patient's Relationship to Responsible Party ☐ 1. Self ☐ 2. Spouse ☐ 3. Child ☐ 4. Other

| Insurance Comany Name | Plan | Carrier Code |

| Subscriber/Member # | Location | Group # |

| Insurance Address | | Physician's Provider # |

| City | State | ZIP |

| Employer's Name or Number | Insured SSN |

Diagnosis/Signs/Symptoms in ICD-9 Format (Highest Specificity)

REQUIRED

ICD-9 codes are the internationally accepted method of describing the clinical picture of the patient. All diagnoses should be provided by the ordering physician or his or her authorized designee. The following is a partial list of of common diagnoses in ICD-9 format. Most third party payers require an ICD-9 code to indicate the medical necessity of the test(s) and or profile(s) ordered. For a complete list of all ICD-9 codes, please refer to a current ICD-9 manual.

V76.2	Routine Cervical Pap Smear	616.0	Cervicitis	626.8	Abnormal Bleeding
V15.89	High Risk Cervical Screening	616.10	Vaginitis	627.1	Postmenopausal Bleeding
V22.2	Pregnancy	617.0	Endometriosis, Uterus	627.3	Atrophic Vaginitis
079.4	Human Papillomavirus	622.1	Dysplasia, Cervix	795.0	Abnormal Cervical Pap Smear
180.0	Malignant Neoplasm, Cervix	623.0	Dysplasia, Vagina		

COLLECTION METHOD

Liquid Based Prep

192055 ☐ Thin Prep Pap Test

192039 ☐ Thin Prep Pap Test w/reflex to HPV Hybrid Capture when ASC-US or SIL

192047 ☐ Thin Prep Pap Test w/reflex to high-risk only HPV Hybrid Capture when ASC-US

Pap Smear
009100 ☐ 1 Slide   009191 ☐ 2 Slides

Pap Smear and Maturation Index
009209 ☐ 1 Slide   190074 ☐ 2 Slides

SOURCE OF SPECIMEN

☐ Cervical
☐ Endocervical
☐ Vaginal

Date LMP

___/___/___
Mo   Day   Year

COLLECTION TECHNIQUE

☐ Spatula
☐ Brush
☐ Broom
☐ Other

_____

PATIENT HISTORY

☐ Pregnant
☐ Lactating
☐ Oral Contraceptives
☐ Postmenopausal
☐ Hormone Replacement Therapy

☐ PMP Bleeding
☐ Postpartum
☐ IUD
☐ Postcoital Bleeding
☐ DES Exposure
☐ Previous Abnormal Pap Test

☐ Other _____

PREVIOUS TREATMENT

☐ None
☐ Colposcopy and Bx
☐ Cryosurgery
☐ LEEP
☐ Laser Vaporization
☐ Conization
☐ Hysterectomy
☐ Radiation
☐ Chemotherapy

Date/Results

_____
_____
_____
_____
_____
_____
_____

Figure 8-5. Cytology request form.

cytology request by checking the box labeled Maturation Index (see Figure 8-5). Numerous factors affect the results of the maturation index; therefore it is important to indicate on the cytology request the presence of abnormal bleeding, hormone treatment, or treatment with digitalis, corticosteroids, or thyroid medication.

Cytology Report

The Bethesda System (TBS) is the standard for reporting the results of a Pap test on the cytology report (Figure 8-6). This system was developed by the National Cancer Institute in Bethesda, Maryland. It provides a detailed cytologic description rather than a numerical result (as

GYN CYTOLOGY REPORT

RIVERVIEW MEDICAL LABORATORY
DEPARTMENT OF PATHOLOGY
2501 GRANT AVENUE
ST. LOUIS, MO 63146
(314) 555-3443

PATIENT: Heather Jones
PATIENT NO: 45876
DOB: 10/20/65
SUBMITTING: T. Woodside, MD

Date of Specimen: 7/01/05	**SPECIMEN TYPE**	
Date Received: 7/02/05	☒ Thin Prep	☐ Conventional Pap Smear
Date Reported: 7/06/05		

Performed By: Richard McVay, Cytotechnologist   **Checked By:** Melissa Wagner, Pathologist

SPECIMEN ADEQUACY	GENERAL CATEGORIZATION
☒ Satisfactory for Evaluation ☐ Unsatisfactory for Evaluation	☐ Negative for Intraepithelial Lesion or Malignancy (*see Interpretation/Result*) ☒ Epithelial Cell Abnormality (*see Interpretation/Result*) ☐ Other (*see Interpretation/Result*)

INTERPRETATION/RESULT

A. BENIGN CELLULAR CHANGES

☐ Infection:
- ☐ Trichomonas vaginalis
- ☐ Fungal organisms morphologically compatible
   w/ Candida species
- ☐ Cellular changes associated with herpes
   simplex virus
- ☐ Bacterial infection morphologically compatible
   with gardnerella
- ☐ Cytoplasmic inclusions suggestive of chlamydia

☐ Reactive changes
- ☐ Without inflammation
- ☐ With inflammation
- ☐ Atrophy with inflammation (atrophic vaginitis)
- ☐ Radiation effect
- ☐ Repair
- ☐ Hyperkeratosis
- ☐ Parakeratosis

B. EPITHELIAL CELL ABNORMALITIES

☒ Squamous Cell
- ☒ Atypical Squamous Cells of Undetermined Significance (ASC-US)
- ☐ Atypical Squamous Cells of Higher Risk (ASC-H)
- ☐ Low Grade Squamous Intraepithelial Lesion (LSIL)
- ☐ High Grade Squamous Intraepithelial Lesion (HSIL)
- ☐ Squamous Cell Carcinoma

☐ Glandular Cell
- ☐ Atypical Glandular Cells of Undetermined Significance (AGUS)
- ☐ Adenocarcinoma

Figure 8-6. Cytology report form (Bethesda system).

with the previous class I through V system). For this reason, the Bethesda System is a more effective means of communicating the results of the Pap test to the physician.

The Bethesda system separates the cytology report into the following categories:

1. **Specimen Type.** This category identifies whether the specimen is a conventional cell sample (Pap smear) or a liquid-based cell sample (Thin Prep).
2. **Specimen Adequacy.** This category refers to the quality of the specimen collected by the physician.

The specimen is described using one of the following classifications:

a. **Satisfactory for Evaluation.** This indicates that the specimen was of sufficient sampling and quality for a comprehensive assessment of the cells.
b. **Unsatisfactory for Evaluation.** This indicates that the overall sampling or quality of the specimen was inadequate. A reason is given for the inability to evaluate the Pap slide, such as too few cells were collected or the presence of blood or inflammation is obscuring the cells.

3. **General Categorization.** This category provides the medical office with a quick review of the report. The following classifications are used to categorize the specimen:
   a. **Negative for Intraepithelial Lesion or Malignancy.** This indicates that the epithelial cells were normal and that there were no precancerous or cancerous findings. This classification is also assigned to a specimen that exhibits certain benign (noncancerous) changes. Benign changes can be caused by vaginal infections such as bacterial vaginosis, chlamydia, trichomoniasis, candidiasis, and herpes. Benign changes can also be caused by inflammation resulting from the normal cell repair process, radiation, and chemotherapy. Any benign findings of importance (e.g., vaginal infections) are described in detail in the Interpretation/Result section of the cytology report.
   b. **Epithelial Cell Abnormality.** This classification indicates abnormal cell changes. The abnormality is described in detail in the Interpretation/Result section of the report.
   c. **Other.** This classification is used to indicate that no abnormality was found in the cells but the findings indicate some increased risk. For example, the presence of normal appearing endometrial cells in a postmenopausal woman may indicate an abnormality of the endometrium. These findings are described in detail in the Interpretation/Result section of the report.
4. **Interpretation/Result.** This part of the report provides the physician with a detailed description of findings. This includes any significant benign changes (e.g., vaginal infections), as well as any abnormal changes in the epithelial cells. Table 8-1 lists and describes the findings most frequently reported.

5. **Automated Review.** This category indicates if the specimen was evaluated using an automated computer-imaging device. Both the name of the device and the results are specified in this section.
6. **Ancillary Testing.** This category is used if an additional test method is used to evaluate the specimen. For example, if abnormal cells are detected on the Pap slide, an HPV (human papillomavirus) test may be performed. The name of the test method and the results would be then be reported under this category.

Bimanual Pelvic Examination

After obtaining the smear for the Pap test, the physician withdraws the speculum and performs a bimanual pelvic examination. The physician inserts the index and middle fingers of a lubricated gloved hand into the vagina. The fingers of the other hand are placed on the woman's lower abdomen. Between the two hands, the physician can palpate the size, shape, and position of the uterus and ovaries and detect tenderness or lumps (Figure 8-7).

Rectal-Vaginal Examination

The last part of the pelvic examination is a rectal-vaginal examination. The physician inserts one gloved finger into the vagina and another gloved finger into the rectum to obtain information about the tone and alignment of the pelvic organs and the **adnexal** region (the ovaries, fallopian tubes, and ligaments of the uterus). The presence of hemorrhoids, fistulas, and fissures can also be noted. During this examination, the physician may want to obtain some fecal material from the rectum to test for occult blood in the stool, which requires a guaiac slide test (e.g., Hemoccult). The medical assistant is responsible for assisting with the collection, as well as testing the specimen for occult blood. This procedure (fecal occult blood testing) is presented in detail in Chapter 13.

TABLE 8-1 Pap Test Results	
Test Result	**Interpretation**
Negative for intraepithelial lesion or malignancy	The epithelial cells were normal and there were no precancerous or cancerous findings.
Atypical squamous cells of undetermined significance (ASC-US)	Cells are only slightly abnormal. The nature and cause of the abnormality cannot be determined. These slightly altered cells usually return to normal on their own, resulting in negative results on subsequent Pap tests.
Atypical squamous cells of higher risk (ASC-H)	Minor abnormal changes in the cells with unknown causes but at risk of progressing to a high-grade lesion (HSIL). Further testing is required to determine if this is a minor condition or one that may progress to HSIL.
Low-grade squamous intraepithelial lesion (LSIL)	Abnormal cells that show definite minor changes but are unlikely to progress to cancer. (A general term for this is *mild dysplasia*). LSIL may be caused by HPV infection, but of a type that is not likely to lead to cervical cancer.
High-grade squamous intraepithelial lesion (HSIL)	Abnormal cell changes that have a higher likelihood of progressing to cancer. Although not cancerous yet, the abnormal cells may become cancerous if treatment is not obtained. (A general term for this is *moderate to severe dysplasia*.) HSIL is often caused by an HPV infection of a type associated with cervical cancer.
Carcinoma	Usually means the patient has cervical cancer. Most women with cervical cancer also test positive for HPV infection.

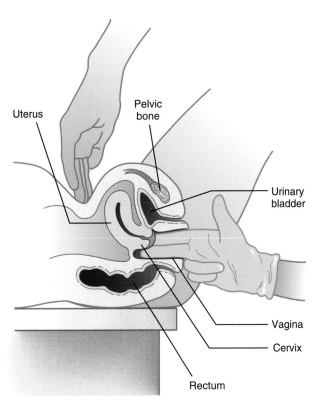

Figure 8-7. The bimanual pelvic examination.

PROCEDURE 8-1 (vertical sidebar)

PROCEDURE 8-1 Breast Self-Examination Instructions

Outcome Instruct an individual in the procedure for performing a breast self-examination.

Equipment/Supplies:
- Small pillow

1. **Procedural Step.** Greet and identify the patient. Introduce yourself, and inform the patient that you will be showing her how to perform a breast self-examination. Discuss with her the purpose of a breast self-examination and when to examine the breasts. (See the Patient Teaching feature on Breast Self-Examination.)

2. **Procedural Step.** Explain to the patient that a complete breast self-examination should be performed in three ways: before a mirror, lying down, and in the shower.
   Principle. Using three methods results in a thorough examination, making it more likely that breast changes will be detected.

Instruct the patient in the procedure for performing a breast self-examination as follows:

Before a mirror

3. **Procedural Step.** Remove clothing from the waist up. Stand in front of a large mirror with your arms relaxed at your sides. Observe each breast for the following:
   - Change in size or shape
   - Swelling, puckering, or dimpling of the skin
   - Change in skin texture
   - Retraction of the nipple
   - Changes in size or position of one nipple compared to the other

   Principle. Puckering and dimpling of the skin or retraction of the nipple may mean that a tumor is pulling the skin inward.

Continued

PROCEDURE 8-1   Breast Self-Examination Instructions—Cont'd

4. Procedural Step. Raise your arms over your head and repeat the same inspection listed in procedural step 3.

Principle. When the arms are moved at the same time into the same positions, both breasts and nipples should react to the movement in the same way. A change in one breast (e.g., dimpling or puckering of the skin) and not the other should be reported to your physician.

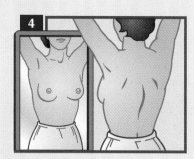

5. Procedural Step. Rest your palms on your hips and press down firmly to flex your chest muscles. Repeat the inspection in procedural step 3.

Principle. Flexing the chest muscles allows abnormalities to become more apparent.

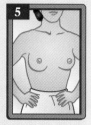

6. Procedural Step. Gently squeeze the nipple of each breast with your fingertips and look for a discharge.

Lying Down

7. Procedural Step. To examine the right breast, lie on your back and place a small pillow (or folded towel) under your right shoulder. Place your right hand behind your head.

Principle. The purpose of this step is to flatten the breast and distribute the breast tissue more evenly on the chest, making it easier to palpate the breast tissue.

8. Procedural Step. Extend your left hand with the fingers held flat. The pads of the middle three fingers of the left hand are used to perform the examination. The finger pads include the top third of each finger. Do not use the tips of the fingers. Use small rotating motions (about the size of a dime) and continuous firm pressure with the finger pads.

Principle. The finger pads are more sensitive than the fingertips, making it easier to detect an abnormality.

9. Procedural Step. Use one of the following patterns to move around the breast: circular, vertical strip, or wedge. Choose the pattern that is easiest for you. Once you have chosen a pattern, use the same pattern each time you examine your breasts.

Circular

a. Visualize the breast as a clock face.
b. Start at the outside top edge of the breast.
c. Proceed clockwise around the entire outer rim of the breast until your fingers return to the starting point.
d. Move in about an inch toward the nipple and make the same circling motion again.
e. Move around the breast in smaller and smaller circles until you reach the nipple.

Vertical Strip

a. Mentally divide the breast into strips.
b. Start in the underarm area and slowly move your fingers downward until they are below the breast.
c. Move your fingers about an inch toward the middle and slowly move back up.
d. Repeat until the entire breast has been examined.

Wedge

a. Mentally divide your breast into wedges similar to the pieces of a pie.
b. Starting at the outer edge of the breast, move your fingers toward the nipple and back to the edge of the breast.
c. Check your entire breast, covering one small wedge-shaped section at a time.

Principle. Using a specific pattern ensures that the entire breast is examined.

PROCEDURE 8-1

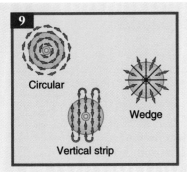

Circular

Wedge

Vertical strip

In the Shower

13. **Procedural Step.** Gently lather each breast.
    Principle. Fingers glide easily over wet, soapy skin, making it easier to detect changes in the breast.

14. **Procedural Step.** Place your right hand behind your head. Extend your left hand with the fingers held flat. With the finger pads of the middle three fingers, use small rotating motions (about the size of a dime) and continuous firm pressure with the finger pads to examine the right breast. Use your preferred pattern (circular, vertical strip, or wedge) to palpate for lumps, hard knots, and thickening. Be sure to examine the area between the breast and underarm, including the underarm itself.
    Principle. The upright position makes it easier to examine the upper and outer portions of the breast.

15. **Procedural Step.** Repeat the procedure on the left breast. Place the left arm behind the head and use the right fingers to examine the left breast.

10. **Procedural Step.** Making sure to hold the middle three fingers of your hand together with the thumb extended, use your finger pads and the pattern you selected to thoroughly examine the right breast. Press firmly enough to feel the different breast tissues. The breast should be palpated for lumps, hard knots, and thickening.

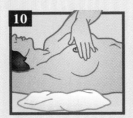

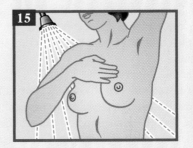

11. **Procedural Step.** Be sure to examine the entire chest area from your collarbone to the base of a properly fitted bra and from the breastbone to the underarm. Pay special attention to the area between the breast and underarm, including the underarm itself. A ridge of firm tissue in the lower curve of the breast is normal. Continue the examination until every part of the breast has been examined, including the nipple.
    Principle. An enlarged node in the armpit can also be a sign of breast cancer even if nothing can be felt in the breast.

12. **Procedural Step.** Repeat this procedure on the left breast. Place a small pillow (or folded towel) under the left shoulder and place your left hand behind your head. Use the finger pads of the right hand to examine the left breast.

16. **Procedural Step.** Instruct the patient to report lumps and other changes to the physician immediately. Reassure the patient that most breast lumps are not cancerous, but the only way to know for sure is to see the physician as soon as possible.

17. **Procedural Step.** Chart the procedure. Include the date and time and the type of instructions given to the patient. If you gave a printed instruction sheet or educational brochure to the patient, document this as well.

PROCEDURE 8-1

CHARTING EXAMPLE	
Date	
9/7/05	11:00 a.m. Instructions provided for a
	BSE. Pt given a BSE educational brochure.
	———————————————— Y. Wu, RMA

PROCEDURE 8-2 Assisting With a Gynecologic Examination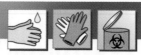

Outcome Assist with a gynecologic examination.

The following procedure describes the medical assistant's role in assisting with a gynecologic examination consisting of breast and pelvic examinations, including a Pap test.

Equipment/Supplies:

- Disposable gloves
- Examining gown and drape
- Disposable vaginal speculum
- Water-based lubricant
- Gauze pads
- Hemoccult slide and developing solution
- Tissues
- Cytology request form
- Biohazard specimen transport bag

Direct Smear Method

- Glass slides with frosted edge
- Cytology fixative
- Plastic spatula
- Endocervical brush
- Slide container

Liquid-Prep Method

- Thin Prep vial
- Plastic spatula and endocervical brush or cytology broom

1. **Procedural Step.** Sanitize your hands.
2. **Procedural Step.** Assemble the equipment. Complete as much of the cytology request form as possible. Some information on the form requires input from the patient, such as the LMP, and must be completed later. Prepare the collection materials as follows:

   Pap Smear Method

   Using a lead pencil, identify the slides on the frosted edge with the patient's name, the date, and the source of the specimen using the following abbreviations: V (vaginal), C (cervical), and E (endocervical).

   Liquid-Prep Method

   Label the vial with the date, the patient's name, and her identification number. The identification number is located on the cytology request form.

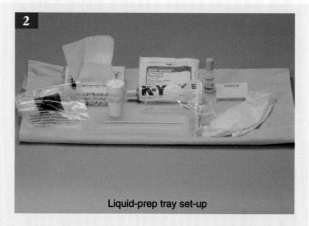

Liquid-prep tray set-up

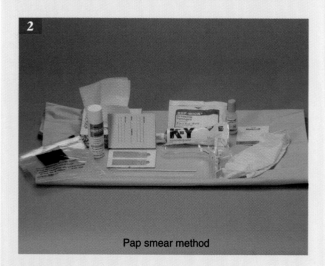

Pap smear method

3. **Procedural Step.** Greet and identify the patient. Introduce yourself. Ask the patient if she needs to empty her bladder before the examination. If a urine specimen is needed, instruct the patient in the proper collection of the specimen.

   Principle. An empty bladder makes the pelvic examination easier and is more comfortable for the patient.

4. **Procedural Step.** Escort the patient to the examining room and ask her to be seated. Seat yourself so that you are facing the patient. Ask the patient if she has any problems or concerns, and record the information in the patient's chart. Ask the patient the necessary questions to complete the rest of the cytology request form.

5. **Procedural Step.** Measure the patient's vital signs, height, and weight, and chart the results.

6. **Procedural Step.** Instruct the patient to undress completely and put on the examining gown with the opening in front. Leave the room to give her privacy.

7. **Procedural Step.** Assist the patient onto the examining table into a sitting position. Place the patient's chart in a convenient location for review by the physician. Inform the physician that the patient is ready.

8. **Procedural Step.** Assist the patient into a supine position and properly drape her for the breast examination.

9. **Procedural Step.** Assist the patient into the lithotomy position for the pelvic examination.

10. **Procedural Step.** Prepare the vaginal speculum and hand it to the physician.

    Pap Smear Method

    Moisten the speculum with warm water.

    Liquid Prep Method

    Lubricate the speculum with a water-based lubricant.

    Principle. Preparing the vaginal specumlum facilitates insertion of it into the vagina.

11. **Procedural Step.** Adjust and focus the light for the physician. Reassure the patient and help her relax the abdominal muscles during the examination by telling her to breathe deeply, slowly, and evenly through the mouth.

    Principle. Visualization of the vagina and cervix requires direct light. If the patient is relaxed, the examination proceeds more smoothly and is more comfortable for her.

12. **Procedural Step.** Apply gloves and assist with the collection of the Pap specimen as follows:

    a. **Direct Smear Method**

    (1) Hold each slide so the physician can smear the specimen on it.

    (2) Fix each slide immediately after collection by flooding it with 95% ethyl alcohol or by spraying it with a cytology fixative. The slide should be sprayed lightly with a continuous motion from a distance of 5 to 6 inches.

    (3) Allow the slides to air dry for 5 to 10 minutes, and then place them in a protective slide container.

b. **Liquid-Prep Spatula and Brush Method**

    (1) Remove the cap from the Thin Prep vial and hold it so the physician can insert the spatula in the vial.

    (2) Rinse the plastic spatula in the liquid preservative by vigorously swirling it around in the solution ten times.

    (3) Discard the spatula in a regular waste container and place the cap on the vial until the physician has collected the next specimen.

    (4) Remove the cap from the Thin Prep vial and hold it so the physician can insert the endocervical brush in the vial.

    (5) Rinse the brush in the liquid preservative by rotating it in the solution ten times while pushing the brush against the vial wall. Next swirl the brush in the solution to further release material.

    (6) Discard the brush in a regular waste container. Tighten the cap so the torque line on the cap passes the torque line on the vial.

c. **Liquid-Prep Broom Method**

    (1) Remove the cap from the Thin Prep vial and hold it so the physician can insert the broom in the vial.

    (2) Rinse the broom in the liquid preservative by pushing the broom vigorously into the bottom of the vial ten times. This motion forces the broom bristles apart, releasing the specimen into the solution. Next swirl the broom vigorously in the liquid preservative to further relese material.

    (3) Discard the broom in a regular waste container. Tighten the cap so the torque line on the cap passes the torque line on the vial.

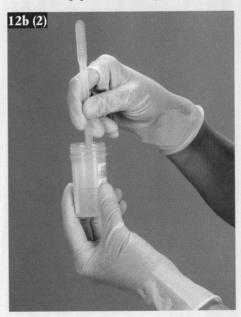

12b (2)

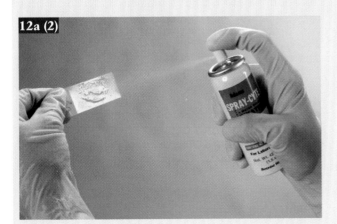

12a (2)

PROCEDURE 8-2

Continued

PROCEDURE 8-2   Assisting With a Gynecologic Examination—Cont'd

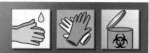

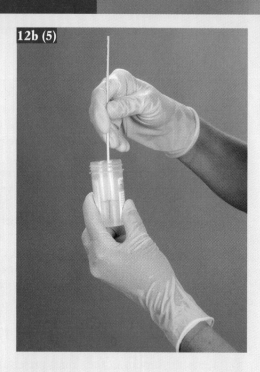

12b (5)

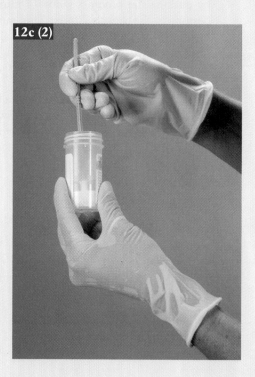

12c (2)

13. Procedural Step. Apply lubricant to a gauze square. Hold it out so the physician can apply lubricant to his or her gloves in order to perform the bimanual and rectal-vaginal examinations. Assist with the collection of the fecal specimen for the fecal occult blood test.

Principle. Applying lubricant to a gauze (rather than directly to the physician's gloved fingers) prevents the opening of the tube of lubricant from touching the physician's gloves and contaminating the contents of the tube.

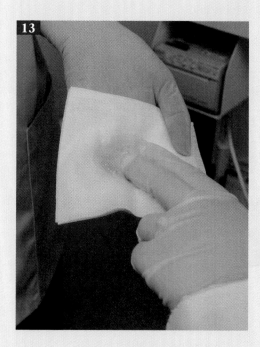

13

14. Procedural Step. After the examination, assist the patient into a sitting position and allow her the opportunity to rest for a moment. Offer the patient tissues to remove excess lubricant from the perineum. Assist the patient off the examining table.

Principle. Patients (especially geriatric) frequently become dizzy after being on the examining table and should be allowed to rest before sitting up.

15. Procedural Step. Instruct the patient to get dressed. Tell the patient how and when she will be notified of Pap test results.

16. Procedural Step. Test the fecal occult blood specimen and chart the results.

17. Procedural Step. Prepare the Pap specimen for transport to the laboratory. Place the Thin Prep vial in a biohazard specimen transport bag and seal the bag. Insert the cytology requisition into the outside pocket of the bag and tuck the top of the requisition under the flap. Place the bag in the appropriate location for pickup by the laboratory.

18. Procedural Step. Chart the transport of the Pap specimen to an outside laboratory.

19. Procedural Step. Clean the examining room.

CHARTING EXAMPLE

Date	
9/7/05	10:00 a.m. Hemoccult: negative.
	Instructions provided for BSE. Thin Prep
	Pap specimen to Medical Center Laboratory
	for cytology. ———————— Y. Wu, RMA

PROCEDURE 8-2

Vaginal Infections

The vagina provides a warm, moist environment, which tends to encourage the growth of various organisms, which can result in a vaginal infection, or *vaginitis*. If an unusual vaginal discharge is present, suggesting a vaginal infection, a specimen is obtained to identify the invading organism. A specimen of the discharge is collected at the medical office and is either evaluated there or placed in a transport medium that is picked up by a lab courier and transported to an outside medical laboratory for evaluation. The patient should be instructed not to douche before coming to the medical office because the physician will be unable to observe the discharge or to obtain a specimen for microbiologic analysis.

The medical assistant is responsible for assembling the appropriate supplies for the collection and evaluation of the suspected invading organism. She or he must be sure to label all specimens with the patient's name, the date, and the source of the specimen. If the specimen will be transported to an outside medical laboratory for evaluation, a laboratory request form must be completed; it must indicate the source of the specimen, the physician's clinical diagnosis, the microbiologic examination requested, and other pertinent information such as medications the patient is taking. The physician's clinical assessment of the patient's signs and symptoms, along with the results of the laboratory evaluation of the specimen, are used to diagnose the presence of a vaginal infection.

Medical assistants should protect themselves from infection with a pathogen while assisting with the collection and evaluation of the specimen by practicing good techniques of medical asepsis. Methods used to identify the invading organism and the supplies required for the collection and evaluation of organisms that cause common vaginal infections are presented next.

Highlight on Sexually Transmitted Diseases

Sexually transmitted diseases (STDs) are among the most common infectious disease in the United States today. Each year more than 15 million new cases of STDs are reported in the United States. If this trend continues, at least one in four Americans will contract an STD at some time in their life. Sexually transmitted diseases are most prevalent among teenagers and young adults; nearly two thirds of STDs are contracted by individuals between 15 and 25 years of age.

STDs are spread most often by sexual contact (vaginal, anal, or oral) with an infected person. They are less commonly spread by skin-to-skin contact and by the use of contaminated needles among drug users. More than 20 sexually transmitted diseases have been identified. The most common STDs are chlamydia, gonorrhea, herpes, HPV, hepatitis, HIV, and syphilis.

A sexually transmitted disease sometimes causes no symptoms at all, particularly in women. With or without symptoms, an STD can be spread to someone else. If symptoms develop, they may be so mild that they go unnoticed, or they may be confused with symptoms of other diseases. Because of this, sexually transmitted diseases may go undetected and untreated. Unfortunately, if not treated, many STDs result in serious complications such as infertility. In addition, some STDs can be passed from an infected mother to her baby before or during birth.

When diagnosed early, most sexually transmitted diseases can be treated effectively and many can be cured. Antibiotics can cure STDs caused by bacteria, such as chlamydia, gonorrhea, and syphilis. Medications have been developed to control the symptoms of STDs caused by viruses such as herpes and HPV; however, they cannot eliminate the virus from the body.

All sexually transmitted diseases can be prevented. The best way to prevent STDs is to practice abstinence or to have a mutually monogamous sexual relationship with an uninfected partner. If an individual's lifestyle does not follow one of these patterns, the following can be done to reduce the risk of contracting an STD:

- Before having a sexual relationship, partners should discuss their sexual histories with each other and also get tested for STDs.
- Use a condom during sexual intercourse. If the condom is not used correctly, however, an individual could still contract an STD.
- Limit the number of sexual partners. The risk of an STD increases with each new partner, particularly if it is not known how many previous partners they have had.

Sexually active individuals who are not in a monogamous relationship should have regular health checkups and ask to be tested for sexually transmitted diseases. These individuals should also learn to recognize the symptoms of STDs and check themselves for signs of STD infection once each month. Common symptoms associated with STDs are as follows: an unusual discharge from the penis or vagina; itching, redness, or soreness of the genitals; sores or blisters on or around the genitals and/or anus; and pain or burning during urination.

If an individual thinks he or she has an STD, a physician should be consulted as soon as possible. If an individual has been treated for a sexually transmitted disease and still has symptoms, he or she should return to the physician for further evaluation. It is possible to have more than one STD at a time and to become reinfected with the same sexually transmitted disease.

An individual diagnosed with an STD should inform his or her partner immediately so the partner can be tested. It is also important for an infected person to take all prescribed medication and to abstain from intercourse until a physician has determined that he or she is no longer contagious.

Trichomoniasis

Trichomonas vaginalis, the causative agent of trichomoniasis (trich), is a pear-shaped protozoan with four flagella, which allow for the motility of the organism (Figure 8-8). Trichomoniasis is usually, but not always, spread through sexual intercourse. Symptoms of this infection include a profuse, frothy vaginal discharge that is usually yellowish green and has an unpleasant odor; itching and irritation of the vulva and vagina; dyspareunia; and dysuria. The cervix may exhibit small red spots, a condition known as "strawberry cervix."

Trichomonas may be identified at the medical office by a wet preparation, which involves placing a small amount of the discharge on a microscope slide using a sterile swab, adding a drop of isotonic saline to it, and then placing a coverslip over the mixture to protect it (Figure 8-9). The slide is then examined under the microscope and observed for the presence of the lashing movements of the flagella and the motility of the organism.

If the physician prefers to have an outside laboratory evaluate the specimen, it must be placed in a tube containing a transport medium. It is important that the specimen be transported as soon as possible (within 24 hours) to prevent it from dying, which would impede visualization of the motility of the organism.

The treatment of trichomoniasis involves the oral administration of metronidazole (Flagyl). Both the woman and her sexual partner must be treated at the same time to prevent reinfection because the partner may harbor the organism without displaying noticeable symptoms.

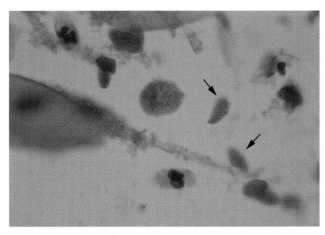

Figure 8-8. *Trichomonas vaginalis* under a microscope. (From Mahon C, Manuselis G: *Textbook of diagnostic microbiology,* ed 2, Philadelphia, 2000, Saunders.)

Candidiasis

Candida albicans is a yeastlike fungus normally found in the intestinal tract and is therefore a frequent contaminant of the vagina; however, it usually does not produce symptoms indicating a vaginal infection. Conditions such as pregnancy, diabetes mellitus, and prolonged antibiotic therapy produce changes in the vagina that may precipitate a candidal infection of the vagina, commonly referred to as a yeast infection. Symptoms of candidiasis include white patches on the mucous membrane of the vagina, along with a thick, odorless cottage cheese–like discharge, vulval irritation, and dysuria. The discharge is extremely irritating and usually results in burning and intense itching.

Candida may be identified microscopically in the medical office by placing a specimen of the vaginal discharge on a slide using a sterile swab and adding a drop of a 10% solution of potassium hydroxide (KOH). The KOH dissolves cellular debris present in the smear and allows better visualization of yeast buds, spores, or hyphae (fungus filaments), indicating the presence of *Candida albicans* (Figure 8-10).

If the specimen is to be transported to a medical laboratory for identification, it must be placed in a transport medium to prevent drying and death of the organism.

The treatment of candidiasis consists of the application of vaginal ointments or suppositories such as miconazole (Monistat), clotrimazole (Gyne-Lotrimin), nystatin (Mycostatin) or the oral administration of fluconazole (Diflucan). Candidiasis has a tendency to recur; therefore the woman should be instructed to contact the medical office if the symptoms of the yeast infection reappear.

Wet Preparation

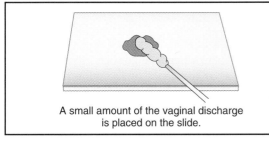

A small amount of the vaginal discharge is placed on the slide.

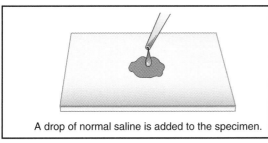

A drop of normal saline is added to the specimen.

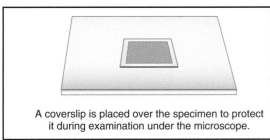

A coverslip is placed over the specimen to protect it during examination under the microscope.

Figure 8-9. Preparing a wet preparation for the identification of *Trichomonas vaginalis.*

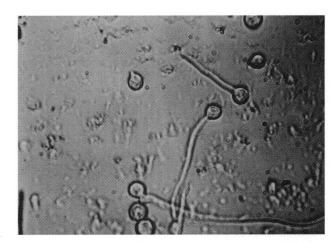

Figure 8-10. *Candida albicans* under a microscope. (From Mahon C, Manuselis G: *Textbook of diagnostic microbiology,* ed 2, Philadelphia, 2000, Saunders.)

Chlamydia

Chlamydia is caused by the bacterium *Chlamydia trachomatis*. It is a gram-negative intracellular bacterium; that is, it grows and multiplies in the cytoplasm of the host cell. Chlamydia is the most frequently reported and fastest spreading STD in the United States, particularly among female adolescents and young adults.

Most women with chlamydia have no symptoms, and therefore are not aware of having the condition. Because of this, many women do not seek medical care until serious complications have occurred. After infection, chlamydia first attacks the cervix, resulting in cervicitis. If symptoms do occur, they may include one or more of the following: dysuria, itching and irritation of the genital area, and a yellowish odorless vaginal discharge. These symptoms usually appear 1 to 3 weeks after the patient has been infected.

If not treated, chlamydia can spread further into the female reproductive tract and cause pelvic inflammatory disease (PID). The symptoms of PID include lower abdominal pain, fever, nausea and vomiting, dyspareunia, a vaginal discharge, and bleeding between periods. Complications of PID are very serious and include chronic pelvic pain, scarring of the fallopian tubes, ectopic pregnancy, and infertility.

Symptoms of a chlamydial infection in men include mild dysuria and a thin watery discharge from the penis. Men are more likely to have symptoms than women; however, the symptoms may appear only early in the day and be so mild that they are ignored. If the infection is not treated, it can cause epididymitis, a painful condition of the testicles that could result in infertility.

When diagnosed early, chlamydia can be treated successfully with antibiotics. The antibiotics most often used are azithromycin (Zithromax) and doxycycline. The patient's partner should also be tested for chlamydia so that if treatment is needed, it can be administered as soon as possible.

Chlamydia is most frequently diagnosed using a DNA-based detection test known as the DNA-probe test. This test is able to detect the presence of the genes of chlamydia bacteria. The physician collects a specimen using a sterile swab. The specimen is collected from the endocervical canal of a female patient and from the urethra of a male patient. Male patients should be instructed not to void for 1 hour before the collection of the specimen to prevent chlamydia organisms from being washed out of the urethra. After collection, the specimen is placed in a tube containing a transport medium to preserve the specimen until it reaches the laboratory. See the box entitled Chlamydia and Gonorrhea Specimen Collection for detailed instructions on how to collect a chlamydia specimen.

Gonorrhea

Gonorrhea is caused by the bacterium *Neisseria gonorrhoeae,* which is a gram-negative diplococcus. Gonorrhea is an infection of the genitourinary tract that is transmitted through sexual intercourse. Chlamydia often occurs in association with gonorrhea; approximately 25% to 40% of patients infected with gonorrhea also have chlamydia.

Women who have contracted gonorrhea may have no symptoms or may exhibit dysuria and a yellow vaginal discharge. The symptoms of gonorrhea (if they occur) appear 2 to 10 days after infection and may be so mild that they are ignored. As the disease progresses, it can spread further into the reproductive tract, resulting in PID. As previously described, PID can lead to serious complications such as infertility.

Men who have contracted gonorrhea exhibit more symptoms than do women, including dysuria and a whitish discharge from the penis, which may progress to a thick and creamy discharge. The burning and pain experienced during urination is often severe, which usually prompts an infected male to seek early treatment. If not treated, gonorrhea may cause epididymitis, which could lead to infertility.

Gonorrhea can be effectively treated with antibiotics. In recent years gonorrhea bacteria have become resistant to the antibiotics typically used to treat the disease. Because of this, newer types of antibiotics have been developed. One of the most effective antibiotics used to treat gonorrhea is ceftriaxone, which is administered in one dose through an injection.

A DNA-probe test is most frequently used by the medical office to diagnose gonorrhea. This test detects the presence of the genes of the gonorrhea bacterium. Before the development of the DNA-probe test, a culture test was most often used to diagnose gonorrhea. Although still used, the disadvantage of this method is that gonorrhea is difficult to culture. Special procedures must be performed following the collection of the

What Would You DO?
What Would You *Not* DO?

Case Study 2

Dagny Fairchild comes to the office. She is 16 years old and her father is a lawyer and her mother is a chemical engineer. Her boyfriend was diagnosed 2 weeks ago with chlamydia. Dagny was hesitant to come in because she doesn't have any symptoms and her boyfriend always uses a condom. She is very worried about her parents finding out that she is sexually active and what they will think if she has one of "those diseases." Dagny is also afraid and extremely embarrassed about what will be "done to her" to determine if she has chlamydia. She tells Yin-Ling that she is thinking of leaving the office and not seeing the doctor at all. (Note: Dagny lives in a state that allows minors to receive health care services without parental consent.)

specimen to make sure the organism remains alive during transport to the laboratory. This includes an atmosphere of carbon dioxide, as well as a specially enriched Thayer-Martin culture medium. Most offices now prefer the DNA-probe test, which is just as accurate as the culture test, but it is much easier to prepare the specimen for transport to the laboratory. The procedure for obtaining a specimen for the DNA-probe test is outlined in the box entitled below.

Chlamydia and Gonorrhea Specimen Collection

DNA-Based Detection Test

The following outline gives the procedure for collecting a specimen for the DNA test. Both the chlamydia and gonorrhea tests can be performed from the same specimen.

1. The medical assistant assembles supplies needed to collect the specimen. This includes a vaginal speculum, clean disposable gloves, and the DNA-probe collection kit. The collection kit includes cotton-tipped swabs and a tube of transport medium.
2. The transport tube must be labeled with the following information: patient's name and identification number, date and time of collection, and the physician's name and phone number.

3. The physician collects the specimen as follows:
   Female Patient: The physician inserts a vaginal speculum into the vagina. Using a cotton-tipped swab, the physician first removes excess mucus or discharge from the cervix. Next the physician collects the specimen by inserting another cotton-tipped swab into the endocervical canal and rotating it for 5 to 10 seconds. This ensures a good sampling of the specimen.
   Male Patient: The patient must not urinate for 1 hour before the collection to prevent any urethral discharge from being washed away. The physician inserts a small-tipped cotton swab 2 to 4 centimeters into the penis. The swab is gently rotated for 3 to 5 seconds to dislodge cells and to ensure contact with all urethral surfaces.
4. The physician withdraws the swab.
5. The medical assistant should make sure that the transport medium is at the bottom of the tube. The medical assistant unscrews the cap and holds the tube for the physician.

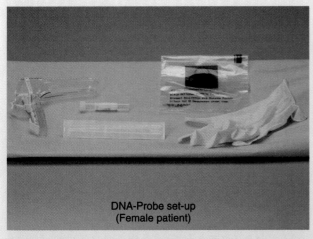

DNA-Probe set-up
(Female patient)

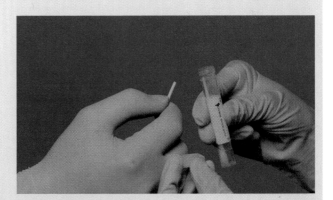

6. The physician inserts the swab into the transport tube and breaks off the shaft of the swab at the score line.
7. The medical assistant places the cap on the tube and twists it until it clicks into place. The tube is then placed in a biohazard specimen transport bag along with the lab requisition for pick up by the laboratory.

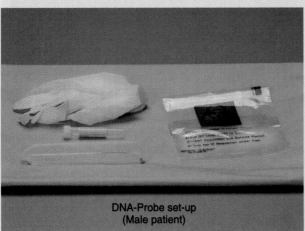

DNA-Probe set-up
(Male patient)

PRENATAL CARE

Obstetrics

Obstetrics is the branch of medicine that deals with the supervision of women's health during pregnancy, childbirth, and the puerperium. **Prenatal** refers to the care of the pregnant woman before delivery of the infant. Prenatal care consists of a series of scheduled medical office visits for the promotion of the health of both mother and fetus through prevention of disease and early detection, diagnosis, and treatment of problems common to pregnancy (e.g., anemia, urinary tract infection, and preeclampsia). Early detection of medical problems helps prevent serious complications in the mother and the fetus.

Obstetric Terminology

The medical assistant should know the common terms related to obstetrics. These terms are listed and defined below:

Braxton Hicks contractions	Intermittent and irregular painless uterine contractions that occur throughout pregnancy. They occur more frequently toward the end of pregnancy and are sometimes mistaken for true labor pains.
Dilation (of the cervix)	The stretching of the external os from an opening of a few millimeters to an opening large enough to allow the passage of an infant (approximately 10 cm).
Effacement	The thinning and shortening of the cervical canal from its normal length of 1 to 2 cm to a structure with paper-thin edges in which there is no canal at all. Effacement occurs late in pregnancy or during labor, or both. The purpose of effacement, along with dilation, is to permit the passage of the infant into the birth canal.
Embryo	The child in utero from the time of conception to the beginning of the first trimester.
Engagement	The entrance of the fetal head or the presenting part into the pelvic inlet.
Fetus	The child in utero, from the third month after conception to birth; during the first 2 months of development, it is called an embryo.
Fundus	The dome-shaped upper portion of the uterus between the fallopian tubes.
Gestation	The period of intrauterine development from conception to birth; the period of pregnancy. The average pregnancy lasts about 280 days, or 40 weeks, from the date of conception to childbirth.
Gestational age	The age of the fetus between conception and birth.
Infant	A child from birth to 12 months of age.
Multigravida	A woman who has been pregnant more than once.
Multipara	A woman who has completed two or more pregnancies to the age of viability regardless of whether they ended in live infants or stillbirths.
Nullipara	A woman who has not carried a pregnancy to the point of fetal viability (20 weeks of gestation).
Position	The relation of the presenting part of the fetus to the maternal pelvis.
Postpartum	Occurring after childbirth.
Preeclampsia	A major complication of pregnancy, the cause of which is unknown, characterized by increasing hypertension, albuminuria, and edema. If the condition is neglected or not treated properly, preeclampsia may develop into eclampsia, which could cause maternal convulsions and coma. Preeclampsia generally occurs between the twentieth week of pregnancy and the end of the first week postpartum.
Presentation	Indication of the part of the fetus that is closest to the cervix and will be delivered first. A cephalic presentation is a delivery in which the fetal head is presenting against the cervix. A breech presentation is a delivery in which the buttocks or feet are presented instead of the head.

Primigravida	A woman who is pregnant for the first time.
Primipara	A woman who has carried a pregnancy to fetal viability (20 weeks of gestation) for the first time, regardless of whether the infant was stillborn or alive at birth.
Puerperium	The period of time (usually 4 to 6 weeks) after delivery in which the uterus and the body systems are returning to normal.
Quickening	The first movements of the fetus in utero as felt by the mother, which usually occurs between the sixteenth and twentieth weeks of gestation and is felt consistently thereafter.
Toxemia	A condition that can occur in pregnant women that includes preeclampsia and eclampsia. If preeclampsia goes undiagnosed or is not satisfactorily controlled, it could develop into eclampsia, which is characterized by convulsions and coma.
Trimester	Three months, or one third, of the gestational period. The 9 months of pregnancy are divided into three trimesters, each consisting of 3 months. From conception to 3 months is the first trimester; from 4 to 6 months is the second trimester; and from 7 to 9 months is the third trimester.

Prenatal Visits

The medical office visits for prenatal and postpartal care of the pregnant woman can be grouped into three major categories as follows:
1. First prenatal visit
2. Return prenatal visits
3. Six-weeks-postpartum visit
Each category is presented in this section.

The First Prenatal Visit

The first prenatal visit generally occurs after the woman has missed her second menstrual period; if problems exist, the woman is seen after missing her first menstrual period. The first visit is often a stressful experience, and the medical assistant plays an important role in relaxing the patient and relieving her anxiety.

The first prenatal visit requires more time than subsequent prenatal visits; therefore sufficient time should be scheduled to allow a complete and accurate initial assessment of the pregnant woman. The components of the first prenatal visit vary, depending on the medical office, but they generally include the following:
1. Completion of a prenatal record form.

2. Initial prenatal examination, consisting of a complete physical examination. Of particular importance are the breast, abdominal, and pelvic examinations. Pelvic measurements may be taken at this time or during a return prenatal visit.
3. Prenatal patient education.
4. Laboratory tests.

The Prenatal Record

The prenatal record provides information regarding the past and present health of the patient and also serves as a data base and flow sheet for subsequent prenatal visits. The prenatal record is essential in helping identify high-risk patients. The medical assistant is usually responsible for collecting a portion of the information required for the prenatal record. Many types of printed prenatal record forms are available (see Figure 8-11 for one example). The form used in your medical office will be based on the physician's preference and the method used for conducting the prenatal examination.

Obtaining and recording information in the prenatal record from one visit to the next provides an opportunity for the medical assistant to develop a rapport with the patient. It is also an excellent time to relay information to her regarding various aspects of the prenatal and postnatal period, such as an explanation of the changes taking place in her body, the signs and symptoms of labor, nutrition of the infant (breast feeding and bottle feeding), and care of the newborn infant. The prenatal record form should be completed in a quiet setting that is free from distractions. This gives the patient the confidence to discuss areas of concern openly which helps ensure a complete and accurate prenatal history.

During the first prenatal visit, the medical assistant should relay his or her name and position to the patient to help build a supportive relationship with her, as well as to allow her to ask for the medical assistant by name when contacting the medical office.

The prenatal record is similar to and contains much of the same information as the health history described in Chapter 1. Particular attention is given to factors that may influence the course of pregnancy, as will be described in the following paragraphs.

Past Medical History

The past medical history focuses on conditions that could affect the health of the mother and fetus such as kidney disease, liver disease, heart disease, hypertension, sexually transmitted diseases, phlebitis, diabetes, tuberculosis, thyroid disorders, drug allergies, alcohol and tobacco intake, drug addiction, previous abnormal Pap tests, infertility problems, surgeries, and so on. In addition, the medical assistant solicits information from the patient regarding immunizations and childhood diseases

PRENATAL HEALTH HISTORY

PATIENT INFORMATION

Date: _____ EDD: _____   Referred By: _____

Name: _____   Phone (home): _____
      LAST   FIRST   MIDDLE   Phone (work): _____

Address: _____   Emergency Contact: _____

_____   Phone: _____
      CITY   STATE   ZIP

Date of Birth: ____/____/____ Age: ____ Marital Status: _____

Occupation: _____

Education: ☐ High School   ☐ College   ☐ Post-graduate

PAST MEDICAL HISTORY

	○ Neg + Pos	DETAIL POSITIVE REMARKS INCLUDE DATE AND TREATMENT			○ Neg + Pos	DETAIL POSITIVE REMARKS INCLUDE DATE AND TREATMENT
1. DIABETES				16. D (Rh) SENSITIZED		
2. HYPERTENSION				17. PULMONARY (TB, ASTHMA)		
3. HEART DISEASE				18. RHEUMATIC FEVER		
4. AUTOIMMUNE DISORDER				19. BLEEDING TENDENCY		
5. KIDNEY DISEASE/UTI				20. GYN SURGERY		
6. NEUROLOGIC/EPILEPSY						
7. PSYCHIATRIC				21. OPERATIONS/HOSPITALIZATIONS (YEAR AND REASON)		
8. HEPATITIS/LIVER DISEASE						
9. VARICOSITIES/PHLEBITIS						
10. THYROID DYSFUNCTION				22. ANESTHETIC COMPLICATIONS		
11. TRAUMA/DOMESTIC VIOLENCE				23. HISTORY OF ABNORMAL PAP		
12. BLOOD TRANSFUSION				24. UTERINE ANOMALY/DES		

	AMT/DAY PREPREG.	AMT/DAY PREG.	# YEARS USE			
				25. INFERTILITY		
				26. SEXUALLY TRANSMITTED DISEASE		
13. TOBACCO						
14. ALCOHOL						
15. STREET DRUGS				27. OTHER		

IMMUNIZATIONS:

Mark an X next to those you have had.

☐ Influenza   ☐ Chickenpox

☐ Hepatitis B   ☐ Pneumococcal

☐ Hib   ☐ Tuberculin Test

☐ Polio   ☐ Tetanus Booster

☐ MMR

ALLERGIES:

List all allergies (foods, drugs, environment).   ☐ None

_____

_____

_____

_____

_____

MENSTRUAL HISTORY

Menarche: Age of Onset _____   GYN Disorders (List): _____

Frequency: Q _____ Days   _____

Duration: _____ Days   _____

Amount of Flow: ☐ Small ☐ Moderate ☐ Large   On contraceptive at conception? ☐ Yes ☐ No

Figure 8-11. Example of a prenatal record form.

to provide the physician the information needed to assess her antibody protection against such diseases.

Rubella, if contracted during pregnancy, can be dangerous to the developing fetus; the earlier in pregnancy the infection occurs, the greater is the chance of birth defects. The infant may be born with heart defects, cataracts, mental retardation, and deafness. Patients who do not have antibody protection against rubella are given a rubella immunization within 6 weeks of delivery. The rubella vaccination cannot be given to a pregnant woman because it may be harmful to the fetus. These patients should be told to avoid exposure to children with rubella during their pregnancy.

Menstrual History

A menstrual history is obtained from the patient. It includes the date of the onset of menstruation, the menstrual interval cycle, the duration, the amount of flow

OBSTETRIC HISTORY

G _____ (Total Pregnancies) T _____ (Term) P _____ (Preterm) A _____ (Abortions) L _____ (Living Children)

PREVIOUS PREGNANCIES:

DATE MONTH/ YEAR	WEEKS GEST.	LENGTH OF LABOR	BIRTH WEIGHT	SEX M/F	TYPE DELIVERY	ANES.	MATERNAL COMPLICATIONS	INFANT COMPLICATIONS

PRESENT PREGNANCY HISTORY

NAUSEA		ABDOMINAL PAIN	
VOMITING		URINARY COMPLAINTS	
FATIGUE		VAGINAL BLEEDING	
BREAST CHANGES		VAGINAL DISCHARGE	
INDIGESTION		PRURITIS	
CONSTIPATION		ACCIDENTS	
PERSISTENT HEADACHES		SURGERY	
DIZZINESS		X-RAYS	
VISUAL DISTURBANCE		RUBELLA EXPOSURE	
EDEMA (SPECIFY AREA)		OTHER VIRAL INFECTIONS	

LMP ____ / ____ / ____   Mo   Day   Year

Amount of Flow: ☐ Small ☐ Moderate ☐ Large

CURRENT MEDICATIONS: (Include prescription, OTC, herbal, and vitamins). ☐ None

Medication _____ **Frequency** _____

INITIAL PHYSICAL EXAMINATION

DATE ____ / ____ / ____

1. HEENT	☐ NORMAL ☐ ABNORMAL	12. VULVA	☐ NORMAL	☐ CONDYLOMA	☐ LESIONS
2. FUNDI	☐ NORMAL ☐ ABNORMAL	13. VAGINA	☐ NORMAL	☐ INFLAMMATION	☐ DISCHARGE
3. TEETH	☐ NORMAL ☐ ABNORMAL	14. CERVIX	☐ NORMAL	☐ INFLAMMATION	☐ LESIONS
4. THYROID	☐ NORMAL ☐ ABNORMAL	15. UTERUS SIZE	_____ WEEKS		☐ FIBROIDS
5. BREASTS	☐ NORMAL ☐ ABNORMAL	16. ADNEXA	☐ NORMAL	☐ MASS	
6. LUNGS	☐ NORMAL ☐ ABNORMAL	17. RECTUM	☐ NORMAL	☐ ABNORMAL	
7. HEART	☐ NORMAL ☐ ABNORMAL	18. DIAGONAL CONJUGATE	☐ REACHED	☐ NO	_____ CM
8. ABDOMEN	☐ NORMAL ☐ ABNORMAL	19. SPINES	☐ AVERAGE	☐ PROMINENT	☐ BLUNT
9. EXTREMITIES	☐ NORMAL ☐ ABNORMAL	20. SACRUM	☐ CONCAVE	☐ STRAIGHT	☐ ANTERIOR
10. SKIN	☐ NORMAL ☐ ABNORMAL	21. SUBPUBIC ARCH	☐ NORMAL	☐ WIDE	☐ NARROW
11. LYMPH NODES	☐ NORMAL ☐ ABNORMAL	22. GYNECOID PELVIC TYPE	☐ YES	☐ NO	

COMMENTS (Number and explain abnormals): _____

EXAM BY _____

Figure 8-11, cont'd. Example of a prenatal record form.   *Continued*

(recorded as small, moderate, or large), and any gynecologic disorders. The patient should be asked if she was using a method of contraception when she became pregnant.

Obstetric History

A thorough obstetric history is a component of the prenatal record and provides the opportunity to obtain information from the patient related to previous pregnancies. Information that is obtained and explored includes gravidity, parity, and other information related to previous pregnancies.

Gravidity and parity provide data with respect to the pregnancy, and the medical assistant should develop skill in recording this information. **Gravidity (G)** is recorded using one digit, which indicates the number of times a woman has been pregnant, regardless of the duration of the pregnancy and including the current pregnancy. For example, a woman who is pregnant for the second time,

PATIENT'S NAME _____

INTERVAL PRENATAL HISTORY

Date 20__	Weeks Gestation	Height of Fundus (cm)	Weight	B/P	Urine Glucose	Urine Protein	FHT	Vaginal Examination	Presentation	Edema	Discharge	Bleeding	Contractions	Fetal Activity	NST	Next Appt.	Initials

PLANS/EDUCATION   **(COUNSELED ☑)**

☐ ANESTHESIA PLANS _____
☐ TOXOPLASMOSIS PRECAUTIONS (CATS/RAW MEAT) _____
☐ CHILDBIRTH CLASSES _____
☐ PHYSICAL/SEXUAL ACTIVITY _____
☐ LABOR SIGNS _____
☐ NUTRITION COUNSELING _____
☐ BREAST OR BOTTLE FEEDING _____
☐ NEWBORN CAR SEAT _____
☐ POSTPARTUM BIRTH CONTROL _____
☐ ENVIRONMENTAL/WORK HAZARDS _____

☐ TUBAL STERILIZATION _____
☐ VBAC COUNSELING _____
☐ CIRCUMCISION _____
☐ TRAVEL _____
☐ LIFESTYLE, TOBACCO, ALCOHOL _____
REQUESTS _____
_____
_____

TUBAL STERILIZATION   **DATE**   **INITIALS**
CONSENT SIGNED   ___/___/___   _____

Figure 8-11, cont'd. Example of a prenatal record form.

but had a spontaneous abortion during the first pregnancy would be recorded as **G: 2.** A woman who is pregnant for the second time (and did not have a spontaneous abortion) would also be recorded as **G: 2.**

Parity refers to the condition of having borne offspring regardless of the outcome. It is recorded using four abbreviations and digits, which represent the following pregnancy outcomes:

A. Term birth (T). Delivery after 37 weeks regardless of whether the child was born alive or stillborn.

B. Preterm birth (P). Delivery between 20 and 37 weeks regardless of whether the child was born alive or stillborn.

C. Abortion (A). The termination of the pregnancy before the fetus reached the age of viability (20 weeks). An abortion can be spontaneous or elective.

D. Living children (L). Number of living children.

For example, a woman has been pregnant four times with the following outcomes: a spontaneous abortion, a full-term stillbirth, a preterm birth of a healthy child, and a full-term birth of a healthy child. The recording would be as follows:

G: 4 *(pregnancies);* **T: 2** *(term);* **P: 1** *(preterm);*
A: 1 *(abortion);* **L: 2** *(living children)*

LABORATORY		PATIENT'S NAME _____			
INITIAL LABS	**DATE**	**RESULTS**		**REVIEWED**	**COMMENTS**
BLOOD TYPE	/ /	A B AB O			
Rh FACTOR	/ /	☐ Pos ☐ Neg			
Rh ANTIBODY SCREEN	/ /	☐ Pos ☐ Neg			
HCT/HGB	/ /	_____ % _____ g/dL			
RUBELLA ANTIBODY TITER	/ /	Immune Nonimmune			
VDRL	/ /	☐ NR ☐ R			
HBsAg (HEPATITIS B)	/ /	☐ Pos ☐ Neg			
HIV	/ /	☐ Pos ☐ Neg ☐ Declined			
URINE CULTURE/SCREEN	/ /				
PAP TEST	/ /	☐ Normal ☐ Abnormal			
CHLAMYDIA (DNA PROBE)	/ /	☐ Pos ☐ Neg			
GONORRHEA (DNA PROBE)	/ /	☐ Pos ☐ Neg			
7–20 WEEK LABS (WHEN INDICATED/ELECTED)	**DATE**	**RESULTS**		**REVIEWED**	**COMMENTS**
ULTRASOUND #1 (7–13 WEEKS)	/ /	EDD:			
ULTRASOUND #2 (18–20 WEEKS)	/ /	EFW:			
TRIPLE SCREEN (15–20 WEEKS)	/ /				
CVS	/ /				
AMNIOCENTESIS	/ /				
24–28 WEEK LABS (WHEN INDICATED)	**DATE**	**RESULTS**		**REVIEWED**	**COMMENTS**
HCT/HGB	/ /	_____ % _____ g/dL			
GCT (24–28 WKS)	/ /	1 Hour _____			
GTT (IF SCREEN ABNORMAL)	/ /	_____ FBS _____ 1 Hour _____ 2 Hour _____ 3 Hour			
D (Rh) ANTIBODY SCREEN	/ /				
D IMMUNE GLOBULIN (RhIG) GIVEN (28 WKS)	/ /	SIGNATURE			
32–36 WEEK LABS	**DATE**	**RESULTS**		**REVIEWED**	**COMMENTS**
HCT/HGB (32 WKS)	/ /	_____ % _____ g/dL			
ULTRASOUND #3 (34 WKS)	/ /	EFW:			
GROUP B STREP (35–37 WKS)	/ /	☐ Pos ☐ Neg			
ADDITIONAL LAB TESTS	**DATE**	**RESULTS**		**REVIEWED**	**COMMENTS**
	/ /				
	/ /				
	/ /				
	/ /				
	/ /				

Figure 8-11, cont'd. Example of a prenatal record form.

Multiple births (twins, triplets) count as only one pregnancy and one delivery. For example, if a woman had been pregnant two times and had a set of full-term healthy twins and a set of preterm healthy triplets, the recording would be **G: 2 T: 1 P: 1 A: 0 L: 5.**

If a woman is a multigravida, information about each pregnancy is obtained and includes the length of the pregnancy, hours of labor, type of delivery (vaginal or cesarean section), type of anesthesia, sex and weight of the newborn, and maternal or infant complications. The obstetric history assists in identifying areas that may need to be investigated further or monitored during the prenatal period. Women with previous complications, such as premature labor, gestational diabetes, or postpartum hemorrhaging, are at risk for having these problems again.

Present Pregnancy History

The present pregnancy history establishes a baseline for the present health status of the prenatal patient. In addition, the patient is queried regarding any warning signs that may be present, such as persistent headaches, visual disturbances, abdominal pain, vaginal bleeding, or discharge that may place the mother or fetus in jeopardy. The patient is also asked if she has experienced any of the early signs of pregnancy such as nausea, vomiting, fatigue, and breast changes.

All prescribed or over-the-counter medications the patient is taking must also be recorded. Certain medications cross the placental barrier and could be harmful to the developing fetus. Therefore the patient should be instructed not to take any medications without first checking with the physician.

In the space provided under the present pregnancy history, the medical assistant will also need to record the first day of the patient's last menstrual period (LMP). The LMP is used to calculate due date, or **expected date of delivery (EDD),** by using Nägele's rule: Add 7 days to the first day of the LMP, subtract 3 months, and add 1 year (EDD = LMP + 7 days −3 months + 1 year). For example, if the first day of the patient's LMP was June 10, 2004, the EDD is March 17, 2005. The problem is set up as follows:

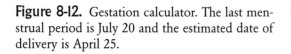

	6	10	2004	(LMP)
	−3 +	7 +	1	(Applying Nägele's rule)
	3	17	2005	(Delivery date)

Using Nägele's rule, approximately 4% of patients deliver spontaneously on the EDD; the majority of patients deliver during the period extending from 7 days before to 7 days after the EDD.

Gestation calculators are commercially available that can be used to determine the delivery date by lining up an arrow and the date of the LMP, using a movable inner cardboard wheel (Figure 8-12). These calculators require less time to determine the EDD than using Nägele's rule, and they provide information on the probable size (length and weight) of the fetus on any given date. The accuracy of gestation calculators is comparable to that of Nägele's rule. If the patient is unsure of the date of her LMP, the physician estimates the length of gestation by other methods such as fundal height measurement and sonography.

Interval Prenatal History

The interval prenatal history is also included in the prenatal record form; its purpose is to update the record. During every return visit, essential data are collected and recorded in this section during, including weight, blood pressure, urine testing results, fundal height measurement, and fetal heart rate. A general inquiry is made regarding the occurrence of additional signs of pregnancy such as fetal movement or Braxton Hicks contractions, as well as how the patient is feeling and any concerns or symptoms since the last prenatal visit.

This information is recorded and assists the medical staff in planning, implementing, and evaluating individual needs. Particular attention is focused on risk factors such as hypertension, thrombophlebitis, and uterine bleeding, which could influence the course of the pregnancy.

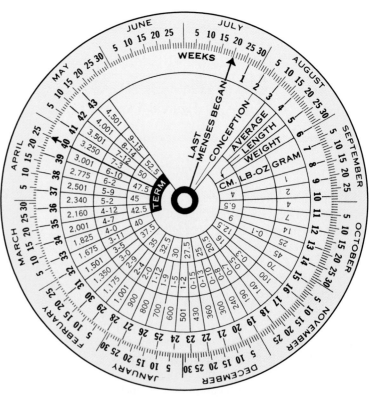

Figure 8-12. Gestation calculator. The last menstrual period is July 20 and the estimated date of delivery is April 25.

Initial Prenatal Examination

Purpose

The initial prenatal examination is of particular importance because it results in confirmation of the pregnancy and establishes a baseline for the woman's state of health. It includes a thorough gynecologic examination (breast and pelvic examinations) and a general physical examination of the other body systems, although the latter may be performed during a subsequent prenatal visit, depending on the medical office routine.

Women often have little or no medical supervision during their child-bearing years; therefore the physical examination is of particular importance in establishing a baseline for the woman's general state of health and in identifying high-risk prenatal patients. Conditions such as obesity, hypertension, severe varicosities, and uterine size inappropriate for the due date can be diagnosed by the physician, and necessary treatment or monitoring can be instituted to help prevent complications.

Preparation of the Patient

Once the patient arrives at the medical office and the prenatal record form has been completed, the medical assistant is responsible for taking and recording the patient's vital signs, height, and weight to provide a data base for subsequent prenatal visits. The patient is then asked to disrobe completely and put on an examining gown with the opening in front. The medical assistant must make sure to give complete and thorough instructions so the patient knows exactly what is expected. The patient should be asked if she needs to empty her bladder because an empty bladder facilitates the examination and is more comfortable for her. If the office policy is such that a specimen is needed for urine testing at the initial prenatal visit, the patient will be required to void.

Special precautions should be taken in assisting the prenatal patient onto and off the examination table. The medical assistant should make sure to support the patient as she gets onto and off the table to ensure her safety and comfort. This is especially important as the pregnancy progresses and the patient becomes more awkward and off-balance.

The medical assistant is responsible for setting up the tray required for the examination. The setup includes the equipment and supplies required for the procedures to be performed. During the prenatal examination, the medical assistant is responsible for positioning the patient as required for each aspect of the examination, as well as assisting the physician as necessary. Table 8-2 lists the procedures commonly included in the prenatal examination and the purpose, implications, and (when applicable) the patient's position. Most of the procedures included in the initial prenatal examination are presented elsewhere in the text; the number of the chapter that contains the step-by-step procedure is included in Table 8-2.

TABLE 8-2 Components of the Initial Prenatal Examination	
Procedure	**Purpose and Implications**
Vital signs (Chapter 4) Temperature Pulse Respiration Blood pressure	To provide a baseline for subsequent prenatal visits. The blood pressure drops slightly during the first and second trimesters and returns to normal or slightly above normal during the last trimester. An elevation in the blood pressure during the pregnancy is used in conjunction with other signs and symptoms to assess possible problems such as pregnancy-induced hypertension or preeclampsia. Patient position: sitting
Weight (Chapter 5)	To provide a baseline weight measurement for comparison with all future weight measurements at subsequent prenatal visits. The medical assistant charts the patient's weight on a flow sheet at each prenatal visit, and any deviations from expected progressions will be evaluated by the physician. Measuring and recording the maternal weight gain or loss are helpful in assessing fetal development and to some extent the mother's nutrition and state of health. A sudden unexplained weight gain may indicate preeclampsia of pregnancy.
Physical examination (Chapter 5)	To establish a baseline for the woman's general state of health to be certain the patient is entering pregnancy in the best possible physical condition. The physical examination includes an examination of the patient's eyes, ears, nose, and throat; chest, lungs, and heart; breasts; abdomen; reproductive organs; rectum; and extremities. Of particular importance are the breast, abdominal, and pelvic examinations, which are outlined in a separate category.

Continued

TABLE 8-2	Components of the Initial Prenatal Examination—cont'd
Procedure	**Purpose and Implications**
Breast examination (Chapter 8)	To check for lumps, swelling, dimpling, puckering, and changes in skin texture. To check for the breast changes that take place during pregnancy, such as tenderness and fullness and darkening of the nipple and areolae. Patient position: supine.
Abdominal examination (Chapter 8)	To detect masses or lumps other than the developing fetus. The abdomen is inspected for scars and striations, and the initial measurement of the fundal height is made to provide a baseline for future fundal height measurements. Patient position: supine.
Pelvic examination (Chapter 8)	To provide data to confirm the pregnancy and to determine the length of gestation. To estimate gestational age of the developing embryo (At 7 weeks, the uterus is the size of an egg; at 10 weeks it is the size of an orange; and at 12 weeks it is the size of a grapefruit). To identify pelvic characteristics and any abnormalities that may result in complications during the pregnancy or delivery. The pelvic examination generally includes the following: a. Inspection of the external genitalia b. Speculum examination of the vagina and cervix c. Pap test d. Specimen for chlamydia and gonorrhea tests e. Vaginal specimen if an infection is suspected f. Bimanual examination Patient position: lithotomy.
Rectal-vaginal examination (Chapter 8)	To assess the strength and irregularity of the posterior vaginal wall and the posterior cervix. The anus is inspected for hemorrhoids and fissures, and the rectum is inspected for herniation and masses. Patient position: lithotomy.
Pelvic measurements (Chapter 8)	To verify that the size and shape of the pelvis are within normal limits to allow the full-term fetus to pass safely through the pelvic inlet in the normal vaginal route of delivery; if not, a cesarean section will be required. Some physicians delay taking the pelvic measurements until later in the pregnancy. At that time, the prenatal patient's perineal muscles are more relaxed, allowing the pelvic measurements to be taken with less patient discomfort and more accuracy.

Patient Education

At the conclusion of the initial prenatal examination and after the patient is dressed, the physician talks with her regarding instructions on diet, weight gain, rest, sleep, clothing, employment, exercise, travel, intercourse, bowel function, dental care, smoking, alcohol, and drugs. Many offices have a prenatal guidebook designed especially for this purpose that is given to each patient to use as a reference. Some offices also use a series of teaching films that the patient views during the return prenatal visit while waiting to see the physician. The physician usually prescribes a daily vitamin supplement to be taken during the prenatal period to ensure that the mother and fetus obtain an adequate supply of vitamins and minerals.

When the physician is finished talking with the patient, the medical assistant is responsible for scheduling the next prenatal visit and for making sure the patient understands the instructions for maintaining health and preventing disease during the pregnancy. The medical assistant should tell the patient to report the occurrence of any warning signs during the pregnancy (see the Warning Signs during Pregnancy box) and not to take any medications without first checking with the physician. The patient should also be encouraged to contact the medical office should any questions or problems arise.

Laboratory Tests

A number of laboratory tests are ordered by the physician to assist in the assessment of the patient's state of health and to detect problems that may put the pregnancy at risk. Several of the tests, such as the Pap test and the chlamydia and gonorrhea tests, require the physician to collect the specimens at the medical office and then have them transported to an outside laboratory for evaluation. The specimen required for the prenatal blood tests must be obtained through a venipuncture to provide a sufficient quantity of blood for the number of tests ordered. The blood specimen is collected either at the medical office or at an outside laboratory.

Warning Signs During Pregnancy

Signs of Infection
Fever
Vaginal discharge
Dysuria
Increased frequency of urination
Marked decrease in urinary output

Signs of Spontaneous Abortion
Vaginal bleeding
Persistent low back pain
Abdominal pain and cramping

Signs of Preeclampsia
Severe, persistent headache
Dizziness
Blurred vision
Sudden swelling of hands, feet, or face
Sudden rapid weight gain
Abdominal pain

Signs of Placental or Fetal Problems
Vaginal spotting or bleeding
Abdominal pain and cramping
Back pain
Noticeable decrease in the baby's activity
No fetal movement

Signs of Preterm Labor
Regular or frequent contractions (more than 4 to 6 per hour)
Recurring low, dull backache
Menstrual-like cramping
Unusual pressure in the pelvis, low back, abdomen, or thighs

It is important to have these initial tests completed as soon as possible to provide the physician with the test results by the time of the next scheduled prenatal visit. Based on the results of the prenatal examination and the laboratory tests, the physician may order additional tests to assess the patient's condition. Certain tests and procedures are scheduled later in the pregnancy, such as the glucose challenge test and the group B streptococcus test. The prenatal laboratory tests that are usually performed on a pregnant woman are listed next.

Urine Tests

Urinalysis. A complete urinalysis is performed, including physical, chemical, and microscopic analyses of the urine; a clean-catch midstream urine specimen is generally required for the test. If bacteria are found in the urine specimen, the physician usually requests a urine culture and sensitivity test to determine the possible presence of a urinary tract infection. A pregnancy test may also be performed on the urine specimen, if ordered by the physician.

Swab Tests

Pap Test. A Pap test is done for the detection of abnormalities of cell growth to diagnose precancerous or cancerous conditions of the cervix. This test can also be used for hormonal assessment (MI) and to assist in the detection of vaginal infections.

Chlamydia and Gonorrhea. These specimens are taken from the endocervical canal and sent to the laboratory to rule out chlamydia and gonorrhea. Chlamydia can be passed from an infected woman to her baby during childbirth, resulting in conjunctivitis and pneumonia in the newborn. If a gonorrheal infection is present at the time of delivery, the *Neisseria gonorrhoeae* organism could infect the infant's eyes and cause *ophthalmia neonatorum,* and if not treated, could lead to blindness. For this reason, most states require that pregnant women be tested for gonorrhea and that the eyes of the newborns be treated with silver nitrate to kill the gonococcal bacteria immediately after birth. A patient who is diagnosed with chlamydia or gonorrhea requires immediate treatment with an appropriate antibiotic to prevent problems for both herself and her baby.

Trichomoniasis and Candidiasis. If an excessive irritating vaginal discharge is present, the physician obtains a specimen to rule out trichomoniasis and candidiasis. It is important to control candidiasis before delivery to prevent the development of thrush, a yeastlike infection of the infant's mucous membrane of the mouth or throat.

Group B Streptococcus. Group B streptococcus (GBS) is a common bacterium often found in the vagina and rectum of healthy adult women. Normally, one out of four pregnant women carries this bacteria. Group B streptococcus is not harmful to a pregnant woman, but it can cause life-threatening infections in the newborn. While passing through the birth canal a newborn can become infected with the bacteria carried by the mother. Once infected, the baby may develop an infection of the blood (septicemia), pneumonia, or meningitis.

To prevent GBS infection of the newborn, a pregnant woman is tested for the bacteria between 35 and 37 weeks of the pregnancy. Using two swabs, the physician collects specimens from the vagina and the rectum. The specimen swabs are then placed in a transport tube and sent to the laboratory to be cultured for GBS bacteria. If group B streptococcus is found, intravenous antibiotics are administered to the woman every 4 hours during labor until delivery. In most cases, this prevents the newborn from becoming infected with group B streptococcus. In situations where the newborn does become infected with GBS, antibiotics are administered immediately and the baby is closely monitored.

Case Study 3

Johanna Kruger is 24 years old and pregnant with her first baby. She is at the office for her first prenatal visit. She is quite upset. Her best friend just had her first baby and the baby died 24 hours later from a group B strep infection. Johanna is afraid that the same thing will happen to her baby. She wants to be tested for GBS as soon as possible. She has some antibiotics at home and is thinking of taking them. Johanna is worried because she has been experiencing some problems with her pregnancy. She is sick all day, her breasts hurt, and yesterday she had some spotting. Johanna is hesitant to tell all of this to the physician because he might think she worries too much.

Blood Tests

Complete Blood Count (CBC).
The CBC is a basic screening test used to assist in assessing the patient's state of health. It includes a hemoglobin, hematocrit, white blood count, red blood count, differential white cell count, platelet count, and red blood cell indices; of particular importance with respect to the prenatal patient are the hemoglobin and hematocrit evaluations, which are described here.

Hemoglobin and Hematocrit.
Low hemoglobin or hematocrit values are seen in cases of anemia. Prenatal patients have a tendency to develop anemia because there is an increased demand for and correlating increased production of red blood cells during pregnancy; therefore the physician carefully reviews the results of these tests. If the hemoglobin or hematocrit value is low, further hematologic evaluation is usually required. If necessary, therapy is instituted, which usually consists of an iron supplement and nutritional counseling. The hemoglobin and hematocrit values are checked again at approximately 32 weeks of gestation as a precaution against anemia before delivery.

Rh Factor and ABO Blood Type.
These tests are performed to anticipate ABO and Rh incompatibilities. If the patient is Rh-negative, the father's blood type must also be evaluated. If the father's blood type is Rh-positive, the possibility of an Rh incompatibility may exist. This warrants the performance of an Rh antibody titer test, as well as repeat antibody titers throughout the pregnancy to determine whether the mother's antibody level is increasing. An increased Rh antibody level could be dangerous to the developing fetus. It can result in severe anemia, jaundice, brain damage, heart failure, and sometimes death of the fetus.

Glucose Challenge Test.
A glucose challenge test (GCT) is performed between 24 and 28 weeks of gestation to screen for gestational diabetes mellitus (GDM). This test works by assessing the body's response to a measured glucose solution. The patient does not need to fast for this test and there is no preparation required other than arriving at the laboratory at the scheduled time. To perform the GCT, the patient is asked to drink 50 grams of a glucose solution and her glucose level is measured 1 hour later. A woman with a glucose level of less than 140 mg/dL does not have GDM and requires no further testing. If the glucose level is greater than 140 mg/dL, the test is abnormal. Not all women with elevated results have diabetes, however, and further testing using the 3-hour GTT must be performed before a final diagnosis can be made.

Serology Test for Syphilis.
The microorganism that causes syphilis, *Treponema pallidum,* is able to cross the placental barrier and infect the fetus; this could result in intrauterine death or could cause the fetus to be born with congenital syphilis. Children with congenital syphilis are often born with deformities and may become blind, deaf, paralyzed, or insane. The tests most commonly employed to screen for the presence of syphilis are the VDRL (Venereal Disease Research Laboratory) test and the RPR (rapid plasma reagin) test. The test results are reported as nonreactive, weakly reactive, or reactive. Because these tests are screening tests, a weakly reactive or reactive test result warrants more specific testing to arrive at a diagnosis for syphilis. Examples of these tests are the FTA-ABS (fluorescent treponemal antibody absorption) test and the MHA-TTP (microhemagglutination-*treponema pallidum*) test.

A prenatal serology test for syphilis is mandated by most states and should be performed early in the pregnancy, before fetal damage occurs. A patient who has contracted syphilis requires treatment with an appropriate antibiotic.

Rubella Antibody Titer.
This test assesses the level of antibody against rubella (German measles) in the patient's blood and is used to determine whether the woman is immune to rubella. If the mother contracts rubella during pregnancy, serious congenital abnormalities can occur in the fetus. Those patients who lack immunity should be immunized against rubella within 6 weeks of delivery.

Rh Antibody Titer (on Rh-Negative Blood Specimens).
This test detects the amount of circulating Rh antibodies against red blood cells. These antibodies can occur in a pregnant woman who is Rh-negative and is carrying an Rh-positive fetus; therefore an Rh antibody titer is performed in all Rh-negative blood specimens. Repeat antibody titer levels are also performed during the pregnancy to determine whether the woman's antibody level is increasing. As previously indicated, an increased Rh antibody level could be dangerous to the developing fetus. As a preventive measure, Rh-negative patients with the potential of having an Rh-positive baby and who test negative for Rh antibodies are given two injections of Rh

Highlight on Gestational Diabetes Mellitus

GDM Defined

Gestational diabetes mellitus (GDM) is a condition in which a pregnant woman who has never had diabetes mellitus develops an elevated glucose level (hyperglycemia). Every year approximately 2% to 5% of pregnant women in the United States are diagnosed with this condition. Because most women with GDM have no symptoms, the American Diabetes Association recommends that all pregnant women be screened for gestational diabetes mellitus during the second trimester of the pregnancy. The screening test used is the glucose challenge test (GCT), which is performed between 24 and 28 weeks of pregnancy.

Cause of GDM

GDM develops from a physical interaction between the mother and her fetus. The placenta of the fetus produces hormones to preserve the pregnancy. These hormones are excreted into the mother's circulatory system in increasing amounts during the second trimester of pregnancy. Unfortunately these hormones counteract the effect of the mother's insulin, which results in a condition known as insulin resistance. In most cases, the mother's pancreas responds to insulin resistance by producing additional insulin to keep the blood glucose at a normal level. Some women, however, are unable to produce enough extra insulin, which causes an elevation of their blood glucose level and results in gestational diabetes mellitus.

Problems for the Baby

If GDM is not treated or if it is poorly controlled, problems can occur in the baby. The extra glucose crosses the placenta and enters the baby's circulatory system. To lower the elevated glucose level, the baby's pancreas produces large amounts of insulin. The increased insulin converts the extra glucose into fat, resulting in the development of a large baby with a condition known as macrosomia. Babies with macrosomia may be too large to be born vaginally, and therefore may require a cesarean birth. Although the baby does not have diabetes, he or she is at risk for developing type 2 diabetes later in life. Other problems that can occur at birth include hypoglycemia, breathing difficulties, and jaundice.

Problems for the Mother

Problems that a mother with GDM develops include an increased incidence of preeclampsia, infection, postpartum bleeding, and injury to the birth canal if the baby is delivered vaginally. Another problem is the development of polyhydramnios (excess amount of amniotic fluid), which causes the uterus to stretch and take up more space in the abdominal cavity. This can result in breathing difficulties for the mother during the pregnancy. Gestational diabetes mellitus almost always goes away after delivery. This is because once the placenta is removed, the hormones causing the problem are also removed. The mother's insulin can then work normally without resistance. Some women, however, go on to develop type 2 diabetes later in life.

Risk Factors for GDM

Certain factors put some women at greater risk for developing gestational diabetes mellitus. These women are usually screened earlier and more often for GDM during the pregnancy. Risk factors for GDM include:

- Obesity
- Family history of diabetes mellitus
- Previous birth of a baby heavier than 9 pounds
- Previous birth of a baby who was stillborn or had a birth defect
- Previous GDM diagnosis
- Over 25 years old
- Polyhydramnios
- Belong to an ethnic group known to have higher rates of GDM (Hispanic, African American, Native American, Asian, Pacific Islanders)

Treatment

If a woman is diagnosed with GDM, the treatment is focused on keeping her glucose at a safe level. This includes special meal plans, exercise, daily blood glucose testing, and insulin injections, if needed. If the blood glucose is controlled during pregnancy, most women with GDM are able to prevent maternal or fetal complications.

---

immune globulin (RhoGAM). The Rh immune globulin prevents the formation of the Rh antibodies in the mother, which avoids Rh incompatibility complications during the next pregnancy. The first injection is given at 28 weeks of pregnancy and the second injection is administered within 72 hours of delivery.

Hepatitis B and HIV. The Centers for Disease Control and Prevention (CDC) recommends that pregnant women have a blood test to screen for the hepatitis B virus. The name of the test is the HBsAg test. Women who have pos-

itive HBsAg test results have an increased risk of spontaneous abortion or preterm labor. In addition, the mother may transmit hepatitis B to the infant, particularly during delivery or in the first few days of life. This risk can be greatly reduced by administering hepatitis immunoglobulin and the hepatitis B vaccine to the newborn infants of women who have tested positive for hepatitis B. It is also recommended that testing for HIV (the AIDS virus) be offered to all pregnant women, particularly those at risk for contracting AIDS. Babies born to women who are HIV positive are at risk of developing the disease.

Return Prenatal Visits

Return prenatal visits provide the opportunity for a continuous assessment of health of the mother and the fetus. During each visit, essential data are collected and recorded in the prenatal record, resulting in an updated record at each visit, as discussed in this section. If signs or symptoms of a pathologic condition are present, the physician performs selected aspects of the physical examination as necessary to diagnose and treat the condition. In addition, diagnostic and laboratory tests may be ordered to assist in diagnosis and treatment. The usual schedule of visits for prenatal care is listed below. The patient who exhibits complications is seen more frequently for closer monitoring.

- Every 4 weeks for the first 28 weeks
- Every 2 weeks until 36 weeks
- Weekly thereafter until delivery

The return prenatal visit also provides the opportunity for the physician and the medical assistant to lend support to the mother, to provide her with ongoing prenatal education to reduce apprehension and anxiety, and to ensure that the mother is well informed and prepared during her pregnancy, childbirth, and the postpartum period. The medical assistant plays an important role in prenatal education and should take the necessary time with each patient to provide appropriate information and to allow the patient to ask questions. Procedure 8-3 outlines the medical assistant's role in the return prenatal visit.

The patient is asked to collect a first-voided morning urine specimen on the day of each return visit to be brought to the medical office for testing. A responsibility of the medical assistant is to instruct the patient in the proper collection techniques and care and handling of the specimen until it reaches the office. The medical assistant is responsible for testing the specimen for glucose and protein, using a reagent strip, and for recording results in the prenatal record. A positive reaction to glucose may indicate the development of gestational diabetes mellitus or a prediabetic condition, and a positive reaction to protein may indicate a urinary tract infection or preeclampsia. Further testing is usually needed to arrive at a final diagnosis and to institute treatment.

During the return visit the physician performs one or more of the following procedures, depending on the stage of the pregnancy: (1) palpation of the woman's abdomen to measure fundal height, (2) measurement of the fetal heart rate, and (3) a vaginal examination. These procedures are discussed in detail in the following paragraphs.

Fundal Height Measurement

The pregnant uterus rises gradually into the abdominal cavity, and the fundus is palpable between the eighth and thirteenth weeks of the pregnancy. The first fundal height measurement, which is usually performed during the first prenatal visit, is used as a guideline for all subsequent measurements. The physician measures the fundal height by placing one end of a flexible, nonstretchable centimeter tape measure on the superior aspect of the symphysis pubis and measuring to the crest or top of the uterine fundus (Figure 8-13). The measurement is then recorded on a flow chart in the patient's prenatal record. By 20 weeks the fundus reaches the lower border of the umbilicus, and between 36 and 37 weeks it reaches the tip of the sternum. During

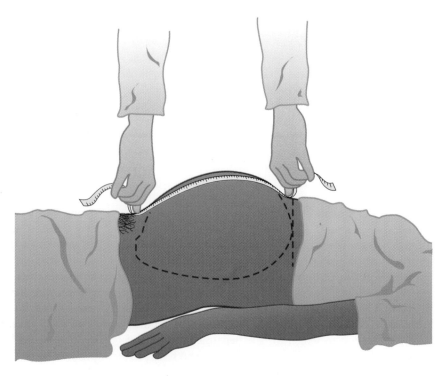

Figure 8-13. Measurement of fundal height. The physician places one end of a centimeter tape measure on the superior aspect of the symphysis pubis and measures to the top of the uterine fundus.

the first and second trimesters, measuring the fundal height provides a rough estimate of the duration of the pregnancy (Figure 8-14). The fundal height measurement is considered accurate to within 4 weeks using McDonald's rule:

Calculation of the duration of the pregnancy using McDonald's rule:

Height of the fundus (in centimeters) × 8/7 =
　　　　　　　　　duration of the pregnancy in weeks.
　　　Example: 21 cm × 8/7 = 24 weeks.

Height of the fundus (in centimeters) × 2/7 =
　　　　　　　　duration of the pregnancy in lunar months.
　　　Example: 21 cm × 2/7 = 6 months.

Because fetal weights vary considerably during the third trimester, it is difficult to use fundal height measurements as an estimate of the duration of the pregnancy in the last trimester.

In addition to assessing the duration of the pregnancy, the fundal height measurements permit variations from normal to become apparent and are used to assess whether fetal development is progressing normally. Growth that is too rapid or too slow must be evaluated further by the physician as a possible indication of high-risk conditions such as multiple pregnancies, polyhydramnios, ovarian tumor, intrauterine growth retardation (IUGR), intrauterine death, and an error in estimating the fetal progress.

Fetal Heart Tones

The normal fetal heart rate falls between 120 and 160 beats per minute with a regular rhythm. A very slow or rapid fetal heart rate usually indicates fetal distress. The **fetal heart tones (FHT)** refers to the heartbeat of the fetus as heard through the mother's abdominal wall. The fetal heart tones can be heard with a Doppler fetal pulse detector between the tenth and twelfth weeks of gestation. The Doppler fetal pulse detector converts ultrasonic waves into audible sounds of the fetal pulse.

The Doppler device consists of a main control unit and a probe (Figure 8-15, *A*). The probe head contains a transducer and electronic components, which generate the sound waves. The probe head is delicate and must be handled carefully, making sure not to drop or knock the head to prevent damaging it.

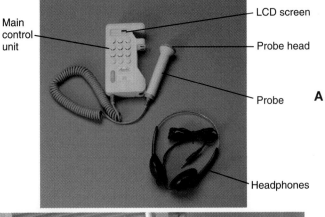

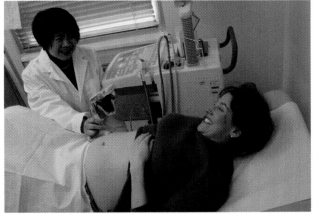

Figure 8-14. Fundal height showing gestational age in weeks.

Figure 8-15. A, The parts of a Doppler device. **B,** The probe of the Doppler device is moved across the abdomen to detect the fetal pulse.

Because air is a poor conductor of sound, an ultrasound coupling gel must first be spread on the mother's abdomen in the area to be examined. The gel is usually applied by the medical assistant and its purpose is to increase conductivity of the sound waves between the abdomen and the transducer.

The physician places the head of the probe into the gel on the mother's abdomen and slowly moves it until the fetal heart tones are located. The Doppler device amplifies the fetal heart tones and they are broadcast through a built-in loudspeaker in the main unit. A volume control provides adjustment of the sound level as required. (Fetal heart tones sound like the hoofbeats of a galloping horse, and when the probe is over the placenta, a windlike sound is heard.) The Doppler device may also have an LCD screen, which provides a digital display of the fetal pulse rate. Stereo headphones come with the Doppler device to allow private listening. The loudspeaker is muted when the headphones are connected (Figure 8-15, *B*).

Following the procedure, the medical assistant should remove excess gel from the mother's abdomen with a paper towel. The probe head is cleaned using a damp cloth and a mild detergent. The Doppler device should be properly stored in its carrying case to prevent it from becoming damaged.

Vaginal Examination

In the absence of vaginal bleeding, vaginal examinations may be performed at any time during the pregnancy; however, in a normal pregnancy, there is usually no need to perform a vaginal examination until the patient nears term. The vaginal examination is usually begun approximately 2 to 3 weeks from the EDD and is performed to confirm the presenting part and to determine the degree, if any, of cervical dilation and effacement. The purpose of dilation and effacement is to permit the passage of the infant from the uterus into the birth canal (Figure 8-16).

Special Tests and Procedures

The pregnancy can be evaluated with one or more of the following special tests and procedures: triple screen test, obstetric ultrasound scan, amniocentesis, and fetal heart rate monitoring. These are not considered routine procedures; however, they involve little or no risk to the mother or the fetus. Because some of these tests may be performed in the obstetric medical office, the medical assistant should have a general knowledge of these procedures.

What Would You DO? What Would You *Not* DO?

Case Study 4

Wynita Lopez is at the office with her husband. She is 32 years old and 18 weeks pregnant. It took Wynita a long time, almost 6 years, to get pregnant. She is excited and happy about being pregnant, but at the same time, very sad and confused. Her test results on her triple screen test came back indicating the possibility that her baby has Down syndrome. A repeat test was done with the same results. Wynita just got finished having an ultrasound that showed a normal baby, but Wynita and her husband understand that the only way to know for sure is to have an amniocentesis. Wynita does not know what to do. She is afraid of having an amniocentesis because of the chance of miscarriage. She also knows her triple screen test could be a false-positive. Wynita is not sure what her decision would be if the baby did have Down syndrome. Her husband is visibly distressed and wants Wynita to make all the decisions, saying he will be supportive of whatever she decides. Right now she wants as much information as she can get about all of this before she makes a decision. She feels "safer" being at the medical office and doesn't want to go home just yet.

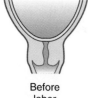
Before labor

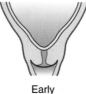
Early effacement

Complete effacement

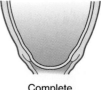
Complete dilation

Figure 8-16. Effacement and dilation occur to permit the passage of the infant into the birth canal. The cervical canal will shorten from its normal length of 1 to 2 cm to a structure with paper-thin edges in which there is no canal at all. The cervix will dilate from an opening a few millimeters wide to an opening large enough to allow the passage of the infant (approximately 10 cm).

Triple Screen Test

The triple screen test is a laboratory test available to pregnant women between 15 and 20 weeks of pregnancy. Its purpose is to screen for the presence of certain fetal abnormalities, which include neural tube defects, Down syndrome, trisomy 18, and ventral wall defect. Because the triple screen test has a high incidence of false-positive test results, it is not a mandatory prenatal test; however, the American College of Obstetricians and Gynecologists believes that this test should be offered to all pregnant women regardless of maternal age.

The triple screen test measures the level of the following three substances normally produced by the baby and placenta and excreted into the mother's blood in the second trimester of pregnancy: alphafetoprotein (AFP), unconjugated estriol (uEST), and human chorionic gonadotropin (hCG).

Alphafetoprotein is a glycoprotein produced by the fetus. During pregnancy, some AFP crosses from the amniotic fluid to the mother's bloodstream. When the neural tube of the fetus is not properly formed, increased amounts of AFP appear in the maternal blood. Hence, elevated AFP levels indicate the possibility of a neural tube defect in the fetus, such as spina bifida (incomplete closure of the spinal column) and anencephaly (incomplete closure of the brain).

A lower serum level of AFP and estriol, along with a higher level of hCG, is associated with an increased risk of having a baby with Down syndrome. A woman who is carrying a baby with trisomy 18 may have lower blood levels of AFP, estriol, and hCG than women with unaffected babies.

The triple screen test is a screening test; therefore abnormal test results always require further testing, such as ultrasound or amniocentesis, to determine whether a fetal abnormality actually exists.

Obstetric Ultrasound Scan

An obstetric ultrasound (US) scan is a diagnostic imaging technique, similar to sonar, used to view the fetus in utero. It allows continuous viewing of the fetus and shows fetal movement. The procedure is performed by a physician or an ultrasound technologist. The primary purpose of an ultrasound scan is to evaluate the health of the fetus and to determine gestational age. This is accomplished by

---

▶▶ PATIENT **TEACHING**

Obstetric Ultrasound Scan

- Emphasize the importance of preparing properly for the examination.
- Provide the patient with educational materials on obstetric ultrasound.
- Answer questions patients have about an obstetric ultrasound scan.

What is an ultrasound scan?

An ultrasound scan is performed to look at the baby in the uterus with the use of sound waves. During the examination, a gel is spread over your abdomen, and a scanning device is moved lightly over the area. The baby's image is displayed on a monitor similar to a television screen. During the examination, pictures of your baby will be taken and you will be given a copy for your baby album. If you choose, you may bring a standard VHS tape for the ultrasonographer to record your baby on videotape. The ultrasound examination usually takes no longer than 30 minutes.

Why is an ultrasound scan performed?

Ultrasound scanning is used to determine the age and position of the unborn baby, the location of the placenta, and the number of babies present, and overall to help the physician monitor and manage the pregnancy.

What preparation is needed?

To prepare for an abdominal ultrasound, you will need to drink 32 ounces of fluid 1 hour before the examination. Drink all the water within 15 to 20 minutes, and do not void until the examination has been completed. You should wear comfortable clothing. A two-piece outfit is recommended so that you do not have to undress completely.

Is an ultrasound scan safe?

There are no known side effects or risks to either mother or fetus during an ultrasound examination. Ultrasound does not use x-rays. No long-term risks have been detected. The procedure is painless and the only discomfort is from a full bladder, which will make you want to go to the bathroom. Once the examination is completed, you will have the opportunity to do so.

Can I learn the sex of my baby through an ultrasound scan?

Although an ultrasound scan is not just performed to determine the sex of the baby, it is sometimes possible (usually by 20 weeks) to tell whether the baby is a boy or girl, depending on the position of the baby in the uterus. Because not all parents want to know their baby's sex in advance, you will not automatically be told the baby's sex if it is determined, but you will be given the opportunity to make the choice of knowing or not knowing.

viewing the image of the fetus and by taking various measurements of the image such as the crown-rump length (CRL); biparietal diameter (BPD), which is a side-to-side measurement of the fetal head; femur length (FL); and abdominal circumference (AC).

Obstetric ultrasound scanning uses high-frequency sound waves that are directed into the uterus through a transducer. When the sound waves reach the uterus, they "bounce" back to the transducer, similar to an echo. These reflected sound waves are then converted into an image, or *sonogram* (Figure 8-17), that is displayed on a monitor screen. The monitor is usually positioned so the mother can observe the image on the screen if she wishes. There are two methods for performing an ultrasound scan: the transabdominal method and the endovaginal method, which are described next.

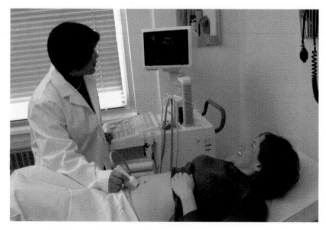

Figure 8-17. Obstetric ultrasound scan.

Transabdominal Ultrasound Scan. Transabdominal is the ultrasound scanning method performed most often. The patient must have a full bladder for this examination. This is accomplished by instructing the patient to consume 32 ounces of fluid approximately 1 hour before the procedure. A full bladder acts as an "acoustic window" through which the sound waves can travel to provide a clear visualization of the uterus. In addition, a full bladder holds the uterus stable and pushes away any bowel that might interfere with the image. The patient lies on an examining table in a supine position and is draped with the abdomen exposed. A coupling agent, in the form of a liquid gel, is applied to the patient's abdomen to increase the transmission of the sound waves. An abdominal probe (containing a transducer) is placed into the gel and the probe is slowly moved over the patient's abdomen, and the image of the fetus is displayed on the screen of the monitor (see Figure 8-17).

Endovaginal Ultrasound Scan. In the very early states of the pregnancy (up to 12 weeks), endovaginal scanning is preferred over transabdominal scanning. The patient must have an empty bladder for this scan, which makes the examination more comfortable. The patient is placed in the lithotomy position and a vaginal probe is placed in the patient's vagina. The image of the embryo is displayed on the screen of the monitor. An endovaginal ultrasound scan provides clearer visualization of the uterus in the beginning of the pregnancy because the probe is situated in the vagina, which places it closer to the uterus.

Although an obstetric ultrasound scan can be performed at any time during the pregnancy, it is often performed between 7 and 12 weeks of the pregnancy and then again between 18 and 20 weeks. A third scan is sometimes done around 34 weeks of the pregnancy. Table 8-3 outlines this schedule and what can be assessed at these times.

TABLE 8-3	Purpose of Obstetric Ultrasound Scanning

Between 7 and 13 Weeks
- To confirm the pregnancy by detecting the fetal heart motion
- To determine gestational age by taking measurements of the embryo and embryonic sac
- To detect an ectopic pregnancy

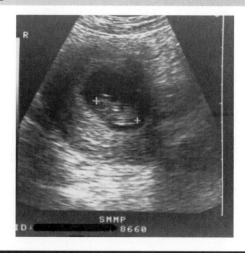

Embryo at approximately 9 weeks gestation. (From Greer I et al.: *Mosby's color atlas and text of obstetrics and gynecology,* St. Louis, 2001, Mosby.)

TABLE 8-3 Purpose of Obstetric Ultrasound Scanning—cont'd

Between 18 and 20 Weeks
- To determine fetal growth, size, and weight by taking measurements of the fetus
- To detect the presence of multiple fetuses
- To examine the brain, spinal cord, heart, lungs, gastrointestinal tract, reproductive organs, kidneys, bladder, bowel, and extremities of the fetus
- To detect congenital abnormalities
- To determine the location of the placenta
- To determine the cause of bleeding or spotting

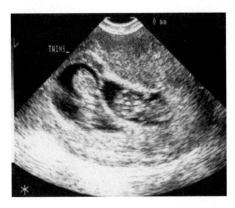

Twins.

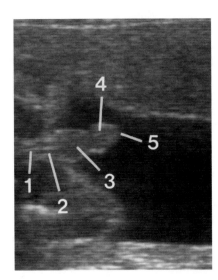

Erect fetal penis. *1,* urethra; *2,* corpus cavernosum; *3,* shaft; *4,* glans; *5,* foreskin. (From Callen P: *Ultrasonography in obstetrics and gynecology,* ed 4, Philadelphia, 2000, Saunders.)

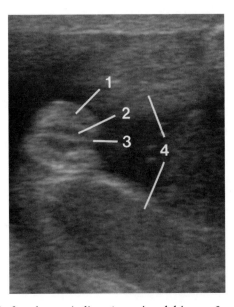

External female genitalia. *1,* major labium; *2,* minor labium; *3,* vaginal cleft; *4,* thighs. (From Callen P: *Ultrasonography in obstetrics and gynecology,* ed 4, Philadelphia, 2000, Saunders.)

At 34 Weeks
- To evaluate fetal growth, size, and weight by taking measurements of the fetus
- To verify the location of the placenta
- To confirm fetal presentation in uncertain cases

Other Purposes
- To diagnose uterine and pelvic abnormalities during pregnancy
- To view the fetus, placenta, and amniotic fluid during tests such as amniocentesis and chorionic villus sampling
- To confirm intrauterine death

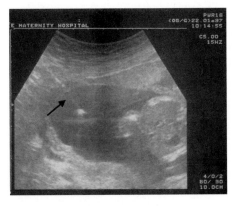

Amniocentesis being performed under ultrasound guidance. (From Greer I et al.: *Mosby's color atlas and text of obstetrics and gynecology,* St. Louis, 2001, Mosby.)

Amniocentesis

Amniocentesis is a diagnostic procedure that can be performed between 15 and 18 weeks of the pregnancy. Amniocentesis aids in prenatal diagnosis of certain genetically transmitted errors of metabolism, congenital abnormalities, and chromosomal disorders such as Down syndrome. It is also used to detect fetal jeopardy or distress and, later in the pregnancy, to assess fetal lung maturity. Amniocentesis can also determine whether the baby is a boy or girl.

To perform the procedure, the physician inserts a long, thin needle through the mother's abdomen and into the amniotic sac surrounding the fetus (Figure 8-18). An obstetric ultrasound scan is always performed in conjunction with amniocentesis so that the physician can view the position of the fetus, placenta, and amniotic fluid. This allows the physician to know the exact place to insert the needle. The physician withdraws a sample (about a tablespoon) of fluid, which contains fetal cells. The fluid is then sent to a laboratory for study. It usually takes between 1 and 3 weeks to evaluate the amniotic fluid and report the results.

Although the complication rate for an amniocentesis is extremely low, it is not risk free. There is a slight risk of bleeding, leakage of fluid, and infection of the amniotic fluid. There is also a slight possibility of miscarriage. Because of these risks, amniocentesis is offered only to women whose pregnancies are at risk for fetal abnormalities.

These include women who are 35 years of age or older or who have a child with a genetic or neural tube defect; women who have abnormal triple screen test results; and when one parent has a chromosomal abnormality or is a carrier for a metabolic disease.

Fetal Heart Rate Monitoring

Fetal heart rate (FHR) monitoring is performed later in the pregnancy to obtain information on the physical condition of the fetus. Specific conditions that may warrant this procedure are fetal growth that is not progressing well, decreased amniotic fluid, decreased fetal activity, elevation of the mother's blood pressure, gestational diabetes, and an overdue baby.

To perform the procedure, an electronic microphone is strapped to the mother's abdomen to amplify the fetal heartbeat. A gel is usually applied under the microphone to make the sounds clearer. The fetal heartbeat is heard and also displayed on a screen and printed on special paper.

There are two kinds of fetal heart rate monitoring procedures: the nonstress test and the contraction stress test. The *nonstress test (NST)* monitors changes in the fetal heart rate in response to the baby's spontaneous movements. The mother is instructed to press a button when she feels the baby move. In a normal test, the baby's heart rate increases when the baby moves. To prepare for the NST, the mother must be instructed to eat a light meal within 2 hours of the procedure to stimulate fetal movement.

If the results of the nonstress test are abnormal, a *contraction stress test (CST)* may be performed. This test is similar to the NST, except that mild contractions of the uterus are stimulated for a short period of time. The CST is used to evaluate the response of the baby's heart rate to the contractions in order to determine whether the baby will be able to withstand the stress of repeated contractions during labor. If the results of the test are abnormal, further evaluation is required to evaluate the well-being of the baby and to determine how and when delivery of the baby should be carried out.

Medical Assisting Responsibilities

The medical assistant has many important responsibilities in the return prenatal examination, which are outlined in Procedure 8-3. The medical assistant is responsible for assembling the equipment and supplies required for the examination, for obtaining information to update the prenatal record, for preparing the patient for the examination, and for assisting the physician during the examination. The physician depends on the medical assistant to have the urine test results and certain measurements, such as blood pressure and weight, completed and recorded in advance to allow him or her the opportunity to review these measurements before examining the patient.

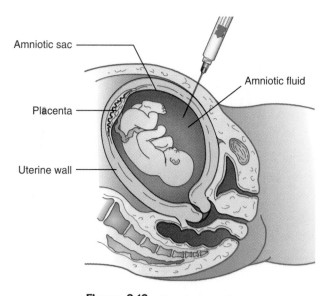

Amniotic sac

Amniotic fluid

Placenta

Uterine wall

Figure 8-18. Amniocentesis.

PROCEDURE 8-3   Assisting With a Return Prenatal Examination

Outcome Assisting with a Return Prenatal Examination

Equipment/Supplies:

- Centimeter tape measure
- Doppler fetal pulse detector
- Ultrasound coupling gel
- Paper towel
- Disposable vaginal speculum

- Disposable gloves
- Water-based lubricant
- Gauze pads
- Examining gown and drape

1. **Procedural Step.** Sanitize your hands.
2. **Procedural Step.** Set up the tray for the prenatal examination. The equipment and supplies depend on the procedures to be included in the examination, which may include one or more of the following:
   a. Fundal height measurement
   b. Measurement of fetal heart tones
   c. Examination of the legs, feet, and face for edema and development of varicosities
   d. Taking a specimen for the diagnosis of a vaginal infection
   e. Vaginal examination

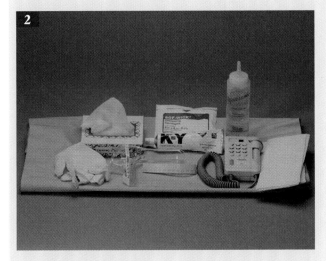

3. **Procedural Step.** Greet and identify the patient. Introduce yourself, and explain the procedure. Obtain the urine specimen that the patient has collected at home. Determine whether the patient has taken the necessary precautions to preserve the specimen before bringing it to the medical office.
   Principle. Specimens that have been left standing out produce inaccurate test results.

4. **Procedural Step.** Escort the patient to the examining room and ask her to be seated. Seat yourself so that you are facing the patient. Ask the patient if she has experienced any problems since the last prenatal visit, and record information in the appropriate section in her prenatal record.
   Principle. The physician investigates any unusual or abnormal signs or symptoms relayed by the patient.

5. **Procedural Step.** Measure the patient's blood pressure, and chart the results in the prenatal record. If the blood pressure is elevated, allow the patient to relax, then measure the blood pressure again.
   Principle. Taking the blood pressure again gives the opportunity to determine whether the elevation was due to emotional excitement.

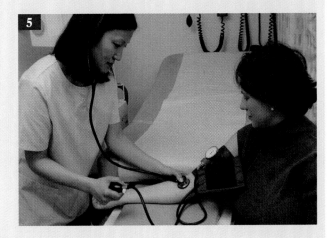

Continued

PROCEDURE 8-3

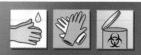

PROCEDURE 8-3   Assisting with a Return Prenatal Examination—Cont'd

6. **Procedural Step.** Weigh the patient and chart the results in the prenatal record.
Principle. Maternal weight gain or loss assists in assessing fetal development, as well as the mother's nutrition and state of health.

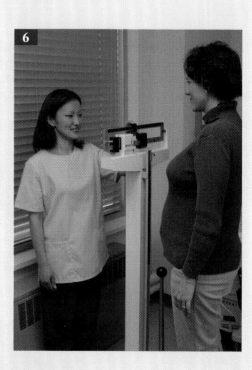

7. **Procedural Step.** Ask the patient if she needs to empty her bladder before the examination.
Principle. An empty bladder makes the examination easier and more comfortable for the patient.

8. **Procedural Step.** Instruct and prepare the patient for the examination. Have her remove her outer clothing to expose the abdominal area. If the physician will be performing a vaginal examination, the patient must also remove her panties; otherwise she may leave them on. Leave the room to give the patient privacy.

9. **Procedural Step.** Using a reagent strip, test the urine specimen for glucose and protein, and chart the results. *Note:* The urine specimen may be tested at any time before the physician examines the patient; however, a convenient time to test the specimen is while the patient is disrobing.
Principle. The prenatal patient's urine must be tested at every visit to assist in the early detection and prevention of disease.

10. **Procedural Step.** Assist the patient onto the examining table into a sitting position.
Principle. The medical assistant should make sure to provide for the safety of the prenatal patient while she is getting onto the examining table.

11. **Procedural Step.** Place the patient's chart in a convenient location for review by the physician. Inform the physician that the patient is ready to be examined.
Principle. Before going into the room, the physician will want to review the measurements taken by the medical assistant.

12. **Procedural Step.** Assist the patient into a supine position and properly drape her. Provide support and reassurance to the patient to help her relax during the examination.
Principle. The patient should be properly draped so that she is warm and comfortable.

13. **Procedural Step.** Assist the physician as required for the prenatal examination as follows:
a. Fundal Height Measurement: Hand the physician the tape measure for the determination of the fundal measurement.

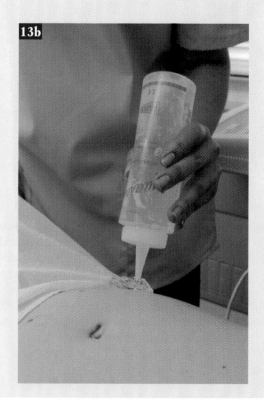

PROCEDURE 8-3

b. Fetal Heart Tones: Apply a liberal amount of coupling gel to the mother's abdomen. Turn on the Doppler fetal pulse detector and hand it to the physician. Once the physician is finished, remove excess gel from the patient with a paper towel. Clean the probe head of the Doppler device with a damp cloth and a mild detergent. Place the probe head back in its holder.

c. Vaginal Specimen: Assist the patient into the lithotomy position if a specimen is to be taken for the detection of a vaginal infection. Assist with the collection of the specimen as required.

d. Vaginal Examination: Assist the patient into the lithotomy position if a vaginal examination is to be performed.

14. Procedural Step. After the examination, assist the patient into a sitting position and allow her the opportunity to rest for a moment. If a vaginal examination was performed, offer the patient tissues to remove excess lubricating jelly from the perineum. Assist her off the examining table to prevent falls. Instruct the patient to get dressed.
Principle. The patient may become dizzy after being on the examining table and should be allowed to rest before getting off.

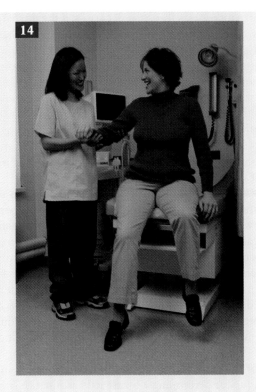

15. Procedural Step. Provide prenatal patient teaching and further explanation of the physician's instructions as required to meet individual patient needs.

16. Procedural Step. Clean the examining room in preparation for the next patient and, if necessary, prepare specimens for transport to an outside medical laboratory.

PROCEDURE 8-3

Six-Weeks-Postpartum Visit

The **puerperium** includes the period of time in which the body systems are returning to their prepregnant or nearly prepregnant state, which usually extends for 4 to 6 weeks after delivery. During this time numerous changes take place in the woman's body. The involution of the uterus (i.e., the process by which it returns to its normal size and state) occurs; this includes healing of any injuries sustained to the birth canal during delivery.

During the puerperium, the patient experiences a vaginal discharge shed from the lining of the uterus, known as **lochia.** Lochia consists of blood, tissue, white blood cells, mucus, and some bacteria. The color of the lochia is an indication of the progress of the healing of the uterus. For the first 3 days after delivery, the lochia

consists almost entirely of blood and because of its red color is termed *lochia rubra.* By approximately the fourth day postpartum, the amount of blood decreases and the discharge becomes pink or brownish and is known as *lochia serosa.* By the tenth day postpartum, the flow should decrease and the lochia should become yellowish-white; this is known as *lochia alba.* Lochia usually continues in consistently decreasing amounts (from moderate to scant to occasional spotting) and becomes more pale in color until the third week following delivery, when it usually disappears altogether. However, it would not be considered unusual for the discharge to last the entire 6 weeks.

The patient should be instructed to contact the medical office under the following circumstances: if the amount of discharge increases rather than decreases; if the discharge is absent within the first 2 weeks after delivery; if it changes to red after having been yellowish white, which indicates bleeding; or if it takes on a foul odor, which indicates infection. Menstruation usually begins approximately 2 months after delivery in the nonnursing mother and 3 to 6 months after delivery in the nursing mother.

During the puerperium the patient should be encouraged to avoid fatigue, to avoid lifting heavy objects, and to consume a nutritious, well-balanced diet that helps maintain health and promote healing.

The physician will want to see the patient at the medical office at the end of the 6-week period. The purpose of the 6-weeks-postpartum visit is to evaluate the general physical condition of the patient, to make sure there are no residual problems from childbearing, and to provide the patient with education regarding methods of birth control and infant care. During this visit the patient is queried about problems or abnormalities related to vaginal discharge, urinary or bowel function, and breast feeding if she is nursing. This information is recorded in the patient's chart. The postpartum visit provides an excellent opportunity for the medical assistant to instruct the patient in the technique for performing a breast self-examination and to educate her in the importance of returning to the medical office annually for a Pap test.

During the postpartal examination, the physician evaluates the patient's general appearance, performs breast and pelvic examinations, and checks to determine whether the muscle tone has returned to the muscles of the abdominal wall. During the puerperium, atypical cells may be sloughed off into the cervical and vaginal mucus as part of the normal healing process. Because of this, the Pap test is not included in the postpartum visit. If the patient has problems with hemorrhoids or varicosities, the physician discusses any further treatment required. If the patient does not have antibody protection to rubella, as has been evidenced through the prenatal laboratory tests, she receives rubella immunization at this time (if it was not administered in the hospital). In addition, hemoglobin and hematocrit determinations are usually performed on the postpartum patient to screen for anemia caused by blood loss during delivery and the puerperium.

The responsibilities of the medical assistant during the postpartum visit include measuring and recording the patient's vital signs and weight and preparing the patient for the examination. The patient is required to disrobe completely for this examination and to put on an examining gown with the opening in front. Table 8-4 lists the procedures commonly included in the 6-weeks-postpartum visit and the purpose of each.

TABLE 8-4	Six-Weeks-Postpartum Examination
Procedure	**Purpose**
Vital signs (Chapter 4) 　Temperature 　Pulse 　Respiration 　Blood pressure	To make sure the vital signs fall within normal limits and that the blood pressure has returned to its normal prepregnant level.
Weight (Chapter 5)	To determine whether the patient's weight has returned to its prepregnant measurement. If not, nutritional counseling may be indicated.
Breast examination (Chapter 8)	To make sure the breasts are not sore or tender and no cysts or lumps are present. In the nonnursing mother, the breasts will be examined to determine whether they have returned to their prepregnant size. In the nursing mother, the nipples will be examined for cracks, redness, soreness, and fissures.
Pelvic examination (Chapter 8)	To make sure involution of the uterus is complete and to determine whether the cervix has healed. To make sure the episiotomy (if performed) and any injuries sustained by the birth canal have healed. To make sure no abnormal vaginal discharge is present.
Rectal-vaginal examination (Chapter 8)	To make sure the pelvic floor has regained its muscle tone. To determine whether hemorrhoids are present.
Evaluation of the patient's general physical condition (Chapter 5)	To make sure the body systems have returned to their prepregnant state.

MEDICAL Practice and the LAW

Mature Minor

A difficult and complex issue facing policy makers today involves whether a minor should be able to obtain health care services without a parent's consent. A minor is an individual who has not reached the age of majority; in most states minors reach majority at 18 years of age (at that time, individuals are legally able to make their own decisions regarding health care).

Over the past three decades, many states have passed legislation permitting minors to receive some health care services without parental consent. These include contraceptive services, testing and treatment for sexually transmitted diseases, prenatal care and delivery services, treatment for alcohol and drug abuse, and outpatient mental health care. States that have passed such legislation reason that some minors might avoid seeking the care that they need for certain conditions if they had to have their parent's consent. The one major exception to this is abortion. Most states have laws that require the involvement of at least one parent in a minor's decision to have an abortion.

In recent years, some states have given minors even greater authority to make health care decisions for themselves by adopting what is known as the *mature minor rule.* This allows an individual in the middle to late teens who exhibits the intelligence and maturity to understand the nature and consequences of a medical treatment to consent to such treatment without parental consent.

It is important for the medical assistant to become familiar with the laws in his or her state regarding a minor's right to consent to health care. This will help in making appropriate decisions with respect to minors. For example, if a state does not allow a minor to obtain prenatal care without parental consent, the medical assistant would not be permitted to make an appointment for a minor who is pregnant; rather it would have to be scheduled by the minor's parent. Consent by minors to health care services will continue to be a complex issue; therefore the medical assistant must keep up-to-date with changes in his or her state.

What Would You DO?
What Would You *Not* DO? RESPONSES

Case Study 1

What Did Yin-Ling Do?

❑ Reassured Mrs. Wooster that the doctor is there to help her and stressed that he will be pleased that she has come to the office for an examination.

❑ Commended Mrs. Wooster on performing a breast self-examination at home and encouraged her to continue performing a BSE each month. Asked her if she had any questions on how to perform a BSE.

❑ Told Mrs. Wooster that some breast changes are normal and others are not normal, and the only way to know for sure is to be examined by the doctor.

❑ Told Mrs. Wooster that it is important to have a yearly examination even if her periods are normal. Explained to her that some conditions can be present without symptoms. Took plenty of time with her so she would feel comfortable coming back for a yearly examination.

❑ Gave Mrs. Wooster a patient information brochure on mammograms and explained the mammogram procedure to reduce her apprehension. Explained that the procedure is not painful, but there may be some minor discomfort. Provided

her with some tips on reducing discomfort that may occur, such as avoiding caffeine several days before the procedure and having the office schedule the mammogram a week after her menstrual period.

What Did Yin-Ling Not Do?

❑ Did not criticize Mrs. Wooster for waiting so long to schedule a GYN exam.

❑ Did not tell Mrs. Wooster that there is no discomfort involved with a mammogram.

What Would You Do?/What Would You *Not* Do? Review Yin-Ling's response and place a checkmark next to the information you included in your response. List additional information you included in your response below.

_____
_____
_____
_____

Continued

Case Study 2

What Did Yin-Ling Do?

❑ Stressed to Dagny how important it is that she be seen by the doctor. Explained that she could be infected with chlamydia and not know it because chlamydia often has no symptoms, especially in women.

❑ Explained to Dagny that state law allows her to be treated for a sexually transmitted disease without permission from her parents. Told her the law was created to encourage minors to seek treatment for STDs.

❑ Commended Dagny on practicing safe sex. Relayed to her that if a condom is not used correctly, or if it tears, she might not be protected from getting a sexually transmitted disease. That is another reason she should be tested.

❑ Explained to Dagny what will occur during the examination and what the doctor will be doing. Relayed techniques that Dagney could use to relax during the procedure.

What Did Yin-Ling Not Do?

❑ Did not tell Dagny everything would be all right and that she probably doesn't have chlamydia.

❑ Did not ask Dagny if she knew how her boyfriend got chlamydia.

❑ If Dagny still insisted on leaving, did not try to prevent her from doing so.

What Would You Do?/What Would You *Not* Do? Review Yin-Ling's response and place a checkmark next to the information you included in your response. List additional information you included in your response below.

_____

_____

_____

_____

Case Study 3

What Did Yin-Ling Do?

❑ Tried to calm Johanna by telling her that it is normal for her to be worried and concerned. Explained that the purpose of her prenatal visits are so that the doctor can keep a close watch on her and catch any problems that might occur.

❑ Reassured Johanna that she doesn't need to be afraid to tell the doctor any of her concerns because he is there to help her and her baby.

❑ Told Johanna that it is very important not to take any medications during her pregnancy without first checking with the doctor because some medications could be harmful to her baby.

❑ Told Johanna that her problems and concerns would be relayed to the doctor and that he would want to talk to her about them. Explained that the doctor would also talk with her about being tested for group B *streptococcus.*

What Did Yin-Ling Not Do?

❑ Did not tell Johanna that it was all right to take the antibiotics.

What Would You Do?/What Would You *Not* Do? Review Yin-Ling's response and place a checkmark next to the information you included in your response. List additional information you included in your response below.

_____

_____

_____

_____

Case Study 4

What Did Yin-Ling Do?

❑ Escorted Mr. and Mrs. Lopez to a private room in the office. Tried to relax them and told them that whatever they choose to do will be the right decision for them. Reassured them that they could stay at the office for as long as they wanted.

❑ Gave Mrs. Lopez the information she requested that was available at the office and provided her with a list of resources approved by the physician that she could contact for further information.

❑ Asked Mr. and Mrs. Lopez if they had any more questions they wanted to ask the doctor.

What Did Yin-Ling Not Do?

❑ Did not give Mr. and Mrs. Lopez advice on what they should do.

What Would You Do?/What Would You *Not* Do? Review Yin-Ling's response and place a checkmark next to the information you included in your response. List additional information you included in your response below.

_____

_____

_____

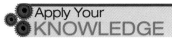

Apply Your KNOWLEDGE

Choose the best answer for the following questions.

Gynecology

1. Ashley Jacobs is 24 years old and has come to the office for her first GYN examination. While taking her medical history, Yin-Ling Wu, RMA, obtains the following information. Which of these puts Ashley at an increased risk for breast cancer?
   A. She is taking birth control pills
   B. She started her periods at age 13
   C. Her older sister has breast cancer
   D. She has irregular periods and dysmenorrhea

2. Yin-Ling helps Ashley into the lithotomy position for the pelvic examination. All of the following should be done when placing a patient in this position EXCEPT:
   A. Positioning the stirrups so they are level with the examining table
   B. Pulling the stirrups out 1 foot from the table
   C. Positioning the patient's buttocks 10 inches from the edge of the table
   D. Making sure the patient's knees are bent and relaxed

3. Since Ashley is having a ThinPrep Pap test done, Yin-Ling prepares the disposable plastic vaginal speculum by:
   A. Lightly spraying it with a cytology fixative
   B. Lubricating it with KY jelly
   C. Polishing it with Windex
   D. Moistening it with warm water

4. Miss Jacobs asks Yin-Ling why a Pap test is being performed. Yin-Ling tells her:
   A. To diagnose vaginal infections
   B. For the early detection of cervical cancer
   C. To evaluate the cause of infertility
   D. For the early detection of ovarian cancer

5. After the GYN examination, Yin-Ling instructs Ashley on how to perform a breast self-examination. Yin-Ling explains to her that she should perform a BSE once a month:
   A. Any day during the month
   B. Approximately 2 to 3 days after the start of her menstrual period
   C. Approximately 2 to 3 days after her menstrual period ends
   D. On the day she receives her electric bill

6. Rachel Purdy comes to the office with the symptoms of a yeast infection. Yin-Ling Wu, RMA, is assembling the supplies that will be needed to prepare a vaginal specimen for the microscopic examination of candidiasis. She will need to have ready:
   A. A slide and normal saline
   B. A live turkey
   C. A collection and transport tube
   D. A slide and a 10% KOH solution

7. Mrs. Purdy has been diagnosed with candidiasis. Dr. Papanicolaou writes a prescription for Mrs. Purdy to treat her condition. A drug used to treat this vaginal infection is:
   A. Miconazole (Monistat)
   B. Azithromycin (Zithromax)
   C. Penicillin (Amoxil)
   D. Metronidazole (Flagyl)

Prenatal

1. Amanda Delaney, who is 33 years old, has come to the office for her first prenatal visit. Amanda asks Yin-Ling Wu, RMA, what is going to happen during the visit. Yin-Ling would relay all of the following EXCEPT:
   A. Measurement of vital signs and weight
   B. Breast and pelvic examination
   C. Transabdominal ultrasound scan
   D. Measurement of fundal height

2. Yin-Ling obtains information from Amanda for the prenatal record. Amanda has been pregnant before and has a 6-year-old daughter. During the interview, Amanda relays the following information to Yin-Ling. Which statement does NOT provide information for the Obstetric History?
   A. "My daughter weighed 6 pounds and 8 ounces at birth"
   B. "My daughter was born 3 weeks early"
   C. "I was in labor for 8 hours with my daughter"
   D. "I breastfed my daughter for 6 months"

Continued

3. After the prenatal examination, Amanda asks to talk with Yin-Ling in private. She tells Yin-Ling that she is upset that she is being tested for gonorrhea. She says that she has been happily married for 12 years and can't understand why the doctor would think she has gonorrhea. Which of the following is the best response to help calm down Amanda?
   A. "You may have contracted gonorrhea without knowing it, from a toilet seat in a public restroom"
   B. "Gonorrhea can cause a serious eye infection in the newborn, which could lead to blindness"
   C. "You may be happily married, but we don't know if the same is true for your husband"
   D. "There is a state law that says we have to test all pregnant women for gonorrhea"

4. While proofreading the prenatal testing schedule just typed by the medical transcriber, Yin-Ling Wu, RMA, notices a mistake in the schedule. Which of the following should she ask the transcriber to correct?
   A. Endovaginal Ultrasound: 7 to 13 weeks
   B. Triple Screen Test: 15 to 20 weeks
   C. 1-hour GTT: 18 to 24 weeks
   D. GBS Test: 35 to 37 weeks

5. Amanda Delaney has come to the office for a return prenatal visit. She is now 4 months pregnant. The responsibilities of Yin-Ling Wu, RMA, during this visit include all of the following EXCEPT:
   A. Documenting any problems Amanda has experienced since the last visit
   B. Testing Amanda's urine specimen for glucose and protein
   C. Measuring Amanda's weight and blood pressure
   D. Placing Amanda in the lithotomy position for a vaginal exam

6. During Amanda's prenatal visit, Dr. Braxton listens for fetal heart tones using a Doppler device. He determines the fetal heart rate to be 145. What does this indicate?
   A. The heart rate is too fast; the fetus may be in distress
   B. The heart rate is within normal limits
   C. The heart rate is too slow; the fetus may not be receiving enough oxygen
   D. The baby is going to have red hair

7. Amanda is scheduled to have a transabdominal ultrasound scan performed at her next prenatal visit. Which of the following should Yin-Ling relay to Amanda regarding this exam?
   A. You need to drink 32 ounces of fluid 1 hour before the scan
   B. You may have some spotting following the scan
   C. You need to fast for 12 hours before the scan
   D. You will find out if the baby is a boy or girl

8. Amanda delivers a healthy 8-pound, 3-ounce baby boy on her due date. Toward the end of her pregnancy, Yin-Ling Wu, RMA, talked with Amanda regarding instructions on postpartum care. Which of the following instructions would Yin-Ling NOT have included in the discussion?
   A. Call the office if you have an increase in the amount of vaginal discharge
   B. Make an appointment to come in 6 weeks after delivery
   C. Do not use any type of birth control
   D. Eat nutritiously and rest as much as possible

CERTIFICATIONREVIEW

❑ **Gynecology** is the branch of medicine that deals with diseases of women' reproductive organs. A gynecologic examination includes breast and pelvic examinations. The purpose of the examination is to assess the health status of the female reproductive organs and to detect early signs of disease, leading to early diagnosis and treatment.

❑ **During the breast examination,** the physician inspects the breasts and nipples for swelling, dimpling, puckering, and change in skin texture. The nipples are checked for abnormalities and the breasts and axial lymph nodes are palpated for lumps. Women should perform a breast self-examination at home each month starting at age 20, approximately 2 to 3 days after the menstrual period ends.

❑ **The purpose of the pelvic examination** is to assess the size, shape, and location of the reproductive organs and to detect the presence of disease. The pelvic examination consists of an inspection of the external genitalia, vagina, and cervix; collection of a specimen for a Pap test; bimanual pelvic examination; and a rectal-vaginal examination.

❑ **The purpose of the Pap test** is early detection and treatment of cervical cancer. It is also used to detect abnormal cells that might develop into cancer if not treated. Abnormal cytologic findings on the Pap test indicate the need for further tests such as colposcopy, cervical biopsy, and endocervical curettage.

❑ **The purpose of the bimanual pelvic examination** is to determine the size, shape, and position of the uterus and ovaries and detect tenderness or lumps. The purpose of the rectal-vaginal examination is to obtain information about the tone and alignment of the pelvic organs and the adnexal region and to collect a fecal specimen for occult blood testing. The presence of hemorrhoids, fistulas, and fissures can also be noted during this examination.

❑ **Trichomoniasis** is a vaginal infection caused by a protozoan and is most commonly spread through sexual intercourse. Symptoms include a profuse, frothy, yellowish-green vaginal discharge with an unpleasant odor, itching and irritation of the vulva and vagina, and dysuria. The cervix may exhibit small red spots; this is known as "strawberry cervix."

❑ **Candidiasis** is a vaginal infection caused by a yeastlike fungus. Conditions such as pregnancy, diabetes mellitus, and prolonged antibiotic therapy may precipitate a candidal infection, commonly referred to as a yeast infection. Symptoms of candidiasis include white patches on the mucous membrane of the vagina, along with a thick, odorless cottage cheese–like discharge that results in burning and intense itching.

❑ **Chlamydia** is caused by a bacterium and is the most frequently reported and fastest spreading STD in the United States. Most women with chlamydia have no symptoms. Women with symptoms have dysuria; itching and irritation of the genital area; an odorless thick, yellowish-white vaginal discharge; dull abdominal pain; and bleeding between menstrual periods. If not treated, chlamydia can lead to PID, which can result in infertility.

❑ **Gonorrhea** is an infection of the genitourinary tract and is caused by a bacterium that is transmitted through sexual intercourse. Women who have contracted gonorrhea may be asymptomatic or may exhibit dysuria and a yellow vaginal discharge. As the disease progresses, it may spread to the lining of the uterus, resulting in PID.

❑ **Obstetrics** is the branch of medicine that deals with the supervision of women during pregnancy, childbirth, and the puerperium. Prenatal refers to the care of the pregnant woman before delivery of the infant to promote health of both mother and fetus through the prevention of disease and early detection, diagnosis, and treatment of problems common to pregnancy.

❑ **The first prenatal examination** consists of the completion of a prenatal record form, an initial prenatal examination, prenatal patient education, and laboratory tests.

❑ **The prenatal record** provides information regarding the past and present health of the patient and also serves as a data base and flow sheet for subsequent prenatal visits. The past medical history focuses on conditions that could affect the health of the mother and fetus. The menstrual history provides information on the patient's menstrual cycle. The obstetric history provides information from the patient related to previous pregnancies. The present pregnancy history establishes a baseline for the present health status of the patient. The purpose of the interval prenatal history is to update the prenatal record at each return visit.

❑ **The expected date of delivery (EDD)** can be determined using Nägele's rule and a gestation calculator. Approximately 4% of patients deliver spontaneously on the EDD, and the majority of patients deliver during the period from 7 days before to 7 days after the EDD.

❑ **The purpose of the initial prenatal examination** is to confirm the pregnancy and to establish a baseline for the woman's state of health. It includes a thorough gynecologic examination (breast and pelvic) and a general physical examination of the other body systems.

Continued

CERTIFICATIONREVIEW—Cont'd

❏ **A number of laboratory tests** are ordered to assist in the overall initial assessment of the patient's health and to detect problems that might put the pregnancy at risk. Prenatal laboratory tests that are performed include a complete urinalysis, Pap test, chlamydia and gonorrhea tests, tests for trichomoniasis and candidiasis (if warranted), group B streptococcus tests, complete blood count, Rh factor and ABO blood type, glucose challenge test, serology test for syphilis, rubella antibody titer, Rh antibody titer, hepatitis B test, and HIV test.

❏ **Return prenatal visits** provide the opportunity for a continuous assessment of the health of both mother and fetus. During the return visit the physician performs one or more of the following procedures: palpation of the woman's abdomen to measure fundal height, measurement of the fetal heart rate, and a vaginal examination.

❏ **The triple screen test** is performed between 15 and 20 weeks of pregnancy to screen for certain fetal abnormalities. Abnormal test results may indicate the possibility of a neural tube defect, Down syndrome, trisomy 18, and ventral wall defect.

❏ **Obstetric ultrasound scanning** is used to view the fetus in utero. It is used most frequently to evaluate the health of the fetus and to determine gestational age. There are two methods for performing an ultrasound scan based on gestational age: endovaginal scan (up to 12 weeks) and the transabdominal scan (after 12 weeks).

❏ **Amniocentesis** is performed to diagnose certain genetically transmitted errors of metabolism, congenital abnormalities, and chromosomal disorders such as Down syndrome. Fetal heart rate monitoring is performed to obtain information on the physical condition of the fetus.

❏ **The puerperium** includes the period of time in which the body systems are returning to the prepregnant or nearly prepregnant state, which usually extends for 4 to 6 weeks after delivery. The physician will want to see the patient at the medical office at the end of the 6-week period. The purpose of this postpartum visit is to evaluate the general physical condition of the patient, to make sure there are no residual problems from childbearing, and to provide the patient with education regarding methods of birth control and infant care.

Terminology Review

Abortion The termination of the pregnancy before the fetus reached the age of viability.

Adnexal Adjacent.

Amenorrhea The absence or cessation of the menstrual period. Amenorrhea occurs normally before puberty, during pregnancy, and after menopause.

Atypical Deviation from the normal.

Braxton Hicks contractions Intermittent and irregular painless uterine contractions that occur throughout pregnancy. They occur more frequently toward the end of pregnancy and are sometimes mistaken for true labor pains.

Cervix The lower narrow end of the uterus that opens into the vagina.

Colposcopy Examination of the cervix using a colposcope (a lighted instrument with a magnifying lens).

Cytology The science that deals with the study of cells, including their origin, structure, function, and pathology.

Dilation (of the cervix) The stretching of the external os from an opening a few millimeters wide to an opening large enough to allow the passage of an infant (approximately 10 cm).

Dysmenorrhea Pain associated with the menstrual period.

Dyspareunia Pain in the vagina or pelvis experienced by a woman during sexual intercourse.

Dysplasia The growth of abnormal cells. Dysplasia is a precancerous condition that may or may not develop into cancer.

EDD Expected date of delivery, or due date.

Effacement The thinning and shortening of the cervical canal from its normal length of 1 to 2 cm to a structure with paper-thin edges in which there is no canal at all. Effacement occurs late in pregnancy or during labor, or both. The purpose of effacement along with dilation is to permit the passage of the infant into the birth canal.

Embryo The child in utero from the time of conception to the beginning of the first trimester.

Endocervix The mucous membrane lining the cervical canal.

Engagement The entrance of the fetal head or the presenting part into the pelvic inlet.

External os The opening of the cervical canal of the uterus into the vagina.

Fetal heart rate (FHR) The number of times per minute the fetal heart beats.

Fetal heart tones (FHT) The sounds of the heartbeat of the fetus heard through the mother's abdominal wall.

Fetus The child in utero from the third month after conception to birth; during the first 2 months of development, it is called an embryo.

Fundus The dome-shaped upper portion of the uterus between the fallopian tubes.

Gestation The period of intrauterine development from conception to birth; the period of pregnancy. The average pregnancy lasts about 280 days, or 40 weeks, from the date of conception to childbirth.

Gestational age The age of the fetus between conception and birth.

Gravidity The total number of pregnancies a woman has had regardless of duration, including a current pregnancy.

Gynecology The branch of medicine that deals with the diseases of reproductive organs of women.

Infant A child from birth to 12 months of age.

Internal os The internal opening of the cervical canal into the uterus.

Lochia A discharge from the uterus after delivery that consists of blood, tissue, white blood cells, and some bacteria.

Menopause The permanent cessation of menstruation, which usually occurs between the ages of 35 and 58.

Menorrhagia Excessive bleeding during a menstrual period, in the number of days or the amount of blood or both. Also called dysfunction uterine bleeding (DUB).

Metrorrhagia Bleeding between menstrual periods.

Multigravida A woman who has been pregnant more than once.

Multipara A woman who has completed two or more pregnancies to the age of fetal viability regardless of whether they ended in live infants or stillbirths.

Nullipara A woman who has not carried a pregnancy to the point of fetal viability (20 weeks of gestation).

Obstetrics The branch of medicine concerned with the care of the woman during pregnancy, childbirth, and the postpartal period.

Parity The condition of having borne offspring regardless of the outcome.

Perimenopause Before the onset of menopause, the phase during which the woman with regular periods changes to irregular cycles and increased periods of amenorrhea.

Perineum The external region between the vaginal orifice and the anus in a female and between the scrotum and the anus in a male.

Position The relation of the presenting part of the fetus to the maternal pelvis.

Postpartum Occurring after childbirth.

Preeclampsia A major complication of pregnancy, the cause of which is unknown, characterized by increasing hypertension, albuminuria, and edema. If this condition is neglected or not treated properly, it may develop into eclampsia, which could cause maternal convulsions and coma. Preeclampsia generally occurs between the twentieth week of pregnancy and the end of the first week postpartum.

Prenatal Before birth.

Presentation Indication of the part of the fetus that is closest to the cervix and will be delivered first. A cephalic presentation is a delivery in which the fetal head is presenting against the cervix. A breech presentation is a delivery in which the buttocks or feet are presented instead of the head.

Preterm birth Delivery occurring between 20 and 37 weeks regardless of whether the child was born alive or stillborn.

Terminology Review—cont'd

Primigravida A woman who is pregnant for the first time.

Primipara A woman who has carried a pregnancy to fetal viability (20 weeks of gestation) for the first time, regardless of whether the infant was stillborn or alive at birth.

Puerperium The period of time, usually 4 to 6 weeks after delivery, in which the uterus and the body systems are returning to normal.

Quickening The first movements of the fetus in utero as felt by the mother, which usually occurs between the sixteenth and twentieth weeks of gestation and is felt consistently thereafter.

Risk factor Anything that increases an individual's chance of developing a disease. Some risk factors (e.g., smoking) can be avoided, but others cannot (e.g., age and family history).

Term birth Delivery occurring after 37 weeks regardless of whether the child was born alive or stillborn.

Toxemia A condition that can occur in pregnant women that includes preeclampsia and eclampsia. If preeclampsia goes undiagnosed or is not satisfactorily controlled, it could develop into eclampsia, characterized by convulsions and coma.

Trimester Three months, or one third, of the gestational period of pregnancy.

Vulva The region of the external female genital organs.

ON THE WEB

For active weblinks to each website visit http://evolve.elsevier.com/Bonewit/.

For Information on Sexually Transmitted Diseases:

National Institute of Allergy and Infectious Diseases

Centers for Disease Control Division of Sexually Transmitted Diseases
(located under Disease Facts and Information)

Planned Parenthood

American Social Health Association

Herpes Information

HPV Information

For Information on Women's Health:

The National Women's Health Information Center

The Universe of Women's Health

Female Health Today

For Information on Contraceptives:

Planned Parenthood

Ultimate Birth Control Links

Reproductive Health Online

For Information on Menopause:

North American Menopause Society

Menopause Online

For Information on Pregnancy and Childbirth:

Childbirth

StorkNet's Pregnancy Guide

Lamaze International

LaLeche League

Learning Objectives	Procedures
Pediatric Office Visits	
1. List the components of the well-child visit.	Carry an infant using the following positions:
2. State the usual schedule for well-child visits.	▪ Cradle
3. Explain the purpose of the sick-child visit.	▪ Upright
4. List the procedures performed by the medical assistant during pediatric office visits.	
5. Explain why it is important to develop a rapport with the pediatric patient.	
Growth Measurements	
1. State the importance of measuring the child's weight, height (or length), and head circumference during each office visit.	Plot pediatric growth values on a growth chart. Measure the weight and length of an infant. Measure the head and chest circumference of an infant.
2. State the functions served by a growth chart.	
Pediatric Blood Pressure Measurement	
1. State the importance of measuring a child's blood pressure.	Measure the blood pressure of a child.
2. List the three factors that determine if a child has hypertension.	
Collection of a Urine Specimen	
List the reasons for collecting a urine specimen from a child.	Collect a urine specimen using a pediatric urine collector.
Pediatric Injections	
1. State the range for the gauge and length of needles used for IM and SC pediatric injections.	Locate the following pediatric IM injection sites: ▪ Dorsogluteal
2. Explain the use of each of the following pediatric injection sites: dorsogluteal, vastus lateralis, and deltoid.	▪ Vastus lateralis ▪ Deltoid Administer an intramuscular injection to an infant. Administer a subcutaneous injection to an infant.
Immunizations	
1. Describe the schedule for immunization of infants and children recommended by the American Academy of Pediatrics.	Read and interpret a vaccine information statement. Record information on a pediatric vaccine administration record.
2. State the information that must be provided to parents as required by the NCVIA.	
3. List the information that must be recorded in the medical record after administering an immunization.	
Newborn Screening Test	
1. Explain the purpose of a newborn screening test.	Collect a specimen for a newborn screening test.
2. List the symptoms of PKU.	
3. State what occurs if PKU is left untreated.	

CHAPTER 9

The Pediatric Examination

Chapter Outline

INTRODUCTION TO THE PEDIATRIC EXAMINATION
PEDIATRIC OFFICE VISITS
Developing Rapport
Carrying the Infant
Growth Measurements
  Weight
  Length and Height
  Head and Chest Circumference
  Growth Charts
Pediatric Blood Pressure Measurement
  Special Guidelines for Children
  Correct Cuff Size
  Cooperation of the Child
  Blood Pressure Classifications
Collection of a Urine Specimen
Pediatric Injections
  Type of Needle
  Intramuscular Injection Sites
Immunizations
  National Childhood Vaccine Injury Act
Newborn Screening Test

National Competencies

Clinical Competencies
Patient Care
- Prepare and maintain examination and treatment areas.
- Prepare patient for and assist with routine and specialty examinations.
- Prepare patient for and assist with procedures, treatments, and minor office surgeries.
- Maintain medication and immunization records.

General Competencies
Patient Instruction
- Instruct individuals according to their needs.
- Provide instruction for health maintenance and disease prevention.

Key Terms

adolescent

immunity (ih-MYOO-nih-tee)

immunization (IM-yoo-nih-ZAY-shun)

infant

length

pediatrician (PEE-dee-uh-TRIH-shun)

pediatrics (pee-dee-AT-riks)

preschooler (PREE-skool-er)

school-age child

toddler (TOD-ler)

toxoid (TOKS-oid)

vaccine (vak-SEEN)

vertex (VER-teks)

Introduction to the Pediatric Examination

Pediatrics is the branch of medicine that deals with the care and development of children and the diagnosis and treatment of diseases in children. A **pediatrician** is a medical doctor who specializes in pediatrics. Many physicians in general practice also handle pediatric patients. It is essential that the medical assistant develop the skills needed to assist the physician in the care and treatment of children.

PEDIATRIC OFFICE VISITS

There are two broad categories of pediatric patient office visits. The first is the *well-child visit* (also termed health maintenance visit), in which the physician progressively evaluates the growth and development of the child. A physical examination is performed during each well-child visit and is directed toward discovering any abnormal conditions commonly associated with the stage of development reached by the child. See Table 9-1 for an outline of normal development during infancy. The child will also receive necessary immunizations during these visits.

Another important component of the well-child visit is anticipatory guidance. *Anticipatory guidance* is the process of providing parents with information to prepare them for anticipated developmental events and to assist them in promoting their children's well-being (Table 9-2). Topics that are commonly included are safety, nutrition, sleep, play, exercise, development, and discipline. See Table 9-3 for a presentation of child safety guidelines by age group.

The interval between well-child visits depends on the medical office, but it frequently follows this schedule after birth: 1 month, 2 months, 4 months, 6 months, 9 months, 12 months, 15 months, 18 months, 24 months, and yearly thereafter.

The second category of pediatric patient office visits is the *sick child visit*. The child is exhibiting the signs and symptoms of disease, and the physician evaluates the patient's condition to arrive at a diagnosis and to prescribe treatment.

During both well-child and sick child visits, the medical assistant performs many of the same procedures that have been presented in previous chapters (e.g., measurement of temperature, pulse, respiration and blood pressure; measurement of weight and height; measurement of visual acuity; and assisting with the physical examination). Procedures specifically related to the pediatric patient and variations in procedures previously presented are discussed in this chapter.

Text continued on p. 340

TABLE 9-1	Milestones of Gross and Fine Motor Development in Infancy	
Average Age (Mo)	**Gross Motor**	**Fine Motor**
1	Turns head from side to side	Grasping reflex present
2	Holds head at 45-degree angle when prone	Holds rattle briefly
3	Begins rolling over	Grasps rattle or dangling objects
4	Slight head lag when pulled to sitting position	Brings objects to mouth
5	No head wobble when held in sitting position	Transfers objects from hand to hand
6	Sits without support	Manipulates and examines large objects with hands
7	Stands while holding on	Reaches for, grabs, and retains object
8	Pulls self to stand	Grasps objects with thumb and finger
9	Crawls backwards	Begins to show hand preference
10	Creeps on hands and knees	Hits cup with spoon
11	Walks using furniture for support	Picks up small objects with thumb and forefinger (pincer grasp)
12	Stands alone easily	Puts three or more objects into a container
12-16	Walks alone easily	Turns two or three pages in a large cardboard book

From Leahy JM, and Kizilay PE: *Foundations of nursing practice,* Philadelphia, 1998, Saunders.

TABLE 9-2	Anticipatory Guidance	
ANTICIPATORY GUIDANCE IN INFANCY		
Issue	**Rationale**	**Guidance**
Thumb sucking and pacifiers	Sucking is a major pleasure for the infant. Benefits such as decreased crying and increased relaxation have been identified by meeting the infant's need for nonnutritive sucking. Infants generally find their fingers or hands to suck on to meet this need without a pacifier. As the need for nonnutritive sucking decreases, so does the need for the pacifier or thumb, unless their use is treated as reinforcement by parents to relieve infant distress.	Explore parents' feelings regarding the infant's need for a pacifier. If pacifiers are to be used, review safety considerations (e.g., preferably constructed in one piece, have a flange with at least two ventilation holes and large enough to prevent aspiration; remove from infant when not in use; never secure to infant by tying with a cord around the neck). Thumb sucking is generally abandoned by the age when dental problems may become an issue (when permanent teeth erupt). If a pacifier is used, try removing it around 6 mo old, when the infant is not yet old enough to remember or miss it for long. If pacifiers are used beyond the first year, unless you are meticulous about sterilizing them they can be very unhygienic as the child toddles around with them; this is a good reason to discontinue pacifier use.

From Leahy, JM, and Kizilay, PE: *Foundations of Nursing Practice,* Philadelphia, 1998, Saunders.

Continued

TABLE 9-2	Anticipatory Guidance—cont'd	
ANTICIPATORY GUIDANCE IN INFANCY		
Issue	**Rationale**	**Guidance**
Teething	Teething seldom causes discomfort in an infant younger than 4 mo. At 5 or 6 mo, as the first tooth emerges, drooling, chewing on hard objects, and some irritability may accompany the minor inflammation of the gums. Most discomfort is felt by the infant with the eruption of the first molars at age 12 to 15 mo.	Believing that an infant younger than 4 mo of age is irritable for long periods because of "teething" may cause a parent to neglect a real illness. Medical attention should be sought for any infant experiencing fever, diarrhea, vomiting, or loss of appetite; these are not symptoms of teething. Avoid teething gels because they contain anesthetics that may cause untoward effects in the infant if overused. Provide something cold to bite on (e.g., a frozen gel-filled teething ring).
Separation and stranger fear	Around 8 mo, infants have sufficient capacity to recognize their primary caregivers and find comfort in their presence. Because they have not yet developed the task of object permanence, infants experience great displeasure when their caregivers leave them alone or with an unfamiliar substitute. This behavior may continue into toddlerhood.	Accustom the infant to new persons, especially those that may be called on to babysit (the more frequent the exposure, the less likely the fear). Give infants opportunities to explore strangers at their own pace to allow a "warm-up" of adjustment. Talk to infants when leaving them and greet them when you return. This can aid the development of object permanence and reassure them that you will always return. Use a transitional object (e.g., your scarf, a toy) to reassure them of your continued presence.
Spoiling and limit setting	When infants' needs are not promptly met, they become anxious, quick to fuss or cry, and slow to accept comfort; therefore the less you meet the infants' needs, the more demanding they become. As infants become more mobile toward the latter half of the first year, parents need to set limits to provide for their safety; however, there is no substitute for vigilant parental monitoring.	Prompt attention to the crying infant often is greeted by the infant's smile and comfort. Delaying attention to the crying infant leads to an encounter with a miserably distressed infant who does not settle down easily, has a stomach full of air from excessive crying, and will most likely start crying again before long. Set limits for older infant through consistent and age-appropriate methods. A negative voice and stern eye-to-eye contact may be all that is needed. A quiet period for the infant in the playpen may be warranted. Parents who express concern about disciplining an infant stage should recognize that the earlier it is started, the easier it is to maintain throughout childhood.

From Leahy, JM, and Kizilay, PE: *Foundations of Nursing Practice,* Philadelphia, 1998, Saunders.

TABLE 9-2	Anticipatory Guidance—cont'd

ANTICIPATORY GUIDANCE IN INFANCY

Issue	Rationale	Guidance
Injury prevention	Unintentional injury is the second leading cause of death in infancy. Common risks associated with this developmental stage include: Choking or suffocation Falls Motor vehicle crash injuries Burns	Parents and caregivers should know CPR, especially techniques for infants and children. Parents should review the home and environmental safety checklist.
Crying and colic	Colicky infants are those who cry for long periods (>3 hr daily) with legs drawn up. Colic has no known cause but has been associated with intolerance to cow's milk formula or ingestion of milk products by breast-feeding mothers and passive smoking. As infants cry, they swallow more air, distend the abdomen, cry some more, and pass flatus, and the cycle continues. Periods of crying up to 2 hr per day are a normal part of the infant's temperament.	Reassurance should be given to parents that the crying is a release of energy for the infant. Parents should always initially respond to the infant's cry to determine the cause. When no cause for the crying episodes can be identified, time of onset should be noted; successful responses to the infant are changing position, massaging the abdomen, swaddling in blanket, taking for car ride, or placing the infant in wind-up swing. Continued long periods of crying should be reported to the health care provider. Avoid smoking near the infant. Provide small frequent feedings; burp during and after feeding; have the infant sit upright for half an hour after feeding.

ANTICIPATORY GUIDANCE IN TODDLERHOOD

Issue	Rationale	Guidance
Toilet training	The ability to control elimination requires muscular maturation and cognitive maturity. The toddler needs to understand instructions and the purpose of this task for which there is no tangible reward other than that of "pleasing" a caregiver. 84% of 3-year-olds are dry throughout the day, and 66%, throughout the night.	Most parents initiate toilet training between 20 and 24 mo. Parents should be informed that "successful" toilet training at a very early age is usually because the parent is "trained" to recognize the child's readiness and places the child on the potty at the appropriate time. Teach parents to record the toddler's pattern and signals of elimination for several weeks prior to starting. Have parents obtain a sturdy potty chair, if possible, so the child can independently sit and get up, or a sturdy step stool to access toilet with adult supervision. Have parents dress child in loose clothing to aid access and prevent accidents. Inform parents that when the child signals that a bowel movement or voiding may be on the way, they should casually suggest to the child that he or she may want to sit on the potty.

Continued

TABLE 9-2	Anticipatory Guidance—cont'd	
ANTICIPATORY GUIDANCE IN TODDLERHOOD—cont'd		
Issue	**Rationale**	**Guidance**
Toilet training—cont'd		Encourage parents not to force the child to sit on the potty or to show disappointment if attempts are unsuccessful. Explain to parents that accidents will happen and will need to be taken in stride. Nagging and punishing a child for being uncooperative or for having "accidents" will mean certain failure; the toddler will become overwhelmed and confused about what is expected.
Temper tantrums	Temper tantrums are common toward the end of the second year. Tantrums are the result of excessive frustration; for example, when a child becomes overwhelmed with emotion and feelings of tension, an explosive outburst is a means of release. Tantrums often involve screaming, thrashing, and breath-holding spells.	Parents should be taught that a temper tantrum is like an "emotional blown fuse," which is not something that the toddler can control. Parents need to recognize a balance between a frustration level that their child can tolerate and that is useful for learning and the amount of frustration that will cause the fuse to blow. During a tantrum, a parent should be instructed to protect child from harm but not to overpower him or her because this physical restriction may heighten the anger. Reassure parents that breath-holding spells, although alarming to watch, do not result in physical harm. The body's natural reflex to breathe will allow the child to take in air before damage can occur.
Stress, anxiety, and fear	Toddlers live on an emotional see-saw, with most of the stress and tears arising from the basic contradiction of wanting to be independent and to be protected and loved by their caregivers. Toddlers need a balance of autonomy yet protection from separation anxiety. A toddler feels anxious when his or her feelings become uncontrollable, leading to crying or temper tantrums.	Inform parents to recognize cues from the toddler that indicates an impending problem (e.g., excessive clinginess, less adventurous behavior, increased shyness). Instruct parents to offer more affection, attention, and protection for several days until the toddler regains a normal sense of independence and adventure.
Bedtime struggles	As many as 50% of children between the ages of 1 and 2 yr engage in fussing or bedtime struggles lasting for more than an hour. Sometimes these struggles are associated with family stress, such as illness or change in normal routines.	Inform parents that they are not alone with this struggle—it is very common. Inform parents that if they continue to coddle, rock, or nurse their toddlers to sleep at this age, it will be harder to institute a different bedtime routine. Instruct parents to alter the routine by providing about 20 min of sedentary activity, such as quiet conversation or storytelling.

From Leahy, JM, and Kizilay, PE: *Foundations of Nursing Practice*, Philadelphia, 1998, Saunders.

TABLE 9-2	Anticipatory Guidance—cont'd		
	ANTICIPATORY GUIDANCE IN TODDLERHOOD—cont'd		
Issue	**Rationale**		**Guidance**
Bedtime struggles—cont'd	Most struggles are caused by continued infancy routines of "being put to sleep" by nursing, rocking, or coddling.		Have parents keep a night light on if it makes the child more comfortable. Tell parents to finish their sedentary time with a pleasant "goodnight," and if child begins to cry and continues for several minutes, they should go back in the room, repeat "goodnight" and leave again; this performance should be repeated every few minutes for as long as it takes toddler to settle down. Any sleep problem that persists over several months should be referred to the child's health care provider.
Unintentional injuries	Unintentional injury is the leading cause of death and disability in toddlerhood. Toddlers are especially vulnerable to unintentional injuries because of their activity level, developing motor skills, and inability to perceive dangerous situations. Common risks associated with this developmental stage include: Drowning Burns or scalds Motor vehicle injuries Falls Poisoning		Parents and caregivers should know CPR. Home and environmental safety checklist should be reviewed with parents and caregivers. Reinforce with parents and caregivers the importance of vigilant child monitoring and supervision during this highly vulnerable developmental stage.
Play activities	Play is the "work" of the young; it helps children to use their muscles and gain mastery over what they think, see, and do—a form of learning. Pretending or imaginative play emerges during this period—the toddler reenacts past experiences through retained mental pictures of things seen or heard; for example, a little boy might dip a sock in the dog's water bowl and use it to clean his toy truck after having observed his father wash the car a month ago.		Inform parents that providing a safe place, safe toys or play equipment, and time is all that is needed to promote healthy play by toddlers. If the toddler gets frustrated, the toys or activities may be too advanced, or he or she may be asking for assistance or guidance. Boredom will ensue if the play space and the activities are not varied from time to time. Inform parents that toys need not be expensive; children at this age are content to play with household objects, such as plastic bowls and wooden spoons. Instruct parents to be responsible consumers: when purchasing toys, they should (1) inspect them for small pieces or loose parts that may present a choking hazard, (2) determine if they are appropriate for their child's age, and (3) not sacrifice safety and quality for price.

Continued

TABLE 9-2 Anticipatory Guidance—cont'd

ANTICIPATORY GUIDANCE FOR THE PRESCHOOL CHILD

Issue	Rationale	Guidance
Aggression	A hostile act may be intended to hurt somebody or to establish dominance and is usually triggered by the social conflicts that arise during cooperative play. Children between 2 and 5 yr old who fight the most tend to be the most sociable and competent. A decline in physical aggression is often accompanied by an increase in verbal aggression, usually in the form of name calling. Even in a normal child, aggression can get out of hand and become dangerous. Since the 1950s, research has correlated televised violence with children's aggressive behavior.	Parents can often reduce aggressive tendencies by the way they act or react to the situation. Teach parents to deal with misbehavior by reasoning with the child, reinforcing good behavior, and being consistent in their approach to discipline. Spanking causes a child to suffer frustration, pain, and humiliation, and it is poor role modeling—the child sees hitting as an acceptable solution to a problem. Encourage parents to monitor their child's television viewing by limiting time allowed for viewing and selecting shows that are educational and prosocial.
Fearfulness	Preschoolers have an inability to distinguish "pretend" from reality as part of normal development. Preschoolers have an intense sense of fantasy and are more likely to be frightened by something that looks "scary" than by something that can cause real harm. Common fears of this age-group include separation from parent, dark, animals, and noises—especially those in the dark. Sometimes the anxiety is grounded in reality: for example, a child who was bitten by a dog may fear that it will happen again.	Parents can often reduce fears by instilling a sense of trust and normal caution without being overprotective. Teach parents to avoid ridiculing their child but to provide reassurance and encourage open expression of feelings. Have parents avoid coercion and logical persuasion because developmentally the child is unable to process such statements as "Pet the nice parrot—it won't hurt you," or "Lions are only found in a zoo." Encourage parents to seek out modeling behavior and expose their child to it; by observing fearlessness in other children, their child will gradually overcome the perceived threat.
Daycare or preschool	Preschoolers can thrive physically, intellectually, and emotionally in daycare and preschool settings that have small groups, high adult-to-child ratios, and a stable, competent, and involved staff. Preschoolers develop best when they have a balance between structured activities and freedom to explore on their own. Parents may feel less stress knowing that their child is being well cared for while they are earning the income needed or fulfilling personal achievements.	Teach parents strategies for choosing a good program for their child that includes the following: Provides a safe, clean setting Welcomes parents who visit unannounced Has warm and friendly personnel that are responsive to the children Fosters social skills, self-esteem, and respect for others Helps parents improve their parenting skills Teach parents to avoid programs that: Employ staff members who are not educated, trained in CPR, or experienced in child care or child education Are not licensed by the state Have no written plan for meals or emergencies Have poor ventilation or lighting or no smoke alarms, fire extinguishers, or first-aid kits

From Leahy, JM, and Kizilay, PE: *Foundations of Nursing Practice,* Philadelphia, 1998, Saunders.

TABLE **9-2**	Anticipatory Guidance—cont'd		
ANTICIPATORY GUIDANCE FOR THE PRESCHOOL CHILD—cont'd			
Issue	**Rationale**		**Guidance**
Sleep disorders	Approximately one in four preschoolers suffers from night terrors or nightmares. Night terrors are identified by abrupt awakening from deep sleep in a state of panic; the child is not really awake and will quiet down quickly and not remember the incident in the morning. Night terrors do not indicate underlying emotional problems and are thought to be an effect of very deep sleep states. Persistent nightmares, especially those that cause fear and anxiety to the child during the day, may indicate excessive stress in the child.		Explain to parents that these are common sleep problems in preschoolers. Teach parents to set up a pleasant, relaxed bedtime ritual to share with their child, such as recalling a happy family outing or event. Recommend that parents leave a small light on that does not produce shadows on the wall. Encourage parents to provide their child with comfort and reassurance every time an episode occurs.

Unintentional injuries	Unintentional injury continues to be the leading cause of death and disability in preschool children.
	
	Nightmares usually come toward the early morning and are vividly remembered by the child.
	
	Preschoolers are no longer content with their home environment and venture outside of the home, often with less supervision than in previous years.
	
	Common risks associated with this developmental stage include:
	    Motor vehicle injuries
	    Burns or scalds
	    Drowning
	    Falls
	    Poisoning
			Parents and caregivers should know CPR.
			
			Home and environmental safety checklist should be reviewed with parents and caregivers.
			
			Reinforce with parents and caregivers the importance of vigilant child monitoring and supervision.

ANTICIPATORY GUIDANCE IN SCHOOL-AGE CHILDREN			
School anxiety or phobia	Adjusting to grade school is a significant change for a 6-year-old, even if preschool was attended; no longer is the focus play, the sessions are full days, and the expectations are high. Major tasks occur in first and second grade as children learn to read and write and have to meet the teacher's expectations. Competing with schoolmates for the teacher's attention and approval can cause strain and anxiety. Children sometimes resist attending school by becoming physically sick—abdominal pain or complaints of headache last until the child is allowed to stay home for the day.		Encourage parents to communicate regularly with the child's teacher to stay well informed on progress and to identify problems early. Have parents spend time each evening reviewing the child's day and homework assignments and providing guidance and security when indicated. Inform parents that school adjustments take place not only in first grade but every time there is a change in grade, teacher, and classmates and when other stressful events are happening around the child. If anxiety or other school difficulties persist, suggest that the parent have the child evaluated by a health care provider or refer for counseling.

Continued

TABLE **9-2**	Anticipatory Guidance—cont'd	
ANTICIPATORY GUIDANCE IN SCHOOL-AGE CHILDREN—cont'd		
Issue	**Rationale**	**Guidance**
Dental problems	As primary teeth are shed and secondary teeth erupt, the child is at risk for malocclusion, a condition where the upper and lower teeth malalign, predisposing the child to permanent jaw and dental problems. Dental caries are a significant health problem in all age groups; however, because school-age children are relied on to independently perform self-care activities, dental hygiene measures often are neglected. Tooth evulsion, or loss due to trauma, is common because children participate in more risky and challenging physical activities (e.g., contact sports, inline skating) than when they were younger.	Orthodontic referrals for braces are usually made during early adolescence after all primary teeth are shed; however, in the case of malocclusion, prompt referral should be made as soon as a problem is evident. Stress to parents the importance of dental checkups every 6 months and daily oral hygiene measures to prevent dental caries. In addition to brushing and using fluoride supplements, school-age children should floss their teeth regularly; medical assistants can provide instruction and reinforce teaching in this area. Instruct parents and children about what to do if a permanent tooth is traumatically knocked out; tell them to hold the tooth by the crown and avoid touching the root; if it is dirty, rinse under running water, then insert the root end into the socket and seek medical care immediately. Always stress the importance of wearing protective gear, including mouth shields, when playing contact sports and other physical activities to minimize injuries.
Sleeptalking or sleepwalking	Approximately one in six children experiences an episode of sleepwalking during the school-age years, with few who walk persistently. Sleepwalking and talking occur 1 to 2 hr after onset of sleep and are associated with neurologic immaturity or anxiety-provoking daytime experiences. Almost all children outgrow this behavior and do not develop persistent sleeping problems.	Inform parents of the self-limiting nature of this problem and have them focus on maintaining safety for the child who wanders from bed at night by keeping doors securely locked. Guiding the sleepwalking child back to bed before ready may result in the child getting up again during the night; remain with the child until he or she returns to bed or awakens from the trance. If these behaviors suddenly develop in the child, have parents try to identify a stressor or exciting event that the child recently experienced as the possible cause. Instruct parents to prevent their children from watching action-packed television or videos prior to sleep and to encourage more sedentary activities like reading and playing a card game.

From Leahy, JM, and Kizilay, PE: *Foundations of Nursing Practice,* Philadelphia, 1998, Saunders.

TABLE 9-2	Anticipatory Guidance—cont'd	
ANTICIPATORY GUIDANCE IN SCHOOL-AGE CHILDREN—cont'd		
Issue	**Rationale**	**Guidance**
Sex education	Ideally, the preteen years are the time when parents need to be available to answer their child's questions regarding sex. Many parents are extremely uncomfortable discussing sex with their children because they are ignorant about the topic themselves. As they enter puberty, children have many questions about sex and often have no place to get answers; they turn to misinformed peers for information. Medical assistants are in a good position to educate parents and children about sexuality but only after examining their own beliefs and attitudes about such issues.	Introduce the subject of sex education to parents of preteens and assess their knowledge and comfort level with the topic. Ask parents if they are willing to introduce the topic of sex to their children, and if not, would they allow you to do so. Approach the topic initially from a physiological perspective, informing them about the outward changes that will occur as they go through puberty; then advance to more social and emotional issues when they are ready. A matter-of-fact tone should be used when presenting information to children so they can observe the lack of spirited emotion attached to the subject. Reinforce to them that no person has a right to touch them in places that make them feel uncomfortable.

TABLE 9-3	Child Safety Guidelines	
Age	**Common Injury**	**Prevention Strategies**
Infancy	Motor vehicle crash	Use infant car restraints that meet safety standards. Infants weighing <20 lb (9 kg) face rear in center back seat of car (never in passenger front seat because of danger of airbag deployment). Install restraint and secure infant appropriately according to manufacturer's guidelines.
	Falls	Never leave child unattended on bed, changing table, or other high place. Keep cribs away from windows; put mattress in lowest position. Use safety gates at top and bottom of staircases.
	Burns and scalds	Never hold child while handling hot foods, liquids, or cigarettes. Keep water heater temperature at 110-120°F (43.3-48.9°C). Test water prior to bathing. Use outlet covers; keep electric cords out of reach. Use sunscreen with sun protection factor (SPF) ≥30; expose child to sun gradually.
	Drowning	Hold on to infant at all times during bath. Never leave infant unattended in bath or near water.

From Leahy JM, and Kizilay PE: *Foundations of Nursing Practice,* Philadelphia, 1998, Saunders.

Continued

TABLE **9-3**	Child Safety Guidelines—cont'd	
Age	**Common Injury**	**Prevention Strategies**
Infancy—cont'd	Choking and suffocation	Avoid propping bottles for feeding. Keep small objects out of reach. Keep plastic bags and balloons out of reach. Check all toys for loose parts. Do not tie pacifier around neck. Keep cribs away from drapery and dangling cords. Learn CPR.
	Poisoning	Use cabinet latches on all low cabinets. Keep house plants out of reach. Keep syrup of ipecac handy. Post poison control center phone number by the telephone.
Toddler	Motor vehicle crash	Switch to toddler car restraint when child weighs >40 lb (18 kg). Do not put children <12 yr in front seat to avoid injuries from airbag deployment. Hold child's hand when crossing street. Begin teaching proper street crossing and safety rules. Set a good example when crossing streets.
	Falls	Continue infant guidelines. Switch to youth bed when child can climb over crib rails or leave the rails down. Install guards on windows that open more than 4 in.
	Burns and scalds	Continue infant guidelines. Avoid placing hot objects within child's reach. Restrict child from cooking areas. Cook on back burners of stove and turn pot handles inward. Avoid using tablecloths. Keep matches and lighters out of reach. Begin teaching the meaning of "hot"
	Drowning	Supervise continually in bath and near lakes, ocean, rivers, and pools. Begin teaching water safety and swimming. Keep away from toilets and buckets of water.
	Choking	Continue infant guidelines. Cut foods well and instruct not to talk or run while eating. Avoid feeding hard candies, peanuts, raw vegetable sticks, raisins, and frankfurters.
	Poisoning	Continue infant guidelines. Use cabinet latches on all high and low cabinets. Avoid taking pills in child's presence.
Preschool	Motor vehicle crash	Continue toddler guidelines. Use regular car safety restraints for children ≥40 lb or 4 yr old.
	Falls	Continue toddler guidelines. Supervise playground activities. Ensure padded ground in playground areas. Use approved helmet and knee and elbow pads for bicycling and skating.
	Burns and scalds	Continue toddler guidelines. Teach stop, drop, roll, and cool in event of flame burns. Run home fire safety drills.
	Choking	Instruct not to talk or run while eating. Instruct to chew food well. Learn CPR.
	Poisoning	Continue toddler guidelines.

From Leahy JM, and Kizilay PE: *Foundations of Nursing Practice,* Philadelphia, 1998, Saunders.

TABLE 9-3 Child Safety Guidelines—cont'd

Age	Common Injury	Prevention Strategies
School age	Motor vehicle crash	Remember that these children are most at risk for pedestrian injury.
		Use specially designed car restraints until the child weighs at least 60 lb or is 8 yr old.
		Stress street crossing safety guidelines.
		Stress bicycling, skating, and motorized vehicle safety.
	Falls	Continue preschool guidelines.
	Burns and scalds	Continue preschool guidelines.
	Drowning	Continue supervision when in and around water.
		Teach swimming and proper diving guidelines if not already done.
	Choking and suffocation	Continue preschool guidelines.
		Learn CPR.
	Poisoning	Monitor for signs of depression or despondency, which may lead to intentional ingestion.
	Firearm injury	Store all guns unloaded and out of reach.
		Install trigger latches on all firearms.
		Have child attend hunting safety classes if appropriate.
Adolescence	Motor vehicle crash	Monitor for signs of alcohol use and counsel to avoid drinking and driving.
		Instruct teen to avoid riding with an impaired driver.
		Continue to stress safety restraint use.
		Have teen attend driver education classes.
	Falls	Instruct regarding proper use of protective gear to prevent sports-related injuries.
	Burns	Instruct regarding dangers of smoking and smoking in bed.
	Drowning	Instruct regarding dangers of diving into unknown (shallow) bodies of water to prevent head injury.
		Stress attending boating or Coast Guard safety course.
	Choking	Continue stressing not talking while eating, especially if alcohol impaired.
		Learn CPR.
	Poisoning	Continue school-age guidelines.
	Firearm injury	Continue school-age guidelines.

What Would You DO?
What Would You Not DO?

Case Study 1

My-Lai Chang comes into the office with Christopher Chang, her 2-month-old son. Christopher is here for his 2-month well-child visit. Mrs. Chang is very distraught. She says that Christopher has episodes of nonstop crying every day that last 2 to 3 hours at a time. She is breastfeeding Christopher and says that the crying is worse after he nurses. Although Mrs. Chang realizes that Christopher has colic, she feels very guilty because it seems like it's "her milk" that is making it worse. She is also having problems with sore nipples and engorgement. She really wanted to breastfeed Christopher, but she is thinking of stopping because it just seems too hard to do. Christopher measures in the 50th percentile for both weight and length. Mrs. Chang is worried that he is not growing enough and thinks it's because she's not producing enough milk.

Developing a Rapport

The medical assistant must establish a rapport with the pediatric patient. If the medical assistant gains the child's trust and confidence, the child is likely to cooperate during an examination or procedure. Interacting with children requires special techniques, depending on the age of the child. For example, toddlers and preschoolers often respond well to making a game of the procedure. Explaining the purpose of an instrument (e.g., the stethoscope) to a school-age child and allowing him or her to hold the instrument or even to help during the procedure may overcome fears in that age-group (Figure 9-1).

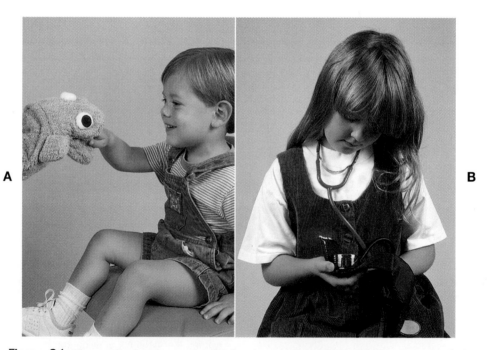

Figure 9-1. The medical assistant should develop a rapport with children to gain their trust and cooperation. Making a game of the procedure **(A)** and explaining the purpose of the stethoscope and allowing the child to hold it **(B)** help the child overcome fears.

The medical assistant should always explain the procedure to children who are able to understand. Each child must be approached at his or her level of understanding. To do this, the medical assistant should know what to expect from a child at a particular age, in terms of both motor and social development. It should be kept in mind, however, that each child has his or her own rate of development. The descriptions of normal development based on age are meant to serve as a guide only and may have to be modified to meet individual needs. It is also important to realize that it is normal for an ill child to regress to an earlier level of behavior. Table 9-4 outlines techniques that can be used with various age-groups to gain their cooperation during an examination or procedure.

TABLE 9-4 Techniques for Interaction with Children

Technique	Infant (Birth-1 yr)	Toddler (1-3 yr)	Preschooler (3-6 yr)	School Age (6-12 yr)	Adolescent (12-18 yr)
Avoid sudden motion and loud or abrupt noises.	♥				
Limit the number of strangers in the room.	♥				
Use distractions, bright objections, rattles, and talking to gain cooperation.	♥				
Physically restrain the child if necessary to ensure safety.	♥	♥	♥		
Allow physical contact with the parent during the procedure.	♥	♥	♥		
Encourage the parent to comfort the child after the procedure.	♥	♥	♥		
Use play to explain the procedure (e.g., dolls, puppets).		♥	♥		
Perform procedures quickly, if possible.		♥	♥		
Use concrete terms, rather than abstract terms.		♥	♥		
Avoid words that have more than one meaning (e.g., *shot*).		♥	♥		
Give the child permission to cry, yell, or otherwise express pain verbally.		♥	♥		
Praise the child for cooperative behavior.		♥	♥	♥	
Allow the child to handle the equipment, if possible.			♥	♥	
Make sure the child understands the body part to be involved.			♥	♥	
Try to describe how the procedure will feel.			♥	♥	
Tell the child about any discomfort that may be felt, but don't dwell on it.			♥	♥	
Stress the benefits of anything the child may find pleasurable afterwards (e.g., stickers, feeling better).			♥	♥	
Give the child choices when possible (e.g., arm to use).			♥	♥	
Suggest ways to maintain control (e.g., counting, deep breathing, relaxation).			♥	♥	
Use drawing and diagrams to illustrate the parts of the body that will be involved.			♥	♥	
Encourage participation such as holding an instrument during the procedure.			♥	♥	
Include the child in the decision-making process.				♥	♥
Discuss risks of the procedure.					♥
Provide information about appearance changes that might result.					♥
Give the child educational brochures and/or have them view videos about the procedure.					♥
Ask the parent to step out if the child does not want the parent in the examining room.					♥

Carrying the Infant

The medical assistant needs to lift and carry the infant in order to perform various procedures, such as measurement of length and weight. The infant should be lifted and carried in a manner that is both safe and comfortable. These positions include the cradle and upright positions, which are described here.

Cradle Position. The medical assistant slides the left hand and arm under the infant's back and grasps the baby's arm from behind. The thumb and fingers should encircle the infant's forearm. The infant's head, shoulders, and back are supported by the medical assistant's arm. Next the medical assistant slips the right arm up and under the baby's buttocks. The infant is cradled in the arm with the child's body resting against the medical assistant's chest (Figure 9-2).

Upright Position. The medical assistant slips the right hand under the infant's head and shoulders. The fingers should be spread apart to support the infant's head and neck. The left forearm is then slipped under the infant's buttocks to help support the baby's weight. The infant should be allowed to rest against the medical assistant's chest with the cheek resting on the medical assistant's shoulder (Figure 9-3).

Growth Measurements

One of the best methods to evaluate the progress of a child is to measure his or her growth. The weight, height (or length), and head circumference (up to age 3 years) of a child should be measured during each office visit and plotted on a growth chart.

Weight

A child's weight is often used to determine nutritional needs and the proper dosage of a medication to administer to the child. Therefore the medical assistant should exercise care in measuring weight. Infants are weighed in a recumbent position as is outlined in Procedure 9-1. Older children are weighed in a standing position, as presented in Chapter 5.

Length and Height

Another measure of a child's growth is length, or height (stature). Length is measured in children younger than 24 months. The recumbent length is a measurement from the vertex of the head to the heel of the infant in a supine position, as is outlined in Procedure 9-1. Two people are needed to accurately determine the length of an infant. The parent's help can be requested; however, the medical assistant should be sure to provide the parent with thorough instructions on what is to be done. Older children have their height measured in a standing position (Figure 9-4), as presented in Chapter 5.

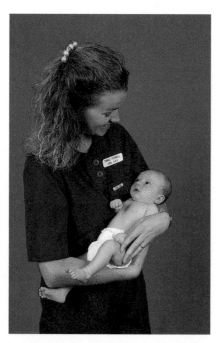

Figure 9-2. Traci holds the baby in the cradle position.

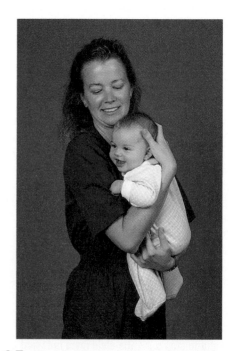

Figure 9-3. Traci holds the infant in the upright position.

Head and Chest Circumference

Infancy is a period of rapid brain growth. Because of this, the head circumference is one of the most important measurements to obtain. The head circumference for a newborn ranges between 32 and 38 centimeters, or 12½ and 15 inches. A 4-inch (10-cm) increase in head circumference occurs within the first year of life.

The head circumference of children under 3 years of age should be routinely measured and plotted on a head circumference growth chart. Measurement of head circumference is an important screening measure for microencephaly and macroencephaly.

At birth a newborn's head circumference is about 2 cm larger than his or her chest circumference. The chest grows at a faster rate than the cranium, and between 6 months and 2 years of age, the measurements are about the same. After age 2, the chest circumference is greater than the head circumference. The measurement of the chest circumference is valuable in a comparison with the head circumference but not necessarily by itself. The chest circumference is not typically measured on a routine basis, but only when a heart or lung abnormality is suspected.

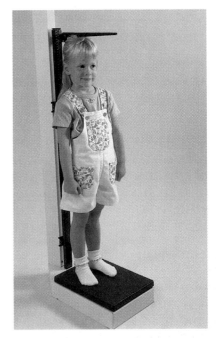

Figure 9-4. Measuring the height of a child.

Highlight on Childhood Obesity

An epidemic of childhood obesity is occurring in the United States; the incidence of obesity in children has doubled over the past 20 years. Approximately 25% of Americans under the age of 19 are overweight or obese, which equates to 1 of every 4 children. A child is considered overweight if his or her weight falls in the 90th to 95th percentile for age, gender, and height on the National Center for Health Statistics (NCHS) growth charts. When a child's weight exceeds the 95th percentile for age, gender, and height, he or she is considered obese.

The primary causes of childhood obesity are overeating and inadequate exercise. Other causes include hormonal and genetic problems, but these are much less likely, occurring in only 5% of obese children. The risk of obesity tends to be greater among children who have obese parents. After age 3, the likelihood that obesity will persist into adulthood increases as the child gets older. Once a child reaches the age of 6, the probability is more than 50% that obesity will persist into adulthood, and 70% to 80% of obese adolescents remain obese as adults.

Some of the problems associated with childhood obesity include high blood pressure, type 2 diabetes, orthopedic problems caused by increased stress on weight-bearing joints, skin disorders such as dermatitis, sleep apnea, low self-esteem, social isolation, and feelings of rejection and depression. Some authorities feel that the social and psychological problems are the most significant consequences of childhood obesity.

It is much easier to prevent childhood obesity than to treat it once it has occurred. Authorities believe that the primary focus should be on educating parents as to the problems associated with childhood obesity and helping them employ preventive measures. Examples of guidelines for preventing childhood obesity include:

- Provide a healthy diet, with 30% or fewer calories coming from fat.
- Encourage active play.
- Don't use food for reward, comfort, or bribes.
- Limit television, video, and computer time.
- Limit the amount of "junk" food kept in the home.
- Don't make the child eat when he or she is not hungry.
- Don't offer dessert as a reward for finishing meal.
- Encourage child to drink water instead of sweet beverages.
- Don't frequently eat at fast-food restaurants.

The treatment of childhood obesity is difficult and the success rate is not particularly high. Children seem to be most successful at losing weight and keeping it off when the entire family is involved. Parents should eat healthy meals and snacks with their children. The most successful diets are those that use ordinary foods in controlled portions, rather than diets that require the avoidance of specific foods. Parents should also spend time being active with their children. Activities should stress self-improvement rather than competition.

Procedure 9-2 outlines the procedure for measuring the head and chest circumference of an infant.

Growth Charts

Growth charts should be part of every child's permanent record. The National Center for Health Statistics (NCHS) developed growth charts to assist physicians in determining if the growth of a child is normal. The charts can be used to identify children with growth or nutritional abnormalities. The medical assistant is usually responsible for plotting the child's measurements on the growth chart (see Procedure 9-3).

Growth charts provide a means of comparing a child's weight and length (or height) with that of other children of the same age. For example, let's say the medical assistant calculates the growth percentile of an 18-month-old boy and finds that he is in the 25th percentile for weight and the 80th percentile for length. This means that 75% of 18-month-old boys weigh more than he does, and 25% weigh less than he does. It also means that 20% of 18-month-old boys are taller, and 80% are shorter. Although comparing a child with other children of the same age is one use of growth charts (particularly by parents), it is not the most important use.

The primary use of growth charts is to look at the child's growth pattern. If a child has always hovered around a certain percentile in both height and weight, there is no need for concern. For example, if a child is in the 20th percentile for weight, but has always been in this percentile, he is very likely growing normally. There would be more of a concern if the child had been in the 75th percentile and then dropped to the 20th percentile. The physician will investigate any significant change or rapid rise or drop in a child's growth pattern.

Text continued on p. 354

What Would You DO?
What Would You *Not* DO?

Case Study 2

Wanda Tilley comes to the office with her 10-year-old daughter, Courtney. Courtney has a skin condition on her legs that needs to be evaluated by the physician. Courtney has been obese since she was 4 years old. Mrs. Tilley is also obese and is not too concerned about Courtney's weight. She says that Courtney must have inherited her "fat gene" and there's not much that can be done about it. Courtney's favorite activities are playing video games and reading. She would really like to join the community swim team, but she's too embarrassed for anyone to see her in a bathing suit. Courtney says the other kids are always making fun of her at school. She says that they call her two-ton Tilley and double-roll and they don't want to sit with her at lunch. Courtney wants her mom to home-school her because she's getting to the point where she can't take it anymore. She doesn't want the doctor to examine her because he'll see how fat she is and say bad things about it.

PROCEDURE 9-1   Measuring the Weight and Length of an Infant

Outcome Measure the weight and length of an infant.

Equipment/Supplies:
- Pediatric balance scale (table model)

1. **Procedural Step.** Sanitize your hands.
2. **Procedural Step.** Greet the child's parent, and identify the child. Introduce yourself, and explain the procedure.
3. **Procedural Step.** Unlock the pediatric scale, and place a clean paper protector on it. Check the balance scale for accuracy, making sure to compensate for the weight of the paper.
   Principle. The paper protector prevents cross-contamination and reduces the spread of disease from one patient to another.
4. **Procedural Step.** Remove the infant's clothing, including the diaper.

Principle. Bulky diapers tend to increase the child's weight considerably. In addition, growth charts for infants and young children base their percentiles on the weight of the child without clothing.

5. **Procedural Step.** Gently place the infant on his or her back on the table of the scale. Place one hand slightly above the infant as a safety precaution.
6. **Procedural Step.** Balance the scale as follows:
   a. Move the lower weight to the notched groove that does not cause the indicator point to drop to the bottom of the calibration area. Make sure the lower weight is seated firmly in its groove.

b. Slowly slide the upper weight along its calibration bar by tapping it gently until the indicator point comes to a rest at the center of the balance area.

Principle. Not seating the lower weight firmly in its groove results in an inaccurate reading.

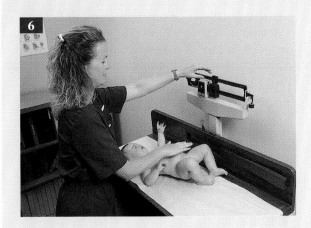

7. **Procedural Step.** Read the results in pounds and ounces while the infant is lying still. (*Note:* The result on the pictured scale is 15 pounds and 2 ounces.)

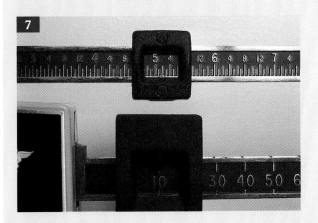

8. **Procedural Step.** Return the balance to its resting position and lock the scale.
9. **Procedural Step.** Place the **vertex** (top) of the infant's head against the headboard at the zero mark. Ask the parent to hold the infant's head in this position.

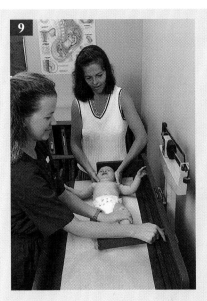

10. **Procedural Step.** Straighten the infant's knees and place the soles of his or her feet firmly against the upright foot board (to create a right angle).
11. **Procedural Step.** Read the infant's length in inches (to the nearest ⅛ inch) from the measure and return the footboard to its resting position. (*Note:* The result on this scale is 25½ inches.)

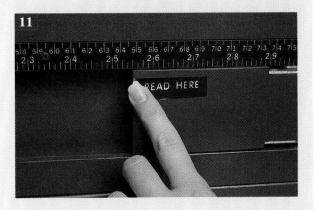

12. **Procedural Step.** Gently remove the infant from the table and hand him or her to the parent.
13. **Procedural Step.** Chart the results.

CHARTING EXAMPLE

Date	
8/10/05	9:30 a.m. Wt. 15 lb 2 oz. Length 25 ½ in. —————————————— T. Powell, CMA

PROCEDURE 9-1

PROCEDURE 9-2 Measuring Head and Chest Circumference of an Infant

Outcome Measure the head and chest circumference of an infant.

Equipment/Supplies:
• Flexible nonstretch tape measure

Measurement of Head Circumference

1. **Procedural Step.** Sanitize your hands, and assemble the equipment.
2. **Procedural Step.** Position the infant. The infant should be placed on his or her back on the examining table. An alternative position is to have the parent hold the child.
3. **Procedural Step.** Position the tape measure around the infant's head at the greatest circumference. This is usually accomplished by placing the tape slightly above the eyebrows and pinna of the ears and around the occipital prominence at the back of the skull.

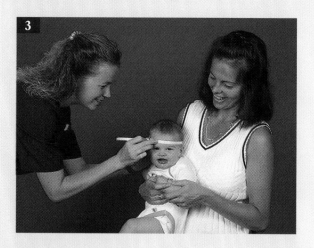

4. **Procedural Step.** Read the results in centimeters (or inches) to the nearest ½ cm (or ¼ inch). Chart the results.

CHARTING EXAMPLE

Date	
8/10/05	10:00 a.m. Head circumference: 42 ½ cm. —
	———————— T. Powell, CMA

Measurement of Chest Circumference

1. **Procedural Step.** Position the infant on his or her back on the examining table.
2. **Procedural Step.** Encircle the tape around the infant's chest at the nipple line. It should be snug but not so tight that it leaves a mark.

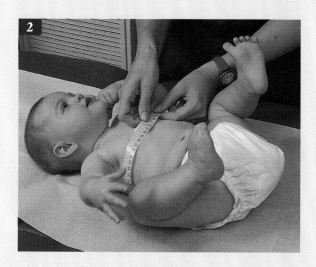

3. **Procedural Step.** Read the results in centimeters (or inches) to the nearest 0.5 cm (or ¼ inch). Chart the results.

CHARTING EXAMPLE

Date	
8/15/05	10:00 a.m. Chest circumference: 42 cm. —
	———————— T. Powell, CMA

PROCEDURE 9-3 Calculating Growth Percentiles

Outcome Plot a pediatric growth value on a growth chart.

Equipment/Supplies:
- Pediatric growth chart

1. **Procedural Step.** Select the proper growth chart.
2. **Procedural Step.** Locate the child's age in the horizontal column at the bottom of the chart and draw an (imaginary) vertical line on the chart.
3. **Procedural Step.** Locate the growth value in the vertical column under the appropriate category (weight, length or stature, and head circumference) and draw an (imaginary) horizontal line on the chart.
4. **Procedural Step.** Find the site at which the two lines (extending from these values) intersect on the graph and place a dot on this site.
5. **Procedural Step.** To determine the percentile in which the child falls, follow the curved percentile line upward to read the value located on the right side of the chart. Interpolation is needed if the value does not fall exactly on a percentile line. (Interpolation means that you must estimate a percentile that falls between a larger and smaller known percentile.)
6. **Procedural Step.** Chart the results. Include the date and time and each growth percentile.

Note: The weight (15 lb, 2 oz) length (25½ inches), and head circumference (42½ cm) of the child in Procedures 9-1 and 9-2 have been plotted on a growth chart. This child is 5 months old. Locate these values on the appropriate growth chart to make sure you obtain the same percentiles.

CHARTING EXAMPLE

Date	
10/22/05	10:30 a.m. Weight: 55%. Length: 70%. ————
	Head Circum: 67% ———— T. Powell, CMA

Continued

PROCEDURE 9-3

PROCEDURE 9-3 Calculating Growth Percentiles—Cont'd

Birth to 36 months: Girls
Length-for-age and Weight-for-age percentiles

NAME _____

RECORD# _____

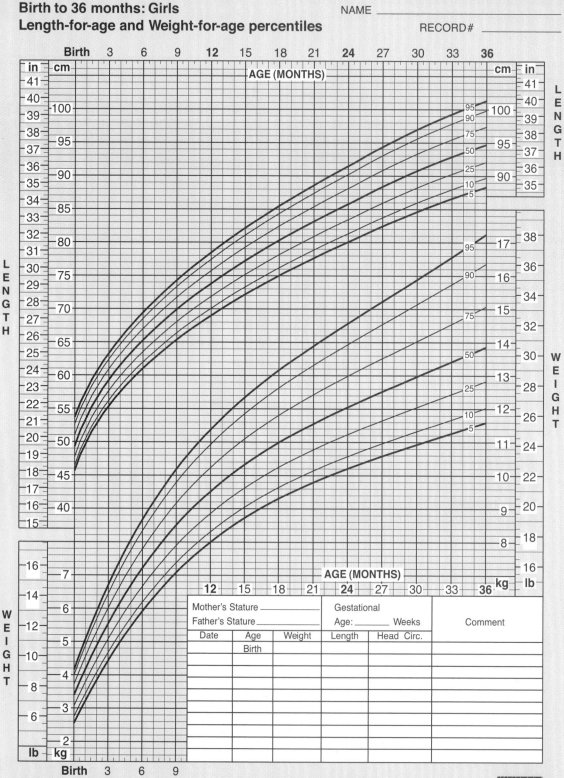

Published May 30, 2000 (modified 4/20/01).
SOURCE: Developed by the National Center for Health Statistics in collaboration with
the National Center for Chronic Disease Prevention and Health Promotion (2000).
http://www.cdc.gov/growthcharts

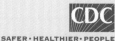

SAFER · HEALTHIER · PEOPLE™

PROCEDURE 9-3 Calculating Growth Percentiles—Cont'd

Birth to 36 months: Girls
Head circumference-for-age and
Weight-for-length percentiles

NAME _____

RECORD# _____

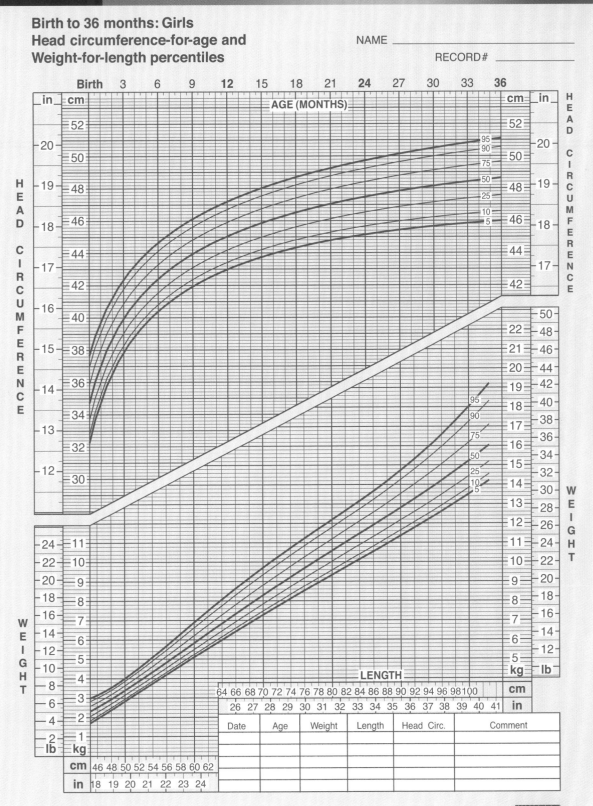

AGE (MONTHS)

HEAD CIRCUMFERENCE

WEIGHT

LENGTH

Date	Age	Weight	Length	Head Circ.	Comment

Published May 30, 2000 (modified 10/16/00).

SOURCE: Developed by the National Center for Health Statistics in collaboration with the National Center for Chronic Disease Prevention and Health Promotion (2000).
http://www.cdc.gov/growthcharts

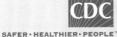

SAFER·HEALTHIER·PEOPLE™

PROCEDURE 9-3

Continued

PROCEDURE 9-3 Calculating Growth Percentiles—Cont'd

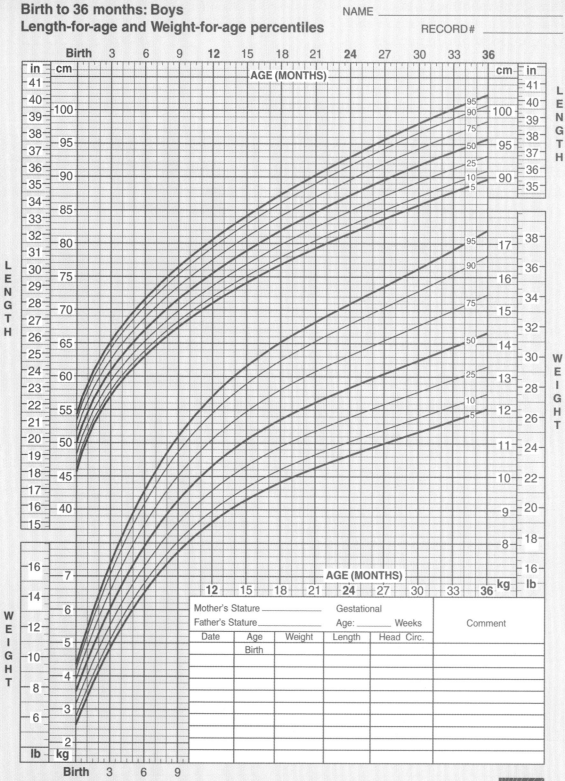

Birth to 36 months: Boys
Length-for-age and Weight-for-age percentiles

NAME _____

RECORD# _____

Published May 30, 2000 (modified 4/20/01).
SOURCE: Developed by the National Center for Health Statistics in collaboration with
the National Center for Chronic Disease Prevention and Health Promotion (2000).
http://www.cdc.gov/growthcharts

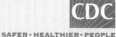

SAFER · HEALTHIER · PEOPLE™

PROCEDURE 9-3

PROCEDURE 9-3 Calculating Growth Percentiles—Cont'd

Birth to 36 months: Boys
Head circumference-for-age and
Weight-for-length percentiles

NAME _____

RECORD# _____

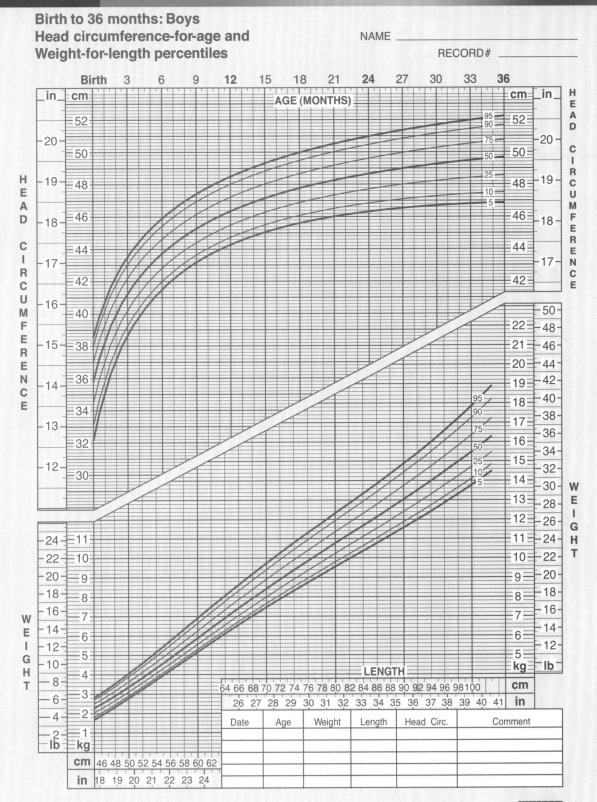

Published May 30, 2000 (modified 10/16/00).
SOURCE: Developed by the National Center for Health Statistics in collaboration with
the National Center for Chronic Disease Prevention and Health Promotion (2000).
http://www.cdc.gov/growthcharts

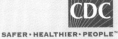

SAFER·HEALTHIER·PEOPLE™

PROCEDURE 9-3

Continued

PROCEDURE 9-3 Calculating Growth Percentiles—Cont'd

2 to 20 years: Girls
Stature-for-age and Weight-for-age percentiles

NAME _____

RECORD# _____

Mother's Stature _____		Father's Stature _____		
Date	Age	Weight	Stature	BMI*

***To Calculate BMI**: Weight (kg) ÷ Stature (cm) ÷ Stature (cm) x 10,000
or Weight (lb) ÷ Stature (in) ÷ Stature (in) x 703

AGE (YEARS)

Published May 30, 2000 (modified 11/21/00).
SOURCE: Developed by the National Center for Health Statistics in collaboration with
the National Center for Chronic Disease Prevention and Health Promotion (2000).
http://www.cdc.gov/growthcharts

SAFER·HEALTHIER·PEOPLE™

PROCEDURE 9-3 Calculating Growth Percentiles—Cont'd

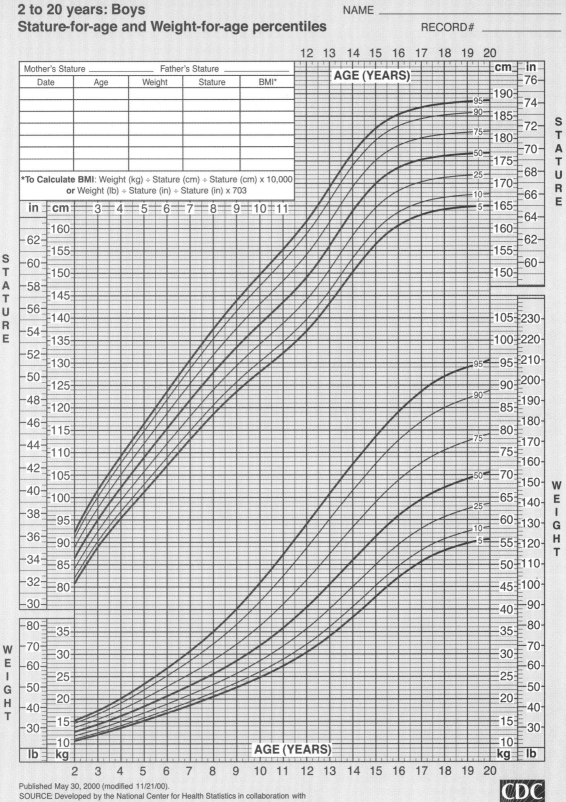

2 to 20 years: Boys
Stature-for-age and Weight-for-age percentiles

NAME _____

RECORD# _____

Mother's Stature _____ Father's Stature _____

Date	Age	Weight	Stature	BMI*

*To Calculate BMI: Weight (kg) ÷ Stature (cm) ÷ Stature (cm) x 10,000
or Weight (lb) ÷ Stature (in) ÷ Stature (in) x 703

AGE (YEARS)

STATURE

WEIGHT

Published May 30, 2000 (modified 11/21/00).
SOURCE: Developed by the National Center for Health Statistics in collaboration with
the National Center for Chronic Disease Prevention and Health Promotion (2000).
http://www.cdc.gov/growthcharts

SAFER·HEALTHIER·PEOPLE™

PROCEDURE **9-3**

Pediatric Blood Pressure Measurement

The American Academy of Pediatrics recommends that all children 3 years of age and older have their blood pressure measured annually. Measuring pediatric blood pressure helps to identify children at risk for developing hypertension as adults. High blood pressure in children can be caused by kidney disease and, to a lesser degree, by heart disease. Once the condition is treated, the blood pressure usually returns to normal. Overweight children usually have higher blood pressure than those of normal weight. A prescribed special diet and regular physical activity may lower blood pressure in these children.

Special Guidelines for Children

The procedure for measuring blood pressure in children is the same as that for adults and is presented in Chapter 4. Some special pediatric guidelines must be taken into consideration, and they are described next.

Correct Cuff Size

The most important criterion in obtaining an accurate pediatric blood pressure measurement is selecting the correct cuff size. If the cuff is too small, the reading may be falsely high. If the cuff is too large, the reading may be falsely low. Blood pressure cuffs come in a variety of sizes and are measured in centimeters (cm). The size of a cuff refers to its inner inflatable bladder, rather than its cloth cover. Table 9-5 lists the range of cuff sizes commercially available. It is important to realize that the name of the cuff (e.g., child, adult) does not necessarily imply it is

appropriate for that age. For example, an 8-year-old overweight child may need an adult-sized cuff.

For an accurate blood pressure measurement, the bladder of the cuff should encircle 80% to 100% of the arm. The child's arm circumference should be assessed midpoint between the acromion process (shoulder) and the olecranon process (elbow). Figure 9-5 shows how to determine the correct pediatric cuff size.

Cooperation of the Child

Another important factor to consider when taking pediatric blood pressure is preparing the child for the procedure. It is important to gain the child's cooperation and to make sure that the child is relaxed. Apprehension can

TABLE 9-5	Acceptable Bladder Dimensions for Arms of Different Sizes	
Cuff	Bladder Length (cm)	Arm Circumference Range at Midpoint (cm)
Newborn	6	<6
Infant	15	6–15
Child	21	16–21
Small adult	24	22–26
Adult	30	27–34
Large adult	38	35–44
Adult thigh	42	45–52

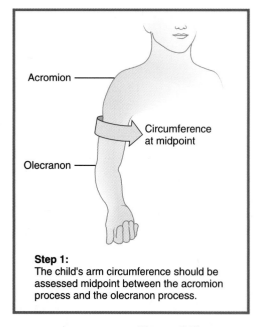

Step 1:
The child's arm circumference should be assessed midpoint between the acromion process and the olecranon process.

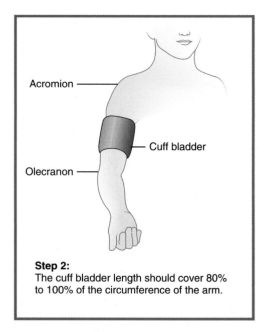

Step 2:
The cuff bladder length should cover 80% to 100% of the circumference of the arm.

Figure 9-5. Determination of proper cuff size.

cause the blood pressure to be falsely high. To reduce a child's anxiety level, carefully explain the procedure to the child and, if appropriate, allow him or her to handle the equipment before measuring blood pressure. The blood pressure should be measured after the child has been sitting quietly for 3 to 5 minutes (Figure 9-6).

Blood Pressure Classifications

Blood pressure varies depending on the age of the child, as well as his or her height and gender. The National High Blood Pressure Education Program (NHBPEP) recently prepared a set of tables that physicians use to determine if a child's blood pressure is higher than the average among children of the same age and height. If a child has a blood pressure that is higher than 90% to 95% of most other children of same age, height, and gender, then the child may have high blood pressure.

These tables (one for boys and one for girls) allow precise classification of blood pressure according to body size, which avoids misclassifying children at the extreme ends

of normal growth. For example, a very tall child will not be mistakenly diagnosed as having hypertension and, on the other hand, hypertension will not be missed in a very short child. The NHBPEP tables used by physicians to assist in the diagnosis of hypertension in children can be found at the National Heart, Lung, and Blood Institute website: www.nhlbi.nih.gov/health/prof/heart/hbp/hbp_ped.htm.

Blood pressure varies throughout the day in children as a result of normal fluctuations in physical activity and emotional stress. If a child's blood pressure is elevated, two more readings must be taken at different visits before the physician can make a diagnosis of hypertension.

Collection of a Urine Specimen

A urine specimen may be required from a pediatric patient as part of a general physical examination to assist in the diagnosis of a pathologic condition or to evaluate the effectiveness of therapy.

The collection of a urine specimen from a child who exhibits bladder control is performed using the technique outlined in Chapter 16. Collecting a urine specimen from an infant or young child who cannot urinate voluntarily involves a pediatric urine collector. Pediatric urine collectors are designed to be used with both sexes. The urine collector consists of a clear plastic bag containing a soft sponge ring coated with a pressure-sensitive adhesive around the opening. The adhesive firmly attaches the urine collector to the genitalia. Procedure 9-4 outlines the procedure for applying a pediatric urine collector.

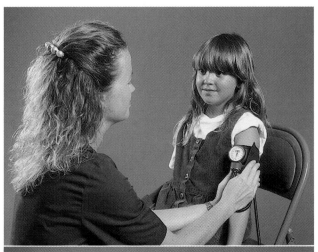

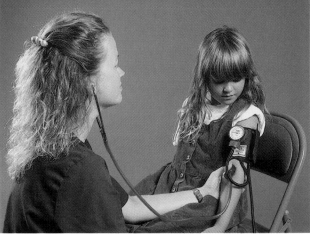

Figure 9-6. Traci measures the blood pressure of a pediatric patient.

PROCEDURE 9-4   Applying a Pediatric Urine Collector

Outcome Apply a pediatric urine collector.

Equipment/Supplies:
- Disposable gloves
- Personal antiseptic wipes
- Pediatric urine collector bag
- Urine specimen container and label
- Regular waste container

1. **Procedural Step.** Sanitize your hands.
2. **Procedural Step.** Assemble the equipment.

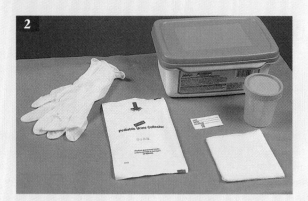

3. **Procedural Step.** Greet the child's parent, and identify the child. Introduce yourself, and explain the procedure.
4. **Procedural Step.** Apply gloves. Position the child. The child should be placed on the back with the legs spread apart. The medical assistant may need another individual to hold the child's legs apart.
   Principle. This position facilitates cleansing of the genitalia and permits proper application of the urine collector bag.
5. **Procedural Step.** Cleanse the child's genitalia.
   Female: Using a front-to-back motion (pubis to anus), cleanse each side of the meatus with a separate wipe. With a third wipe cleanse directly down the middle (directly over the urinary meatus). Allow the area to dry completely.
   Male: If the child is not circumcised, retract the foreskin of the penis. Cleanse the area around the meatus and the urethral opening (meatal orifice) in a manner similar to that used to cleanse the female patient. Be sure to use a separate wipe for each swipe. Cleanse the scrotum last, using a fresh wipe. Allow the area to dry completely.
   Principle. The urinary meatus and surrounding area must be cleansed to prevent contaminants such as baby powder, fecal material, and microorganisms from entering the urine specimen, which could affect the test results. A front-to-back motion must be used to prevent drawing microorganisms from the anal area into the area being

cleansed. The area must be completely dry to ensure an airtight adhesion of the collection bag to prevent leakage of urine.

6. **Procedural Step.** Remove the paper backing from the urine collector bag, thereby exposing the adhesive surface of the sponge ring. Firmly attach the bag in the following manner:
   Female: Place the bottom of the adhesive sponge ring on the perineum and work upward. Firmly press the sponge ring to the skin surrounding the external genitalia, making sure there is no puckering. The opening of the bag should be directly over the urinary meatus. The excess of the bag should be positioned toward the child's feet.

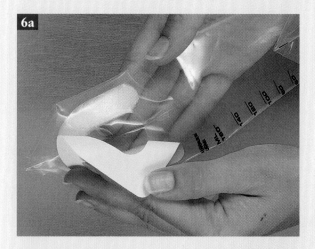

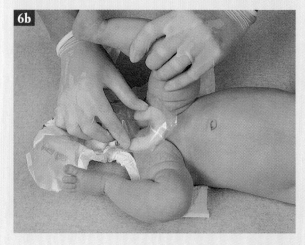

Male: Position the bag so the child's penis and scrotum are projected through the opening of the bag. Press the adhesive surface of the sponge ring firmly to the skin surrounding the penis and scrotum, making sure there is no puckering. Position the excess of the bag positioned towards the child's feet.

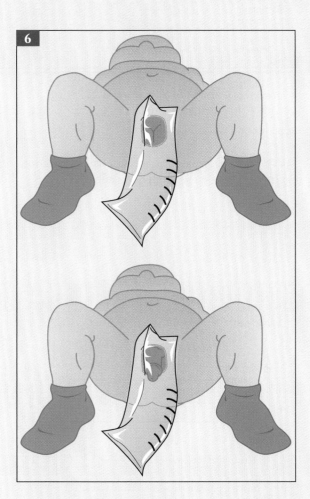

Principle. The sponge ring must be attached securely with no puckering to prevent leakage.

7. **Procedural Step.** Loosely diaper the child. Check the urine collector bag every 15 minutes until a urine specimen is obtained.
Principle. The diaper helps hold the urine collector bag in place.

8. **Procedural Step.** Once the child has voided, gently remove the urine collector bag.
Principle. The bag must be removed gently because pulling the adhesive away too quickly may cause discomfort and irritation of the child's skin.

9. **Procedural Step.** Clean the genital area with a personal antiseptic wipe. Rediaper the child.

10. **Procedural Step.** Transfer the urine specimen into a urine specimen container and tightly apply the lid. Label the container with the child's name, the date, the time of collection, and the type of specimen (i.e., urine). Dispose of the collector bag in a regular waste container. (*Note:* The urine collector bag can be used as a urine container to transport the specimen to the laboratory. This is accomplished by folding the adhesive sponge ring in half along its vertical axis and pressing the adhesive surfaces firmly together to ensure a tight seal.)

11. **Procedural Step.** Based on the medical office routine, test the urine specimen or prepare it for transfer to an outside laboratory, making sure to include a completed laboratory request form. If the specimen cannot be tested or transferred immediately, preserve it by placing it in the refrigerator.
Principle. Changes take place in a urine specimen that is left sitting out at room temperature.

12. **Procedural Step.** Remove the gloves, and sanitize your hands.

13. **Procedural Step.** Chart the procedure. Include the date, the time of collection, and the type of specimen (i.e., urine). If the specimen is to be transported to an outside laboratory, indicate this information, including the laboratory tests ordered.

CHARTING EXAMPLE

Date	
8/12/05	10:15 a.m. Urine specimen collected for culture. Picked up by Medical Center Lab on 8/12/05. ———————— T. Powell, CMA

PROCEDURE 9-4

Pediatric Injections

Administering an injection to a child is an important responsibility. The experience a child has with early injections influences his or her attitude toward later ones. If the child is old enough to understand, the procedure should be explained. The medical assistant should be honest and attempt to gain the child's trust and cooperation. The child should be told the truth about the injection—that it will hurt but only for a short time. It is also advisable to explain that the medicine will help him or her get better. Another person should be present to assist. The assistant can help position the child and can divert or restrain him or her if necessary. If the child struggles and fights excessively, however, the medical assistant should delay the injection and consult the physician.

The administration of injections is presented in Chapter 11. Before undertaking the study of pediatric injections, the medical assistant should review this chapter thoroughly, concentrating on the location of injection sites and the procedures for preparing and administering injections. The same basic technique is used to administer an injection to an adult and a child. Variations in procedure are explained in the following section.

Type of Needle

The gauge and length of the needle used for intramuscular injections vary, depending on the consistency of the medication to be administered and the size of the child. Thick or oily preparations require a larger needle lumen, and the needle must be long enough to reach muscle tissue. A needle length ranging from ⅝ inch to 1 inch is generally used to administer an IM injection to a child, and the gauge of the needle generally ranges between 22 and 25 depending on the viscosity of the medication.

The length of the needle used to administer a pediatric subcutaneous injection ranges between ⅜ inch and 1 inch, and the gauge of the needle ranges between 23 and 25.

Intramuscular Injection Sites

There are variations in pediatric injection sites based on the age of the child. The specific site to be injected is stated in the package insert accompanying the medication. Until the child is walking, the gluteus muscle is small, not well developed, and covered with a thick layer of fat. Moreover, an injection in the dorsogluteal site may come dangerously close to the sciatic nerve. The danger is increased if the child is squirming or fighting. Because serious trauma can result from incorrect administration of an injection in this area, it is recommended that the dorsogluteal site not be used until the child has been walking for at least a year (Figure 9-7).

The vastus lateralis muscle site is recommended instead for injections of infants and young children. It is located on the anterior surface of the midlateral thigh, away from

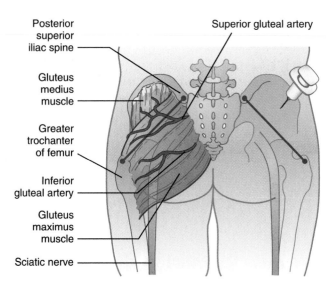

Figure 9-7. Dorsogluteal intramuscular injection site. (Courtesy Wyeth Laboratories, Philadelphia.)

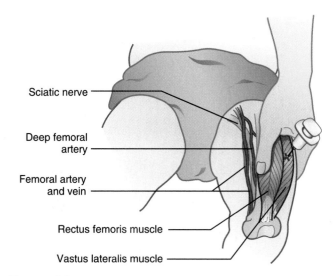

Figure 9-8. Vastus lateralis intramuscular injection site. (Courtesy Wyeth Laboratories, Philadelphia.)

major nerves and blood vessels, and it is large enough to accommodate the injected medication (Figure 9-8). The length of the needle used depends on the overall size of the thigh. It should be long enough to penetrate the muscle belly for proper absorption to take place. A 1-inch needle is often used. To administer the injection, the infant is placed on the back. The thigh is grasped in order to compress the muscle tissue and to stabilize the extremity. The injection is administered following the procedure outlined in Chapter 11.

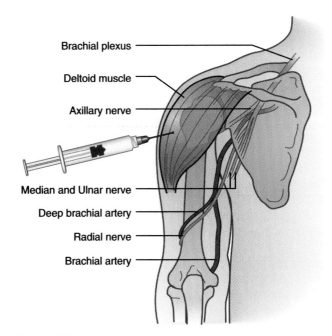

Figure 9-9. Deltoid intramuscular injection site. (Courtesy Wyeth Laboratories, Philadelphia.)

The deltoid muscle is shallow and can accommodate only a very small amount of medication. In addition, repeated injections to this site are painful. To administer the injection, the deltoid muscle mass should be grasped at the injection site and compressed between the thumb and fingers. The needle should be inserted pointing slightly upward toward the shoulder (Figure 9-9).

After giving the injection, the medical assistant or the child's parent should hold the infant and provide comfort and show approval so that the child associates something other than pain with this procedure.

Immunizations

Immunity is the resistance of the body to the effects of harmful agents such as pathogenic microorganisms and their toxins. The process of becoming immune or rendering an individual immune through the use of a **vaccine** or toxoid is known as active, artificial **immunization.** Immunizations build the body's defenses and protect an individual from attack by certain infectious diseases.

Immunizations should be administered to infants and young children during well-child visits according to an immunization schedule (Figure 9-10). The American Academy of Pediatrics recommends following the schedule outlined in the accompanying box. This schedule is

intended as a guide to be used with any modifications needed to meet the requirements of an individual or group.

The medical assistant should be familiar with every immunization that is given including its use, common side effects, route of administration, dosage, and method of storage. With each vaccine and toxoid the drug manufacturer includes a package insert that contains valuable information about the drug. Drug references, such as the *Physician's Desk Reference,* also can be used to locate information on immunizations. Immunizations administered to infants and children, along with the routes of administration and common minor problems, are listed in Table 9-6.

Parents should be provided with an immunization record card (Figure 9-11) at their baby's first well-child visit. They should be instructed to bring this card to every visit so that their child's immunizations can be recorded. Parents should be informed of the possible normal side effects of each immunization and given instructions on how to respond if they occur.

National Childhood Vaccine Injury Act

The National Childhood Vaccine Injury Act (NCVIA), which became effective in 1988, requires that parents be provided with information about the benefits and risks of childhood immunizations. To help medical offices comply with these regulations, the Centers for Disease Control developed a set of vaccine information statements. A vaccine information statement (VIS) explains, in lay terminology, the benefits and risks of a vaccine. See Figure 9-12 for a DTaP vaccine information statement.

The NCVIA requires that the appropriate VIS be given to the child's parent or guardian before the child receives a dose of any vaccine listed in Table 9-6. The medical assistant must make sure to give the parent or guardian enough time to read the VIS before the immunization is administered. In addition, the medical assistant must chart the following information in the patient's medical record: the date each VIS was provided and the publication date of the VIS, which is located at the bottom of the VIS.

Vaccine information statements are also available for influenza, pneumococcal polysaccharide, hepatitis A, meningococcal, and Lyme disease vaccines. Their use is encouraged, but not required, since these vaccines are not administered to children on a routine basis.

The NCVIA also requires that the following information be recorded in each patient's medical record following the administration of the vaccine: the date of administration of the vaccine, the manufacturer and lot number of the vaccine, the signature and title of the health care provider who administered the vaccine, and the address of the medical office where the vaccine was administered. See Figure 9-13 for an example of a pediatric vaccine administrative record.

PATIENT TEACHING

Childhood Immunizations

- Encourage parents to have their children immunized.
- Emphasize to parents the importance of maintaining an immunization record card that documents all of their children's immunizations.
- Provide parents with educational materials on the importance of immunizations.
- Answer questions patients have about childhood immunizations.

What is immunity?

Immunity is the resistance of the body to microorganisms that cause disease. When an individual has an infection, the body responds by producing disease-fighting substances known as antibodies. Antibodies usually remain in the body even after the individual has recovered from the disease. This protects the individual from getting that disease again.

How do immunizations prevent disease?

The microorganisms that cause disease or their toxins are weakened or killed and made into vaccines. These vaccines are then injected into the body. The body reacts to these vaccines the same way that it responds to the disease itself, by producing antibodies. These antibodies last for a long time, often for life, to defend the body against disease.

What childhood diseases can be prevented through immunization?

The reduction of childhood disease by immunization during the past 40 years has been dramatic. Eleven diseases can be prevented by routine immunization: hepatitis B, diphtheria, tetanus, pertussis, *Haemophilus influenzae* type b infections, polio, measles, mumps, rubella (German measles), chickenpox (varicella), and pneumococcal infections (meningitis and blood infections). Except for tetanus, all these diseases are contagious. They can be spread from child to child and from one community to another. When children are not protected against them, serious outbreaks of disease can still occur.

Haven't most of these diseases been eliminated in the United States?

Although most of the vaccine-preventable diseases have been reduced to very low levels in the United States, this is not true worldwide. Some of these diseases are quite prevalent in other countries. An infected traveler can bring these diseases into the United States without knowing it. If Americans were not immunized, these diseases could quickly spread throughout the population and cause an epidemic. Only when a disease has been eradicated worldwide, is it safe to stop vaccinating for that particular disease.

Do immunizations have side effects?

Vaccines are among the safest and most reliable medications available. However, minor side effects may occur following administration of an immunization. They do not last long and may include a slight fever and irritability; redness, swelling, and soreness at the injection site; and a mild rash. On rare occasions, the effects can be more serious; therefore if any unusual symptoms occur following immunization, it is important to contact the physician immediately. Overall the benefits of vaccines to prevent childhood diseases are greater than the possible risks for almost all children.

Are immunizations required by law?

Every state has laws requiring vaccination against some or all of these diseases before children enter school. Children who get their vaccinations not only benefit from the protection these vaccinations provide, but they also contribute to the well-being of everyone by reducing the chance for disease to spread.

What Would You DO? What Would You Not DO?

Case Study 3

Stacy Jones, a legal secretary, brings her 5-year-old son, Matthew, in for a kindergarten physical. Stacy has read the vaccine information statements for the DTaP, IPV, and MMR immunizations that Matthew will be getting at this visit and has some questions. She wants to know why polio isn't given orally anymore. She also wants to know why children are immunized against chickenpox since it's such a harmless disease. She is somewhat annoyed by all this because she thinks that children are receiving too many unnecessary injections these days. Matthew is extremely afraid of "shots" and says that no one with a needle is getting anywhere near him. Stacy is rather protective of Matthew and knows that he will be hard to handle. She wants to know if this set of immunizations could just be skipped. She says that most of these diseases don't even exist anymore and that she noticed, from reading the vaccine sheets, that there are a lot of possible side effects.

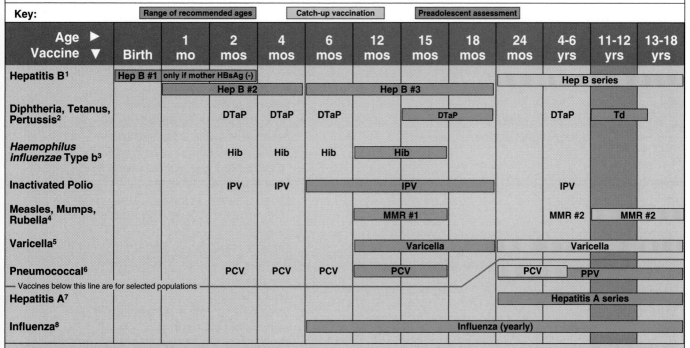

Recommended Childhood Immunization Schedule, United States 2003

This schedule indicates the recommended ages for routine administration of currently licensed childhood vaccines, as of December 1, 2002, for children through age 18 years. Any dose not given at the recommended age should be given at any subsequent visit when indicated and feasible. ☐ Indicates age groups that warrant special effort to administer those vaccines not previously given. Additional vaccines may be licensed and recommended during the year. Licensed combination vaccines may be used whenever any components of the combination are indicated and the vaccine's other components are not contraindicated. Providers should consult the manufacturers' package insert for detailed recommendations.

1. Hepatitis B Vaccine (Hep B). All infants should receive the first dose of hepatitis B vaccine soon after birth and before hospital discharge; the first dose may also be given by age 2 months if the infant's mother is HBsAg-negative. Only monovalent hepatitis B vaccine can be used for the birth dose. Monovalent or combination vaccine containing Hep B may be used to complete the series; four doses of vaccine may be administered if combination vaccine is used. The second dose should be given at least 4 weeks after the first dose, except for Hib-containing vaccine which cannot be administered before age 6 weeks. The third dose should be given at least 16 weeks after the first dose and at least 8 weeks after the second dose. The last dose in the vaccination series (third or fourth dose) should not be administered before age 6 months.

Infants born to HBsAg-positive mothers should receive hepatitis B vaccine and 0.5 mL hepatitis B immune globulin (HBIG) within 12 hours of birth at separate sites. The second dose is recommended at age 1–2 months. The last dose in the vaccination series should not be administered before age 6 months. These infants should be tested for HBsAg and anti-HBs at 9–15 months of age.

Infants born to mothers whose HBsAg status is unknown should receive the first dose of hepatitis B vaccine series within 12 hours of birth. Maternal blood should be drawn as soon as possible to determine the mother's HBsAg status; if the HBsAg test is positive, the infant should receive HBIG as soon as possible (no later than age 1 week). The second dose is recommended at age 1–2 months. The last dose in the vaccination series should not be administered before age 6 months.

2. Diphtheria and tetanus toxoids and acellular pertussis vaccine (DTaP). The fourth dose of DTaP may be administered as early as age 12 months, provided 6 months have elapsed since the third dose and the child is unlikely to return at age 15–18 months. **Tetanus and diphtheria toxoids (Td)** is recommended at age 11–12 years if at least 5 years have elapsed since the last dose of tetanus and diphtheria toxoid-containing vaccine. Subsequent routine Td boosters are recommended every 10 years.

3. Haemophilus influenzae type b (Hib) conjugate vaccine. Three Hib conjugate vaccines are licensed for infant use. If PRP-OMP (PedvaxHIB® or ComVax® [Merck]) is administered at ages 2 and 4 months, a dose at age 6 months is not required. DTaP/Hib combination products should not be used for primary immunization in infants at age 2, 4 or 6 months, but can be used as boosters following any Hib vaccine.

4. Measles, mumps, and rubella vaccine (MMR). The second dose of MMR is recommended routinely at age 4–6 years but may be administered during any visit, provided at least 4 weeks have elapsed since the first dose and that both doses are administered at or after age 12 months. Those who have not previously received the second dose should complete the schedule by the 11–12 year old visit.

5. Varicella vaccine. Varicella vaccine is recommended at any visit at or after age 12 months for susceptible children (i.e. those who lack a reliable history of chickenpox). Susceptible persons aged ≥ 13 years should receive two doses, given at least 4 weeks apart.

6. Pneumococcal vaccine. The heptavalent **pneumococcal conjugate vaccine (PCV)** is recommended for all children aged 2–23 months and for certain children aged 24–59 months. **Pneumococcal polysaccharide vaccine (PPV)** is recommended in addition to PCV for certain high-risk groups. See *MMWR* 2000;49(RR-9);1–38.

7. Hepatitis A vaccine. Hepatitis A vaccine is recommended for children and adolescents in selected states and regions, and for certain high-risk groups; consult your local public health authority. Children and adolescents in these states, regions, and high risk groups who have not been immunized against hepatitis A can begin the hepatitis A vaccination series during any visit. The two doses in the series should be administered at least 6 months apart. See *MMWR* 1999;48(RR-12);1–37.

8. Influenza vaccine. Influenza vaccine is recommended annually for children age ≥ 6 months with certain risk factors (including but not limited to asthma, cardiac disease, sickle cell disease, HIV, diabetes, and household members of persons in groups at high risk; see *MMWR* 2002;51 (RR-3);1–31), and can be administered to all others wishing to obtain immunity. In addition, healthy children age 6–23 months are encouraged to receive influenza vaccine if feasible because children in this age group are at substantially increased risk for influenza-related hospitalizations. Children aged ≤12 years should receive vaccine in a dosage appropriate for their age (0.25 mL if age 6–35 months or 0.5 mL if aged ≥3 years). Children aged ≤ 8 years who are receiving influenza vaccine for the first time should receive two doses separated by at least 4 weeks.

For additional information about vaccines, vaccine supply, and contraindications for immunization, please visit the National Immunization Program Website at www.cdc.gov.nip or call the National Immunization Hotline at 800-232-2522 (English) or 800-232-0233 (Spanish). Approved by the Advisory Committee on Immunization Practices (www.cdc.gov/nip/acip), the American Academy of Pediatrics (www.aap.org), and the American Academy of Family Physicians (www.aafp.org).

Figure 9-10. Immunization schedule.

TABLE **9-6**	Childhood Immunizations

Immunization		Route of Administration	Common Minor Problems Following Administration
Hep B	Hepatitis B vaccine	IM	Mild to moderate fever Soreness at the injection site
DTaP	Diphtheria and tetanus toxoids and acellular pertussis vaccine	M	Fever, irritability, tiredness, and poor appetite Redness or swelling at the injection site Soreness or tenderness at the injection site (Occurs 1 to 3 days after the injection)
Hib	Haemophilus influenzae type b conjugate vaccine	M	Fever higher than 101° F Redness, warmth, or swelling at the injection site (Occurs within a day after the injection; lasts 2 to 3 days)
IPV	Inactivated polio vaccine	IM or SC	Soreness at the injection site
MMR	Measles, mumps, and rubella vaccine	SC	Fever Mild rash
Varicella	Chickenpox vaccine	SC	Fever, mild rash Soreness or swelling at the injection site
PCV	Pneumococcal conjugate vaccine	IM	Fever higher than 100.4° F Irritability and drowsiness Loss of appetite

Newborn Screening Test

A newborn screening test is performed on the infant to screen for the presence of certain metabolic and endocrine diseases. These diseases include phenylketonuria (PKU), hypothyroidism, galactosemia, homocystinuria, and sickle cell anemia. The most important of these is the PKU, which is described in the following paragraphs.

Phenylketonuria is a congenital hereditary disease caused by a lack of the enzyme *phenylalanine hydroxylase*. This enzyme is needed to convert phenylalanine, an amino acid, into tyrosine, which is an amino acid needed for normal metabolic functioning. Without this enzyme, phenylalanine accumulates in the blood and, if the accumulation is left untreated, causes mental retardation and other abnormalities such as tremors and poor muscle coordination. In most cases, upon early detection, a special low-phenylalanine diet and close periodic monitoring can prevent adverse effects. Normal development usually occurs if treatment is started before the child reaches 3 to 4 weeks of age. To promote the best development of cognitive abilities, most authorities recommend lifelong dietary restriction of phenylalanine.

All states require by law that infants undergo PKU screening. The best time to perform the test is between 1 and 7 days after birth. Although PKU is not a common condition (affecting 1 in every 12,000 births), early diagnosis and treatment lead to a better prognosis.

Phenylalanine can be detected in the blood of an afflicted child only after the child has been on an intake of breast or formula milk. Infants taking formula can be tested earlier than breast-fed babies because formula contains phenylalanine, whereas the "first breast-milk," or colostrum, does not. Therefore the test results of breast-fed babies are usually invalid until the mother begins producing milk.

The newborn screening test is performed on capillary blood obtained from the plantar surface of the infant's heel. The blood specimen is placed on a special filter paper attached to the newborn screening test card (Figure 9-14) and mailed to an outside laboratory for analysis. The results are ready in a few days. If one of the newborn screening test results is positive, further testing is performed.

IMMUNIZATION RECORD

Name _____

Birthdate _____

Immunization	DATE	DATE	DATE	DATE	DATE
Heb B (Hepatitis B)					
DTaP (Diphtheria, Tetanus, and Pertussis)					
Hib (Haemophilius Influenzae Type b)					
IPV (Inactivated Polio Vaccine)					
MMR (Measles, Mumps, Rubella)					
Varicella (Chickenpox)					
PCV (Pneumococcal Conjugate Vaccine)					
Tuberculin (Mantoux) **RESULT**					
Tetanus Booster					
Other					

Figure 9-11. Immunization record card.

DIPHTHERIA, TETANUS AND PERTUSSIS VACCINE

What You Need to Know

1. Why get vaccinated?

Diphtheria, tetanus, and pertussis are serious diseases caused by bacteria. Diphtheria and pertussis are spread from person to person. Tetanus enters the body through cuts or wounds.

DIPHTHERIA causes a thick covering in the back of the throat.
• It can lead to breathing problems, paralysis, heart failure, and even death.

TETANUS (Lockjaw) causes painful tightening of the muscles, usually all over the body.
• It can lead to "locking" of the jaw so the victim cannot open his mouth or swallow. Tetanus leads to death in about 1 out of 10 cases.

PERTUSSIS (Whooping cough) causes coughing spells so bad that it is hard for infants to eat, drink, or breathe. These spells can last for weeks.
• It can lead to pneumonia, seizures (jerking and staring spells), brain damage, and death.

Diphtheria, tetanus, and pertussis vaccine (DTaP) can help prevent these diseases. Most children who are vaccinated with DTaP will be protected throughout childhood. Many more children would get these diseases if we stopped vaccinating.

DTaP is a safer version of an older vaccine called DTP. DTP is no longer used in the United States.

2. Who should get DTaP vaccine and when?

Children shoud get <u>5 doses</u> of DTaP vaccine, one dose at each of the following ages:

2 months	15–18 months
4 months	4–6 years
6 months	

DTaP may be given at the same time as other vaccines.

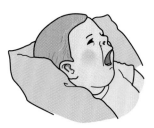

3. Some children should not get DTaP vaccine or should wait

• Children with minor illnesses, such as a cold, may be vaccinated. But children who are moderately or severely ill should wait until they recover before getting DTaP vaccine.

• Any child who had a life-threatening allergic reaction after a dose of DTaP should not get another dose.

• Any child who suffered a brain or nervous systyem disease within 7 days after a dose of DTaP should not get another dose.

• Talk with your doctor if your child:
  – had a seizure or collapsed after a dose of DTaP,
  – cried non-stop for 3 hours or more after a dose of DTaP,
  – had a fever over 105°F after a dose of DTaP.

Ask your health care provider for more information. Some of these children should not get another dose of pertussis vaccine, but may get a vaccine without pertussis, called **DT**.

4. Older children and adults

DTaP should not be given to anyone 7 years of age or older because pertussis vaccine is only licensed for children under 7.

But older children, adolescents, and adults still need protection from tetanus and diphtheria. A booster shot called **Td** is recommended at 11–12 years of age, and then every 10 years. There is a separate Vaccine Information Statement for Td vaccine.

Diptheria/ Tetanus/ Pertussis 7/30/2001

Figure 9-12. Vaccine information statement for DTaP. (Courtesy Centers for Disease Control and Prevention, Atlanta, Georgia.)

Continued

5. What are the risks from DTaP vaccine?

Getting diphtheria, tetanus, or pertussis disease is much riskier than getting DTaP vaccine.

However, a vaccine, like any medicine, is capable of causing serious problems, such as severe allergic reactions. The risk of DTaP vaccine causing serious harm, or death, is extremely small.

Mild Problems (Common)
• Fever (up to about 1 child in 4)
• Redness or swelling where the shot was given (up to about 1 child in 4)
• Soreness or tenderness where the shot was given (up to about 1 child in 4).
These problems occur more often after the fourth and fifth doses of the DTaP series than after earlier doses. Sometimes the fourth or fifth dose of DTaP vaccine is followed by swelling of the entire arm or leg in which the shot was given, lasting 1–7 days (up to about 1 child in 30).
Other mild problems include:
• Fussiness (up to about 1 child in 3)
• Tiredness or poor appetite (up to about 1 child in 10)
• Vomiting (up to about 1 child in 50)

These problems generally occur 1–3 days after the shot.

Moderate Problems (Uncommon)
• Seizure (jerking or staring) (about 1 child out of 14,000)
• Non-stop crying, for 3 hours or more (up to about 1 child out of 1,000)
• High fever, over 105°F (about 1 child out of 16,000)

Severe Problems (Very Rare)
• Serious allergic reactions (less than 1 out of a million doses)
• Several other severe problems have been reported after DTaP vaccine. These include:
  – Long-term seizures, coma, or lowered consciousness
  – Permanent brain damage.
  These are so rare it is hard to tell if they are caused by the vaccine.

Controlling fever is especially important for children who have had seizures, for any reason. It is also important if another family member has had seizures. You can reduce fever and pain by giving your child an *aspirin-free* pain reliever when the shot is given, and for the next 24 hours, following the package instructions.

6. What if there is a moderate or severe reaction?

What should I look for?

Any unusual conditions, such as a serious allergic reaction, high fever or unusual behavior. Serious allergic reactions are extremely rare with any vaccine. If one were to occur, it would most likely be within a few minutes to a few hours after the shot. Signs can include difficulty breathing, hoarseness or wheezing, hives, paleness, weakness, a fast heart beat or dizziness. If a high fever or seizure were to occur, it would usually be within a week after the shot.

What should I do?

• Call a doctor, or get the person to a doctor right away.
• Tell your doctor what happened, the date and time it happened, and when the vaccination was given.
• Ask your doctor, nurse, or health department to file a Vaccine Adverse Event Reporting System (VAERS) form, or call VAERS yourself at 1-800-822-7967.

7. The National Vaccine Injury Compensation Program

In the rare event that you or your child has a serious reaction to a vaccine, a federal program has been created to help pay for the care of those who have been harmed.

For details about the National Vaccine Injury Compensation Program, call **1-800-338-2382** or visit the program's website at **http://www.hrsa.gov./bhpr/vicp**

8. How can I learn more?

• Ask your health care provider. They can give you the vaccine package insert or suggest other sources of information.

• Call your local or state health department's immunization program.

• Contact the Centers for Disease Control and Prevention (CDC):
  – Call **1-800-232-2522** (English)
  – Call **1-800-232-0233** (Español)
  – Visit the National Immunization Program's website at **http://www.cdc.gov/nip**

U.S. DEPARTMENT OF HEALTH AND HUMAN SERVICES
Centers for Disease Control and Prevention
National Immunization Program

Figure 9-12, cont'd. Vaccine information statement for DTaP. (Courtesy Centers for Disease Control and Prevention, Atlanta, Georgia.)

PEDIATRIC VACCINE ADMINISTRATION RECORD

Name _____
(first)   (MI)   (last)

DOB _____

Physician _____

Address _____
_____

SITE ABBREVIATIONS:

RVL: Right vastus lateralis

LVL: Left vastus lateralis

RD: Right deltoid

LD: Left deltoid

Vaccine	Date Dose and VIS Given	Vaccine Manufacturer	Vaccine Lot Number	Exp. Date	Site	VIS Pub. Date	Signature of Vaccine Administrator
DTaP 1							
DTaP 2							
DTaP 3							
DTaP 4							
DTaP 5							
Hib 1							
Hib 2							
Hib 3							
Hib 4							
IPV 1							
IPV 2							
IPV 3							
IPV 4							
MMR 1							
MMR 2							
Hep B 1							
Hep B 2							
Hep B 3							
Mantoux							Reaction
Varicella 1							
Varicella 2							
PCV 1							
PCV 2							
PCV 3							
PCV 4							
Other							
Other							

Figure 9-13. Pediatric vaccine administration record.

PROCEDURE 9-5 Newborn Screening Test

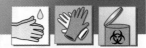

Outcome Collect a capillary blood specimen for a newborn screening test.

Equipment/Supplies:
- Disposable gloves
- Infant heel warmer or warm compress
- Antiseptic wipe
- Sterile 2 × 2 gauze pad
- Sterile lancet
- Newborn screening test card
- Mailing envelope
- Biohazard sharps container

1. Procedural Step. Sanitize your hands, and assemble the equipment.

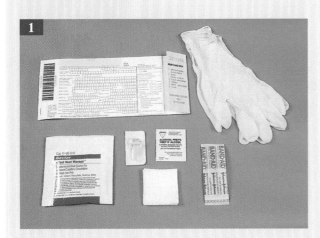

2. Procedural Step. Greet the infant's parent, and identify the infant. Introduce yourself, and explain the procedure.

3. Procedural Step. Complete the information section of the newborn screening card.

4. Procedural Step. Apply gloves. Select an appropriate puncture site. The lateral and medial curves of the plantar surface of the heel can be used.
Principle. The lateral and medial curves of the heel are used to avoid calcaneal complications.

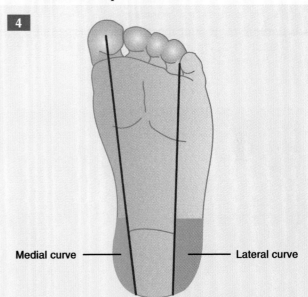

Medial curve ————   ———— Lateral curve

The shading indicates the appropriate
area for making the puncture.

5. Procedural Step. Warm the puncture site with a commercially available infant heel warmer or a warm compress for approximately 5 minutes.
Principle. Warming the puncture site increases capillary circulation and promotes bleeding.

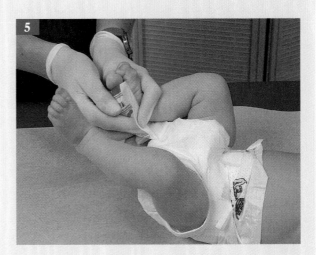

PROCEDURE 9-5

Continued

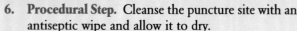

PROCEDURE 9-5 Newborn Screening Test—Cont'd

6. **Procedural Step.** Cleanse the puncture site with an antiseptic wipe and allow it to dry.

7. **Procedural Step.** Grasp the infant's foot around the puncture site and, without touching the cleansed site, make a puncture with the sterile lancet. The puncture should be made at a right angle to the lines of the skin. Dispose of the lancet in a biohazard sharps container.

Principle. Touching the site after cleansing will contaminate it, and the cleansing process will have to be repeated.

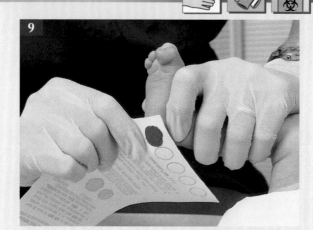

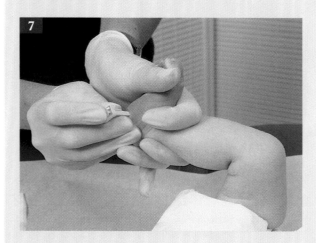

8. **Procedural Step.** Wipe away the first drop of blood with a gauze pad.

Principle. The first drop of blood is diluted with alcohol and tissue fluid and is not a suitable specimen.

9. **Procedural Step.** Encourage a large drop of blood to form by exerting gentle pressure without excessively squeezing the area. Place the backside of the filter paper (side opposite the circles) next to the baby's heel. Touch the drop of blood to the center of the first circle on the test card and completely fill the first circle with the blood specimen. The proper amount of specimen is obtained when the blood can be observed soaking completely through the filter paper from one side to the other.

Principle. Excessive squeezing will cause dilution of the blood sample with tissue fluid, leading to inaccurate test results.

10. **Procedural Step.** Repeat step 9 until all the circles on the card are completely filled with blood.

Principle. The circles must be completely filled to ensure enough of a blood sample to perform the test. Most repeat tests are required because of inadequate blood specimens.

11. **Procedural Step.** Hold a piece of gauze over the puncture site and apply pressure to control the bleeding. Remain with the infant until the bleeding stops.

12. **Procedural Step.** Remove the gloves and sanitize your hands.

13. **Procedural Step.** Allow the test card to dry for 2 hours at room temperature on a nonabsorbent surface. Cards should not be stacked together while drying.

14. **Procedural Step.** After the blood is completely dry, place the test card in its protective envelope and mail it to an outside laboratory for testing within 48 hours.

Principle. The test card should be mailed within 48 hours to ensure accurate test results.

15. **Procedural Step.** Chart the procedure. Include the date and time, the type of procedure, the puncture site location, and information regarding transfer to an outside laboratory.

CHARTING EXAMPLE

Date	
8/15/05	9:30 a.m. Blood specimen collected from ® medial heel. Sent to Newborn Screening Lab on 8/15/05 for newborn screening test.
	—————————————— T. Powell, CMA

PROCEDURE 9-5

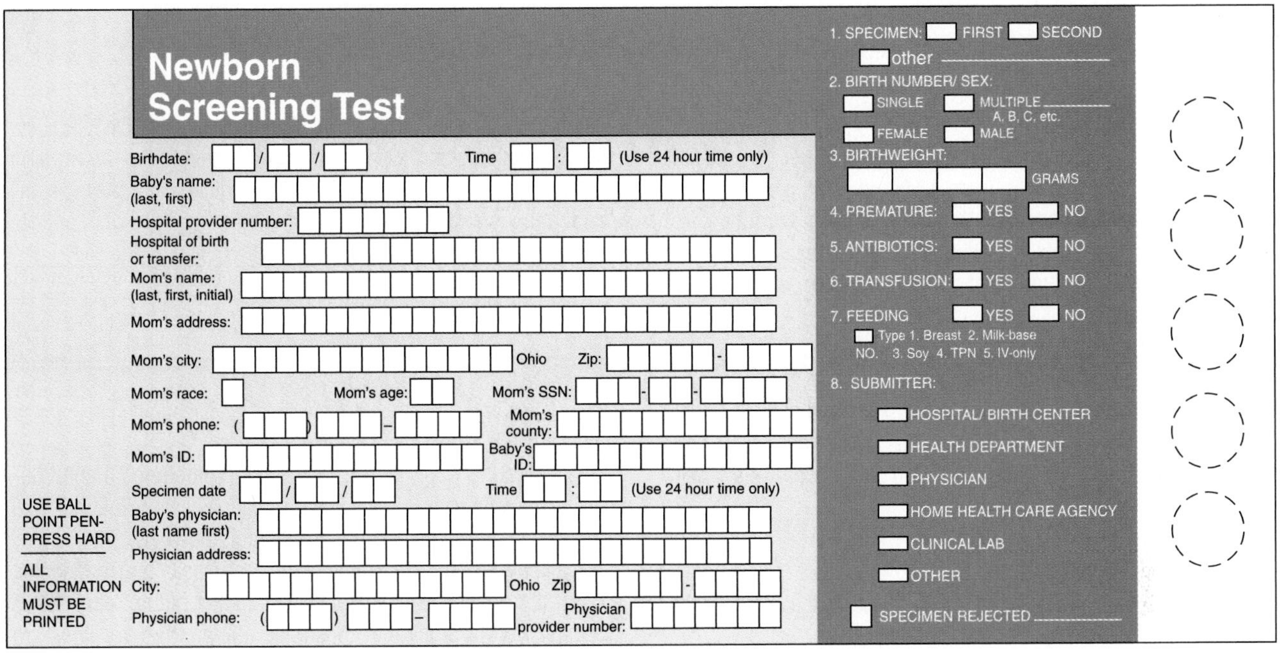

Newborn Screening Test

Birthdate: ☐☐ / ☐☐ / ☐☐   Time ☐☐ : ☐☐ (Use 24 hour time only)

Baby's name: (last, first)

Hospital provider number:

Hospital of birth or transfer:

Mom's name: (last, first, initial)

Mom's address:

Mom's city: _____ Ohio   Zip: ☐☐☐☐☐-☐☐☐☐

Mom's race: ☐   Mom's age: ☐☐   Mom's SSN: ☐☐☐-☐☐-☐☐☐☐

Mom's phone: (☐☐☐) ☐☐☐-☐☐☐☐   Mom's county:

Mom's ID: Baby's ID:

Specimen date ☐☐ / ☐☐ / ☐☐   Time ☐☐ : ☐☐ (Use 24 hour time only)

Baby's physician: (last name first)

Physician address:

City: _____ Ohio Zip ☐☐☐☐☐-☐☐☐☐

Physician phone: (☐☐☐) ☐☐☐-☐☐☐☐   Physician provider number:

USE BALL POINT PEN-PRESS HARD

ALL INFORMATION MUST BE PRINTED

1. SPECIMEN: ☐ FIRST ☐ SECOND ☐ other _____

2. BIRTH NUMBER/ SEX:
☐ SINGLE   ☐ MULTIPLE _____ A, B, C, etc.
☐ FEMALE   ☐ MALE

3. BIRTHWEIGHT: _____ GRAMS

4. PREMATURE: ☐ YES ☐ NO

5. ANTIBIOTICS: ☐ YES ☐ NO

6. TRANSFUSION: ☐ YES ☐ NO

7. FEEDING ☐ YES ☐ NO
☐ Type 1. Breast 2. Milk-base NO. 3. Soy 4. TPN 5. IV-only

8. SUBMITTER:
☐ HOSPITAL/ BIRTH CENTER
☐ HEALTH DEPARTMENT
☐ PHYSICIAN
☐ HOME HEALTH CARE AGENCY
☐ CLINICAL LAB
☐ OTHER

☐ SPECIMEN REJECTED _____

Figure 9-14. Newborn screening test card.

MEDICAL Practice and the LAW

Children are not small adults. They must be treated as individuals, according to their developmental level. Pediatric patients, except for emancipated minors, cannot give written or verbal consents. Make sure a parent or *legal* guardian is available for consent. For example, a babysitter or grandparent cannot give consent for treatment without written permission from a parent or legal guardian. Similarly, patient information can be given only to a parent or legal guardian.

If your office sees pediatric patients, you have a responsibility to be aware of developmental needs and milestones of children at various ages. This is necessary for accurate developmental assessment.

What Would You DO?
What Would You *Not* DO? *RESPONSES*

Case Study 1
What Did Traci Do?

❑ Listened patiently to Mrs. Chang and allowed her to vent her frustrations.

❑ Reassured Mrs. Chang that her milk is very nutritious for Christopher. Gave her a brochure on breastfeeding that included information on what to do for sore nipples and engorgement.

❑ Gave Mrs. Chang the names and phones number of community resources for nursing mothers.

❑ Told Mrs. Chang that Christopher's weight and length do not fall in the underweight category on his growth chart. Showed her Christopher's growth chart so she could see that Christopher is progressing normally.

What Did Traci Not Do?

❑ Did not tell Mrs. Chang to cheer up because the colic would eventually go away on its own.

❑ Did not give a personal opinion on whether Mrs. Chang should breastfeed or bottle-feed her baby.

What Would You Do?/What Would You *Not* Do? Review Traci's response and place a checkmark next to the information you included in your response. List additional information included in your response.

_____
_____
_____
_____

Case Study 2
What Did Traci Do?

❑ Explained to Mrs. Tilly that childhood obesity has doubled in the past 20 years and has become a serious health concern.

❑ Told Mrs. Tilly that she could have a big impact on Courtney's life by preparing healthy meals and eating them with her and also by becoming involved in activities with Courtney such as taking walks.

❑ Spent some time talking with Courtney about her interests and complimented Courtney on her achievements.

❑ Encouraged Courtney to join the swim team and told her that lots of people don't like to be seen in a bathing suit and encouraged her not to let that stand in her way of doing something she wants to do.

❑ Reassured Courtney that the doctor wants to help her and that he would never say anything bad about her weight.

What Did Traci Not Do?

❑ Did not agree with Mrs. Tilly that there is nothing that can be done about Courtney's weight problem.

❑ Did not tell Courtney that she needs to lose weight or she might develop serious health problems such as diabetes.

What Would You Do?/What Would You *Not* Do? Review Traci's response and place a checkmark next to the information you included in your response. List additional information included in your response.

_____
_____
_____
_____

Case Study 3
What Did Traci Do?

❑ Explained to Stacy that it is rare, but sometimes a child develops polio from getting the oral polio vaccine. Told her that this does not occur with the injectable polio vaccine.

❑ Explained to Stacy that chickenpox is usually a mild disease, but it can be serious especially in young infants and adults.

❑ Explained to Stacy that most side effects from vaccines are mild and the complications from the diseases far outweigh the possible side effects.

❑ Told Stacy that these diseases have been reduced to very low levels in this country, but they still occur in other countries. Explained that infected travelers can bring these diseases to the United States and infect individuals who are not immunized.

❑ Reminded Stacy that these immunizations are required for Matthew to start kindergarten.

❑ Talked with Matthew on his level about why he needs to be immunized.

❑ Told Matthew that they would play a game so it wouldn't hurt much. Taught him to hold up his finger and pretended that it was a birthday candle; when the injection was given, told him to keep blowing out the candle until he was told to stop.

❑ Told Matthew that he could choose a prize from the treasure chest after he had his immunizations.

What Did Traci Not Do?

❑ Did not ignore or minimize Stacy's concerns.

❑ Did not tell Stacy that the answers to all her questions are in the vaccine information sheets that she was just given.

❑ Did not tell Stacy it would be all right to skip Matthew's immunizations.

❑ Did not refer to the immunizations as "shots" when talking with Matthew.

❑ Did not tell Matthew that it would not hurt when he gets his immunizations.

What Would You Do?/What Would You *Not* Do? Review Traci's response and place a checkmark next to the information you included in your response. List additional information included in your response.

_____
_____
_____
_____

Apply Your KNOWLEDGE

Choose the best answer for the following questions.

1. Trisha Jordan, a surgical nurse, brings her 6-month-old daughter, Amy, to the office for a well-child visit. To prepare the exam room for her visit, Traci Powell, CMA, would have available all of the following EXCEPT:
   A. A pediatric balance scale
   B. A growth chart for Girls: Birth to 36 Months
   C. A blood pressure cuff and stethoscope
   D. A cm tape measure

2. All of the following immunizations will be given to 6-month-old Amy at this visit EXCEPT:
   A. DTaP   C. Hib
   B. MMR   D. IPV

3. Traci Powell, CMA, measures Amy's weight and length and calculates her growth values. Amy is in the 75th percentile for weight and the 25th percentile for length. Traci notices that Amy has been in approximately these same percentiles since birth. Which of the following will Dr. Immunity most likely relay to Mrs. Jordan regarding Amy's growth?
   A. Amy needs to have some growth evaluation tests
   B. You have a short fat baby
   C. Amy is growing normally
   D. You need to stop breastfeeding

4. Traci asks Mrs. Jordan some questions regarding Amy's stage of development. Which of the following should Amy be able to do now that she is 6 months old?
   A. Sit without support
   B. Ride a bike
   C. Stand alone
   D. Pick up small objects

5. John Whitmore, a stay-at-home dad, brings his 6-year-old daughter, Samantha, to the office for her kindergarten physical. Samantha is to receive an MMR immunization at this visit. Mr. Whitmore wants to know what vaccines are in an MMR. Traci Powell, CMA, tells him that MMR includes:
   A. Meningitis, mumps, and rubella
   B. Measles, mumps, and rubella
   C. Measles, mumps, and roseola
   D. Measles, mononucleosis, and rat-fever

6. Samantha is also scheduled for a DTaP immunization during this visit. Mr. Jordan wants to know if this immunization has side effects. Which of the following should Traci Powell, CMA, relay to Mr. Jordan?
   A. Amy may be fussy and tired 1 to 3 days after the injection
   B. The vaccine may cause a slight fever 1 to 3 days after the injection
   C. There may be some swelling and redness at the injection site
   D. All of the above

7. Samantha is very upset about having to get "shots." A developmentally appropriate approach that Traci could use to reduce Samantha's anxiety level might be:
   A. Tell Samantha that she is a "big girl" and should not cry
   B. Have Samantha count from ten to one backwards while the injections are being administered
   C. Have Samantha's father give her the injections
   D. Have Samantha read the VISs for these vaccines so she will understand why she needs them

8. Samantha is crying after receiving her immunizations. Traci Powell, CMA, would respond to her behavior by:
   A. Telling Samantha that she is disappointed because she thought Samantha would be braver about this
   B. Leaving the room and letting Samantha's father handle the situation
   C. Giving Samantha a hug and letting her pick a prize from the treasure chest
   D. Having the doctor do a tap-dance for Samantha to cheer her up

9. After administering the DTaP injection, Traci is required by the NCVIA to record all of the following in Samantha's chart EXCEPT:
   A. The expiration date of the vaccine
   B. The lot number of the vaccine
   C. The manufacturer of the vaccine
   D. The date the injection was administered

Continued

10. Cecila Morales, a radiologic technician, comes in with her newborn son, Sandro, who is 1 week old. Sandro had a PKU test done in the hospital, but now must have another one done at the medical office. Mrs. Morales wants to know why the PKU test has to be repeated. Traci Powell, CMA, is aware that Mrs. Morales is breastfeeding and includes all of the following statements in her explanation EXCEPT:

A. Breast-fed babies can be tested earlier for PKU than formula-fed babies
B. The PKU test is not accurate until the baby is consuming milk
C. The first few days after delivery a nursing mother produces colostrum, which is not "true" milk
D. Colostrum causes invalid PKU test results

CERTIFICATION REVIEW

❑ **Pediatrics** is the branch of medicine that deals with the care and development of children and the diagnosis and treatment of diseases in children. A pediatrician is a medical doctor who specializes in pediatrics.

❑ **There are two categories of pediatric office visit:** the well-child visit and the sick child visit. The purpose of the well-child visit is to receive necessary immunizations and to observe for abnormal conditions associated with the child's stage of development. The sick child visit is to diagnose the condition of a child who is exhibiting the signs and symptoms of disease.

❑ **To evaluate the progress of a child,** the weight, height (or length), and head circumference are measured during each visit and plotted on a growth chart. The child's weight is used to determine nutritional needs and the proper dosage of a medication to administer to the child. Growth charts provide a means for assessing the child's rate of growth; the physician investigates any significant change or rapid rise or drop in the child's growth pattern.

❑ **Blood pressure** should be measured in children 3 years of age and older to identify children at risk for developing hypertension as adults. To obtain an accurate pediatric blood pressure measurement, the correct cuff size must be used. Blood pressure varies depending on the age of the child, as well as his or her height and gender.

❑ **A urine specimen** may be required from a pediatric patient as part of a general physical examination to assist in the diagnosis of a pathologic condition or to evaluate the effec-

tiveness of therapy. Collecting a urine specimen from an infant or young child who cannot urinate voluntarily involves the use of a pediatric urine collector.

❑ **Administering an injection to a child** uses the same basic technique as that used to administer an injection to an adult. The vastus lateralis muscle is the recommended intramuscular injection site for infants and young children. It is large enough to accommodate the injected medication. The dorsogluteal site should not be used until the child has been walking for at least a year.

❑ **Immunity** is the resistance of the body to the effects of harmful agents such as pathogenic microorganisms and their toxins. Immunizations build the body's defenses and protect an individual from attack by certain infectious diseases.

❑ **The National Childhood Vaccine Injury Act (NCVIA)** requires that parents be provided with information about the benefits and risks of childhood immunizations through VISs (Vaccine Information Sheets) developed by the Centers for Disease Control and Prevention.

❑ **Phenylketonuria (PKU)** is a congenital hereditary disease. If left untreated, PKU can result in mental retardation and other abnormalities. Most states require that infants undergo PKU screening because early diagnosis and treatment can lead to a better prognosis. In addition to the PKU test, other tests are performed on the blood specimen to screen for congenital hypothyroidism, galactosemia, and homocystinuria.

Terminology Review

Adolescent An individual from 12 to 18 years of age.

Immunity The resistance of the body to the effects of a harmful agent such as a pathogenic microorganism and its toxins.

Immunization (active, artificial) The process of becoming immune or of rendering an individual immune through the use of a vaccine or toxoid.

Infant A child from birth to 12 months of age.

Length (recumbent) The measurement from the vertex of the head to the heel of the foot in a supine position.

Pediatrician A medical doctor who specializes in the care and development of children and the diagnosis and treatment of children's diseases.

Pediatrics The branch of medicine that deals with the care and development of children and the diagnosis and treatment of children's diseases.

Preschooler A child from 3 to 6 years of age.

School-age child A child from 6 to 12 years of age.

Toddler A child from 1 to 3 years of age.

Toxoid A toxin (poisonous substance produced by a bacterium) that has been treated by heat or chemicals to destroy its harmful properties. It is administered to an individual to prevent an infectious disease by stimulating the production of antibodies in that individual.

Vaccine A suspension of attenuated (weakened) or killed microorganisms administered to an individual to prevent an infectious disease by stimulating the production of antibodies in that individual.

Vertex The summit, or top, especially the top of the head.

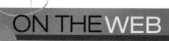

ON THE WEB

For active weblinks to each website visit http://evolve. elsevier.com/Bonewit/.

For Information on Child Health:

KidsHealth

Healthy Kids

ParentCenter

Pediatric on Call

Kids Source Online

American Academy of Pediatrics

For Information on Childhood Conditions:

Attention-Deficit Hyperactive Disorder

Attention Deficit Disorder Association

Cerebral Palsy

American Academy for Cerebral Palsy and Developmental Medicine

Child Abuse

American Professional Society on the Abuse of Children

Cystic Fibrosis

Cystic Fibrosis Foundation

Dental Health

The Tooth Fairy Online

Diabetes

Children with Diabetes

Down Syndrome

National Down Syndrome Society

Spina Bifida

Spina Bifida Association of America

Sudden Infant Death Syndrome

SIDS Alliance

For Information on Immunizations:

Centers for Disease Control and Prevention: Vaccine Information Statements

Immunization Action Coalition: Vaccine Information Statements

American Academy of Pediatrics Childhood Immunization Support Program

The Children's Hospital of Philadelphia Vaccine Education Center

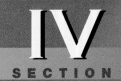
Advanced Clinical Procedures

10 Minor Office Surgery

11 Administration of Medication

Learning Objectives	Procedures

Surgical Asepsis

1. Identify procedures that require the use of surgical asepsis.
2. Describe the medical assistant's responsibilities during a minor surgical procedure.
3. List the guidelines to follow to maintain surgical asepsis during a sterile procedure.
4. Identify and explain the use and care of instruments commonly used for minor office surgery.

Apply and remove sterile gloves.
Open a sterile package.
Add an article to a sterile field.
Pour a sterile solution.

Wound Healing

1. Explain the difference between a closed and an open wound, and give examples.
2. List and explain the three phases of the healing process.
3. List and describe the different types of wound drainage.
4. List the functions of a dressing.

Change a sterile dressing.

Sutures

1. Explain the method used to measure the diameter of suturing material.
2. Describe the two types of sutures (absorbable and nonabsorbable), and give examples of their uses.
3. Categorize suturing needles according to type of point and shape.

Remove sutures.
Remove surgical staples.
Apply and remove adhesive skin closures.
Set up a tray for each of the following surgical procedures:
  Suture insertion
  Sebaceous cyst removal
  Incision and drainage of a localized infection
  Needle biopsy
  Ingrown toenail removal
  Colposcopy
  Cervical punch biopsy
  Cryosurgery
Assist the physician with minor office surgery.

Medical Office Surgical Procedures

1. Explain the purpose of and procedure for the following minor surgical operations: sebaceous cyst removal, incision and drainage of a localized infection, needle biopsy, ingrown toenail removal, colposcopy, cervical punch biopsy, and cryosurgery.
2. Explain the principles underlying each step in the minor office surgery procedures.

Bandaging

1. State the functions of a bandage, and list the guidelines for applying a bandage.
2. Identify the common types of bandage used in the medical office.
3. Explain the use of a tubular gauze bandage.

Apply the following bandage turns:
  Circular
  Spiral
  Spiral-reverse
  Figure-eight
  Recurrent
Apply a tubular gauze bandage.

Minor Office Surgery

Chapter Outline

INTRODUCTION TO MINOR OFFICE SURGERY
Surgical Asepsis
Instruments Used in Minor Office Surgery
  Care of Surgical Instruments
Commercially Prepared Sterile Packages
Wounds
  Wound Healing
Sterile Dressing Change
Sutures
  Types of Sutures
  Suture Size and Packaging
  Suture Needles
  Insertion of Sutures
  Suture Removal
  Surgical Skin Staples
  Adhesive Skin Closures
Assisting With Minor Office Surgery
  Tray Setup
  Skin Preparation
  Local Anesthetic
  Assisting the Physician
Medical Office Surgical Procedures
  Sebaceous Cyst Removal
  Surgical Incision and Drainage of Localized Infections
  Needle Biopsy
  Ingrown Toenail Removal
  Colposcopy
  Cervical Punch Biopsy
  Cryosurgery
Bandaging
  Guidelines for Application
  Types of Bandages
  Bandage Turns
  Tubular Gauze Bandages

National Competencies

Clinical Competencies
Patient Care
- Prepare patient and assist with procedures, treatments, and minor office surgeries.

General Competencies

Legal Concepts
- Identify and respond to issues of confidentiality.
- Perform within legal and ethical boundaries.

Patient Instruction
- Provide instruction for health maintenance and disease prevention.

abrasion (ah-BRAY-shun)
abscess (AB-sess)
absorbable suture (ab-SOR-ba-bul SOO-chur)
approximation (ah-PROKS-ih-MAY-shun)
bandage
biopsy (BYE-op-see)
capillary action (KAP-ill-air-ee AK-shun)
colposcope (KOL-poe-skope)
colposcopy (kol-POS-koe-pee)
contaminate (kon-TAM-in-ate)
contusion (kon-TOO-shun)
cryosurgery (KRY-oh-SURJ-er-ee)
exudate (EKS-oo-date)
fibroblast (FYE-broh-blast)
forceps (FORE-seps)
furuncle (FYOOR-un-kul)
hemostasis (hee-moe-STAY-sis)
incision (in-SIH-shun)
infection (in-FEK-shun)
infiltration (in-fill-TRAY-shun))
inflammation (in-flah-MAY-shun)
laceration (Lass-ur-AY-shun)
ligate (LIH-gate)
local anesthetic (LOE-kul an-es-STET-ik)
Mayo (MAY-oe) tray
needle biopsy (NEE-dul BYE-op-see)
nonabsorbable suture (non-ab-SOR-ba-bul SOO-chur)
postoperative (post-OP-er-uh-tiv)
preoperative (pree-OP-er-uh-tiv)
puncture (PUNK-shur)
scalpel (SKAL-pul)
scissors
sebaceous cyst (suh-BAY-shus SIST)
serum (SEER-um)
sterile (STARE-ul)
surgical asepsis (SUR-jih-kul ay-SEP-sis)
sutures (SOO-churz)
swaged (SWAYJD) needle
wound

Introduction to Minor Office Surgery

Various types of minor surgical operations are performed in the medical office, such as insertion of sutures, sebaceous cyst removal, incision and drainage of infections, needle biopsies, cervical biopsies, and ingrown toenail removal. The physician explains the nature of the surgical procedure and any risks to the patient and offers to answer questions. The medical assistant is responsible for explaining the patient preparation required for the procedure and for obtaining the patient's signature on a written consent to treatment form, which grants the physician permission to perform the surgery (Figure 10-1).

Additional responsibilities of the medical assistant involve preparing the treatment room, preparing the patient, preparing the minor surgery tray, assisting the physician during the procedure, administering postoperative care to the patient, and cleaning the treatment room after the procedure.

The treatment room must be spotlessly clean, and the medical assistant should make sure the physician has adequate lighting for the procedure. The patient is positioned and draped according to the procedure to be performed. The skin is prepared as specified by the physician. Hair around the operative site is a contaminant and may need to be removed by shaving. The skin is cleansed and an appropriate antiseptic is applied to the area to reduce the number of microorganisms present.

The medical assistant prepares the minor surgery tray using **sterile** technique. The specific instruments and supplies included in each setup vary somewhat, depending on the type of surgery to be performed and the physician's preference. Therefore the medical assistant must become familiar with the instruments and supplies required for each surgical procedure performed in the medical office.

During the minor surgery, the medical assistant is present to assist the physician as needed and to lend support to the patient. The medical assistant should become completely familiar with every surgical procedure and learn to anticipate the physician's needs to help the procedure go quickly and smoothly.

After the minor surgery, the medical assistant should remain with the patient as a safety precaution to prevent accidental falls and other injuries and to make sure the patient understands the postoperative instructions. The medical assistant then removes and properly cares for all used instruments and supplies and cleans the treatment room in preparation for the next patient.

Surgical Asepsis

Surgical asepsis, also known as sterile technique, refers to practices that keep objects and areas sterile, or free from all living microorganisms. Surgical asepsis protects the patient from pathogenic microorganisms that may enter the body

---

(attach label or complete blanks)

First name: _____   Last name: _____

Date of Birth: _____ Month _____ Day _____ Year

Account Number: _____

Procedure Consent Form

I, _____ , hereby consent to have

Dr. _____ perform _____ .

I have been fully informed of the following by my physician:

1. The nature of my condition.
2. The nature and purpose of the procedure.
3. An explanation of risks involved with the procedure.
4. Alternative treatments or procedures available.
5. The likely results of the procedure.
6. The risks involved with declining or delaying the procedure.

My physician has offered to answer all questions concerning the proposed procedure.

I am aware that the practice of medicine and surgery is not an exact science, and I acknowledge that no guarantees have been made to me about the results of the procedure.

Patient _____   Date _____
(or guardian and relationship)

Witnessed _____   Date _____

Figure 10-1. A consent to treatment form.

and cause disease. It is always employed under the following circumstances: when caring for broken skin, such as open wounds and suture punctures; when a skin surface is being penetrated, as by a surgical incision or the administration of an injection (the needle must remain sterile); and when a body cavity is entered that is normally sterile, such as during the insertion of a urinary catheter. Sterility of instruments and supplies is achieved through the use of disposable sterile items or by sterilizing reusable articles.

A sterile object that touches any unsterile object is automatically considered contaminated and must not be used. A medical assistant who is in doubt or has a question concerning the sterility of an article should consider it contaminated and replace it with a sterile article.

Sterility of the hands cannot be attained. Sanitizing the hands renders them medically aseptic and must be performed before and after every surgical procedure using proper technique (see Chapter 2). To prevent contamination of sterile articles, sterile gloves must be worn while picking up or transferring articles during a sterile procedure. Procedures 10-1 and 10-2 describe the procedure for applying and removing sterile gloves.

Guidelines for Surgical Asepsis

1. Take precautions to prevent sterile packages from becoming wet. Wet packages draw microorganisms into the package owing to the **capillary action** of the liquid, resulting in contamination of the sterile package. If a sterile package that has been prepared at the medical office becomes wet, it must be resterilized; if a disposable sterile package becomes wet, it must be discarded.
2. A 1-inch border around the sterile field is considered contaminated or unsterile because this area may have become contaminated while the sterile field was being set up.
3. Always face the sterile field. If you must turn your back to it or leave the room, a sterile towel must be placed over the sterile field.
4. Hold all sterile articles above waist level. Anything out of sight might become contaminated. The sterile articles should also be held in front of you and should not touch your uniform.
5. To avoid contamination, place all sterile items in the center, not around the edges, of the sterile field.
6. Be careful not to spill water or solutions on the sterile field. The area beneath the field is contaminated, and microorganisms will be drawn up onto the field by the capillary action of the liquid, resulting in contamination of the field.
7. Do not talk, cough, or sneeze over a sterile field. Water vapor from the nose, mouth, and lungs will be carried out by the air and contaminate the sterile field.
8. Do not reach over a sterile field. Dust or lint from your clothing may fall onto it or your unsterile clothing may accidentally touch it.
9. Do not pass soiled dressings over the sterile field.
10. Always acknowledge if you have contaminated the sterile field so that proper steps can be taken to regain sterility.

Specific guidelines must be observed during a sterile procedure to maintain surgical asepsis. See the accompanying box on Guidelines for Surgical Asepsis.

Instruments Used in Minor Office Surgery

A variety of surgical instruments are used for minor office surgery. Most instruments are made of stainless steel and have either a bright, highly polished finish or a dull finish. The medical assistant should become familiar with the name, use, and proper care of all instruments used in the medical office. Some of the common instruments are described here and are illustrated in Figure 10-2.

Scalpels

A **scalpel** is a small straight surgical knife consisting of a handle and a thin, sharp blade that has a convex edge. It is used to make surgical incisions and can divide tissue with the least possible trauma to the surrounding structures. Both reusable and disposable scalpels are available; scalpels that have a reusable handle and a disposable blade are used most frequently.

Scissors

Scissors are cutting instruments that have either straight (str) or curved (cvd) blades. Both blade tips may be sharp (s/s), both may be blunt (b/b), or one tip may be blunt and the other sharp (b/s). The two parts of a pair of scissors come together at a hinge joint known as a box lock. The type of scissors employed depends on the intended use. The various types of scissors are listed and described next.

- *Operating scissors* have straight delicate blades with sharp cutting edges and are used to cut through tissue. They are available with sharp/sharp, blunt/blunt, or blunt/sharp tips.
- *Suture scissors* are used to remove sutures. The hook on the tip aids in getting under a suture, and the blunt end prevents puncturing of the tissues.
- *Bandage scissors* are inserted beneath a dressing or bandage to cut it for removal. The flat blunt prow can be inserted beneath a dressing without puncturing the skin.
- *Dissecting scissors* have thick blades with a fine cutting edge used to divide tissue and are available with either straight or curved blades. Both blade tips of dissecting scissors are blunt.

Forceps

Forceps are two-pronged instruments for grasping and squeezing. Some forceps have a spring handle (e.g., thumb, tissue, splinter, and dressing forceps) that provides the proper tension for grasping tissue. As you will note from Figure 10-2, some varieties have toothed clasps on the handle, known as ratchets, to hold the tips securely together (e.g., Allis tissue forceps, hemostatic forceps, and sponge forceps). The ratchets are designed to allow closure of the instrument at three or more positions. The various types of forceps are listed and described next.

- *Thumb forceps* have serrated tips and are used to pick up tissue or to hold tissue between adjacent surfaces. Serrations are sawlike teeth that grasp tissue and prevent it from slipping out of the jaws of the instrument.
- *Tissue forceps* have teeth to prevent them from slipping and are used to grasp tissue. Tissue forceps are identified by the number of apposing teeth on each jaw

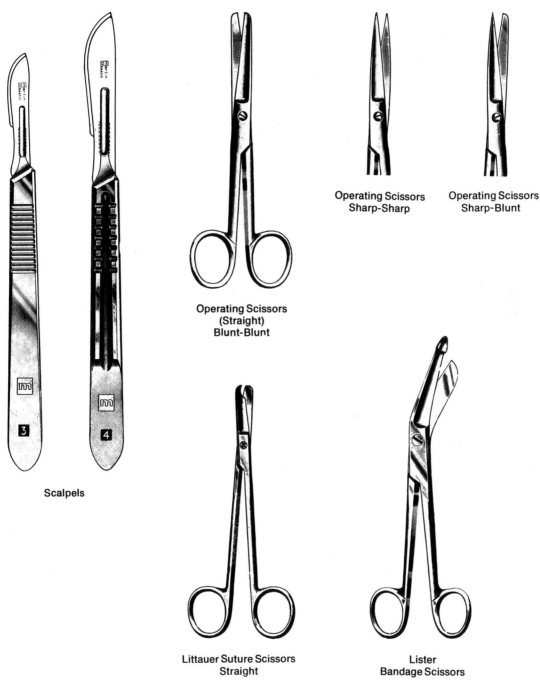

Scalpels

**Operating Scissors
(Straight)
Blunt-Blunt**

**Operating Scissors
Sharp-Sharp**

**Operating Scissors
Sharp-Blunt**

**Littauer Suture Scissors
Straight**

**Lister
Bandage Scissors**

Figure 10-2. Instruments used in minor office surgery. (Courtesy Elmed, Addison, Ill.)

Continued

(e.g., 1 × 2, 2 × 3, 3 × 4). The teeth should approximate tightly when the instrument is closed.

- *Splinter forceps* have sharp points that are useful in removing foreign objects, such as splinters, from the tissues.
- *Dressing forceps* are used in the application and removal of dressings. They have blunt ends that contain coarse cross striations used for grasping.
- *Hemostatic forceps* have serrated tips, ratchets, and box locks and are available with either straight or curved blades. Hemostats are used to clamp off blood vessels and to establish **hemostasis** until the vessels can be closed with sutures. The ratchets keep the hemostat tightly shut when it is closed. They should mesh together smoothly when the instrument is closed; if they spring back open, the instrument is in need of repair. The serrations on a hemostat prevent the blood vessel from slipping out of the jaws of the instrument.
- *Sponge forceps,* as the name implies, have large serrated rings on the tips for holding sponges. A sponge is a porous, absorbent pad, such as a 4-inch gauze pad, used to absorb fluids, apply medication, or cleanse an area.

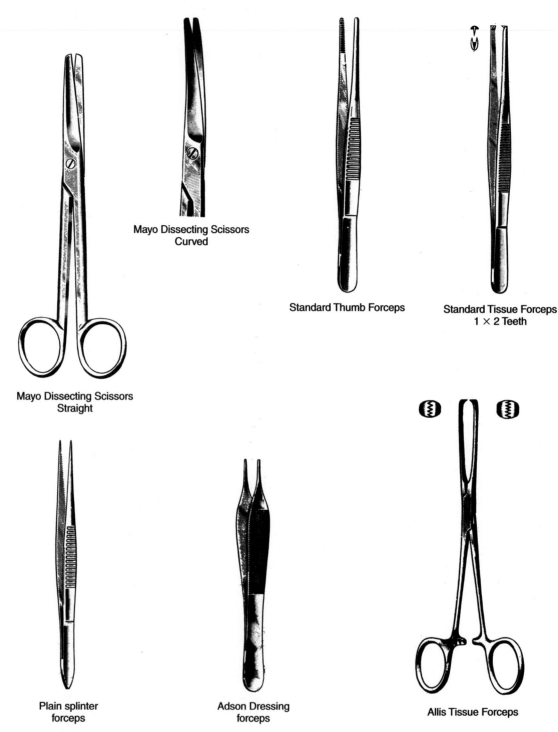

Figure 10-2, cont'd. Instruments used in minor office surgery. (Courtesy Elmed, Addison, Ill.)

Miscellaneous Instruments

Various miscellaneous instruments used in the medical office are listed and described next.

- *Needle holders* have serrated tips, ratchets, and box locks; they are used to grasp a curved needle firmly to insert it through the skin flaps of an incision.

- *Towel clamps* have two sharp points to hold the edges of a sterile towel in place.
- *Retractors* are used to hold tissues aside to improve the exposure of the operative area.
- *Probes* are long slender instruments used to explore wounds or body cavities.

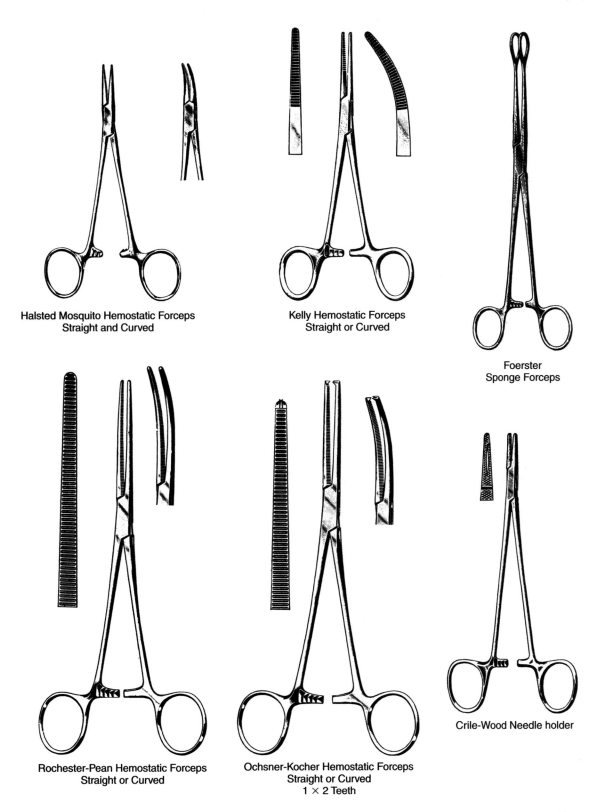

Halsted Mosquito Hemostatic Forceps
Straight and Curved

Kelly Hemostatic Forceps
Straight or Curved

Foerster
Sponge Forceps

Rochester-Pean Hemostatic Forceps
Straight or Curved

Ochsner-Kocher Hemostatic Forceps
Straight or Curved
1 × 2 Teeth

Crile-Wood Needle holder

Figure 10-2, cont'd. Instruments used in minor office surgery. (Courtesy Elmed, Addison, Ill.)

Continued

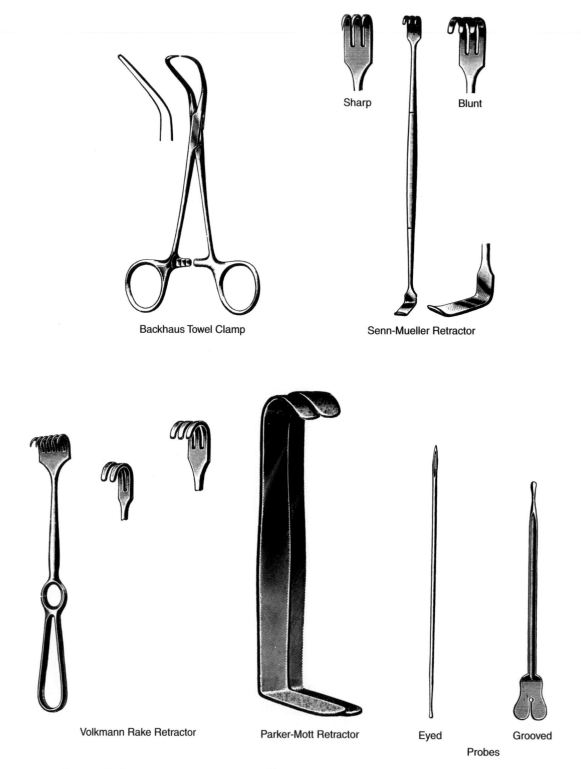

Sharp   Blunt

Backhaus Towel Clamp

Senn-Mueller Retractor

Volkmann Rake Retractor   Parker-Mott Retractor   Eyed   Grooved

Probes

Figure 10-2, cont'd. Instruments used in minor office surgery. (Courtesy Elmed, Addison, Ill.)

Gynecologic Instruments

Gynecologic surgical procedures are often performed in the medical office; therefore the medical assistant should be familiar with terms related to gynecologic instruments. These are listed and described next.

- A *speculum* is an instrument used to open or distend a body orifice or cavity to permit visual inspection.
- A *tenaculum* is a hooklike instrument used to grasp and hold body parts. For example, a uterine tenaculum is used to grasp and hold the cervix.

GYNECOLOGIC INSTRUMENTS

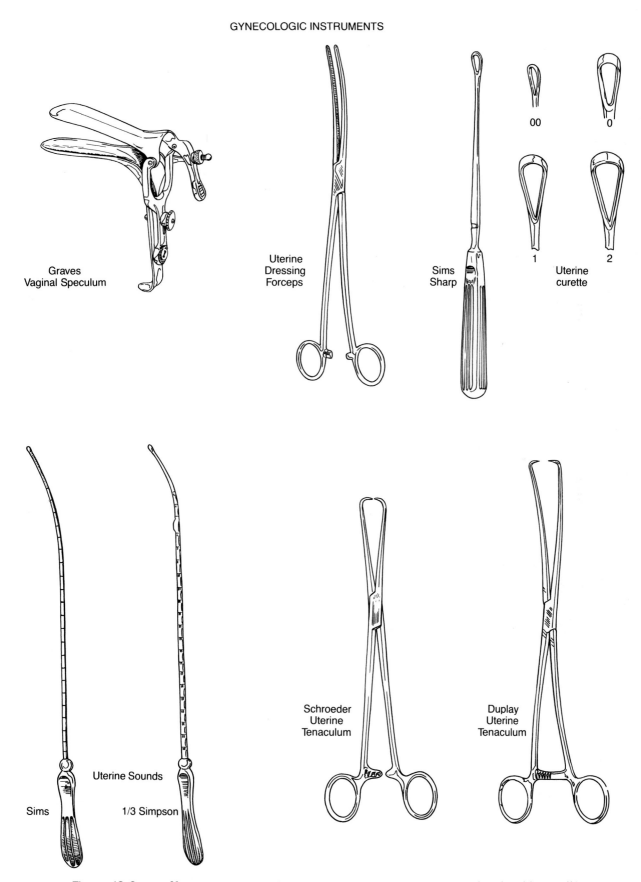

Graves
Vaginal Speculum

Uterine
Dressing
Forceps

Sims
Sharp

00

0

1

2

Uterine
curette

Uterine Sounds

Sims

1/3 Simpson

Schroeder
Uterine
Tenaculum

Duplay
Uterine
Tenaculum

Figure 10-2, cont'd. Instruments used in minor office surgery. (Courtesy Elmed, Addison, Ill.)

- A *sound* is a long slender instrument that is introduced into a body passage or cavity as a means of dilating strictures or to detect the presence of foreign bodies.
- A *curette* is a spoon-shaped instrument used to remove material from the wall of a cavity or other surface.

Care of Surgical Instruments

Surgical instruments are expensive, delicate yet durable, and will last for many years if handled and maintained properly. The care an instrument receives depends to a large degree on the parts of the instrument (e.g., box lock, ratchet, cutting edge, serrations). The medical assistant works with instruments while setting up a sterile tray, performing certain procedures such as suture removal and sterile dressing change, and cleaning up after minor office surgery and during the sanitization and sterilization process. During each of these procedures, the following guidelines must be followed to prolong the life span of each instrument and to ensure its proper functioning:

1. Always handle instruments carefully. Dropping an instrument on the floor or throwing an instrument into a basin could damage it.

2. Do not pile instruments in a heap because they will become entangled and might be damaged when separated.
3. Keep sharp instruments separate from the rest of the instruments to prevent damaging or dulling the cutting edge. Also keep delicate instruments, such as lensed instruments, separate to protect them from damage.
4. To prolong the proper functioning of the ratchet, keep instruments with a ratchet in an open position when not in use.
5. Rinse blood and body secretions off an instrument as soon as possible to prevent them from drying and hardening on the instrument.
6. When performing procedures that require surgical instruments, always use the instrument for the purpose for which it was designed. Substituting one type of instrument for another could damage it.
7. Sanitize and sterilize instruments using proper technique.

Commercially Prepared Sterile Packages

Commercially prepared disposable packages are frequently used and may contain one particular article (such as sterile dressing) or a complete sterile setup (such as one for the removal of sutures). The directions for opening the package are clearly stated on the outside of the package; follow them carefully to prevent contamination of the sterile contents. Procedure 10-2 describes opening a sterile package.

One type of commercially prepared package is the peel-apart package (commonly referred to as a peel-pack). This type of sterile package has an edge with two flaps that can be pulled apart in the following manner: Grasp each unsterile flap between your bent index finger and extended thumb and, rolling your hands outward, pull the package apart (Figure 10-3, *A*). The inside of the wrapper and the contents are sterile and, to prevent contamination, they must not be touched with the bare hands.

The medical assistant can place the contents of the peel-pack directly on the sterile field by stepping back slightly from the field and then gently ejecting or "flipping" the contents onto it (Figure 10-3, *B*). Stepping back prevents the unsterile outer wrapper and the medical assistant's hands from crossing over the sterile field, which would result in contamination.

The contents of the package can also be removed with a sterile gloved hand. This technique is useful during minor office surgery when the physician needs additional supplies such as gauze pads, sutures, and so on. The medical assistant opens the sterile package and the physician removes the sterile contents from the package using his or her gloved hand (Figure 10-3, *C*).

The inside of the package can be used as a sterile field by opening the peel-apart package completely and laying it flat on a clean dry surface (Figure 10-3, *D*).

Text continued on p. 392

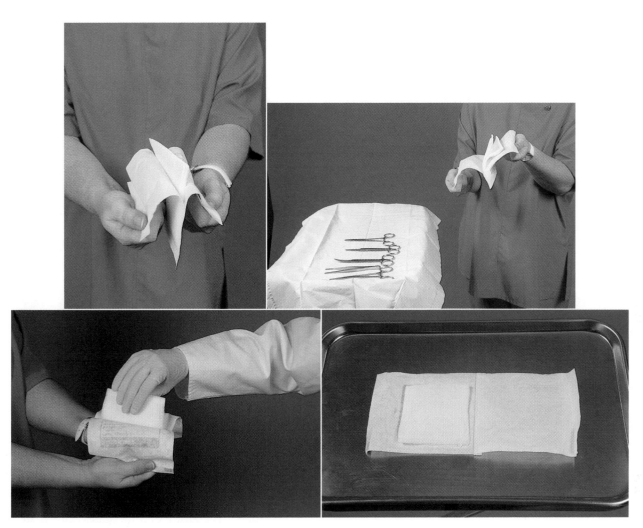

Figure 10-3. Methods for removing the sterile contents of a peel-apart package so that sterility is maintained.

PROCEDURE 10-1 | Applying Sterile Gloves

Outcome Apply and remove sterile gloves.

The medical assistant must wear sterile gloves to perform a sterile procedure, such as a dressing change, or to assist the physician during minor office surgery. The medical assistant must learn to put on the gloves using the principles of surgical asepsis so as not to contaminate them.

Equipment/Supplies:
- Sterile gloves

1. **Procedural Step.** Remove all rings; sanitize your hands.
   Principle. Rings may cause the gloves to tear. The warm, moist environment inside gloves provides ideal growing conditions for the multiplication of transient microorganisms on the hands. Sanitizing the hands removes these microorganisms and prevents the transmission of pathogens.

2. **Procedural Step.** Place the glove package on a clean flat surface. Open the glove package without touching the inside of the wrapper. The tops of the gloves are turned down to form a cuff.
   Principle. The hands are not sterile and the inside of the wrapper is sterile.

Continued

PROCEDURE 10-1

3. **Procedural Step.** Pick up the first glove on the inside of the cuff with the fingers of the opposite hand, making sure not to touch the outside of the glove with your ungloved hand.

Principle. The inside of the cuff will be lying next to your skin and does not remain sterile. Therefore it is permissible to pick up the glove by the cuff. The outside of the glove is sterile and touching it will contaminate it. If a glove becomes contaminated, you must obtain a new pair of gloves and repeat the procedure, beginning with step 2.

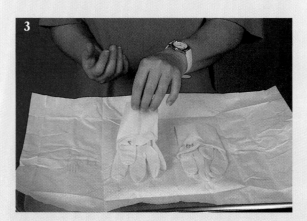

4. **Procedural Step.** Pull the glove on. Allow the cuff to remain turned back on itself.

5. **Procedural Step.** Pick up the second glove by slipping your sterile gloved fingers under its cuff.

Principle. The area under the cuff is sterile and may be touched by the sterile gloved hand.

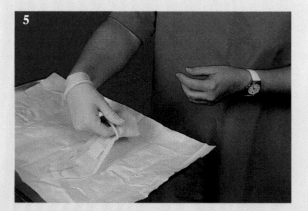

6. **Procedural Step.** Pull the glove on and turn back the cuff.

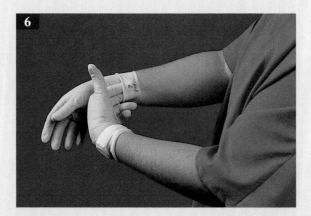

7. **Procedural Step.** Turn back the cuff of the first glove by reaching under the cuff with the other gloved hand. Do not allow the sterile glove to come in contact with the inside of the cuff. Adjust the gloves to a comfortable position. Inspect the gloves for tears.

Principle. The area under the folded cuff is sterile and may be touched by the sterile gloved hand. The inside of the cuff has previously been touched by your clean hands and is not sterile. If a tear is present, a new pair of gloves must be applied.

PROCEDURE 10-2   Removing Sterile Gloves

Outcome Gloves must be removed in a manner that protects the medical assistant from contaminating the clean hands with pathogens that might be on the outside of the gloves. This is accomplished by not allowing the bare hands to come in contact with the outside of the gloves.

Equipment/Supplies:

• Sterile gloves

1. **Procedural Step.** With your gloved left hand, grasp the outside of the right glove 1 to 2 inches from the top. (*Note:* It does not matter which glove is removed first—you may start with the left glove if you prefer.)

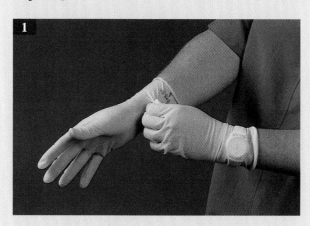

2. **Procedural Step.** Slowly pull the right glove off the hand. It will turn inside out as it is removed from your hand.

3. **Procedural Step.** Pull the right glove free and scrunch it into a ball with your gloved left hand.

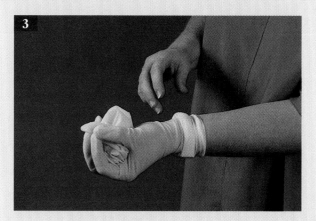

4. **Procedural Step.** Place the index and middle fingers of the right hand on the *inside* of the left glove. Do not allow your clean hand to touch the outside of the glove.

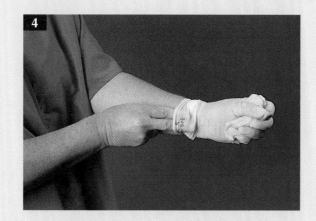

5. **Procedural Step.** Pull the second glove off the left hand. It will turn inside out as it is removed from your hand, enclosing the balled-up right glove. Discard both gloves in an appropriate waste container.

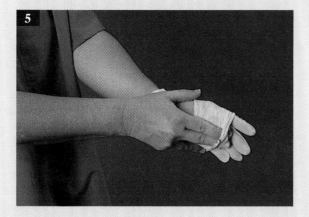

6. **Procedural Step.** Sanitize your hands thoroughly to remove any microorganisms that may have come in contact with your hands.

PROCEDURE 10-2

PROCEDURE 10-3 Opening a Sterile Package

Outcome Open a sterile package.

A sterile package that has been wrapped following the procedure for wrapping presented in Chapter 3 is opened using the procedure outlined here. The sterile package may be in the form of a commercially prepared disposable package or a pack that has been assembled and sterilized at the medical office; in both cases the inside of the sterile wrapper serves as the sterile field.

Equipment/Supplies:
• Sterile package

1. **Procedural Step.** Sanitize your hands.
2. **Procedural Step.** Assemble the equipment.
3. **Procedural Step.** Check the sterilization indicator to make sure the wrapped package is sterile.
   Principle. Sterilization indicators are used to determine the effectiveness of the sterilization process.

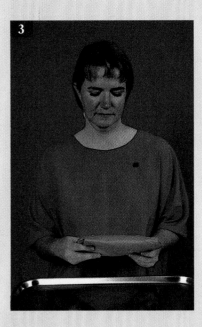

4. **Procedural Step.** Place the wrapped package on the table so that the top flap of the wrapper will open away from you.
5. **Procedural Step.** Loosen and remove the fastener on the wrapped package and discard it in a waste container.
6. **Procedural Step.** Open the first flap away from the body. Handle only the outside of the wrapper.
   Principle. The medical assistant should open the sterile package so as not to reach over the sterile contents. Otherwise, dust or lint from unsterile clothing may fall on the contents of the package and cause contamination.

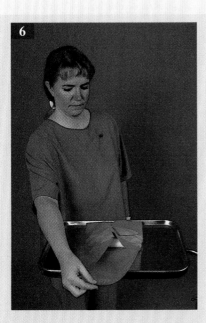

7. **Procedural Step.** Without crossing over the sterile field, open the left and right flaps.

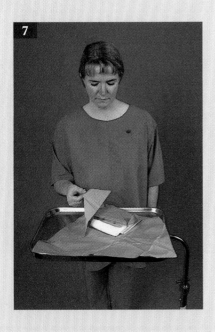

8. Procedural Step. Open the flap closest to the body by lifting it toward you. Make sure to touch only the outside of the wrapper.

9. **Procedural Step.** Adjust the sterile wrapper by the corners as needed to make sure it lies in proper position on the tray or table.

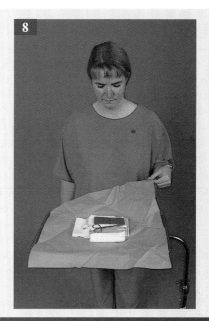

PROCEDURE 10-4

PROCEDURE 10-4   Pouring a Sterile Solution

Outcome   Pour a sterile solution. The medical assistant may need to pour a sterile solution, such as an antiseptic, into a container located on a sterile field. To do so, follow the steps of surgical asepsis outlined in the following procedure.

Equipment/Supplies:
*   Sterile solution
*   Sterile container
*   Sterile towel

1. **Procedural Step.** Read the label to make sure you have the correct solution.
2. **Procedural Step.** Check the expiration date on the solution. Do not use an outdated solution.
3. **Procedural Step.** Palm the label of the bottle.
    Principle. Palming the label prevents the solution from dripping on the label and obscuring it.
4. **Procedural Step.** Remove the cap by touching only the outside, and place the cap on a flat surface with the open end up.
    Principle. Handling the cap by the outside prevents contamination of the inside. Placing the cap with the open end up prevents contamination of the inside of the cap by the unsterile surface.
5. **Procedural Step.** Rinse the lip of the bottle by pouring a small amount of solution into a separate container.
    Principle. Rinsing the lip washes away any microorganisms that may be on it.
6. **Procedural Step.** Pour the proper amount of solution into the sterile container at a height of approximately 6 inches. Do not allow the neck of the bottle

to come in contact with the sterile container, and be careful not to splash solution onto the sterile field.
Principle. Pouring from a height of approximately 6 inches reduces splashing.

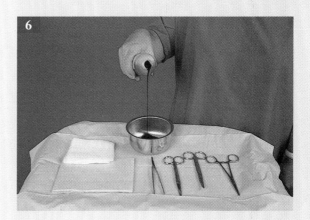

7. **Procedural Step.** Replace the cap on the container without contaminating it. Read the label again to make sure you have poured the correct solution.

Wounds

A **wound** is a break in the continuity of an external or internal surface caused by physical means. Wounds can be accidental or intentional (as when the physician makes an incision during a surgical operation). There are two basic types of wound: closed and open.

A *closed wound* involves an injury to the underlying tissues of the body without a break in the skin surface or mucous membrane; an example is a contusion, or bruise. A **contusion** results when the tissues under the skin are injured and is often caused by a blunt object. Blood vessels rupture, allowing blood to seep into the tissues, which results in a bluish discoloration of the skin. After several days, the color of the contusion turns greenish yellow as a result of oxidation of blood pigments. Bruising commonly occurs with injuries such as fractures, sprains, strains, and black eyes.

Open wounds involve a break in the skin surface or mucous membrane that exposes the underlying tissues; examples include incisions, lacerations, punctures, and abrasions.

- An **incision** is a clean, smooth cut caused by a sharp instrument such as a knife, razor, and a piece of glass. Deep incisions are accompanied by profuse bleeding; in addition, damage to muscles, tendons, and nerves may occur.
- A **laceration** is a wound in which the tissues are torn apart, rather than cut, leaving ragged and irregular edges. Lacerations are caused by dull knives, large objects that have been driven into the skin, and heavy machinery. Deep lacerations result in profuse bleeding, and a scar often results from the jagged tearing of the tissues.
- A **puncture** is a wound made by a sharp-pointed object piercing the skin layers–for example, a nail, splinter, needle, wire, knife, bullet, and animal bite. A puncture wound has a very small external skin opening, and for this reason bleeding is usually minor. A tetanus booster may be administered with this type of wound because the tetanus bacteria grow best in a warm anaerobic environment, like the one in a puncture.
- An **abrasion** or scrape is a wound in which the outer layers of the skin are scraped or rubbed off, resulting in an oozing of blood from ruptured capillaries. Abrasions are often caused by falling on gravel and floors (floor burn). These falls can result in skinned knees and elbows.

Figure 10-4 illustrates the specific wounds just described.

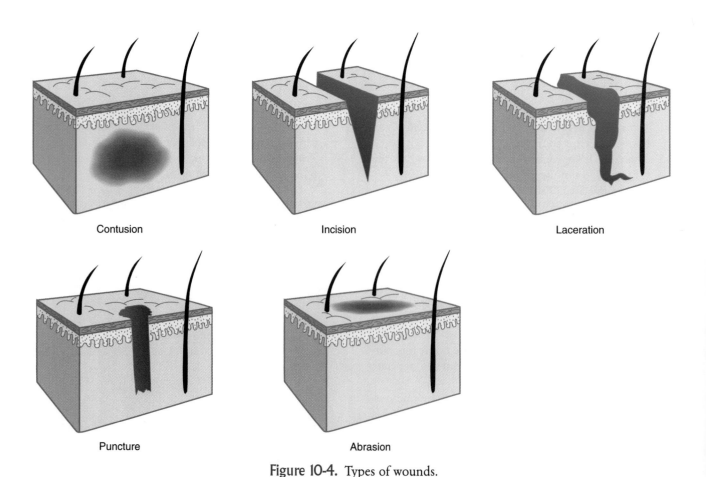

Contusion   Incision   Laceration

Puncture   Abrasion

Figure 10-4. Types of wounds.

Wound Healing

The skin is a protective barrier for the body and is considered its first line of defense. Once the surface of the skin has been broken, it is easy for microorganisms to enter and cause infection. The body has a natural healing process that works to destroy invading microorganisms and to restore the structure and function of the damaged tissues, as is described next.

Phases of Wound Healing

Wound healing takes place in three phases, which are described here and illustrated in Figure 10-5.

Phase 1. Phase 1, also called the *inflammatory phase,* begins as soon as the body is injured. This phase lasts approximately 3 to 4 days. During this phase, a fibrin network forms, resulting in a blood clot that "plugs" up the opening of the wound and stops the flow of blood. The blood clot eventually becomes the scab. The inflammatory process also occurs during this phase. **Inflammation** is the protective response of the body to trauma such as cuts and abrasions and to the entrance of foreign matter such as microorganisms. During inflammation, the blood supply to the wound increases, which brings white blood cells and nutrients to the site to assist in the healing process. The four local signs of inflammation are redness, swelling, pain, and warmth. The purpose of inflammation is to destroy invading microorganisms and to remove damaged tissue debris from the area so that proper healing can occur.

Phase 2. Phase 2 is also called the *granulation phase* and typically lasts from 4 to 20 days. During this phase **fibroblasts** migrate to the wound and begin to synthesize collagen. Collagen is a white protein that provides strength to the wound. Therefore, as the amount of collagen increases, the wound becomes stronger and the chance that the wound will open decreases. There is also a growth of new capillaries during this phase to provide the damaged tissue with an abundant supply of blood. As the capillary network develops, the tissue becomes a translucent red color. This tissue is known as *granulation tissue.* Granulation tissue consists primarily of collagen and is fragile, shiny, and bleeds easily.

)) PATIENT **TEACHING**

Wound Care

Explain the following to the patient regarding wounds:

- The type of wound that the patient has: incision, laceration, puncture, or abrasion.
- The purpose of suturing the wound: to close the skin and protect against further contamination, to facilitate healing, and to leave a smaller scar.
- If a tetanus toxoid has been administered, explain the purpose of this immunization: to protect against tetanus (lockjaw).

Teach the patient how to care for the wound, as follows:

- Keep the dressing clean and dry. If it becomes wet, contact the medical office to schedule a sterile dressing change.
- Apply an ice bag for swelling (if prescribed by the physician).
- Immediately report any signs that the wound is infected. These include fever, persistent or increased pain, swelling, drainage, and red streaks radiating away from the wound.
- Return as instructed by the physician for the removal of sutures.
- Teach the patient how to apply an ice bag (if prescribed by the physician).

Give the patient written instructions on wound care to refer to at home.

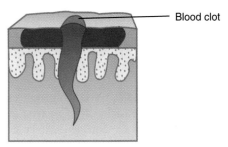

Phase 1: Inflammatory Phase

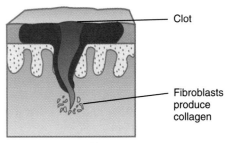

Phase 2: Granulation Phase

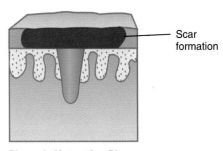

Phase 3: Maturation Phase

Figure 10-5. Phases of wound healing.

Phase 3. Phase 3, also known as the *maturation phase,* begins as soon as granulation tissue forms and can last for up to 2 years. During this phase, collagen continues to be synthesized and the granulation tissue eventually hardens to white scar tissue. Scar tissue is not true skin and does not contain nerves or have a blood supply.

The medical assistant should always inspect the wound when providing wound care. The wound should be observed for signs of inflammation and the amount of healing that has taken place. This information should be charted in the patient's record.

Wound Drainage

The medical term for drainage is exudate. An **exudate** is material, such as fluid and cells, that has escaped from blood vessels during the inflammatory process. The exudate is deposited in tissue or on tissue surfaces and, therefore, is often present in a wound. When providing wound care, the medical assistant should always inspect the wound for drainage and chart this information in the patient's record. There are three major types of exudates: serous, sanguineous, and purulent.

Serous Exudate. A serous exudate consists chiefly of **serum,** which is the clear portion of the blood. Serous drainage is clear and watery. An example of a serous exudate is the fluid in a blister from a burn.

Sanguineous Exudate. A sanguineous exudate is red and consists of red blood cells. This type of drainage results when capillaries are damaged, allowing the escape of red blood cells, and is frequently seen in open wounds. A bright red sanguineous exudate indicates fresh bleeding and a dark exudate indicates older bleeding.

Purulent Exudate. A purulent exudate contains pus, which consists of leukocytes, dead liquefied tissue debris, and dead and living bacteria. Purulent drainage is usually thick and has an unpleasant odor. It is white in color, but may acquire tinges of pink, green, or yellow depending on the type of infecting organism. The process of pus formation is *suppuration.*

In addition to the exudates just described, mixed types of exudates are often observed in a wound. A *serosanguineous exudate* consists of clear and blood-tinged drainage and is commonly seen in surgical incisions. A *purosanguineous exudate* consists of pus and blood and is often seen in a new wound that is infected.

Sterile Dressing Change

Surgical asepsis must be maintained when one is caring for and applying a dry sterile dressing (abbreviated DSD) to an open wound. The medical assistant must take care to prevent infection in clean wounds and to decrease infection in wounds already infected. The function of a sterile

dressing is to protect the wound from contamination and trauma, to absorb drainage, and to restrict motion, which may interfere with proper wound healing. The size, type, and amount of dressing material used during a sterile dressing change depend on the size and location of the wound and the amount of drainage.

Sterile folded *gauze pads* are used in the medical office for a sterile dressing change. This type of dressing is good at absorbing drainage; however, the gauze has a tendency to stick to the wound when the drainage dries. Gauze pads come in a variety of sizes including 4×4, 3×3, and 2×2; the 4×4 size is used most frequently.

Nonadherent pads are also used as a sterile dressing; they have one surface impregnated with agents that prevent the dressing from sticking to the wound. One brand of this type of material is Telfa pads. The nonadhering side, which is shiny, is placed next to the wound. Telfa dressings are often used to cover burned skin.

Procedure 10-5 presents the procedure for changing a sterile dressing.

PROCEDURE 10-5 Changing a Sterile Dressing

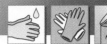

Outcome Change a sterile dressing.

Equipment/Supplies:
Side Table
- Clean disposable gloves
- Antiseptic swabs
- Sterile gloves

- Plastic waste bag
- Adhesive tape and scissors

Sterile Field
- Sterile dressing
- Thumb forceps

1. **Procedural Step.** Sanitize your hands.
2. **Procedural Step.** Assemble the equipment, and prepare the sterile field using surgical asepsis. Items are either contained in a prepackaged sterile setup or placed onto a sterile field. Position the waterproof waste bag in a location convenient for disposal of contaminated items.

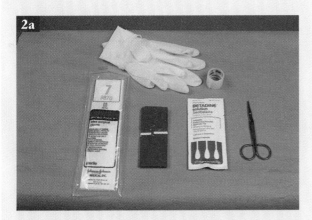

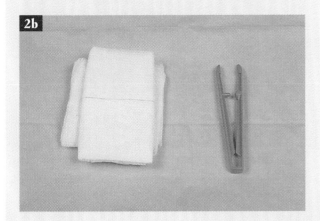

3. **Procedural Step.** Greet and identify the patient. Introduce yourself, and explain the procedure. Instruct the patient not to move during the procedure and not to talk, laugh, sneeze, or cough over the sterile field. Adjust the light so that it is focused on the dressing.
   Principle. By moving, the patient may accidentally contaminate the sterile field or touch the wound. Microorganisms are carried in water vapor from the mouth, nose, and lungs and can be transferred onto the sterile field.

4. **Procedural Step.** Apply clean gloves. Loosen the tape on the dressing, and pull it toward the wound. Carefully and gently remove the soiled dressing. If the dressing is stuck to the wound, it can be loosened by moistening it with a normal saline solution. Do not pass the soiled dressing over the sterile field. Place the soiled dressing in the waste bag without allowing the dressing to touch the outside of the bag.
   Principle. Gentle tape removal avoids unnecessary stress on the wound. Passing the soiled dressing over the sterile field will contaminate the field.

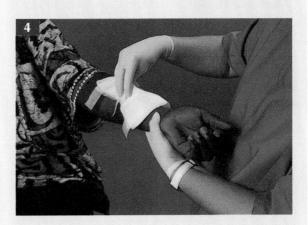

5. **Procedural Step.** Inspect the wound and observe for the following: amount of healing, presence of inflammation, presence of drainage, including the amount (scant, moderate, or profuse) and type of drainage.
   Principle. Drainage is classified as *serous* (containing serum); *sanguineous* (red and composed of blood); *serosanguineous* (containing serum and blood); *purulent* (containing pus and appearing

PROCEDURE 10-5

Continued

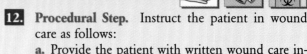

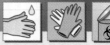

PROCEDURE 10-5   Changing a Sterile Dressing—Cont'd

white with tinges of yellow, pink, or green, depending on the type of infecting microorganism). Purulent drainage is usually thick and has an unpleasant odor.

6. **Procedural Step.** Open the pouch containing the sterile antiseptic swabs and place it in a convenient location.

7. **Procedural Step.** Using the antiseptic swabs, cleanse the wound. Cleanse the wound from the top to the bottom, working from the center to the outside of the wound. Use a new swab for each cleansing motion. Discard each contaminated swab in the waste bag after use.

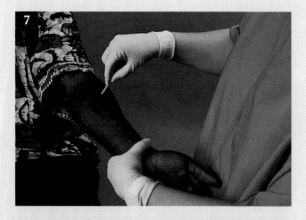

8. **Procedural Step.** Remove the gloves, and discard them in the waste bag without contaminating yourself.

9. **Procedural Step.** Open a package of sterile gloves and apply them.

10. **Procedural Step.** Pick up the sterile dressing with your gloved hand or sterile forceps. Place the sterile dressing over the wound by dropping it in place. Discard the gloves or forceps in the waste bag.
    Principle. Dropping the dressing over the wound prevents the transfer of microorganisms from the skin to the center of the wound.

11. **Procedural Step.** Apply adhesive tape to hold the dressing in place. The tape must be long enough to adhere to the skin but not so long that it will loosen when the patient moves. The strips of tape should be evenly spaced, with strips at each end of the dressing.

12. **Procedural Step.** Instruct the patient in wound care as follows:
    a. Provide the patient with written wound care instructions.
    b. Explain the wound care instructions, and ask the patient if he or she has any questions. Tell the patient to keep the wound clean and dry and to contact the office if signs of inflammation occur.
    c. Ask the patient to sign the instruction sheet on the appropriate line.
    d. Witness the patient's signature by signing your name in the appropriate space on the form. Include today's date.
    e. Give a signed copy of the wound care instructions to the patient, and file a copy in the patient's medical record.

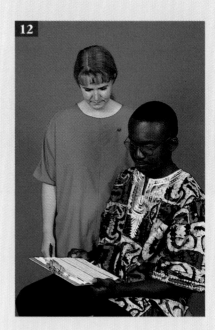

13. **Procedural Step.** Return the equipment. Tightly secure the bag containing the soiled dressing and contaminated articles, and dispose of it in a biohazard waste container.
    Principle. Contaminated items must be disposed of properly to prevent the spread of infection.

14. **Procedural Step.** Sanitize your hands.
15. **Procedural Step.** Chart the procedure. Include the date and time, location of the dressing, condition of the wound, type and amount of drainage, care of the wound, and any problems the patient experienced with the wound. Also chart the instructions given to the patient on wound care.

CHARTING EXAMPLE

Date	
9/20/05	10:30 a.m. Dressing changed (L) ant forearm.
	Scant amt of serous drainage noted. Sl
	redness around incision line. Sutures intact
	and suture line in good approximation. Incision
	cleaned c̄ Betadine and DSD applied. No
	complaints of pain or discomfort. Explained
	wound care. Written instructions provided.
	Signed copy filed in chart. To return in 2 days
	for suture removal. ——— T. Browning, CMA

Sutures

The insertion and removal of **sutures** are commonly performed in the medical office. Sutures may be required to close a surgical incision or to repair an accidental wound. They **approximate,** or bring together, the edges of the wound with surgical stitches and hold them in place until proper healing can occur. Sutures also protect the wound from further contamination and minimize the amount of scar formation. A **local anesthetic** is necessary to numb the area before the sutures are inserted.

Types of Sutures

Sutures are available in two types: absorbable and nonabsorbable.

Absorbable sutures consist of surgical gut or synthetic materials such as polyglycolic acid (Dexon) and polyglactin 910 (Vicryl) (Figure 10-6, *A*). Surgical gut is made from the submucosa of sheep or cow intestine. This type of suturing material is gradually digested by tissue enzymes and absorbed by the body's tissues from 5 to 20 days after insertion, depending on the kind of surgical gut employed. Plain surgical gut has a rapid absorption time, whereas chromic surgical gut is treated to slow down its rate of absorption in the tissues. Absorbable sutures are frequently used to suture subcutaneous tissue, fascia, intestines, bladder, and peritoneum and to **ligate,** or tie off, vessels. Since the suturing of this type of tissue is generally done during surgery performed by the physician in a hospital setting with the patient under a general anesthetic, the medical office may not stock absorbable suture material.

Nonabsorbable sutures (Figure 10-6, *B*) are not absorbed by the body and either remain permanently in the body tissues and become encapsulated by fibrous tissue or are removed (e.g., skin sutures). Nonabsorbable sutures are used to suture skin; therefore this type of suture is frequently used in the medical office.

Nonabsorbable sutures are made from materials that are not affected by tissue enzymes. These materials include silk, cotton, nylon, polyester fiber, polypropylene, stainless steel, and surgical skin staples.

Suture Size and Packaging

Sutures are measured by their gauge, which refers to the diameter of the suturing material. The size ranges from numbers below 0 (pronounced "aught") to numbers above 0. The diameter of the suture material increases with each number above 0 and decreases with each number below 0. If the size of a particular suture material ranges from 6-0 to 4, the available sizes include 6-0, 5-0, 4-0, 3-0, 2-0, 0, 1, 2, 3, and 4; size 6-0 are very fine sutures; and size 4 are very heavy sutures. For example, size 2-0 (00) sutures have a smaller diameter than size 0 sutures.

Nonabsorbable sutures with a smaller gauge (5-0 to 6-0) are used for suturing incisions in more delicate tissue such as the face and neck whereas heavy sutures are used for firmer tissue such as the chest and abdomen. Finer sutures also leave less scar formation and are used when cosmetic results are desired.

Sutures come in individual packages that consist of an outer peel-apart package and a sterile inner packet. They are labeled according to the type of suture material (e.g., surgical silk), the size (e.g., 4-0), and the length of the suturing material (e.g., 18 inches). The type and size of material used are based on the nature and location of the tissue being sutured and the physician's preference. For example, to repair a laceration of the arm, the physician might use a 4-0 surgical silk suture. The physician informs the medical assistant of the type and size of sutures needed.

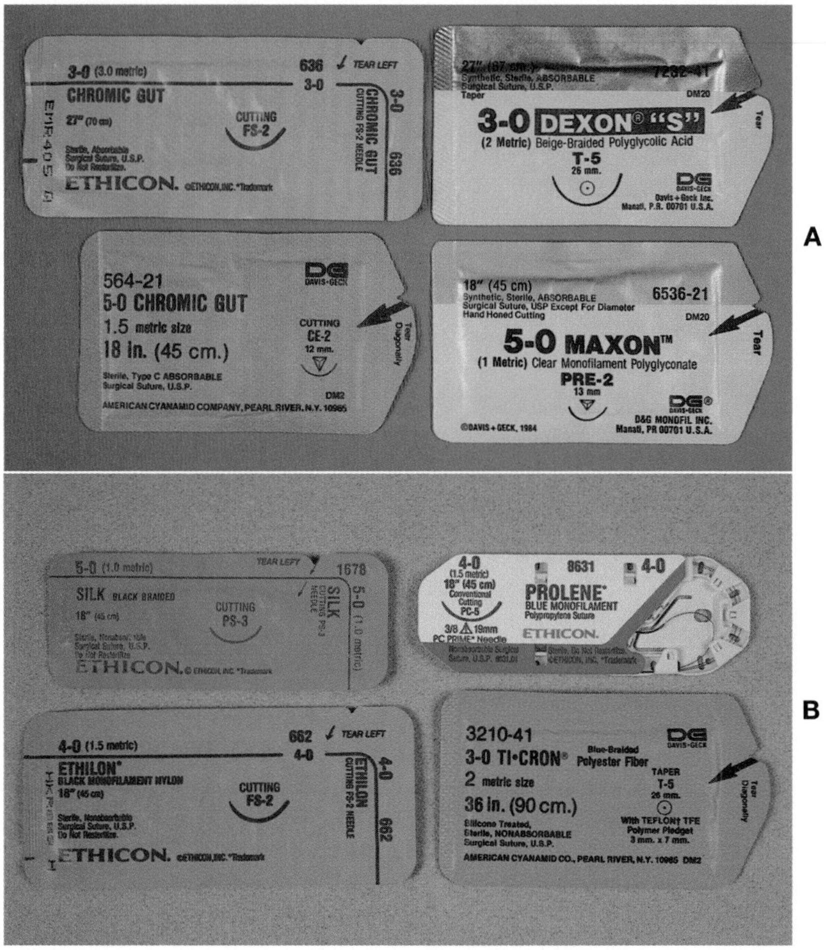

Figure 10-6. Swaged suture packets. **A,** Absorbable sutures. **B,** Nonabsorbable sutures.

Suture Needles

Needles used for suturing are categorized according to both their type of point and their shape. A needle with a sharp point is a *cutting needle* and one with a round point is a *noncutting needle*. Cutting needles (Figure 10-7, *A*) are used for firm tissues such as skin; the sharp point helps push the needle through the tissue. Noncutting needles are used to penetrate tissues that offer a small amount of resistance, such as the viscera, subcutaneous tissue, muscle, and peritoneum.

A suture needle is either curved or straight (see Figure 10-7, *A*). *Curved needles* permit the physician to dip in and out of the tissue. A needle holder must be used with a curved needle. A *straight needle* is used when the tissue can be displaced sufficiently to permit the needle to be pushed and pulled through the tissue. Straight needles do not require the use of a needle holder.

Some needles have an eye through which the suture material is inserted, and some needles are **swaged** (Figure 10-7, *B*). Swaged means the suture and needle are one continuous unit; in other words, the needle is permanently attached to the end of the suture. Swaged needles are used frequently because they offer several advantages over eyed needles. One advantage is that the suture material does not slip off the needle, as might occur with suture material threaded through the eye of a needle. Another advantage is that tissue trauma is reduced because a swaged needle has only a single strand of suture that must be pulled through the tissue, compared with a double strand in an eyed needle. Therefore the swaged needle can be pulled through the tissue with less resulting trauma. Swaged suture packets are labeled to specify the gauge, type, and length of suture material, as well as the type of needle point (cutting or noncutting) and the needle shape (curved or straight) (see Figure 10-6).

Insertion of Sutures

The medical assistant may be responsible for preparing the suture tray and for assisting the physician during the insertion of the sutures. The physician designates the size and type of suture material and needle required. Since sutures, needles, and suture-needle combinations (swaged needles) are contained in peel-apart packages, they can be added to the sterile field by flipping them onto the sterile field or by placing them there with a sterile gloved hand (Figure 10-8).

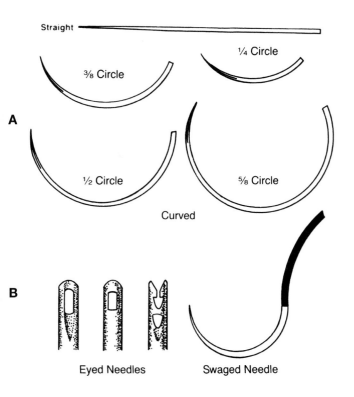

Straight

3/8 Circle

1/4 Circle

1/2 Circle

5/8 Circle

Curved

A

B

Eyed Needles

Swaged Needle

Figure 10-7. Common suture needles. **A,** Needles with a cutting point. **B,** Eyed needles and a swaged needle. (**A,** from *Perspectives on sutures,* courtesy Davis & Geck, Danbury CT. **B,** from Nealon TF, Jr: *Fundamental skills in surgery,* ed 4, Philadelphia, 1994, Saunders.)

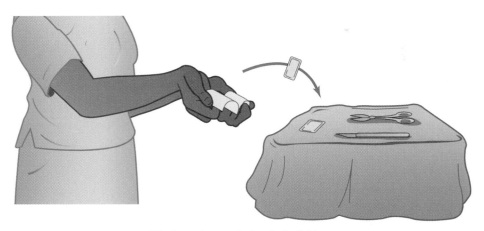

Flipping sutures onto the sterile field.

Figure 10-8. Adding sutures to a sterile field.

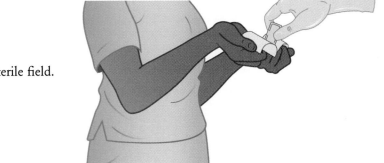

The physician removing the sutures with a sterile gloved hand.

Items Placed to the Side of the Sterile Field

Insertion of sutures:

- Clean disposable gloves
- Antiseptic solution
- Surgical scrub brush
- Antiseptic swabs
- Sterile gloves
- Local anesthetic
- Alcohol wipe to cleanse the vial
- Tetanus toxoid with needle and syringe

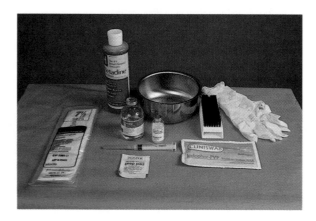

Items Included on the Sterile Field

Insertion of sutures:

- Fenestrated drape
- Syringe and needle
- Hemostatic forceps
- Thumb forceps
- Tissue forceps
- Dissecting scissors
- Operating scissors
- Needle holder
- Suture
- Sterile 4 × 4 gauze

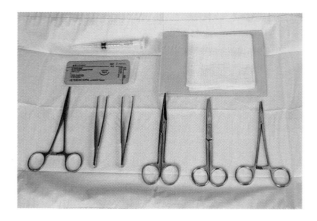

Suture Removal

When the wound has healed so that it no longer needs the support of nonabsorbable suture material, the sutures must be removed. The length of time the sutures remain in place depends on their location and the amount of healing that must occur. Some areas of the body, such as the head and neck, have a good blood supply; the sutures do not need to remain there as long as they do in other areas because this area heals more rapidly.

Sutures must always be left in place long enough for proper healing to take place. The physician decides on the length of time, but in general, skin sutures inserted in the head and neck are removed in 3 to 5 days, and sutures inserted in other areas, such as the skin of the arms, legs, and hands, are removed in 7 to 10 days.

Surgical Skin Staples

Surgical skin staples are often used to close wounds. Stapling is the fastest method of closure of long skin incisions. In addition, trauma to the tissue is reduced because the tissue does not have to be handled very much when inserting the staples.

Surgical staples are stainless steel and are inserted into the skin using a special skin stapler. Skin staplers are available as reusable or disposable devices. The skin stapler holds a cartridge that contains a prescribed number and size of staples (Figure 10-9).

The physician inserts the staples by gently approximating the tissues with tissue forceps. The skin stapler is then held

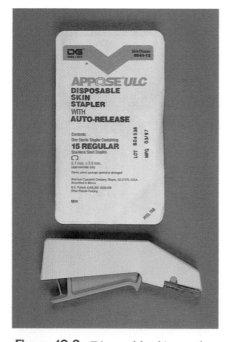

Figure 10-9. Disposable skin stapler.

over the site and the staple is inserted into the skin. Skin stapling produces excellent cosmetic results, and the staples are easy to remove with a specially designed staple remover.

The medical assistant is frequently responsible for removing sutures and staples. This procedure should only be done after a written or verbal order has been given to the medical assistant by the physician. Procedure 10-6 presents the method used to remove sutures and skin staples.

Adhesive Skin Closures

Adhesive skin closures may be used for wound repair to approximate the edges of a laceration or incision. Skin closures consist of sterile, nonallergenic tape that is commercially available in a variety of widths and lengths and is strong enough to approximate a wound until healing takes place. Brand names for adhesive skin closures are Steri-Strip (3M Corporation) and Proxi-Strip (Johnson and Johnson) (Figure 10-10).

Adhesive skin closures may be used when not much tension exists on the skin edges. The strips of tape are applied transversely across the line of incision to approximate the skin edges. The advantages of adhesive skin closures are that they eliminate the need for skin sutures and a local anesthetic, they are easy to apply and remove, and they result in less scarring than skin sutures.

The medical assistant is frequently responsible for applying and removing adhesive skin closures. Procedure 10-7 outlines this procedure.

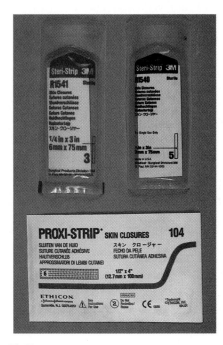

Figure 10-10. Adhesive skin closures in different sizes.

What Would You DO?
What Would You Not DO?

Case Study 1

Kerry Ventura brings her son Cory, age 6, to the medical office. Cory got a new bike for his birthday and just learned how to ride it without training wheels. While going around a corner, he lost his balance and fell and cut his left knee. The incision is about an inch and one-half long. Cory is going to need sutures to approximate the wound. Mrs. Ventura is very upset and blames herself. She says that she should have been watching him more closely. Mrs. Ventura wants to know why Steri-Strips can't be used to close the incision. She says that it would be a lot less painful for Cory than having stitches. When asked to sign the consent to treatment form for Cory, Mrs. Ventura says she doesn't want to sign the form until her husband has a chance to read it. She says that right now he's in Japan for 2 weeks on a business trip.

PROCEDURE 10-6 Removing Sutures and Staples

Outcome Remove sutures and staples.

Equipment/Supplies:
- Antiseptic swabs
- Clean disposable gloves
- Sterile 4 × 4 gauze
- Surgical tape

For Suture Removal

Suture removal kit, which includes:
- Suture scissors

- Thumb forceps
- Sterile 4 × 4 gauze

For Staple Removal

Staple remover kit, which includes:
- Staple remover
- Sterile 4 × 4 gauze

Continued

PROCEDURE 10-6 Removing Sutures and Staples—Cont'd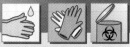

1. **Procedural Step.** Sanitize your hands, and assemble the equipment.

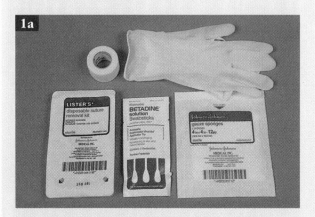

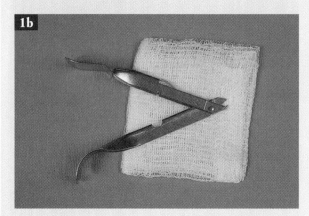

2. **Procedural Step.** Greet and identify the patient. Introduce yourself, and explain the procedure.

3. **Procedural Step.** Position the patient as required. Adjusted the light so that it is focused on the wound. Check to make sure the sutures (or staples) are intact and the incision line is approximated and not gapping. Check that the incision line is not infected. If the incision line is not approximated or if redness, swelling, or a discharge is present, do not remove the sutures; notify the physician.
Principle. The sutures (or staples) should not be removed unless the incision line is approximated and free from infection.

4. **Procedural Step.** Open the suture or staple removal kit, making sure to keep the contents of the kit sterile. Most kits are opened by peeling back a top cover, which exposes a plastic tray that holds the necessary instruments and supplies.

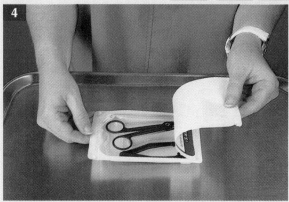

5. **Procedural Step.** Apply clean gloves. Cleanse the incision line with an antiseptic swab to destroy microorganisms and to remove any dried exudate encrusted around the sutures or staples. Clean the wound from the top to the bottom, working from the center to the outside of the wound. Use a new swab for each cleansing motion. Allow the skin to dry.
Principle. Dried exudate must be removed to allow unimpeded removal of the sutures or staples.

6. **Procedural Step.** Remove the sutures or staples. Tell the patient that he or she will feel a pulling or tugging sensation as each suture (or staple) is removed, but that it will not be painful. Count the number of sutures or staples removed. Check the patient's chart to make sure the same number are removed as were inserted by the physician.

To remove sutures:

a. Using the sterile thumb forceps provided in the kit, pick up the knot of the first suture.

b. Place the curved tip of the suture scissors under the suture. Using the sterile suture scissors, cut the suture below the knot on the side of the suture closest to the skin. Cut the suture as close to the skin as possible.

c. Using a smooth, continuous motion, gently pull the suture out through the outer skin orifice. Remove the suture without allowing any portion that was previously outside to be pulled through the skin. Place the suture on the 4 × 4 gauze included in the suture kit.

d. Continue in this manner until all the sutures have been removed.

PROCEDURE 10-6

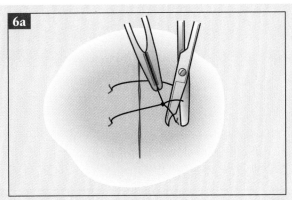

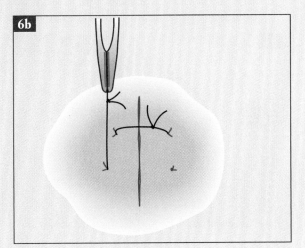

(From Nealon TF: *Fundamental skills in surgery,* ed 4, Philadelphia, 1994, Saunders.)

Principle. To prevent infection, the suture must be removed without pulling any portion that has been outside the skin back through the skin.

To remove staples:

a. Gently place the bottom jaws of the staple remover under the staple to be removed.

b. Firmly squeeze the staple handles until they are fully closed.

c. Carefully lift the staple remover upward to remove the staple from the incision line. Place the staple on the 4 × 4 gauze included in the staple kit.

d. Continue in this manner until all the staples have been removed.

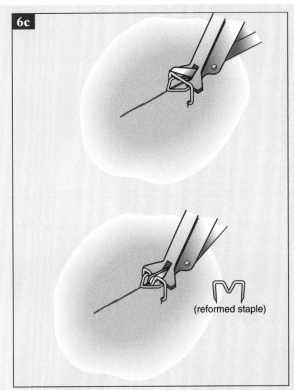

(reformed staple)

(Courtesy Ethicon, Somerville, NJ.)

7. **Procedural Step.** Cleanse the site with an antiseptic swab. Some physicians want the medical assistant to apply adhesive skin closures after removing the sutures or staples to provide additional support to the wound as it continues to heal.

8. **Procedural Step.** Apply a dry sterile dressing if indicated by the physician.

9. **Procedural Step.** Properly dispose of all contaminated supplies in a biohazard waste container.

10. **Procedural Step.** Remove the gloves, and sanitize your hands.

11. **Procedural Step.** Chart the procedure. Include the date and time, the status of the sutures (or staples) and incision line, the number of sutures (or staples) removed, the location of the site, and care of the wound (i.e., application of an antiseptic or dressing). Chart any instructions given to the patient.

CHARTING EXAMPLE	
Date	
9/20/05	10:30 a.m. Sutures intact and incision line in good approximation. No signs of infection. Sutures x6 removed from (R) ant forearm. Incision line cleaned c̄ Betadine and DSD applied. Instructions provided on dressing care. ———————— T. Browning, CMA

PROCEDURE 10-7 Applying and Removing Adhesive Skin Closures

Outcome Apply and remove adhesive skin closures.

Equipment/Supplies:

- Clean disposable gloves
- Sterile gloves
- Antiseptic solution
- Surgical scrub brush
- Antiseptic swabs
- Tincture of benzoin
- Sterile cotton-tipped applicator
- Adhesive skin closure strips
- Sterile 4 × 4 gauze pads
- Surgical tape

Application of Adhesive Skin Closures

1. **Procedural Step.** Sanitize your hands, and assemble the equipment.

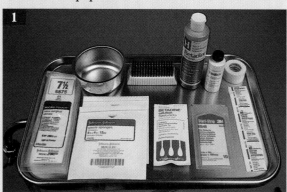

2. **Procedural Step.** Greet and identify the patient.
3. **Procedural Step.** Introduce yourself, and explain the procedure.
4. **Procedural Step.** Position the patient as required. Adjust the light so that it is focused on the wound. Apply clean gloves. Inspect the wound for signs of redness, swelling, and drainage. (*Note:* Chart this information in the patient's record at the end of the procedure.)
5. **Procedural Step.** Gently scrub the wound using an antiseptic solution (e.g., Betadine solution) and a sterile gauze pad or a surgical scrub brush. Clean at least 3 inches around the wound, making sure to remove all debris, skin oil, and exudates. Allow the skin to dry or pat dry with gauze squares. (*Note:* Change gloves as needed to maintain cleanliness.)

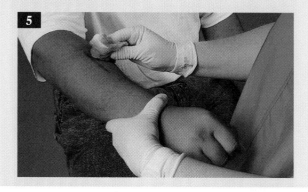

6. **Procedural Step.** Cleanse the site using antiseptic swabs such as Betadine or alcohol swabs. Clean the wound from the top to the bottom, working from the center to the outside of the wound. Use a new swab for each cleansing motion. Allow the skin to dry.

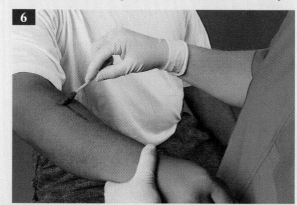

7. **Procedural Step.** If dictated by the medical office policy, using a sterile cotton-tipped applicator, apply a thin coat of tincture of benzoin to the skin parallel to the wound. Do not allow the tincture of benzoin to touch the wound. Allow the skin to dry. Remove gloves and sanitize your hands.
   Principle. Tincture of benzoin facilitates adhesion of the strips to the skin.

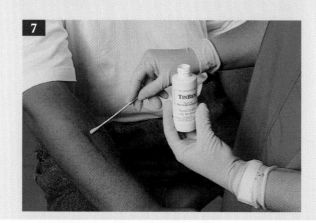

8. **Procedural Step.** Open the plastic peel-apart package of strips using sterile technique as follows:
   a. Grasp each flap of the package between the thumbs and pull the package apart.
   b. Peel back the package until it is completely open.
   c. Lay the opened package flat on a clean dry surface. The inside of the package serves as the sterile field.

9. **Procedural Step.** Apply sterile gloves. Fold the card of strips along its perforated tab and tear off the tab, which exposes the ends of the strips, making them easier to grasp. Peel a strip of tape off the card at a 45-degree angle to the card.

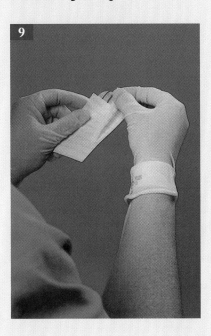

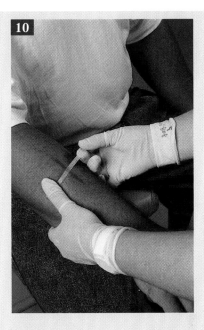

11. **Procedural Step.** Apply the next strip midway between the middle (first) strip and one end of the wound. Apply a third strip between the middle strip and the other end of the wound. Continue applying the strips at ⅛-inch intervals until the edges of the wound are approximated. If at any time the skin surfaces become moist with perspiration, blood, or serum, wipe the area dry with a sterile gauze pad before applying the next strip.
   Principle. Applying the strips in this manner facilitates good approximation of the wound. Spacing the strips at ⅛-inch intervals allows proper drainage of the wound.

10. **Procedural Step.** Check to make sure the skin surface is dry. Position the first strip over the center of the wound as follows:
   a. Secure one end of the strip of tape to the skin on one side of the wound by pressing down firmly on the tape.
   b. Stretch the strip transversely across the line of the incision until the edges of the wound are approximated exactly. If necessary, use your gloved hand to assist in bringing the edges of the wound together.
   c. Secure the strip on the skin on the other side of the wound by pressing down firmly on the tape.
   Principle. Approximating the wound exactly facilitates good healing and minimizes scar formation.

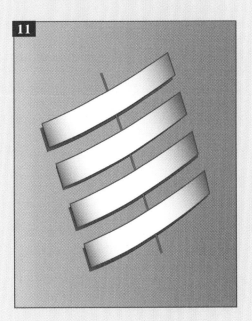

PROCEDURE 10-7

Continued

PROCEDURE 10-7 Applying and Removing Adhesive Skin Closures—Cont'd

12. **Procedural Step.** Apply two closures approximately ½ inch from the ends of the strips and parallel to the wound (ladder fashion).
Principle. Applying a strip along each edge redistributes the tension and assists in holding the strips firmly in place.

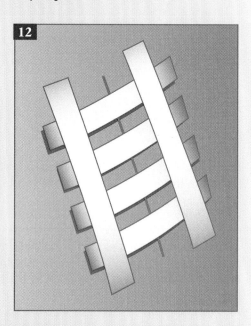

13. **Procedural Step.** Apply a dry sterile dressing over the strips if indicated by the physician (see Procedure 10-5).
14. **Procedural Step.** Remove the gloves, and sanitize your hands.
15. **Procedural Step.** Instruct the patient in wound care as follows:
   a. Provide the patient with written wound care instructions.
   b. Explain the wound care instructions and ask the patient if he or she has any questions.
   c. Ask the patient to sign the instruction sheet on the appropriate line.
   d. Witness the patient's signature by signing your name in the appropriate space on the form. Include today's date.
   e. Give a signed copy of the wound care instructions to the patient and file a copy in the patient's medical record.
Principle. An instruction sheet signed by the patient provides legal documentation that wound care instructions were provided to the patient.

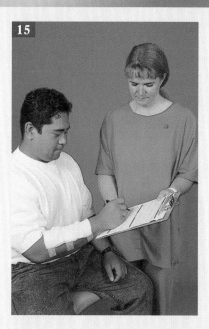

16. **Procedural Step.** Chart the procedure. Include the date and time, the appearance of the wound, wound preparation, the number of strips applied, the location of the wound, and care of the wound. Chart instructions given to the patient about wound care.

CHARTING EXAMPLE

Date	
9/20/05	10:30 a.m. Incision approx 5 cm long located on ℝ post forearm. Redness noted on edge of wound. Sl amt of serous drainage noted. Wound scrubbed c̄ Betadine sol and Betadine antiseptic applied. Applied Steri-Strips x4. Incision in good approximation. Applied DSD. Explained wound care. Written instructions provided. Signed copy filed in chart. To return in 5 days for removal of strips. ——————————————— T. Browning, CMA

Removal of Adhesive Skin Closures

1. **Procedural Step.** Sanitize your hands. Greet and identify the patient. Introduce yourself, and explain the procedure.

2. **Procedural Step.** Position the patient as required. Adjusted the light so that it is focused on the wound. Check to made sure the skin closures are intact and the incision line is approximated and not gapping. Check that incision line is not infected. If the incision line is not approximated or if redness, swelling, or a discharge is present, do not remove the skin closures; notify the physician.

3. **Procedural Step.** Position a 4 × 4 gauze pad in a convenient location. Apply clean gloves.

4. **Procedural Step.** Remove the skin closures as follows:

   a. Peel off each half of the strip of tape from the outside toward the wound margin. Never pull the strips away from the wound because tension on the wound site could disrupt the healing process.

   b. Gently lift the strip away from the wound surface. Place the strip on a 4 × 4 gauze pad.

   c. Continue in this manner until all the skin closures have been removed.

5. **Procedural Step.** Cleanse the site with an antiseptic swab. Apply a dry sterile dressing if indicated by the physician (see Procedure 10-5).

6. **Procedural Step.** Properly dispose of all contaminated supplies. Remove the gloves, and sanitize your hands.

7. **Procedural Step.** Chart the procedure. Include the date and time, the status of the skin closures, the number of skin closures removed, the location of the site, and care of the wound. Chart any instructions given to the patient.

CHARTING EXAMPLE	
Date	
9/20/05	10:30 a.m. Skin closures intact and in good approximation. No signs of infection. Strips x 4 removed from Ⓡ post forearm. Incision line cleaned c̄ Betadine and DSD applied. Instructions provided on dressing care.
	— T. Browning, CMA

PROCEDURE 10-7

Assisting With Minor Office Surgery

Tray Setup

Assisting with minor office surgery requires a thorough knowledge of the instruments and supplies for each tray setup and the type of assistance required by the physician during the surgery. The medical assistant must be able to work quickly and efficiently and to anticipate the physician's needs.

The instruments and supplies for the surgery must be set on a sterile field. Many offices maintain index cards indicating the appropriate instruments and supplies for each minor office surgery tray setup. The card may also include information regarding the type of skin preparation, the position of the patient, the physician's glove size, the type of suture material, preoperative instructions, and postoperative instructions. The index cards are generally kept in a file box and are filed alphabetically by the type of surgery. The medical assistant should pull the card before setting up for the minor office surgery and use it as a guide to make sure all the required articles are placed on the sterile field. The medical assistant may set up the sterile tray either before or after preparing the patient's skin. The sterile tray setup must not be permitted to become contaminated. If the medical assistant must turn away from the sterile tray or leave the room after setting up, a sterile towel must be placed over the tray to maintain sterility.

Methods Used to Set Up a Sterile Tray

A common method used to set up a sterile tray is to use prepackaged sterile setups wrapped in disposable sterilization paper or muslin that are prepared by the medical office through autoclave sterilization (Procedure 10-3). These setups are labeled according to use (e.g., suture pack, cyst removal pack) and contain most of the instruments and supplies required for the minor office surgery indicated on the label. The medical assistant opens the wrapped package on a flat surface, such as a **Mayo tray;** the inside of the wrapper is sterile and serves as the sterile field. Several additional articles not contained in the prepackaged setup (e.g., an antiseptic, sterile 4 × 4 gauze pads, disposable syringes and needles, and sutures) may need to be added to the sterile field once the package is opened. The antiseptic is added to the sterile field according to Procedure 10-4 previously outlined in this chapter. Items in peel-apart packages are added by flipping them onto the sterile field or by placing them on the field using a sterile gloved hand.

Another method used to set up a sterile tray is to place all the necessary articles on the sterile field by flipping them onto the sterile field from peel-apart packages. With this method, the sterile field is prepared by placing a sterile towel over a tray such as a Mayo tray or other flat surface. The sterile towel must be handled by the corners only so as not to contaminate it. It must not be fanned through the air but laid down gently and slowly to prevent airborne contamination.

Side Table

Some articles required for minor office surgery are not placed on the sterile field but are set on an adjacent table or counter. These articles, such as a surgical scrub brush, are not sterile and must *not* be placed on the sterile field. The local anesthetic, which is a sterile solution, is in a vial that is not sterile and therefore must not be placed on the sterile field. The physician needs to apply gloves to perform the surgery. Although the gloves are sterile, the outside wrapper is not; therefore the package of gloves must not be placed on the sterile field. In addition, it is easier for the physician to apply gloves from a side table or counter. To facilitate applying the gloves, the medical assistant opens the outside wrapper for the physician.

Skin Preparation

The patient's skin must be prepared prior to the minor office surgery because the skin contains an abundance of microorganisms. If these microorganisms were to enter the body, a wound infection could develop. It is not possible to sterilize skin, because chemical agents required to kill all living microorganisms are too strong to be placed on the skin surfaces. Therefore the operative site and an area surrounding it must be cleaned and prepared in such a way as to remove as many microorganisms as possible to reduce the risk of surgical wound contamination.

Shaving the Site

Hair supports the growth of microorganisms, and the physician may therefore want the medical assistant to shave the skin at and around the operative site. Disposable shave prep trays are commercially available and include several gauze sponges, a measured amount of antiseptic soap, a container for soapy water, and a disposable safety razor. The skin should be pulled taut as it is shaved, and the medical assistant must be careful to prevent nicks. Once all the hair has been removed, the shaved area should be rinsed and dried thoroughly.

Cleansing the Site

The site must next be cleaned with an antiseptic solution such as povidone-iodine (Betadine Surgical Scrub) or chlorhexidine gluconate (Hibiclens) (Figure 10-11). The medical assistant should scrub the area with a surgical scrub brush using a firm circular motion, moving from the inside outward. The area is then rinsed using gauze pads saturated with water and is blotted dry with sterile gauze.

Antiseptic Application

Once the patient's skin has been shaved (if required) and cleansed, an antiseptic is applied to the operative area, followed by the application of a sterile drape. The antiseptic decreases the number of microorganisms on the patient's skin; a common antiseptic is Betadine. A disposable sterile fenestrated drape (Figure 10-12) is most commonly used. It has an opening that is placed directly over the operative site. A fenestrated drape covers a wide area of skin around the operative area, leaving only the operative site exposed. This provides a sterile area around the operative site and thereby decreases contamination of the patient's surgical wound.

Local Anesthetic

Minor office surgeries often require the use of a local anesthetic; local anesthetics frequently used in the medical office include lidocaine hydrochloride (Xylocaine) and procaine hydrochloride (Novocaine). The physician injects

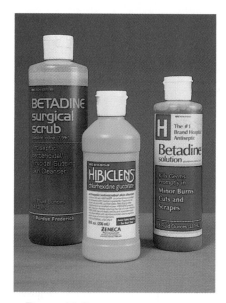

Figure 10-11. Cleansing solutions.

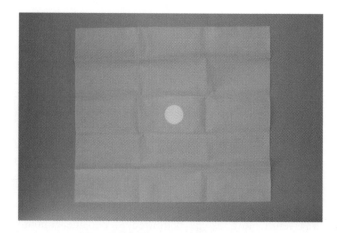

Figure 10-12. Fenestrated drape.

the local anesthetic into the tissue surrounding the operative site, a process termed **infiltration,** to produce a loss of sensation in that area and thereby prevent the patient from feeling pain during the surgery. Local anesthetics begin working in 5 to 15 minutes and have a duration of action of from 1 to 3 hours, depending on the type of anesthetic.

Some physicians prefer to use a local anesthetic containing *epinephrine.* Epinephrine is a vasoconstrictor that prolongs the local effect of the anesthetic and decreases the rate of systemic absorption of the local anesthetic. It accomplishes this by constricting the blood vessels at the operative site. The physician will inform the medical assistant as to the type, strength, and amount of the local anesthetic needed for the minor office surgery. For example, Xylocaine is available in 0.5, 1.0, 1.5, and 2.0% solutions. The physician may order 1 ml of Xylocaine 2.0% with epinephrine to suture a laceration of the forearm.

Preparing the Anesthetic

The local anesthetic is drawn up into the syringe according to the procedure presented in Chapter 11. The vial must first be cleansed using an alcohol wipe. The correct amount of anesthetic solution is then withdrawn into the syringe. This may be performed by either the medical assistant or the physician. The medical assistant withdraws the anesthetic into the syringe and hands it to the physician, who has not yet applied gloves. The physician injects the anesthetic into the patient's tissues and then applies gloves to begin the surgery.

The physician may prefer to draw the anesthetic solution into the syringe after he or she has applied gloves. The medical assistant should first show the label of the vial to the physician and then hold the vial securely while the physician withdraws the medication (Figure 10-13). The medical assistant must hold the vial, because the outside of the vial is medically aseptic and cannot be touched by the physician's sterile gloved hand.

If the medical assistant prepares the anesthetic injection, the needle and syringe are not placed on the sterile field but are assembled off to the side. If the physician withdraws the anesthetic, the needle and syringe are placed on the sterile field.

Highlight on the History of Surgery

Surgery evolved from very primitive beginnings. The first record of a surgical operation dates back to 350,000 BC. Primitive humans believed that headaches were caused by demons that had gained entrance to the head and were unable to get out. To release the demons, a hole was chiseled through the patient's skull with a sharp flint. Early operating instruments consisted of sharpened flints and crude hammers. Sharpened animal teeth were used for blood-letting and drainage of abscesses. Ancient records show that suturing materials consisted of dried gut, dried tendon, strips of hide, horsehair, and fibers from tree bark. To help form a clot, bleeding wounds were covered with materials such as rabbit fur, shredded tree bark, egg yolk, and cobwebs.

As late as the early 1800s, surgical instruments were still almost nonexistent. Kitchen knives and penknives doubled as scalpels, and table forks were used as retractors. Physicians would use household pincushions to hold their suturing needles. The same sponges were used for every patient to wipe away blood and other secretions. Because of these conditions, the most trivial operations were likely to be followed by infection, and death occurred in up to half of all surgical operations. Joseph Lister, an English surgeon, was one of the first individuals to advocate the use of antiseptics during surgery. Lister insisted on the use of antiseptics on the hands of his surgical team, instruments, wounds, and dressings. Lister's ideas were ridiculed by many surgeons, but in 1879 his antiseptic principles were, at long last, formally adopted by the medical profession. Today Joseph Lister is known as the father of modern surgery.

Anesthetic agents, such as ether and chloroform, were discovered in the mid-1800s. Before this time, various methods were used to subdue and restrain patients during surgery, such as having the patient consume alcohol before the operation and strapping the patient to the operating table. With the advent of anesthetics, new surgical procedures never before considered possible came into existence. This resulted in new demands for surgical instruments, as well as the necessity for smaller and more delicate instruments.

The late 1800s and early 1900s saw dramatic advances in surgical operations and techniques. The most notable include the invention of the steam sterilizer, which permitted sterilization of surgical instruments and supplies; the use of surgical gowns, caps, masks, and gloves during surgery; the monitoring of a patient's condition while under anesthesia; the development of stainless steel, which provided a superior material for manufacturing surgical instruments; and the establishment of standards for manufacturing and packaging sutures. Other discoveries important to surgery during this time included the discovery of x-rays by Wilhelm Roentgen, the discovery of penicillin by Alexander Fleming, the discovery by William Halsted that cocaine could be used as a local anesthetic, and the development of endoscopic instruments such as the laryngoscope, bronchoscope, and sigmoidoscope for viewing internal structures of the body.

The breakthroughs in surgical technology established through the ages laid the foundation for present-day complex surgical procedures such as laser surgery, open-heart surgery, and microsurgery. It is incredible indeed to think that it all started with a sharpened flint!

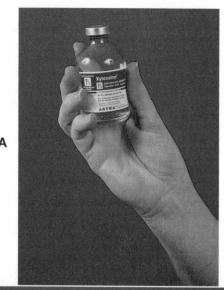

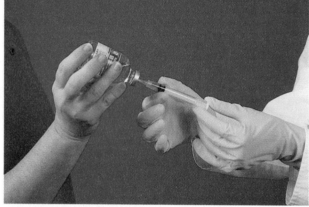

Figure 10-13. Drawing up the local anesthetic. **A,** Trudy holds up the vial so that the physician can verify the name and strength of the local anesthetic. **B,** Trudy holds the vial securely while the physician withdraws the medication.

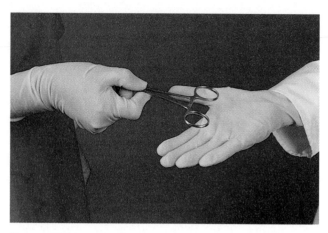

Figure 10-14. Trudy hands a hemostat to the physician in its functional position.

Assisting the Physician

The type of assistance required by the physician during minor office surgery is based on the type of surgery and physician's preference.

Some physicians want the medical assistant to apply sterile gloves and assist directly by handing instruments and supplies from the sterile field. An instrument should be handed to the physician in a firm, confident manner so that the instrument does not slip out of the physician's hand and drop on the floor. The instrument should be placed in the physician's hand in its functional position, that is, the position in which it is to be used (Figure 10-14). If the instrument is handed correctly, the physician should not have to reposition the instrument to use it.

The medical assistant is responsible for adding any instruments or supplies to the sterile field that the physician

requires after the surgery has begun, such as another hemostat, additional 4 × 4 gauze pads, and sutures. This is generally accomplished using peel-apart packages and either flipping the contents onto the sterile field or holding the package open and allowing the physician to remove the contents with a gloved hand. In assisting with minor office surgery, it is essential to know all steps in the procedure so that the physician's needs are anticipated and the surgery proceeds smoothly and efficiently.

The physician may obtain a tissue specimen that is sent to the laboratory for histologic examination. The specimen must be placed in an appropriate-sized container with a preservative. The medical assistant is responsible for labeling the specimen container with the patient's name, the date, and the type of specimen. The medical assistant must also complete a laboratory requisition to accompany the specimen; this is known as a biopsy requisition (Figure 10-15).

Once the minor office surgery is completed, the physician may want the medical assistant to place a dry sterile dressing over the surgical wound to protect it from contamination or injury or to absorb drainage. The medical assistant is also responsible for assisting the patient and cleaning the examining room.

Procedure 10-8 describes the medical assistant's responsibilities while assisting with minor office surgery. Specific instruments and supplies required for the minor office surgery depend on the type of surgery being performed and the physician's preference. Knowing the name and function of the surgical instruments shown in Figure 10-2 enables the medical assistant to set up for each type of minor surgery performed in the medical office. If the medical office uses prepackaged sterile setups, the medical assistant will have already assembled the instruments and supplies in the package during the sanitization and sterilization process; however, the instruments and supplies should be checked after the pack is opened to make sure all the sterile articles are included.

DIAGNOSTIC PATHOLOGY ASSOCIATES, INC

HISTOPATHOLOGY/CYTOPATHOLOGY REQUISITION

BILL TO: ☐ ACCOUNT ☐ PATIENT	☐ MEDICARE ☐ MEDICAID	☐ BLUE SHIELD ☐ OTHER	PATIENT NAME (LAST, FIRST, MIDDLE INITIAL)		PATIENT ID	ROOM NO.

SEX	BIRTHDATE / /	DATE COLLECTED	TIME COLLECTED A.M. P.M.	REQUESTING PHYSICIAN	SPECIAL INSTRUCTIONS

RESPONSIBLE PARTY NAME	RESPONSIBLE PARTY ADDRESS	CITY, STATE, ZIP

PHONE	MEDICAID ID NUMBER	MEDICARE HIC NUMBER	INSURANCE COMPANY NAME

INSURANCE COMPANY ADDRESS	GROUP NUMBER	CONTRACT NUMBER	COVERAGE CODE	PATIENT/INSURED RELATIONSHIP ☐ SELF ☐ SPOUSE ☐ DEPEND.

PATIENT AUTHORIZATION: I AUTHORIZE THE RELEASE OF ANY MEDICAL INFORMATION NECESSARY TO PROCESS A CLAIM, I PERMIT A COPY OF THIS AUTHORIZATION TO BE USED IN PLACE OF THE ORIGINAL AND REQUEST PAYMENT OF ANY MEDICAL INSURANCE BENEFITS EITHER TO ME OR TO THE PARTY WHO ACCEPTS ASSIGNMENT. | SIGNED X_____ | DATE _____

TISSUE EXAM: ☐ GROSS & MICROSCOPIC ☐ GROSS ONLY SPECIMEN TYPE: ☐ BIOPSY ☐ SCRAPING ☐ BRUSHING ☐ WASHING ☐ FLUIDS ☐ FINE NEEDLE ☐ OTHER _____	SOURCE OF SPECIMEN: ☐ PHONE REPORT (NEXT WORKING DAY) COPIES TO: _____	CLINICAL DIAGNOSIS: PATIENT HISTORY:

Figure 10-15. Biopsy requisition. (Courtesy Diagnostic Pathology Associates, Columbus, Ohio.)

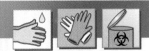

PROCEDURE 10-8   Assisting With Minor Office Surgery

Outcome Set up a surgical tray and assist with minor office surgery.

Equipment/Supplies:
- Instruments and supplies for the type of surgery to be performed

Preparing the Tray

1. **Procedural Step.** Determine the type of minor office surgery to be performed. The physician instructs the medical assistant as to the type of surgery as well as any additional information needed to set up for the surgery, such as the appropriate anesthetic and suture material. If the medical office maintains a minor office surgery filing system, pull the file card that indicates the instruments and supplies required for the type of surgery to be performed.

2. **Procedural Step.** Prepare the examining room. Make sure the room is clean and well lighted.

3. **Procedural Step.** Sanitize your hands.

4. **Procedural Step.** Set up nonsterile articles on a side table or counter.
   Principle. Articles that are not sterile cannot be placed on the sterile field because they would contaminate it.

5. **Procedural Step.** Sanitize your hands, and set up the minor office surgery tray on a clean, dry, flat surface, using the principles of surgical asepsis. The sterile tray can be set up as follows:

   Prepackaged Setup:
   a. Select the appropriate package from the supply shelf, and place it on a Mayo tray or other flat surface.
   b. Open the setup using the inside of the wrapper as the sterile field.
   c. Add other articles to the sterile field that are needed for the surgery but not contained in the sterile package.

   Transferring Articles to a Sterile Field:
   a. Pick up the folded sterile towel by two corner ends and allow it to unfold; make sure it does not touch an unsterile surface.
   b. Lay the sterile towel down gently and slowly over the Mayo tray, making sure it does not

Continued

PROCEDURE 10-8 Assisting With Minor Office Surgery—Cont'd

brush against an unsterile surface such as your uniform. Do not allow your arms to pass over the towel as you lay it down because this would result in contamination of the sterile field.

c. Transfer instruments and supplies to the sterile filed from wrapped or peel-apart packages.

Principle. The principles of surgical asepsis must be followed to prevent contamination of the sterile field.

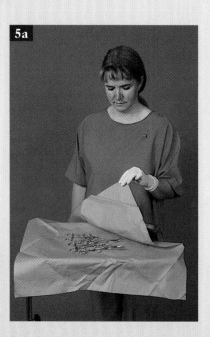

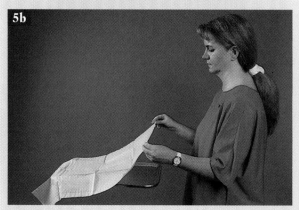

6. **Procedural Step.** Apply a sterile glove and arrange the articles neatly on the sterile field. Do not allow one article to lay on top of another. Check to make sure all the instruments and supplies required for the surgery are available on the sterile field.

Principle. Instruments and supplies can be located quickly and efficiently on a neat and orderly sterile field. Sterile gloves must be used to prevent contamination of the sterile articles.

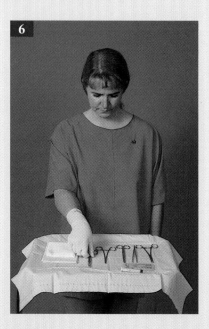

7. **Procedural Step.** Cover the tray setup with a sterile towel by picking up the towel by two corner ends and placing it gently and slowly over the setup. Do not allow your arms to pass over the sterile field as you lay it down.

Principle. The towel prevents the sterile tray from becoming contaminated. The towel must be picked up by the corner ends to prevent contaminating it and should be moved slowly and not fanned through the air to prevent airborne contamination. Passing the arms over the sterile field results in contamination of the field.

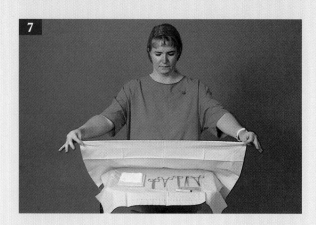

Preparing the Patient

8. **Procedural Step.** Greet and identify the patient. Introduce yourself. Explain the procedure, and prepare the patient for the minor office surgery. Try to allay the patient's fear or anxiety. Ask the patient if he or she needs to void before the surgery. Provide instructions to the patient on any clothing that must be removed and putting on an examination gown, if required. Enough clothing must be removed to completely expose the operative area. Instruct the patient not to move during the procedure and not to talk, laugh, sneeze, or cough over the sterile field.

   Principle. Minor office surgery is often a frightening experience for the patient, and reassurance should be offered to reduce apprehension. The amount of clothing that must be removed will depend on the type of minor office surgery being performed. By moving, the patient may accidentally contaminate the sterile field or touch the operative site. Microorganisms are carried in water vapor from the mouth, nose, and lungs and can be transferred onto the sterile field.

9. **Procedural Step.** Position the patient. The type of position is determined by the type of minor office surgery to be performed. The patient is positioned in such a way as to provide the best possible exposure and accessibility to the operative site. *Note:* If a difficult position must be maintained, such as the knee-chest position, the patient should not be positioned until the physician is ready to begin the minor office surgery.

10. **Procedural Step.** Adjust the light so that it is focused on the operative site.

11. **Procedural Step.** Apply clean disposable gloves. Prepare the patient's skin as specified by the physician. The skin at and around the operative site may need to be shaved. The skin should be pulled taut as it is shaved. The area is then rinsed and dried thoroughly.

    Cleanse the patient's skin with an antiseptic solution and a surgical scrub brush using a firm, circular motion and moving from the inside outward. Do not return to an area just cleansed. The area is then rinsed using gauze pads saturated with water and blotted dry with a sterile gauze pad.

    Cleanse the site using antiseptic swabs such as Betadine or alcohol swabs. Allow the skin to dry. Remove the gloves, and sanitize your hands.

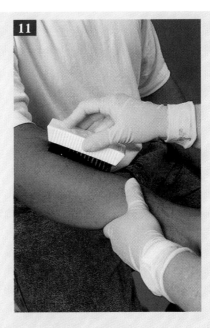

12. **Procedural Step.** Check to make sure everything is prepared for the minor office surgery and inform the physician that the patient is ready.

Assisting the Physician

13. **Procedural Step.** Assist the physician as required during the minor office surgery, following the principles of surgical asepsis. The physician will inject the local anesthetic, drape the patient, and perform the surgery.

    The responsibilities of the medical assistant may include:

    a. Uncover the sterile tray setup by picking up the sterile towel covering it. The towel should be picked up by two corner ends and removed slowly and gently without allowing the arms to pass over the sterile field.

    b. Withdraw the local anesthetic into a syringe and hand it to the physician or hold the vial while the physician withdraws the local anesthetic.

    c. Open the outer glove wrapper for the physician to facilitate the application of sterile gloves.

    d. Adjust the light as needed by the physician for good visualization of the operative site.

    e. Restrain patients such as children.

    f. Relax and reassure the patient during the minor office surgery.

PROCEDURE 10-8

Continued

g. Hand instruments and supplies to the physician. (Sterile gloves required.)

h. Keep the sterile field neat and orderly. (Sterile gloves required.)

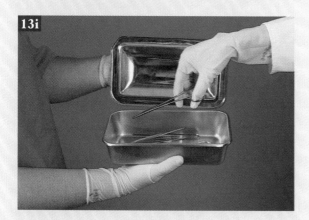

i. Hold a basin in which the physician can deposit soiled instruments and supplies, such as hemostats and gauze sponges. (Clean gloves required.)

j. Retract tissue from an area to allow the physician the best access and visibility of the operative site. (Sterile gloves required.)

k. Sponge blood from the operative site. (Sterile gloves required.)

l. Add instruments and supplies to the sterile field as required by the physician.

m. Hold the specimen container to accept a specimen received from the physician. (Clean gloves required.) Do not touch the inside of the container because it is sterile. Label the specimen container with the patient's name, the date, and the type of specimen.

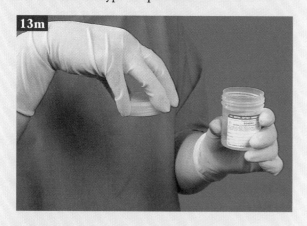

14. **Procedural Step.** Apply a sterile dressing to the surgical wound, if ordered by the physician (see Procedure 10-5).

    Principle. The sterile dressing protects the wound from contamination and injury and absorbs drainage.

15. **Procedural Step.** Stay with the patient as a safety precaution and to assist and instruct the patient. The patient may need to rest before getting off the examining table. Help the patient off the table to prevent falls. Instruct the patient to dress, offering assistance if needed. Make sure postoperative instructions regarding any type of medical care to be administered at home are understood. Relay information regarding the return visit for postoperative care, such as the removal of sutures or a dressing change. If the patient has a wound or if sutures have been inserted, he or she should be told to keep the area clean and dry and to report any signs of inflammation such as redness, swelling, discharge, or increase in pain. Any instructions given must be charted in the patient's medical record.

    Principle. The patient (especially an elderly one) may become dizzy after the minor office surgery and should be allowed to rest before getting off the examining table. Patient instructions must be charted to protect the physician legally, in the event that the patient fails to follow instructions and causes harm or damage to the operative site.

16. **Procedural Step.** If a specimen was collected, it must be transferred to the laboratory in a tightly closed, properly labeled specimen container. Complete a biopsy request form to accompany the specimen. Record information in the patient's chart, including the date the specimen was picked up or sent to the laboratory, as well as the name of the laboratory.

    Principle. Recording information regarding transport of the specimen documents that the specimen was sent to the laboratory.

17. **Procedural Step.** Clean the examining room. Handle the instruments carefully so as not to damage them. Be especially careful with sharp instruments to prevent cutting yourself. Blood and body secretions should be rinsed off the instruments immediately to prevent them from drying and hardening. The instruments must then be sanitized and sterilized when it is convenient to do so; follow the procedures presented in Chapter 3. Discard disposable articles contaminated with blood or other potentially infectious materials in a biohazard waste container.

Principle. Surgical instruments are expensive and must be handled carefully to prolong their life span. Hardened blood and secretions on an instrument are difficult to remove. Disposable articles must be discarded in an appropriate manner to prevent the spread of infection.

PROCEDURE 10-8

CHARTING EXAMPLE

Date	
9/25/05	2:00 p.m. Applied DSD to (R) post forearm.
	Instructed patient on suture care. Written
	instructions provided. Signed copy filed in
	chart. To return in 5 days for removal of
	sutures. Sebaceous cyst specimen sent to
	Medical Center Laboratory for biopsy on
	9/25/05. ———————— T. Browning, CMA

What Would You DO?
What Would You *Not* DO?

Case Study 2

Abbey Mendy is having a sebaceous cyst removed from her neck. She wants to know why the antiseptic applied to her neck is orange, and if it is going to permanently stain her skin. During the procedure Abbey reaches her hand up to adjust her hair and accidentally touches the physician's gloved hand. After the procedure, a sterile dressing is applied to her neck and she is given an appointment to return to have her sutures removed. Abbey becomes alarmed when she is told that the cyst will be sent to the lab for a biopsy. She wants to know if the physician is not telling her everything about her condition and that maybe he thinks she has cancer. Abbey asks if her neighbor can take out her sutures. She says that he has worked as a veterinary assistant for the past 8 years and has lots of experience in removing stitches.

Medical Office Surgical Procedures

The most common surgical procedures performed in the medical office are presented on the following pages. A discussion of the procedure and the items required for each tray setup are included. The medical assistant should take into account, however, that the instruments and supplies may vary slightly from those listed here, based on the physician's preference.

Sebaceous Cyst Removal

A **sebaceous cyst** is a thin, closed sac or capsule that contains secretions from a sebaceous, or oil, gland. It forms when the outlet of the gland becomes obstructed. The built-up secretion of sebum from the gland causes swelling, and the lining of the cyst consists of the stretched sebaceous gland. Sebaceous cysts are soft to firm in consistency and are generally elevated and filled with an odorous cheesy material. This type of cyst can occur anywhere on the body except on the palms of the hands and the soles of the feet—these areas do not contain sebaceous glands. Sebaceous cysts tend to occur most frequently on the scalp, face, ears, neck, and back.

A sebaceous cyst is usually painless and nontender, although it may become infected; to avoid this, the cyst should be excised by the physician. If it is already infected, the physician does not excise the cyst but drains it and performs the removal at a later time. A sebaceous cyst is removed as follows:

1. A local anesthetic is used to numb the area.
2. The physician makes an incision, removes the cyst, and sutures the surgical incision (Figure 10-16).
3. The cyst is placed in a specimen container with a preservative and sent to the laboratory for examination by a pathologist.
4. A sterile dressing is then applied to the operative site.

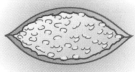

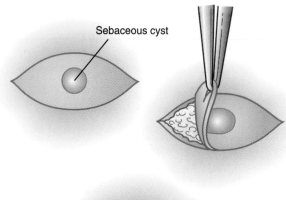

Figure 10-16. Sebaceous cyst removal. The physician makes an incision, removes the cyst, and sutures the surgical incision. (From Nealon TF, Jr: *Fundamental skills in surgery,* ed 4, Philadelphia, 1994, Saunders.)

Items Placed to the Side of the Sterile Field

Sebaceous cyst removal:

- Clean disposable gloves
- Antiseptic solution
- Surgical scrub brush
- Antiseptic swabs
- Sterile gloves
- Local anesthetic
- Alcohol wipe to cleanse the vial
- Specimen container with preservative and label
- Laboratory request form
- Surgical tape

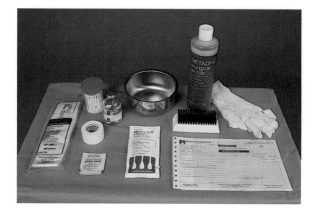

Items Included on the Sterile Field

Sebaceous cyst removal:

- Fenestrated drape
- Needle and syringe for drawing up the local anesthetic
- Scalpel and blade
- Dissecting scissors
- Hemostatic forceps
- Tissue forceps
- Thumb forceps
- Operating scissors
- Needle holder
- Sutures
- Sterile 4 × 4 gauze

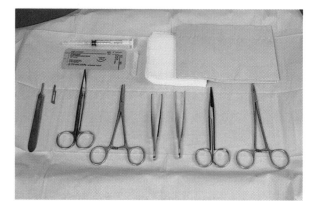

Surgical Incision and Drainage of Localized Infections

An **abscess** is a collection of pus in a cavity surrounded by inflamed tissue (Figure 10-17). It is caused by a pathogen that invades the tissues, usually by way of a break in the skin. An abscess serves as a defense mechanism of the body to keep an infection localized by walling off the microorganisms, preventing them from spreading through the body. A **furuncle,** also known as a boil, is a localized staphylococcal infection that originates deep within a hair follicle. Furuncles produce pain and itching. The skin initially becomes red and then turns white and necrotic over the top of the furuncle. Erythema and induration usually surround it.

Localized infections, such as abscesses, furuncles, and infected sebaceous cysts, that do not rupture and drain naturally may need to be incised and drained by the physician as follows:

1. A local anesthetic is generally used for the procedure.
2. A scalpel is used to make the incision. Then either a rubber Penrose drain or a gauze wick is inserted into the wound to keep the edges of the tissues apart, which facilitates drainage of the exudate. The exudate contains pathogenic microorganisms; therefore the medical assistant should be careful to avoid contact with the exudate while assisting with the minor surgery.
3. A sterile dressing of several thicknesses is applied over the operative site to absorb the drainage.

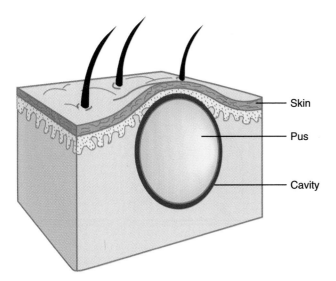

Figure 10-17. An abscess is a collection of pus in a cavity surrounded by inflamed tissue. (From Nealon TF, Jr: *Fundamental skills in surgery*, ed 4, Philadelphia, 1994, Saunders.)

4. The patient may be instructed to apply warm moist compresses at home to promote healing.

Items Placed to the Side of the Sterile Field

Incision and drainage:

- Clean disposable gloves
- Antiseptic solution
- Surgical scrub brush
- Antiseptic swabs
- Sterile gloves
- Local anesthetic
- Alcohol wipe to cleanse the vial
- Rubber Penrose drain or gauze wick
- Iodoform packing material
- Surgical tape

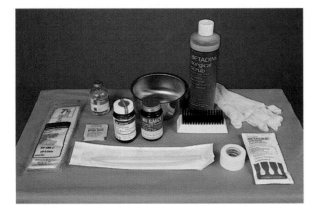

Items Included on the Sterile Field

Incision and drainage:

- Fenestrated drape
- Needle or syringe for drawing up the anesthetic
- Scalpel and blade
- Dissecting scissors
- Hemostatic forceps
- Tissue forceps
- Thumb forceps
- Operating scissors
- Sterile 4 × 4 gauze

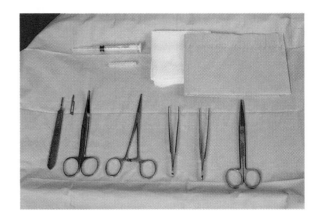

Needle Biopsy

A **biopsy** is the removal and examination of tissue from the living body. The tissue is usually examined under a microscope. Biopsies are most often performed to determine whether a tumor is malignant or benign; however, a biopsy may also be used as a diagnostic aid for other conditions, such as infections. A **needle biopsy** is a type of biopsy in which tissue from deep within the body is obtained by the insertion of a biopsy needle through the skin. A biopsy needle consists of an outer needle for making the puncture and a forked inner needle for obtaining the tissue specimen (Figure 10-18, *A*). The inner needle detaches tissue from a part of the body and brings it to the surface through its lumen (Figure 10-18, *B*).

The advantage of a needle biopsy is that a sample of tissue can be obtained that might otherwise require a major surgical operation. The procedure is performed under a local anesthetic, and, since an incision is not required, the patient does not have to undergo the discomfort and inconvenience of an operative recovery. The tissue specimen is placed in a container with a preservative and sent to the laboratory for examination by a pathologist. A small dressing, placed over the needle puncture site, is usually sufficient to protect the operative site and promote healing. After the procedure, the patient should be observed for any evidence of complications related to the procedure.

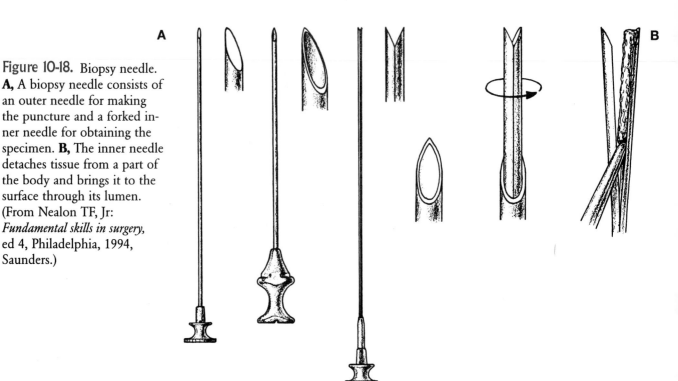

Figure 10-18. Biopsy needle. **A,** A biopsy needle consists of an outer needle for making the puncture and a forked inner needle for obtaining the specimen. **B,** The inner needle detaches tissue from a part of the body and brings it to the surface through its lumen. (From Nealon TF, Jr: *Fundamental skills in surgery,* ed 4, Philadelphia, 1994, Saunders.)

Needle Biopsy Setup

The items required for a needle biopsy are listed here.

Items Placed to the Side of the Sterile Field
Needle biopsy:
- Clean disposable gloves
- Antiseptic solution
- Surgical scrub brush
- Antiseptic swabs
- Sterile gloves
- Local anesthetic
- Alcohol wipe to cleanse the vial
- Specimen container with preservative and label
- Laboratory request form
- Surgical tape

Items Included on the Sterile Field
Needle biopsy:
- Fenestrated drape
- Needle and syringe for drawing up the local anesthetic
- Biopsy needle
- Sterile 4 × 4 gauze

Ingrown Toenail Removal

An ingrown toenail occurs when the edge of the toenail grows deeply into the nail groove and penetrates the surrounding skin, resulting in pain and discomfort to the patient (Figure 10-19, *A*). Ingrown toenails are caused by external pressure, such as from tight shoes, or from trauma, improper nail trimming, or infection. The protruding nail

acts as a foreign body, usually resulting in secondary infection and inflammation. In mild cases, this condition is treated by inserting a small piece of cotton packing under the toenail to raise the nail edge away from the tissue of the nail groove (Figure 10-19, *B*). In severe and recurring cases, part of the nail must be surgically removed, which relieves pain by decreasing the nail pressure on the soft tissues.

Ingrown Toenail Removal Setup

The items required for the removal of an ingrown toenail are listed here.

Items Placed to the Side of the Sterile Field
Ingrown toenail removal:
- Clean disposable gloves
- Antiseptic solution
- Surgical scrub brush
- Antiseptic swabs
- Sterile gloves
- Local anesthetic
- Alcohol wipe to cleanse the vial
- Surgical tape

Items Included on the Sterile Field
Ingrown toenail removal:
- Fenestrated drape
- Needle and syringe for drawing up the local anesthetic
- Surgical toenail scissors
- Hemostatic forceps
- Operating scissors
- Sterile 4 × 4 gauze

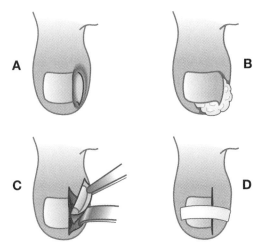

Figure 10-19. Ingrown toenail. **A,** The edge of the toenail grows deeply into the nail groove. **B,** In mild cases, treatment consists of inserting a small piece of cotton packing under the toenail. **C,** In severe and recurring cases, a wedge of the nail is surgically removed, and, **D,** a strip of surgical tape is applied over the area. (From Nealon TF, Jr: *Fundamental skills in surgery,* ed 4, Philadelphia, 1994, Saunders.)

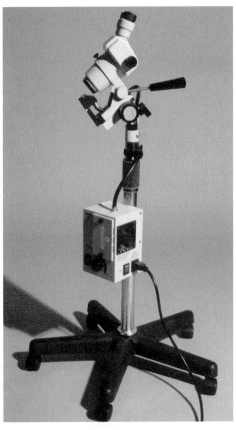

Figure 10-20. A colposcope. (From Apgar BS, Brotzman GL, Spitzer M: *Colposcopy: principles and practice—an integrated textbook and atlas,* Philadelphia, 2002, Saunders.)

Procedure

An ingrown toenail is removed as follows:

1. Before the surgical procedure is performed, the affected foot must be soaked in tepid water containing an antibacterial skin solution for 10 to 15 minutes to soften the nail plate and decrease the possibility of bacterial infection.
2. The patient is placed in a reclining position with the foot adequately supported, and the toe is shaved to remove hair, which would act as a contaminant.
3. An antiseptic is applied to the affected toe, which is then numbed using a local anesthetic.
4. Using surgical toenail scissors, the physician surgically removes a wedge of the nail (Figure 10-19, *C*).
5. A sterile gauze dressing or a strip of surgical tape is applied over the area to protect the operative site and to promote healing (Figure 10-19, *D*).

Colposcopy

Colposcopy is the visual examination of the vagina and cervix by means of a lighted instrument with a binocular magnifying lens, known as a **colposcope** (Figure 10-20). The purpose of colposcopy is to examine the vagina and cervix to determine areas of abnormal tissue growth. Colposcopy is performed following abnormal Pap test results, to evaluate a vaginal or cervical lesion observed during a pelvic examination, or after treatment for cancer of the cervix. The lens of the colposcope is positioned at the opening of the vagina. The lens magnifies tissue, thereby facilitating the inspection of cervical cells and the obtaining of a biopsy. For a routine colposcopic examination, a magnification of ×16 is generally used. The colposcope may be placed on an adjustable stand or attached to the side of the examining table and swung out prior to use.

Colposcopy Setup

The items required for colposcopy are listed here.

Items Placed to the Side of the Sterile Field

Colposcopy:
- Colposcope
- Sterile gloves
- Normal saline
- Acetic acid (3%)
- Lugol's iodine solution

Items Included on the Sterile Field

Colposcopy:
- Vaginal speculum
- Long, sterile cotton-tipped applicators
- Uterine tenaculum
- Uterine dressing forceps

Procedure

Colposcopy is performed as follows:

1. The patient is assisted into a lithotomy position and prepared as for the pelvic examination.
2. The physician inserts a vaginal speculum into the vagina.
3. A long, cotton-tipped applicator moistened with saline is used to wipe the cervix to remove the mucus film that normally covers it. The saline also provides better visualization of the cervical epithelium because dry cervical epithelium is not transparent and therefore does not allow satisfactory viewing of the vascular pattern of the cervix.
4. The colposcope is focused on the cervix and the physician inspects the saline-moistened cervix.
5. The cervix is swabbed with acetic acid, using a long, cotton-tipped applicator. The acetic acid dissolves cervical mucus and other secretions; furthermore, the acetic acid provides the best contrast between normal and abnormal tissue, allowing easier visualization of dysplastic and neoplastic epithelium.
6. The cervical epithelium may also be stained with Lugol's iodine solution using a long, cotton-tipped applicator. This provides another means to identify unhealthy epithelium. The healthy epithelium of the cervix contains glycogen, which is able to absorb the iodine causing the epithelium to stain a dark brown color. Conversely, abnormal epithelium, such as would constitute a malignancy, does not contain glycogen and therefore is unable to absorb the iodine.
7. If an abnormal area is observed, the physician will obtain a cervical biopsy using punch biopsy forceps which is described next.

Cervical Punch Biopsy

A cervical biopsy is performed in combination with colposcopy to remove a cervical tissue specimen for examination by a pathologist. The purpose of the biopsy is to determine whether the specimen is benign or malignant. Cervical biopsies are often performed following abnormal Pap test results. The procedure is usually performed a week after the end of the menstrual period, when the cervix is the least vascular. To prepare for the procedure, the patient should be told not to douche, use vaginal creams, or have intercourse for 2 days before the examination.

Cervical Punch Biopsy Setup

The items required for a cervical punch biopsy are listed here.

Items Placed to the Side of the Sterile Field

Cervical punch biopsy:
- Colposcope
- Sterile gloves
- Lugol's iodine solution
- Monsel's solution
- Specimen container with preservative and label
- Laboratory request form
- Sanitary pad

Items Included on the Sterile Field

Cervical punch biopsy:
- Vaginal speculum
- Long, sterile cotton-tipped applicators
- Cervical punch biopsy forceps
- Uterine dressing forceps
- Uterine tenaculum
- Sterile 4 × 4 gauze

Procedure

A cervical biopsy is performed as follows:

1. The patient is positioned and draped in a lithotomy position. An anesthetic is not needed; because the cervix has few pain receptors, the patient experiences little discomfort from the procedure.
2. The physician inserts a vaginal speculum into the vagina for proper visualization of the cervix.
3. To assist in obtaining the specimen, the physician may stain the cervix with Lugol's solution.
4. The colposcope is focused on the cervix and and the physician inspects the cervix.
5. Using cervical biopsy punch forceps, the physician obtains several tissue specimens (Figure 10-21, *A*) from the abnormal cervical epithelium (Figure 10-21, *B*).
6. The specimen is placed in a container with a preservative and is sent to the laboratory for examination by a pathologist.
7. If bleeding occurs, the physician controls it with gauze packing, a hemostatic solution (e.g., Monsel's solution), or electrocautery.
8. The patient is given a sanitary pad at the office following the procedure to absorb any discharge.
9. The patient should be informed that a minimum amount of bleeding may follow the procedure; however,

---

What Would You DO?
What Would You *Not* DO?

Case Study 3

Sadira Wisal has been referred to the office for a colposcopy by her family physician. Her last Pap test came back as abnormal and a repeat Pap test 3 months later was also abnormal. While having her vital signs taken, Sadira bursts into tears. She tearfully explains that she's afraid that she has cancer and that no one at her regular physician's office told her what to expect from this procedure. Sadira doesn't understand why she has to have this procedure done and she doesn't know what the doctor will be doing during the procedure. She says that she feels stupid, but she doesn't even know what a cervix is. Sadira also worries that the procedure will affect her ability to have children.

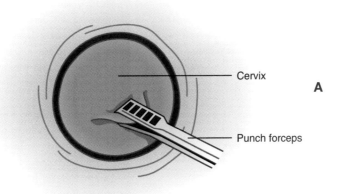

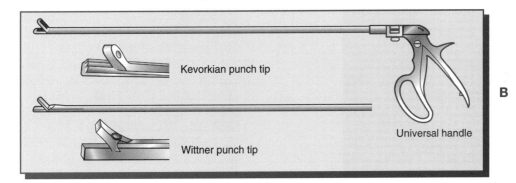

Figure 10-21. Cervical punch biopsy. **A,** Obtaining a tissue specimen from the cervix using cervical biopsy punch forceps. **B,** Cervical biopsy punch forceps. (Courtesy Elmed, Addison, Ill.)

the patient should be instructed to contact the physician if bleeding is heavier than normal menstrual bleeding.

10. A foul-smelling gray-green vaginal discharge may occur several days after the procedure and continue for a period of up to 3 weeks. The patient should be informed that this discharge results from normal healing of cervical tissue and will gradually diminish as the healing progresses.

Cryosurgery

Cervical

Cervical cryosurgery, also known as **cryotherapy,** is often used to treat chronic cervicitis and cervical erosion through the use of freezing temperatures. The procedure can be performed without an anesthetic, although occasionally a mild analgesic is necessary immediately afterward. The cryosurgery unit consists of a long metal probe attached to a cooling-agent tank (Figure 10-22). The principal cooling agents are liquid nitrogen, nitrous oxide, and carbon dioxide gas; of these, liquid nitrogen is used most often. The probe is placed in contact with

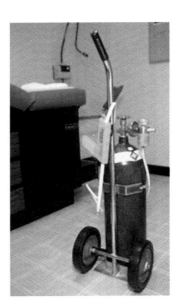

Figure 10-22. Cryosurgery unit. (From Zakus S: *Clinical skills for medical assistants,* ed 4, Philadelphia, 2001, Saunders.)

the infected area, and the cooling agent flows through the probe, freezing the cervical tissue to $-40°$ to $-80°$ C. This causes the cells to die and slough off so that the cervical covering can eventually be replaced with new, healthy epithelial tissue. The regeneration of cervical tissue occurs within approximately 4 to 6 weeks after the procedure.

Cryosurgery Setup

The items required for cryosurgery are listed here.

Items Placed to the Side of the Sterile Field

Cryosurgery:

• Cryosurgery unit
• Sanitary pads

Items Included on the Sterile Field

Cryosurgery:

• Vaginal speculum
• Acid-saline solution
• Long, cotton-tipped applicators

Procedure

Cryosurgery is performed as follows:

1. The patient is draped and assisted into the lithotomy position.
2. The physician inserts a vaginal speculum for proper visualization of the cervix.
3. The cervix is swabbed with an acid-saline solution to remove mucus and other contaminants.
4. The metal probe is placed in contact with the affected area, and the cryosurgery unit is turned on.
5. The cooling agent is permitted to flow over the cervical area for approximately 3 minutes. During the procedure, the patient may experience some pain resembling menstrual cramping that usually lasts about 30 minutes.
6. Once the procedure has been completed, the medical assistant should assist the patient as necessary and observe her for signs of discomfort or vertigo.
7. The patient is given a sanitary pad at the office following the procedure to absorb any discharge.
8. On the first postoperative day, the patient will develop a heavy, clear, watery vaginal discharge, which usually reaches its maximum by the sixth day.
9. The patient should be told to use sanitary pads, rather than tampons, at home. In addition, a vaginal cream may be prescribed to promote wound healing and the formation of new epithelial tissue.
10. The patient should be told that continuation of the discharge for approximately 4 weeks is normal, but that the development of a foul odor should be reported to the physician.
11. The patient should be informed that the next menstrual period will be heavier than normal and may involve some cramping.
12. The patient is usually instructed to abstain from intercourse for 4 weeks following the procedure and to douche with a solution of dilute vinegar and water.
13. The patient will be required to schedule a return visit 6 weeks following the procedure to make sure proper wound healing has taken place.

Skin Lesions

In the medical office, cryosurgery may also be used to remove benign skin lesions, such as common warts. Only a small amount of cooling agent is required for skin lesions, therefore the cryosurgery unit is considerably smaller than the one just described for cervical cryosurgery. Most physicians use liquid nitrogen contained in a small, pressurized stainless steel canister with an attached probe. The physician applies the liquid nitrogen to the skin lesion until it turns white, which indicates that freezing of the tissue has taken place. During the procedure, the patient feels a slight burning or stinging sensation as the cooling agent is applied. Following cryosurgery, a blister develops and dries to a scab in a week to 10 days and eventually sloughs off. The patient should be told to keep the area clean and dry until the scab has sloughed off. In some cases, the treatment may not result in complete destruction of the lesion; two or more treatments may be required to remove the lesion.

Bandaging

A **bandage** is a strip of woven material used to wrap or cover a part of the body. The function of the bandage may be to apply pressure to control bleeding; to protect a wound from contamination; to hold a dressing in place; or to protect, support, or immobilize an injured part of the body.

Guidelines for Application

The bandage should be applied so that it feels comfortable to the patient, and it must be fastened securely with metal clips or adhesive tape. Guidelines for applying a bandage follow.

1. Observe the principles of medical asepsis during the application of a bandage.
2. Be sure that the area to which a bandage is applied is clean and dry.
3. Do not apply a bandage directly over an open wound. To prevent contamination of the wound, first apply a sterile dressing and then the bandage. The bandage should extend at least 2 inches (5 cm) beyond the edge of the dressing,
4. To prevent irritation, do not allow the skin surfaces of two body parts (for example, two fingers) to touch. In addition, the patient's perspiration provides a moist environment that encourages the growth of microorganisms. A piece of gauze should be inserted between the two body parts.
5. Be sure that joints and prominent parts of bones are padded to prevent the bandage from rubbing the skin and causing irritation.

6. Bandage the body part in its normal position with joints slightly flexed to avoid muscle strain.

7. Apply the bandage from the distal to the proximal part of the body to aid the venous return of blood to the heart.

8. As you apply the bandage, ask the patient if it feels comfortable. The bandage should fit snugly enough that it does not fall off but not so tightly that it impedes circulation. If possible, leave the fingers and toes exposed when bandaging an extremity. This provides the opportunity to check them for signs of impairment in circulation. Signs indicating that the bandage is too tight include coldness, pallor, numbness, cyanosis of the nailbeds, swelling, pain, and tingling sensations. If any of these signs occurs, loosen the bandage immediately.

9. If a bandage roll is dropped during the procedure, obtain a new bandage and begin again.

Types of Bandages

Three basic types of bandages are used in the medical office. A *roller bandage* is a long strip of soft material wound on itself to form a roll. It ranges from ½ to 6 inches (1.3 to 15.2 cm) wide and from 2 to 5 yards (1.83 to 4.57 m) long. The width used depends on the part being bandaged. Roller bandages are usually made of sterilized gauze. Gauze is porous and lightweight, molds easily to a body part, and is relatively inexpensive and easily disposed of. However, since it is made of loosely woven cotton, it may slip and fray easily. *Kling gauze* is a special type of gauze that stretches; this allows it to cling, and, as a result, it molds and conforms better to the body part than does regular gauze.

Elastic bandages are made of woven cotton that contains elastic fibers. One brand name of elastic bandages is the Ace bandage. Although elastic bandages are expensive, they can be washed and used again. The medical assistant must be extremely careful when applying an elastic bandage because it is easy to apply it too tightly and impede circulation. Elastic adhesive bandages may also be used; these have an adhesive backing to provide a secure fit.

Bandage Turns

Five basic bandage turns are used, alone or in combination. The type of turn used depends on which body part is to be bandaged and whether the bandage is used for support or immobilization or for holding a dressing in place.

The *circular turn* is applied to a part of uniform width, such as toes, fingers, or the head. Each turn completely overlaps the previous turn. Two circular turns are used to anchor a bandage at the beginning and end of a spiral, spiral-reverse, figure-eight, or recurrent turn (Figure 10-23).

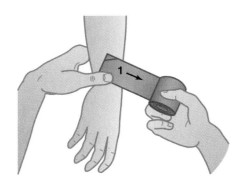

1. Place the end of the roller bandage on a slant.

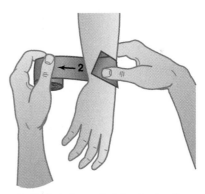

2. Encircle the part while allowing the corner of the bandage to extend.

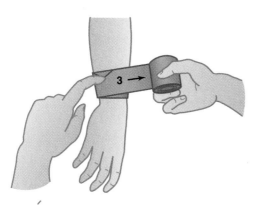

3. Turn down the corner of the bandage.

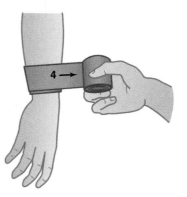

4. Make another circular turn around the part.

Figure 10-23. The procedure for anchoring a bandage.

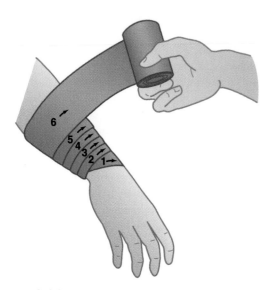

Figure 10-24. The procedure for making the spiral turn.

The *spiral turn* is applied to a part of uniform circumference, such as the fingers, arms, legs, chest, or abdomen. Each spiral turn is carried upward at a slight angle and should overlap the previous turn by one half to two thirds the width of the bandage (Figure 10-24).

The *spiral-reverse turn* is useful for bandaging a part that varies in width, such as the forearm or lower leg. Reversing each spiral turn allows for a smoother fit and prevents gaping due to the variation in the contour of the limb. The thumb is used to make the reverse halfway through each spiral turn. The bandage is then directed downward and folded on itself while it is kept parallel to the lower edge of the previous turn. Each turn should overlap the previous one by two thirds of the width of the bandage. The reverse turn is used as often as necessary to provide a uniform fit (Figure 10-25).

The *figure-eight turn* is generally used to hold a dressing in place or to support and immobilize an injured joint,

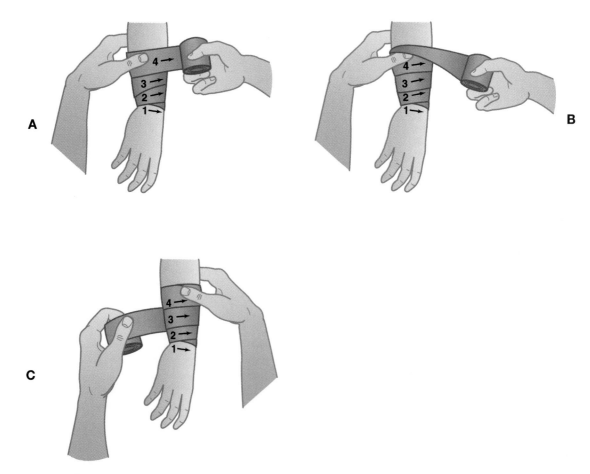

Figure 10-25. The procedure for making the spiral-reverse turn. **A,** Encircle the part while keeping the bandage at a slant. **B,** Reverse the spiral turn using the thumb and direct the bandage downward and fold it on itself. **C,** Keep the bandage parallel to the lower edge of the previous turn.

such as the ankle, knee, elbow, or wrist. The figure-eight consists of slanting turns that alternately ascend and descend around the part and cross over one another in the middle, resembling the figure 8. Each turn overlaps the previous one by two thirds of the width of the bandage (Figure 10-26).

The *recurrent turn* is a series of back-and-forth turns used to bandage the tips of fingers or toes, the stump of an amputated extremity, or the head. The bandage is anchored by using two circular turns and then is passed back and forth over the tip of the part to be bandaged, first on one side and then on the other side of the first center turn. Each turn should overlap the previous turn by two thirds of the width of the bandage (Figure 10-27).

Tubular Gauze Bandage

A tubular gauze bandage consists of seamless elasticized gauze fabric dispensed in a roll. It is used to cover round body parts such as fingers, toes, arms, and legs and fits like a sleeve. This type of bandage is easier to apply than a roller bandage, and it also adheres more securely to the body part. Tubular gauze is not sterile and therefore should not be applied over open wounds; however, it can be applied over a sterile dressing to hold it in place. The gauze is available in varying widths; selection of the width is based on the body part to be bandaged. See Table 10-1 for a list of tubular gauze widths and the body parts each size can be used to bandage.

The gauze is applied by means of a plastic or metal framelike applicator, which comes in different sizes. The applicator must be somewhat larger than the part to be bandaged to allow the gauze to slide easily over the body part. To assist in selecting the proper gauze width, each applicator is marked with a size that corresponds to the size on the tubular gauze bandage box. Procedure 10-9 outlines the method to apply a tubular gauze bandage to a finger.

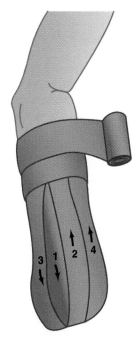

Figure 10-27. The procedure for using the recurrent turn to bandage the end of a stump.

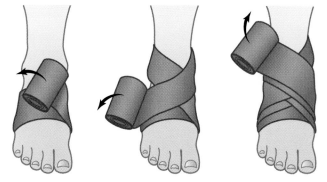

Figure 10-26. The procedure for applying an elastic bandage around the ankle using a figure-eight turn. (From Leake MJ: *A manual of simple nursing procedures,* Philadelphia, 1971, Saunders.)

TABLE **10-1**	Tubular Gauze Bandage Widths and Recommended Application Sites
Width	**Recommended Application Sites**
$^5/_8$ inch	Fingers and toes of infants
	Small fingers and toes of adults
1 inch	Hands and feet of infants
	Fingers and toes of adults
	Over bulky dressings
$1^1/_2$ inches	Arms and legs of infants
	Arms and feet of children
	Small hands, arms, and feet of adults
$2^5/_8$ inches	Legs, thighs, and heads of children
	Arms and lower legs of adults
	Small thighs and small heads of adults
$3^5/_8$ inches	Legs, thighs, lower legs, shoulders, arms, and heads of adults
	Trunks of infants
5 inches	Large heads and small trunks of adults
7 inches	Trunks of adults

PROCEDURE **10-9** Applying a Tubular Gauze Bandage

Outcome Apply a tubular gauze bandage.

Equipment/Supplies:
- Applicator
- Roll of tubular gauze
- Adhesive tape
- Bandage scissors

1. **Procedural Step.** Sanitize your hands. Greet and identify the patient. Introduce yourself, and explain the procedure.

2. **Procedural Step.** Assemble the equipment. The applicator selected should be somewhat larger than the part to be bandaged. The proper gauze width must be used to ensure a secure fit.
   Principle. The applicator should be larger than the body part to allow the gauze to slide easily over the body part.

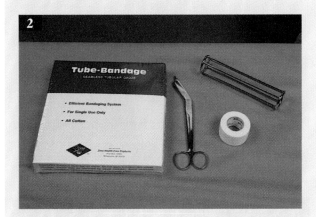

3. **Procedural Step.** Place the gauze bandage on the applicator as follows:
   a. Pull a sufficient length of gauze from the dispensing box roll.
   b. Spread apart the open end of the gauze, using your fingers.
   c. Slide the gauze over one end of the applicator. Continue loading the applicator by gathering enough gauze on the applicator to complete the bandage.
   d. Cut the roll of gauze near the opening of the box.

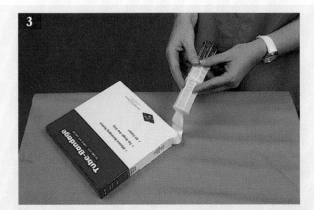

4. **Procedural Step.** Place the applicator over the proximal end of the patient's finger.

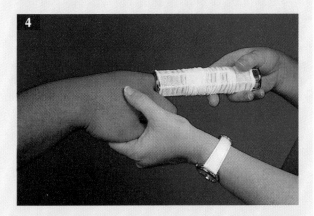

5. **Procedural Step.** Move the applicator from the proximal end to the distal end of the patient's finger, while leaving the bandage on the length of the finger. The bandage should be held in place at the base of the patient's fingers with your fingers.
   Principle. The bandage should be held in place to prevent it from sliding, which would not ensure complete coverage of the affected part.

PROCEDURE 10-9

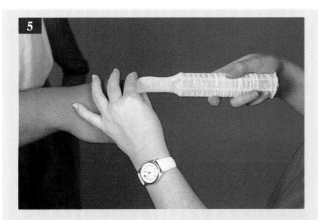

5

6. Procedural Step. Pull the applicator 1 to 2 inches past the end of the patient's finger. Continue to hold the bandage in place with your fingers.
Principle. The bandage must extend beyond the length of the patient's finger in order to secure it at the distal end.

7. Procedural Step. Rotate the applicator one full turn to anchor the bandage.
Principle. Anchoring the bandage holds it securely in place.

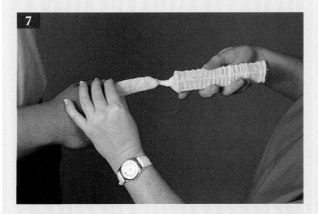

7

8. Procedural Step. Move the applicator forward again toward the proximal end of the patient's finger.
Principle. Moving the applicator forward applies a second layer of bandaging material to the patient's finger.

9. Procedural Step. Move the applicator forward approximately 1 inch past the original starting point of the bandage and anchor it using another rotating motion.
Principle. Anchoring the bandage holds it securely in place.

10. Procedural Step. Repeat this procedure for the number of layers desired. Finish the last layer at the proximal end. Cut unused gauze from the applicator and remove the applicator.

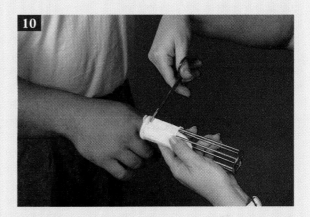

10

11. Procedural Step. Apply adhesive tape at the base of the finger to secure the bandage.

12. Procedural Step. Sanitize your hands, and record the procedure. Include the date and time and location of the bandage application and any instructions given to the patient.

CHARTING EXAMPLE	
Date	
9/30/05	10:00 a.m. Tubular gauze bandage applied
	to Ⓡ index finger. Explained bandage care.
	——————————— T. Browning, CMA

PROCEDURE 10-9

MEDICAL Practice and the LAW

Surgical procedures are invasive and painful, and they have the potential for harmful complications, and therefore, lawsuits.

Before having a surgical procedure performed, the patient must sign a consent to treatment form. It is the medical assistant's responsibility to witness the patient's signature, but it is the physician's responsibility to inform the patient of the procedure to be performed, and its risks, alternative procedures, and benefits. The physician may delegate some or all of these tasks to the medical assistant, but *do not* accept this responsibility. Patients cannot sign for themselves if they are minors or if they are impaired by drugs or disease such as Alzheimer's. In these cases, consent must be obtained from the legal guardian or next of kin. Before asking a patient to sign a consent to treatment form, ask if he or she has any questions. If so, make sure the information is given before the consent is signed. Make sure you know what procedures require informed consent in your office.

During the procedure, your duty is to assist the physician and maintain surgical asepsis. If this is broken, you must inform the physician and remedy the situation. There is no such thing as "almost sterile."

After the surgical procedure, the medical assistant must give the patient home-care instructions. Home care must be performed exactly to ensure proper healing. Instructions should be given verbally, demonstrated, and given in writing. Written instructions must be in the correct language, and at the patient's reading level. Pictures included with the written instructions can clarify difficult points. Many offices purchase preprinted instructions for common surgical procedures. Make sure the signs of infection are listed on these sheets, along with instructions to call the physician if they occur, or if any other problems or questions arise.

What Would You DO?
What Would You *Not* DO? *RESPONSES*

Case Study 1

What Did Trudy Do?

❑ Tried to calm and reassure Mrs. Ventura. Told her that children at this age are prone to accidents and that she shouldn't blame herself.

❑ Told Mrs. Ventura that Cory's wound could not be held together effectively with Steri-Strips. Explained that sutures would help the wound heal better.

❑ Told Mrs. Ventura that the doctor could not perform the procedure unless she signs the consent form. Explained that Cory's wound should be sutured as soon as possible to prevent infection and to minimize scarring.

❑ Asked Mrs. Ventura if she would like to talk with the doctor again about any questions she might have about the procedure before signing the form.

What Did Trudy Not Do?

❑ Did not prepare Cory for the suture insertion procedure until Mrs. Ventura signed the consent to treatment form.

What Would You Do?/What Would You *Not* Do? Review Trudy's response and place a checkmark next to the information you included in your response. List additional information you included in your response below.

_____
_____
_____
_____

Case Study 2

What Did Trudy Do?

❑ Explained to Abbey that the antiseptic contains iodine, which appears orange when it is applied to the skin. Assured her that the iodine would not stain her skin permanently and that it would wear off in a few days.

❑ Calmly and discreetly opened a new pair of sterile gloves so that the physician could reapply sterile gloves. Reminded Abbey not to move during the procedure.

❑ Told Abbey that all tissues removed from patients are routinely sent to the lab for a biopsy. Reassured her that the physician has told her everything he knows about her condition.

❑ Made it very clear to Abbey that her neighbor is not permitted to remove her sutures. Stressed to her that the physician needs to check her incision before the sutures are removed to make sure proper healing has occurred.

What Did Trudy Not Do?

❑ Did not scold Abbey for contaminating the physician's sterile gloved hand.

What Would You Do?/What Would You *Not* Do? Review Trudy's response and place a checkmark next to the information you included in your response. List additional information you included in your response below.

_____
_____
_____
_____

Case Study 3

What Did Trudy Do?

❑ Listened empathetically to Sadira, and tried to calm and reassure her.

❑ Spent some time going over the colposcopy procedure and what to expect.

❑ Answered as many of Sadira's questions as possible. Reassured her that a lot of people don't know what a cervix is and that she was asking some very good questions.

❑ Asked the physician to spend some time talking with Sadira before the procedure to answer the questions that Trudy was not qualified to answer.

❑ Made sure that Sadira understood all of the information about the procedure before asking her to sign a consent to treatment form.

What Did Trudy Not Do?

❑ Did not tell Sadira that her family physician and staff should have spent some time explaining the procedure to her so that she didn't have to worry so much.

❑ Did not tell Sadira that she did not have cancer.

What Would You Do?/What Would You *Not* Do? Review Trudy's response and place a checkmark next to the information you included in your response. List additional information you included in your response below.

_____
_____
_____
_____

Apply Your KNOWLEDGE

Choose the best answer for the following questions.

1. Dr. Xylocaine will be suturing a large laceration on Seth James's left thigh. Trudy Browning, CMA, is assisting the physician. Trudy explains to Mr. James that he should not talk during the procedure. He asks her, "Why?" Trudy explains:
   A. It is easier for the physician to concentrate when it is quiet.
   B. The local anesthetic will work faster.
   C. The wound will not heal properly.
   D. Microorganisms from the mouth can contaminate the sterile field.

2. After opening and setting up the sterile suture insertion tray for Mr. James's laceration, Trudy Browning, CMA, notices that she forgot to bring in sutures. Trudy should:
   A. Leave the room and obtain the sutures as quickly as possible.
   B. Send Mr. James out to get the sutures.
   C. Cover the tray with a sterile towel and leave to get the sutures.
   D. Leave to get the sutures and then set up a new sterile suture tray after returning.

3. Dr. Xylocaine has started suturing Mr. James's laceration. He asks Trudy Browning, CMA, for more sterile gauze. Of the following methods, Trudy would best maintain surgical asepsis by:
   A. Using her bare hands to place the gauze on the sterile field
   B. Opening the sterile package and allowing Dr. Xylocaine to remove the gauze with his gloved hand
   C. Applying clean gloves and adding the sterile gauze to the tray
   D. Handing a sterile gauze package to Dr. Xylocaine

4. Dr. Xylocaine tells Mr. James to return to the office in 10 days to have his sutures removed. Trudy Browning, CMA, realizes that by that time Mr. James would be in which of the following phases of the healing process?
   A. Phase 1, or the inflammatory phase
   B. Phase 2, or the granulation phase
   C. Phase 3, or the maturation phase
   D. Phase 4, or the final phase

5. Mr. James returns to the office to have his sutures removed. Upon inspection of Mr. James's sutures, Trudy Browning, CMA, notices that he has a small gaping area at the bottom of his laceration with greenish-yellow, foul-smelling drainage. She would document this as:
   A. Laceration well approximated with serous drainage
   B. Laceration unapproximated at distal end with serosanguineous drainage
   C. Laceration gaping with sanguineous drainage
   D. Purulent drainage noted from unapproximated area at distal end of laceration

6. Dr. Xylocaine tells Trudy not to remove the sutures and to apply Steri-Strips to the gaping area of Mr. James's laceration. To prepare the area for the application, Trudy would:
   A. Cleanse the laceration with normal saline and allow it to dry.
   B. Cleanse the laceration with phenol and then apply tincture of benzoin directly on the laceration.
   C. Cleanse the laceration with Betadine and then apply tincture of benzoin on each side of the laceration.
   D. Wipe the laceration clean with sterile gauze and apply the Steri-Strips.

7. Eric Link is 16 years old and has come to the office with his mother to have surgery on his ingrown toenail. Before starting the procedure, Trudy Browning, CMA, must:
   A. Inform Eric of the risks of the procedure and have him sign a consent to treatment form.
   B. Obtain verbal consent from Eric's mother for the surgery.
   C. Make sure that Eric is not allergic to bee stings.
   D. Be certain that Eric's mother has discussed the procedure with Dr. Xylocaine and has signed a consent to treatment form.

8. Before the surgical procedure is started, which of the following would be appropriate to do preoperatively for Eric's ingrown toenail?
   A. Soak his foot in tepid water and an antiseptic solution.
   B. Scrub his foot and toe with a surgical scrub sponge moistened with 90% ethyl alcohol.
   C. Ask him to wiggle his big toe.
   D. Trim as much of the toenail away as possible.

Apply Your KNOWLEDGE—Cont'd

9. Dr. Xylocaine will use Betadine to cleanse the area of the toe before making an incision. He asks Trudy Browning, CMA, to pour some Betadine into the basin on the sterile field. Which of the following would represent an ERROR in technique when pouring the Betadine into the sterile basin?
   A. Placing the bottle cap on a flat surface with the open end facing down
   B. Palming the label of the Betadine bottle
   C. Making sure the Betadine is not expired
   D. Pouring the solution from a height of 6 inches

10. After Eric's surgery, Trudy Browning, CMA, is teaching him signs that might indicate that he has an infection at his surgical site. These would include all of the following EXCEPT:
    A. Bruising
    B. Warmth
    C. Edema
    D. Redness

CERTIFICATION REVIEW

❑ **Surgical asepsis** refers to practices that keep objects and areas sterile or free of all living microorganisms. It is always employed when caring for broken skin, when a skin surface is being penetrated, and when a body cavity is entered that is normally sterile.

❑ During a sterile procedure **specific guidelines** must be followed. Do not allow sterile packages to become wet. A 1-inch border around the sterile field is considered contaminated. Always face the sterile field. Hold all sterile articles above waist level. All sterile items should be placed in the center of the sterile field. Do not spill water or solutions on the sterile field. Do not talk, cough, or sneeze over a sterile field. Do not reach over a sterile field. Do not pass soiled dressings over a sterile field. Always acknowledge if you have contaminated the sterile field.

❑ **A wound** is a break in the continuity of an external or internal surface caused by physical means. The two basic types of wounds are closed and open. A closed wound involves an injury to the underlying tissue without a break in the skin surface, such as a contusion. An open wound involves a break in the skin surface that exposes the underlying tissues; examples include incisions, lacerations, punctures, and abrasions.

❑ **The body has a natural healing process** that works to destroy invading microorganisms and to restore the structure and function of the damaged tissue. Wound healing takes places in three phases: the inflammatory phase, the granulation phase, and the maturation phase.

❑ **The function of a sterile dressing** is to protect a wound from contamination and trauma, to absorb drainage, and to restrict motion, which may interfere with proper wound healing.

❑ **Sutures** are available in two types: absorbable and nonabsorbable. Absorbable sutures consist of surgical gut or synthetic materials that are gradually digested by tissue enzymes and absorbed by the body's tissues. Nonabsorbable sutures are not absorbed by the body and either remain permanently in the body tissues or are removed. They are made from silk, cotton, nylon, polyester fiber, polypropylene, stainless steel and surgical skin staples.

❑ **Needles for suturing** are categorized as cutting needles (having a sharp point) or noncutting needles (having a round point). Cutting needles are used for skin, and noncutting needles are used to penetrate tissues that offer a small amount of resistance, such as the viscera, subcutaneous tissue, muscle, and peritoneum. A swaged needle is one in which the suture and needle are one continuous unit.

Continued

CERTIFICATION REVIEW—Cont'd

❏ **Surgical skin staples** are often used to close wounds. Stapling is the fastest method of closing long skin incisions. In addition, trauma to the tissue is reduced because the tissue does not have to be handled very much when inserting the staples.

❏ **Adhesive skin closures** may be used for wound repair to approximate the edges of a laceration or incision. They are used when not much tension exists on the skin edges. The advantages of adhesive skin closures are that they eliminate the need for skin sutures and a local anesthetic, they are easy to apply and remove, and they result in less scarring than skin sutures.

❏ **The instruments and supplies for a minor office surgery** depend on the surgery to be performed. Many offices maintain index cards that indicate the appropriate instruments and supplies for each minor office surgery tray setup.

❏ **The patient's skin must be prepared** prior to the minor office surgery because the skin contains an abundance of microorganisms. Skin preparation involves shaving the site, scrubbing the site with an antiseptic cleansing solution, and applying an antiseptic.

❏ **The use of a local anesthetic,** such as Xylocaine, is often required for minor office surgery. Xylocaine with epinephrine prolongs the local effect of the anesthetic and decreases the rate of systemic absorption by constricting blood vessels at the operative site.

❏ **A sebaceous cyst** is a thin, closed sac or capsule that contains secretions from a sebaceous, or oil, gland. It forms when the outlet of the gland becomes obstructed. A sebaceous cyst is usually painless and nontender, although it may become infected; to avoid this, the cyst should be excised by the physician.

❏ **An abscess** is a collection of pus in a cavity surrounded by inflamed tissue. An abscess serves as a defense mechanism of the body to keep an infection localized by walling off the microorganisms, preventing them from spreading through the body. A furuncle (boil) is a localized staphylococcal infection that originates deep within a hair follicle.

❏ **A biopsy is** the removal and examination of tissue from the living body. It is most often performed to determine whether a tumor is malignant or benign. A needle biopsy is a type of biopsy in which tissue from deep within the body is obtained by the insertion of a biopsy needle through the skin. The advantage of a needle biopsy is that a sample of tissue can be obtained that might otherwise require a major surgical operation.

❏ **An ingrown toenail** occurs when the edge of the toenail grows deeply into the nail groove and penetrates the surrounding skin, resulting in pain and discomfort to the patient. The protruding nail acts as a foreign body, usually resulting in secondary infection and inflammation.

❏ **Colposcopy** is the visual examination of the vagina and cervix by means of a colposcope, a lighted instrument with a binocular magnifying lens. The purpose of colposcopy is to examine the vagina and cervix to determine areas of abnormal tissue growth. Colposcopy is performed following an abnormal cytology report from a Pap test, to evaluate a vaginal or cervical lesion observed during a pelvic examination, and after treatment for cancer of the cervix.

❏ **A cervical punch biopsy** is usually performed in combination with colposcopy to remove a cervical tissue specimen to determine if it is benign or malignant. Cervical biopsies are often performed after an abnormal Pap test result.

❏ **Cervical cryosurgery** is often used to treat chronic cervicitis and cervical erosion through the use of freezing temperatures. A cooling agent is applied to the infected area, which causes the cells to die and slough off so that the cervical covering can eventually be replaced with new, healthy epithelial tissue.

❏ **A bandage** is a strip of woven material used to wrap or cover a part of the body. The function of the bandage may be to apply pressure to control bleeding, to protect a wound from contamination, to hold a dressing in place, or to protect, support, or immobilize an injured part of the body.

Terminology Review

Abrasion A wound in which the outer layers of the skin are damaged; a scrape.

Abscess A collection of pus in a cavity surrounded by inflamed tissue.

Absorbable suture Suture material that is gradually digested by tissue enzymes and absorbed by the body.

Approximation The process of bringing two parts, such as tissue, together, through the use of sutures or other means.

Bandage A strip of woven material used to wrap or cover a part of the body.

Biopsy The surgical removal and examination of tissue from the living body. Biopsies are generally performed to determine whether a tumor is benign or malignant.

Capillary action The action that causes liquid to rise along a wick, a tube, or a gauze dressing.

Colposcope A lighted instrument with a binocular magnifying lens used to examine the vagina and cervix.

Colposcopy The visual examination of the vagina and cervix using a colposcope.

Contaminate As it relates to sterile technique, to cause a sterile object or surface to become unsterile.

Contusion An injury to the tissues under the skin that causes blood vessels to rupture, allowing blood to seep into the tissues; a bruise.

Cryosurgery The therapeutic use of freezing temperatures to destroy abnormal tissue.

Exudates A discharge produced by the body's tissues.

Fibroblast An immature cell from which connective tissue can develop.

Forceps A two-pronged instrument for grasping and squeezing.

Furuncle A localized staphylococcal infection that originates deep within a hair follicle. Also known as a boil.

Hemostasis The arrest of bleeding by natural or artificial means.

Incision A clean cut caused by a cutting instrument.

Infection The condition in which the body, or part of it, is invaded by a pathogen.

Infiltration The process by which a substance passes into and is deposited within the substance of a cell, tissue, or organ.

Inflammation A protective response of the body to trauma and the entrance of foreign matter. The purpose of inflammation is to destroy invading microorganisms and to repair injured tissue.

Laceration A wound in which the tissues are torn apart, leaving ragged and irregular edges.

Ligate To tie off and close a structure such as a severed blood vessel.

Local anesthetic A drug that produces a loss of feeling and an inability to perceive pain in only a specific part of the body.

Mayo tray A broad, flat metal tray placed on a stand and used to hold sterile instruments and supplies once it has been covered with a sterile towel.

Needle biopsy A type of biopsy in which tissue from deep within the body is obtained by the insertion of a biopsy needle through the skin.

Nonabsorbable suture Suture material that is not absorbed by the body and either remains permanently in the body tissue and becomes encapsulated by fibrous tissue or is removed.

Postoperative After a surgical operation.

Preoperative Preceding a surgical operation.

Puncture A wound made by a sharp pointed object piercing the skin.

Scalpel A surgical knife used to divide tissues.

Scissors A cutting instrument.

Sebaceous cyst A thin, closed sac or capsule that contains fatty secretions from a sebaceous gland.

Serum The clear, straw-colored part of the blood that remains after the solid elements have been separated out of it.

Sterile Free of all living microorganisms and bacterial spores.

Surgical asepsis Practices that keep objects and areas sterile or free from microorganisms.

Sutures Material used to approximate tissues with surgical stitches.

Swaged needle A needle with suturing material permanently attached to its end.

Wound A break in the continuity of an external or internal surface caused by physical means.

ON THE WEB

For active weblinks to each website visit
http://evolve.elsevier.com/Bonewit/.

For Information on Surgery and Emergency Medicine:

The American College of Surgeons

American Red Cross

Ethicon Incorporated

Federal Emergency Management Agency

Learning Objectives	Procedures

Introduction to the Administration of Medication
1. Explain the difference between administering, prescribing, and dispensing medication.
2. State the common routes for administering medication.
3. List and describe the six sections of the PDR.
4. List and describe the categories of information in a drug package insert.
5. Describe the FDA's responsibilities with respect to drugs.
6. List and define the four names of drugs.
7. Classify drugs according to preparation.
8. Classify drugs according to the action they have on the body.
9. List the guidelines for writing metric and apothecary notations.
10. List and describe the five schedules for controlled drugs.
11. List and explain the parts of a prescription.
12. Explain the purpose of a medication record.
13. Describe the factors that affect the action of drugs in the body.
14. List and describe the possible adverse effects of medication.
15. List the guidelines for preparing and administering medication.

Research a drug using the *Physician's Desk Reference*.
Interpret a drug package insert.
Calculate drug dosage.
Complete a prescription form.
Complete a medication record form.

Oral Administration
1. Explain why the oral route is most frequently used to administer medication.
2. State where the absorption of most oral medications take place.

Prepare and administer oral medications.

Parenteral Administration
1. State the advantages and disadvantages of the parenteral route of administration.
2. Identify the parts of a needle and syringe, and explain their functions.
3. State the ranges of both gauge and length of needles for the following injections: intradermal, subcutaneous, and intramuscular.
4. State the purpose of safety engineered syringes.
5. Describe the dispensing units available for injectable medications.
6. State which tissue layers of the body are used for intradermal, subcutaneous, and intramuscular injections.
7. List the medications commonly administered through the following routes: subcutaneous and intramuscular.
8. Explain the reason for administering medication with the Z-track method.

Reconstitute a powdered drug for parenteral administration.
Withdraw medication from a vial.
Withdraw medication from an ampule.
Locate appropriate subcutaneous injection sites.
Administer a subcutaneous injection.
Locate the following intramuscular injection sites: dorsogluteal, deltoid, vastus lateralis, and ventrogluteal.
Administer an intramuscular injection.
Administer an injection using the Z-track method.
Administer an intradermal injection.

Tuberculin Testing
1. List the symptoms of active tuberculosis.
2. Explain the purpose of tuberculin testing.
3. Explain the significance of a positive reaction to a tuberculin test.
4. List the diagnostic procedures that might be performed following a positive tuberculin test.

Administer a Mantoux test and read the test results.
Administer a tine test and read the test results.
Complete a tuberculosis test record card.

Allergy Testing
1. Define an allergy and name common allergens.
2. Explain what occurs during an allergic reaction.
3. List the guidelines for direct skin allergy testing.
4. State the purpose of the following types of allergy tests:
   - Patch Testing
   - Skin-Prick Testing
   - Intradermal Skin Testing
   - RAST Testing

Perform allergy skin testing.

CHAPTER 11

Administration of Medication

Chapter Outline

INTRODUCTION TO ADMINISTRATION OF MEDICATION
Food and Drug Administration
Drug Nomenclature
Classification of Drugs Based on Preparation
  Liquid Preparations
  Solid Preparations
Classification of Drugs Based on Action
Systems of Measurement for Medication
  Metric System
  Apothecary System
  Household System
Converting Units of Measurement
Controlled Drugs
The Prescription
  Parts of a Prescription
  Generic Prescribing
  Completing a Prescription Form
The Medication Record
Factors Affecting Drug Action
  Therapeutic Effect
  Undesirable Effects of Drugs
Guidelines for Preparation and Administration of Medication
Oral Administration
Parenteral Administration
  Parts of a Needle and Syringe
  Safety Engineered Syringes
  Preparation of Parenteral Medication
  Storage
  Reconstitution of Powdered Drugs
  Subcutaneous Injections
  Intramuscular Injections
  Intradermal Injections

Tuberculin Testing
  Tuberculosis
  Purpose of Tuberculin Testing
  Tuberculin Test Reactions
  Tuberculin Testing Methods
  Administering a Tuberculin Test
  Reading Tuberculin Test Results
Allergy Testing
  Allergy
  Allergic Reaction
  Diagnosis and Treatment
  Types of Allergy Tests

National Competencies

Clinical Competencies
Patient Care
▪ Apply pharmacology principles to prepare and administer oral and parenteral medications.

General Competencies
Legal Concepts
▪ Document appropriately.
▪ Demonstrate knowledge of federal and state health care legislation and regulations.

Key Terms

adverse reaction (AD-vers ree-AK-shun)
allergen (AL-er-jen)
allergy (AL-er-jee)
ampule (AM-pyool)
anaphylactic reaction (an-uh-ful-AK-tik ree-AK-shun)
  controlled drug
conversion (kon-VER-shun)
cubic centimeter (KYOO-bik SEN-tih-mee-ter)
DEA number
dose
drug
gauge (GAYJ)
induration (in-dur-AY-shun)
inhalation (in-hal-AY-shun) administration
inscription (in-SKRIP-shun)
intradermal (in-tra-DER-mal in-JEK-shun) injection
intramuscular (in-tra-MUS-kyoo-lar) injection
intravenous injection (in-tra-VEE-nus)
oral (OR-ul) administration
parenteral (par-EN-ter-al)
pharmacology (far-ma-KOL-oh-jee)
prescription
signatura (sig-na-CHUR-ah)
subcutaneous (sub-kyoo-TAY-nee-us) injection
sublingual (sub-LIN-gwal) administration
subscription (sub-SKRIP-shun)
superscription (soo-per-SKRIP-shun)
topical (TOP-ih-kul) administration
vial (VIE-ul)
wheal (WEE-ul)

Introduction to Administration of Medication

Pharmacology is the study of drugs, and includes the preparation, use, and action of drugs in the body. A **drug** is a chemical that is used for the treatment, prevention, or diagnosis of disease. Most drugs are produced synthetically, but they can also be obtained from other sources such as animals, plants, and minerals.

In the medical office medication may be administered, prescribed, or dispensed. Medication that is *administered* is actually given to the patient at the office. Medication is *prescribed* when a physician provides the patient with a handwritten or computer-generated prescription for a drug to be filled at a pharmacy. Prescriptions can also be telephoned or faxed to the pharmacy by the physician, depending on the preference of the patient. *Dispensed* medication is given to the patient at the office to be taken at home; for example, the physician gives the patient drug samples to take home.

An important responsibility of the medical assistant is the administration of medication. (One should check the laws of the state to make sure that it is legally permissible for the medical assistant to administer medication.) The medical assistant should administer medication only under the direction of the physician. In all states it is unlawful to administer medication in the medical office without the consent of the physician.

Common routes of administration of medication are oral, sublingual, inhalation, rectal, vaginal, topical, intradermal, subcutaneous, intramuscular, and intravenous. The route of administration depends on the type of drug being given, the dosage form, the intended action, and the rapidity of response desired. The route by which medication is most commonly administered in the medical office is the parenteral route. **Parenteral** refers to sites outside the gastrointestinal tract; this term is most commonly used to refer to the administration of medication by injection.

The medical assistant is obligated to become familiar with the drugs that are most frequently used in his or her office. It is essential to know their indications, adverse reactions, route of administration, dosage, and storage. With each drug (including drug samples and injectable medications), the manufacturer includes a *package insert (PI)*, which contains valuable information regarding the drug. In addition, many drug references are available. The *Physician's Desk Reference (PDR)* is frequently used in the medical office. The *PDR* contains information on most major prescription pharmaceutical products available in the United States. The drug information in the *PDR* consists of the actual drug package insert. See Figure 11-1 for guidelines for using the *Physician's Desk Reference*. These guidelines will not only assist in learning how to use the *PDR*, they will also provide the necessary information for understanding how to interpret drug package inserts.

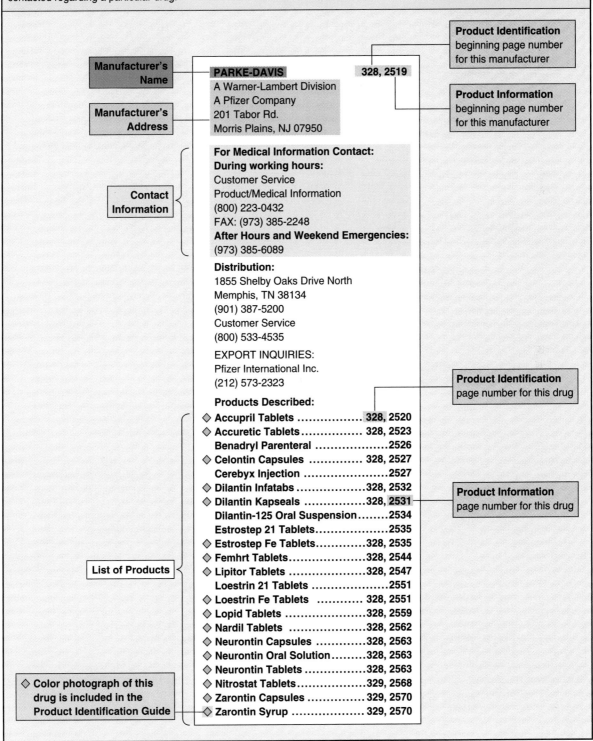

GUIDELINES FOR USING THE PHYSICIAN'S DESK REFERENCE

The *Physician's Desk Reference* (PDR) is published anually by the Medical Economics Company with the cooperation of the pharmaceutical manufacturers whose products are included in it. This reference includes essential information on most major prescription pharmaceutical products available in the United States. The PDR is divided into color-coded sections which are described below.

SECTION 1: MANUFACTURER'S INDEX
(Color Code: White)

The Manufacturer's Index lists pharmaceutical manufacturers in alphabetical order along with a list of drugs that are manufactured by each company. This index provides all of the necessary information should the manufacturer need to be contacted regarding a particular drug.

Product Identification
beginning page number for this manufacturer

Product Information
beginning page number for this manufacturer

Manufacturer's Name

PARKE-DAVIS 328, 2519
A Warner-Lambert Division
A Pfizer Company
201 Tabor Rd.
Morris Plains, NJ 07950

Manufacturer's Address

Contact Information

For Medical Information Contact:
During working hours:
Customer Service
Product/Medical Information
(800) 223-0432
FAX: (973) 385-2248
After Hours and Weekend Emergencies:
(973) 385-6089

Distribution:
1855 Shelby Oaks Drive North
Memphis, TN 38134
(901) 387-5200
Customer Service
(800) 533-4535

EXPORT INQUIRIES:
Pfizer International Inc.
(212) 573-2323

Product Identification
page number for this drug

List of Products

Products Described:
◇ Accupril Tablets 328, 2520
◇ Accuretic Tablets 328, 2523
   Benadryl Parenteral 2526
◇ Celontin Capsules 328, 2527
   Cerebyx Injection 2527
◇ Dilantin Infatabs 328, 2532
◇ Dilantin Kapseals 328, 2531
   Dilantin-125 Oral Suspension 2534
   Estrostep 21 Tablets................... 2535
◇ Estrostep Fe Tablets............ 328, 2535
◇ Femhrt Tablets................... 328, 2544
◇ Lipitor Tablets 328, 2547
   Loestrin 21 Tablets 2551
◇ Loestrin Fe Tablets 328, 2551
◇ Lopid Tablets 328, 2559
◇ Nardil Tablets 328, 2562
◇ Neurontin Capsules 328, 2563
◇ Neurontin Oral Solution........ 328, 2563
◇ Neurontin Tablets 328, 2563
◇ Nitrostat Tablets.................. 329, 2568
◇ Zarontin Capsules 329, 2570
◇ Zarontin Syrup 329, 2570

Product Information
page number for this drug

◇ **Color photograph of this drug is included in the Product Identification Guide**

Figure 11-1. Guidelines for using the *Physician's Desk Reference.*

Continued

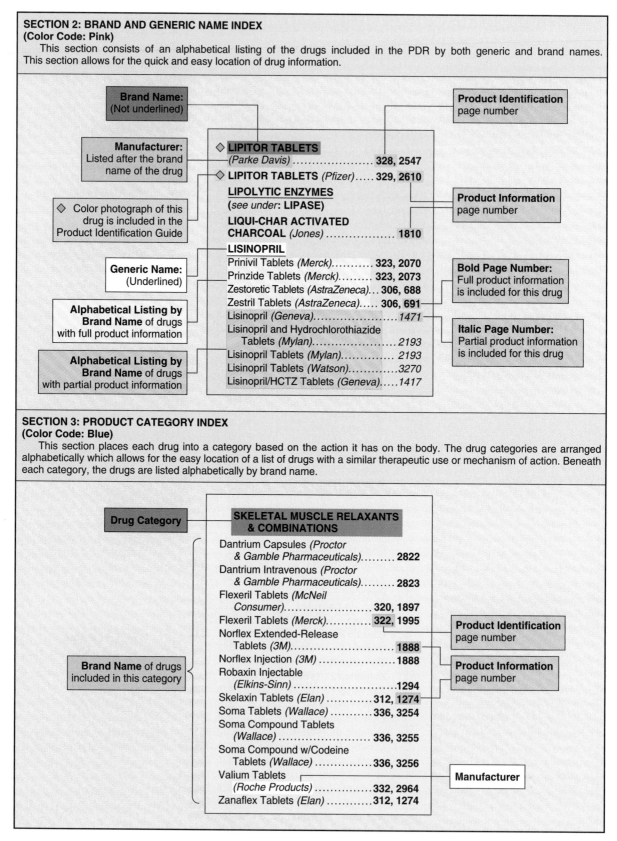

Figure 11-1, cont'd. Guidelines for using the *Physician's Desk Reference.*

SECTION 4: PRODUCT IDENTIFICATION GUIDE
(Color Code: Gray)

This section provides a full-color (actual size) photograph of the tablets and capsules included in the PDR. The drugs are arranged alphabetically by manufacturer. A variety of other dosage forms are also illustrated, but are shown in less than actual size (e.g., inhalers, injectable drugs in vials). This section provides valuable assistance in identifying a drug.

SECTION 5: PRODUCT INFORMATION
(Color Code: White)

This index makes up the main section of the PDR and contains product information on approximately 3,000 drug products. The drugs are arranged alphabetically by manufacturer; under the manufacturer, the drugs are listed alphabetically by brand name. The information included in this section consists of the actual drug package inserts. The following information is included for each medication:

DESCRIPTION: This category consists of a general description of the drug and includes the following information: brand name (with pronunciation), generic name, drug category, dosage form (e.g., tablets, capsules), route of administration, chemical name and structural formula, and the inactive ingredients contained in the drug. This category also indicates if the product requires a prescription (Rx) or if it is available over-the-counter (OTC). The symbol C and a Roman numeral appearing next to the drug it indicates that it is a scheduled drug and that a prescription written for this drug requires the physician's DEA number.

CLINICAL PHARMACOLOGY: This category describes how the drug functions in the body to produce its therapeutic effect. Also included is an analysis of the absorption, distribution, metabolism, excretion of the drug after it enters the body.

INDICATIONS AND USAGE: This category presents a list of the conditions that the drug has been formally approved to treat by the Food and Drug Administration (FDA).

CONTRAINDICATIONS: This category includes situations in which the drug should not be used because the risk of using the drug in these situations outweighs any possible benefit. Contraindications include administration of the drug to patients known to have a hypersensitivity (allergy) to it and use of the drug in patients who have a substantial risk of being harmed by it because of their particular age, sex, concurrent use of another drug, disease state or condition (e.g., pregnancy).

WARNINGS: This category describes serious adverse reactions and potential safety hazards that may occasionally occur with the use of the drug and what shoul be done if they occur.

PRECAUTIONS: This category includes information regarding any special care that needs to be taken by the physician for the safe and effective use of the drug. Information typically presented in this category includes:

- **General Precautions:** Lists any disease states or situations may require special consideration when the drug is being taken.
- **Information for Patients:** Includes information that should be relayed to the patient to ensure safe and effective use of the drug.
- **Laboratory Tests:** Indicates the laboratory tests that may be helpful in following the patient's response to the drug or in identifying possible adverse reactions to the drug.
- **Drug Interactions:** Lists any known interactions of this drug with other drugs that can affect the proper functioning of the drug.
- **Laboratory Test Interactions:** Includes any laboratory tests that may be affected when taking the medication.
- **Pregnancy:** Indicates the pregnancy category of the drug.

ADVERSE REACTIONS: This category describes the unintended and undesirable effects that may occur with the use of the drug. Some adverse reactions are harmless, and therefore often tolerated by the patient in order to obtain the therapeutic effect of the drug. Other adverse reactions may be harmful to the patient and warrant discontinuing the medication.

OVERDOSAGE: This category describes symptoms associated with an overdosage of the drug, as well as the complications that can occur and the treatment to institute for an overdosage.

DOSAGE AND ADMINISTRATION: This category lists the recommended adult dosage, the usual dosage range of the drug and the route of administration (e.g., by mouth, sublingual, IM). Also included is information about the intervals recommended between doses, the usual duration of treatment, and any modification of dosage needed for special groups such as children, the elderly, and patients with renal or hepatic disease.

HOW SUPPLIED: This category indicates the dosage forms that are available (e.g., 20 mg tablets), the units in which the dosage form is available (e.g., bottles of 100; 5 ml multiple-dose vial), information to help identify the dosage form (shape and color), and the handling and storage conditions for the drug.

SECTION 6: DIAGNOSTIC PRODUCT INFORMATION

This section includes product information on diagnostic products. They are listed alphabetically by manufacturer and provide information on the use of these products. An example of diagnostic product included in this section is Tubersol which is used to perform tuberculin testing.

Additional information included in the Physician's Desk Reference is listed below:

- **FDA Drug Information Centers**
- **Key to Controlled Substances Categories**
- **Key to FDA Use-In-Pregnancy Ratings**

Figure 11-1, cont'd. Guidelines for using the *Physician's Desk Reference.*

Food and Drug Administration

The United States Food and Drug Administration (FDA) is a federal agency in the Department of Health of Human Services (DHHS). The FDA is responsible for determining if new food products, drugs, vaccines, medical devices, cosmetics, and other products are safe before they are released for human use.

The FDA determines the safety and effectiveness of both prescription and nonprescription (OTC) drugs. Pharmaceutical manufacturers are required to submit new drug applications to the FDA for review and approval before products can be released for human use.

The FDA is also responsible for determining if a medication will be available with or without a prescription. Medications that require a prescription have been determined by the FDA to be safe and effective when used under the guidance of a physician. Prescription medication labels must bear the following statement: *Caution: Federal law prohibits dispensing without a prescription.*

Nonprescription medications, on the other hand, are drugs that the FDA determines to be safe and effective for use without physician supervision. Nonprescription medications have a low incidence of adverse reactions when the consumer follows the directions and warnings on the label. Examples of nonprescription medications include mild pain relievers, topical antibiotics, topical corticosteroids, cold medications, and laxatives.

What Would You DO? What Would You *Not* DO?

Case Study 1

Carol Okasinski, 56 years old, is a new patient. She was a patient of another physician in the community; however his receptionist was often rude to her, and she finally decided not to go there anymore. Mrs. Okasinski is obese and has hypertension, type 2 diabetes, osteoarthritis in her hands and knees, and problems with depression. While filling in the health history form, she says she can't fill in the names of the medications she is taking. She is on a lot of medications prescribed by her previous doctor. She says she couldn't get the childproof pill containers open because of the arthritis in her hands so she had her husband throw away the childproof containers and transfer each medication into an easy-to-open plastic container. She knows when to take her medications, but she doesn't know the names of them or why she is taking them. She has brought in a bag with all her medications in their plastic containers.

Drug Nomenclature

Each drug has four names: the chemical, generic, official, and brand, or trade, name. Each of these is described below.

The *chemical name* provides a precise description of the drug's chemical composition; pharmaceutical manufacturers and pharmacists are most concerned with the chemical makeup of a drug.

The *generic name* is assigned by the pharmaceutical manufacturer who develops the drug, before it receives official approval by the FDA. The generic name is often a shortened derivative of the chemical name.

The *official name* is the name under which the drug is listed in official publications such as the *United States Pharmacopeia (USP)* and the *National Formulary (NF)*. Official publications set specific standards to regulate the strength, purity, packaging, safety, labeling, and dosage form of each drug. The generic name is frequently used for the official name.

The *brand name* is the name under which a pharmaceutical manufacturer markets a drug. Because a drug may be manufactured by more than one pharmaceutical company, it may have several brand names. For example, the generic name of a common analgesic is *acetaminophen;* brand names for this drug include Tylenol, Tempra, Apacet, Genapap, Panadol, and Liquiprin.

The medical assistant should be familiar with both the generic and brand names of the medications commonly prescribed and administered in the medical office.

Classification of Drugs Based on Preparation

Drugs are available in two basic forms: liquid and solid. A medication may be available in both liquid and solid forms, which permits it to be administered to different types of patients. For example, a liquid preparation of an antibiotic is administered to young children, and the solid preparation (e.g., tablets, capsules) of the same medication is administered to older children and adults. The following list includes the common categories of drugs based on preparation.

Liquid Preparations

Elixir A drug that is dissolved in a solution of alcohol and water. Elixirs are sweetened and flavored and are taken orally. *Example:* Dimetapp Elixir.

Emulsion A mixture of fats or oils in water. *Example:* Soyacol Emulsion.

Liniment A drug combined with oil, soap, alcohol, or water. Liniments are applied externally, using friction, to produce a feeling of heat or warmth. *Example:* Heet Liniment.

Lotion
An aqueous preparation that contains suspended ingredients. Lotions are used to treat external skin conditions. They work to soothe, protect, and moisten the skin and to destroy harmful bacteria. *Example:* Caladryl Lotion.

Solution
A liquid preparation that contains one or more completely dissolved substances. The dissolved substance is known as the solute, and the liquid in which it is dissolved is known as the solvent. *Example:* Polysporin Ophthalmic Solution.

Spirit
A drug combined with an alcoholic solution that is volatile (a substance that is volatile evaporates readily). *Example:* aromatic spirit of ammonia.

Spray
A fine stream of medicated vapor, usually used to treat nose and throat conditions. *Example:* Dristan Nasal Spray.

Suspension
A drug that contains solid insoluble drug particles in a liquid; the preparation must be shaken before administration. *Example:* Amoxicillin Oral Suspension.

Suspension
A pressurized form in which solid aerosol or liquid drug particles are suspended in a gas to be dispensed in a cloud or mist. *Example:* Proventil Inhalation Aerosol.

Syrup
A drug dissolved in a solution of sugar, water, and sometimes a flavoring to disguise an unpleasant taste. *Example:* Robitussin Cough Syrup.

Tincture
A drug dissolved in a solution of alcohol or alcohol and water. *Example:* tincture of iodine.

Solid Preparations

Tablet
A powdered drug that has been pressed into discs. Some tablets are *scored,* that is, they are marked with an indentation so they can be broken into halves or quarters for proper dosage. *Example:* Tylenol Tablets.

Chewable tablet
A powdered drug that has been flavored and pressed into a disc. Chewable tablets are often used for antacids, antiflatulents, and children's medication. *Example:* Pepto-Bismol Chewable Tablets.

Sublingual tablet
A powdered drug that has been pressed into a disc and is designed to dissolve under the tongue, which permits its rapid absorption into the bloodstream. *Example:* nitroglycerin sublingual tablets (Nitrostat).

Enteric-coated tablet
Tablets coated with a substance that prevents them from dissolving until they reach the intestines. The coating protects the drug from being destroyed by gastric juices and prevents it from irritating the stomach lining. To prevent the active ingredients from being released prematurely in the stomach, enteric-coated tablets must not be crushed or chewed. *Example:* Ecotrin Enteric-Coated Aspirin.

Capsule
A drug contained in a gelatin capsule that is water soluble and functions to prevent the patient from tasting the drug. *Example:* Benadryl Capsules.

Sustained-release capsules
Capsules that contain granules that dissolve at different rates to provide a gradual and continuous release of medication. This reduces the number of doses that must be administered. *Example:* Contac 12-Hour Sustained-Release Capsules. (Sustained-release medication also comes in other preparations such as tablets and caplets.)

Caplet
A drug contained in an oblong tablet with a smooth coating to make swallowing easier. *Example:* Advil Caplets.

Lozenge
A drug contained in a candylike base. Lozenges are circular and are designed to dissolve on the tongue. *Example:* Chloraseptic Throat Lozenges.

Cream
A drug combined in a base that is generally nongreasy, resulting in a semisolid preparation. Creams are applied externally to the skin. *Example:* Hydrocortisone Topical Cream.

Ointment
A drug with an oil base, resulting in a semisolid preparation. Ointments are applied externally to the skin and are usually greasy. *Example:* Cortisporin Topical Ointment.

Suppository
A drug mixed with a firm base, such as cocoa butter, that is designed to melt at body temperature. A suppository is shaped into a cylinder or a cone for easy insertion into a body cavity, such as the rectum or vagina. *Example:* Preparation H Suppositories.

Transdermal patch
A patch with an adhesive backing, which contains a drug, that is applied to the skin. The drug enters the circulation after being absorbed through the skin. *Example:* nitroglycerin patches (Nitro-Dur).

Classification of Drugs Based on Action

Drugs can also be classified according to the action they have on the body. The medical assistant should know in which category a particular drug belongs, as well as its primary use and major therapeutic effects. See Table 11-1 for classifications and examples of drugs based on action that are commonly administered and prescribed in the medical office.

Text continued on p. 455

TABLE 11-1 — Classification of Drugs Based on Action

Drug Category	Primary Use and Major Therapeutic Effects	Commonly Prescribed Drugs	
		Generic	**Brand**
Analgesics (opioid)	**Used to** manage moderate to severe pain. **Works by** altering the perception of and response to painful stimuli. **Vicodin** VICODIN 500/5 mg **Darvocet-N** DARVOCET-N 50 50/325 mg DARVOCET-N 100 100/650 mg	codeine/APAP hydrocodone/APAP hydrocodone/ASA meperidine oxycodone oxycodone/APAP oxycodone/ASA propoxyphene propoxyphene N/APAP tramadol	► Tylenol w/ Codeine (III) ► Vicodin (III) Lortab (III) Demerol (II) ► OxyContin (II) Percocet (II) Percodan (II) Darvon (IV) ► Darvocet-N (IV) ► Ultram
Analgesics/antipyretics	**Used to** manage mild to moderate pain and to reduce fever. **Works by** relieving pain and reducing fever. **Naprosyn** NAPROSYN 250 250 mg NAPROSYN 375 mg NAPROSYN 500 mg	acetaminophen aspirin **NSAID** ibuprofen naproxen	Tylenol* Bayer* Ecotrin* Advil* Motrin* Aleve* Anaprox Naprosyn
Anesthetics (local)	**Used to** produce local anesthesia through a loss of feeling to a part of the body. **Works by** preventing initiation and conduction of normal nerve impulses in a body part.	lidocaine dibucaine	Xylocaine Nupercainal Ointment*
Antacids	**Used to** treat heartburn, hyperacidity, indigestion, and GERD, and to promote healing of ulcers. **Works by** neutralizing gastric acid to relieve gastric pain and irritation.	aluminum hydroxide/ magnesium hydroxide calcium carbonate sodium bicarbonate/ASA	Maalox* Mylanta* Tums* Alka-Seltzer*
Antianemics	**Iron Supplements** **Used to** prevent or cure iron-deficiency anemia. **Works by** increasing the amount of iron in the body.		Feosol* DexFerrum

*Available OTC (over-the-counter).
► Top-100 most prescribed drugs.
(II) Schedule II drug.
(III) Schedule III drug.
(IV) Schedule IV drug.

TABLE **11-1** Classification of Drugs Based on Action—cont'd

Drug Category	Primary Use and Major Therapeutic Effects	Commonly Prescribed Drugs	
		Generic	Brand
Antianemics—cont'd	**Vitamin B$_{12}$ Injection** **Used to** treat pernicious anemia. **Works by** increasing the amount of vitamin B$_{12}$ in the body. **Used to** relieve or prevent angina attacks.	ferrous sulfate iron dextran cyanocobalamin	InFed Cobex Cyanoject
Antianginals	**Works by** increasing the blood supply to myocardial tissue. **Imdur** 60 mg **Nitrostat** 0.3 mg 0.4 mg 0.6 mg	**Nitrates** isosorbide dinitrate isosorbide mononitrate nitroglycerin **Beta Blockers** atenolol propranolol **Calcium Channel Blockers** amlodipine bepridil diltiazem nifedipine verapamil	Sorbitrate ▶ Imdur Nitro-Bid Nitro-Dur Nitrostat ▶ Tenormin Inderal ▶ Norvasc Vascor ▶ Cardizem Adalat Procardia-XL Calan Isoptin Verelan
Antianxiety agents	**Used to** treat anxiety. **Work at** many levels in the CNS to produce an anxiolytic (anxiety-relieving) effect. **Xanax** 0.25 mg 0.5 mg 1 mg 2 mg	alprazolam buspirone chlordiazepoxide diazepam lorazepam	▶ Xanax (IV) BuSpar Librium (IV) Valium (IV) ▶ Ativan (IV)
Anticholinergics	**Used to** preoperatively decrease oral and respiratory secretions. **Works by** blocking the effects of acetylcholine in the autonomic nervous system.	atropine	Atro-Pen
Anticoagulants	**Used to** prevent and treat venous thrombosis, pulmonary embolism, and MI by preventing clot extension and formation. **Works by** delaying or preventing blood coagulation. **Coumadin** 1 mg 2 mg	warfarin heparin	▶ Coumadin

Continued

TABLE 11-1 Classification of Drugs Based on Action—cont'd

Drug Category	Primary Use and Major Therapeutic Effects	Commonly Prescribed Drugs	
		Generic	Brand
Anticonvulsants	**Used to** prevent or relieve seizures. **Works by** decreasing the incidence and severity of seizures.	carbamazepine	Tegretol
		clonazepam	► Klonopin (IV)
		gabapentin	► Neurontin
		phenytoin	► Dilantin
		divalproex	► Depakote
		valproic acid	Depakene

Neurontin

100 mg   300 mg   400 mg

Antidepressants	**Used to** prevent, cure, or alleviate depression. Also **Used to** treat anxiety disorders (panic attacks) and OCD. **Works by** inhibiting the reuptake of neurotransmitter(s) in the CNS.	**Selective Serotonin Reuptake Inhibitors (SSRIs)**	
		citalopram	► Celexa
		fluoxetine	► Prozac
		paroxetine	► Paxil
		sertraline	► Zoloft
		Miscellaneous	
		amitriptyline	Elavil
		buproprion	► Wellbutrin-SR
		nefazodone	► Serzone
		venlafaxine	► Effexor XR

Prozac

10 mg   20 mg

Wellbutrin-SR

100 mg   150 mg

Antidiabetics	**Oral Hypoglycemics** **Used to** manage non-insulin-dependent type 2 diabetes mellitus. **Works by** stimulating the release of insulin from the pancreas and increasing the sensitivity to insulin.	glimepiride	► Amaryl
		glipizide	► Glucotrol XL
		glyburide	DiaBeta
			Micronase
		metformin	► Glucophage
		pioglitazone	► Actos
		rosiglitazone	► Avandia

Antidiarrheals	**Insulins** **Used to** manage diabetes mellitus. **Works by** reducing blood glucose levels.	regular insulin	Humulin R* Novolin R*
		NPH insulin	► Humulin N* Novolin N*
		NPH/regular insulin	► Humulin 70/30* Novolin 70/30*
		insulin glargine	Lantus
		insulin lispro	Humalog

Amaryl

2 mg   4 mg

Glucotrol XL

5 mg   10 mg

*Available OTC (over-the-counter).
► Top-100 most prescribed drugs.
(II) Schedule II drug.
(III) Schedule III drug.
(IV) Schedule IV drug.

TABLE 11-1 Classification of Drugs Based on Action—cont'd

Drug Category	Primary Use and Major Therapeutic Effects	Commonly Prescribed Drugs	
		Generic	Brand
	Used to control and relieve diarrhea. **Works by** inhibiting peristalsis, reducing fecal volume, and preventing the loss of fluids and electrolytes. **Lomotil** 2.5/0.025 mg	bismuth subsalicylate diphenoxylate/ atropine kaolin/pectin loperamide	Pepto-Bismol* Lomotil (V) Kaopectate* Imodium*
Antidysrhythmics	**Used to** control or prevent a wide variety of cardiac dysrhythmias. **Works by** decreasing myocardial excitability and slowing conduction velocity. **Inderal** 10 mg 20 mg 40 mg 60 mg 80 mg	procainamide propranolol	Pronestyl Inderal
Antiemetics	**Used to** prevent or relieve nausea and vomiting. **Works by** depressing the chemoreceptor trigger zone in the CNS to inhibit nausea and vomiting.	dronabinol ondansetron prochlorperazine promethazine meclizine	Marinol (III) Zofran Compazine Phenergan Bonine*
Antiflatulents	**Used to** relieve discomfort of excess gas and bloating in the GI tract. **Works by** causing coalescence of gas bubbles in the intestinal tract.	simethicone	Gas-X* Mylanta Gas*
Antifungals	**Used to** treat fungal infections. **Works by** killing or inhibiting growth of susceptible fungi. **Diflucan** 50 mg 100 mg 200 mg	amphotericin B clotrimazole fluconazole ketoconazole miconazole nystatin terconazole	Fungizone Gyne-Lotrimin* ▶ Diflucan Nizoral Monistat* Mycostatin* Terazol
Antigout agents	**Used to** prevent attacks of gout. **Works by** inhibiting production of uric acid. **Zyloprim** 100 mg 300 mg	allopurinol colchicine	Zyloprim Colchicine tablets
Anthelmintics	**Used to** treat worm infections (pinworms, roundworms, hookworms). **Works by** destroying worms.	mebendazole	Vermox
Antihistamines	**Used to** relieve symptoms associated with allergies (decreased sneezing; rhinorrhea; itchy eyes, nose and throat). **Works by** blocking effects of histamine at histamine receptor sites. **Allegra** 60 mg 180 mg	cetirizine brompheniramine chlorpheniramine fexofenadine hydroxyzine loratadine promethazine diphenhydramine	▶ Zyrtec Dimetaine* Chlor-Trimetron* Teldrin* ▶ Allegra Atarax Vistaril Claritin* Phenergan Benadryl*

TABLE **11-1**	Classification of Drugs Based on Action—cont'd		
	Primary Use and Major Therapeutic	**Commonly Prescribed Drugs**	
Drug Category	**Effects**	**Generic**	**Brand**
Antihypertensives	***Used to*** manage hypertension. ***Works by*** causing systemic vasodilation to lower blood pressure.	**Angiotensin-Converting Enzyme (ACE) Inhibitors**	
		benazepril	▶ Lotensin
	Accupril	*captopril*	Capoten
		enalapril	▶ Vasotec
	5 mg / 10 mg	*lisinopril*	▶ Prinivil
		quinapril	▶ Accupril
	20 mg / 40 mg	*ramipril*	▶ Altace
		Peripherally Acting Adrenergic Blockers	
		clonidine	▶ Catapres
		doxazosin	Cardura
		prazosin	Minipress
	Cozaar	**Angiotensin II Receptor Antagonists**	
		candesartan	Atacand
	25 mg / 50 mg	*irbesartan*	▶ Avapro
		losartan	▶ Cozaar
		valsartan	▶ Diovan
	Toprol XL	**Beta Blockers**	
		atenolol	Tenormin
	50 mg / 100 mg	*metoprolol*	Lopressor
			▶ Toprol XL
	200 mg	*propranolol*	Inderal
		Calcium Channel Blockers	
		amlodipine	▶ Norvasc
		diltiazem	▶ Cardizem
		felodipine	Plendil
	Cardizem	**Vasodilator**	
		hydralazine	Apresoline
	30 mg / 60 mg	**Miscellaneous**	
		amlodipine/ benazepril	▶ Lotrel
	90 mg / 120 mg	*bisoprolol/ hydrochlorothiazide*	Ziac
		losartan/ hydrochlorothiazide	▶ Hyzaar
		nadolol/bendro- flumethiazide	Corzide

*Available OTC (over-the-counter).
▶ Top-100 most prescribed drugs.
(II) Schedule II drug.
(III) Schedule III drug.
(IV) Schedule IV drug.

TABLE 11-1	Classification of Drugs Based on Action—cont'd		
Drug Category	**Primary Use and Major Therapeutic Effects**	**Commonly Prescribed Drugs**	
		Generic	**Brand**
Anti-impotence agents	**Used to** treat erectile dysfunction. **Works by** promoting an increased blood flow to the penis.	*sildenafil*	▶ Viagra

Viagra

25 mg   50 mg   100 mg

Anti-infectives	**Used to** treat infections. **Works by** killing or inhibiting growth of bacteria.	**Pencillins**	
		amoxicillin	▶ Amoxil
			▶ Trimox
		amoxicillin/ clavulanate	▶ Augmentin
		benzathine penicillin	Bicillin
		penicillin V	▶ Veetids
		procaine penicillin	Wycillin
		Macrolides	
		azithromycin	▶ Zithromax
		clarithromycin	▶ Biaxin
		erythromycin	Ery-Tab
			Pediazole
		Cephalosporins	
		cefaclor	Ceclor
		cefprozil	▶ Cefzil
		ceftriaxone	Rocephin
		cephalexin	▶ Keflex
		Fluoroquinolones	
		ciprofloxacin	▶ Cipro
		levofloxacin	▶ Levaquin
		ofloxacin	Floxin
		Tetracyclines	
		doxycycline	▶ Doryx, Vibramycin
		tetracycline	Sumycin, Achromycin
		Aminoglycosides	
		gentamicin	Garamycin
		kanamycin	Kantrex
		neomycin	Neobiotic
		tobramycin	Tobrax
		Sulfonamides	
		sulfamethoxazole	Gantanol
		trimethoprim/ sulfamethoxazole	Bactrim
		Miscellaneous	
		chloramphenical	Chloromycetin
		mupirocin	▶ Bactroban
		nitrofurantoin	▶ Macrobid
			Macrodantin
		vancomycin	Vancocin

Amoxil

125 mg   250 mg

250 mg

500 mg

Zithromax

250 mg   250 mg

Keflex

250 mg   500 mg

Cipro

250 mg   500 mg

750 mg

Macrobid

100 mg

Continued

	Primary Use and Major Therapeutic Effects	Commonly Prescribed Drugs	
Drug Category		Generic	Brand
Anti-inflammatory agents	**Used to** relieve signs and symptoms of osteoarthritis and rheumatoid arthritis in adults. **Works by** decreasing pain and inflammation.	aspirin	Bayer* Ecotrin*
		celecoxib	▶ Celebrex
		etodolac	Lodine
		ibuprofen	Advil* Motrin*
		indomethacin	Indocin
		nabumetone	Relafen
		naproxen	Aleve* Anaprox Naprosyn
		rofecoxib	▶ Vioxx
		valdecoxib	Bextra

Celebrex

100 mg   200 mg

Vioxx

12.5 mg   25 mg

	Primary Use and Major Therapeutic Effects	Generic	Brand
Antimanics	**Used to** treat bipolar affective disorders. **Works by** altering cation transport in nerves and muscles.	lithium	Eskalith Eskalith CR

Eskalith   Eskalith CR

300 mg   450 mg

Antimigraines	**Used** in the acute treatment of migraine attacks. **Works by** causing vasoconstriction in large intracranial arteries.	sumatriptan	▶ Imitrex
Antineoplastics	**Used to** treat tumors. **Works by** preventing development, growth, or proliferation of malignant cells.	cyclophosphamide methotrexate	Cytoxan Mexate Folex
Antiparkinson agents	**Used to** treat symptoms of Parkinson's disease. **Works by** restoring the balance between acetylcholine and dopamine in the CNS.	carbidopa/levodopa	Sinemet

Sinemet

10/100 mg   25/100 mg

50/200 mg   25/250 mg

*Available OTC (over-the-counter).
▶ Top-100 most prescribed drugs.
(II) Schedule II drug.
(III) Schedule III drug.
(IV) Schedule IV drug.

Drug Category	Primary Use and Major Therapeutic Effects	Commonly Prescribed Drugs	
		Generic	Brand
Antiprotozoals	***Used to*** treat protozoal infections. ***Works by*** destroying protozoa.	*metronidazole*	Flagyl
	Flagyl 250 mg 500 mg 375 mg		
Antipsychotics	***Used to*** treat psychotic disorders. ***Works by*** blocking dopamine and serotonin receptors in the CNS.	*haloperidol* *olanzapine* *risperidone*	Haldol ▶ Zyprexa ▶ Risperdal
	Risperdal 1 mg 2 mg 3 mg 4 mg		
Antiretrovirals	***Used to*** manage HIV infections and to reduce maternal/fetal transmission of HIV. ***Works by*** inhibiting replication of retroviruses.	*zidovudine*	Retrovir
	Retrovir 100 mg		
Antispasmodics	***Used to*** control hypermotility in irritable bowel syndrome, spastic colitis, spastic bladder, and pylorospasm. ***Works by*** preventing or relieving spasms of the GI and GU tracts.	*dicyclomine* *hyoscyamine*	Bentyl Levsin
Antituberculars	***Used to*** treat tuberculosis. ***Works by*** killing or inhibiting growth of mycobacteria.	*isoniazid* *pyrazinamide* *rifampin*	*Isotamine (INH)* *PMS-Pyrazinamide* *Rifadin*
Antitussives	***Used in*** the prevention or relief of coughs caused by minor viral URIs or inhaled irritants. ***Works by*** suppressing the cough reflex by a direct effect on the cough center in the CNS.	*benzonatate* *chlorpheniramine/ hydrocodone* *dextromethorphan* *guaifenesin/codeine*	Tessalon Tussionex (III) Robitussin DM* Robitussin A-C (V)
Antiulcers	***Used to*** manage ulcers, GERD, heartburn, indigestion, and gastric hyperacidity. ***Works by*** preventing accumulation of acid the stomach.	**Gastric Pump Inhibitors** *esomeprazole* *lansoprazole* *omeprazole* **H2-Receptor Antagonist** *cimetidine* *famotidine* *ranitidine*	Nexium ▶ Prevacid Prilosec* Tagamet* Pepcid AC* Zantac*
	Prevacid 15 mg 30 mg		

Continued

TABLE **11-1** Classification of Drugs Based on Action—cont'd

Drug Category	Primary Use and Major Therapeutic Effects	Commonly Prescribed Drugs	
		Generic	Brand
Antivirals	**Used to** manage herpes infections. **Works by** inhibiting viral replication.	*acyclovir* *valacyclovir*	Zovirax ► Valtrex

Valtrex

500 mg   1 g

| Bone resorption inhibitors | **Used to** treat and prevent osteoporosis. **Works by** inhibiting resorption of bone. | *alendronate* *raloxifene* *risedronate* | ► Fosamax ► Evista Actonel |

Fosamax

5 mg   10 mg

40 mg

| Bronchodilators | **Used to** manage reversible airway obstruction caused by asthma or COPD. **Works by** relaxing the smooth muscle of the respiratory tract resulting in bronchodilation. | *albuterol* *montelukast* *salmeterol* *theophylline* *zafirlukast* | ► Proventil ► Singulair ► Serevent Bronkodyl Accolate |

Singulair

4 mg   5 mg

10 mg

| Cardiac glycosides | **Used to** treat CHF and cardiac arrhythmias. **Works by** increasing the strength and force of myocardial contractions and slowing heart rate. | *digitoxin* *digoxin* | Crystodigin Lanoxicaps ► Lanoxin |

Lanoxicaps

0.1 mg

| CNS stimulants | **Used to** treat narcolepsy and manage ADHD. **Works by** increasing the level of catecholamines in the CNS. | *dextroamphetamine* *dextroamphetamine/ saccinarate and sulfate* *methylphenidate* | Dexedrine (II) ► Adderall (II) Ritalin (II) ► Concerta (II) |

Adderal (II)

5 mg   10 mg

20 mg   30 mg

*Available OTC (over-the-counter).
► Top-100 most prescribed drugs.
(II) Schedule II drug.
(III) Schedule III drug.
(IV) Schedule IV drug.

TABLE **11-1** Classification of Drugs Based on Action—cont'd

Drug Category	Primary Use and Major Therapeutic Effects	Commonly Prescribed Drugs	
		Generic	**Brand**
Contraceptives (hormonal)	*Used to* prevent pregnancy and regulate the menstrual cycle. *Works by* inhibiting ovulation.	**Oral Contraceptives**	
		ethinyl estradiol/ norethindrone	Mircette ▶ Ortho-Novum
		ethinyl estradiol/ norgestimate	▶ Ortho Tri-Cyclen
		ethinyl estradiol/ levonorgestrel	▶ Alesse
		Injectable Contraceptives	
		medroxy-progesterone	▶ Depo-Provera
		Transdermal Contraceptives	
		ethinyl estradiol/ norelgestromin	Ortho Evra
		Vaginal Ring Contraceptives	
		ethinyl estradiol/ etonogestrel	NuvaRing
Corticosteroids	**Systemic Corticosteroids** *Used to* treat inflammation, allergies, asthma, autoimmune disorders, and replacement therapy in adrenal insufficiency. *Works by* suppressing inflammation and modifying normal immune response.	cortisone fluticasone hydrocortisone methylprednisolone triamcinolone	Cortone ▶ Flovent Cortef Medrol Depo-Medrol Aristocort
	Nasal Corticosteroids *Used to* treat chronic nasal inflammatory conditions (e.g., allergic rhinitis). *Works by* suppressing inflammation and reducing hypersecretions of the respiratory tract.	beclomethasone fluticasone mometasone prednisone triamcinolone	Vancenase ▶ Flonase ▶ Nasonex Deltasnoe Nasacort
Decongestants	*Used to* decrease nasal congestion. *Works by* producing vasoconstriction in respiratory tract mucosa.	oxymetazoline phenylephrine pseudoephedrine	Afrin*, Dristan* Neo-Synephrine* Sudafed*
Diuretics	*Used to* manage hypertension, edema in CHF, and renal disease. *Works by* removing excess fluid from the body by increasing urine output.	**Loop Diuretics** bumetanide furosemide	Bumex ▶ Lasix
		Thiazide Diuretics chlorthalidone hydrochlorothiazide	Hygroton Esidrix HydroDiuril
		Potassium-Sparing Diuretics spironolactone triamterene	Aldactone Dyrenium

Ortho-Novum

7/7/7

1/35

Lasix

20 mg   40 mg   80 mg

HydroDiuril

25 mg   50 mg

Continued

TABLE 11-1 Classification of Drugs Based on Action—cont'd

Drug Category	Primary Use and Major Therapeutic Effects	Commonly Prescribed Drugs	
		Generic	Brand
Electrolyte replacements	**Used to** treat or prevent electrolyte depletion. **Works by** replacing electrolytes in the body.	**Potassium Supplements** *potassium chloride*	▶ K-Dur ▶ Klor-Con

Klor-Con

600 mg   750 mg

Drug Category	Effects	Generic	Brand
Emetics	**Works by** inducing vomiting.	*syrup of ipecac*	
Expectorants	**Used to** manage coughs by expelling mucus. **Works by** decreasing viscosity of bronchial secretions to promote clearance of mucus from the respiratory tract.	*guaifenesin*	Robitussin* Naldecon*
Hormone replacements	**Used to** treat moderate to severe vasomotor symptoms of menopause. **Works by** restoring hormonal balance.	*conjugated estrogens* *conjugated estrogen/ progesterone* *estradiol/ norethindrone*	▶ Premarin ▶ Prempro Activella

Premarin

0.3 mg   0.625 mg

0.9 mg   1.25 mg   2.5 mg

Drug Category	Effects	Generic	Brand
Immunizations	**Used to** prevent (vaccine-preventable) diseases. **Works by** stimulating the body to produce antibodies.	*diphtheria, tetanus toxoids and acellular pertussis vaccine* *Haemophilus b conjugate vaccine* *hepatitis A vaccine* *hepatitis B vaccine* *inactivated polio vaccine*	Acel-Imune Daptacel Infanrix Tripedia ActHIB HibTITER Havrix Vaqta Engerix-B Recombivax HB IPOL

*Available OTC (over-the-counter).
▶ Top-100 most prescribed drugs.
(II) Schedule II drug.
(III) Schedule III drug.
(IV) Schedule IV drug.

TABLE **11-1**	Classification of Drugs Based on Action—cont'd		
	Primary Use and Major Therapeutic	**Commonly Prescribed Drugs**	
Drug Category	**Effects**	**Generic**	**Brand**
Immunizations—cont'd		*influenza virus vaccine types A & B*	Fluogen
			FluShield
		measles, mumps, and rubella vaccine	Fluzone
			M-R-Vax II
			M-M-R II
		pneumococcal 7-valent conjugate vaccine	Pneumovax II
			Prevnar
Immuno-suppressants	**Used to** treat severe rheumatoid arthritis and to prevent and treat rejection of transplanted organs.	*rubella vaccine*	
		varicella vaccine	Meruvax II
		cyclosporine	Varivax
	Works by inhibiting body's normal immune response.		Sandimmune
		methotrexate	Neoral
Laxatives	**Used to** relieve constipation.		Rheumatrex
	Works by promoting defecation of a normal, soft stool.	*bisacodyl*	
		docusate	Dulcolax*
Lipid-lowering agents	**Used to** lower cholesterol to reduce risk of MI and stroke.	*phenolphthalein*	Colace*
		psyllium	Phenolax*
	Works by inhibiting an enzyme needed to synthesize cholesterol in the body.	*atorvastatin*	Metamucil*
		fluvastatin	▶ Lipitor
		lovastatin	Lescol
	Lipitor	*pravastatin*	Mevacor
		simvastatin	▶ Pravachol
			▶ Zocor

Lipitor

PD 155
10
20

10 mg   20 mg

S P

712
40 mg

Muscle relaxants (skeletal)	**Used to** treat acute painful musculoskeletal conditions.	*carisoprodol*	▶ Soma
		cyclobenzaprine	Flexeril
	Works by relaxing skeletal muscles.	*metaxalone*	Skelaxin
		methocarbamol	Robaxin

Flexeril

10 mg

Ophthalmic anti-infectives	**Used to** treat eye infections.	*dexamethasone/ tobramycin*	TobraDex
	Works by destroying bacteria.	*polymyxin/bacitracin*	Polysporin
		polymyxin/neomycin	Neosporin
		polymyxin/ trimethoprim	Polytrim
		tobramycin	Tobrex

Continued

TABLE **11-1**	Classification of Drugs Based on Action—cont'd		
Drug Category	**Primary Use and Major Therapeutic Effects**	**Commonly Prescribed Drugs**	
		Generic	**Brand**
Otic preparations	**Used to** treat ear conditions.	**Anti-infective (relives ear pain)**	
		benzocaine	Auralgan
		Anti-infective (treatment of otitis externa)	
		neomycin/polymyxin/ hydrocortisone	Cortisporin Otic
		ofloxacin	Floxin Otic
		Cerumenolytics (softens cerumen)	
		carbamide peroxide	Debrox
Platelet inhibitors	**Used to** reduce incidence of a heart attack (MI) and stroke. **Works by** interfering with ability of platelets to adhere to each other.	*clopidogrel* *salicylates*	► Plavix Aspirin*
Sedatives and hypnotics	**Used for** the short-term treatment of insomnia. **Works by** promoting sleep by CNS depression. **Ambien** 5 mg 10 mg	*flurazepam* *phenobarbital* *temazepam* *zolpidem*	Dalmane (IV) Luminal (IV) Restoril (IV) ► Ambien (IV)
Smoking deterrents	**Used to** manage nicotine withdrawal to give up cigarette smoking. **Works by** providing nicotine during controlled withdrawal from cigarette smoking.	*nicotine*	Nicorette Gum* Nicotrol Inhaler Nicoderm Patch* Commit Lozenges*
Thrombolytic agents	**Used** for the acute management of coronary thrombosis (MI). **Works by** dissolving existing clots.	*alteplase* *anistreplase* *reteplase* *streptokinase*	Activase Eminase Retavase Streptase
Thyroid preparations	**Thyroid Hormones** **Used to** replace or substitute therapy in diminished or absent thyroid functioning of many causes. **Works by** increasing basal metabolism rate. **Levoxyl** 0.05 mg	*levothyroxine*	► Levoxyl ► Synthroid

*Available OTC (over-the-counter).
► Top-100 most prescribed drugs.
(II) Schedule II drug.
(III) Schedule III drug.
(IV) Schedule IV drug.

TABLE 11-1	Classification of Drugs Based on Action—cont'd		
	Primary Use and Major Therapeutic Effects	Commonly Prescribed Drugs	
Drug Category		**Generic**	**Brand**
Thyroid preparations— cont'd	**Antithyroid Agents** *Used to* treat hyperthyroidism. *Works by* inhibiting thyroid hormone synthesis, thereby reducing the basal metabolism rate.	*methimazole*	Tapazole
Vasopressors	*Used to* treat severe allergic reactions and cardiac arrest. *Works by* increasing blood pressure, and cardiac output and dilating the bronchi.	*epinephrine*	Adrenalin EpiPen
Weight control agent	*Used to* manage obesity. **Appetite Suppressants** *Works by* suppressing the appetite center in the CNS.	*diethylpropion* *phentermine* *sibutramine* *orlistat*	Tenuate (IV) Fastin (IV) ► Meridia (IV) Xenical

Meridia

5 mg   10 mg   15 mg

Lipase Inhibitors
Works by inhibiting the action of lipase to decrease absorption of dietary fats.

Systems of Measurement for Medication

Three systems of measurement are used in the United States for prescribing and administering medication: the metric system, the apothecary system, and the household system. The metric system is the most common because it is more accurate and easier to use. Some physicians occasionally use the apothecary system; therefore the medical assistant should be familiar with this system. The third system of measurement, the household system, is the least accurate and is generally used only when a patient takes liquid medication at home.

Systems of measurement have units of weight, volume, and length. *Weight* refers to the heaviness of an item, and *volume* refers to the amount of space occupied by a substance. *Length* is a unit of linear measurement of the distance from one point to another. Although length is not used to administer medication, it is used in other aspects of the medical office. For example, the head circumference

of infants is measured in centimeters (cm), a metric unit of linear measurement.

To prepare and administer medication properly and to avoid medication errors, the medical assistant must have a thorough knowledge of the specific units of measurement for these three systems and must be able to convert within each, as well as from one system to another. A basic discussion of the metric, apothecary, and household systems is presented next. A more thorough study of these systems, including conversion of units and dose calculation, is included in the *Student Mastery Manual* (Chapter 11).

Metric System

The metric system was developed in France in the latter part of the eighteenth century in an effort to simplify measurement. Most European countries are required by law to use this system for the measurement of weight, volume, and length. Overall the metric system is used for most scientific and medical measurements. Pharmaceutical companies use the metric system to measure and label medications.

The metric system employs a uniform decimal scale based on units of 10, making it very flexible and logical. The basic metric units of measurement are the gram, liter, and meter. The *gram* is a unit of weight used to measure solids, the *liter* is a unit of volume used to measure liquids, and the *meter* is a linear unit used to measure length or distance. The metric units used most often in the administration of medication in the medical office are the milligram, gram, milliliter, and cubic centimeter. Because a *cubic centimeter (cc)* is the amount of space occupied by 1 milliliter (ml), these two units can be used interchangeably (i.e., 1 ml = 1 cc).

Prefixes added to the words *gram, liter,* and *meter* designate smaller or larger units of measurement in the metric system. The same prefixes are used with all three units. For example, *milli* is used as follows: *milli*gram, *milli*liter, and *milli*meter. Each prefix changes the value of the basic unit of measurement by the same amount. The prefix *milli* describes a unit that is 1/1000 of the basic unit. Therefore 1 gram is equal to 1000 milligrams, 1 liter is equal to 1000 milliliters, and 1 meter is equal to 1000 millimeters. The box entitled Metric Notation Guidelines lists the metric units of measurement and equivalent values in different units.

Specific guidelines are used in the medical notation of metric units and doses, which are also presented in the box. To read prescriptions and medication orders, to record medication administration, and, most important, to avoid medication errors, the medical assistant must be familiar with and be able to follow these guidelines.

Apothecary System

The apothecary system is older and less accurate than the metric system. It was brought to the United States from England during the eighteenth century. Pharmacists used this system during the colonial period to compound and measure medications. This system is gradually being phased out in favor of the metric system. Until that process is completed, however, the medical assistant must be familiar with this system and be able to use it to administer medication.

The basic unit of weight in the apothecary system is the *grain*, derived from the weight of a large grain of wheat,

---

Metric Notation Guidelines

Follow these guidelines when using the metric notation of measurement and dosage.

1. The units of metric measurement are written using the following abbreviations:

   Weight
   > microgram: mg or μg
   > milligram: mg
   > gram: g
   > kilogram: kg

   Volume
   > milliliter: ml
   > cubic centimeter: cc
   > liter: L

2. Do not use a period with the abbreviation of metric units because it might be mistaken for another letter or symbol.
   > *Correct:*   mg
   >   ml
   > *Incorrect:*   mg.
   >   ml.

3. Use Arabic numerals (e.g., 1, 2, 3, 4) to express the quantity of the dose.
   > *Correct:*   4 mg
   > *Incorrect:*   iv mg

4. Place the numeral that expresses the quantity of the dose in front of the abbreviation. To make it easier to read, leave a (single) space between the quantity and the abbreviation.
   > *Correct:*   5 ml
   > *Incorrect:*   ml 5 and 5mL

5. Write a fraction of a dose as a decimal.
   > *Correct:*   0.5 g
   > *Incorrect:*   ½ g

6. If the dose is a fraction of a unit, place a zero before the decimal point as a means of focusing on the fractional dose. This reduces the possibility of misreading the dose as a whole number.
   > *Correct:*   0.5 g (this reduces the possibility of not seeing the decimal point and reading the dose as 5 grams)
   > *Incorrect:*   .5 g

7. Do not place a decimal point and a zero after a whole number. The decimal point may be overlooked, resulting in a tenfold overdose error.
   > *Correct:*   1 ml (this reduces the possibility of not seeing the decimal point and reading the dose as 10 ml)
   > *Incorrect:*   1.0 ml

Metric System: Conversion of Equivalent Values

Weight
> 1000 micrograms   =   1 milligram
> 1000 milligrams   =   1 gram
> 1000 grams   =   1 kilogram

Volume
> 1000 milliliters   =   1 liter
> 1000 liters   =   1 kiloliter
> 1 milliliter   =   1 cubic centimeter

which was used to balance the material being weighed. The next largest unit of measurement is the *scruple;* however, this unit is not used to administer medication. The remaining units, in order of increasing weight, are *dram, ounce,* and *pound.* The pound is not generally used in the administration of medication. The medical assistant should note, however, that in the apothecary system the pound is equal to 12 ounces, in contrast to the more familiar *avoirdupois* pound used to measure body weight, which is equal to 16 ounces.

Measures of liquid volume in the apothecary system correlate closely with measures of dry weight in the same system. The smallest unit of measurement is the *minim,* meaning "the least." A minim is approximately equivalent to a volume of water that weighs 1 grain. A minim glass or a syringe calibrated in minims must be used to measure with this unit. The remaining units of liquid volume in the apothecary system, in order of increasing volume, are *fluid dram, fluid ounce, pint, quart,* and *gallon.* The basic unit of linear measurement is the *inch,* followed by *foot, yard,* and *mile.* Most Americans are familiar with apothecary units of measurement because of their use in everyday life. For example, milk is available in pints, quarts, and gallons, and height is measured in feet and inches.

The box entitled Apothecary Notation Guidelines lists the units of measurement in the apothecary system and equivalent values in different units. It also includes guidelines for the medical notation of apothecary units.

Household System

The household system is more complicated and less accurate for administering liquid medication than either the metric or the apothecary system. Nevertheless, most individuals are familiar with this system because of its frequent use in the United States. This system of measurement may be the only one the patient can understand and therefore safely use to take liquid medication at home. For example, most patients are more comfortable measuring medication in drops and teaspoons than in minims and milliliters. In addition, the patient is more likely to have household measuring devices on hand than to have metric measuring devices. If a precise measurement is needed, however, the metric system must be used, and the medical assistant should instruct the patient in the use of the metric measuring device.

Apothecary Notation Guidelines

Follow these guidelines when using the medical notation of apothecary units and dosage.

1. The units of apothecary measurement are usually written with abbreviations and symbols as follows:

   Weight
   > grain: gr
   > dram: dr or ꝫ
   > ounce: oz or ℥

   Volume
   > minim: ♏
   > fluid dram: fꝫ, fluid ounce: f℥
   > pint: pt
   > quart: qt
   > gallon: gal

2. When writing symbols and abbreviations to express apothecary units, use lowercase roman numerals to express the dose quantity.
   > *Correct:* ℥ v̄ī *(6 ounces)*
   > *Incorrect:* 6 ℥; ℥6

3. Place the roman numeral expressing dose quantity *after* the symbol or abbreviation.
   > *Correct:* ꝫ īi (2 drams); gr v (5 grains)
   > *Incorrect:* ii ꝫ; v gr

4. A line may be placed over the roman numerals. Dots are placed above the line for emphasis as a safeguard against error.
   > *Correct:* f ꝫ ïïï (3 fluid drams)
   > *Incorrect:* f ꝫ iii

5. Write ss to designate one half of a dose and place it after the apothecary symbol or abbreviation.
   > *Correct:* gr ss
   > *Incorrect:* gr ½

6. Write fractions (other than ½) in Arabic numerals and place them after the apothecary symbol or abbreviation.
   > *Correct:* gr ¼
   > *Incorrect:* gr 0.25; ¼ gr

   Note: If abbreviations and symbols are not used to express apothecary units of measurement, Arabic numerals must be used to express dose quantity and are placed before the unit of measurement. *Example:* ¼ grain.

Apothecary System: Conversion of Equivalent Values

Weight

60 grains	= 1 dram
8 drams	= 1 ounce
12 ounces	= 1 pound

Volume

60 minims	= 1 fluid dram
8 fluidrams	= 1 fluid ounce
16 fluidounces	= 1 pint
2 pints	= 1 quart
4 quarts	= 1 gallon

TABLE **11-2**	Household System: Conversion of Common Values

Abbreviations

drop:	gtt
teaspoon:	tsp
tablespoon:	tbsp
ounce:	oz
cup:	c

Volume

60 gtt	=	1 tsp
3 tsp	=	1 tbs
6 tsp	=	1 oz
2 tbs	=	1 oz
6 oz	=	1 teacup
8 oz	=	1 glass

Volume is the only household unit of measurement used to administer medication. The basic unit of liquid volume in the household system is the *drop (gtt),* which is approximately equal to 0.6 ml in the metric system and 1 minim in the apothecary system. These units cannot be considered exact equivalents because the size of the drop varies based on temperature, the viscosity of the liquid, and the size of the dropper. The remaining units, in order of increasing volume, are *teaspoon, tablespoon, ounce (fluid ounce), cup,* and *glass.* Table 11-2 lists the units of liquid volume measurement in the household system and equivalent values in different units.

Converting Units of Measurement

Changing from one unit of measurement to another is known as **conversion.** Conversion is required when medication is ordered in a unit of measurement that differs from the medication's label. The dose quantity must be mathematically translated or converted to the unit of measurement of the medication on hand. For example, if the physician orders 5 grams of an oral solid medication and the medication label expresses the drug

TABLE **11-3**	Conversion Charts for Systems of Measurement

CONVERSION CHART FOR METRIC AND APOTHECARY SYSTEMS (COMMON APPROXIMATE EQUIVALENTS)

Metric System to Apothecary System			Apothecary System to Metric System		
Weight			**Weight**		
60 mg	=	1 gr	15 gr	=	1000 mg (1 g)
21 g	=	15 gr	10 gr	=	600 mg
24 g	=	1 dr	$7\frac{1}{2}$ gr	=	500 mg
30 mg	=	1 oz	5 gr	=	300 mg
1 kg	=	2.2 lb	3 gr	=	200 mg
			$1\frac{1}{2}$ gr	=	100 mg
			1 gr	=	60 mg
Volume			$\frac{3}{4}$ gr	=	50 mg
0.06 ml	=	1 ℳ	$\frac{1}{2}$ gr	=	30 mg
1 ml (cc)	=	15 ℳ	$\frac{1}{4}$ gr	=	15 mg
4 ml	=	1 f ʒ	$\frac{1}{6}$ gr	=	10 mg
30 ml	=	1 f ℥	$\frac{1}{8}$ gr	=	8 mg
500 ml	=	1 pt	$\frac{1}{12}$ gr	=	5 mg
1000 ml (1 L)	=	1 qt	$\frac{1}{15}$ gr	=	4 mg
			$\frac{1}{20}$ gr	=	3 mg
			$\frac{1}{30}$ gr	=	2 mg
			$\frac{1}{40}$ gr	=	1.5 mg
			$\frac{1}{50}$ gr	=	1.2 mg
			$\frac{1}{60}$ gr	=	1 mg
			$\frac{1}{100}$ gr	=	0.6 mg
			$\frac{1}{120}$ gr	=	0.5 mg
			$\frac{1}{150}$ gr	=	0.4 mg
			$\frac{1}{200}$ gr	=	0.3 mg
			$\frac{1}{300}$ gr	=	0.2 mg
			$\frac{1}{600}$ gr	=	0.1 mg

TABLE 11-3 Conversion Charts for Systems of Measurement—cont'd

EQUIVALENCES IN HOUSEHOLD, APOTHECARY, AND METRIC UNITS (VOLUME)

Household	Apothecary	Metric
1 gtt	= 1 ♏	= 0.06 ml
15 gtt	= 15 ♏	= 1 ml (1 cc)
1 tsp	= 1 f ℥	= 5 (4) ml*
1 tsp	= 4 f ℥	= 15 ml
2 tsp	= 1 f ℥	= 30 ml
1 oz	= 1 f ℥	= 30 ml
1 teacup	= 6 f ℥	= 180 ml
1 glass	= 8 f ℥	= 240 ml

*The American standard teaspoon is accepted as 5 ml; however, 4 ml can be used as the equivalent to provide a more accurate conversion.

PUTTING It All Into PRACTICE

MY NAME IS Theresa Cline, and I work for four physicians in a family practice medical office. I have worked there ever since I graduated from college in 1983. There was one experience that I will never forget relating to the administration of an injection because it taught our entire office staff a very valuable lesson. It involved a woman who came to our office because she had lacerated her wrist while using a butcher knife. After the wound was sutured, I proceeded to give her a tetanus injection because she was past due for one. Shortly thereafter she became very nauseated and dizzy, and I made her lie down on the examining table. She asked me to get her a cold drink of water and I left the room to do so. Apparently, while I was gone she must have tried to sit up or turn over because she rolled off the table and struck the back of her head on the floor. She sustained a laceration to her scalp, which also had to be sutured. Owing to her persistent symptoms of severe nausea, vomiting, and headache, it was decided that she should be admitted to the hospital for neurologic observation and x-ray studies.

The vitally important lesson that this experience taught everyone in our office was that you must never leave a patient alone, not even for a minute to get something, if there is the slightest indication that he or she is not feeling perfectly fine. Another staff member should be called to obtain whatever is needed. From that point on, this has been our office policy and procedure.

strength in milligrams, the medical assistant would need to convert the grams into milligrams to know how much medication to administer. Converting units of measurement can be classified into the following categories: (1) conversion of units within a measurement system and (2) conversion of units from one measurement system to another.

Converting units within a measurement system allows a quantity to be expressed in two different but equal units of measurement within *one* system. An example of converting units of weight within the metric system is as follows: 1 gram is equal to 1000 milligrams. Converting from one measurement system to another allows a quantity written in one measurement system to be expressed in an equivalent unit of measurement in *another* system. An example of a conversion from the apothecary system to the metric system is as follows: 1 grain (apothecary system) is equivalent to 60 milligrams (metric system).

Conversion requires the use of a conversion table to indicate the equivalent values of various units of measurement. Conversion tables of equivalent values in these three measurement systems are included in this chapter:

Metric conversion–Box on p. 456
Apothecary conversion–Box on p. 457
Household conversion–Table 11-2

Tables used to convert from one system to another consist of approximate rather than exact equivalents, and a 10% error usually occurs in making these conversions. Conversion tables used to convert from one system to another are presented in Table 11-3.

The medical assistant must be very careful when using conversion tables to avoid errors in interpolation. The numbers on conversion tables are small and close together; it is easy to misread the chart from one column to the other. To reduce this possibility, a straightedge should be used when reading a conversion table.

Controlled Drugs

By means of federal and state legislation, restrictions are placed on drugs that have potential for abuse. These drugs are known as **controlled** drugs. They are classified into five categories, called schedules, which are based on their abuse potential. See Table 11-4 for a list, description, and examples of the schedules for controlled drugs.

TABLE **11-4**	Classification of Controlled Drugs		
		Examples	
Classification	**Description**	**Generic**	**Brand**
Schedule I	High potential for abuse. No accepted medical use. Use may lead to severe physical or psychological dependence. Not available for prescribing. May be used for research with appropriate limitations.	GHB heroin LSD marijuana MDMA (Ectasy) mescaline methaqualone (Quaalude) phencyclidine (PCP) psilocybin	
Schedule II	High potential for abuse. Accepted medical use in U.S. Abuse may lead to severe psychological or physical dependence. Prescription must be in writing in indelible ink or typed. Emergency telephone order permitted only for immediate amount needed to treat the patient. Written prescription must be provided to pharmacist within 7 days. No refills allowed. Manufacturer's label marked C-II.	**Analgesics** cocaine codeine fentanyl hydrocodone hydromorphone meperidine methadone morphine oxycodone oxycodone/APAP oxycodone/ASA **CNS Stimulants** dextroamphetamine methylphenidate methamphetamine **Sedatives/Hypnotics** amobarbital glutethimide pentobarbital secobarbital	 Sublimaze Hycodan Dilaudid Demerol Dolophine Roxanol OxyContin Percocet Percodan Dexedrine, Adderall Ritalin Desoxyn Amytal Doriden Nembutal Seconal
Schedule III	Intermediate potential for abuse. Accepted medical use in U.S. Abuse may lead to low to moderate physical dependence and moderate to high psychological dependence. Telephone and fax orders permitted. If authorized by physician, prescription can be refilled up to 5 times within 6 months from issue date. Prescription expires 6 months from issue date. Manufacturer's label marked C-III.	**Anabolic Steroids** oxandrolone oxymetholone **Analgesics** buprenorphine butalbital compound codeine in combination with a nonopioid analgesic hydrocodone in combination with a nonopioid analgesic **CNS Stimulant** benzphetamine **Male Hormone** testosterone **Sedative/Hypnotic** butabarbital	 Anavar Oranabol Buprenex Fiorinal Tylenol w/ codeine Soma w/ codeine Empirin w/ codeine Vicodin Lortab Lorcet Tussionex Didrex Androderm Delatestryl Butisol

TABLE 11-4 | Classification of Controlled Drugs—cont'd

Classification	Description	Examples Generic	Brand
Schedule IV	Low potential for abuse. Accepted medical use in U.S. Abuse may lead to limited physical or psychological dependence. Telephone and fax orders permitted. If authorized by physician, prescription can be refilled up to 5 times within 6 months of issue date. Prescription expires 6 months from issue date. Manufacturer's label marked C-IV.	**Analgesics** butorphanol pentazocine propoxyphene **Antianxiety Agents** alprazolam buspirone chlordiazepoxide clorazepate diazepam halazepam lorazepam meprobamate oxazepam **Anticonvulsant** clonazepam **CNS Stimulants** modafinil pemoline **Sedative/Hypnotics** chloral hydrate ethchlorvynol flurazepam midazolam phenobarbital temazepam triazolam zaleplon zolpidem **Weight Control Agents** diethylpropion phentermine sibutramine	Stadol Talwin Darvon Darvocet-N Xanax BuSpar Librium Tranxene Valium Paxipam Ativan Equanil Serax Klonopin Provigil Cylert Noctec Placidyl Dalmane Versed Luminal Restoril Halcion Sonata Ambien Tenuate Fastin Meridia
Schedule V	Very low potential for abuse. Accepted medical use in U.S. Abuse may lead to low physical or psychological dependence. Telephone and fax orders permitted. Prescribing polices determined by state and local regulations. In most states: • Number of refills determined by the physician. • Prescription expires 1 year from issue date. • Some are available without prescription to patients > 18 yr. Manufacturer's label marked C-V.	cough suppressants with small amounts of codeine antidiarrheals containing paregoric diphenoxylate/ atropine	Robitussin A-C Cheracol syrup Parepectolin Kapectolin PG Lomotil

To administer prescribe or dispense controlled drugs, the physician must register every year with the Drug Enforcement Administration (DEA). The physician is assigned a registration number known as the **DEA number.** Every time a prescription for a controlled drug is written, the physician must put his or her DEA number in the appropriate space on the prescription blank.

The Prescription

A **prescription** is a physician's order authorizing the dispensing of a drug by a pharmacist. Prescriptions can be authorized in different forms including handwritten, computer-generated, and telephoned or faxed to a pharmacy.

Abbreviations and symbols are usually used to write a prescription. They are also used to record medication information in the patient's chart. Common abbreviations

TABLE 11-5	Common Abbreviations and Symbols Used in Medication Documentation		
Abbreviation or Symbol	**Meaning**	**Abbreviation or Symbol**	**Meaning**
a͞a	of each	OD	right eye
ac	before meals	OS	left eye
AD	right ear	OTC	over-the-counter
ad lib	as desired	OU	in each eye
aq	water	℥ or oz	ounce
admin	administer, administration	p̄	after
AM or a.m.	morning	pc	after meals
APAP	acetaminophen	Pt or pt	patient
AS	left ear	per	by
ASA	aspirin	PM or p.m.	evening
AU	in each ear	po or PO	by mouth
bid	twice a day	prn	as needed
c̄	with	qAM	every morning
cap(s)	capsule(s)	qd	every day
cc	cubic centimeter	qh	every hour
DAW	dispense as written	q (2, 3, 4) h	every (2, 3, 4) hours
dil	dilute	qid	four times a day
ℨ or dr	dram	qod	every other day
elix	elixir	qs	of sufficient quantity
g	gram	Rx	take
gr	grain	s̄	without
gtt(s)	drop(s)	SC or SQ	subcutaneous
h or hr	hour	SL	sublingual
hs	at bedtime	sol	solution
ID	intradermal	ss	one half
IM	intramuscular	STAT	immediately
INH	inhalation	tab(s)	tablet(s)
IV	intravenous	tbsp	tablespoon
kg	kilogram	tid	three times a day
L	liter	tsp	teaspoon
liq	liquid	#	number
♏	minim	×	times
med(s)	medication(s)	∅	no, none
mg	milligram	ī	one
min	minute	īī	two
ml	milliliter	īīī	three
NPO	nothing by mouth	īv̄	four
		v̄	five

used in the medical office for writing prescriptions are included in Table 11-5.

The medical assistant should make sure that all prescription pads are kept in a safe place and out of reach of individuals who may want to obtain drugs illegally. The stock supply of prescription pads should be locked in a drawer.

Parts of a Prescription

A prescription is written on a specially designed form. It includes directions to the pharmacist for filling the prescription and instructions to the patient for taking the medication (Figure 11-2). The specific information that the prescription must include is:

- **Date.** A pharmacist cannot fill a prescription unless the date the prescription was issued is indicated on the form. The reason for this is that a prescription expires after a certain length of time. In most states, a prescription for a drug (with the exception of controlled drugs) expires 1 year from the date of issue. After this time, the prescription (or any refills left on the prescription) cannot be filled.
- **Physician's name, address, telephone number, and fax number.** This information is preprinted on the prescription form. It identifies the physician issuing the prescription and provides the necessary information should the pharmacist have a question and need to contact the medical office.
- **Patient's name and address.** This information is important for insurance billing and in properly dispensing the medication.
- **Patient's age.** The patient's age is important to the pharmacist when he or she double-checks the physician's order to make sure the proper dose is being dispensed. The most common errors in dosage occur among children and the elderly, who may not require the standard dose of a drug because these age-groups metabolize drugs differently. The patient's age also allows the pharmacist to double-check that the drug is age-appropriate for the patient. For example *ciprofloxacin* (e.g., Cipro) should not be taken by children and adolescents because this antibiotic can damage cartilage in individuals younger than 18 years of age.
- **Superscription.** The superscription consists of the symbol Rx. This symbol comes from the Latin word *recipe* and means "take."
- **Inscription.** The inscription states the name of the drug and the dosage (*Example:* Amoxil 250 mg). Most drugs are available in various dosages; therefore it is important that the correct dosage be prescribed. *Example:* Amoxil comes in the following dosages: 125 mg, 250 mg, and 500 mg.
- **Subscription.** The subscription gives directions to the pharmacist. At present, it is generally used to designate the number of doses to be dispensed. To prevent a prescription from being altered illegally, it is recommended

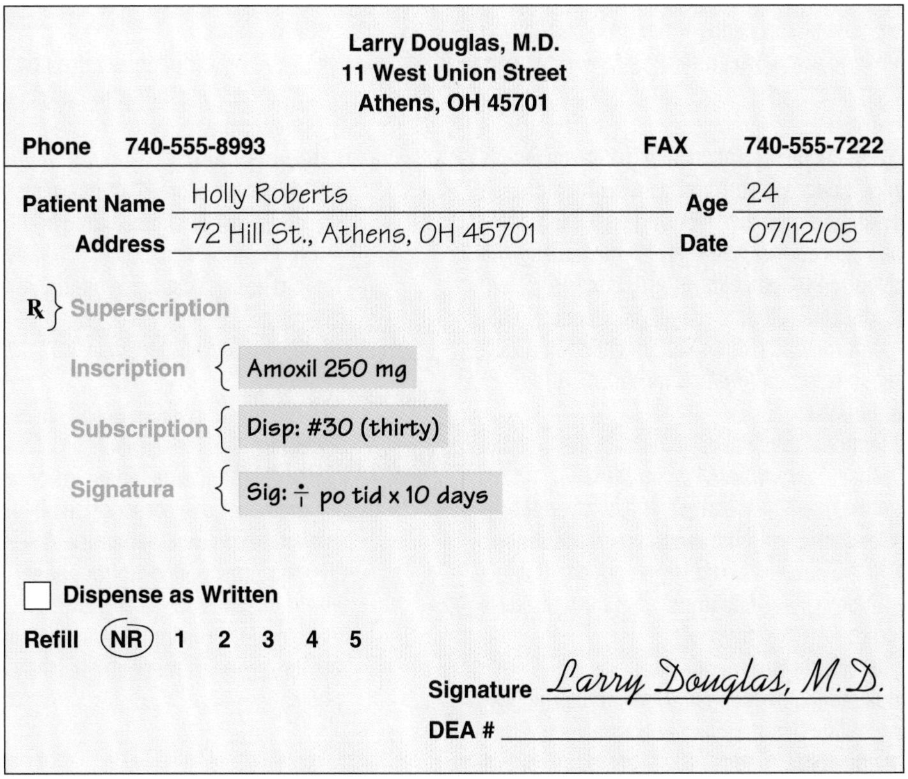
Larry Douglas, M.D.
11 West Union Street
Athens, OH 45701
Phone 740-555-8993 FAX 740-555-7222
Patient Name Holly Roberts Age 24
Address 72 Hill St., Athens, OH 45701 Date 07/12/05
℞ } Superscription
Inscription { Amoxil 250 mg
Subscription { Disp: #30 (thirty)
Signatura { Sig: ī po tid x 10 days
☐ Dispense as Written
Refill (NR) 1 2 3 4 5
Signature Larry Douglas, M.D.
DEA #

Figure 11-2. An example of a prescription.

that both numbers and letters be used to indicate the quantity to be dispensed. *Example:* #30 (thirty).

- **Signatura.** The signatura (abbreviated Sig.) is a Latin term that means "write" or "label" and indicates the information to be included on the medication label. It consists of directions to the patient for taking the medication. The name of the medication is also included on the label so the patient can identify the medication.

- **Refill.** This part of the prescription indicates the number of times the prescription may be refilled.
- **Physician's signature.** A prescription cannot be filled unless it is signed by the physician.
- **DEA number.** The number assigned to the physician by the Drug Enforcement Administration must appear on the prescription for a controlled drug. See Table 11-4 for examples of controlled drugs.

Guidelines for Completing a Prescription Form

- Work in a quiet, well-lit area that is free of distractions.
- Use an indelible black ink pen to write on the form.
- Print all information on the form.
- Make sure that all information is spelled correctly.
- Review the metric notation guidelines presented in the box on p. 456. (Most prescriptions are written in metric units.)
- Always ask the physician if you have questions about the prescription.
- Be sure to complete all of the required information on the form; it includes the following:
  1. **Patient's name, address, and age**
     - Clearly print all of this information on the form. Never leave the address and age categories blank.
  2. **Date**
     - Indicate today's date on the prescription form.
  3. **Name of the medication**
     - The physician may prescribe the medication using either the generic or the brand name.
     - Make sure to spell the name of the drug correctly. If you are unsure, use a drug reference to find the correct spelling of a drug.
  4. **Medication dosage**
     - Never leave a decimal point "naked." If the dosage is a fraction of a unit, a zero *must* be placed before the decimal point as a means of focusing on the fractional dose. This reduces the possibility of misreading the dose as a whole number. *Example:* 0.5 ml (*not* .5 ml).
     - Never place a zero after a decimal point because the decimel point may be overlooked, resulting in a ten-fold overdose error. *Example:* 5 mg (*not* 5.0 mg).
  5. **Quantity to dispense**
     - Use both numbers and letters to indicate the quantity to be dispensed. *Example:* Disp: #30 (thirty).
     - Make sure the quantity is correct. The number of prescribed pills should match the duration of treatment. *Example:* If the patient has been prescribed 3 tablets a day for 7 days, the quantity should be written as follows: Disp: #21 (twenty-one).
  6. **Directions for taking the medication**
     - Clearly indicate the directions for taking the medication. Many authorities recommend writing the directions without abbreviations. *Example:* Sig: Take 1 capsule 3 times a day for 10 days.

- If abbreviations are used, be sure to use only *commonly accepted* abbreviations and make sure to print the information clearly. *Example:* Sig:†̄ cap po tid x 10 days.

7. **Refills**
   - Never leave this category blank.
   - If there are no refills, indicate this clearly on the form. The method for doing this will be based on the setup of the preprinted form.

     Example: Refill: (NR) 1 2 3 4 5
     (on this form the information is circled)

     Example: Refill: Ø
     (on this form the information is written in)

8. ***Dispense as written***
   - If the physician does not allow a substitution (e.g., generic equivalent) for this medication, check this category.

9. **DEA number**
   - If the prescription is for a controlled drug, be sure to clearly indicate the physician's DEA number on the form.

10. **Group practice**
    - If there is more than one physician in the practice, circle (or check) the name of the physician prescribing the medication. This will avoid confusion if the pharmacist cannot read the physician's signature.

    Example:

    James Ortman, MD, (Mark Rothstein, MD,) Richard Bontrager, MD

- Give the prescription to the physician to review and sign.
- Document the prescription order in the patient's medication record if directed by the physician. Some offices use multiple-copy prescription pads. In this case, file the copy of the prescription in the patient's medical record.
- Give the prescription to the patient. Provide the patient with guidelines for taking the medication (see Patient Teaching for Prescription Medications).
- Ask the patient if he or she has any questions about the medication

Generic Prescribing

Generic prescribing means that the physician writes the prescription using the generic rather than the brand name of the drug. Because a number of pharmaceutical manufacturers may produce the same generic drug and sell it under different brand names, price competition often results. If the physician prescribes a drug using its generic name, the pharmacist is permitted to fill it with the drug that offers the best savings to the patient. In addition, most states allow the pharmacist the option of filling the prescription with a chemically equivalent generic drug, even if the prescription has been prescribed by brand name. If the physician wants the prescription be filled with a specific brand of drug, instructions must be indicated on the prescription form such as "Dispense as Written (DAW)," or words of a similar meaning (see Figure 11-2).

Completing a Prescription Form

The physician is responsible for having accurate and pertinent information on the prescription form. If delegated by the physician, a prescription form can be completed by the medical assistant and then signed by the physician. The physician must thoroughly review the prescription before signing it to make sure all of the information is correct. If the medical assistant is delegated this responsibility, he or she must carefully follow some very important guidelines, which are presented in the box on p. 464.

The Medication Record

The medical office may use a preprinted form to record the medications (Rx and OTC) that a patient is taking; vitamin supplements and herbal products the patient is taking should also be recorded on the form. A medication record form (Figure 11-3) includes detailed information about each medication so that the physician can tell at a glance what medications and how much the patient is taking. The medication record is part of the patient's medical record. The medical assistant may be responsible for documenting medication information on this form. Care must be taken to ensure the information is correct and clearly written.

MEDICATION RECORD									
Patient John Walsh						ALLERGY Ø			
Birthdate 6/10/49									

DATE	MEDICATION AND DOSAGE	FREQUENCY	RX	OTC	REFILLS			STOP
2/18/03	Cipro 250mg	ẗ q 12 h po x 10 days	X					2/28/03
6/10/03	Prevacid 15mg	ẗ qd po	X					7/10/03
6/10/03	Lipitor 10mg	ẗ qd po	X		1/6/04			
6/10/03	Prozac 20mg	ẗ qd po	X		1/6/04			
12/3/03	Tobrex Ophthalmic Solution	ẗ gtt q3h OD	X					12/10/03
2/5/04	Echinacea	ẗ qd po		X				
3/15/04	Nitrostat 0.4mg	ẗ prn pain SL Rep q 5 min prn pain, not to exceed 3 tabs	X					
3/15/04	Inderal 40mg	ẗ bid po	X					
3/15/04	St Joseph ASA Enteric Coated 81 mg	ẗ qd po		X				

Figure 11-3. An example of a medication record.

A medication record form typically includes the following information:

- Patient's name and date of birth
- Any drug allergies
- Date the medication was prescribed (Rx) or date the patient started taking the medication (OTC)

- Name and dosage of the medication
- Frequency of administration of the medication
- Route of administration
- Prescription or OTC medication category
- Refills (Rx medication only)
- Date the patient stopped taking the medication

‖ PATIENT **TEACHING**

Prescription Medications

To avoid adverse reactions, teach patients the proper guidelines for taking prescription medication. They include the following:

Know the names of all your medications, both prescription and nonprescription. Nonprescription drugs are known as over-the-counter (OTC) drugs; they are drugs, including vitamin supplements and herbal products, that can be purchased without a prescription.

Know why you are taking each medication. It is important to know the desired therapeutic outcome and the common side effects of each medication, as well as guidelines ("do's and don'ts") to follow when taking the medication.

Take your medication exactly as prescribed, at the right times and in the right amounts. The medication may not work properly if it is not taken as directed. If the dose is too small, the drug may not produce its intended therapeutic effect; exceeding the recommended dosage could result in a toxic effect.

Inform the physician if new symptoms or adverse effects develop when you are taking the medication. The physician may need to change your dosage or prescribe a different medication. There are usually alternative medications that the physician can prescribe to treat your condition.

Take the medication for the prescribed duration of time, even after you begin to feel better. If you don't complete the entire course of drug therapy, your condition may recur. For example, not taking all of a prescribed antibiotic may cause an infection to return, and it may be worse than the first infection.

Be sure to tell the physician if you decide not to take your medication. Otherwise, the physician may think your medication is not working. Not taking a medication prescribed by the physician could be serious because it may allow your condition to worsen.

Do not take additional medications, including OTC medications, without checking with the physician. All drugs, including OTC medications, are designed to have an effect on the body. Some combinations of drugs cause serious reactions. In some cases, one drug cancels the effects of another and prevents it from working.

Never take a medication that was prescribed for someone else. Physicians prescribe medication based on an individual's age, weight, sex, and condition. Taking a medication prescribed for someone else can have serious results.

Keep all medications in their original containers to avoid taking the wrong medication by mistake. Store your medications in their original containers from the pharmacy. Basic information about your medication is on the original container. Medications that are not clearly marked may be taken inadvertently by the wrong person.

Store your medications in a safe place, away from the reach of children. Ask for child-resistant safety closures and make sure the caps of the bottles are closed tightly. Accidental drug poisoning in children is a common and preventable problem. Also, do not take your medication in front of small children because they may want to mimic your behavior.

Store medications in a cool, dry place, or as stated on the label. Don't store capsules or tablets in the bathroom or kitchen because heat or moisture may cause the medication to break down.

Discard unused portions of prescription medications and outdated OTC medications. Medications should be discarded by flushing them down the toilet. Medications that are past their expiration date may produce adverse effects in the body.

What Would You **DO?**
What Would You *Not DO?*

Case Study 2

Linda Cardwell calls the medical office. Her daughter Rachel, 9 years old, was seen in the office 10 days ago. Rachel was diagnosed with strep throat and the physician ordered Amoxil 250 mg tid × 7 days. Mrs. Cardwell says that after 3 days of taking the medication, Rachel was much better, so she stopped giving her the Amoxil because it was causing her to have diarrhea. Mrs. Cardwell says that her 12-year-old son started feeling achy all over and she gave him the Amoxil for 2 days, and it seemed to help. She also says that her husband started complaining of sinus problems, so she also gave him the Amoxil for 2 days. Mrs. Cardwell says that now Rachel's throat is hurting again and she has a fever. She wants to know if Rachel has developed another case of strep throat. Mrs. Cardwell says she doesn't know what to do because she doesn't have any Amoxil left to give Rachel.

Factors Affecting Drug Action

Therapeutic Effect

Each drug has an intended therapeutic effect, in other words, the reason the patient takes the medication. Certain factors affect the therapeutic action of drugs in the body, causing patients to respond differently to the same drug. Because of this, the drug therapy may need to be adjusted to meet these variations, which include the following:

Age. Children and elderly people tend to respond more strongly to drugs than do young and middle-age adults. The physician may calculate smaller doses for very young and old patients.

Route of Administration. Medications administered by different routes are absorbed at different rates. Drugs administered orally are absorbed slowly because they must first be digested. Parenterally administered drugs are absorbed more quickly than orally administered drugs because they are injected directly into the body.

Size. A patient's body size has an effect on drug action. A thin person may require a smaller quantity of a drug, and an obese person may require more.

Time of Administration. A drug administered through the oral route is absorbed more rapidly when the stomach is empty than when it contains food. A drug may not produce the desired effect or may be absorbed too slowly if it is taken when food is present. However, some drugs irritate the stomach's lining and therefore must be taken with food. The drug package insert or a drug reference should always be consulted to determine when a drug should be taken.

Tolerance. A patient taking a certain drug over a period of time may develop a tolerance to it. This means that the same dose of a drug no longer produces the desired effect after prolonged administration. The physician should be notified to determine whether a change of drug or dosage is needed.

Undesirable Effects of Drugs

A drug may cause undesirable effects, which may occur immediately or be delayed hours or even days following administration of the medication. Undesirable effects of drugs include those discussed in the following section.

Adverse Reactions

The majority of drugs produce unintended and undesirable effects known as **adverse reactions.** Adverse reactions are secondary effects that occur along with the therapeutic effect of the drug. Some adverse reactions, referred to as *side effects,* are harmless and therefore often tolerated by the patient in order to obtain the therapeutic effect of the drug. For example, most patients are willing to tolerate the dry mouth and drowsiness that may accompany an antihistamine in order to obtain its therapeutic effect. Other adverse reactions, such as a drop in blood pressure or an allergic reaction, can be harmful to the patient and warrant discontinuing the medication.

Drug Interactions

When certain medications are used at the same time, drug interactions may produce undesirable effects. The medical assistant should inquire about other medications the patient is taking and record this information in the patient's chart for review by the physician.

Allergic Drug Reaction

The patient may exhibit an allergic reaction to a drug. The reaction is often mild and may take the form of a rash, rhinitis, or pruritus. Occasionally a patient has a severe allergic reaction that occurs suddenly and immediately. It is then known as an **anaphylactic reaction.**

An anaphylactic reaction is the least common but the most serious type of allergic reaction. Symptoms begin with sneezing, urticaria (hives), itching, *angioedema, erythema,* and disorientation. Erythema is the reddening of the skin caused by dilation of superficial blood vessels in the skin. Angioedema is a localized urticaria of the deeper tissues of the body.

If not treated, the symptoms of anaphylaxis quickly increase in severity and progress to dyspnea, cyanosis, and

MEMORIES From EXTERNSHIP

THERESA CLINE: I can clearly remember the first time I gave an injection at my externship site. I was worried that I would forget how to give an injection and look stupid in front of my externship supervisor and the patient. What made things even worse is that the patient was a woman with very thin arms. I was giving her a flu shot and I was so scared that the needle would hit her bone even though I was only using a one-inch needle. When I walked into the room, my supervisor told the woman that I was a student and asked her if it was all right if I gave her the flu injection. The woman laughed and said, "Well, I guess so." That made me feel even more nervous. The patient then asked if it was my first shot. I told her "yes" and she said, "Just don't hurt me." When it came time to give the injection, everything that I had ever learned about injections came back to me. I gave the injection and the woman told me I did a good job and that she didn't even feel it. That made me feel so good! My supervisor said, "If you can give a shot to her, you can give a shot to anyone." Every injection after that was a "piece of cake." I've learned just to take a deep breath before each difficult situation encountered in the office and everything will work out.

shock. Blood pressure decreases, and the pulse becomes weak and thready. Convulsions, loss of consciousness, and death may occur if treatment is not initiated promptly.

To prevent an anaphylactic reaction to a drug or to reduce its danger, the medical assistant should stay with the patient after administration of the medication. The medical assistant should be especially alert for signs of an anaphylactic reaction after administering allergy skin tests or a penicillin or allergy injection. If a reaction occurs, the physician should be notified immediately so he or she can begin treatment immediately. Treatment generally consists of one or more injections of epinephrine, depending on the severity of the reaction. Epinephrine goes to work immediately to reverse the life-threatening symptoms of anaphylaxis. Once the patient is stabilized, he or she is usually given an injection of an antihistamine. The antihistamine takes longer to begin working but helps alleviate urticaria, itching, angioedema, and erythema. The medical assistant must make sure that an ample supply of epinephrine is on hand at all times. Many offices maintain emergency carts for this purpose.

Idiosyncratic Reaction

An idiosyncratic reaction is an abnormal or peculiar response to a drug that is unexplained and unpredictable. Elderly patients are most prone to idiosyncratic reactions to drugs and therefore should be monitored very closely when they are taking a new medication.

Guidelines for Preparation and Administration of Medication

To prevent medication errors, the medical assistant should follow these guidelines when preparing and administering any drug:

1. Work in a quiet, well-lit atmosphere that is free of distractions.
2. Always ask if you have a question about the medication order.
3. Know the drug to be given.
4. Select the proper drug. Check the label of the medication three times: as it is taken from its storage location, before preparing the medication, and after preparing the medication. Do not use a drug if the label is missing or is difficult to read.
5. Do not use a drug if the color has changed, if a precipitate has formed, or if it has an unusual odor.
6. Check the expiration date before preparing the drug for administration.
7. Prepare the proper dose of the drug. The term **dose** refers to the quantity of a drug to be administered at one time. Each medication has a *dosage range,* or range of quantities of the drug that can produce therapeutic effects. It is important to administer the exact dose of the drug. If the dose is too small, it will not produce a therapeutic effect, and a dose that is too large could be harmful or even fatal to the patient.
8. Be sure to correctly identify the patient so that the drug is administered to the intended patient.
9. Before administering the medication, check the patient's records or question the patient to make sure that he or she is not allergic to the medication.
10. If you are giving an injection, determine the appropriate route and site at which to administer the injection; the route and site are dictated by the type of injection being given. For example, an allergy injection is given through the subcutaneous route and an antibiotic injection is given through the intramuscular route. The site must be free from abrasions, lesions, bruises, and edema.
11. Use the proper technique to administer the medication.
12. Stay with the patient after administering the medication.
13. Document information properly in the patient's chart immediately after administering the drug. Make sure the recording is clear and legible to avoid confusion by others who will read it. Include the date and time, the name of the medication, the dose given, the route of administration, the site of administration, and any unusual observations or patient reactions. Sign the recording with your name and credentials. If you administer a medication that contains a fraction of a gram, place a 0 before the decimal point (e.g., 0.5 mg, *not* .5 mg) so that the dosage is not misread as 5 mg. On the other hand, a decimal point and a zero should *never* be placed after a whole number. The decimal point may be overlooked and misread, resulting in a tenfold overdose error (e.g., 20 mg, *not* 20.0 mg).
14. Always follow the seven "rights" of preparing and administering medication in the medical office:

Right drug	Right dose
Right time	Right patient
Right route	Right technique
Right documentation	

Oral Administration

The oral route is the most convenient and the most used method of administering medication. **Oral administration** means that the drug is given by mouth in either a solid form (such as a tablet or capsule) or a liquid form (such as a suspension or a syrup). Absorption of most oral medication takes place in the small intestine, although some may be absorbed in the mouth and stomach.

Many patients find it easier to swallow a tablet or capsule with a glass of water. Water should not be offered after the patient has received a cough syrup, however, because the water would dilute the medication's beneficial effects. Unless the patient has a malabsorption problem or is unable to swallow, the oral route is considered the safest and most desirable route for administering medication. Procedure 11-1 outlines the procedure for the administration of oral medications.

PROCEDURE 11-1   Administering Oral Medication

Outcome Administer oral solid and liquid medications.

Equipment/Supplies:
- Medication ordered by the physician
- Medicine cup
- Medication tray

1. **Procedural Step.** Sanitize your hands.
2. **Procedural Step.** Assemble the equipment.
3. **Procedural Step.** Work in a quiet, well-lit atmosphere.
   Principle. Good lighting aids the medical assistant in reading the medication label.
4. **Procedural Step.** Select the correct medication from the shelf. Compare the medication with the physician's instructions. Check the drug label three times: while removing the medication from storage, while preparing the medication, and after preparing the medication. Check the expiration date.
   Principle. If the medication is outdated, consult the physician because it may produce undesirable effects for which the medical assistant could be held responsible. To prevent a drug error, the medication should be carefully compared with the physician's instructions.
5. **Procedural Step.** Calculate the correct dose to be given, if necessary.
6. **Procedural Step.** Remove the bottle cap, touching the outside of the lid only.
   Principle. Touching the inside of the lid will contaminate it.
7. **Procedural Step.** Check the drug label and pour the medication.
   Solid Medications. Pour the correct number of capsules or tablets into the bottle cap. Transfer the medication to a medicine cup, being careful not to touch the inside of the cup.

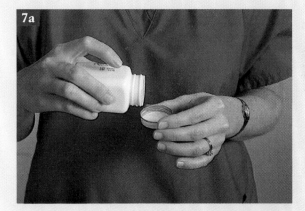

Principle. Pouring the medication into the lid prevents contamination of the medication and lid.

Liquid Medications. Place the lid of the bottle upside down on a flat surface with the open end facing up. Palm the surface of the label. With the opposite hand, place the thumbnail at the proper calibration on the medicine cup, and hold the cup at eye level. Pour the medication and read the dose at the lowest level of the meniscus. (The meniscus is the curved surface of the liquid in a container. When a liquid is poured into a medicine cup, capillary action will cause the liquid in contact with

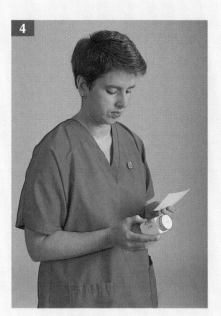

Continued

PROCEDURE 11-1 Administering Oral Medication—Cont'd

the cup to be drawn upward, resulting in a curved surface in the middle.)
Principle. Placing the bottle cap with the open end up prevents contamination of the inside of the cap.

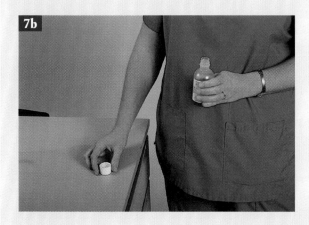

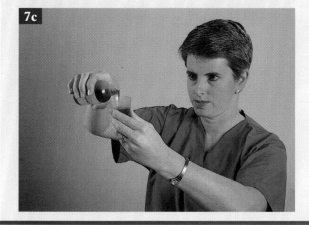

Palming the medication label prevents the medication from dripping on the label and obscuring it.

8. **Procedural Step.** Replace the bottle cap, and check the drug label to make sure it is the correct medication. Return the medication to its storage location.

9. **Procedural Step.** Greet and identify the patient. Introduce yourself and explain the procedure. Explain the purpose of administering the medication.
Principle. It is crucial that no error be made in patient identity.

10. **Procedural Step.** Hand the medicine cup containing the medication to the patient, along with a glass of water. (If the medication is a cough syrup, do not offer water.)
Principle. Water helps the patient swallow the medication.

11. **Procedural Step.** Remain with the patient until the medication is swallowed. If the patient experiences any unusual reaction, notify the physician.

12. **Procedural Step.** Sanitize your hands.

13. **Procedural Step.** Chart the procedure. Include the date and time, the name of the medication, the dosage given, the route of administration, and any significant observations or patient reactions. The Latin abbreviation *po,* which means "by mouth," can be used to indicate the route of administration.

CHARTING EXAMPLE

Date	
2/12/05	9:30 a.m. Acetaminophen, 650 mg, po.
	————————————————— T. Cline, CMA

Parenteral Administration

The parenteral route of drug administration has several advantages. Medications given subcutaneously, intramuscularly, and intravenously are absorbed more rapidly and completely than those given orally. In some cases, the parenteral route is the only way a drug can be given. For example, if the patient is unconscious or has a gastric disturbance such as nausea or vomiting, the parenteral route would be used. If the state laws permit, the medical assistant is usually responsible for administering subcutaneous,

intramuscular, and intradermal injections. **Intravenous injections** are given when an immediate effect is needed; in the medical office, they are usually administered by the physician in an emergency situation.

The parenteral route also has disadvantages, such as pain and the possibility of infection as a result of breaking the skin. The medical assistant can minimize pain by inserting and withdrawing the needle quickly and smoothly, and by withdrawing the needle at the same angle as for insertion.

If injections are given repeatedly (e.g., allergy injections), the sites should be rotated to prevent the overuse of one site, which may cause irritation and tissue damage. Rotating sites also allows better absorption of the drug. When recording the procedure in the patient's chart, the medical assistant must include the site of the injection (e.g., right upper arm, left dorsogluteal). This assists in proper site rotation for patients who receive repeated injections. In addition, the information provides a reference point should a problem arise with the injection site.

Medical asepsis must be used when parenteral medications are administered. In addition, the needle and the inside of the syringe must remain sterile. These practices reduce the danger of microorganisms entering the patient's body during the administration of medication. The medical assistant must be sure to follow the OSHA Standard when administering medication as a means of protecting oneself from bloodborne pathogens (see Chapter 2). Procedure 11-2 describes how to prepare an injection.

Parts of a Needle and Syringe

Needle

The needle consists of several parts (Figure 11-4). The *hub* of the needle fits onto the top of the syringe. The *shaft* is inserted into the body tissue. The opening in the shaft of the needle, known as the *lumen,* is continuous with the needle hub. Medication flows from the syringe and through the lumen of the needle. The *point* of the needle is located at the end of the needle shaft. The point is sharp so that it can penetrate body tissues easily. The top of the needle is slanted and is called the *bevel.* The bevel is designed to make a narrow, slitlike opening in the skin. This narrow opening closes quickly when the needle is removed to prevent leakage of medication, and it also heals quickly.

Each needle has a certain **gauge;** needle gauges for administering medication range between 18 and 27. The gauge of a needle is determined by the diameter of the lumen: As the size of the gauge increases, the diameter of the lumen decreases. Thus a needle with a gauge of 23 has a smaller lumen diameter than a needle with a gauge of 21. Thick or oily preparations must be given with a large lumen because they are too thick to pass through a smaller one. A needle with a larger lumen makes a larger needle track in the tissues. To reduce pain and tissue damage, a needle with the smallest gauge appropriate for the solution and route of administration is always chosen. The length of the needle ranges between 3/8 and 3 inches; the length used is based on the type of injection being given. For instance, the needle used to give an intramuscular injection must be longer than one used for a subcutaneous injection so that it penetrates deeply enough to reach the muscle tissue.

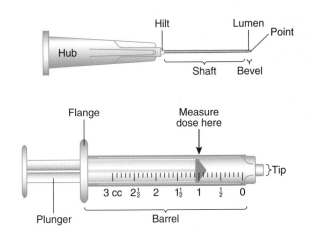

Figure 11-4. Diagram of a needle and a 3-cc syringe, with parts identified.

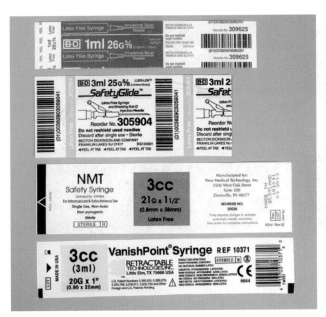

Figure 11-5. Examples of syringe and needle packages labeled according to contents.

Syringe

The syringe is used for inserting fluids into the body. It is made of plastic and must be disposed of after one use. The syringe with an attached needle is packaged in a cellophane wrapper or a rigid plastic container. Information regarding the syringe's capacity and the needle's length and gauge is printed on the wrapper of the syringe and needle (Figure 11-5). Syringes and needles are also available in separate packages. In this case, the medical assistant must attach a needle to the syringe before drawing medication into the syringe.

The parts of a syringe are the barrel, flange, and plunger (see Figure 11-4). The *barrel* of the syringe holds the medication and contains calibrated markings to measure the proper amount of medication. Most syringes are calibrated in cubic centimeters; the unit of measurement used most often to administer parenteral medication. The medical assistant should become familiar with reading the graduated scales on syringes. At the end of the barrel is a rim known as the *flange*, which helps in injecting the medication. The flange also prevents the syringe from rolling when it is placed on a flat surface. The *plunger* is a movable cylinder that slides back and forth in the barrel. It is used to draw medication into the syringe when preparing an injection and to push medication out of the syringe when administering an injection.

Various types of syringes are available to administer injections. The choice is based on the type of injection being given (e.g., tuberculin skin test, allergy injection, antibiotic injection) and amount of medication being administered. The types of syringes used most often in the medical office include hypodermic, insulin, and tuberculin (Figure 11-6).

Hypodermic syringes are available in 2-, 2.5-, 3-, and 5-cc sizes and are calibrated in cubic centimeters. They are commonly used to administer intramuscular injections.

The insulin syringe is designed especially for the administration of an insulin injection, and the barrel is calibrated in units. The most common type is the U-100 syringe, which is calibrated into 100 units in increments of 2.

Tuberculin syringes are employed to administer a very small dose of medication, such as when administering a tuberculin test. The tuberculin syringe has a capacity of 1 cc, and the calibrations are divided into tenths (0.10) and hundredths (0.01) of a cubic centimeter.

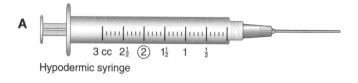

A
Hypodermic syringe

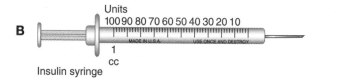

B
Insulin syringe

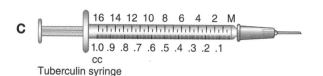

C
Tuberculin syringe

Figure 11-6. Various types of syringe used to administer injections. **A,** Hypodermic. **B,** Insulin (U-100). **C,** Tuberculin.

Syringes are also available with capacities of 10, 20, 30, 50, and 60 cc; however, they are not used for administering medication but rather for medical treatments such as irrigating wounds and draining fluid from cysts.

Safety Engineered Syringes

OSHA stipulates requirements to reduce needlestick and other sharps injuries among health care workers. As discussed in Chapter 2, employers are required to evaluate and implement commercially available safer medical devices that reduce occupational exposure to the lowest extent feasible.

Safer medical devices include safety engineered syringes. *Safety engineered syringes* incorporate a built-in safety feature to reduce the risk of a needlestick injury. Figure 11-7 illustrates types of safety engineered syringes and the methods for using them.

Preparation of Parenteral Medication

Medication used for injections is available in various types of dispensing unit: vials, ampules, and prefilled syringes and cartridges.

Vials

A **vial** is a closed glass container with a rubber stopper; a soft metal or plastic cap protects the rubber stopper and must be removed the first time the medication is used. An injectable medication may be available in a single-dose vial, a multiple-dose vial, or both (Figure 11-8).

Before the medication can be withdrawn, some vials require mixing (e.g., reconstituting a powdered drug or mixing a vial that separates upon standing). Vials that require mixing should be rolled between the hands rather than shaken because shaking will cause the medication to foam, thus creating air bubbles that may enter the syringe when the medication is withdrawn.

To remove medication from a vial, an amount of air exactly equal to the amount of liquid to be removed is injected into the vial. The air should be inserted above the fluid level to avoid creating bubbles in the medication. If air is not injected first, a partial vacuum will be created and it will be difficult to remove the medication. During the withdrawal of medication, the needle opening should be inserted below the fluid level to prevent the entrance of air bubbles. Air bubbles can be removed by tapping the barrel of the syringe with the fingertips. If the bubbles are allowed to remain, they take up space that the medication should occupy, which would prevent the patient from receiving the full dose of medication.

Ampules

An **ampule** is a small, sealed glass container that holds a single dose of medication (see Figure 11-8). An ampule has a constriction in the stem, known as the neck, that helps in opening it. Before opening, make sure that there is no medication in the stem by tapping it lightly.

A colored ring around the neck indicates where the ampule is prescored for easy opening. The ampule is opened by holding it firmly with gauze and breaking off the stem with a strong steady pressure.

A hazard with medication in ampules is the possibility of small glass particles getting into the ampule as the stem is broken off. When the medication is withdrawn into the syringe, the glass particles might also be withdrawn.

To prevent this problem, a needle with a filter should be used that filters out small glass particles (Figure 11-9).

The needle opening is inserted into the base of the ampule below the fluid level to withdraw medication. To prevent contamination, the needle should not be permitted to touch the outside of the ampule. Air should never be injected into the ampule because it could force out some of the medication.

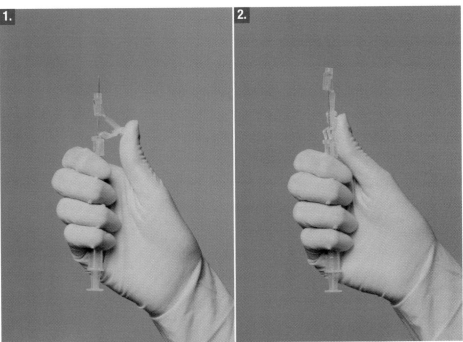

A. Safety Engineered Syringes Hinged Shield Syringe
(Becton-Dickinson Safety Glide Syringe)

1. After administering the injection, push the lever of the hinged-shield forward.

2. Continue pushing until the needle tip is fully covered by the shield and then discard the syringe in a biohazard sharps container.

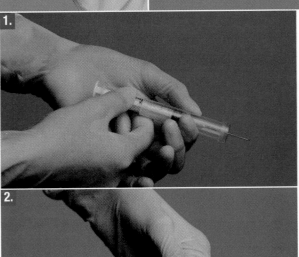

B. Sliding Shield Syringe
(Monoject Safety Syringe)

1. After administering the injection, extend the sliding shield forward fully until a click is heard.

2. Lock the shield by twisting it in either direction until a click is heard. Discard the syringe in a biohazard sharps container.

Figure 11-7. Safety engineered syringes.

Continued

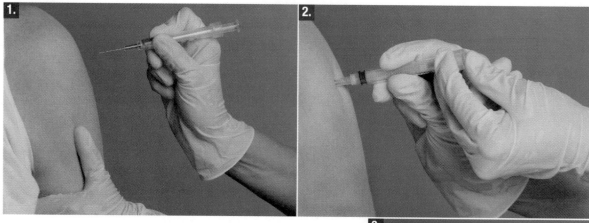

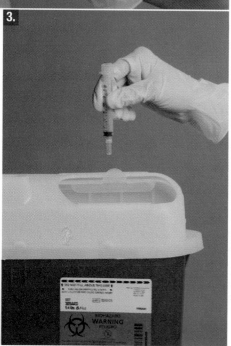

C. Retractable Needle
(Vanish Point Syringe)

1. Administer the injection following proper technique.

2. After administering the medication, continue depressing the plunger with the thumb. Use firm pressure past the point of initial resistance.
   This action delivers the full dose of medication to the patient and then activates the needle retraction device causing the needle to automatically retract from the patient's skin and into the barrel of the syringe.

3. Discard the syringe in a biohazard sharps container.

Figure 11-7, cont'd. Safety engineered syringes.

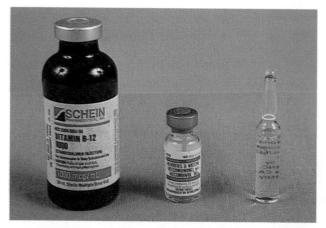

Figure 11-8. The multiple-dose vial *(left)* and the single-dose vial *(middle)* consist of a closed glass container with a rubber stopper. The ampule *(right)* consists of a small, sealed glass container that holds a single dose of medication.

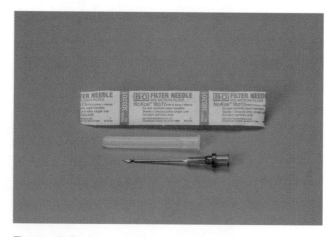

Figure 11-9. Filter needle used to withdraw medication from an ampule.

Prefilled Syringes and Cartridges

Some drugs come in *prefilled disposable syringes,* or cartridges. Using this type of dispensing unit does not require drawing up the medication. The name of the drug, the dose, and the expiration date are printed on the syringe or cartridge (Figure 11-10). An example is the Tubex Injector, which consists of a reusable device that holds a Tubex sterile cartridge-needle unit. The procedure for administering an injection using the Tubex Injector is presented in Figure 11-11.

Storage

The medical assistant should always read the drug package insert to determine the proper method for storing each parenteral medication because improper storage may alter the effectiveness of the medication.

Reconstitution of Powdered Drugs

Some parenteral medications are stable for only a short time in liquid form; therefore these medications are prepared and stored in powdered form and require the addition of a liquid before administration. The process of adding a liquid to a powdered drug is known as reconstitution. The liquid used to reconstitute a powdered drug is known as the *diluent* and usually consists of sterile water or normal saline. The powdered drug is contained in a single-dose or multiple-dose vial and is accompanied by specific instructions for reconstitution. An example of a parenteral medication that requires reconstitution is the measles, mumps, and rubella (MMR) immunization (Figure 11-12). The procedure for reconstituting powdered drugs is outlined in Procedure 11-3.

Subcutaneous Injections

A **subcutaneous injection** is made into the subcutaneous tissue, which consists of adipose (fat) tissue and is located just under the skin (see Figure 11-13). Subcutaneous tissue is located all over the body; however, certain sites are more commonly used. They are located where bones and

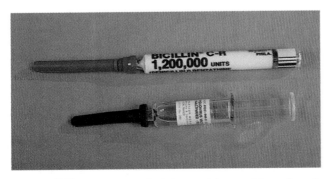

Figure 11-10. *Top,* A prefilled disposable cartridge of medication. Disposable cartridges must be inserted into a specially designed syringe for administration of the injection. *Bottom,* A prefilled disposable syringe.

blood vessels are not near the surface of the skin. These sites include the upper lateral part of the arms, the anterior thigh, the upper back, and the abdomen (Figure 11-14). Absorption of medication from a subcutaneous injection occurs mainly through capillaries, resulting in a slower absorption rate than with intramuscular injections. To ensure proper absorption, tissue that is grossly adipose, hardened, inflamed, or edematous should not be used as an injection site.

The needle length varies from $\frac{1}{2}$ to $\frac{5}{8}$ inch, and the gauge ranges from 23 to 25. Elderly and dehydrated patients tend to have less subcutaneous tissue, and obese patients have more. The length of the needle should be adjusted accordingly to make sure the medication is administered into the subcutaneous tissue and not into muscle tissue.

Subcutaneous tissue is sensitive to irritating solutions and large volumes of medications; therefore drugs given subcutaneously must be isotonic, nonirritating, nonviscous, and water soluble. The amount of medication injected through the subcutaneous route should not exceed 1 cc. More than this amount results in pressure on sensory nerve endings, causing discomfort and pain.

Medications commonly administered through the subcutaneous route include epinephrine, insulin, and allergy injections. Patients who receive allergy injections must wait in the medical office for 15 to 20 minutes following the injection to be observed for unusual reactions. Procedure 11-4 outlines the administration of a subcutaneous injection.

Intramuscular Injections

Intramuscular injections are made into the muscular layer of the body, which lies below the skin and subcutaneous layers (see Figure 11-13). The amount of medication that can be injected into muscle tissue is more than the amount that can be injected into subcutaneous tissue. An amount up to 3 cc can be injected into the gluteal or vastus lateralis muscles, although older and very thin adults are able to tolerate only 2 cc or less in these sites.

Absorption is more rapid by this route than by the subcutaneous route because there are more blood vessels in muscle tissue. Medication that is irritating to subcutaneous tissue is often given intramuscularly because there are fewer nerve endings in deep muscle tissue. Most parenteral medications administered in the medical office are given through the intramuscular route; examples include immunizations, antibiotics, injectable contraceptives, vitamin B_{12}, and corticosteroids.

The length of the needle varies from 1 to 3 inches; a $1\frac{1}{2}$-inch needle is typically used for an average-sized adult. The gauge of the needle ranges from 18 to 23, depending on the viscosity of the medication. Procedure 11-5 outlines the technique for the administration of an intramuscular injection.

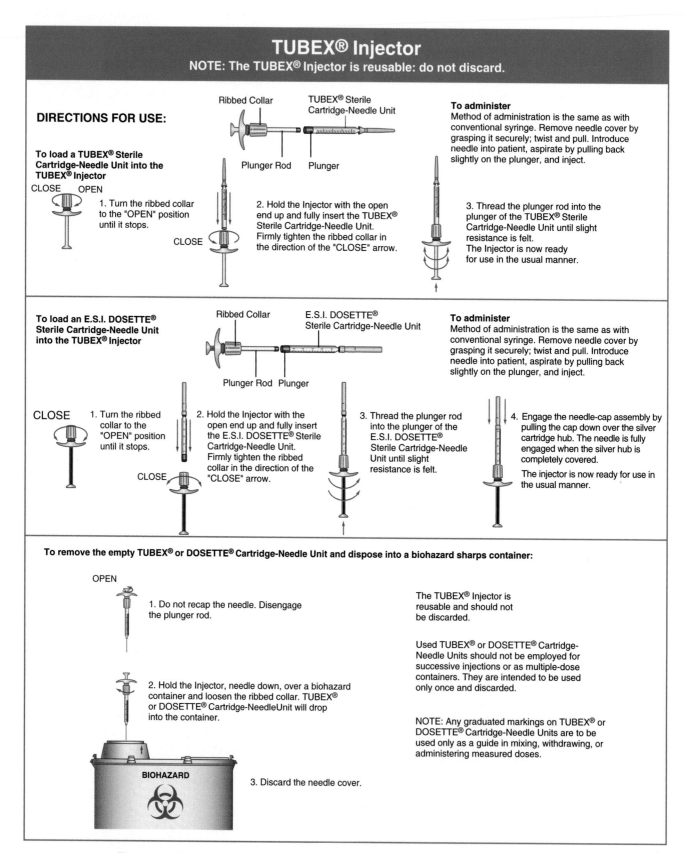

Figure 11-11. Procedure for administering an injection using a Tubex Injector. (Courtesy ESI Lederle, Division of American Home Products Corporation, St. Davids, PA.)

Intramuscular Injection Sites

The sites chosen for intramuscular injections are away from large nerves and blood vessels. The medical assistant should practice locating these sites to become familiar with them. The area should always be fully exposed to permit clear visualization of the injection site. Intramuscular injection sites are described in the following sections.

Dorsogluteal Site

The dorsogluteal site is often used to administer intramuscular injections. In adults and children older than 3 years of age, the gluteal muscles are well developed and can ab-

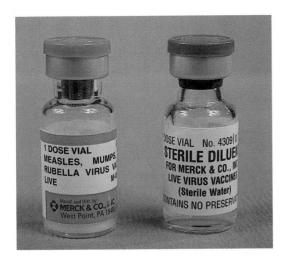

Figure 11-12. The measles, mumps, and rubella (MMR) vaccine is a parenteral medication that requires reconstitution before administration. The vial on the left contains the medication in powdered form, and the vial on the right contains the sterile diluent.

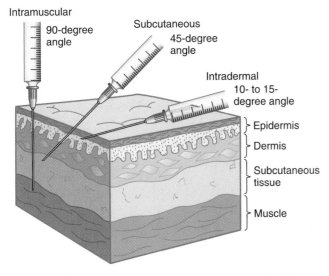

Figure 11-13. Angle of insertion for intradermal, subcutaneous, and intramuscular injections.

sorb a large amount of medication. The patient should lie on the abdomen with the toes pointed inward, which aids in relaxation of the gluteal muscles. The medication is injected into the upper outer quadrant of the gluteal area, in the area located above and outside a diagonal line drawn from the greater trochanter to the posterior superior iliac spine. These landmarks should be identified through palpation. The medical assistant must be *extremely* careful to maintain the proper boundary lines to avoid injection into the sciatic nerve or superior gluteal artery (Figure 11-15).

Deltoid Site

The deltoid area is easily accessible and can be used when the patient is sitting or lying down. This site is small because major nerves and blood vessels surround it, and large amounts of medication (no more than 1 cc) and repeated injections should not be given in this area. The medication is injected into the deltoid muscle.

The medical assistant should make sure that the entire arm is exposed by having the patient's sleeve completely pulled up or by removing the sleeve from the arm if it cannot be pulled up. A tight sleeve constricts the arm and causes unnecessary bleeding from the puncture site.

The deltoid site is located by palpating the lower edge of the acromion process, which forms the base of a triangle in line with the midpoint of the lateral side of the arm, opposite the axilla (see Figure 11-15). This site may also be located by placing your four fingers horizontally across the deltoid muscle with the top finger along the acromion process. The injection site is located three finger widths below the acromion process.

Vastus Lateralis Site

The vastus lateralis is used because it is away from major nerves and blood vessels and is a relatively thick muscle (see Figure 11-15). This site is particularly desirable for infants and children younger than 3 years of age whose gluteal muscles are not yet well developed. The area is bounded by the midanterior thigh on the front of the leg and the midlateral thigh on the side. The proximal boundary is a

---

What Would You DO?
What Would You Not DO?

Case Study 3

Danielle Roush, 16 years old, has come to the office with her mother. Danielle is complaining of a painful sore throat, fever, and aching in both of her ears. The physician diagnoses her with strep throat and otitis media, and orders 2 cc of an antibiotic to be given deep IM. Danielle says that she's a basketball player and on the varsity team at her high school. She says that she is always too embarrassed to change or take a shower in front of the other girls because she's so skinny. Danielle would like to have the injection in her arm because it would be too embarrassing to have it in the buttocks.

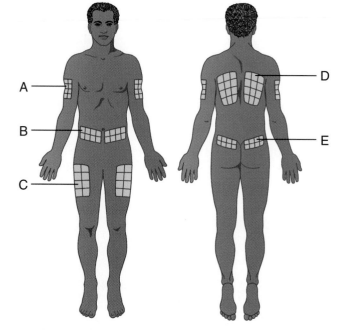

Figure 11-14. Common sites for subcutaneous injections. **A,** Upper outer arm; **B,** lower abdomen; **C,** upper outer thigh; **D,** upper back; and **E,** flank region.

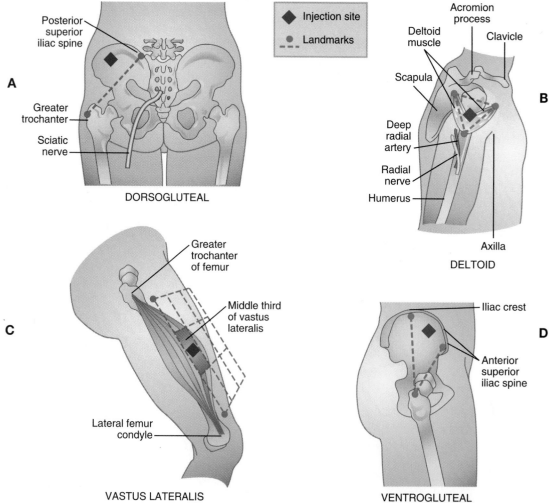

Figure 11-15. Sites of intramuscular injections. **A,** Dorsogluteal muscle; **B,** deltoid muscle; **C,** vastus lateralis; and **D,** ventrogluteal muscle. (From Leahy JM, Kizilay PE: *Foundations of Nursing Practice: A Nursing Process Approach.* Philadelphia, 1988, W. B. Saunders.)

hand's breadth below the greater trochanter, and the distal boundary is a hand's breadth above the knee. It is easier to give an injection in the vastus lateralis if the patient is lying down, but a sitting position can also be used.

Ventrogluteal Site

The ventrogluteal site is growing in acceptability as an IM injection site because the subcutaneous layer is relatively small, and the muscle layer is thick. The site is located away from major nerves and blood vessels. Through palpation, the greater trochanter of the femur, the anterior superior iliac spine, and the iliac crest can be located. If the injection is being made into the patient's left side, the palm of the right hand is placed on the greater trochanter, and the index finger is placed on the anterior superior iliac spine. The middle finger is spread posteriorly as far as possible away from the index finger, to touch the iliac crest. The hand position is reversed if the injection is being made into the patient's right side. The triangle formed by the fingers is the area into which the injection is given.

An injection into the ventrogluteal site can be administered when the patient is lying prone or on one side (see Figure 11-15).

Z-Track Method

Medications that are irritating to subcutaneous and skin tissue or that discolor the skin must be given intramuscularly using the Z-track method; one medication that is administered by this method is iron dextran. The dorsogluteal, ventrogluteal, and vastus lateralis sites can all be used as areas to administer a Z-track injection.

The Z-track method is very similar to the intramuscular injection procedure, except that the skin and subcutaneous tissue at the injection site are pulled to the side before the needle is inserted. This causes a zigzag path through the tissues once the skin is released, preventing the medication from reaching the subcutaneous layer or skin surface by sealing off the needle track (Figure 11-16). The procedure for administering medication using the Z-track method is outlined in Procedure 11-6.

Text continued on p. 489

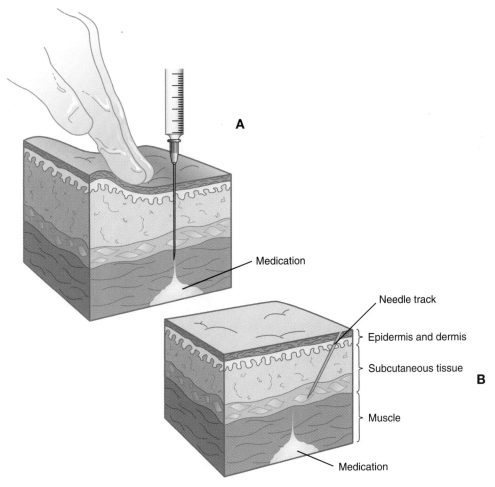

Figure 11-16. The Z-track intramuscular injection method. **A,** The skin and subcutaneous tissue are pulled to the side before the needle is inserted. **B,** This causes a zigzag path through the tissue once the skin is released, which seals off the needle track.

PROCEDURE 11-2   Preparing the Injection

Outcome Prepare an injection from an ampule and a vial.

Equipment/Supplies:

- Medication ordered by the physician
- Appropriate needle and syringe
- Antiseptic wipe
- Medication tray

1. **Procedural Step.** Sanitize your hands.
2. **Procedural Step.** Assemble the equipment.
3. **Procedural Step.** Work in a quiet and well-lit atmosphere.

   Principle. Good lighting aids the medical assistant in reading the medication label.

4. **Procedural Step.** Select the proper medication. Compare the medication with the physician's instructions. Check the drug label three times: while removing the medication from storage, before withdrawing the medication into the syringe, and after preparing the medication. Check the expiration date.

   Principle. The medication should be carefully identified to prevent the administration of the wrong medication. Outdated medication should not be used because it could produce undesirable effects.

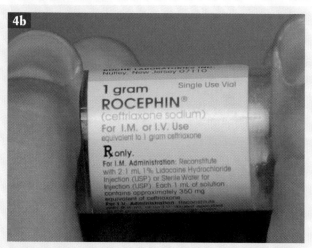

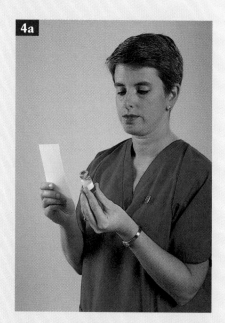

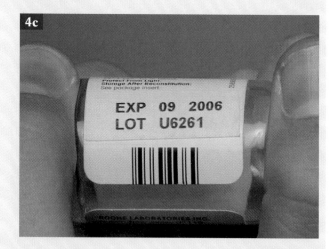

5. **Procedural Step.** Calculate the correct dose to be given, if necessary. If you have any questions regarding the administration of the medication, check the package insert accompanying the drug.

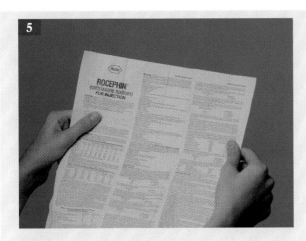

6. **Procedural Step.** Open the syringe and needle package. If necessary, assemble the needle and syringe.
Principle. Disposable needles and syringes may come together already assembled in a package, or in separate packages that require assembly of the needle and syringe.

7. **Procedural Step.** Check to make sure that the needle is attached firmly to the syringe by loosening the guard on the needle, grasping the needle at the hub, and tightening it. Break the seal on the syringe by moving the plunger back and forth several times.

8. **Procedural Step.** Check the drug label again to make sure it is the correct medication.

9. **Procedural Step.** Withdraw the medication following the steps below.

Withdrawing Medication From a Vial

a. **Procedural Step.** Remove the soft metal or plastic cap protecting the rubber stopper of the vial. Open the antiseptic; wipe and cleanse the rubber stopper.
Principle. Cleansing the top of the vial removes dust and bacteria.

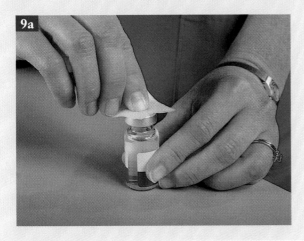

b. **Procedural Step.** Remove the needle guard. Pull back on the plunger to draw an amount of air into the syringe equal to the amount of medication to be withdrawn from the vial.
Principle. Air must first be injected into the vial to prevent the formation of a partial vacuum in the vial, which would make it difficult to remove medication.

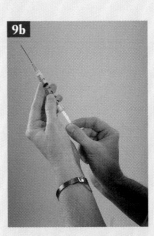

c. **Procedural Step.** Place the vial in an upright position on a flat surface. Using moderate pressure, insert the needle through the center of the rubber stopper at a 90-degree angle, until it reaches the empty space between the stopper and fluid level. Be careful not to bend the needle. Push down on the plunger to inject the air into the vial, making sure to keep the needle opening above the fluid level. (*Note:* If you are using a retractable safety syringe, do not push too hard on the plunger to avoid activating the retracting mechanism prematurely.)
Principle. The air must be inserted above the fluid level to avoid creating air bubbles in the medication.

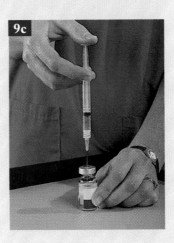

PROCEDURE 11-2

Continued

PROCEDURE **11-2**　Preparing the Injection—Cont'd

d. **Procedural Step.** Invert the vial while holding onto the syringe and plunger. Hold the syringe at eye level, and withdraw the proper amount of medication. Keep the needle opening below the fluid level. *Principle.* The needle opening must be below the fluid level to prevent the entrance of air bubbles into the syringe.

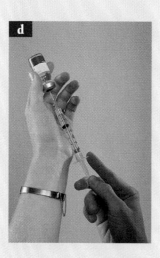

e. **Procedural Step.** Remove any air bubbles in the syringe by holding the syringe in a vertical position and tapping the barrel with the fingertips until they disappear.
Principle. Air bubbles take up space the medication should occupy.

f. **Procedural Step.** Remove any air remaining at the top of the syringe by slowly pushing the plunger forward and allowing the air to flow back into the vial. Carefully remove the needle from the rubber stopper and replace the needle guard. *Principle.* The needle must remain sterile. The needle guard prevents the needle from becoming contaminated.

g. **Procedural Step.** Check the drug label for the third time, and return the medication to its proper storage location.

Withdrawing Medication From an Ampule

a. **Procedural Step.** Remove the needle from the syringe and attach a filter needle.

b. **Procedural Step.** Open the antiseptic wipe and cleanse the neck of the ampule.
Principle. Cleansing the neck of the ampule removes dust and bacteria.

c. **Procedural Step.** Tap the stem of the ampule lightly to remove any medication in the neck of the ampule.

d. **Procedural Step.** Place a piece of gauze around the neck of the ampule. Hold the base of the ampule between the first two fingers and the thumb of one hand. Hold the neck of the vial between the first two fingers and the thumb of the other hand. Apply a strong steady pressure with the thumbs and break off the stem by snapping it quickly and firmly away from the body. Discard the stem in a biohazard sharps container.

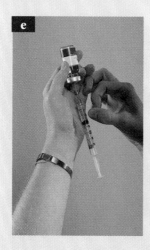

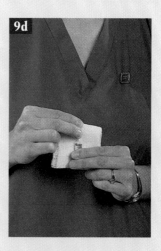

e. Procedural Step. Remove the needle guard. Insert the filter needle opening below the fluid level.
Principle. The filter needle prevents glass particles from being withdrawn into the syringe.

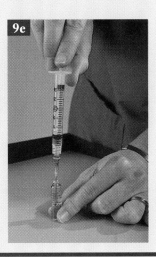

f. Procedural Step. Withdraw the proper amount of medication by pulling back on the plunger. Be sure to keep the needle opening below the fluid level to prevent the entrance of air bubbles into the syringe.
Principle. Air bubbles take up space the medication should occupy, resulting in an inaccurate measurement of medication.

g. Procedural Step. Remove the needle from the ampule. If air bubbles are in the syringe, hold the syringe in a vertical position and tap the barrel with the fingertips until they disappear. Remove the air at the top of the syringe by slowly pushing the plunger forward. Do not eject the fluid.

h. Procedural Step. Replace the needle guard. Remove the filter needle from the syringe and discard it in a biohazard sharps container. Reapply the needle (and guard) for administering the medication.

i. Procedural Step. Check the drug label for the third time and dispose of the glass ampule in a biohazard sharps container.

PROCEDURE 11-3 Reconstituting Powdered Drugs

Outcome Reconstitute a powdered drug for parenteral administration.

Equipment/Supplies:
- Medication ordered by the physician
- Appropriate needle and syringe
- Antiseptic wipe
- Medication tray

1. **Procedural Step.** Follow steps 1 through 8 of Procedure 11-2.
2. **Procedural Step.** From the vial of the powdered drug, withdraw an amount of air equal to the amount of liquid to be injected into the vial.
   Principle. Removing air from the powdered drug vial allows room for injection of the diluent.
3. **Procedural Step.** Inject the air removed from the powdered drug vial into the vial of diluent.
   Principle. Air must be injected into the vial to prevent formation of a partial vacuum in the vial, which would make it difficult to remove the diluent.
4. **Procedural Step.** Invert the diluent vial and withdraw the proper amount of liquid into the syringe. Remove air bubbles from the syringe and carefully remove the needle from the vial.
5. **Procedural Step.** Insert the needle into the powdered drug vial and inject the diluent into the vial. Remove the needle from the vial and replace the needle guard.

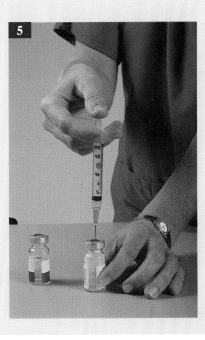

Continued

PROCEDURE **11-3**   Reconstituting Powdered Drugs—Cont'd

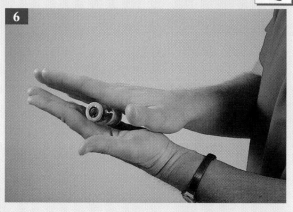
6

6. **Procedural Step.** Roll the vial between the hands to mix the powdered drug and liquid (unless indicated otherwise by the drug package insert).
   Principle. Shaking the vial may cause the formation of air bubbles.
7. **Procedural Step.** Label multiple-dose vials with the date of preparation and your initials.
8. **Procedural Step.** Follow steps 9 (a through g) of Procedure 11-2.
9. **Procedural Step.** Store multiple-dose vials as indicated by the manufacturer's instructions. Because reconstituted drugs are stable for a short time, carefully check the date of preparation on the multiple-dose vial before administering it again.

PROCEDURE **11-4**   Administering a Subcutaneous Injection

Outcome Administer a subcutaneous injection.

Equipment/Supplies:
- Medication ordered by the physician
- Appropriate needle and syringe
- Antiseptic wipe
- Sterile 2 × 2 gauze pad
- Disposable gloves
- Biohazard sharps container

1. **Procedural Step.** Sanitize your hands and prepare the injection (see Procedure 11-2).
2. **Procedural Step.** Greet and identify the patient. Introduce yourself and explain the procedure and purpose of the injection.
   Principle. It is crucial that no error be made in patient identity. An apprehensive patient may need reassurance.
3. **Procedural Step.** Select an appropriate injection site. The upper arm, thigh, back, and abdomen are recommended sites for a subcutaneous injection. See Figure 11-14.
   Principle. The entire area should be exposed to ensure a safe and comfortable injection.
4. **Procedural Step.** Prepare the injection site. Cleanse the area with an antiseptic wipe. Using a circular motion, start with the injection site and move outward. Do not touch the site after cleansing it.
   Principle. Using a circular motion carries contaminants away from the injection site. Touching the site after cleansing will contaminate it, and the cleansing process will need to be repeated.

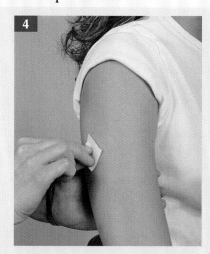
4

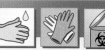

5. **Procedural Step.** Allow the area to dry completely.
   Principle. If the area is not permitted to dry, the antiseptic may enter the tissues when the skin is pierced, resulting in irritation and patient discomfort.

6. **Procedural Step.** Apply gloves, and remove the needle guard. Position your nondominant hand on the area surrounding the injection site. The skin may be held taut, or the area surrounding the injection site may be grasped and held in a cushion fashion.

   Principle. Gloves provide a barrier against bloodborne pathogens. In normal adults, the needle will enter the subcutaneous tissue when the skin is held taut. Grasping the area around the injection site is recommended for a thin or dehydrated patient. It will ensure that the subcutaneous tissue, and not muscle tissue, is entered.

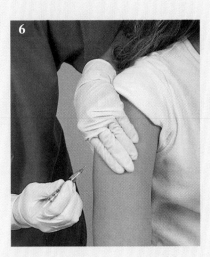

7. **Procedural Step.** Hold the barrel of the syringe between your thumb and index finger. Insert the needle quickly and smoothly at a 45-degree or 90-degree angle, depending on the length of the needle. With a ½-inch needle, a 90-degree angle should be used; with a ⅝-inch needle, a 45-degree angle should be used. Insert the needle to the hub.

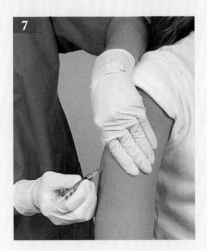

   Principle. Inserting the needle quickly and smoothly minimizes tissue trauma and pain. Needle length determines the angle of insertion to ensure placement of the medication in subcutaneous tissue.

8. **Procedural Step.** Remove your hand from the skin.

   Principle. Medication injected into compressed tissue causes pressure against nerve fibers and is uncomfortable for the patient.

9. **Procedural Step.** Hold the syringe steady and pull back gently on the plunger to determine whether the needle is in a blood vessel, in which case blood will appear in the syringe. If blood appears, withdraw the needle, prepare a new injection, and begin again.

   Principle. Moving the syringe once the needle has entered the tissue causes patient discomfort. Drugs intended for subcutaneous administration but injected into a blood vessel are absorbed too quickly, and undesirable results may occur.

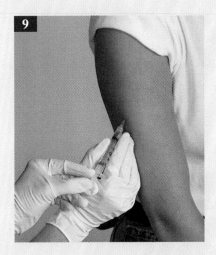

10. **Procedural Step.** Inject the medication slowly and steadily by depressing the plunger.

    If you are using a retractable safety syringe, activate it at this time following the steps outlined in Figure 11-7 and continue to step 12.

    Principle. Rapid injection creates pressure and destroys tissue, which are uncomfortable for the patient.

11. **Procedural Step.** Place the antiseptic wipe or a gauze pad gently over the injection site and quickly remove the needle, keeping it at the same angle as for insertion.

    Principle. Withdrawing the needle quickly and at the same angle as for insertion reduces patient discomfort. The antiseptic wipe or gauze pad placed over the injection site helps prevent tissue movement as the needle is withdrawn, reducing patient

Continued

PROCEDURE 11-4

PROCEDURE 11-4   Administering a Subcutaneous Injection—Cont'd

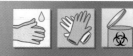

discomfort. Using a gauze pad prevents a stinging sensation from the alcohol.

12. **Procedural Step.** Apply gentle pressure to the injection site with the antiseptic wipe or gauze pad. If you are using a safety syringe with a shield, activate the safety feature at this time following the steps outlined in Figure 11-7.
    Principle. Gentle pressure helps distribute the medication so that it is completely absorbed. Avoid vigorous massaging because it could damage underlying tissue.

13. **Procedural Step.** Properly dispose of the needle and syringe in a biohazard sharps container.
    Principle. Proper disposal is required by the OSHA Standard to prevent accidental needlestick injuries.

14. **Procedural Step.** Remove the gloves, and sanitize your hands.

15. **Procedural Step.** Chart the procedure. Include the date and time, the name of the medication, the dosage given, the route of administration, the in-

jection site used, and any significant observations or patient reactions.

16. **Procedural Step.** Stay with the patient to make sure he or she is not experiencing any unusual reactions. (*Note:* If an allergy injection has been given, the patient should remain at the medical office for at least 15 minutes to make sure that a reaction does not occur.) If the patient experiences an unusual reaction, notify the physician immediately.

CHARTING EXAMPLE	
Date	
2/17/05	3:30 p.m. Ragweed allergy inj, 0.20 cc, SC Ⓡ upper arm. Arm checked 15 min. after admin. No reaction noted. —————— T. Cline, CMA

PROCEDURE 11-5   Administering an Intramuscular Injection

Outcome Administer an intramuscular injection.

Equipment/Supplies:
- Medication ordered by the physician
- Appropriate needle and syringe
- Antiseptic wipe
- Sterile 2 × 2 gauze pad
- Disposable gloves
- Biohazard sharps container

1. **Procedural Step.** Sanitize your hands and prepare the injection (see Procedure 11-2).

2. **Procedural Step.** Greet and identify the patient. Introduce yourself and explain the procedure.
   Principle. Make sure that you are giving the medication to the right patient. Explain the purpose of the injection. Assistance may be needed for restraining infants and children.

3. **Procedural Step.** Select an appropriate injection site. See Figure 11-15 for the recommended intramuscular injection sites. Remove the patient's clothing as necessary to make sure the entire area is exposed.

Principle. Major nerves and blood vessels may lie in close proximity to the intramuscular injection sites. The medical assistant should develop skill and accuracy in locating the proper sites.

4. **Procedural Step.** Prepare the injection site. Cleanse the area with an antiseptic wipe. Using a circular motion, start with the injection site and move outward. Do not touch the site after cleansing it.
   Principle. Using a circular motion carries contaminants away from the injection site. Touching the site after cleansing will contaminate it, and the cleansing process will need to be repeated.

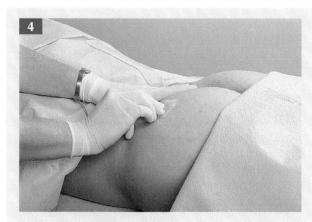

5. **Procedural Step.** Allow the area to dry completely.
   Principle. If the area is not permitted to dry, the antiseptic may enter the tissues when the skin is pierced, resulting in irritation and patient discomfort.

6. **Procedural Step.** Apply gloves and remove the needle guard. Using the thumb and first two fingers of the nondominant hand, stretch the skin taut over the injection site.
   Principle. Gloves provide a barrier against blood-borne pathogens. Stretching the skin taut permits easier insertion of the needle and helps ensure that the needle enters muscle tissue.

7. **Procedural Step.** Hold the barrel of the syringe like a dart and insert the needle quickly and smoothly at a 90-degree angle to the patient's skin with a firm motion. Insert the needle to the hub.
   Principle. The needle is inserted at a 90-degree angle to ensure that it reaches muscle tissue. Inserting the needle quickly and smoothly minimizes tissue trauma and pain.

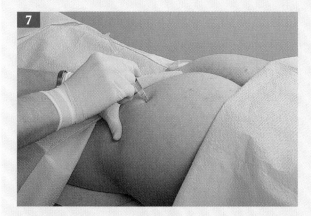

8. **Procedural Step.** Hold the syringe steady, and pull back gently on the plunger to determine whether the needle is in a blood vessel. If blood appears, withdraw the needle, prepare a new injection, and begin again.

Principle. Moving the syringe once the needle has penetrated the tissue causes patient discomfort. If drugs intended for intramuscular administration are injected into a blood vessel, the result is faster absorption of the medication. This may produce undesirable results.

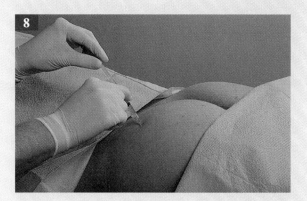

9. **Procedural Step.** Inject the medication slowly and steadily by depressing the plunger. If you are using a retractable safety syringe, activate it at this time following the steps outlined in Figure 11-7, and continue to step 11.
   Principle. Rapid injection creates pressure and destroys tissue, thus causing discomfort for the patient.

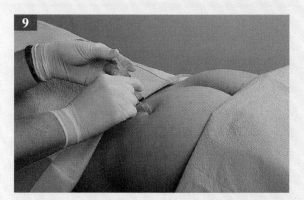

10. **Procedural Step.** Place the antiseptic wipe or gauze pad gently over the injection site, and remove the needle quickly, keeping it at the same angle as for insertion.
    Principle. Withdrawing the needle quickly and at the same angle as for insertion reduces patient discomfort. Placing the antiseptic wipe or gauze pad over the injection site helps prevent tissue movement as the needle is withdrawn, also reducing patient discomfort. Using a gauze pad prevents a stinging sensation from the alcohol.

PROCEDURE 11-5

Continued

PROCEDURE 11-5   Administering an Intramuscular Injection—Cont'd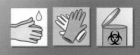

11. **Procedural Step.** Apply gentle pressure to the injection site with an antiseptic wipe or gauze pad. If you are using a safety syringe with a shield, activate the safety feature at this time following the steps outlined in Figure 11-7.
Principle. Gentle pressure helps distribute the medication so that it is absorbed by the muscle tissue. Avoid vigorous massaging because it could damage underlying tissues.

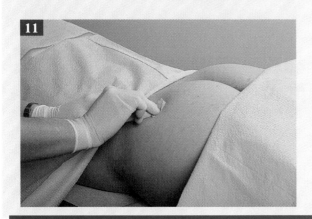

12. **Procedural Step.** Properly dispose of the needle and syringe in a biohazard sharps container.
Principle. Proper disposal is required by the OSHA Standard to prevent accidental needlestick injuries.
13. **Procedural Step.** Remove the gloves, and sanitize your hands.
14. **Procedural Step.** Chart the procedure. Include the date and time, the name of the medication, the dosage given, the route of administration, the injection site used, and any significant observations or patient reactions.
15. **Procedural Step.** Stay with the patient to make sure he or she is not experiencing any unusual reactions. If the patient experiences an unusual reaction, notify the physician immediately.

CHARTING EXAMPLE	
Date	
2/20/05	9:30 a.m. Rocephin 1 gram, IM, Ⓛ dorsogluteal.
	Tolerated injection well. ——————— T. Cline, CMA

PROCEDURE 11-6   Z-Track Intramuscular Injection Technique

Outcome Administer an intramuscular injection using the Z-track method.

Equipment/Supplies:
• Medication ordered by the physician
• Appropriate needle and syringe
• Antiseptic wipe
• Disposable gloves
• Biohazard sharps container

1. **Procedural Step.** Follow steps 1 through 5 of the intramuscular injection procedure (see Procedure 11-5).
2. **Procedural Step.** Apply gloves, and remove the needle guard. With the nondominant hand, pull the skin away laterally from the injection site approximately 1 to 1½ inches.
3. **Procedural Step.** Insert the needle quickly and smoothly at a 90-degree angle.

4. **Procedural Step.** Aspirate to determine whether the needle is in a blood vessel.
5. **Procedural Step.** Inject the medication slowly and steadily.
6. **Procedural Step.** After injecting the medication, wait 10 seconds before withdrawing the needle to allow initial absorption of the medication.
7. **Procedural Step.** Withdraw the needle quickly keeping it at the same angle as for insertion.
8. **Procedural Step.** Release the traction on the skin in order to seal off the needle track; doing so prevents the medication from reaching the subcutaneous tissue and skin surface.

9. **Procedural Step.** Do not apply pressure to the site because it could cause the medication to seep out.
10. **Procedural Step.** Complete the procedure by following steps 12 through 15 of Procedure 11-2.

CHARTING EXAMPLE	
Date	
2/20/05	10:30 a.m. Iron dextran 100 mg, IM, Z-track into ⓡ dorsogluteal. No complaints of discomfort. —————————— T. Cline, CMA

Intradermal Injections

An **intradermal injection** is given into the dermal layer of the skin, at an angle almost parallel to the skin (see Figure 11-13). Absorption is slow; therefore only a small amount of medication may be injected (0.01 to 0.2 cc). The sites most often used for an intradermal injection are areas where the skin is thin, such as the anterior forearm and the middle of the back. The upper arm is also used to administer an intradermal injection.

The needle used is short, usually $3/8$ to $5/8$ inch long, and the lumen has a small diameter, usually 25 to 27 gauge. A tuberculin syringe is often used for administering the injection. The capacity of the syringe is small (1 cc), and the calibrations are divided into tenths and hundredths of a cubic centimeter. The fine calibrations allow a very small amount of medication to be administered, which is required with an intradermal injection. Procedure 11-7 outlines the technique for the administration of an intradermal injection.

The most frequent use of intradermal injections is to administer a skin test such as an allergy test or a tuberculin test. The medication for the appropriate test is placed into the skin layers, and a small raised area known as a **wheal**

is produced at the injection site, owing to distention of the skin (Figure 11-17). At a time dictated by the type of test being administered, the results are read and interpreted. For example, the majority of allergy tests can be read and interpreted at the medical office a short time (usually 15 to 20 minutes) after administration of the test, whereas tuberculin testing requires 48 hours before the results can be read.

The skin testing medication interacts with the body tissues; if no reaction occurs, the wheal disappears within a short time, and the only visible sign left is the puncture site. If a reaction to the skin test occurs, induration results, indicating a positive reaction. Erythema may also be present at the test site; however, for most skin tests, the extent of induration is the only criterion used to assess a positive reaction.

Tuberculin Testing

Tuberculosis

Tuberculosis (TB) is an infectious disease that usually attacks the lungs, although it can occur in almost any other part of the body, particularly the brain and kidneys. The causative agent of tuberculosis is the tubercle bacillus *(Mycobacterium tuberculosis)*, which is a rod-shaped bacterium. Symptoms of active pulmonary tuberculosis include fatigue, weakness, unexplained weight loss, low-grade fever, night sweats, a cough that produces mucopurulent sputum, and occasional hemoptysis (coughing up blood) and chest pain.

Tuberculosis is not a highly contagious disease, and many people who are infected with the tubercle bacillus do not develop the disease because their body defenses protect them. This protective mechanism involves building a fibrous wall around the TB organisms to encapsulate them. Some of the TB bacteria may remain alive inside the capsule in a dormant or inactive state. During this time, the patient experiences no symptoms and cannot spread the disease to others. The individual is said to have a *latent tuberculosis infection (LTBI)* and usually has a positive reaction to a tuberculin test.

Latent tuberculosis may develop into active tuberculosis shortly after infection or even many years after infection.

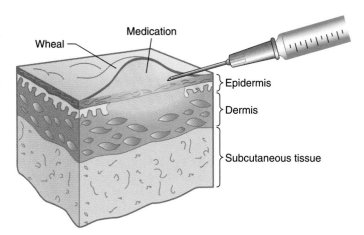

Figure 11-17. Intradermal injections are used to administer skin tests. Enough medication must be deposited in the skin layers to form a wheal.

The TB bacteria break out of the capsule and cause the symptoms of active tuberculosis. This occurs in approximately 10% of individuals with LTBI. It is most apt to occur when the body defenses are weakened, such as during a serious illness, or in patients who have an immune disorder such as AIDS.

Purpose of Tuberculin Testing

The purpose of tuberculin testing is to detect the presence of a tuberculin infection. The tuberculin test is recommended for patients who have close day-to-day contact with someone who has active tuberculosis, individuals who have symptoms of tuberculosis, and individuals with lowered immunity such as HIV. The test is also recommended as a screening measure to assist in the early detection of unsuspected cases of tuberculosis before the patient becomes symptomatic. In this way, appropriate therapeutic measures can be instituted, leading to early treatment, which also helps prevent the spread of the disease. Tuberculin testing is usually part of a regular health screen, or it may be required as a prerequisite for employment, college entrance, entrance into the military service, and so on.

The medical assistant is responsible for administering the tuberculin test and for interpreting the test results. Although tuberculin testing is relatively easy to perform, the procedure must be followed exactly to ensure accurate results. A patient with a tuberculous infection may fail to react to the test if it is not performed correctly.

Tuberculin Test Reactions

The substance used in the test is tuberculin, which consists of a purified protein derivative (PPD) extracted from a culture of tubercle bacilli (the causative agent of tuberculosis), to test for sensitivity to the microorganism. When introduced into the skin of an individual with an active or latent case of tuberculosis, tuberculin causes a localized thickening of the skin, resulting in **induration.** Induration is an abnormally hard spot caused by an accumulation of small sensitized lymphocytes that occurs in the area in which the tuberculin was injected into the skin. Tuberculin test reactions are based on the amount of induration present and are interpreted according to the manufacturer's instructions that accompany the test.

A positive reaction to a tuberculin test indicates the presence of a tuberculous infection; however, it does not

---

Highlight on Tuberculosis

Tuberculosis has made an unwelcome comeback in the United States among certain high-risk groups. Until recently public health officials considered tuberculosis a disease that had been conquered. Worldwide eight million people are infected with tuberculosis every year, and an estimated three million die from this disease annually. In addition, outbreaks of drug-resistant strains of tuberculosis have appeared in patients in hospitals, prisons, and community health clinics across the country.

Although any part of the body can be infected, the TB organism prefers body tissues with high oxygen concentrations, such as the lungs. That is why approximately 85% of individuals with TB have *pulmonary tuberculosis.* Tuberculosis is not highly contagious, and prolonged contact with an infected individual is usually required before the disease develops. This is because the natural defense mechanisms in the upper respiratory tract prevent most inhaled TB organisms from reaching the lungs.

Individuals at greatest risk for contracting tuberculosis from infected patients are young children whose immune systems are not fully developed, the elderly whose immune systems are diminished, and individuals with immune deficiency diseases such as AIDS. There has also been an increase in environments conducive to the transmission of tuberculosis, which include long-term care facilities such as nursing homes and prisons.

The tuberculin test is used to identify individuals infected with the TB organism. A positive reaction occurs 2 to 10 weeks after infection with tuberculosis. Most authorities believe that the Mantoux tuberculin test method is more specific and accurate than the tine test. This is because the Mantoux test uses a known amount of tuberculin (0.10 ml of PPD), compared with the tine test in which the tuberculin cannot be as precisely controlled. Because of this, authorities recommend that the tine test be used only for screening individuals at low risk for tuberculosis infection.

Fortunately, active tuberculosis can be treated if it is diagnosed early. Antibiotics have been available since the 1940s to cure tuberculosis and thereby help prevent its spread. Unless antibiotic drug resistance occurs, most patients are able to leave the hospital shortly after beginning drug therapy. Discharge, however, does not mean that the patient is cured. Compared with most other infectious diseases, treatment for tuberculosis is lengthy, typically lasting 6 months to 1 year. After 2 to 4 weeks of drug therapy, the disease is no longer contagious and the patient can resume a normal lifestyle. If the patient does not comply with the drug therapy regimen, however, some of the TB organisms will survive and the patient will be at risk for a recurrence of the disease. Many physicians recommend treating individuals with LTBI to prevent it from developing into active tuberculosis.

Tuberculosis is a reportable disease; therefore physicians must notify the local health department of cases of tuberculosis. The physician is also required to keep public health officials informed of the patient's compliance with the drug therapy regimen. To help prevent the spread of tuberculosis, public health officials conduct investigations to locate people who may have been infected by people known to have TB.

differentiate between the active and latent forms of the infection. Therefore a positive reaction warrants further diagnostic procedures before the physician can make a final diagnosis. Additional procedures used to detect an active tuberculous infection include a chest x-ray and microbiologic examination of the patient's sputum for tubercle bacilli.

Tuberculin Testing Methods

Two methods can be used for tuberculin testing: the *Mantoux* test and the *tine* test. The Mantoux test is the most common method. The Mantoux test is administered using an intradermal needle and syringe. The tine test is typically used only to screen individuals at low risk for tuberculosis. The tine test uses a sterile plastic unit containing four stainless-steel tines for puncturing the skin. The Mantoux test and the tine test have similar guidelines for administering and reading the tests, which are presented next. Information specific to each test are presented following these general guidelines.

Administering a Tuberculin Test

1. Use the anterior forearm, approximately 4 inches below the bend in the elbow, as the site of administration of the test. Avoid the following areas because they make the test harder to perform and interfere with good visualization and palpation of test reactions:
   - hairy areas of the skin
   - areas with visible veins
   - scar tissue
   - red or swollen areas
   - bruised areas
   - areas with dermatitis or other skin irritations
2. Cleanse the skin thoroughly with an antiseptic wipe and allow it to dry completely before administering the test
3. Be sure to deposit the tuberculin into the superficial layers of the skin. If blood appears at the puncture site once the test has been administered, it is not significant and will not interfere with the test.
4. Once the test has been administered, you must read the results within 48 to 72 hours.

Reading Tuberculin Test Results

1. Read the test results in good lighting.
2. Instruct the patient to flex the arm at the elbow.
3. Use both inspection and palpation to read the test results. If induration is present, rub your finger lightly from the area of normal skin (without induration) to the indurated area to assess its size. Then measure the area of induration in millimeters. The extent of induration present is the only criterion used to determine a positive reaction. If erythema is present without induration, the results are interpreted as negative.
4. Record all reactions in millimeters. If no induration is present, record 0 mm.

Mantoux Test

The Mantoux test is administered through an intradermal injection using a tuberculin syringe with a capacity of 1.0 ml and a short ($\frac{3}{8}$ to $\frac{1}{2}$ inch) needle with a gauge of 26 to 27. The standard injected dose is 0.10 ml of PPD solution containing 5 TU (tuberculin units). Brand names for Mantoux tests include Tubersol and Aplisol.

It is important that the medical assistant draw up the proper amount of tuberculin solution. Injecting too much of the solution might elicit a reaction not caused by a tuberculous infection, and injecting too little of the solution results in insufficient solution being injected into the skin to elicit a reaction. This will invalidate the test because if no reaction occurs, it cannot be accepted as a negative reaction.

The medical assistant must make sure to inject the solution into the superficial skin layers to form a wheal. If the injection is made into the subcutaneous layer, a wheal will not form and the test will yield a false-negative result, whereas a too-shallow injection may cause leakage of the tuberculin solution onto the skin. In either case, the medical assistant must repeat the test at a site at least 2 inches away.

The medical assistant should not apply pressure to the site after injecting the solution because the solution is not intended to be absorbed into the tissues. In addition, applying pressure may cause leakage of the tuberculin solution through the needle puncture site. The wheal will disappear on its own within a few minutes and should not be covered with an adhesive bandage.

Mantoux Test Results

The test results must be read in good lighting within 48 to 72 hours. The diameter of induration should be measured horizontally to the long axis of the forearm, and the results should be recorded in millimeters. Results should never be recorded as positive or negative. Mantoux tuberculin test results are interpreted as follows:

Positive reaction. The following reactions might indicate tuberculous infection:
- *Vesiculation* is the formation of vesicles, which are fluid-containing lesions of the skin. If vesiculation is present, the test is interpreted as strongly positive and warrants further diagnostic procedures to determine whether active tuberculosis is present.
- *Induration of 10 mm or more* constitutes a positive reaction and warrants further diagnostic procedures to determine whether active tuberculosis is present.
- *Induration of 5 mm* should be interpreted as a positive reaction for an individual who lives in close contact with a person with infectious tuberculosis; an HIV-infected individual; and an individual at risk for HIV infection, but whose HIV status is unknown.

Doubtful reaction. Induration measuring 5 to 9 mm means that retesting is recommended, using a different site of injection.

Negative reaction. Induration of less than 5 mm constitutes a negative reaction.

The procedure for administering and reading a Mantoux test is presented in Procedure 11-7.

Tine Test

The tine test, a multiple puncture test, is convenient and easy to administer; therefore it is especially useful for tuberculin screening. A sterile disposable intradermal test device is used that consists of a stainless-steel disc attached to a plastic handle. Four triangular prongs, or tines, approximately 2 mm long, project from the disc; these tines have been impregnated with tuberculin. The patient is inoculated intradermally to a depth of 1 to 2 mm by simple pressure on the skin, and the tuberculin on the tines is deposited into the skin layers.

The medical assistant frequently administers the tine test in the medical office and is also responsible for reading the test results. If the tine test reaction is positive, most physicians confirm the positive reaction by performing the Mantoux test. The procedure for administering and reading a tine test is presented in Procedure 11-8.

Highlight on Allergens

House Dust

There are many components in house dust to which an individual may be allergic—the most significant of these is the house dust mite. Dust mites thrive in warm humid conditions and feed on scales shed from human skin; therefore they are often found in mattresses, carpets, stuffed animals, and upholstered furniture. An individual who is allergic to house dust reacts to the waste products of these dust mites.

There is no shortage of food for the dust mite, since one person sheds up to 1 gram of scales per day, which is enough to feed thousands of mites for months. *Dermatophagoides pteronyssinus* and *Dermatophagoides farinae* are the most common house dust mites and are present in varying numbers in virtually every home. Mites occur in greatest numbers in bedding, particularly in mattresses; there may be up to 5,000 mites in each gram of dust from a mattress. Sufferers often notice that symptoms become much worse when the bedding is disturbed and allergenic material becomes airborne. Practices that eliminate dust also reduce the number of dust mites in a household.

Insect Stings

It is estimated that one of every 125 Americans is allergic to insect stings. Approximately 40 people in the United States die each year from a severe allergic reaction to insect stings. The incidence of deaths is low because most people know they need to obtain medical attention immediately if an allergic reaction begins.

Almost all insects whose venom can cause allergic reactions belong to a group called Hymenoptera, which includes honeybees and bumblebees, wasps, yellow jackets, and hornets. When a honeybee stings, its stinger remains embedded in the victim's skin, causing the bee to die as it tries to tear itself away. Wasps, yellow jackets, and hornets are more aggressive than bees and can sting repeatedly. Hornets are the most aggressive of the group and may sting even when not provoked. Yellow jackets are close behind in aggressiveness, but wasps usually sting only if someone interferes with them near their nest.

If an insect sting does not cause an allergic reaction within 30 minutes, chances are excellent that no problem will occur. A normal reaction to an insect sting includes localized pain, redness, swelling, and itching lasting 1 to 2 days. Any generalized reaction not arising directly from the area of the sting is almost certain to be an anaphylactic reaction, which begins with such symptoms as sneezing, urticaria, itching, angioedema, erythema, and disorientation and progresses to difficulty in breathing, dizziness, faintness, and loss of consciousness. Medical care should be sought immediately because most fatalities occur within the 2 hours of the sting. Because time is a factor, individuals who are known to have a severe allergy to insect stings are provided with an anaphylactic emergency treatment kit that contains epinephrine in a prefilled syringe and oral antihistamines. They can carry the kit with them so that treatment for a severe allergic reaction can be started as soon as possible.

Penicillin

Penicillin is one of the most common causes of allergic drug reactions. Approximately 2% to 5% of individuals are allergic to penicillin. The reaction may be mild and completely overlooked or confused with the symptoms of the disease being treated with penicillin, or it can be more serious and take the form of severe dermatitis or an anaphylactic reaction. Death as a result of a severe anaphylactic reaction is rare, occurring only in 0.01% of patients being treated with penicillin.

Penicillin was discovered in 1929 by Sir Alexander Fleming but was not used as a therapeutic drug until 1940. By 1944 it was evident that some of the side effects of penicillin were allergic reactions; the first recorded death due to an anaphylactic reaction to penicillin occurred in 1945.

Oral administration of penicillin is safer than a penicillin injection because it has a lower frequency of severe allergic reactions. There have been only six reported deaths from oral administration of penicillin.

Approximately 95% of serious reactions occur within 1 hour following a penicillin injection. The best preventive measure, therefore, is to keep the patient under direct observation for at least 30 minutes after administration of the injection.

Allergy Testing

Allergy

An allergy is an abnormal hypersensitivity of the body to substances that are ordinarily harmless; these substances are known as **allergens.** Allergens enter the body by being inhaled, by being swallowed, by being injected, or by contact with the skin. Almost any substance in the environment can be an allergen. Some common allergens are plant pollens, molds, house dust, animal danders, feather pillows, dyes, soaps, detergents, cosmetics, certain foods and medications, and insect stings.

The exact cause of allergies is not fully understood. In many cases, the tendency to develop allergies seems to be inherited because children of allergic parents tend to exhibit more allergic symptoms than children of nonallergic parents do. Although allergies can develop at any age, children are more apt to develop allergies than are older individuals.

Allergic Reaction

The first time an allergen enters the body of an allergic person, it stimulates the body to produce antibodies to that allergen. These antibodies are usually of a type known as IgE antibodies. After the initial sensitization, allergic antibodies combine with the allergen in the body, resulting in an allergen-antibody reaction. When such a reaction occurs, histamine is released in significant amounts, causing allergic symptoms. Allergen-antibody reactions may involve any system of the body; however, they most frequently affect the respiratory and the integumentary systems. Allergic symptoms can range from mild to very severe, as is the case with the potentially fatal anaphylactic reaction.

Depending on the allergen and the body system affected, allergies appear in different forms in an individual. Table 11-6 lists the common clinical forms and symptoms of allergies.

Diagnosis and Treatment

The best way to prevent allergic symptoms is to identify and avoid the offending allergen or allergens. The first and most important step in this process is the completion of a very careful and detailed medical history by the physician. Of particular importance to the diagnosis of an allergy are the patient's home and work environments, diet, and living habits. The physician also performs a thorough physical examination to detect conditions resulting from allergies, such as nasal polyps, wheezing, skin rashes, and urticaria.

Once the medical history and physical examination have been completed, the physician may order diagnostic tests. Allergy testing is performed to confirm information obtained through the medical history and physical examination. The allergy tests ordered most often are direct skin testing and the radioallergosorbent assay (RAST) test, which are described in more detail in the following section.

The general treatment of allergies includes avoidance of the allergen (if possible); alleviation of the symptoms through drug therapy such as antihistamines, decongestants, bronchodilators, and inhaled steroids; and decreasing the sensitivity of the body to the allergen by the administration of allergy injections, or desensitization injections.

Types of Allergy Tests

The purpose of allergy testing is to determine the specific substances or allergens that are causing the patient's allergic symptoms. The two main categories of allergy tests are the direct skin tests and the RAST test. The medical assistant is often responsible for performing direct skin testing in the medical office. The RAST test is performed by an outside laboratory on a blood specimen. The medical assistant may be responsible for performing a venipuncture to obtain the blood specimen.

Direct Skin Testing

Direct skin testing involves applying extracts of common allergens to the skin and observing the body's reaction to them. The extract is applied either topically to the skin (patch testing) or into the superficial skin layers (skin-prick and intradermal testing). The advantage of direct skin testing is that test results are obtained immediately. This in vivo administration of allergens, however, has the potential to cause adverse reactions, the least common but most serious being an anaphylactic reaction. The medical assistant should have a thorough knowledge of the symptoms of an anaphylactic reaction and alert the physician immediately if the patient begins to exhibit them.

Regardless of the specific type of direct skin test (patch, skin-prick, or intradermal), some general guidelines should be followed:

1. Instruct the patient to discontinue the use of antihistamines for 3 days before the skin testing; otherwise false-negative results may occur.
2. Verify that the area of application is free from hair, scar tissue, and dermatitis to permit good visualization and palpation of test reactions. Recommended sites include the anterior forearm, the upper arm, and the middle of the back. The back is usually used for patch and skin-prick testing, and the upper arm and forearm are typically used for intradermal skin testing.
3. Cleanse the area of application thoroughly with an antiseptic wipe and allow it to dry completely.
4. Wear gloves when the allergy testing involves puncture of the skin, which includes both skin-prick testing and intradermal skin testing. Gloves protect the medical assistant from exposure to bloodborne pathogens, as required by the OSHA Standard.

TABLE 11-6	Clinical Forms of Allergies
Allergic rhinitis	An inflammation of the mucous membrane of the nose caused by allergies. Symptoms include nasal congestion, sneezing, and a runny nose. An individual may have seasonal allergic rhinitis, meaning that the nasal mucosa is inflamed only during certain seasons of the year, as typically occurs with hay fever. On the other hand, an individual may have perennial rhinitis in which the nasal mucosa is inflamed year-round. This type of allergic rhinitis is commonly caused by allergens that are always present in the environment, such as house dust and animal danders.
Hay fever	Caused by an allergy to molds or the pollen of trees, grasses, or weeds. The term *hay fever* is completely misleading, because hay fever is not caused by hay nor does it result in a fever. The term was first used in the early 1800s by English physicians treating patients with allergies to grass pollens. The symptoms of hay fever and the common cold are almost identical. Sufferers of both experience episodes of sneezing, itching and watery eyes, runny and stuffy nose, and a burning sensation of the palate and throat. Hay fever is seasonal, occurring when there is pollen in the air. Depending on the geograhic location, hay fever may occur in the spring, summer, or fall and last until the first frost.
Asthma	A condition characterized by wheezing, coughing, and dyspnea. During an asthmatic attack, the bronchioles constrict and become clogged with mucus, which accounts for many of the symptoms of asthma. Asthma can occur at any age but is more common in children and young adults and, if not treated, can lead to serious complications such as permanent lung damage. It is frequently, but not always, associated with a family history of allergy. Any of the common allergens such as house dust, pollens, molds, or animal danders may trigger an asthmatic attack. Asthmatic attacks also can be caused by nonspecific factors such as air pollutants, tobacco smoke, chemical fumes, vigorous exercise, respiratory infections, exposure to cold, and emotional stress.
Urticaria	Urticaria, or hives, is an outbreak on the skin of welts of varying sizes that are redder or paler than the surrounding skin and are accompanied by intense itching. When the swellings are large and invade deeper tissues, the condition is known as angioedema. Hives may develop on the face or lips or even internally. Allergies to food or drugs (especially penicillin and aspirin) and insect bites often cause hives, but they may also result from an underlying disease or occur after exercise. In many cases, the exact cause of the urticaria cannot be determined.
Contact dermatitis	A rash caused by direct contact with the skin of an allergen such as cosmetics, perfumes, deodorants, rubber, plastics, and clothing treated with certain preservatives or dyes. Symptoms include swelling, blistering, oozing, and scaling. The rash usually occurs only on the area of the body that has been in contact with the allergen. The most common causes of contact dermatitis are poison ivy, poison oak, and sumac.
Eczema	A noncontagious rash accompanied by redness, itching, vesicles, oozing, crusting, and scaling. Eczema is a common allergic reaction in children, but it may also occur in adults, usually in a more severe form. The rash commonly appears on the face, neck, and folds of the elbows and knees. Eczema is frequently associated with allergies, and substances to which a person is allergic may aggravate it. Foods may be important factors, particularly milk, fish, or eggs. Allergens that are inhaled, such as dust and pollen, rarely cause eczema.

5. Space the allergen extracts at least 1 inch apart to provide enough surface area for a sizeable reaction. If not enough surface area is available, large adjacent reactions may run together, making it difficult to read test results.

6. Label the test sites so that the application site of each allergen extract can be later identified when reading results.

7. Make the patient aware that the skin testing may cause a mild allergic reaction, such as a runny nose, sneezing, and mild wheezing 8 to 24 hours following skin-prick and intradermal skin testing. Instruct the patient to contact the physician if a more severe reaction than this occurs.

Patch Testing. Patch testing is primarily used to identify allergens that cause contact dermatitis. Patch testing involves the topical application of each allergen to the skin, using a "patch." A patch consists of a small piece of gauze or filter paper impregnated with the allergen, which is

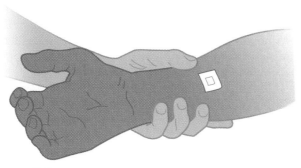

Figure 11-18. Patch testing. A patch consists of a small piece of gauze or filter paper impregnated with the allergen, which is applied to the skin and taped in place.

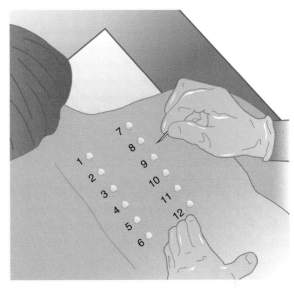

Figure 11-19. Skin-prick testing. Skin-prick testing involves the application of a number of allergen extracts to the skin, followed by the pricking of each with a sterile needle.

TABLE 11-7	Guidelines for Recording Direct Skin Test Results

Patch Test

−	No reaction
+1	Presence of erythema and edema, possibly papules
+2	Presence of erythema, edema, and vesicles, possibly papules
+3	Erythema, vesicles, and severe edema

Skin-Prick Testing and Intradermal Testing

−	No reaction
±1	Induration of 1 mm or less
+1	Induration greater than 1 mm and up to 5 mm in diameter
+2	Induration greater than 5 mm and up to 10 mm in diameter
+3	Induration greater than 10 mm and up to 15 mm in diameter
+4	Induration greater than 15 mm in diameter

applied to the skin and taped in place with hypoallergenic tape (Figure 11-18). Allergens commonly applied include plants, topical drugs, resins, metals, cosmetics, dyes, and chemicals. The patient should be instructed to leave the patches in place, keep them dry, and return to the medical office in 48 hours to have the results read. When the patient returns to the office, the patches are carefully removed and the results are read 20 minutes later. The delayed reading time allows lessening of redness that may occur from the tape removal.

Test results are recorded as positive or negative. Positive reactions are characterized by itching, erythema, and induration, often accompanied by vesiculation. In strongly positive responses, the reaction may extend beyond the margin of the patch. Positive results are further graded on a quantitative 1+ to 3+ scoring system according to the type of reaction (Table 11-7).

Skin-Prick Testing. Skin-prick testing is usually performed to diagnose allergies to common allergens, particularly those that are inhaled, such as house dust, pollens, and molds. Skin-prick testing involves the application of a number of allergen extracts to the skin, followed by pricking each with a sterile needle or other sharp instrument (Figure 11-19). The number of allergen extracts applied during one office visit usually ranges between 20 and 30. Pricking the skin deposits the allergens in the outer layers of the skin to allow each to react with the body tissues.

The following guidelines should be followed for skin-prick testing: The extracts should be placed on the skin in rows in a specific pattern. This, along with labeling the test sites with a felt-tipped pen, tracks the location of each extract. Only a single drop of extract should be placed on the skin; more than this amount may cause the extracts to diffuse and run together. A sterile needle should be passed through the drop, and the point should lightly lift the top layer of skin without causing bleeding. It is important to wipe the needle dry with a sterile swab between each prick to prevent one extract from mixing with the next, leading to inaccurate test results.

The maximum reaction is usually seen in 15 to 20 minutes. During this time, the test sites should be left uncovered and the patient should be instructed not to touch them. The area should not be wiped because this removes the allergen extract, resulting in false-negative results. The results are read (after 15 to 20 minutes) using a millimeter ruler.

Positive reactions are characterized by an area of induration surrounded by redness and itching. Positive results are recorded by measuring the size of the induration in millimeters and converting it to a numerical scale based on the extent of the induration (see Table 11-7). Any redness should be ignored. See Figure 11-17 for an illustration of skin test results. If only a mild reaction occurs, the physician may perform more specific intradermal skin testing.

Intradermal Skin Testing. Intradermal skin testing is similar to skin-prick testing, but it is more specific. The number of skin tests performed during one office visit ranges from 5 to 30. Because there is a greater chance of

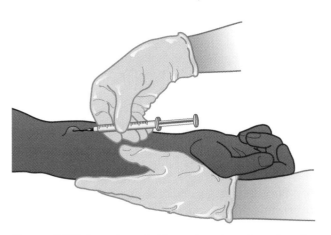

Figure 11-20. Intradermal skin testing. Intradermal testing involves the injection of a small amount of allergen extract into the superficial skin layers through the intradermal route of administration.

adverse allergic reactions to intradermal skin testing, the physician often starts with skin-prick testing in individuals who are suspected of being highly allergic as determined by the medical history and the results of the physical examination.

Intradermal skin testing involves the injection of a small amount (0.02 to 0.05 ml) of allergen extract into the superficial skin layers through the intradermal route of administration (Figure 11-20). A tuberculin syringe is used to administer the test, and the allergen extract is injected until a wheal forms (Procedure 11-7). After 15 to 20 minutes, the test sites are observed for reactions. Positive reactions are characterized by an area of induration surrounded by redness and itching. As with skin-prick testing, positive results are recorded by measuring the size of the induration in millimeters and converting it to a numeric scale based on the amount of induration present (see Figure 11-21 and Table 11-7).

RAST Testing. The RAST (radioallergosorbent test) measures the amount of IgE antibodies in the blood to common allergens. A sample of the patient's blood is sent to an outside laboratory, where it is exposed to radioactively tagged allergens. A radiation detection device is then used to measure the amount of IgE antibodies to the allergens. The advantages of the RAST test over direct skin testing are as follows: The results are not affected by medications (such as antihistamines); there is no danger of adverse allergic reactions because the test is performed in vitro, meaning outside the body; and RAST testing can be performed on patients who have skin eruptions and are unable to undergo direct skin testing because of a lack of an intact skin surface area. On the other hand, RAST testing is expensive and does not provide immediate test results, which are available with direct skin testing.

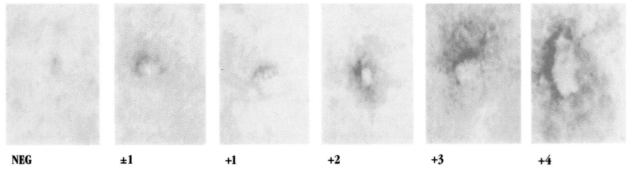

| NEG | ±1 | +1 | +2 | +3 | +4 |

Figure 11-21. Skin-prick and intradermal skin test results. (Copyright and courtesy Hollister-Stier Spokane, Washington.)

PROCEDURE 11-7 Administering an Intradermal Injection

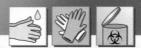

Outcome Administer an intradermal injection and read the test results.

Equipment/Supplies:
- Medication ordered by the physician
- Appropriate needle and syringe
- Antiseptic wipe
- Sterile 2 × 2 gauze pad
- Disposable gloves
- Biohazard sharps container

1. **Procedural Step.** Sanitize your hands and prepare the injection (see Procedure 11-2).
2. **Procedural Step.** Greet and identify the patient. Introduce yourself and explain the procedure.
   Principle. It is crucial that no error be made in patient identity. Explain the purpose of the injection to reassure an apprehensive patient.
3. **Procedural Step.** Select an appropriate injection site. The anterior forearm and the middle of the back are recommended sites for an intradermal injection.
   Principle. The entire area should be exposed to ensure a safe and comfortable injection.
4. **Procedural Step.** Prepare the injection site. Cleanse the area with an antiseptic wipe. Using a circular motion, start with the injection site and move outward. Do not touch the site after cleansing it.
   Principle. Using a circular motion will carry material away from the injection site. Touching the site after cleansing will contaminate it, and the cleansing process will need to be repeated.
5. **Procedural Step.** Allow the area to dry completely.
   Principle. If the area is not permitted to dry, the antiseptic may enter the tissue when the skin is pierced, resulting in irritation and patient discomfort. In addition, the antiseptic may cause a reaction that could be mistaken for a positive test response.
6. **Procedural Step.** Apply gloves, and remove the needle guard. With the nondominant hand, stretch the skin taut at the proposed site of administration. Insert the needle at a 10- to 15-degree angle (almost parallel to the skin), with the bevel upward. The needle should be inserted about ⅛ inch until the bevel of the needle just penetrates the skin. Slight resistance may be felt as the needle is inserted. No aspiration is needed.
   Principle. Gloves provide a barrier against bloodborne pathogens. Stretching the patient's skin taut will permit easier insertion of the needle. The needle should be inserted at an angle almost parallel to the skin, to ensure penetration within the dermal layer of the skin. The needle must be inserted with the bevel facing up to allow proper wheal formation. If the needle is inserted with the bevel facing down, the medication will be absorbed into the underlying tissues and a wheal will not form.

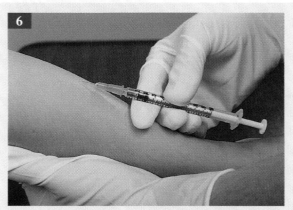

7. **Procedural Step.** Hold the syringe steady, and inject the medication slowly and steadily by depressing the plunger until a firm, tense, white wheal forms (approximately 6 to 10 mm in diameter). Expect to feel a certain amount of resistance as you inject the medication; this helps in indicating that the needle is properly located in the superficial skin layers rather than in the deeper subcutaneous tissue.
   Principle. Moving the syringe once the needle has entered the skin causes patient discomfort. Test results are considered reliable only if a wheal forms.

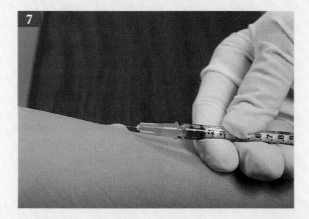

8. **Procedural Step.** Place the antiseptic wipe or gauze pad gently over the injection site and remove the needle quickly and at the same angle as for insertion.
   Principle. Withdrawing the needle quickly and at the angle of insertion reduces patient discomfort. The

PROCEDURE 11-7

Continued

PROCEDURE 11-7   Administering an Intradermal Injection—Cont'd

antiseptic wipe or gauze pad placed over the injection site helps prevent tissue movement as the needle is withdrawn, also reducing patient discomfort.

9. **Procedural Step.** Do not apply pressure to the injection site. If you are using a safety syringe with a shield, activate the safety feature at this time following the steps outlined in Figure 11-7.

   Principle. Applying pressure may cause leakage of the testing solution through the needle puncture site, resulting in inaccurate test results.

10. **Procedural Step.** Properly dispose of the needle and syringe in a biohazard sharps container.

    Principle. Proper disposal of the needle and syringe is required by the OSHA Standard to prevent accidental needlestick injuries.

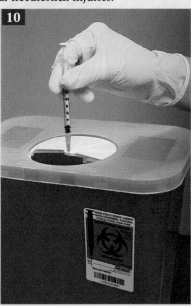

11. **Procedural Step.** Remove gloves and sanitize your hands.

12. **Procedural Step.** Stay with the patient to make sure that he or she is not experiencing any unusual reactions. The medical assistant should be especially careful and alert for any sign of a patient reaction when administering allergy skin tests. If the patient experiences an unusual reaction, notify the physician immediately.

13. **Procedural Step.** Perform *one* of the following, based on the type of skin test being administered:

Allergy Skin Tests

a. Read the test results within 20 to 30 minutes, using inspection and palpation at the site of the injection to assess the presence of and to determine the amount of induration. Interpret the skin test results according to the information outlined in Table 11-7.

b. Chart the procedure. Include the date and time, the injection site used, the names of the skin tests, the skin test results, and any significant observations or patient reactions.

CHARTING EXAMPLE	
Date	
2/15/05	Allergy skin tests, ID, Ⓡ ant forearm.
	Results: House dust +2
	Cat dander +4
	Dog dander –
	Ragweed +4
	Mixed fungi +3
	———————————— T. Cline, CMA

Mantoux Tuberculin Test

a. Inform the patient of the date and time to return to the medical office to have the results read. Results must be read within 48 to 72 hours after the test has been administered.

b. Chart the procedure. Include the date and time, the name of the medication, the dosage given, the manufacturer and lot number, the route of administration, the injection site used, and any significant observations or patient reactions. The lot number indicates the batch in which the medication was made. Should a problem arise with that batch, the drug can be recalled and individuals who received it can be identified.

c. Instruct the patient in the care of the test site as follows:
   • Do not cover the test site with a Band-Aid.
   • Do not scratch the arm. If it itches, apply a cold compress to the test site.
   • Pat the arm dry after washing it. Do not rub it dry.

CHARTING EXAMPLE

Date	
2/15/05	10:00 a.m. Tubersol Mantoux test 5 TU,
	0.10 ml, ID. Connaught Laboratories,
	Lot #: C0832AA. Admin Ⓡ ant forearm.
	Pt to return on 2/17/05 to have results
	read. ————————— T. Cline, CMA

Reading Mantoux Test Results
Equipment/Supplies:
- Millimeter ruler
- Disposable gloves
- Tuberculin test record card

1. **Procedural Step.** Greet and identify the patient. Introduce yourself and explain the procedure.
2. **Procedural Step.** Work in a quiet well-lit atmosphere. Check the patient's chart to determine which arm was used to administer the test.
3. **Procedural Step.** Sanitize your hands and apply gloves.
4. **Procedural Step.** Ask the patient to flex the arm at the elbow.
5. **Procedural Step.** Locate the application site. The result should be read horizontally to the long axis of the forearm, meaning "across" the forearm.
6. **Procedural Step.** Gently rub your finger over the test site and lightly palpate for the presence of induration. If induration is present, the area should be lightly rubbed from the area of normal skin (without induration) to the indurated area to assess the size of the area of induration.
   Principle. Induration is the only criterion used in determining a positive reaction. If erythema is present without induration, the results are interpreted as negative.

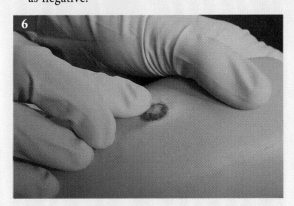

7. **Procedural Step.** Measure the diameter of the induration with a flexible millimeter ruler (supplied by the manufacturer). The results of the Mantoux test are interpreted as follows:

Positive Reaction: Vesiculation or induration of 10 mm or more.
Doubtful Reaction: Induration measuring 5 to 9 mm.
Negative Reaction: Induration of less than 5 mm.

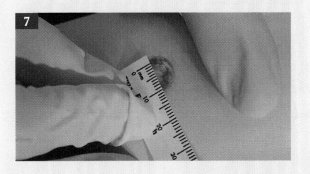

8. **Procedural Step.** Remove gloves and sanitize your hands.
9. **Procedural Step.** Chart the results. Include the date and time, the name of the test (Mantoux), and the test results (recorded in millimeters). If no induration is present, 0 mm should be recorded.
10. **Procedural Step.** Complete a tuberculin test record card and give it to the patient.
    Principle. The record card provides the patient with a permanent record of the test results.

TUBERCULOSIS TEST RECORD

Name		Date Admin: 2/15/05
Carrie Fee		Date Read: 2/17/05

MANTOUX TEST	RESULT		
	Negative	Doubtful	Positive
Tubersol, 5 TU	____ mm	9 mm	____ mm

Logan Family Practice
401 St. George St.
St. Augustine, FL 32084
(904) 555-3933

Performed by _____ T. Cline, CMA _____

CHARTING EXAMPLE

Date	
2/17/05	3:00 p.m. Tubersol Mantoux test: 9mm.
	Pt provided c̄ TB record card. Scheduled
	for TB retesting on 2/28/05. —————
	————————— T. Cline, CMA

PROCEDURE 11-8   Administering and Reading a Tine Test

Outcome Administer a tine test and read the test results.

Equipment/Supplies:
- Tine test
- Antiseptic wipe
- Sterile 2 × 2 gauze pad
- Disposable gloves
- Biohazard sharps container
- Millimeter ruler
- Tuberculin test record card

Administering the Tine Test

1. **Procedural Step.** Sanitize your hands.
2. **Procedural Step.** Greet and identify the patient. Introduce yourself and explain the procedure.
3. **Procedural Step.** Select an appropriate site to administer the tine test. The anterior surface of the forearm, approximately 4 inches below the bend of the elbow, is recommended. Hairy areas of the skin, areas with blemishes, scar tissue, and areas without adequate subcutaneous tissue should be avoided.
   Principle. Hairy areas of the skin and areas with blemishes make it difficult to read the test results.
4. **Procedural Step.** Prepare the site. Cleanse the area with an antiseptic wipe. Allow the area to dry completely. Do not touch the site once it has been cleansed.
   Principle. Touching the site after cleansing contaminates it, and the cleansing process will need to be repeated.

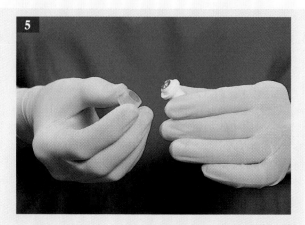

6. **Procedural Step.** Grasp the forearm with the nondominant hand immediately behind the proposed site of administration of the test, and stretch the skin of the forearm tightly to prevent the patient's arm from jerking during administration.
   Principle. If the patient jerked the arm during administration of the test, it could result in a scratch on the arm. Stretching the skin will permit easier insertion of the tines.

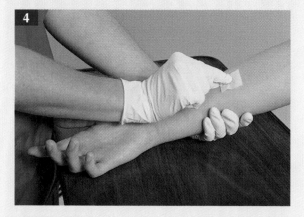

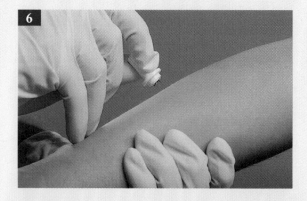

5. **Procedural Step.** Apply gloves. Expose the four tuberculin-coated tines using the following technique: Hold the protective plastic cap with one hand and, with the other hand, use a twisting pulling motion on the cap covering the tines, thereby removing the cap and exposing the tines.
   Principle. Gloves provide a barrier against bloodborne pathogens.

7. Procedural Step. Hold the tine test device in the dominant hand, place the plastic disc (with the four tines) on the patient's skin, and hold for at least 1 second (between 1 and 2 seconds is recommended) to allow the tines to pierce the skin. Exert sufficient pressure so that the four puncture sites and the circular depression from the plastic base are visible on the patient's skin.

Principle. The tines penetrate the skin, thereby introducing the tuberculin on the tines into the patient's skin.

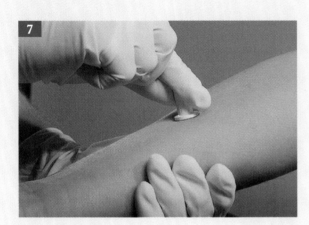

8. Procedural Step. Release the tension from your grasp on the patient's forearm, and withdraw the tine test unit. Do *not* apply pressure to the test site after application of the tines.

Principle. The incidence of bleeding at the test site is reduced if the tension on the forearm is released before the tines are withdrawn. Pressure should not be applied to the test site because the tuberculin is intended to be deposited into the skin layers and not absorbed into the tissues.

9. Procedural Step. Discard the plastic disc in a biohazard sharps container. Local care of the skin is not necessary. Some minor bleeding may occur, but this does not interfere with the test results.

Principle. Once used, the tine test unit is contaminated and should never be reused.

10. Procedural Step. Remove gloves, and sanitize your hands.

11. Procedural Step. Inform the patient of the date and time to return to the medical office to have the results read. Results must be read within 48 to 72 hours after the test has been administered.

12. Procedural Step. Chart the procedure. Include the date and time, the name of the test administered (tine test), the manufacturer and lot number, the site of administration, and any unusual patient reactions.

Principle. Recording the site of administration facilitates locating the test when the patient returns to the medical office to have the test read.

CHARTING EXAMPLE	
Date	
2/20/05	1:15 p.m. Tine test. Lederle Laboratories, Lot # 464-260. Admin Ⓡ ant forearm.
	Pt to return on 2/23 to have results read.
	———————————— T. Cline, CMA

Reading Tine Test Results

1. Procedural Step. Greet and identify the patient. Introduce yourself and explain the procedure.

2. Procedural Step. Work in a quiet well-lit atmosphere. Check the patient's chart to determine which arm was used to administer the test.

3. Procedural Step. Sanitize your hands and apply gloves.

4. Procedural Step. Ask the patient to flex the arm at the elbow.

5. Procedural Step. Locate the application site by referring to the patient's chart. Inspect the patient's arm for the presence of the four-point pattern.

PROCEDURE 11-8

Continued

PROCEDURE 11-8	Administering and Reading a Tine Test—Cont'd

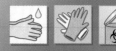

6. **Procedural Step.** Gently rub your finger over the test site and lightly palpate for the presence of induration. If induration is present, the area should be lightly rubbed from the area of normal skin (without induration) to the indurated area to assess the size of the area of induration.

7. **Procedural Step.** Measure the diameter of the largest single reaction around one of the puncture sites with a millimeter ruler (supplied by the manufacturer). The results of the Mantoux test are interpreted as follows:

   Positive Reaction. Vesiculation or induration 2 mm or greater is interpreted as a positive reaction. Most physicians confirm the positive reaction by performing the Mantoux test (before performing further diagnostic procedures).

   Negative Reaction. Induration less than 2 mm constitutes a negative reaction.

   Principle. Vesiculation or induration 2 mm or greater is the only criterion used to determine a positive reaction. Erythema without the presence of vesicles or induration constitutes a negative reaction.

8. **Procedural Step.** Remove gloves and sanitize your hands.

9. **Procedural Step.** Chart the results. Include the date and time, the name of the test (tine), and the test results (recorded in millimeters). If no induration is present, record the results as 0 mm.

10. **Procedural Step.** Complete a tuberculin test record card and give it to the patient.

    Principle. The record card provides the patient with a permanent record of the test results.

TUBERCULOSIS TEST RECORD

Name	Date Admin: 2/ 21 /05
Sarah King	Date Read: 2 /23/05

	RESULT
Tine Test	Negative	Positive
	_0_ mm	_____ mm

Logan Family Practice
401 St. George St.
St. Augustine, FL 32084
(904) 555-3933

Performed by _____ T. Cline, CMA _____

CHARTING EXAMPLE

Date	
2/23/05	3:00 p.m. Tine test: 0 mm. Pt provided
	c̄ TB record card.————— T. Cline, CMA

MEDICAL Practice and the LAW

Medications have the potential to do both great good and great harm. One of the most common sources of lawsuits is medication related, so the medical assistant has a tremendous responsibility to follow all procedures in order to avoid doing harm.

Many patients are prescribed multiple medications from various physicians. When performing a medication evaluation, ask the patient to bring in all medications he or she is currently taking. Be sure to include over-the-counter medications such as aspirin, vitamins, and herbal products.

When administering medications, first check a current medication reference to determine potential adverse effects. See the *Physician's Desk Reference* or package insert for this information. This information may also be available on a computer program. Next check for patient allergies. Check the chart, then ask the patient about allergies before administering the medication. Be sure the patient is informed why the drug is being given, its name, and common side effects. Watch the patient take the drug if given orally. If given parenterally, be sure to use proper technique to prevent injury. Follow the seven "rights" of medication administration and make sure to check the medication label three times before administering any medication. This all may seem cumbersome, but if any steps are omitted and the patient has a serious adverse reaction, you could be held liable.

Controlled drugs have specific laws that regulate their ordering, storing, and dispensing. Failure to adhere to these regulations could cause the physician to lose his or her license. Be aware of drug-seeking behavior of patients, as well as physical symptoms of addiction. You also have a duty to be aware of coworkers' behavior, and report to the physician any individual who appears chemically impaired, or whom you suspect of diverting medications for themselves.

What Would You DO?
What Would You *Not* DO? RESPONSES

Case Study 1
What Did Theresa Do?
- ❏ Asked Mrs. Okasinski what pharmacy she uses. Called the pharmacy and asked them to fax a copy of her medications to the medical office. Used the information from the pharmacy and the Product Identification section of the *PDR* to identify Mrs. Okasinski's medications.
- ❏ Wrote the names of her medications in her chart for the physician to review.
- ❏ Explained to Mrs. Okasinki that when she has her prescriptions filled, she should request non-childproof containers so that she will have be able to use the original containers, which have the name and prescription information on them. This will make it easier to tell her medications apart.
- ❏ After the physician was finished with Mrs. Okasinski, made a list of all the medications she would be taking based upon the physician's order. Went over each medication with Mrs. Okasinski and gave her a copy of the medication list to keep as a reference.

What Did Theresa Not Do?
- ❏ Did not criticize Mrs. Okasinski for taking her medications out of their original containers.

What Would You Do?/What Would You *Not* Do? Review Theresa's response and place a checkmark next to the information you included in your response. List additional information you included in your response below.

_____
_____
_____
_____

Case Study 2
What Did Theresa Do?
- ❏ Explained to Mrs. Cardwell that in order for the infection to be completely eliminated from Rachel's body, she needed to be given all of the medication.
- ❏ Stressed to Mrs. Cardwell that medication prescribed to one person should never be given to someone else because it might cause them to have a bad reaction.
- ❏ Explained to Mrs. Cardwell that if side effects of medication ever occur, it is important to call the medical office for information on what to do.
- ❏ Told Mrs. Cardwell that Rachel needs to be seen by the doctor again and scheduled an appointment for her. Asked if any other family members needed an appointment with the doctor.

What Did Theresa Not Do?
- ❏ Did not tell Mrs. Cardwell that she should have known better than to give Rachel's antibiotic to the other family members.

What Would You Do?/What Would You *Not* Do? Review Theresa's response and place a checkmark next to the information you included in your response. List additional information you included in your response below.

_____
_____
_____
_____

Continued

What Would You DO?
What Would You *Not* DO? *RESPONSES*—Cont'd

Case Study 3

What Did Theresa Do?

❑ Explained to Danielle that if the injection were given in her arm, it wouldn't be absorbed very well and she might not get better.

❑ Explained to Danielle that injections are given to patients every day at the office and that Danielle doesn't need to be embarrassed.

❑ Told Danielle that she would be draped extra well, and that it would only take a minute to give the injection.

What Did Theresa Not Do?

❑ Did not disregard Danielle's concerns.
❑ Did not give the injection in the deltoid.

What Would You Do?/What Would You *Not* Do? Review Theresa's response and place a checkmark next to the information you included in your response. List additional information you included in your response below.

_____

_____

_____

_____

Apply Your
KNOWLEDGE

Choose the best answer to each of the following questions.

1. Cruz Rodriguez is 25 years old, weighs 130 pounds, and receives allergy injections twice a week. Theresa Cline, CMA, is getting ready to administer an allergy injection to Cruz. Which of the following needles does she select to administer his injection?
   A. 27 G and ³⁄₈-inch
   B. 18 G and 1½-inch
   C. 25 G and ⁵⁄₈-inch
   D. 21 G and 1-inch

2. Theresa checks Cruz's chart to determine where his last injection was administered. The chart indicates it was given in his right upper arm. Which would be the best site for Teresa to use to administer today's injection?
   A. Left upper arm
   B. Right upper arm
   C. Right deltoid
   D. Left forearm

3. Theresa cleanses the injection site and prepares to administer the injection. What angle of insertion would Theresa use to administer this injection?
   A. 15-degree angle
   B. 45-degree angle
   C. 90-degree angle
   D. 120-degree angle

4. After administering the injection, Theresa gives Cruz the following instructions:
   A. Do not consume any food or fluid for 1 hour
   B. Elevate your arm above heart level for 5 minutes
   C. Choose a prize from the treasure box
   D. Remain in the waiting room for 15 minutes

5. Courtney Hill is at the medical office for an influenza vaccination. Theresa Cline, CMA, will be administering the injection from a multiple-dose vial. Theresa is not sure where to administer the injection so she consults the drug package insert accompanying the flu vaccine. Which of the following sections contains the information she needs?
   A. Indications and Usage
   B. Contraindications
   C. Dosage and Administration
   D. How Supplied

6. Theresa needs to administer 0.5 ml of the flu vaccine to Courtney. When preparing the medication, how much air should she first inject into the multiple-dose vial?
   A. 0.5 cc
   B. 5 ml
   C. 1 cc
   D. No air is needed since this is a multiple-dose vial

7. After administering the flu vaccine, Theresa performs which of the following:
   A. Asks Courtney if she is allergic to eggs
   B. Applies gentle pressure to the injection site
   C. Vigorously massages the injection site
   D. Places Courtney's arm in a sling

8. Theresa Cline, CMA, is preparing to administer a Tubersol Mantoux test to Christy McWhorter. Theresa injects the tuberculin solution, but a wheal does not form. What should Theresa do next?
   A. Instruct Christy to return in 2 days to have the test results read.
   B. Repeat the test using a tine test at a different site
   C. Burst into tears.
   D. Repeat the Mantoux test at a different site.

9. Christy returns to have her tuberculosis test read. Theresa palpates the site and measures 12 mm of induration. What should Theresa do next?
   A. Record the results as positive.
   B. Record 12 mm of induration.
   C. Inform Christy that she has active tuberculosis.
   D. Record the results as doubtful.

10. Dr. Wheal reviews the test results from Christy's tuberculosis test. What will Dr. Wheal most likely ask Theresa to do?
    A. Schedule Christy for a chest x-ray.
    B. Repeat the test using the tine testing method.
    C. Administer an injection of an antibiotic to Christy.
    D. Take a coffee break.

CERTIFICATION REVIEW

❑ **Pharmacology** is the study of drugs and includes the preparation, use, and action of drugs in the body. Medication that is administered is given to the patient at the office. Medication is prescribed when a physician provides the patient with a written prescription for a drug to be filled at a pharmacy. Dispensed medication is either given or sold to the patient at the office to be taken at home. Common routes of administration of medication are oral, sublingual, inhalation, rectal, vaginal, topical, intradermal, subcutaneous, intramuscular, and intravenous.

❑ **Drug package inserts** are included with each drug manufactured by a pharmaceutical company. The *Physician's Desk Reference* is a drug reference frequently used in the medical office to research information on prescription drugs. The U.S. Food and Drug Administration is responsible for determining the safety and effectiveness of drugs for human use.

❑ **Each drug has four names.** The chemical name of a drug provides a precise description of a drug's chemical composition. The generic name is assigned by the pharmaceutical manufacturer who first develops the drug. The official name is the name under which the drug is listed in official publications. The brand name is the name under which a pharmaceutical manufacturer markets a drug.

❑ **Three systems of measurement** are used in the United States for prescribing and administering medication: the metric system, the apothecary system, and the household system. The metric system is the most common because it is more accurate and easier to use. Conversion is required when medication is ordered in one unit of measurement and the medication label expresses the drug strength in a different unit.

❑ **Controlled drugs** are drugs that have potential for abuse. They are classified into five categories based on their abuse potential. To prescribe or dispense controlled drugs, the physician must register each year with the DEA. The physician is assigned a DEA number that must appear on the prescription of every controlled drug that he or she writes.

❑ **A prescription** is a physician's order authorizing the dispensing of a drug by a pharmacist. The prescription includes directions to the pharmacist for filling the prescription and instructions to the patient for taking the medication. Prescriptions can be authorized in different forms including handwritten, computer-generated, and telephoned or faxed to a pharmacy.

❑ **The therapeutic effect** of a drug is its desired effect. Factors that affect therapeutic action of drugs include age of the patient, route of administration, body size, time of administration, and tolerance to the drug.

Continued

CERTIFICATION REVIEW—Cont'd

❏ **Most drugs produce adverse reactions.** They may be harmless and tolerated in order to obtain the therapeutic effect of the drug. Some adverse reactions are harmful to some patients and warrant discontinuing the medication.

❏ **A patient can have an allergic reaction** to a drug after administration. The reaction is usually mild and may take the form of a rash, rhinitis, or pruritus. Occasionally a severe allergic reaction occurs suddenly and immediately. This reaction is known as an anaphylactic reaction.

❏ **The seven "rights"** of preparing and administering medication in the medical office include the right drug, right dose, right time, right patient, right route, right technique, and the right documentation.

❏ **The oral route** is the most convenient and most widely used method of administering medication. Absorption of most oral medication takes place in the small intestine, although some may be absorbed in the mouth and stomach.

❏ **The parenteral routes** of administration include subcutaneous, intramuscular, and intravenous. With parenteral administration, medications are absorbed more rapidly and completely. In some cases, such as when a patient is unconscious, the parenteral route is the only way a drug can be given.

❏ **The syringe** is used to insert fluids into the body. Various types of syringes are available to administer injections. The types used most often in the medical office are hypodermic, insulin, and tuberculin. Each needle has a certain gauge, which refers to the diameter of the lumen. As the size of the gauge increases, the diameter of the lumen decreases. The length of the needle ranges between $3/8$ inch and 3 inches; the length used is based on the type of injection. Safety engineered syringes incorporate a built-in safety feature to reduce the risk of a needlestick injury.

❏ **The most common dispensing units** for injectable medications include vials, ampules, and prefilled disposable syringes or cartridges that hold a single dose of medication.

❏ **A subcutaneous injection** is made into the subcutaneous tissue, which consists of adipose tissue. The needle length varies from $1/2$ to $5/8$ inch, and the gauge ranges from 23 to 25. The amount of medication injected subcutaneously should not exceed 1 cc. More than this amount causes pain and discomfort to the patient.

❏ **Intramuscular injections** are made into the muscular layer of the body. An amount up to 3 cc may be given intramuscularly. The length of the needle varies from 1 to 3 inches, and the gauge ranges from 18 to 23, depending on the viscosity of the medication. Intramuscular injection sites include the following: dorsogluteal, deltoid, vastus lateralis, and ventrogluteal.

❏ **An intradermal injection** is given into the dermal layer of the skin. The size of the needle ranges from $3/8$ to $5/8$ inch, and the lumen ranges from 25 to 27. The most frequent use of intradermal injections is to administer a skin test such as an allergy test or a tuberculin test (Mantoux test).

❏ **Tuberculosis is an infectious disease** that usually attacks the lungs. The purpose of tuberculin testing is to detect the presence of a tuberculin infection. A positive reaction to a tuberculin test indicates the presence of a tuberculous infection; however, it does not differentiate between the active and dormant states of the infection. A positive reaction warrants further diagnostic procedures before a final diagnosis can be made.

❏ **Allergy skin testing** determines the specific allergens that are causing the patient's allergic symptoms. Direct skin testing involves applying extracts of common allergens to the skin then observing the body's reaction to them. Direct skin testing includes patch testing, skin-prick testing, and intradermal skin testing. The RAST test is performed by an outside laboratory on a blood specimen and measures the amount of antibodies in the blood to common allergens.

Terminology Review

Adverse reaction An unintended and undesirable effect produced by a drug.

Allergen A substance that is capable of causing an allergic reaction.

Allergy An abnormal hypersensitivity of the body to substances that are ordinarily harmless.

Ampule A small sealed glass container that holds a single dose of medication.

Anaphylactic reaction A serious allergic reaction that requires immediate treatment.

Controlled drug A drug that has restrictions placed on it by the federal government because of its potential for abuse.

Conversion Changing from one system of measurement to another.

Cubic centimeter The amount of space occupied by 1 milliliter (1 ml = 1 cc).

DEA number A registration number assigned to physicians by the Drug Enforcement Administration for prescribing or dispensing controlled drugs.

Dose The quantity of a drug to be administered at one time.

Drug A chemical used for the treatment, prevention, or diagnosis of disease.

Gauge The diameter of the lumen of a needle used to administer medication.

Induration An area of hardened tissue.

Inhalation administration The administration of medication by way of air or other vapor being drawn into the lungs.

Inscription The part of a prescription that indicates the name of the drug and the drug dosage.

Intradermal injection Introduction of medication into the dermal layer of the skin.

Intramuscular injection Introduction of medication into the muscular layer of the body.

Intravenous injection Introduction of medication directly into the bloodstream through a vein.

Oral administration Administration of medication by mouth.

Parenteral Administration of medication by injection.

Pharmacology The study of drugs.

Prescription A physician's order authorizing the dispensing of a drug by a pharmacist

Signatura The part of a prescription that indicates the information to print on the medication label.

Subcutaneous injection Introduction of medication beneath the skin, into the subcutaneous or fatty layer of the body.

Sublingual administration Administration of medication by placing it under the tongue, where it dissolves and is absorbed through the mucous membrane.

Subscription The part of the prescription that gives directions to the pharmacist and usually designates the number of doses to be dispensed.

Superscription That part of a prescription consisting of the symbol Rx (from the Latin word *recipe,* meaning "take").

Topical administration Application of a drug to a particular spot, usually for a local action.

Vial A closed glass container with a rubber stopper that holds medication.

Wheal A small raised area of the skin.

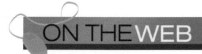

ON THE WEB

For active weblinks to each website visit http://evolve.
elsevier.com/Bonewit/.

For Information on Pharmacology:

Food and Drug Administration

Drug Enforcement Administration

RxList: The Internet Drug Index

Drug Topics

Medline Plus

Health Square

For a Current List of the Top 200 Drugs:

Mosby's Drug Consult

For Information on Alcohol and Drug Abuse:

Alcoholics Anonymous (AA)

**National Institute on Alcohol Abuse and Alcoholism
(NIAAA)**

**National Council on Alcoholism and Drug Dependence
(NCADD)**

**National Clearinghouse for Alcohol and Drug
Information**

Partnership for a Drug Free America

Institute for a Drug-Free Workplace

Al-Anon/Alateen

Mothers Against Drunk Driving (MADD)

For Information on Tuberculosis:

American Lung Association

American Thoracic Society

National Center for TB Prevention

For Information on Allergies:

**American Academy of Allergy, Asthma, and
Immunology**

**National Institute of Allergy and Infectious Diseases
(NIAID)**

Allergy Now

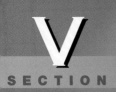

SECTION

Diagnostic Testing

12 Cardiopulmonary Procedures

13 Colon Procedures and Male
    Reproductive Health

14 Radiology and Diagnostic
    Imaging

Electrocardiography

1. Trace the path of the blood through the heart starting with the right atrium.
2. Explain the heart's conduction system.
3. State the purpose of electrocardiography.
4. Identify the following components of the ECG cycle:
   - P wave
   - QRS complex
   - T wave
   - P-R segment
   - S-T segment
   - P-R interval
   - Q-T interval
   - Baseline following the T wave
5. State the purpose of the standardization mark.
6. State the function of the electrodes, amplifier, and galvanometer.
7. List the 12 leads that are included in an electrocardiogram.
8. Describe the function served by each of the following:
   - Three-channel recording
   - Phone transmission
   - Interpretive electrocardiography
9. Identify the following types of artifact and state their causes:
   - Muscle
   - Wandering baseline
   - Alternating current
   - Interrupted baseline

Record a 12-lead electrocardiogram.

Holter Monitor Electrocardiography

1. List the reasons for applying a Holter monitor.
2. List the guidelines for wearing a Holter monitor.
3. Explain the use of the patient diary in Holter monitor electrocardiography.

Instruct a patient in the guidelines for wearing a Holter monitor.
Apply and remove a Holter monitor.

Cardiac Dysrhythmias

Identify the following cardiac dysrhythmias and explain their causes:
- Atrial premature contraction
- Paroxysmal atrial tachycardia
- Atrial flutter
- Atrial fibrillation
- Premature ventricular contraction
- Ventricular tachycardia
- Ventricular fibrillation

Identify cardiac dysrhythmias on a 12-lead ECG.

Pulmonary Function Testing

1. List the different pulmonary function tests.
2. List indications for performing spirometry testing.
3. Describe the following: FVC, FEV_1, and the FEV_1/FVC ratio.
4. Explain the difference between predicted values and measured values.
5. Describe the patient preparation for spirometry.
6. Explain how to calibrate a spirometer.
7. Explain the purpose of post-bronchodilator spirometry.

Perform spirometry testing.

CHAPTER 12

Cardiopulmonary Procedures

Chapter Outline

INTRODUCTION TO ELECTROCARDIOGRAPHY
Structure of the Heart
Conduction System of the Heart
Cardiac Cycle
  Waves
  Baseline, Segments, and Intervals
Electrocardiograph Paper
Standardization of the Electrocardiograph
Electrocardiograph Leads
  Bipolar Leads
  Augmented Leads
  Chest Leads
Maintenance of the Electrocardiograph
Electrocardiographic Capabilities
  Three-Channel Recording Capability
  Telephone Transmission
  Interpretive Electrocardiographs
Artifacts
  Muscle
  Wandering Baseline
  Alternating Current
  Interrupted Baseline

Holter Monitor Electrocardiography
  Electrode Placement
  Activity Diary
  Event Marker
  Evaluating Results
Cardiac Dysrhythmias
  Atrial Premature Contraction
  Paroxysmal Atrial Tachycardia
  Atrial Flutter
  Atrial Fibrillation
  Premature Ventricular Contraction
  Ventricular Tachycardia
  Ventricular Fibrillation
Pulmonary Function Tests
  Spirometry
  Post-Bronchodilator Spirometry

National Competencies

Clinical Competencies
Diagnostic Testing
- Perform electrocardiograms.
- Perform respiratory testing.

Key Terms

amplitude (AM-pli-tood)
artifact (AR-tih-fakt)
atherosclerosis (ath-roe-skler-OH-sus)
baseline
cardiac cycle
dysrhythmia (dis-RITH-mee-ah)
ECG cycle
electrocardiogram (ee-LEK-troe-KAR-dee-oh-gram)
electrocardiograph (ee-LEK-troe-KAR-dee-oh-graf)
electrode (ee-LEK-trode)
electrolyte (ee-LEK-troe-lite)
interval (IN-ter-val)
ischemia (is-KEEM-ee-ah)
normal sinus rhythm
segment
spirometer (spih-ROM-ih-ter)
spirometry (spih-ROM-ih-tree)

Introduction to Electrocardiography

The **electrocardiograph** is an instrument used to record the electrical activity of the heart. The **electrocardiogram (ECG)** is the graphic representation of this activity. The ECG exhibits the amount of electrical activity produced by the heart and the time required for the impulse to travel through the heart.

Electrocardiography is used for the following purposes: to detect an abnormal cardiac rhythm (dysrhythmia); to help diagnose damage to the heart caused by a myocardial infarction; to assess the effect on the heart of digitalis or other cardiac drugs; to determine the presence of electrolyte disturbances; to assess the progress of rheumatic fever; to determine the presence of hypertrophy of the heart chambers; and before surgery to assess cardiac risk during surgery.

An ECG is not able to detect all cardiovascular disorders. In addition, it cannot always detect impending heart disease. The ECG is generally used in combination with other diagnostic and laboratory tests to assess cardiac functioning.

The medical assistant is frequently responsible for recording electrocardiograms in the medical office. Because of this, knowledge and skill must be acquired in the following aspects of electrocardiography: preparation of the patient, operation of the electrocardiograph, identification and elimination of artifacts, labeling the completed ECG, and care and maintenance of the electrocardiograph.

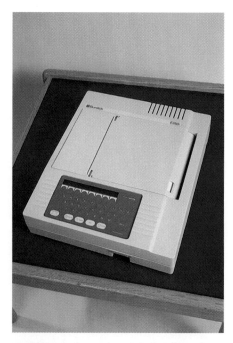

Figure 12-1. A three-channel electrocardiograph.

Electrocardiographs are available in single-channel and three-channel recording formats. Because most medical offices use a three-channel ECG, the information in this chapter focuses on the three-channel electrocardiograph (Figure 12-1).

Structure of the Heart

The human heart consists of four chambers: the right and left atria are the upper chambers, and the right and left ventricles are the lower chambers (Figure 12-2). Blood enters the right atrium from two large veins, the superior vena cava and the inferior vena cava, that bring it back from its circulation through the body. The blood entering the right atrium is deoxygenated, meaning it contains very little oxygen and is high in carbon dioxide.

From the right atrium, the blood enters the right ventricle. It is pumped from here to the lungs by way of the pulmonary artery. It picks up oxygen in the lungs in exchange for carbon dioxide and returns to the left atrium of the heart by way of the pulmonary veins. From the left atrium, the blood enters the left ventricle. This is the most powerful chamber of the heart and serves to pump blood to the entire body. Blood exits from the left ventricle by way of the aorta, which distributes it to all parts of the body to nourish the tissues with oxygen and nutrients.

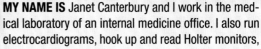

PUTTING It All Into PRACTICE

MY NAME IS Janet Canterbury and I work in the medical laboratory of an internal medicine office. I also run electrocardiograms, hook up and read Holter monitors, and perform pulmonary function tests and assist with stress tests.

One of my most rewarding experiences was when a young woman came into the office with severe chest pains. I immediately helped her back to an examining room. I then ran an electrocardiogram as ordered by the physician. After the physician read the ECG, he indicated the results did not look good and that the patient would have to be transported to the hospital. I went into the patient's room to comfort her. She asked me if she was going to have to go to the hospital. I replied, "Possibly." She immediately said "No!" Then I began to explain to her that it was important to have more tests. She finally agreed to go. After being taken to the hospital by an ambulance, she was later transferred to another hospital for a heart catheterization. A few weeks passed and she came into the office. She hugged me and thanked me for possibly saving her life. It felt so good that I could help make a difference in a patient's life.

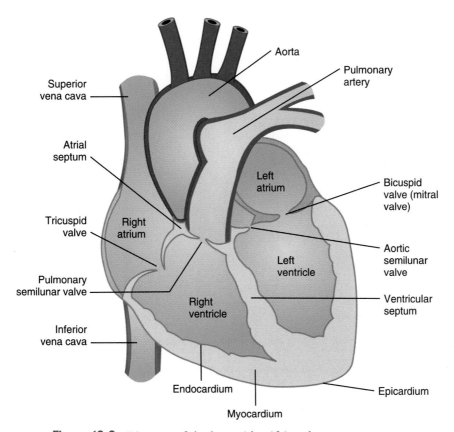

Figure 12-2. Diagram of the heart, identifying the structures.

Conduction System of the Heart

The *sinoatrial (SA) node* is located in the upper portion of the right atrium, just below the opening of the superior vena cava. It consists of a knot of modified myocardial cells that have the ability to send out an electrical impulse without an external nerve stimulus. In this way the SA node initiates and regulates the heartbeat.

Each electrical impulse discharged by the SA node is distributed to the right and left atria and causes them to contract. This contraction forces blood through the

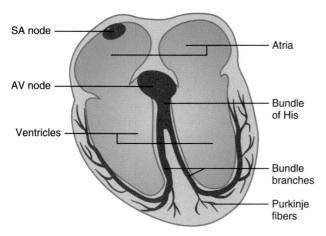

Figure 12-3. Diagram of the heart, identifying the structures involved with the conduction of an electrical impulse through the heart.

open cuspid valves and into the ventricles. The impulse is then picked up by the *atrioventricular (AV) node*, another knot of modified myocardial cells located at the base of the right atrium. The AV node then transmits the electrical impulse to the *bundle of His*. The AV node delays the impulse momentarily to give the ventricles a chance to fill with blood from the atria.

The bundle of His divides into right and left branches known as the *bundle branches*, which then relay the impulse to the *Purkinje fibers*. The Purkinje fibers distribute the impulse evenly to the right and left ventricles, causing them to contract; this forces blood out of the ventricles and into the pulmonary artery and aorta. The entire heart relaxes momentarily. Then a new impulse is initiated by the SA node and the cycle repeats (Figure 12-3).

Cardiac Cycle

The **cardiac cycle** represents one complete heartbeat. It consists of the contraction of the atria, the contraction of the ventricles, and the relaxation of the entire heart (as described previously). The electrocardiograph records the electrical activity that causes these events in the cardiac cycle. The **ECG cycle** is the graphic representation of the cardiac cycle (Figure 12-4).

Waves

The normal ECG cycle consists of a P wave; the Q, R, and S waves (known as the QRS complex); and a T wave. The ECG cycle is recorded from left to right, beginning with the P wave.

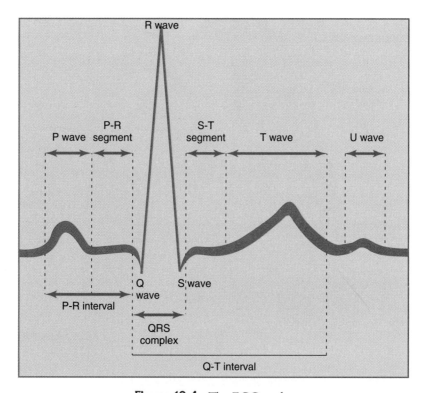

Figure 12-4. The ECG cycle.

P wave	The P wave represents the electrical activity associated with the contraction of the atria, or *atrial depolarization*.
QRS complex	The QRS complex represents the electrical activity associated with the contraction of the ventricles, or *ventricular depolarization*, and consists of the Q wave, the R wave, and the S wave.
T wave	The T wave represents the electrical recovery of the ventricles, or *ventricular repolarization*. The muscle cells are recovering in preparation for another impulse.
U wave	Occasionally a U wave follows a T wave. It is a small wave that is associated in some as yet undefined way with repolarization.

Baseline, Segments, and Intervals

The flat, horizontal line that separates the various waves is known as the **baseline.** The waves deflect either upward (positive deflection) or downward (negative deflection) from the baseline. The baseline is divided into segments and intervals for the purpose of interpretation and analysis of the ECG by the physician. A **segment** is the portion of the ECG between two waves, and an **interval** is the length of a wave or the length of a wave with a segment.

P–R segment	The P–R segment represents the time interval from the end of the atrial depolarization to the beginning of the ventricular depolarization. It is the time needed for the impulse to be delayed at the AV node and then travel through the bundle of His and Purkinje fibers to the ventricles.

S–T segment	The S–T segment represents the time interval from the end of the ventricular depolarization to the beginning of repolarization of the ventricles.
P–R interval	The P–R interval represents the time interval from the beginning of the atrial depolarization to the beginning of the ventricular depolarization.
Q–T interval	The Q–T interval is the time interval from the beginning of the ventricular depolarization to the end of repolarization of the ventricles.
Baseline	The baseline after the T wave (or U wave, if present) represents the period when the entire heart returns to its resting, or polarized, state.

Electrocardiograph Paper

Electrocardiograph paper is divided into two sets of squares for accurate and convenient measurement of the waves, intervals, and segments (Figure 12-5). Each small square is 1 millimeter (mm) high and 1 mm wide. Each large square (made up of 25 small squares) is 5 mm high and 5 mm wide. By measuring the various waves, intervals, and segments of the graph cycle, the physician is able to determine whether the electrical activity of the heart falls within normal limits.

Electrocardiograph paper consists of a black or blue base with a white plastic coating. A black or red graph is printed on top of the plastic coating. A heated stylus moves over the heat-sensitive paper and melts away the plastic coating, resulting in the recording of the ECG cycles. In addition to being heat sensitive, the paper is pressure sensitive and should be handled carefully to avoid making impressions that would interfere with its proper reading.

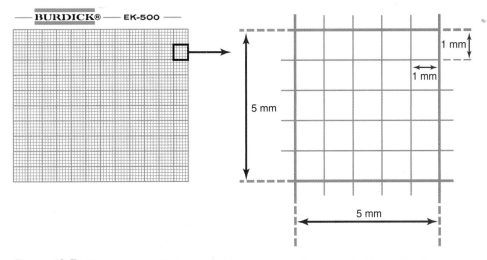

Figure 12-5. Diagram of ECG paper with a section enlarged to indicate the size of the large and small squares.

Standardization of the Electrocardiograph

The electrocardiograph machine must be standardized when recording an ECG. This ensures an accurate and reliable recording. It means that an ECG run on one electrocardiograph will compare with a tracing run on another machine.

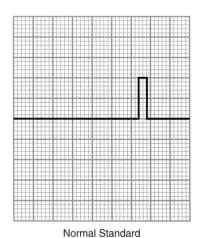

Normal Standard
Standardization mark is
10 mm high

Figure 12-6. Standardization mark.

By international agreement, 1 millivolt (mV) of electricity should cause the stylus to move 10 mm high in amplitude (10 small squares). A three-channel electrocardiograph automatically records standardization marks on the tracing. During the recording, the machine allows 1 mV to enter the electrocardiograph machine, which should result in an upward deflection of 10 mm. The marking on the ECG paper is known as the *standardization mark* (Figure 12-6). The width of the mark made by the machine is approximately 2 mm (two small squares). If the standardization mark is more or less than 10 mm in amplitude, it can be adjusted. The manufacturer's operating manual must be consulted for proper adjustment information. An electrocardiograph must never be adjusted without use of the operating manual.

Electrocardiograph Leads

The standard electrocardiogram consists of 12 leads. Each lead provides and electrical "photograph" of the heart's activity from a different angle. Together the 12 leads, or "photographs" facilitate a thorough interpretation of the heart's activity.

The electrical impulses given off by the heart are picked up by **electrodes** and conducted into the machine through lead wires. Electrodes are made of a substance that is a good conductor of electricity. The impulses given off by the heart are very small. Therefore, to produce a readable ECG, they must be made larger, or

---

Highlight on Stress Testing

Exercise tolerance testing, also called stress testing, is a diagnostic procedure used to evaluate the cardiovascular system. It is usually performed in a hospital under the direction of a cardiologist and an exercise tolerance technician so that emergency equipment and trained personnel are available to deal with unusual situations that might arise.

The purpose of exercise tolerance testing is as follows:

1. To diagnose ischemic heart disease that cannot be detected by a standard resting electrocardiogram. *Ischemic heart disease* is heart disease that occurs as a result of inadequate blood supply to the myocardium, as in a myocardial infarction and angina pectoris.
2. To assist in evaluating the cause of cardiac symptoms, such as chest discomfort and dysrhythmias.
3. To assess the effectiveness of cardiac drug therapy.
4. To follow the course of rehabilitation after a myocardial infarction or a cardiac surgical procedure such as a coronary bypass operation or a coronary stent placement.
5. To determine an individual's fitness for a strenuous exercise program, such as jogging.

Exercise tolerance testing involves the continuous electrocardiographic monitoring of an individual during physical exercise. The patient's blood pressure, heart rate, and physical symptoms are also monitored during the test. The tolerance testing is accomplished by having the patient use a treadmill. The intensity of the physical exertion is gradually increased until the patient's target heart rate is reached unless the signs and symptoms of cardiac ischemia appear, in which case the test is stopped. These symptoms include claudication (severe leg pain), severe dyspnea, chest discomfort or pain, pallor, and dizziness.

The individual's response to the exercise tolerance testing is used to determine normal or abnormal results. For example, a normal response is a gradual increase in the patient's blood pressure as the physical exertion increases, whereas an abnormal response is a sudden increase or decrease of the patient's blood pressure. The electrocardiogram of a normal individual exhibits a shortened P–R interval and a compressed QRS complex. An abnormal tracing indicative of myocardial ischemia results in a depressed S–T segment and an inverted T wave. An abnormal exercise tolerance test usually warrants further testing, such as a coronary angiogram.

amplified, by a device known as an amplifier, located within the electrocardiograph. The amplified voltages are changed into mechanical motion by the *galvanometer* and recorded on the electrocardiograph paper by a heated stylus (Figure 12-7).

There are four limb electrodes, which include the right arm electrode (RA), the left arm electrode (LA), the right leg electrode (RL), and the left leg electrode (LL). The right leg electrode is known as the ground. It is not used for the actual recording but serves as an electrical reference point. The chest leads are abbreviated V or C and use six chest electrodes.

Disposable electrodes are typically used with a three-channel electrocardiograph. A disposable electrode consists of a self-adhesive tab that contains an electrolyte. An **electrolyte** is a substance that facilitates the transmission of the heart's electrical impulse. The electrode is applied to the skin and held in place with its adhesive backing; it is thrown away after use.

Bipolar Leads

The first three leads of the 12-lead ECG are the bipolar leads; they are leads I, II, and III. The bipolar leads use two of the limb electrodes to record the heart's electrical activity. Lead I records the heart's voltage difference between the right arm and the left arm, lead II records the difference between the right arm and the left leg, and lead III records the difference between the left arm and the left leg (Figure 12-8).

Lead II shows the heart's rhythm more clearly than the other leads. Because of this, the physician often requests a *rhythm strip,* which is a longer recording (approximately 12 inches) of lead II.

Augmented Leads

The next three leads are the augmented leads. They include aVR (augmented voltage–right arm), aVL (augmented voltage–left arm), and aVF (augmented voltage–left leg or foot). Lead aVR records the heart's voltage difference between the right arm electrode and a central point between the left arm and left leg. Lead aVL records the heart's voltage difference between the left arm electrode and a central point between the right arm and left leg. Lead aVF records the heart's voltage difference between the left leg electrode and a central point between the right and left arms. Leads I, II, III, aVR, aVL, and aVF record the voltage from side to side or from top to bottom of the heart (see Figure 12-8).

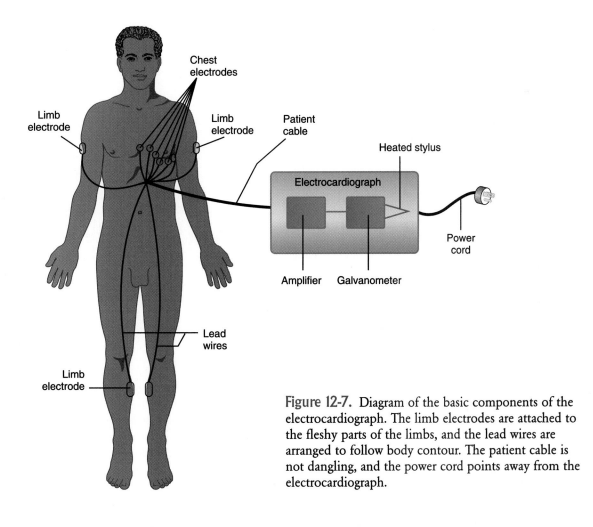

Figure 12-7. Diagram of the basic components of the electrocardiograph. The limb electrodes are attached to the fleshy parts of the limbs, and the lead wires are arranged to follow body contour. The patient cable is not dangling, and the power cord points away from the electrocardiograph.

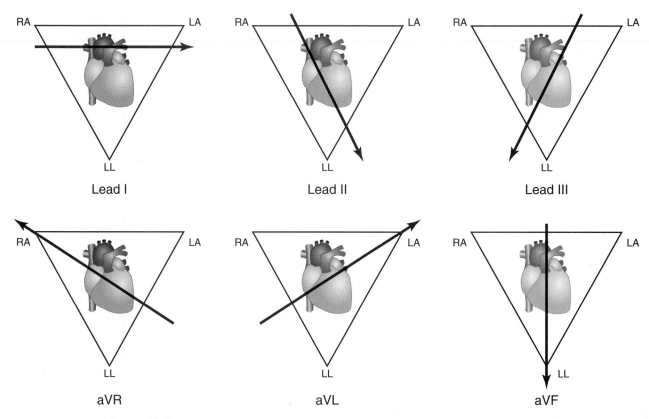

Figure 12-8. Diagram of the heart's voltage for leads I, II, III, aVR, aVL, and aVF.

What Would You DO?
What Would You *Not* DO?

Case Study 1

Camilla Rossi is 22 years old and works at a waffle house. She comes to the office because she has been experiencing some heart problems. Over the past month she's had three episodes of tachycardia, palpitations, trouble breathing, and profuse sweating. She is really scared that she has heart disease. Her grandfather died a year ago from a heart attack and she's afraid she'll be next. The physician orders an ECG but

Camilla is reluctant to have the procedure. She's embarrassed about having to take her top off, and she's worried that she will get shocked by all the wires coming out of the machine. She says that she doesn't have health insurance, and she doesn't know how she would pay for such a fancy test. She wants to know if there's a cheaper way to find out what's wrong with her.

Chest Leads

The last six leads are the chest, or precordial, leads. They are V_1, V_2, V_3, V_4, V_5, and V_6. These leads record the heart's voltage from front to back. The voltage is recorded from a central point "inside" the heart to a point on the chest wall where the electrode is placed. These points correspond to the chest leads. Figure 12-9 shows the proper location of

the six chest leads. The medical assistant should be able to locate them accurately. When first learning to locate the chest leads, it helps to mark their location on the patient's chest with a felt-tipped pen.

Normally the electrocardiogram is recorded with the paper moving at a speed of 25 mm/sec. Occasionally the ECG cycles are close together, making the recording

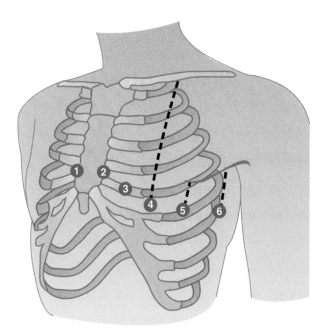

Figure 12-9. Recommended positions for ECG chest leads:
1. V_1, Fourth intercostal space at right margin of sternum
2. V_2, Fourth intercostal space at left margin of sternum
3. V_3, Midway between positions 2 and 4
4. V_4, Fifth intercostal space at junction of left midclavicular line
5. V_5, At horizontal level of position 4 at left anterior axillary line
6. V_6, At horizontal level of position 4 at left midaxillary line

difficult to read. The medical assistant can change the paper speed to 50 mm/sec to spread out the cycles. To alert the physician to the change, he or she must make a notation of it on the recording.

Maintenance of the Electrocardiograph

Electrocardiographs require very little maintenance. The electrocardiograph should be cleaned frequently with a mild detergent and a soft cloth to remove dust and dirt. Commercial solvents and abrasives should not be used because they can damage the finish.

The electrode cables should be cleaned periodically with a cloth saturated with a disinfectant cleaner. The cables should never be immersed in the cleaning solution because this could damage them.

Electrocardiographic Capabilities

Electrocardiographs have a variety of capabilities that permit specific recording options. These capabilities are listed and described next.

Three-Channel Recording Capability

An electrocardiograph with a three-channel recording capability can record electrical activity through three leads simultaneously. This is in contrast to a single-channel electrocardiograph, which records only one lead at a time. The advantage of a three channel electrocardiograph is that an ECG can be produced in less time than would be required if each lead were recorded separately.

The leads that are recorded simultaneously are leads I, II, and III, followed by aVR, aVL, and aVF, followed by V_1, V_2, and V_3, followed by V_4, V_5, and V_6. Recording three leads at one time requires three-channel recording paper, which is designed in a standard 8½-by-11-inch format. This size of the printout fits easily into the patient's chart. Most three-channel electrocardiographs have a *copy capability* that quickly produces an accurate recording of the last ECG recorded. See Figure 12-10 for an example of a three-channel ECG recording that also includes a rhythm strip.

Procedure 12-1 describes how to run a 12-lead three-channel electrocardiogram.

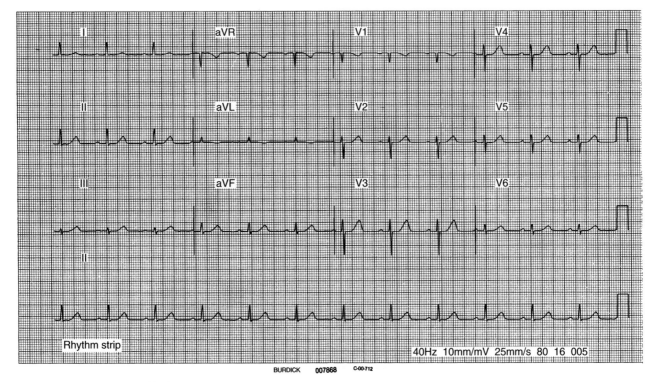

```
Name JANE DOE
ID 12346
34YR Female


13:57 11/22/03
Vent    Durations         Axes
Rate  PR  QRS  QT/QTC    P--QRS--T
 71   188  68  400/423    42  31  71
```

Figure 12-10. A three-channel ECG with a rhythm strip. (Courtesy the Burdick Corporation, Milton, Wisconsin.)

Telephone Transmission

An electrocardiograph with telephone transmission capabilities can transmit a recording over a telephone line to an ECG data interpretation site. The electrocardiograph is equipped with a connector for the attachment of the telephone headset. The recording is interpreted by a cardiologist or a computer at the data reception site, and a printout of the recording along with the interpretation is mailed to the sending office the same day. Patient information and baseline data (e.g., age, sex, height, weight, medications) also need to be relayed to assist in the interpretation. This information is entered on the electrocardiograph and transmitted automatically.

Interpretive Electrocardiographs

An electrocardiograph with interpretive capabilities has a built-in computer program that analyzes the recording as it is being run. Interpretive electrocardiographs provide immediate information on the heart's activity, leading to earlier diagnosis and treatment. Patient data are used in the interpretation of the ECG and must therefore be entered into the computer before running the recording. The data generally required are the patient's age, sex, height, weight, and medications. The computer analysis of the ECG is printed at the top of the recording, along with the reason for each interpretation (Figure 12-11). The results are then reviewed and further interpreted by the physician before diagnosis is made and treatment is initiated.

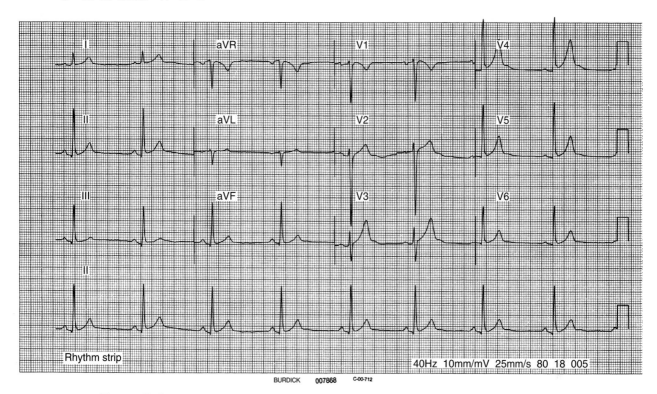

Name JOHN DOE
ID 12345
36YR Male

SINUS BRADYCARDIA
POSSIBLE LEFT VENTRICULAR HYPERTROPHY [VOLTAGE CRITERIA PLUS LAE OR QRS WIDENING]
ABNORMAL ECG

14:04 11/22/03

Vent Rate	Durations			Axes		
	PR	QRS	QT/QTC	P-	-QRS-	-T
48	176	100	428/396	77	75	51

Figure 12-11. An ECG recording with a rhythm strip that has been analyzed by an interpretive electrocardiograph. The computer analysis is printed at the top of the recording, along with the reason for each interpretation. (Courtesy the Burdick Corporation, Milton, Wisconsin.)

Artifacts

The medical assistant is responsible for producing a clear and concise ECG recording that can be easily read and interpreted by the physician. At times structures appear in the recording that are not natural and interfere with the normal appearance of the ECG cycles. They are known as **artifacts** and represent additional electrical activity that is picked up by the electrocardiograph. The medical assistant should be able to identify artifacts and correct them.

There are several types of artifacts; the most common are muscle, wandering baseline, and alternating current (AC) (Figure 12-12).

In some circumstances, as when individuals have trouble holding still or in buildings with older electrical systems, normal methods to eliminate muscle and AC artifacts may not be successful. Electrocardiographs have an *artifact filter* that can reduce artifacts when all else fails.

Because the artifact filter also affects the diagnostic accuracy of the ECG, it should be used as little as possible.

If the medical assistant is unable to correct an artifact, the physician should be consulted. It is possible that the machine is broken. If an electrocardiograph service technician has to be contacted, the medical assistant should have the following information available to aid the service technician in locating the problem:

1. What has already been done to locate and correct the problem
2. Leads in which the artifacts occur
3. A sample of the artifact recorded by the machine

Muscle

A muscle artifact (see Figure 12-12, *A*) can be identified by its fuzzy, irregular baseline. There are two types of muscle artifact: those caused by involuntary muscle

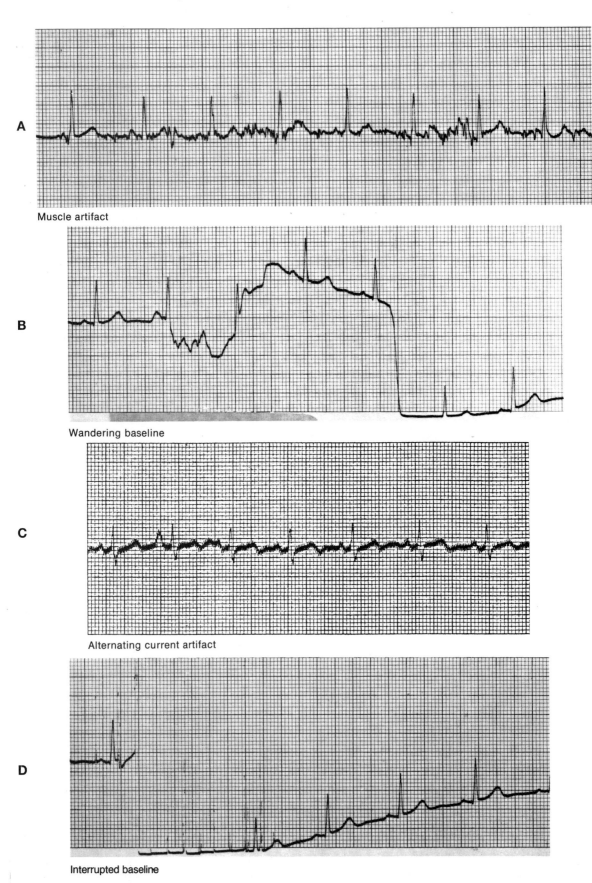

Figure 12-12. A through **D,** Examples of ECG artifacts. (Courtesy the Burdick Corporation, Milton, Wisconsin.)

movement (somatic tremor) and those caused by voluntary muscle movement. Muscle artifacts may be caused by the following:

1. **An apprehensive patient.** To reduce the patient's apprehension and relax muscles, explain the procedure and reassure the patient that having an ECG recorded is a painless procedure.
2. **Patient discomfort.** Make sure the table is wide enough to support the patient's arms and legs adequately. The patient can be made more comfortable by placing a pillow under his or her head. Check to make sure that the room temperature is comfortable for the patient. A temperature that is warm enough for the medical assistant may be too cold for the patient who has removed clothing. This could result in shivering, which would also produce a muscle artifact on the ECG.
3. **Patient movement.** The patient must be instructed to lie still and not talk during the recording.
4. **A physical condition.** Several nervous system disorders, such as Parkinson's disease, prevent relaxation, and the patient trembles continually. The medical assistant must be understanding and try to record while the tremor is at a minimum.

Wandering Baseline

A wandering baseline (see Figure 12-12, *B*) can be caused by the following:

1. **Loose electrodes.** The medical assistant should make sure the disposable adhesive electrodes are attached firmly to the patient's skin. If an electrode pulls loose, it can be reattached with nonallergenic tape. The alligator clips should be attached firmly to the electrodes. To prevent pulling or twisting of the patient cable, it should be well-supported on the table or the patient's abdomen and not be allowed to dangle.
2. **Body creams, oils, or lotions** on the skin in the area where the electrode is applied. The medical assistant should remove these by rubbing with alcohol, using friction.

Alternating Current

Alternating current artifacts (see Figure 12-12, *C*) are caused by electrical interference. Alternating electric current can "leak" or spread out from the power used by electrical appliances in the medical office. This current may be picked up by the patient and carried into the electrocardiograph, where it would show up on the ECG recording as an AC artifact. An AC artifact appears as small straight spiked lines that are consistent. Alternating current artifacts can be caused by the following:

1. **Lead wires not following body contour.** Dangling lead wires can pick up alternating current. Arrange the wires to follow body contour and to lie flat.
2. **Other electrical equipment in the room.** Lamps, autoclaves, radiographic equipment, electrical examining tables, or other electrical equipment that is plugged in may be leaking alternating current. Unplug all nearby electrical equipment.
3. **Wiring in the walls, ceilings, or floors.** Try moving the patient table away from the walls.
4. **Improper grounding of the electrocardiograph.** The machine is automatically grounded when it is plugged in. Make sure the plug is securely in the wall outlet. The right leg electrode is not used for recording the leads but picks up alternating current that has "leaked" onto the patient and carries it into the electrocardiograph. The alternating current is then carried away by the machine's grounding system.

Interrupted Baseline

Occasionally an interrupted baseline (see Figure 12-12, *D*) occurs that may be caused by the metal tip of a lead wire becoming detached or by a broken patient cable. If the latter is the case, the manufacturer should be contacted for directions on replacing the patient cable.

MEMORIES From EXTERNSHIP

JANET CANTERBURY: During externship, I was at an office where electrocardiograms were one of the many procedures that were performed. As I approached my first ECG, I realized that it was a male patient who had a lot of hair on his chest and that I would need to shave his chest. I was very nervous, but the procedure went well. Once the ECG was run, he told me that I did a wonderful job and that it didn't hurt at all to have his chest shaved. It was then that I realized that it wasn't so bad after all. That patient made me feel so good about what I do and helped me feel confident in the procedures I had ahead of me.

PROCEDURE 12-1   Running a 12-Lead, Three-Channel Electrocardiogram

Outcome Record a 12-lead electrocardiogram.

Equipment/Supplies:

- Three-channel electrocardiograph
- Disposable electrodes
- ECG paper

1. **Procedural Step.** Work in a quiet, relaxing atmosphere away from sources of electrical interference.

2. **Procedural Step.** Sanitize your hands. Greet and identify the patient. Introduce yourself, and explain the procedure.
   Principle. Explaining the procedure helps reassure apprehensive patients.

3. **Procedural Step.** Prepare the patient. Ask him or her to remove clothing from the waist up. The lower legs must also be uncovered. Assist the patient into a supine position on the table. The table should support the arms and legs adequately so that they do not dangle. Properly drape the patient's uncovered body parts to prevent exposure and to provide warmth. A pillow can be used to support the patient's head.
   Principle. The chest, upper arms, and lower legs must be uncovered to allow proper placement of the electrodes. The patient should be kept warm, and the arms and legs should not be allowed to dangle; otherwise, muscle artifacts could result.

4. **Procedural Step.** Help the patient relax by explaining the procedure. Tell the patient that having an ECG recording is painless. Explain that he or she must lie still and not talk in order for an accurate recording to be obtained.
   Principle. The patient should be mentally and physically relaxed for an accurate ECG recording; an apprehensive or moving patient produces muscle artifacts.

5. **Procedural Step.** Position the electrocardiograph so that the power cord points away from the patient and does not pass under the table. It is usually easier for the medical assistant to work on the left side of the patient.
   Principle. Proper positioning of the electrocardiograph reduces AC artifacts.

6. **Procedural Step.** Prepare the patient's skin for application of the disposable electrodes. If the patient has oily skin or has used lotion, wipe the area to which the electrode will be applied with alcohol and allow it to dry.
   Principle. The patient's skin must be dry and oil-free so that the adhesive backing of the electrodes will stick to the patient's skin and stay on during the procedure.

7. **Procedural Step.** Apply limb electrodes. Firmly apply the adhesive backing of the electrodes to the fleshy part of each of the four limbs (upper arms and lower legs). The tabs of the arm electrodes should point downward, and the tabs of the leg electrodes should point upward. The adhesive backing of the electrode allows it to adhere firmly to the patient's skin.
   Principle. The tab of the electrodes should be positioned toward the cable to provide a more stable connection when the lead wire is attached to the electrode and to prevent the lead wires from pulling and causing artifacts.

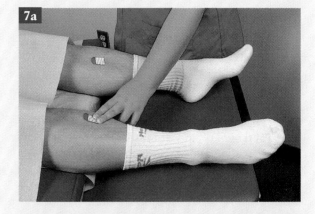

7a

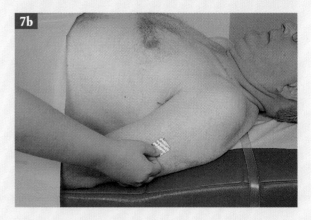

7b

8. **Procedural Step.** Apply the chest electrodes. Properly locate each chest position and apply the electrode with the tab pointing downward. If the patient's chest is hairy, dry shave it at each electrode site before applying the electrode. Continue until all six of the chest electrodes have been applied.

Principle. Positioning the tabs of the electrodes downward prevents the lead wires from pulling and causing artifacts.

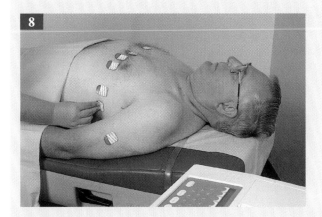

9. **Procedural Step.** Connect the lead wires to the electrodes. This is accomplished by inserting an alligator clip onto the metal tip of each electrode. The alligator clip is then attached to the tab of each electrode. The ends of the lead wires are usually color coded and identified with abbreviations to help the medical assistant connect the proper lead to each electrode. Arrange the lead wires to follow body contour.

Principle. Arranging the lead wires to follow body contour reduces the possibility of AC artifacts.

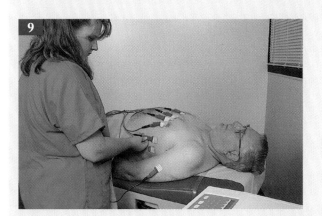

10. **Procedural Step.** Plug the patient cable into the machine. The cable should be supported on the table or on the patient's abdomen to prevent pulling or twisting.

11. **Procedural Step.** Turn on the electrocardiograph. Enter patient data using the soft-touch keypad. Always use your fingertips to enter the data. Pencils or other sharp objects can damage the keyboard. As the data are entered, they will be displayed on the LCD screen. The patient data to be entered generally include the patient's name, a patient identification number, age, sex, height, weight, and medications.

Principle. The patient data and the date, and the time of the recording are printed at the top of the recording. If the electrocardiograph is equipped with interpretive capabilities, this information is also used in the computer-assisted interpretation of the ECG.

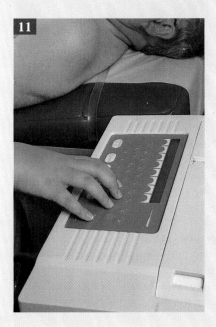

12. **Procedural Step.** Press the AUTO (automatic) button and run the recording. The machine automatically inserts a standardization mark at the beginning of the recording, followed by the recording of the 12-lead electrocardiogram in a three-channel format.

13. **Procedural Step.** After the ECG has been recorded, check the printout to make sure the standardization mark is 10 mm high. If it is more or less than 10 mm, adjust the electrocardiograph as needed and run another ECG. Observe the recording for artifacts. If they appear, correct the problem and run another ECG.

PROCEDURE 12-1

Continued

PROCEDURE 12-1   Running a 12-Lead, Three-Channel
Electrocardiogram—Cont'd

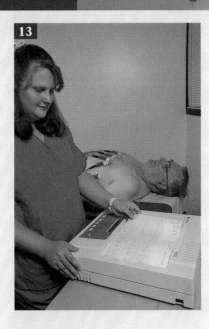

14. **Procedural Step.** Turn the machine off. Disconnect the lead wires. Remove and discard the electrodes.
15. **Procedural Step.** Assist the patient in stepping down from the table.
16. **Procedural Step.** Sanitize your hands. Chart the procedure. Include the date and time and the name of the procedure (12-lead electrocardiogram). Place the recording in the patient's medical record and put the record in the appropriate place to be reviewed by the physician.
17. **Procedural Step.** Return all equipment to its proper storage place.

CHARTING EXAMPLE	
Date	
6/12/05	10:30 a.m. Completed a 12-lead ECG. —————————————— J. Canterbury, CMA

Holter Monitor Electrocardiography

A Holter monitor is a portable ambulatory monitoring system for recording the cardiac activity of a patient for 24 hours. The system is designed so that the patient is able to maintain his or her usual daily activities with minimal inconvenience while being monitored. Holter monitor electrocardiography is an important noninvasive procedure used to diagnose cardiac rhythm and conduction abnormalities. It is most frequently used to evaluate patients with unexplained syncope, to discover intermittent cardiac dysrhythmias not picked up on a routine 12-lead ECG, to assess the effectiveness of antidysrhythmic medications (e.g., digitalis and antianginal drugs), and to assess the effectiveness of an artificial pacemaker.

The Holter monitor consists of electrodes placed on the patient's chest and a special portable magnetic tape recorder that continually monitors the heart's activity (Figure 12-13). The lightweight, battery-powered recorder is held in a protective case, which is worn either on a belt around the patient's waist or hung over the patient's shoulder by a strap. Throughout the 24-hour period, the system continuously records the patient's heartbeat on a magnetic cassette tape.

An increasing number of physicians have Holter monitors in their offices. The medical assistant is responsible for preparing the patient, applying and removing the monitor, and instructing the patient for the procedure (see the box on Holter Monitor Patient Guidelines).

Electrode Placement

A special type of electrode is used with the Holter monitor. It consists of a round electrode plate with an adhesive backing and a central sponge pad that contains an electrolyte gel (Figure 12-14). This type of electrode is disposable and must be discarded after use.

Most Holter monitors are dual-channel systems, which means that two leads are recorded at one time. A dual-channel monitor requires five electrodes, one of which is the ground electrode. Some dual-channel monitors have the ground built into the monitor, in which case only four electrodes are required. The electrodes must be properly placed to ensure an accurate recording. Figure 12-15 shows the electrode positions for the dual-channel Holter monitor. When one is learning to place these leads, it may help to mark their location on the patient's chest with a felt-tipped pen.

The monitor's effectiveness should be checked after hooking up the patient to make sure a clear signal is being relayed from the electrodes to the recorder. This check is performed by attaching one end of an accessory device known as a *test cable* to the recorder and the other end to an electrocardiograph machine. A short baseline strip is then recorded and observed for correct waveforms and the absence of artifacts. If the waveforms are incorrect or if artifacts are present, the patient may not be hooked up properly, or a cable or lead malfunction may exist. The medical assistant should reconnect the leads and reposition the

Holter Monitor Patient Guidelines

The following guidelines must be relayed to the patient to ensure an accurate and reliable electrocardiographic recording.

1. Keep the electrodes and monitor dry to ensure an accurate recording and prevent damage to the recorder. Do not shower, bathe, or swim while wearing the monitor.
2. Do not touch or move the electrodes during the monitoring period to prevent artifacts from appearing in the recording.
3. Do not handle the monitor or take it out of its carrying case.
4. Depress the event marker only momentarily when a significant symptom or event occurs. Overuse of the marker can cause masking of the ECG signals that are being relayed from the electrodes.

5. Do not use an electric blanket while wearing the monitor.
6. Keep a diary of activities, emotional states, and symptoms (e.g., chest pain, nausea, dizziness, anger, excitement) experienced during the monitoring period. With each entry, note the time the activity, feeling, or symptom occurred.
7. Record the following activities in your diary: physical exercise, walking up or down stairs, emotional states, smoking, bowel movements, meals (including alcohol and caffeinated beverages), sexual intercourse, medications consumed, and sleep periods.

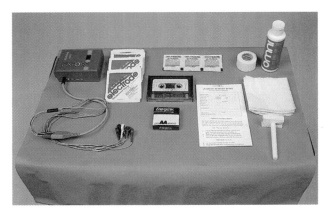

Figure 12-13. Holter monitor and the supplies required for its application.

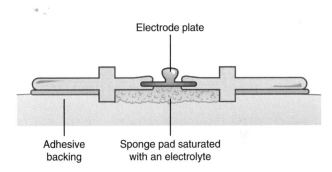

Figure 12-14. Electrode used with a Holter monitor.

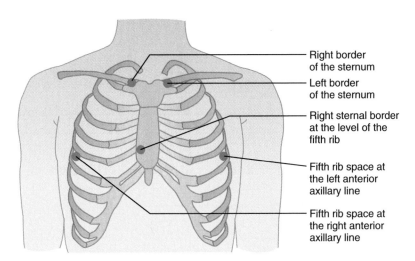

Figure 12-15. Holter monitor electrode positions.

electrodes. If a problem still exists, the monitor may be malfunctioning and need repair.

Activity Diary

An important aspect of the Holter monitor procedure is the completion of an *activity diary* by the patient (Figure 12-16). All activities and emotional states (e.g., stress, anger, excitement) must be recorded during the monitoring period, along with the time of their occurrence. In addition, any physical symptoms experienced by the patient, such as vertigo, syncope, palpitations, chest pain, and dyspnea, must be recorded, along with the time of their occurrence. As a result, any dysrhythmia recorded on the magnetic tape can be compared with reports in the patient's diary to correlate patient symptoms with cardiac activity.

Event Marker

Some monitors have an *event marker* mounted on one end of the recorder; the event marker is used along with the patient diary for patient evaluation. The patient should be told to depress the event marker momentarily when experiencing a symptom. Depressing the marker places an electronic signal on the magnetic tape. This signal will later alert the technician to a significant event on the tape.

Evaluating Results

At the end of the 24-hour period, the Holter monitor system is removed from the patient, and the tape is evaluated either by displaying it on a special Holter scanning screen or by computer analysis. Printouts of any portion of the electrocardiographic recording can be obtained for further study. The tape must be analyzed where a trained technician and Holter scanner or computer are available. This may involve transferring the tape and diary to the cardiac department of a hospital for evaluation. The physician is provided with a written data report of the 24-hour period along with selected printouts of the patient's cardiac activity, including samples of any dysrhythmias or abnormalities exhibited by the patient.

Procedure 12-2 describes how to apply a Holter monitor.

PATIENT ACTIVITY DIARY		
TIME	ACTIVITY	SYMPTOM
AM PM	*Start recording*	
8:30 AM	Ate breakfast Smoked cigarette	
9:15 AM	Driving freeway	Chest pounding
10:35 AM	Argued with boss	Chest pounding
10:45 AM	Took medication	
12:30 PM	Ate lunch	Relaxed
1:15 PM	Walked up two flights of stairs	Stomach burning Pain in left arm

Page 1

PATIENT ACTIVITY DIARY		
TIME	ACTIVITY	SYMPTOM

Page 2

Figure 12-16. Patient's activity diary while wearing a Holter monitor.

PROCEDURE 12-2   Applying a Holter Monitor

Outcome   Apply a Holter monitor.

Equipment/Supplies:
- Holter monitor
- Blank magnetic tape
- Battery
- Carrying case
- Belt or shoulder strap
- Disposable electrodes

- Alcohol swabs
- Gauze
- Razor
- Nonallergenic tape
- Patient diary
- Liquid skin abrasive

1. **Procedural Step.** Assemble the equipment.

2. **Procedural Step.** Prepare the equipment as follows: Remove the old battery from the recorder (if present), and install a new high-quality alkaline battery according to the markings on the battery holder. Insert a blank magnetic tape into the monitor according to the manufacturer's instructions.
   Principle. A new battery must be installed each time the monitor is used to ensure sufficient power throughout the 24-hour monitoring period.

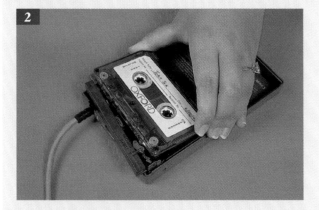

3. **Procedural Step.** Sanitize your hands. Greet and identify the patient.

4. **Procedural Step.** Introduce yourself, and explain the procedure. Tell the patient that the Holter monitor will record the heartbeat without interfering with his or her daily activities. Tell the patient that, because of its small size, the monitor will be fairly inconspicuous. Instruct the patient in the guidelines for wearing a Holter monitor (see the Holter Monitor Patient Guidelines box.
   Principle. The patient must follow the guidelines carefully to ensure an accurate recording.

5. **Procedural Step.** Prepare the patient by asking him or her to remove clothing from the waist up.
   Principle. Clothing must be removed for placement of the chest electrodes.

6. **Procedural Step.** Place the patient in a sitting position.

7. **Procedural Step.** Locate the electrode placement sites (see Figure 12-15), and at each site prepare an area of skin slightly larger than an electrode as follows:
   a. If the patient's chest is hairy, dry shave it at each electrode site.
   b. Swab the skin with an alcohol wipe and allow the area to dry completely.
   c. Slightly abrade the skin with a 4 × 4-inch gauze square moistened with a liquid skin abrasive (e.g., OmniPrep) until the skin is reddened. Rub the skin lightly with four or five small circular motions. On a patient with normal skin, use about the same pressure used to file the fingernails. Use less pressure on patients with sensitive skin or poor skin condition.
   Principle. Shaving the chest improves the adherence of the electrodes and makes them easier to remove. The placement sites must be abraded with gauze to improve the adherence of the electrodes.

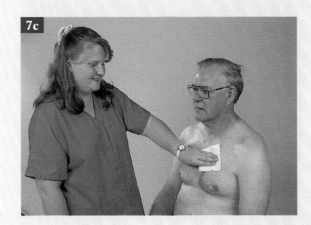

PROCEDURE 12-2

Continued

PROCEDURE 12-2 Applying a Holter Monitor—Cont'd

8. **Procedural Step.** Remove the electrodes from their package. Peel the electrode backing from one of the electrodes. Avoid touching the adhesive to prevent loss of its stickiness. Check to make sure the conducting gel is moist. If it is dry, obtain a new electrode.
   Principle. The conducting gel should be moist to ensure good conduction of electrical impulses.

9. **Procedural Step.** Apply the electrode to the first electrode position site with the adhesive side facing downward. Apply firm pressure beginning at the center of the electrode and moving outward. Ensure a firm seal by running your finger around the outer edge of the electrode until it is firmly attached to the skin.
   Principle. If pressure is applied by starting at one side and moving to the other, some of the conducting gel may be forced out from under the electrode, interfering with good conduction. The electrodes must be firmly attached to prevent distortion of the ECG recording.

10. **Procedural Step.** Repeat steps 8 and 9 until all five electrodes have been applied.
    Principle. The electrodes pick up and conduct the electrical impulses given off by the heart.

11. **Procedural Step.** Attach the lead wires to the electrodes. Form a loop in each lead wire near the electrode, and attach the loop firmly to the patient with surgical tape.
    Principle. The lead wires transmit the electrical impulses to the cardiac monitor. Forming a loop reduces artifacts caused by electrode movement.

12. **Procedural Step.** Place a strip of nonallergenic tape over each electrode. Connect the lead wires to the patient cable.
    Principle. Applying tape facilitates secure attachment of the electrodes by reducing strain and pulling on them.

13. **Procedural Step.** Check the recorder's effectiveness by connecting it to an electrocardiograph machine by way of the test cable and running a short baseline recording.
    Principle. Checking the recorder verifies that the patient is properly hooked up and that no cable or lead malfunction exists.

14. **Procedural Step.** Tell the patient to redress while being careful not to pull on the lead wires. The electrode cable should extend from under the patient's garment or between buttons of the patient's garment.

15. **Procedural Step.** Insert the recorder into its carrying case and strap it over the patient's clothing, using either a waist belt or shoulder strap. Make sure the strap is properly adjusted so the weight of the recorder does not strain or pull on the lead wires.
    Principle. Straining or pulling on the lead wires may cause detachment of the electrodes.

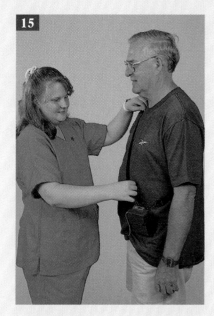

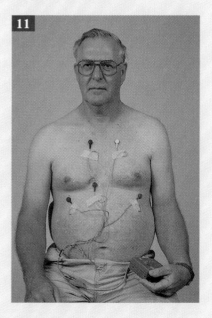

16. **Procedural Step.** Plug the electrode cable into the recorder. Check the time and turn on the recorder according to the manufacturer's instructions. Record the starting time in the patient diary.
Principle. The beginning time must be recorded for later correlation of the patient diary with cardiac activity.

17. **Procedural Step.** Complete the patient information section of the diary notebook. Give the diary to the patient and provide him or her with instructions on completing it.
Principle. The patient diary is used to correlate patient symptoms with cardiac activity.

18. **Procedural Step.** Instruct the patient when to return for removal of the monitor. Be sure to remind the patient not to forget to bring the diary.

19. **Procedural Step.** Sanitize your hands and chart the procedure in the patient's chart. Include the date and time, the name of the procedure (application of a Holter monitor), and the beginning time. Also chart instructions given to the patient.

CHARTING EXAMPLE

Date	
6/15/05	2:00 p.m. Applied Holter monitor. Starting time: 2:15 p.m. Instructed pt on recording data in diary. To return on 6/16/05 at 2:30 p.m. for removal of monitor. ————— J. Canterbury, CMA

PROCEDURE 12-2

⫸ PATIENT TEACHING

Angina Pectoris

Answer questions the patient has about angina pectoris.

What is angina pectoris?
Angina pectoris is actually a symptom rather than a disease. Its name is a Latin term that means "pain in the chest." Angina pectoris occurs when the muscle tissue of the heart does not receive enough oxygenated blood, resulting in discomfort or pain under the sternum.

What causes angina pectoris?
In the majority of patients, the cause of angina is **atherosclerosis.** This is a condition in which fibrous plaques of fatty deposits and cholesterol build up on the inner walls of the coronary arteries, causing a narrowing and obstruction of the lumen of these arteries. This in turn results in a reduction of oxygenated blood flow to the heart. In spite of the narrowing, enough oxygen may still reach the heart for normal needs. However, more oxygen is needed when situations occur that increase the workload of the heart, such as physical activity, emotional stress, a heavy meal, and exposure to cold weather. If the coronary arteries cannot deliver enough oxygen during these times of increased need, angina pectoris results.

Continued

Cardiac Dysrhythmias

The normal ECG graph cycle consists of a P wave, a QRS complex, and a T wave, which repeats in a regular pattern (see Figure 12-4). The term **normal sinus rhythm** refers to an ECG that is within normal limits. This means that the waves, intervals, segments, and cardiac rate fall within normal range. The normal heart rate ranges from 60 to 100 beats per minute. A rate below 60 beats per minute is *sinus bradycardia,* and a rate faster than 100 beats per minute is *sinus tachycardia.*

Each ECG graph cycle is separated from the next one by a flat length of baseline termed the T-P segment. Any change in the baseline distance between graph cycles indicates a cardiac abnormality that falls into one of the following categories: (1) extra beats, (2) an abnormal rhythm, or (3) an abnormal heart rate. The medical assistant should be able to recognize basic cardiac dysrhythmias on an electrocardiographic recording for the purpose of alerting the physician of their presence. The dysrhythmias the medical assistant should be able to identify are presented next, along with brief descriptions and significant clinical aspects.

PATIENT TEACHING—Cont'd

What happens during an angina episode?

Individuals experience angina in different ways, including the following: severe indigestion or burning, heaviness, ache, or squeezing or crushing pressure in the chest. The chest discomfort varies greatly. It can feel only mildly uncomfortable or it may be intense and accompanied by a feeling of suffocation and doom. The pain is usually felt beneath the sternum and may radiate to the neck, throat, jaw, left shoulder, arm, or back. In most cases, the pain lasts no longer than a few minutes and is relieved by resting. Severe and prolonged anginal pain generally suggests a myocardial infarction (heart attack) and requires immediate medical attention.

What type of treatment might be prescribed by the physician?

The goal of treating angina is to reduce the workload of the heart and to increase the oxygen supply to the heart. This is accomplished by resting when an angina attack occurs. In addition, the physician often prescribes medications, the most common one being nitroglycerin. Nitroglycerin is usually taken sublingually. It works by reducing the workload of the heart and increasing the oxygen supply to the heart by dilating the coronary arteries. Nitroglycerin can also be administered through patches worn on the skin or an ointment rubbed into the skin.

What tests might be ordered by the physician?

For patients who exhibit angina pectoris, the physician may order one or more of the following: a 12-lead electrocardiogram, chest x-ray, blood tests, and an exercise tolerance test. These tests assist in detecting coronary artery narrowing and blockage. To determine the exact location and extent of blockage, a more specific test, known as coronary angiography, may be performed. To help prevent more serious heart disease from developing, the physician generally recommends lifestyle changes such as a diet low in cholesterol and saturated fat, weight reduction, smoking cessation, and stress reduction. For patients with severe blockage of the coronary arteries, coronary artery bypass surgery, coronary stent placement, or balloon angioplasty may be recommended.

Provide the patient with educational materials on angina pectoris and coronary artery disease.

Atrial Premature Contraction

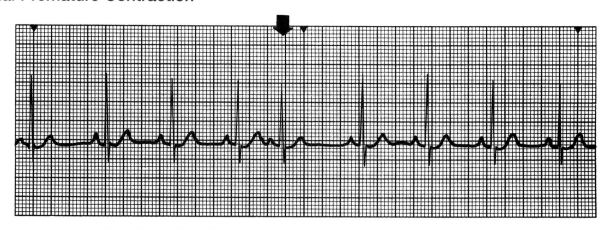

(From Huang, S, et al: *Coronary care nursing.* Philadelphia, 1989, Saunders.)

Description. An atrial premature contraction (APC) is characterized by a beat that comes before the next normal beat is due. The most distinguishing feature is that the P wave of the premature beat has a different shape from the P wave of the normal beat. The APC has a normal QRS complex and a normal T wave, similar to the other ECG graph cycles.

Clinical Aspects. Atrial premature contractions are common in healthy individuals and are often associated with the intake of stimulants such as caffeine and tobacco. They can also be associated with more serious atrial dysrhythmias and structural heart disease.

Paroxysmal Atrial Tachycardia

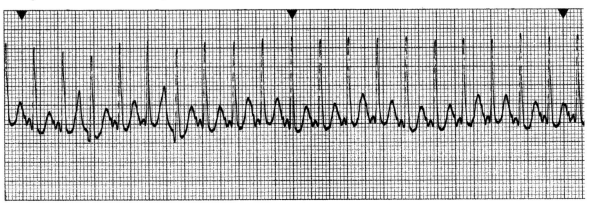

(From Huang, S, et al: *Coronary care nursing.* Philadelphia, 1989, Saunders.)

Description. Paroxysmal atrial tachycardia (PAT) is an abrupt episode of tachycardia with a constant heart rate that usually falls between 150 and 250 beats per minute. PAT is characterized by a rhythm that has a sudden onset and termination. The sudden increase in rate occurs in short bursts and lasts a few seconds only, after which the rate returns to what it was before the PAT occurred. Because of the increase in heart rate, the ECG graph cycles are very close together. With PAT, the patient experiences a sudden pounding or fluttering of the chest associated with weakness, breathlessness, and acute apprehension. Occasionally the patient experiences syncope.

Clinical Aspects. PAT is one of the most common rhythm disorders, often occurring in healthy patients with no underlying heart disease and young adults with normal hearts. It can also occur in individuals with organic heart disease.

Atrial Flutter

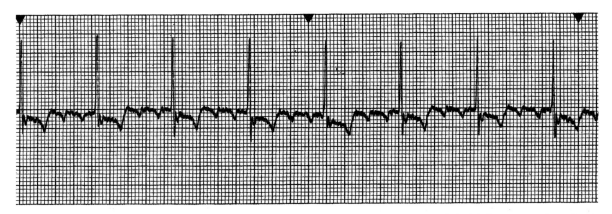

(From Johnson, R, Swartz, MH: *A simplified approach to electrocardiography.* Philadelphia, 1986, Saunders.)

Description. Atrial flutter is a rapid, regular fluttering of the atrium in which the heart rate falls between 250 and 350 beats per minute. More than one P wave precedes each QRS complex, and the P waves appear as saw-toothed spikes between the QRS complexes. The number of waves can range from just 1 extra P wave to as many as 8 falling in rapid succession, but all have the same size and shape. The QRS complexes of an atrial flutter configuration are normal; however, the T wave is usually lost in the P waves.

Clinical Aspects. Atrial flutter rarely occurs in healthy individuals. It is found in patients with underlying heart disease. Atrial flutter is not specific to any particular heart disease; it can occur in patients with mitral valve disease, coronary artery disease, acute myocardial infarction, chronic lung disease, hypertensive heart disease, and pulmonary emboli, and in those who have undergone cardiac surgery.

Atrial Fibrillation

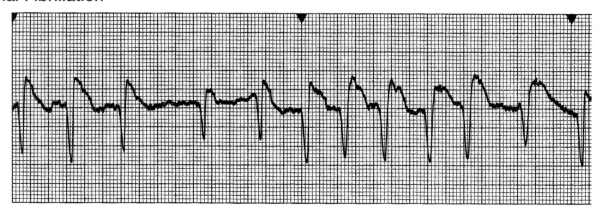

(From Huang, S, et al: *Coronary care nursing.* Philadelphia, 1989, Saunders.)

Description. Atrial fibrillation is characterized by an ECG in which the P waves have no definite pattern or shape. The P waves appear as irregular wavy undulations between the QRS complexes. The QRS complexes in atrial fibrillation are normal but do not have a definite pattern. It is difficult to measure accurately the atrial rate because the P waves are not discernible; however, the atria are contracting between 400 and 500 times per minute. The ventricular rate may be rapid (between 150 and 180 beats per minute) or relatively normal.

Clinical Aspects. Atrial fibrillation is a common dysrhythmia that can occur both in healthy individuals and in patients with a variety of cardiac diseases. In healthy individuals, it can be initiated by emotional stress, excessive alcohol consumption, and vomiting. In individuals under 50 years of age, the common causes of atrial fibrillation are congenital heart disease and rheumatic heart disease with mitral valve involvement. In individuals over 50 years of age, atrial fibrillation is caused by diseases capable of producing **ischemia** or hypertrophy of the atria, such as coronary artery disease, mitral valve disease, and hypertensive heart disease.

Premature Ventricular Contraction

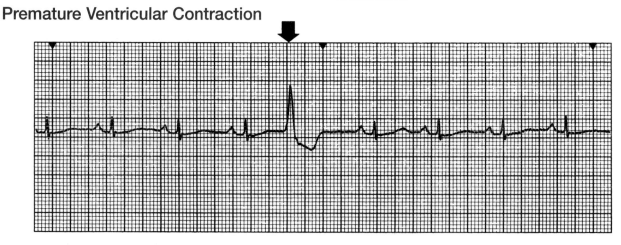

(From Huang, S, et al: *Coronary care nursing.* Philadelphia, 1989, Saunders.)

Description. Premature ventricular contractions (PVCs) are among the most common rhythm disturbances seen on an ECG. The PVC is characterized by a beat that comes early in the cycle, is not preceded by a P wave, has a wide and distorted QRS complex, and has a T wave opposite in direction to the R wave of the QRS complex. Because of the unusual configuration of the QRS complex, the PVC easily stands out from the normal ECG graph cycles. The baseline distance after the PVC is usually longer than the normal distance between the other cycles. In other words, the PVC is followed by a pause before the next normal beat.

Clinical Aspects. PVCs are seen in normal individuals in all age groups and are caused by anxiety, smoking, caffeine, alcohol, and certain medications (e.g., epinephrine, isoproterenol, and aminophylline). PVCs can occur with virtually any type of heart disease but are seen most often in patients with hypertensive heart disease, ischemic heart disease, lung disease with hypoxia, and digitalis toxicity. PVCs are also common in individuals with mitral valve prolapse.

Ventricular Tachycardia

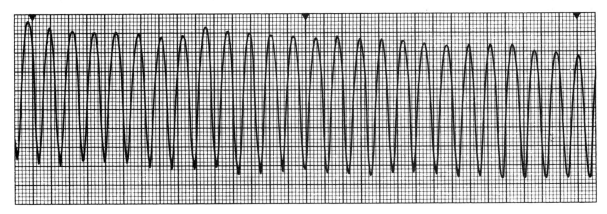

(From Huang, S, et al: *Coronary care nursing.* Philadelphia, 1989, Saunders.)

Description. Ventricular tachycardia consists of a series of three or more consecutive PVCs that occur at a rate of 150 to 250 per minute. The tachycardia may occur paroxysmally and last only a short time, or it may persist for a long time. The QRS complexes are bizarre and widened, and no P waves are present. Sustained ventricular tachycardia is a life-threatening dysrhythmia because the rapid ventricular rate prevents adequate filling time for the heart, leading to reduced cardiac output that often degenerates into ventricular fibrillation and cardiac arrest.

Clinical Aspects. Ventricular tachycardia is usually seen in patients with acute or chronic heart disease. Runs of ventricular tachycardia are indicative of coronary artery disease. Ventricular tachycardia also occurs as a complication of a myocardial infarction.

Ventricular Fibrillation

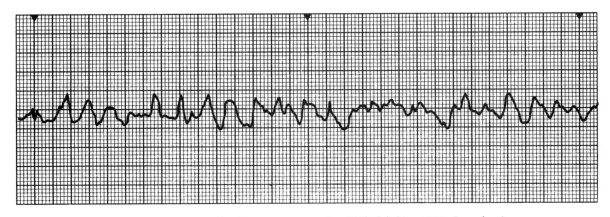

(From Huang, S, et al: *Coronary care nursing.* Philadelphia, 1989, Saunders.)

Description. Ventricular fibrillation is the most serious dysrhythmia. With this type of dysrhythmia, the ventricles do not beat in a coordinated manner but instead they twitch or fibrillate. Because of this, virtually no blood is ejected into the systemic circulation. On an ECG, ventricular fibrillation is characterized by irregular, chaotic undulations of the baseline. There are no recognizable P waves, QRS complexes, or T waves in the irregular line of jagged spikes. Because the ventricles are twitching irregularly, there is no effective ventricular pumping action, resulting in no circulation. Ventricular fibrillation is a serious dysrhythmia that must be treated immediately because it can lead to sudden death.

Clinical Aspects. The most common cause of ventricular fibrillation is an acute myocardial infarction. It can also occur in patients with organic heart disease and cardiac dysrhythmias. It may be preceded by an dysrhythmia such as premature ventricular contractions or ventricular tachycardia, or it may occur spontaneously.

Highlight on Smoking and COPD

Chronic obstructive pulmonary disease (COPD) consists of a group of diseases that includes emphysema, chronic bronchitis, and chronic asthma. It is a chronic, debilitating, and sometimes fatal disease. The primary characteristics associated with COPD are airflow obstruction and shortness of breath.

Currently 16 million people in the United States have been diagnosed with some form of COPD. Smoking tobacco is the primary cause of COPD, specifically emphysema and chronic bronchitis. In the United States, approximately 80% to 90% of the cases of COPD are caused by smoking. According to the American Lung Association, COPD is the fourth leading cause of death in the United States, behind heart disease, cancer, and strokes. Although COPD is much more common in men than in women, the greatest increase in death rates is occurring in females. This is a direct reflection of an increase in the number of women who smoke cigarettes.

Emphysema

Emphysema is most often seen in older people with a long history of smoking. Emphysema is caused by irreversible damage to the alveoli in the lungs from toxins present in cigarette smoke. As alveoli continue to be damaged, the lungs are able to transfer less and less oxygen to the bloodstream. In addition, air becomes trapped in the damaged alveoli, making it difficult to remove during exhalation. Because of this, the primary symptom of emphysema is shortness of breath. Other symptoms include a chronic cough and tiredness. An estimated 2 million people in the United States have emphysema; of these 55% are male and 45% are female. The reason is not yet understood, but fortunately only 10% to 15% of long-term smokers develop emphysema.

Chronic bronchitis is an inflammation of the lining the bronchiole tubes that causes swelling and excess production of mucus. The swelling and excess mucus narrow the bronchiole tubes and restrict airflow into and out of the lungs. Symptoms include a chronic cough, shortness of breath, and coughing up mucus. To be classified as chronic bronchitis, the symptoms must last 3 months or more out of the year for at least 2 years. As the disease progresses, the lips and skin may exhibit cyanosis resulting from a lack of oxygen in the blood. Chronic bronchitis affects people of all ages and often precedes or accompanies emphysema. It is estimated that 12 million Americans have chronic bronchitis.

Damage to the lungs caused by smoking occurs gradually over many years. Because there are no early symptoms, many people don't know they have COPD. By the time a person experiences symptoms, it is usually a sign that irreversible lung damage has already occurred. The first symptoms of COPD include mild shortness of breath on exertion and occasional coughing. The disease slowly becomes more pronounced with severe episodes of dyspnea and coughing even after modest activity. As the disease progresses, the heart can also be affected and the shortness of breath is present all the time, even while sitting quietly. At this point, the individual's quality of life is greatly diminished. When the lungs and heart are no longer able to deliver oxygen to the body's tissues, death occurs.

The best treatment for COPD is for the patient to stop smoking. Continued smoking will make the COPD worse; quitting smoking will slow the disease process. There are programs, support groups, and stop-smoking aids (e.g., nicotine patch) to help individuals quit smoking. Other forms of treatment depend on the patient's condition and degree of lung impairment and may include:

1. Bronchodilators to relax and widen the bronchial tubes to increase airflow. They may be inhaled as aerosol sprays or taken orally.
2. Expectorants to thin the mucus so that is easier to expel.
3. Antibiotics to treat infections that could further interfere with breathing and lung function.
4. Breathing exercises to strengthen the muscles used to breathe.
5. Postural bronchial drainage to remove mucus from the bronchial tubes. The patient lies in positions that allow gravity to drain different parts of the bronchiole tubes.
6. Maintaining overall good health habits, which include proper nutrition, adequate sleep, and regular exercise.
7. Oxygen therapy for patients with low blood oxygen to help with shortness of breath, allowing them to be more active.
8. Special measures include avoiding extremes (heat and cold) of temperature, getting an annual influenza immunization, avoiding individuals with respiratory infections, and reducing exposure to air pollution.
9. Lung transplantation surgery is being performed on some patients who are in the later stages of COPD.

Pulmonary Function Tests

The purpose of a pulmonary function test (PFT) is to assess lung functioning, thus assisting in the detection and evaluation of pulmonary disease. Pulmonary function tests include spirometry, lung volumes, diffusion capacity, arterial blood gas studies, pulse oximetry, and cardiopulmonary exercise tests. The most frequently performed pulmonary function test is spirometry, which is described in detail in the next section. Procedure 12-3 outlines how to use a spirometer.

Spirometry

Spirometry is a simple, noninvasive screening test that is often performed in the medical office. A computerized electronic instrument known as a **spirometer** is used to conduct the test. A spirometer measures how much air is pushed out of the lungs and how fast it is pushed out. The spirometry report is printed out as a table and/or a graph. Spirometry is considered a screening test, and therefore abnormal test results require that the patient undergo additional pulmonary function tests, and possibly a CT scan before a diagnosis can be made. Indications for performing spirometry include the following:

1. Patients who exhibit symptoms of lung dysfunction such as dyspnea
2. Individuals at high risk for lung disease because of smoking or exposure to environmental pollutants such as coal dust, asbestos, and exhaust fumes
3. Patients with lung disease, such as asthma, chronic bronchitis, and emphysema
4. Patients who will undergo surgery (to assess probable lung performance during an operation)
5. Patients who need to be evaluated for lung disability or impairment for a compensation program (e.g., coal miners)

Spirometry Test Results

The results obtained from spirometry testing provide a number of measurements that help the physician assess lung functioning. The most important parameters are described next.

Forced Vital Capacity

Forced vital capacity (FVC) is the maximum volume of air (measured in liters) that can be expired when the patient exhales as forcefully and rapidly as possible and for as long as possible. Forced vital capacity is obtained by having the patient perform a breathing maneuver. The patient is instructed to take a deep breath until the lungs are completely full. Following this, the patient is told to blow all the air out of the lungs and into the mouthpiece as hard and as fast as possible until no more air can be expelled. To be considered an adequate test, the patient must forcibly blow out all the air from the lungs and then continue smooth, continuous exhaling for at least 6 seconds. A minimum of three acceptable efforts should be obtained.

Some patients have difficulty performing the FVC breathing maneuver because they have a physical impairment or poor motivation, or they do not understand the instructions. The medical assistant should be patient and work with these individuals to help them perform the maneuver. If, however, they are unable to perform the maneuver after eight attempts, testing should be discontinued. At this point, fatigue may affect the accuracy of the results and additional efforts are not recommended.

Forced Expiratory Volume After 1 Second

Forced expiratory volume after 1 second (FEV_1) is the volume of air (in liters) that is forcefully exhaled during the first second of the FVC breathing maneuver. The spirometer automatically determines this parameter from the FVC maneuver.

What Would You DO?
What Would You *Not* DO?

Case Study 2

Joel Matthews, 48 years old, is at the office for a biannual checkup. Joel had a mild heart attack 2 years ago. Since then, he has completely changed his life. He's become a vegetarian and practices yoga every morning before going to work. After he gets home, he jogs 10 miles. He also lifts weights every other day and takes herbal vitamin supplements. Since his heart attack he's lost 40 pounds and says that he's never felt better. The only thing he can't seem to do is give up smoking. He started smoking when he was 17 years old and has cut back from 2 packs to 1 pack a day. He keeps trying to stop but says that he's been smoking so long that it might not be possible. Besides, with all the other healthy stuff he's doing, he thinks it probably cancels out the bad effect of the cigarettes. Joel is very concerned that if he does stop smoking, he'll gain back all of the weight that it took him so long to lose.

FEV_1/FVC Ratio

In patients with healthy lungs, 70% to 75% of the air exhaled (FVC) is exhaled in the first second (FEV_1) of the breathing maneuver. This comparison is known as the FEV_1/FVC ratio, and it is expressed as a percentage. For example, a patient with healthy lungs may have a FEV_1/FVC ratio of 85%. This means that 85% of his exhaled air was exhaled during the first second of the breathing maneuver.

In patients with chronic obstructive pulmonary disease (COPD), the FEV_1/FVC ratio falls below 70% to 75%. These patients are unable to move most of their exhaled air out of the lungs during the first second because of an obstruction to the airflow, such as inflammation or damaged lung tissue. Based on the FEV_1/FVC ratio, the obstruction is characterized as mild (61% to 69%), moderate (45% to 60%) or severe (less than 45%). Figure 12-17 illustrates a graph of spirometry parameters in a patient with healthy lungs and in a patient with obstructive pulmonary disease.

Evaluating the Results

To fully evaluate the spirometry test results, certain demographic factors must be taken into consideration. These include the patient's age, sex, weight, and height. These demographic factors are used to calculate the *predicted values*, which is what the results should be for a patient with healthy lungs. Once the test is run, the physician compares the patient's *measured values* with the predicted values.

For example, let's say the FVC predicted value is 6 liters and the FVC measured value is 4 liters. This means that the patient should have been able to exhale 6 liters of air (based on his age, sex, weight, and height), but he was able to exhale only 4 liters of air.

The computerized spirometer automatically calculates predicted values using demographic information entered into the machine by the medical assistant. Both the predicted values and the measured values are then printed on the spirometry report. See Figure 12-18 for an example of these results. Comparing the measured values with the predicted values assists the physician in detecting the presence of pulmonary disease.

Patient Preparation

Patient preparation is essential to obtain accurate test results. To prepare for the test, the patient should be instructed to do the following:

1. Do not eat a heavy meal for 8 hours before the test. (The patient must exert his or her diaphragm muscles and a full stomach may interfere with this action.)
2. Stop smoking at least 8 hours before the test.
3. Do not take bronchodilators for 4 hours before the test.
4. Do not engage in strenuous activity for 4 hours before the test.
5. Wear loose, nonrestrictive clothing to keep the chest area as free as possible, which makes it easier to perform the breathing maneuver.

Calibration of the Spirometer

To ensure accurate and valid test results, the spirometer should be calibrated each day that the machine is used. This is performed by injecting a known quantity of air into the spirometer. A large 3-liter spirometry syringe is used to inject 3 liters of air into the machine. The output should read 3 L, and the reading should not vary by more than 3%. If the machine is not properly calibrated, the medical assistant should consult the operating manual and adjust the machine as required.

Post-Bronchodilator Spirometry

If the results of the spirometry test indicate a possible obstruction, the physician usually orders a post-bronchodilator

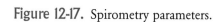

Figure 12-17. Spirometry parameters.

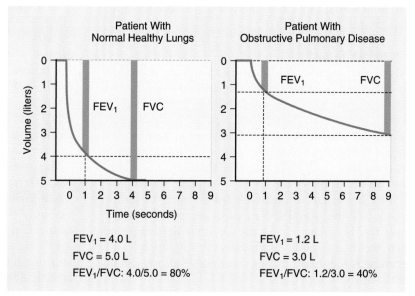

Parameter	Predicted Values	Measured Values
FVC	6.00 liters	4.00 liters
FEV_1	5.00 liters	2.00 liters
FEV_1/FVC	83%	50%

Figure 12-18. Predicted values compared with measured values. This individual exhibits a moderate airflow obstruction.

spirometry test. This test is performed by having the patient inhale a bronchodilator and then running a spirometry test approximately 10 to 15 minutes later. The purpose of this test is to inform the physician as to how treatment will work in patients whose airways are obstructed. If the FVC or FEV_1 parameter increases by at least 15%, the result is reported as positive for bronchodilator responsiveness. This means that the obstruction may be reversible or partially reversible through the use of medication.

What Would You DO?
What Would You *Not* DO?

Case Study 3

Walter Conrad, 62 years old, comes to the office because he has been getting short of breath when he goes up and down stairs. He's worked in the coal mines his whole life and has just retired. The physician orders a pulmonary function test. Walter tries to breathe like he's supposed to during the test, but he just can't seem to do it and he's getting dizzy from trying so hard. He's also having problems with the nose clips. He says they pinch his nose and he feels like he's being smothered. After four attempts, he puts down the spirometer in frustration, and wants to know if he can come back some other time. He says that he's thinking his symptoms aren't that bad after all and maybe he'll just wait and see what happens and come back if it they get worse.

PROCEDURE 12-3   Spirometry Testing

Outcome Provide a spirometry test.

Equipment/Supplies:
- Spirometer
- Disposable tubing
- Disposable mouthpiece
- Disposable nose clips
- Waste container

1. **Procedural Step.** Sanitize your hands. Assemble and prepare the equipment. Calibrate the spirometer according to the manufacturer's instructions. Apply new disposable tubing and a disposable mouthpiece to the spirometer.
   Principle. Calibration of the spirometer ensures accurate and valid test results.

2. **Procedural Step.** Greet and identify the patient. Introduce yourself. Explain the procedure. Tell the patient that he or she will be performing a breathing maneuver several times to see how well his or her lungs are functioning. Ask the patient if he or she prepared properly for the procedure.

3. **Procedural Step.** Measure the patient's weight and height precisely.
   Principle. Precise weight and height measurements are required for the accurate calculation of predicted values.

4. **Procedural Step.** Enter the following data into the computer base of the spirometer: patient's age, sex, weight, height, and any other information required, such as the patient's identification number and whether the patient smokes.
   Principle. Demographic data needs to be entered in order for the computer to calculate the predicted values.

5. **Procedural Step.** Prepare the patient. Have the patient loosen tight clothing such as a necktie or a tight collar. Have the patient sit near the machine. The patient should be seated to prevent dizziness and fainting during the procedure.
   Principle. Tight clothing may make it difficult for the patient to perform the breathing maneuvers.

6. **Procedural Step.** Instruct the patient in the breathing maneuver. The following procedure should be described as well as demonstrated to the patient:
   a. Relax and take the deepest breath possible until your lungs are completely full with air.
   b. Place the mouthpiece in your mouth and seal your lips tightly around it.
   c. Blow out as hard as you can and for as long as possible until your lungs are completely empty. Make sure not to block the opening of the mouthpiece with your tongue.
   d. Remove the mouthpiece from your mouth.
   Principle. The lips must be tightly sealed around the mouthpiece so that all of the air leaving the mouth enters the mouthpiece.

Continued

Spirometry Testing—Cont'd

7. **Procedural Step.** Tell the patient you will repeat the instructions during the test. Encourage the patient to remain calm during the procedure. Gently apply nose clips to the patient's nose. Hand the mouthpiece to the patient and tell him or her to hold it close to the mouth.

   Principle. Fear or anxiety can make the results less reliable. Nose clips prevent air from escaping from the nostrils and makes sure that all breathing is done through the mouth.

8. **Procedural Step.** Begin the test. When the patient is ready, press the enter button on the spirometer. Actively coach the patient as follows:

   a. "Now relax and take in a big breath—in—in—in—more—keep inhaling."

   b. "Put the mouthpiece in your mouth and blow hard. Keep blowing—keep blowing—keep blowing—blow—blow—blow—you're almost there—a little more. That's good. You can stop now."

   c. "Take out the mouthpiece and rest for awhile."

   Principle. Coaching the patient helps to obtain accurate test results.

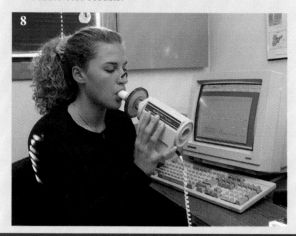

9. **Procedural Step.** If the patient does not perform the breathing maneuver correctly, inform him or her of what modifications are needed for the next effort. Continue until three acceptable efforts have been obtained.

   Principle. Three acceptable efforts must be obtained to ensure valid test results.

10. **Procedural Step.** Gently remove the nose clips from the patient's nose. Remove the mouthpiece and the tubing. Dispose of the mouthpiece, nose clips, and tubing in a regular waste container.

11. **Procedural Step.** Allow the patient to remain seated for a few minutes.

    Principle. The patient may feel light-headed following the procedure.

12. **Procedural Step.** Sanitize your hands. Print the report and label it with the patient's name, date, and your initials. Chart the procedure. Include the date, the time, and the name of the procedure. Place the spirometry report in the patient's medical record and put the record in the appropriate place for review by the physician.

13. **Procedural Step.** Clean the spirometer according to manufacturer's instructions.

CHARTING EXAMPLE

Date	
6/20/05	9:00 a.m. Spirometry test run. Obtained 3 acceptable efforts. Pt stated she was tired following the test. ———————— ————————————— J. Canterbury, CMA

MEDICAL Practice and the LAW

Cardiopulmonary procedures are frightening for many patients because of the potential for unfavorable results. These results must never be given to the patient by the medical assistant. Only a physician can interpret results of electrocardiographic and pulmonary function tests. If results indicate a life-threatening condition, your duty is to calmly notify the physician at once, without alarming the patient. All offices have emergency supplies; be sure you know where they are and how to use them. While you are attending to the machinery and technology, remember the human dignity of the patient, and attend to all of his or her needs for privacy, comfort, respect, and caring.

What Would You DO?
What Would You *Not* DO? RESPONSES

Case Study 1
What Did Janet Do?
- ❏ Tried to reduce Camilla's fears by talking with her calmly and quietly.
- ❏ Explained to Camilla that an ECG is the best screening test available to check for heart problems.
- ❏ Reassured Camilla that she will be draped during the procedure and that she would be exposed as little as possible.
- ❏ Told Camilla that the wires may look a little scary, but they won't shock her. Explained that she won't feel anything when the test is being run.
- ❏ Told Camilla that she could talk with the billing clerk about setting up a payment plan for the test. Provided her with information about community resources that might help her pay for the test.

What Did Janet Not Do?
- ❏ Did not tell Camilla that she was too young to have heart problems.
- ❏ Did not tell Camilla that she needed to act more mature about being tested.

What Would You Do?/What Would You *Not* Do? Review Janet's response and place a checkmark next to the information you included in your response. List additional information you included in your response below.

_____

_____

_____

_____

Case Study 2
What Did Janet Do?
- ❏ Commended Joel on his weight loss and positive lifestyle changes.
- ❏ Shared a positive story with Joel about a patient who stopped smoking and didn't gain weight.
- ❏ Asked Joel if he would like any of the latest information on smoking cessation.

What Did Janet Not Do?
- ❏ Did not agree that Joel's positive lifestyle changes would counteract the bad effects of smoking.

- ❏ Did not lecture Joel on the dangers of smoking because if he has been smoking since age 17 and has been trying to quit, he already knows what they are.

What Would You Do?/What Would You *Not* Do? Review Janet's response and place a checkmark next to the information you included in your response. List additional information you included in your response below.

_____

_____

_____

_____

Case Study 3
What Did Janet Do?
- ❏ Removed the nose clips and emphathized with Mr. Conrad that the test is hard to do and that the nose clips do fit very snugly.
- ❏ Explained to Mr. Conrad that it is normal to feel dizzy and that it is only temporary.
- ❏ Allowed Mr. Conrad to rest for a while. Tried to relax and calm him by talking with him about his family and interests.
- ❏ Talked to Mr. Conrad about the importance of performing the test. Told him that detecting a problem early will help him get the treatment he needs as soon as possible so his condition won't get worse.
- ❏ Asked Mr. Conrad if he would try the test one more time.

What Did Janet Not Do?
- ❏ Did not criticize Mr. Conrad for not being able to perform the test.
- ❏ Did not force Mr. Conrad to stay if he didn't want to but made sure to schedule another PFT for him before he left the office.

What Would You Do?/What Would You *Not* Do? Review Janet's response and place a checkmark next to the information you included in your response. List additional information you included in your response below.

_____

_____

_____

Apply Your KNOWLEDGE

Choose the best answer for each of the following questions.

1. McCabe Waller, 45 years old, has come to the office for a physical examination. Dr. Cardiac has ordered an ECG. Mr. Waller has never had an ECG and asks Janet Canterbury, CMA, what it is. An appropriate response to Mr. Waller would be:
   A. It is a tracing of the muscular activity of the heart
   B. It is a tracing of the electrical activity of the brain
   C. It is an imaging test used to visualize the chambers of the heart
   D. It is a tracing of the electrical activity of the heart

2. Janet makes sure to use proper technique while preparing to run the ECG. Janet does all of the following EXCEPT:
   A. Positions the electrocardiograph on Mr. Waller's left side
   B. Tells Mr. Waller there will be some slight discomfort during the recording
   C. Asks Mr. Waller to lie still and not to talk during the recording
   D. Makes sure the lead wires follow his body contour and do not dangle

3. Janet applies the ten disposable adhesive electrodes to Mr. Waller. Just before running the ECG, she rechecks the electrodes and finds that two of the chest electrodes have come loose. What is the best step for Janet to take to correct this situation?
   A. Remove all of the electrodes and reapply a new set of electrodes
   B. Use nonallergenic tape to secure the loose electrodes
   C. Replace the disposable electrodes with reusable metal electrodes
   D. Ask Mr. Waller to hold the loose electrodes in place while she runs the ECG

4. Janet realizes that it is important for the electrodes to be firmly attached to prevent:
   A. Muscle artifacts
   B. Mr. Waller from escaping
   C. A wandering baseline
   D. Atrial fibrillation

5. After running the ECG, Janet Canterbury, CMA, reviews the recording and notices that it contains three premature ventricular contractions. Janet should:
   A. Shout for help and immediately start CPR on Mr. Waller
   B. Check to make sure all the leads are hooked up correctly
   C. Ask Mr. Waller if he has a living will
   D. Inform Dr. Cardiac that the recording shows a dysrhythmia

6. Mariana Bertilla has come to the office with complaints of an irregular heartbeat, dizziness, and shortness of breath. Dr. Cardiac asks Janet Canterbury, CMA, to run an ECG on Mrs. Bertilla. While recording the ECG, Janet notices that Mrs. Bertilla is shivering and the recording has a fuzzy, irregular baseline. An appropriate action to eliminate this problem would be to:
   A. Cover Mrs. Bertilla with a blanket and rerun the ECG
   B. Unplug all electrical equipment in the room and rerun the ECG
   C. Check to make sure the patient cable is not twisted or dangling
   D. Give Mrs. Bertilla a swig of whiskey to calm her down

7. After running the recording on Mrs. Bertilla, Janet checks to make sure the electrocardiograph machine is properly standardized. This is accomplished by:
   A. Checking the recording to make sure there are no artifacts
   B. Checking the recording to make sure the standardization mark is 10 mm high
   C. Checking the machine to make sure no warning lights are flashing
   D. Checking the recording to make sure it shows a normal sinus rhythm

8. Clement Cooper, 64 years old, has been having some fainting spells lately. His ECG showed a normal sinus rhythm. Dr. Cardiac decides to order a Holter monitor test. To prepare Mr. Cooper for the procedure, Janet Canterbury, CMA, would:
   A. Determine which medications Mr. Cooper should not take during the testing period
   B. Instruct Mr. Cooper to depress the event marker when a significant symptom occurs
   C. Tell Mr. Cooper to take a shower instead of a bath during the testing period
   D. Interpret the recording after the test is completed

9. Mr. Cooper's Holter monitor report indicates that he had intervals of paroxysmal atrial tachycardia during the testing period. The Holter monitor recorded four episodes in 24 hours. Dr. Cardiac checks Mr. Cooper's activity diary to see if he had symptoms at the time of the PAT episodes. Of the following, what symptom would be associated with PAT?
   A. Chest pain
   B. Hiccups
   C. Weakness and breathlessness
   D. Severe headache

10. Albert Newsome, 58 years old, has come to the office. He has a 40-year history of smoking and has mild COPD. Dr. Cardiac wants to assess his lung functioning and asks Janet Canterbury, CMA, to perform spirometry on Mr. Newsome. Which of the following should Janet do during the test?
    A. Ask Mr. Newsome when he last ate
    B. Instruct Mr. Newsome to loosen his necktie
    C. Apply a nose clip to Mr. Newsome's nose
    D. Instruct Mr. Newsome to seal his lips tightly around the mouthpiece
    E. All of the above

CERTIFICATIONREVIEW

❏ **The electrocardiograph** records the heart's electrical activity. An electrocardiogram (ECG) is the graphic representation of this activity.

❏ **The heart consists of four chambers:** the right and left atria and the right and left ventricles. The SA node consists of a knot of modified myocardial cells that have the ability to send out an electrical impulse, which initiates and regulates the heartbeat. The AV node delays the impulse momentarily to give the ventricles a chance to fill with blood. The impulse is then transmitted to the bundle of His, and the Purkinje fibers distribute the impulse evenly to the right and left ventricles, causing them to contract.

❏ **The cardiac cycle** represents one complete heartbeat. It consists of the contraction of the atria, the contraction of the ventricles, and the relaxation of the entire heart. The electrocardiograph records the electrical activity that causes these events in the cardiac cycle.

❏ **The ECG cycle** consists of a P wave, a QRS complex, and a T wave. The P wave represents the contraction of the atria; the QRS complex represents the contraction of the ventricles; and the T wave represents the electrical recovery of the ventricles.

❏ **The electrocardiograph must be standardized** when recording an ECG. This ensures an accurate and reliable recording. A normal standardization mark should be 10 mm high. If it is more or less than this, the electrocardiograph machine must be adjusted.

❏ **The standard ECG consists of 12 leads.** Each lead records the heart's activity from a different angle. The 12 leads are I, II, III, aVR, aVL, aVF, V_1, V_2, V_3, V_4, V_5, and V_6.

❏ **The electrical impulses** given off by the heart are picked up by electrodes and conducted into the machine through lead wires. An electrolyte assists in transmission of the heart's electrical impulses. An electrolyte consists of a chemical substance that promotes conduction of an electrical current.

❏ **An electrocardiograph** with a three-channel recording capability can record three leads simultaneously. An electrocardiograph with telephone transmission capabilities can transmit a recording over a telephone line to an ECG data interpretation site. An electrocardiograph with interpretive capabilities has a built-in computer program that analyzes the recording as it is being run.

❏ **Artifacts** represent additional electrical activity that is picked up by the electrocardiograph. A muscle artifact has a fuzzy, irregular baseline and is caused by voluntary and involuntary muscle movement. A wandering baseline can be caused by electrodes that are too loose and by body creams, oils, or lotions on the skin. Alternating current is caused by electrical interference and is characterized by small, straight spiked lines on the ECG. An interrupted baseline is caused by the metal tip of a lead wire becoming detached or by a broken patient cable.

❏ **Holter monitor electrocardiography** monitors and records the cardiac activity of a patient for 24 hours. It is used to evaluate patients with unexplained syncope, to discover intermittent cardiac dysrhythmias, and to assess the effectiveness of antiarrhythmic medications.

❏ **Normal sinus rhythm** refers to an ECG that is within normal limits. Cardiac abnormalities include extra beats, an abnormal rhythm, and an abnormal heart rate. Cardiac dysrhythmias include atrial premature contraction, paroxysmal atrial tachycardia, atrial flutter, atrial fibrillation, premature ventricular contraction, ventricular tachycardia, and ventricular fibrillation.

❏ **The purpose of a pulmonary function test** is to assess lung functioning, thus assisting in the detection and evaluation of pulmonary disease. The most frequently performed pulmonary function test is spirometry; an instrument known as a spirometer is used to conduct the test. A spirometer measures how much air is pushed out of the lungs and how fast that occurs.

❏ **The most important parameters obtained from spirometry testing** are FVC, FEV_1, and the FEV_1/FVC ratio. The measured values are compared with the predicted values to detect the presence of pulmonary disease. To obtain accurate spirometry test results, it is essential that the following be performed: proper patient preparation, proper calibration of the spirometry machine, and correct performance of the breathing maneuver. Post-bronchodilator spirometry assists the physician in determining how treatment will work for patients with obstructive lung disease.

Terminology Review

Amplitude Refers to amount, extent, size, abundance, or fullness.

Artifact Additional electrical activity picked up by the electrocardiograph that interferes with the normal appearance of the ECG cycles.

Atherosclerosis Buildup of fibrous plaques of fatty deposits and cholesterol on the inner walls of the coronary arteries.

Baseline The flat horizontal line that separates the various waves of the ECG cycle.

Cardiac cycle One complete heartbeat.

Dysrhythmia An irregular heart rhythm. Also termed arrhythmia.

ECG cycle The graphic representation of a heartbeat.

Electrocardiogram (ECG) The graphic representation of the electrical activity of the heart.

Electrocardiograph The instrument used to record the electrical activity of the heart.

Electrode A conductor of electricity, which is used to promote contact between the body and the electrocardiograph.

Electrolyte A chemical substance that promotes conduction of an electrical current.

Interval The length of a wave or the length of a wave with a segment.

Ischemia Deficiency of blood in a body part.

Normal sinus rhythm Refers to an electrocardiogram that is within normal limits.

Segment The portion of the ECG between two waves.

Spirometer An instrument for measuring air taken into and expelled from the lungs.

Spirometry Measurement of an individual's breathing capacity by means of a spirometer.

ON THE WEB

For active weblinks to each website visit http://evolve. elsevier.com/Bonewit/.

For Information on Heart Disease:

American Heart Association

National Heart, Lung, and Blood Institute

Heart Center Online

Heart Information Network

Cardiology Channel

American College of Cardiology

For Information on Lung Disease:

American Lung Association

Pulmonary Channel

Lung Cancer Online

For Information on Smoking Cessation:

Quit Net

Habitual Support Program

National Center for Tobacco-free Kids

Why Quit.com

Learning Objectives

Procedures

Fecal Occult Blood Testing

1. Explain the purpose of a fecal occult blood test.
2. Describe the patient preparation for fecal occult blood testing.
3. Explain the purpose of each type of preparation for FOBT.

Instruct an individual in the procedure for a fecal occult blood test.

Develop a fecal occult blood test.

Flexible Sigmoidoscopy

1. Explain the purpose of a digital rectal examination before a sigmoidoscopic examination.
2. Explain the purpose of a flexible sigmoidoscopy.
3. Describe the patient preparation for a flexible sigmoidoscopy.

Instruct a patient in the preparation for a flexible sigmoidoscopy.

Assist the physician with flexible sigmoidoscopy.

Male Reproductive Health

1. List the symptoms of prostate cancer.
2. Explain how the digital rectal examination is used for the early detection of prostate cancer.
3. Describe how the PSA test is used to screen for the presence of prostate cancer.

Assist the physician with a digital rectal examination.

Instruct the patient in the preparation for a PSA test.

Teach the patient how to perform a testicular self-examination.

CHAPTER 13

Colon Procedures and Male Reproductive Health

Chapter Outline

INTRODUCTION TO COLON PROCEDURES
Fecal Occult Blood Testing
  The Guaiac Slide Test
Flexible Sigmoidoscopy
  Patient Preparation for Sigmoidoscopy
  Digital Rectal Examination
  Flexible Sigmoidoscope
INTRODUCTION TO MALE REPRODUCTIVE HEALTH
Prostate Cancer Screening
  Digital Rectal Examination
  PSA Test
Testicular Self-Examination

National Competencies

Clinical Competencies
Specimen Collection
- Instruct patients in the collection of fecal specimens.

Patient Care
- Prepare and maintain examination and treatment areas.
- Prepare patients for and assist with routine and specialty examinations.

General Competencies
Patient Instruction
- Instruct individuals according to their needs.
- Provide instruction for health maintenance and disease prevention.

Introduction to Colon Procedures

Colon procedures are performed in the medical office and include the fecal occult blood test and the flexible sigmoidoscopic examination, which are presented in this chapter. Some patients may initially be reluctant to perform a fecal occult blood test at home. The medical assistant can help by explaining the purpose of the test to the patient. If the individual understands the beneficial results to be derived from the test, he or she is more likely to participate as required. The medical assistant assists the physician during a sigmoidoscopy and, therefore, he or she should have a thorough knowledge of the responsibilities accompanying this procedure.

Fecal Occult Blood Testing

Blood in the stool can indicate a number of conditions, including hemorrhoids, diverticulosis, polyps, colitis, upper gastrointestinal ulcers, and colorectal cancer. Some of these conditions produce visible red blood on the outside of the stool, making it easy to detect. Blood entering the stool from the upper gastrointestinal tract in an amount of 50 ml or more causes the stool to exhibit **melena,** meaning it is black and tarlike. The dark color is a result of the oxidation of the iron in the blood (heme) by intestinal and bacterial enzymes. If a minute quantity of blood is present, however, it will not be detectable by the unaided eye. This hidden, or nonvisible, blood is termed **occult blood,** and its presence can be determined only through chemical or microscopic analysis.

Colorectal cancer is one of the most common forms of cancer in individuals over the age of 40 years. During the early asymptomatic stages, almost all neoplasms of the colon and rectum bleed a small amount on an intermittent basis, and this takes the form of occult blood. Discovering occult blood is of particular importance for the early diagnosis and treatment of colorectal cancer, which, in turn, increases the patient's survival rate. In most cases, when more pronounced symptoms of colorectal cancer start appearing (e.g., visible bleeding, a change in bowel habits, and abdominal pain), the condition has reached an advanced stage.

The Guaiac Slide Test

Routine screening of stool specimens for occult blood is frequently performed in the medical office. The guaiac slide test is most often used and is commercially available with brand names of Hemoccult and ColoScreen (Figure 13-1). Fecal blood loss in excess of 5 ml per day results in a positive reaction. Patients may normally lose up to 3 ml per day of blood in the feces, owing to minor insignificant abrasions of the nasopharynx and gastrointestinal tract. Thus, to allow for normal blood loss, the test does not show a positive reaction until it reaches 5 ml.

The guaiac slide test is a simple and inexpensive method to screen for the presence of occult blood;

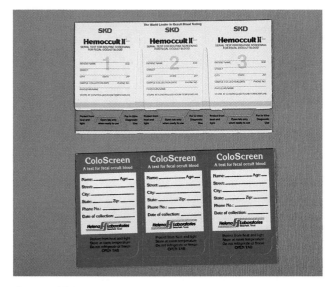

Figure 13-1. Examples of fecal occult blood testing kits. Hemoccult (*top*) and ColoScreen (*bottom*).

however, care must be taken to reduce the occurrence of false-positive or false-negative results. This test is designed to assess the presence of blood in stool specimens collected from three consecutive bowel movements. The purpose of using three specimens is to provide for the detection of blood from gastrointestinal lesions that exhibit intermittent bleeding, meaning they do not bleed every day. Because three stool specimens are required, the patient must collect the specimens at home and return the prepared slides to the medical office for developing. The medical assistant is responsible for providing the patient with instructions on patient preparation and collection, as well as proper care and storage of the slides until they are returned to the medical office.

Although the primary use of the guaiac slide test is to screen for colorectal cancer, other important uses include screening for occult blood for the detection of an upper gastrointestinal ulcer or for disorders causing gastric and intestinal irritation. A positive test result on the guaiac slide test indicates blood in the stool, although the cause of the bleeding must still be determined. Further diagnostic procedures must be performed before the physician can make a final diagnosis; these tests may include flexible sigmoidoscopy, **colonoscopy,** and a double-contrast barium enema radiographic study.

Patient Preparation

Patient preparation plays an important role in ensuring accurate test results. The patient must follow a special diet, beginning 2 days before the test and continuing until all three slides have been prepared. The patient is placed on a high-fiber, meat-free diet. Meat contains animal blood that could lead to a false-positive test result. A high-fiber diet is used because it encourages bleeding from lesions that may bleed only occasionally. In addition, the fiber adds bulk, which promotes bowel elimination and ensures adequate specimen collection.

Certain medications irritate the gastrointestinal tract, which may result in a small amount of bleeding, which could result in a false-positive test result. Medications that irritate the GI tract include aspirin, indomethacin, phenylbutazone, and corticosteroids. In addition, an iron supplement could cause a false-positive result, and a vitamin C supplement (in excess of 250 mg per day) can cause a false-negative result. All of these substances should be discontinued before testing. The box on page 550 lists the specific patient preparation requirements and their purposes.

⚡ PATIENT TEACHING

Patient Preparation for Fecal Occult Blood Testing

Beginning 2 days before obtaining the first stool specimen, the patient should follow the diet modifications listed below. The diet should be followed until all three slides have been prepared.

Meats. Eat no red or rare meat (beef and lamb) or processed meats and liver. Small amounts of well-cooked pork, poultry, and fish are permitted. Red meat contains animal blood that could cause a false-positive test result.

Vegetables. Eat moderate amounts of vegetables, both raw and cooked. Especially advised are lettuce, spinach, corn, and celery. Do not consume horseradish, turnips, broccoli, cauliflower, and radishes. These foods contain **peroxidase,** which could cause a false-positive test result.

Fruits. Eat moderate amounts of apples, bananas, oranges, peaches, pears, and plums. Do not consume melons because they contain peroxidase.

Miscellaneous high-fiber foods. Eat moderate amounts of whole-wheat bread, bran cereal, and popcorn. Foods high in fiber provide roughage to promote bowel elimination and encourage bleeding from lesions that bleed only occasionally.

Medications. Do not take medications that contain aspirin, iron, or vitamin C. In addition, based on the patient's medication therapy, the physician may stipulate additional medication restrictions. Certain medications cause irritation of the gastrointestinal tract, which may result in a small amount of bleeding. (Aspirin and other nonsteroidal anti-inflammatory drugs should be avoided for at least 7 days before and continuing through the test period.)

Special Guidelines

Inform the physician and do not consume any of the food items listed above if you know, from past experience, that they cause you severe gastrointestinal discomfort or serious diarrhea.

Make sure the diet modifications have been followed for 2 days (48 hours) before collecting the first stool specimen.

Do not initiate the test during a menstrual period or in the first 3 days after a menstrual period, or when bleeding from hemorrhoids. These conditions would result in false-positive test results.

Store the slides at room temperature and protect them from heat, sunlight, and fluorescent light to prevent deterioration of the active reagents on the slides.

What Would You DO?
What Would You *Not* DO?

Case Study 1

Beatrice Bernard is 52 years old and has come to the office for a physical examination. The doctor wants Mrs. Bernard to perform a Hemoccult test. After being told the purpose of the test and how to prepare for it, Mrs. Bernard expresses some concerns. She doesn't like the idea of what she has to do to perform the test because it doesn't seem very sanitary to her. She also thinks it will be a lot of work to prepare for the test. She has red meat for dinner at least four times a week and she doesn't understand why she has to eliminate it from her meals. She says she takes a baby aspirin every day for "heart health" and would prefer not to stop taking it. Mrs. Bernard says that she has always taken very good care of herself and she has never had problems with her colon. She also says that there is no history of colon cancer in her family. Mrs. Bernard is too embarrassed to talk about this topic with the doctor. She says she may just throw the test away when she gets home.

Quality Control

Quality control methods must be employed with the guaiac slide test to ensure reliable and valid results. The quality control procedure should be performed after the patient's slide test has been developed, read, and interpreted. The Hemoccult slide test contains an on-slide performance monitor that consists of positive and negative monitor areas. This monitor is located on the developing side of the filter paper under the back flap of the cardboard slide. The positive monitor area contains a control chemical that has been impregnated into the filter paper during the manufacturing process.

The medical assistant should apply 1 drop of the developing solution between the positive and negative performance areas. The results must be read within 10 seconds after application of the developer. If the slide and developer are functional, the positive area will turn blue, whereas the negative area will show no color change. Failure of the expected control results to occur indicates an error, and the test results are not considered valid; possible causes include the use of outdated cards or developing solution, an error in technique, and subjecting the slides to heat, sunlight, or strong fluorescent light. Procedure 13-1 outlines the medical assistant's responsibilities related to fecal occult blood testing. Procedure 13-2 describes the development of a Hemoccult slide test.

Text continued on p. 555

Highlight on Colorectal Cancer

Colorectal cancer (CRC) is the second leading cause of cancer-related deaths in the United States, with the most common being lung cancer. According to the American Cancer Society, every year approximately 150,000 people are diagnosed with colorectal cancer, and approximately 56,000 of them die every year from this disease. As the American population ages, these numbers will increase.

The risk of colorectal cancer begins to increase after age 40 years and reaches a peak from age 60 to 75 years. Other factors that increase the risk of colorectal cancer include a family history of colorectal cancer, personal history of colorectal polyps, and history of inflammatory bowel disease of a long duration (e.g., ulcerative colitis and Crohn's disease). Most colorectal cancer arises from polyps that gradually become malignant over a period of many years. A polyp is a grapelike growth that protrudes from the inner lining of the colon or rectum. Polyps are fairly common in individuals over 50 years of age. Approximately 1 in 20 polyps can become cancerous if not removed.

There are no symptoms during the early stages of colorectal cancer. If colorectal cancer is detected and treated while the patient is still asymptomatic, the patient has an 80% chance of 5-year survival. By comparison, the 5-year survival rate for patients in whom colorectal cancer is diagnosed after the symptoms appear is only 40%.

Symptoms that may occur once colorectal cancer has developed include:

- Bleeding from the rectum
- Blood in the stool
- A change in the shape of the stool (e.g., stools that are narrower than usual)
- A change in bowel habits (e.g., diarrhea, constipation)
- General abdominal discomfort (e.g., aches, pains, or cramps)
- Unexplained weight loss
- Constant fatigue

For the early detection of colorectal cancer, the American Cancer Society (ACS) recommends that all adults 50 years and older who are at average risk for colorectal cancer be screened according to the following schedule:

- Beginning at age 50: Have a fecal occult blood test and a flexible sigmoidoscopy. Repeat the fecal occult blood test annually and the sigmoidoscopy every 5 years,
- *or* have a colonoscopy at 10-year intervals,
- *or* have a double-contrast barium enema every 5 to 10 years.

Individuals who have a family history of colorectal cancer should begin screening at 40 years of age.

The cause of colorectal cancer is unknown, but studies have shown that there is a higher incidence of this disease in countries, such as the United States, whose populations have a diet that is high in meat and animal fat and low in fiber. This finding is supported by the fact that in countries such as Japan, in which the diet is high in fiber and low in fat, the incidence of colorectal cancer is much lower.

PROCEDURE 13-1

PROCEDURE 13-1 Fecal Occult Blood Testing

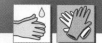

Outcome Instruct an individual in specimen collection for a Hemoccult slide test.

Equipment/Supplies:
- Hemoccult slide testing kit

1. **Procedural Step.** Obtain a Hemoccult slide testing kit. Check the expiration date on the slides. *Principle.* Outdated slides can lead to inaccurate test results.

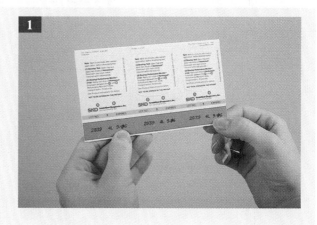

Continued

PROCEDURE 13-1 Fecal Occult Blood Testing—Cont'd

2. **Procedural Step.** Greet and identify the patient. Introduce yourself, and explain the purpose of the test. Tell the patient that the test should not be conducted during a menstrual period or when hemorrhoids are bleeding.
Principle. Bleeding from other (identifiable) sources will invalidate the test results.

3. **Procedural Step.** Instruct the patient in the proper preparation for the test. See the box on p. 550 for the specific guidelines the patient should follow. Tell the patient to begin the diet modifications 2 days before collecting the first stool specimen. Encourage the patient to adhere to the diet modifications.
Principle. The diet modifications may discourage patient compliance. Therefore the medical assistant should reinforce the importance of adhering to the diet requirements. Improper patient preparation can lead to inaccurate test results.

4. **Procedural Step.** Provide the patient with the Hemoccult slide test kit. The kit consists of three identical cardboard slides attached to one another; each slide contains two squares, labeled A and B. Three wooden applicator sticks and written instructions are also included in the testing kit.
Principle. Three slides are provided so that three stool specimens can be collected. The two squares in each slide (A and B) contain filter paper impregnated with guaiac, a chemical necessary for detection of blood in the stool.

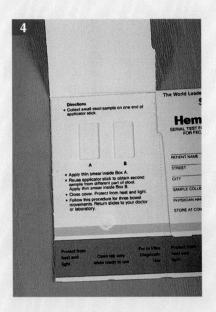

5. **Procedural Step.** Instruct the patient in the completion of the information required on the front flap of each card. This includes the patient's name, address, phone number, and age, and the date of the specimen collection. A ballpoint pen should be used to write this information.

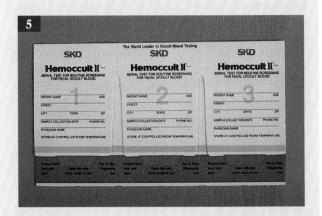

6. **Procedural Step.** Provide instructions on the proper care and storage of the slides. Make it clear that the slides must be stored at room temperature and protected from heat, sunlight, and strong fluorescent light.
Principle. Adverse storage conditions can result in deterioration of the active reagents impregnated on the filter paper, leading to inaccurate test results.

7. **Procedural Step.** Instruct the patient in the initiation of the test by telling him or her to begin the diet modifications and then to collect a stool specimen from the first bowel movement after the 2-day (48-hour) preparatory period.

8. **Procedural Step.** Instruct the patient in the proper collection of the stool specimen:
   a. Using a wooden applicator, obtain a sample of the stool from the commode. The sample may be collected with the aid of a container or toilet tissue.
   b. Open the front flap of the first cardboard slide (located on the left in the series of three).
   c. Spread a very thin smear of the specimen over the filter paper in the square labeled A.
   d. Using the same wooden applicator, obtain another specimen from a different area of the stool.
   e. Spread a thin smear of the specimen over the filter paper in the square labeled B.

f. Close the front flap of the cardboard slide and indicate the date in the space provided.

g. Discard the wooden applicator in a waste container.

Principle. Two squares are included in each slide to allow specimen collection from different parts of the stool because occult blood is not always uniformly distributed throughout the stool (e.g., when bleeding occurs from the lower gastrointestinal tract). Thick specimens prevent adequate light penetration through the filter paper, making it difficult to interpret the test results.

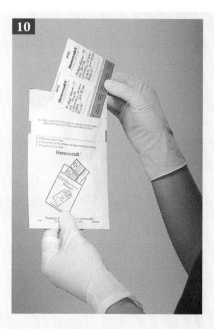

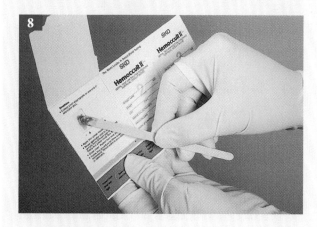

9. **Procedural Step.** Instruct the patient to continue the testing period until all three specimens have been obtained outlined below.

   a. Repeat step 8 after the second bowel movement, using the cardboard slide located in the middle of the series of three.

   b. Repeat step 8 after the third bowel movement, using the cardboard slide located to the right in the series of three.

   c. Allow the completed slides to air-dry overnight.

10. **Procedural Step.** Instruct the patient to place the cardboard slides in the envelope lined with foil, seal carefully, and return them as soon as possible to the medical office. Emphasize to the patient that only the foil-lined envelope can be used to mail the slides; a standard envelope cannot be used.

Principle. Standard paper envelopes are not approved by U.S. postal regulations for mailing fecal occult blood testing slides.

11. **Procedural Step.** Give the patient an opportunity to ask questions; make sure the patient understands the instructions for patient preparation and collection of the stool specimen and for storage of the slides.

Principle. Improper patient preparation and poor collection technique can lead to inaccurate test results.

12. **Procedural Step.** Record in the patient's chart. Include that date and documentation that the Hemoccult test and instructions were given to the patient.

Note: The ColoScreen guaiac slide test uses a procedure similar to that of Hemoccult.

PROCEDURE 13-2   Developing the Hemoccult Slide Test

Outcome Develop a Hemoccult slide test.

Equipment/Supplies:
- Disposable gloves
- Prepared cardboard slides
- Hemoccult developing solution
- Reference card
- Waste container

1. **Procedural Step.** Assemble the equipment. The reference card provides an illustration of positive and negative test results, which can be used as a guide in interpreting results. *Note:* The slides may be developed immediately or stored (at room temperature) for up to 14 days before developing.
2. **Procedural Step.** Check the expiration date on the developing solution bottle. The developing solution contains hydrogen peroxide, should be stored away from heat and light, and should be tightly capped when not in use.
   Principle. Outdated solution should not be used because it can lead to inaccurate test results. The solution should be stored properly because it is flammable and evaporates easily.
3. **Procedural Step.** Sanitize your hands and apply gloves. Open the back flap of the cardboard slides. Apply 2 drops of the developing solution to the guaiac test paper underlying the back of each smear.
   Principle. The developing solution will be absorbed through the filter paper and into the stool specimen.

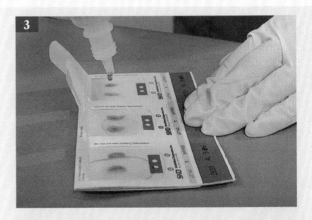

This solution could irritate the skin and eyes; if contact occurs, immediately rinse the area with water.

4. **Procedural Step.** Read the results within 60 seconds. Fecal blood loss in excess of 5 ml per day results in a positive reaction, which is indicated by any trace of blue on or at the edge of the fecal smear. If no detectable color change occurs, the result is considered negative.

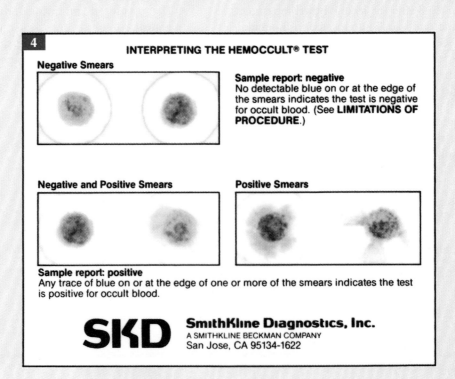

INTERPRETING THE HEMOCCULT® TEST

Negative Smears

Sample report: negative
No detectable blue on or at the edge of the smears indicates the test is negative for occult blood. (See **LIMITATIONS OF PROCEDURE.**)

Negative and Positive Smears

Positive Smears

Sample report: positive
Any trace of blue on or at the edge of one or more of the smears indicates the test is positive for occult blood.

SKD **SmithKline Diagnostics, Inc.**
A SMITHKLINE BECKMAN COMPANY
San Jose, CA 95134-1622

Principle. In the presence of hydrogen peroxide, the heme compound in hemoglobin oxidizes guaiac, causing it to turn blue within 60 seconds after adding the developer. The reading time is important because the color reaction may fade after 2 to 4 minutes.

5. **Procedural Step.** Perform the quality control procedure.
Principle. Quality control procedures ensure the accuracy and reliability of the test results.

6. **Procedural Step.** Properly dispose of the Hemoccult slides in a regular waste container.
Principle. Fecal material is not considered regulated medical waste and, therefore, can be discarded in a regular waste container.

7. **Procedural Step.** Remove gloves and sanitize your hands. Chart the results. Include the date and time, the brand name of the test (Hemoccult), the test results for each slide (recorded as positive or negative).

CHARTING EXAMPLE

Date	
9/08/05	9:00 a.m. Pt provided with a Hemoccult test and instructions for the procedure.
	———————————— M. Baer, CMA
9/14/05	10:30 a.m. Hemoccult test:
	Slide 1: Negative
	Slide 2: Negative
	Slide 3: Positive
	———————————— M. Baer, CMA

PROCEDURE 13-2

Flexible Sigmoidoscopy

Flexible **sigmoidoscopy** is the visual examination of the mucosa of the rectum and lower third of the colon using a flexible fiberoptic **sigmoidoscope.** Sigmoidoscopy may be performed to detect lesions, polyps, hemorrhoids, fissures, infection, and inflammation, or to determine the cause of rectal bleeding. It is especially valuable as a diagnostic procedure for the early detection of symptomatic and asymptomatic colorectal cancer. If an abnormal area is detected, a **biopsy** is taken for histologic examination. Early detection of colorectal cancer leads to early diagnosis and treatment, which in turn increases the chance of survival for individuals with this disease.

Patient Preparation for Sigmoidoscopy

The physician may want the patient to prepare the colon before the sigmoidoscopy. The preparation generally involves eating a light, low-residue meal the evening before the examination. Foods high in residue that should be avoided include raw fruits and vegetables and whole-grain breads and cereals. The patient may also be instructed to take a laxative and/or perform a sodium phosphate (Fleet's) enema or warm tap water cleansing enema the evening before the examination. On the morning of the examination, the patient should consume a light breakfast and perform another enema until the returns are clear. The fecal material must be removed in order for the physician to visualize the mucosa of the colon.

Some physicians prefer that the patient not take a laxative or perform an enema because it may change the ap-

pearance of the intestinal mucosa of the colon, making diagnosis difficult. In this case, the patient is examined after normal defecation. The medical assistant should consult the physician to determine his or her preference.

Digital Rectal Examination

A digital examination of the anal canal and rectum is performed before the sigmoidoscopy. Using a well-lubricated gloved index finger, the physician palpates the rectum for the presence of tenderness, hemorrhoids, polyps, and tumors. Any palpable abnormality will be viewed directly when the **endoscope** is inserted. The digital examination also helps relax the sphincter muscles of the anus and prepares the patient for the insertion of the endoscope.

Flexible Sigmoidoscope

The flexible fiberoptic sigmoidoscope is composed of extremely thin fibers of bendable glass that transmit light and images back to the physician. The image, magnified 10 times by the fiberoptic system, is viewed by the physician through the eye lens located in the handle of the sigmoidoscope. Videoscopes, also available for flexible sigmoidoscopy, permit viewing of the images on a display screen.

Flexible sigmoidoscopes consist of a control head and a long flexible insertion tube attached to a light source (Figure 13-2). The insertion tube is ½ inch in diameter and 65 cm long, which allows the physician to view approximately ⅓ of the colon. To perform the procedure, the distal end of the sigmoidoscope is lubricated and inserted into the anus and rectum, and then slowly advanced into the colon.

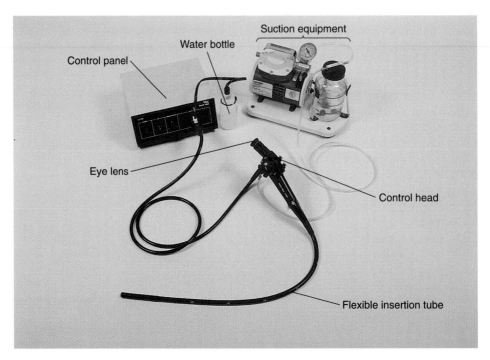

Figure 13-2. Flexible fiberoptic sigmoidoscope.

A small amount of air is usually blown, or **insufflated,** into the colon through tubing attached to the air control valve located on the head of the sigmoidoscope. The function of the air is to distend the lumen of the colon for better visualization.

In addition, suction equipment can be used to remove secretions, such as mucus, blood, and liquid feces, that interfere with proper visualization of the intestinal mucosa. The physician performs the visual examination of the intestinal mucosa as the sigmoidoscope is being inserted and also as it is being withdrawn. Procedure 13-3 outlines the medical assistant's during a flexible sigmoidoscopy.

What Would You DO? What Would You *Not* DO?

Case Study 2

Dr. Frederick Mitchell is 57 years old and is the president of a bank. Two weeks ago, he performed Hemoccult testing at home and two of the three slides were positive. His physician ordered a flexible sigmoidoscopy as a follow-up to help determine if there is a problem. Dr. Mitchell has come to the office for his flexible sigmoidoscopy. Dr. Mitchell says that he was called out of town unexpectedly on business and wasn't able to perform the patient preparation, but says it's fine for the doctor to go ahead and perform the procedure anyway.

PROCEDURE 13-3   Assisting With a Flexible Sigmoidoscopy

Outcome Assist with a sigmoidoscopy.

Equipment/Supplies:
- Flexible sigmoidoscope
- Disposable gloves
- Water-soluble lubricant
- Drape
- Biopsy forceps

- Sterile specimen container with a preservative
- 4 × 4 gauze squares
- Tissue
- Waste container

1. **Procedural Step.** Sanitize your hands.
2. **Procedural Step.** Assemble the equipment. Check to make sure the light source on the sigmoidoscope is working. Label the specimen container with the patient's name, the date, and the source of the specimen.

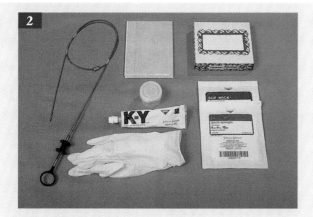

9. **Procedural Step.** Assist the physician as required during the examination. The medical assistant may be responsible for the following:

   a. Lubricating the physician's gloved index finger for the digital examination.

   b. Placing lubricant on the distal end of the sigmoidoscope before insertion into the rectum. The sigmoidoscope should be well lubricated to facilitate insertion.

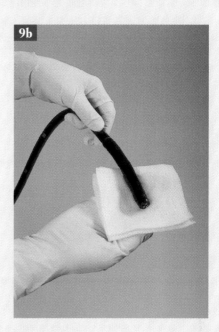

3. **Procedural Step.** Greet and identify the patient and introduce yourself. Ask the patient if he or she has prepared properly for the procedure. Explain the flexible sigmoidoscopy procedure to the patient.
   Principle. The patient must prepare properly to allow the physician to visualize the mucosa of the colon. Explaining the procedure helps reduce patient apprehension.

4. **Procedural Step.** Ask the patient if he or she needs to empty the bladder before the examination. If a urine specimen is needed, the medical assistant requests that the patient void into a specimen container.
   Principle. An empty bladder makes the examination easier and more comfortable for the patient.

5. **Procedural Step.** Instruct and prepare the patient for the examination. Ask him or her to remove all clothing from the waist down and to put on an examining gown with the opening in back.

6. **Procedural Step.** Assist the patient onto the examining table. The Sims position is recommended for flexible sigmoidoscopy.

7. **Procedural Step.** Properly drape the patient so that only the anus is exposed. Some medical offices use fenestrated drapes with the circular opening placed over the anus.
   Principle. Draping the patient reduces exposure and provides warmth.

8. **Procedural Step.** Reassure the patient and help him or her relax the muscles of the anus and rectum by breathing slowly and deeply through the mouth. As the sigmoidoscope is inserted, the patient feels some pressure and the urge to defecate. This pressure is caused by the insertion of the sigmoidoscope, and the patient should be reassured that although it is uncomfortable, it will last only a short time.

   c. Assisting with the suction equipment as required.

   d. Assisting with the collection of a biopsy by handing the biopsy forceps to the physician and holding the specimen container to accept the biopsy. Do not touch the inside of the container because it is sterile.

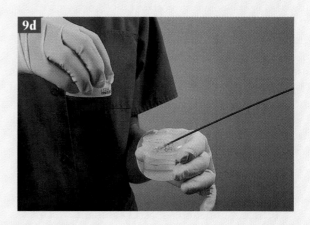

PROCEDURE 13-3

Continued

PROCEDURE 13-3   Assisting With a Flexible Sigmoidoscopy—Cont'd

10.   **Procedural Step.** Once the examination is completed, the medical assistant should apply gloves and clean the patient's anal region of any excess lubricant, using tissue wipes. Discard the tissues in the regular waste container.

11.   **Procedural Step.** Remove gloves and sanitize your hands. Assist the patient off the examining table to. Instruct him or her to get dressed.

12.   **Procedural Step.** If a biopsy was taken, prepare the specimen for transportation to the laboratory. Label the container with the patient's name, date, and source of the specimen. Place the specimen container in a biohazard specimen bag and seal the bag. Insert the biopsy requisition into the outside pocket of the bag and tuck the top of the requisition under the flap. Place the bag in the appropri-

ate location for pickup by the laboratory. Chart the transport of the specimen to an outside laboratory.

13.   **Procedural Step.** Clean the examining room in preparation for the next patient. The sigmoidoscope should be sanitized and disinfected with a high-level disinfectant according to the manufacturer's recommendations.

CHARTING EXAMPLE

Date	
8/15/05	11:00 a.m. Biopsy specimen transported
	to Medical Center Laboratory for pathology.
	— M. Baer, CMA

Introduction to Male Reproductive Health

Two important areas related to male reproductive health are prostate screening and the testicular self-examination. Preventive examinations and tests can detect prostate and testicular cancer early, leading to early treatment, which often results in a cure. Both of these areas are described in the following section.

Prostate Cancer Screening

According to the American Cancer Society, prostate cancer is the second most common cause of cancer deaths in males, lung cancer being the most common. Every year more than 189,000 people are diagnosed with prostate cancer, and approximately 30,000 of them die from this disease. The incidence of prostate cancer increases after age 50 and is found more often in African American males and men with a family history of prostate cancer.

The prostate gland surrounds the urethra and is located just below the bladder and in front of the rectum (Figure 13-3). It is approximately the size and shape of a walnut, and its function is to secrete fluid that transports sperm.

In the early stages, prostate cancer often causes no symptoms. Symptoms that occur once the cancer is more developed include the following:

- Difficulty in urinating
- Weak or interrupted urinary flow
- Pain or burning during urination
- Frequent urination, especially at night
- Blood in the urine
- Pain in the lower back, pelvis, or upper thighs

When prostate cancer is diagnosed early, the chances for a cure are very good. Because of this, the American Cancer Society recommends that men over 50 undergo annual prostate screening. The primary screening tests for prostate cancer are the digital rectal examination (DRE) and the prostate-specific antigen (PSA) test. The American Cancer Society recommends that both of these tests be offered annually to male patients over 50 so that if cancer does develop, it will be found at an early stage. The DRE and PSA test are described below.

Digital Rectal Examination

The digital rectal examination is a quick and simple procedure, which causes only momentary discomfort. During the examination, the physician inserts a lubricated gloved finger into the patient's rectum. Because the prostate gland is located in front of the rectum, the physician is able to palpate the surface of the prostate gland through the rectal wall (see Figure 13-3). The physician palpates the gland to determine if it is enlarged or has an abnormal consistency. Normally the prostate gland should feel soft, whereas malignant tissue is firm and hard. The sensitivity of the DRE is limited, however, because the physician can only palpate the posterior and lateral aspects of the prostate gland.

PSA Test

The PSA (prostate-specific antigen) test is a screening test that measures the amount of PSA in the blood. Prostate-specific antigen is a protein normally produced by the cells of the membrane that covers the prostate gland. The normal range for PSA is 0 to 4 nanograms per milliliter

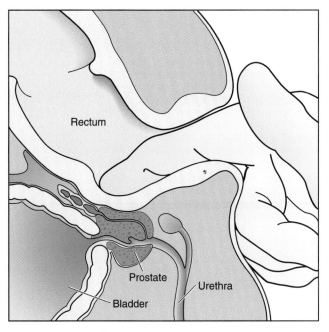

Figure 13-3. Digital rectal examination.

(ng/ml) of blood. The PSA level becomes elevated in men who have a benign or malignant growth in the prostate. A PSA level of 4 to 10 ng/ml is considered slightly elevated; levels between 10 to 20 ng/ml are considered moderately elevated; and a value above 20 ng/ml is considered highly elevated. The higher the PSA level, the more likely that cancer is present.

The PSA level may normally increase after vigorous exercise, such as jogging or biking. Therefore the medical assistant should instruct the patient to engage only in normal activity for 2 days before having blood drawn for a PSA test. The patient should also be instructed not to have sexual intercourse for 2 days before the test because it can change the PSA level.

If the physician determines the likelihood of cancer through prostate screening, further testing is performed to determine if prostate cancer is present and if so, the type of cancer and its location and stage of development. To make this assessment, one or more of the following tests may be performed: transrectal ultrasound (TRUS), biopsy of the prostate gland, bone scan, and CT scan.

Testicular Self-Examination

The purpose of testicular self-examination (TSE) is early detection of testicular cancer. In the past 40 years, testicular cancer among young Caucasian males has more than doubled. Although testicular cancer can develop at any age, it is most common in males between 15 and 40 years old. If detected early, it has a very high cure rate. Most cases of testicular cancer are detected by men themselves, either by accident or when performing a testicular self-examination.

What Would You DO?
What Would You Not DO?

Case Study 3

Peter Bota, a 62-year-old retired Caucasian male, came to the medical office a week ago for a physical examination. The physician performed a DRE but did not palpate anything abnormal. At that visit, Mr. Bota's blood was drawn for a PSA test and the results came back as slightly elevated (8 ng/ml). Mr. Bota has returned to the office and is waiting to talk with the doctor about his test results and possible follow-up testing. Mr. Bota is extremely worried that he has cancer and wants to know the symptoms of prostate cancer. He also wants to know if there's anything he did to cause prostate cancer. He says he doesn't smoke and drinks very little and that he walks his dog twice a day for exercise.

Certain factors increase a man's chance of getting testicular cancer. These risk factors include the following:

- A history of cryptorchidism (undescended testicles)
- Family history of testicular cancer
- Cancer of the other testicle
- Caucasian male (testicular cancer is five times more common in Caucasian males than in African American males).

The testicular self-examination should be performed monthly starting at 15 years of age. A good idea is for the patient to choose an easy-to-remember date each month, such as the first day of the month. The best time to perform

TESTICULAR SELF-EXAMINATION

1
Take a warm bath or shower.

2
Stand in front of a mirror. Look for any swelling of the skin of the scrotum.

3
Place the index and middle fingers of both hands on the underside of one testicle and the thumbs on top of the testicle.

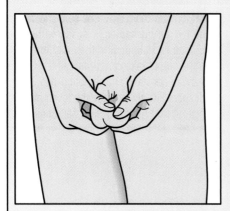

4
Apply a small amount of pressure and gently roll the testicle between the thumb and fingers of both hands, feeling for lumps, swelling, or any change in the size, shape, or consistency of the testicle. A normal testicle should feel smooth, egg-shaped and rather firm. It is also normal for one testicle to be larger or hang lower than the other testicle.

5
Find the epididymis so you do not confuse it with a lump. The epididymis is a soft tubular cord, located behind the testicle which functions in storing and carrying sperm.
(Note: Tenderness in the area of the epididymis is considered normal.)

6
Repeat the examination outlined above on the other testicle.

7
Report any of the following abnormalities to the physician: any unusual lump, a feeling of heaviness in the scrotum, a dull ache in the lower abdomen or groin, enlargement of one of the testicles, tenderness or pain in a testicle, or any change in the way the testicle feels.

Figure 13-4. Testicular self-examination.

the examination is after taking a warm bath or shower. Heat allows the scrotal skin to relax and become soft, making it easier to palpate the underlying testicular tissues.

The most common sign of testicular cancer is a small, hard, painless lump (about the size of a pea) located on the front or side of the testicle. Any abnormalities should be reported to the physician immediately. It does not necessarily mean that the patient has cancer, however; the physician must make that determination. Figure 13-4 outlines the procedure for a testicular self-examination.

MEDICAL Practice and the LAW

Colon procedures can be very embarrassing for the patient. Most colon procedures can be diagnostic for cancer. This combination makes these procedures very stressful for the patient. Professionalism, compassion, and a caring attitude can alleviate many fears. Many invasive procedures require a written informed consent.

While assisting with a flexible sigmoidoscopy, assist the patient and maintain proper positioning as comfortably as possible. Be aware of the patient's condition, and inform the physician if he or she is not tolerating the procedure well.

Malpractice
Malpractice laws require a minimal level of care and of doing good, or beneficence. Malpractice is a type of negligence, which is a tort, or wrong. Torts can be done intentionally or accidentally (negligently), and can be caused by something done or by something that was omitted.

What Would You DO?
What Would You *Not* DO? *RESPONSES*

Case Study 1
What Did Megan Do?

❑ Relayed to Mrs. Bernard that this is not the most fun test to perform, but that if colon cancer is detected early, the cure rate is very high.

❑ Explained to Mrs. Bernard that colon cancer increases after age 40 and that an individual can develop colon cancer without a family history of it.

❑ Told Mrs. Bernard that during the early stages of colon cancer, there are no symptoms, so it's possible to feel fine but still have a problem.

❑ Explained to Mrs. Bernard in more detail the reason for not eating red meat or taking aspirin during the testing period.

❑ Told Mrs. Bernard that disposable gloves could be given to her to take home to wear when she collected the specimens.

❑ Explained to Mrs. Bernard that the doctor talks with patients every day about these types of things and it's important to talk with him about all aspects of her health so that she receives the best care possible.

❑ Told Mrs. Bernard that the office would call her in 3 days to see if she has any questions or is having any problems with the test.

What Did Megan Not Do?

❑ Did not tell Mrs. Bernard that she is getting older and needs to be more concerned about performing health screening tests.

What Would You Do?/What Would You *Not* Do? Review Megan's response and place a checkmark next to the information you included in your response. List additional information you included in your response below.

_____

_____

_____

_____

Case Study 2
What Did Megan Do?

❑ Told Dr. Mitchell that the physician cannot perform a sigmoidoscopy unless the colon has been properly prepared.

❑ Explained that the colon needs to be cleaned out so that the doctor can see the wall of the colon to check for abnormalities.

❑ Went over the preparation instructions with Dr. Mitchell again and gave him another instruction sheet to take home.

❑ Rescheduled his appointment and told him that he would be called the day before the examination to be reminded of his appointment and to see if he has any questions regarding the preparation.

What Did Megan Not Do?

❑ Told Dr. Mitchell that an entire office hour had been scheduled for his examination and that other patients could have been seen during this time.

What Would You Do?/What Would You *Not* Do? Review Megan's response and place a checkmark next to the information you included in your response. List additional information you included in your response below.

_____

_____

_____

_____

Case Study 3
What Did Megan Do?

❑ Listened patiently and tried to reassure and calm Mr. Bota. Told him that doctors don't yet know what causes prostate cancer.

❑ Explained that the PSA test is a *screening* test and that he should not jump to conclusions about the results.

❑ Told Mr. Bota that the physician would talk with him about his test results in just a short while.

❑ Commended Mr. Bota on his healthy lifestyle habits and encouraged him to continue with them.

❑ Gave Mr. Bota some brochures on male reproductive health to read while he waited to be seen by the physician.

What Did Megan Not Do?

❑ Did not tell Mr. Bota that there was nothing to worry about.

What Would You Do?/What Would You *Not* Do? Review Megan's response and place a checkmark next to the information you included in your response. List additional information you included in your response below.

_____

_____

_____

_____

Apply Your KNOWLEDGE

Choose the best answer to each of the following questions.

1. Tess Terrell, a 52-year-old female, comes to the medical office for a complete physical examination. As part of the exam, she is given a Hemoccult test to perform at home. Tess asks Megan Baer, CMA, why she has to do this test. Megan explains to her that the purpose of a Hemoccult test is to:
   A. Screen for the presence of blood in the stool
   B. Determine the presence of parasites in the stool
   C. Detect the presence of polyps in the large intestine
   D. Diagnose colorectal cancer

2. Megan instructs Tess in how to prepare for the Hemoccult test. Megan relays all of the following to her EXCEPT:
   A. Discontinue taking vitamin supplements that contain iron
   B. Eat moderate amounts of broccoli and melon
   C. Start the diet modifications 2 days before collecting the first stool specimen
   D. Do not eat any red meat

3. Tess asks Megan why she must consume a high-fiber diet during the testing period. Megan explains that a high-fiber diet:
   A. Prevents the occurrence of a false-negative test result
   B. Prevents gastrointestinal irritation during the test
   C. Encourages bleeding from intestinal lesions
   D. Prevents constipation during the testing period
   E. All of the above

4. Tess completes the Hemoccult test and returns it to the medical office. Megan develops the slides. After applying the developing solution to the first slide, Megan observes a trace of blue at the edge of the slide. Megan records this as:
   A. Slide 1: Positive
   B. Slide 1: Negative
   C. Slide 1: No reaction
   D. Slide 1: Invalid

5. Dr. Polyp instructs Megan to schedule Tess for a flexible sigmoidoscopy and to instruct Tess in proper bowel preparation. Megan instructs Tess to perform all of the following EXCEPT:
   A. Take a laxative the evening before the exam
   B. Eat a light low-residue meal the evening before the exam
   C. Fast for 12 hours before the exam
   D. Perform a Fleet's enema the evening before the exam

6. Tess arrives at the medical office for her flexible sigmoidoscopy. Megan prepares Tess for the procedure by positioning her in:
   A. Fowler's position
   B. Sims position
   C. Knee-chest position
   D. Prone position

7. During the flexible sigmoidoscopy procedure, Megan assists Dr. Polyp by:
   A. Lubricating Dr. Polyp's gloved finger for the digital rectal examination
   B. Lubricating the distal end of the sigmoidoscope
   C. Assisting with suction equipment
   D. Holding a specimen container to accept a biopsy
   E. All of the above

8. After the sigmoidoscopy, Megan cleans up the examining room. She removes the flexible sigmoidoscope to the back work area and cleans it by:
   A. Rinsing it with hot water
   B. Sanitizing and disinfecting it
   C. Sterilizing it in the autoclave
   D. Soaking it in gasoline

9. Ted Wright, 50 years old, comes to the medical office for a physical examination. Dr. Polyp recommends that he have a DRE and a PSA test. Ted asks Megan Baer, CMA, the purpose of this type of screening. Megan responds by telling Ted that it is:
   A. For the early detection of colorectal cancer
   B. To determine the cause of infertility
   C. To assist in the diagnosis of colitis
   D. For the early detection of prostate cancer

10. Megan draws a blood specimen from Ted for a PSA test. Ted asks Megan what the normal range is for this test. Megan tells him:
    A. 0 to 4 ng/ml
    B. 0 to 10 ng/ml
    C. 5 to 10 ng/ml
    D. 10 to 20 ng/ml

11. Matt Coleman, 22 years old, comes to the medical office to have his cholesterol checked. Dr. Polyp asks Megan Baer, CMA, to instruct Matt in the procedure for a testicular self-examination. All of the following are included in Megan's discussion EXCEPT:
    A. Perform the examination once each month
    B. Refrain from sexual intercourse for 2 days before performing the exam
    C. Take a warm shower before performing the exam
    D. Palpate each testicle for lumps using both hands

12. While taking Matt's medical history, Megan obtains the following information. Which of the following puts Matt at higher risk for testicular cancer?
    A. Matt was born with undescended testicles.
    B. Matt collects old coins.
    C. Matt is a vegetarian.
    D. Matt is of African American heritage.

CERTIFICATION REVIEW

❑ **Blood in the stool** may indicate a number of conditions, including hemorrhoids, diverticulosis, polyps, upper gastrointestinal ulcers, and colorectal cancer. Hidden, or nonvisible, blood in the stool is termed occult blood, and its presence can be determined through fecal occult blood testing.

❑ **Fecal occult blood testing** is routinely performed in the medical office using the guaiac slide test (e.g., Hemoccult and ColoScreen). Patient preparation for the test is important to ensure accurate test results. A positive test result warrants further diagnostic procedures such as flexible sigmoidoscopy, colonoscopy, and a double-contrast barium enema radiographic study.

❑ **Flexible sigmoidoscopy** is the visual examination of the mucosa of the rectum and sigmoid colon via a flexible fiberoptic sigmoidoscope. Sigmoidoscopy may be performed to detect the presence of lesions, polyps, hemorrhoids, fissures, infection, and inflammation, or to determine the cause of rectal bleeding. It is especially valuable in the early detection of colorectal cancer.

❑ **A digital rectal examination** is performed by the physician before the sigmoidoscopy to palpate the rectum for tenderness, hemorrhoids, polyps, or tumors. The digital examination also helps relax the sphincter muscles of the anus for the insertion of the sigmoidoscope.

❑ **The prostate gland** surrounds the urethra and secretes fluid that transports sperm. Beginning at age 50, men should undergo annual prostate screening for the early detection of prostate cancer. The primary screening tests for prostate cancer are the digital rectal examination (DRE) and the PSA test. If the test results indicate the possibility of cancer, further testing is done, which may include one or more of the following: transrectal ultrasound (TRUS), biopsy of the prostate gland, bone scan, and CT scan.

❑ **The purpose of the testicular self-examination (TSE)** is to detect testicular cancer early. Testicular cancer is most common in males between 15 and 40 years of age. The TSE should be performed monthly beginning at 15 years of age. Any abnormality should be reported to the physician immediately.

Terminology Review

Biopsy The surgical removal and examination of tissue from the living body. Biopsies are generally performed to determine whether a tumor is benign or malignant.

Colonoscopy The visualization of the entire colon using a colonoscope.

Endoscope An instrument that consists of a tube and an optical system that is used for direct visual inspection of organs or cavities.

Insufflate To blow a powder, vapor, or gas (such as air) into a body cavity.

Melena The darkening of the stool caused by the presence of blood in an amount of 50 ml or greater.

Occult blood Blood in such a small amount that it is not detectable by the unaided eye.

Peroxidase (as it pertains to the guaiac slide test) A substance that is able to transfer oxygen from hydrogen peroxide to oxidize guaiac, causing the guaiac to turn blue.

Sigmoidoscope An endoscope that is specially designed for passage through the anus to permit visualization of the rectum and sigmoid colon.

Sigmoidoscopy The visual examination of the rectum and sigmoid colon using a sigmoidoscope.

ON THE WEB

For active weblinks to each website visit http://evolve.elsevier.com/Bonewit/.

For Information on Colorectal Cancer:

American Cancer Society

National Cancer Institute

Colorectal Cancer Network

Colon Cancer Alliance

Oncology Channel

For Information on Prostate Cancer:

Prostate Health

Prostate Information

Prostate.com

Prostate.org

Male Health

Learning Objectives

Radiology

1. State the function of radiographs in medicine.
2. Explain the importance of proper patient preparation for a radiographic examination.
3. Describe the following positions used for radiographic examinations:
   - Anteroposterior
   - Posteroanterior
   - Right and left lateral
   - Supine
   - Prone
4. Explain the function of a contrast medium.
5. Describe the purpose of a fluoroscope.
6. Explain the purpose of each of the following types of radiographic examinations:
   - Mammography
   - Upper gastrointestinal
   - Lower gastrointestinal
   - Cholecystography
   - Intravenous pyelography

Diagnostic Imaging

1. Explain the purpose of each of the following diagnostic imaging procedures:
   - Ultrasonography
   - Computed tomography
   - Magnetic resonance imaging

Procedures

Instruct a patient in the proper preparation necessary for each of the following types of radiographic examinations:
- Mammography
- Upper gastrointestinal
- Lower gastrointestinal
- Cholecystography
- Intravenous pyelography

Instruct a patient in the purpose and advance preparation for each of the following diagnostic imaging procedures:
- Ultrasonography
- Computed tomography
- Magnetic resonance imaging

CHAPTER 14

Radiology and Diagnostic Imaging

Chapter Outline

Introduction to Radiology
Contrast Media
Fluoroscopy
Positioning the Patient
Specific Radiographic Examinations
  Mammography
  Gastrointestinal Series
  Cholecystography
  Intravenous Pyelography
  Other Types of Radiographs
Introduction to Diagnostic Imaging
Ultrasonography
Computed Tomography
Magnetic Resonance Imaging

National Competencies

General Competencies
Patient Instruction
- Instruct individuals according to their needs.
- Provide instruction for health maintenance and disease prevention.

Key Terms

contrast medium

echocardiogram (EK-oh-KAR-dee-oh-gram)

enema (EN-em-ah)

fluoroscope (FLOOR-oh-skope)

fluoroscopy (floor-OS-koe-pee)

radiograph (RAY-dee-oh-graf)

radiography (ray-dee-OG-rah-fee)

radiologist (ray-dee-AH-lah-jist)

radiology (ray-dee-AH-lah-jee)

radiolucent (ray-dee-oh-LOO-sent)

radiopaque (ray-dee-oh-PAYK)

sonogram (SON-oh-gram)

ultrasonography (ul-trah-son-AH-grah-fee)

Introduction to Radiology

Wilhelm Konrad Roentgen, a German physicist, discovered x-rays on November 8, 1895, while working with a cathode ray tube. He noticed that these rays could pass through solid materials such as paper, wood, and human skin. Because he did not know what they were, he named them x-rays. The rays have since been renamed roentgen rays after their discoverer; however, they are better known as x-rays.

X-rays are high-energy electromagnetic waves that are invisible and have a short wavelength that enables them to penetrate solid materials. A special radiographic film is placed behind the part being examined, and a shadow or image of the internal body structure photographed is produced on the film. **Radiograph** is the term for the permanent record of the picture produced on the radiographic film.

X-rays are used to visualize internal organs and structures and serve as a diagnostic aid in determining the presence of disease. They are also used therapeutically in the treatment of disease conditions such as malignant neoplasms.

Radiology is the branch of medicine that deals with the use of radiant energy in the diagnosis and treatment of disease. A **radiologist** is a medical doctor who specializes in the diagnosis and treatment of disease with any of various forms of radiant energy, such as x-rays, radium, and radioactive material.

A medical office may have its own radiograph machine, but more often radiographs are taken in a hospital by radiology personnel. Some radiographs, such as a bone study, require no advance preparation, whereas others, such as a lower GI, require a great deal of special preparation. Medical assistants are usually responsible for patient instruction in the type of preparation necessary for a particular radiographic examination and for making sure the patient understands the importance of the preparation. If the patient does not prepare properly, the radiograph may be of poor quality and the procedure may even need to be rescheduled. This section provides an introduction to the study of radiographs, with a focus on the patient preparation necessary for common radiographs.

Contrast Media

Radiography relies on differences in density between various body structures to produce shadows of varying intensities on the radiographic film. For example, there is a difference in density between bone and flesh (bone is denser than flesh). The bone absorbs more x-rays and does not allow them to reach the radiographic film. This leaves that part of the film unexposed and causes white areas to appear on the processed film. If the x-rays penetrate an organ or structure, a black area will appear on the film. For example, because the lungs contain air, x-rays are able to penetrate them easily. As a result, the lungs appear black on the processed film. The ribs, on the other hand, absorb the x-rays and appear as white shadows on the film (Figure 14-1). A structure, such as lung tissue, that permits the passage of x-rays is **radiolucent.** A structure, such as bone, that obstructs the passage of x-rays and causes an image to be cast on the film is **radiopaque.**

In many cases, the natural densities of two adjacent organs or structures are similar. In this instance, a **contrast medium** must be used to make a particular structure visible on the radiograph. Contrast media are usually radiopaque chemical compounds that cause the body tissue or organ to absorb more radiation. This absorption provides a contrast in density between the tissue or organ and the surrounding area. The tissue or organ becomes visible and appears white on the processed radiograph. Substances used as contrast media must be able to be ingested or injected into the body tissues or organs without causing harm to the patient.

Barium sulfate and inorganic iodine compounds are commonly used radiopaque contrast media. Barium sulfate is a chalky compound that is water insoluble and does not allow penetration by x-rays. It is frequently used for examination of the gastrointestinal (GI) tract because barium is not absorbed into the body through the GI tract and does not alter its normal function. Iodine salts are radiopaque and are combined with other compounds for radiographic examination of structures such as the gall-bladder and kidneys. Iodine may sometimes produce an allergic reaction, and before administration, patients should be asked whether they have an allergy to iodine or foods containing iodine. Those patients with known allergies may be given an iodine-sensitivity test as a precautionary measure.

Another type of contrast medium causes the structure to become less dense than the surrounding area. The x-rays can easily penetrate the structure, which appears as a darker area on the radiograph. This type of contrast medium includes substances such as air and carbon dioxide.

What Would You DO?
What Would You *Not* DO?

Case Study 1

Jose Ramirez is a 7-year-old boy with episodes of unexplained abdominal pain and vomiting during the past 6 months. The doctor has scheduled an upper GI at the local hospital. Mrs. Ramirez wants to know how to best prepare Jose for the procedure so he will not be so afraid of the radiograph room and equipment. She asks what she can do so he will drink the barium solution because he will not drink milk and if the barium tastes anything like milk getting him to drink it will be difficult. Mrs. Ramirez wants to know whether Jose can hold his favorite toy (a Tonka truck) during the procedure to help comfort him. She also wants to know whether the barium solution will make him feel sick afterwards.

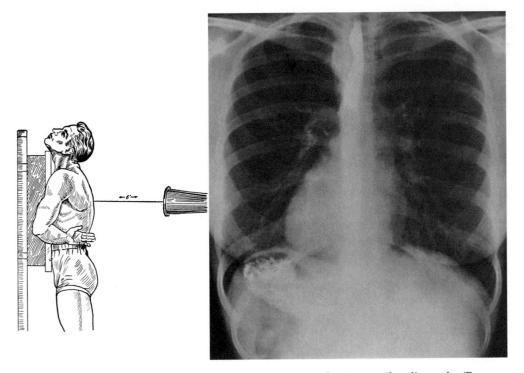

Figure 14-1. Posteroanterior view of chest: position of patient and radiograph. (From Meschan I: *Synopsis of radiologic anatomy with computed tomography,* Philadelphia, 1980, Saunders.)

Fluoroscopy

A **fluoroscope** is an instrument used to view internal organs and structures of the body directly on a display screen. Examination of a patient with a fluoroscope is known as **fluoroscopy.** A radiopaque medium is often used with fluoroscopy to outline various parts of the body. The patient is positioned between the radiographic tube and a fluorescent screen composed of zinc cadmium sulfide crystals. When the x-rays pass through the body and strike the crystals, visible light is emitted so the radiologist can view (on a screen) the action of body organs or structures such as the heart, stomach, and intestines. During fluoroscopy, the radiologist can take radiographs that permit the study of the structure in detail and that also serve as a permanent record.

Positioning the Patient

The position of the patient is determined by the purpose of the examination and the area examined. The patient is generally positioned so that several different views can be taken to provide a complete three-dimensional picture of the part examined. Articles such as jewelry and hairpins must be removed so the image on the radiograph is not obscured. To prevent blurring of the image on the film, patients must maintain the position in which they are placed and not move during the radiographic examination. Blurring prevents good visualization of the part and may warrant retaking of the film. The following types of radiographic views are used, and the methods used to position the patient for each are described.

Anteroposterior view (AP). The x-rays are directed from the front toward the back of the body. The patient is positioned with the anterior aspect of the body facing the radiograph tube and the posterior aspect facing the radiographic film.

Posteroanterior view (PA). The x-rays are directed from the back toward the front of the body. The patient is positioned with the posterior aspect of the body facing the radiograph tube and the anterior aspect facing the radiographic film (see Figure 14–1).

Lateral view. The x-ray beam passes from one side of the body to the opposite side.

Right lateral view (RL). The right side of the body is positioned next to the radiographic film, and the x-rays are directed through the body from the left to the right side.

Left lateral view (LL). The left side of the body is positioned next to the radiographic film, and the x-rays are directed through the body from the right to the left side.

Oblique view. The body is positioned at an angle or in a semilateral position.

Supine position. The patient is positioned on his or her back with the face upward.

Prone position. The patient is positioned face down with the head turned to one side.

Specific Radiographic Examinations

The medical assistant should understand the purpose of commonly performed radiographic examinations and should be able to instruct a patient in the proper preparation for each (Figure 14-2). Frequently performed radiographic examinations and the special advance preparation necessary for each are described. The preparation may vary, depending on the medical office.

PUTTING It All Into **PRACTICE**

MY NAME IS Michelle Shockey, and I work for an orthopedic surgeon in a private practice. I assist the doctor in minor office surgery, dressing changes, joint injections, and cast applications. When the physician performs surgery, I schedule the patients and do their preauthorizations. I have the opportunity to see a variety of problems, from sprains and strains to surgical conditions.

When our patients come to our orthopedic office, they are usually in a lot of pain. Pain plays a big part in how our patients feel on that specific day. We see patients with chronic problems that may never get better. There are also patients who come to our office in pain; but when their visits are over, they feel like they are on top of the world. Seeing a patient go from being unable to walk to being able to run a marathon is the best experience you can encounter.

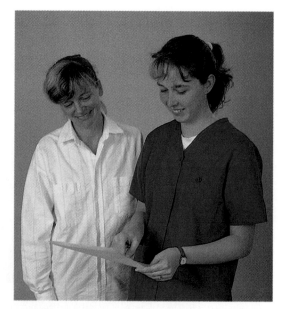

Figure 14-2. Michelle instructs patient in proper preparation for a radiographic examination.

Mammography

Mammography is a radiographic examination of the breasts used to detect many forms of breast disease, such as benign breast masses, breast calcification, fibrocystic breast disease, and particularly breast cancer. It is also used to monitor the effects of surgery and radiation therapy on breast tumors.

Mammography uses low doses of x-rays that pass through the breast and create an image on a film. On the radiograph, an abnormal area appears noticeably different from normal breast tissue. Mammography can be used to detect a breast tumor when the growth is less than 1 cm in diameter (about the size of a pea), and before it is clinically palpable. A malignant lump then can be removed at an early stage, which usually results in conservative treatment with less disfigurement and a high survival rate. In fact, with early diagnosis and treatment, breast cancer survival rates for women can be as high as 94%.

No specific preparation is necessary for mammography. The patient should not wear any lotions, powders, or deodorants because they may contain small amounts of metal that can be seen on the radiograph and may interfere with interpretation. For the mammogram, the patient must remove clothing from the waist up; therefore, the patient should be told to wear a two-piece outfit so the procedure is easier and more comfortable.

A radiology technician generally performs the mammogram. The patient's breast is positioned on the mammography machine, and pressure is applied with a plastic compression paddle that flattens the breast (Figure 14-3). Compression of the breasts is necessary to obtain a clear radiograph and to lower the radiation dosage as much as possible. During the procedure, the patient must hold her breath and remain still momentarily because any type of motion, even breathing, can blur the image and make a repeat radiograph necessary.

Two radiographs are taken of each breast; one from above and one from the side. A radiologist then checks the mammogram (Figure 14-4) and occasionally orders additional images to obtain a more complete view of the breast tissue. After the procedure, the radiologist will study the mammogram for any signs of breast cancer or other breast problems and send a written report of the findings to the patient's physician.

Gastrointestinal Series

Upper Gastrointestinal

An upper GI is an examination of the upper digestive tract using both fluoroscopy and radiography. The examination is helpful in the diagnosis of disorders of the esophagus, stomach, duodenum, and small intestine, such as peptic ulcers or benign and malignant tumors.

Proper patient preparation is important for this procedure. The patient's stomach must be empty at the beginning of the study so food does not obscure the radio-

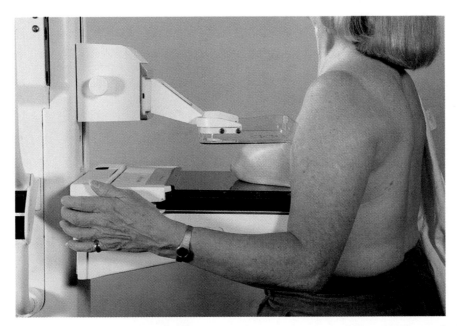

Figure 14-3. Patient positioning for mammography. (From Ballinger PW, Frank ED [eds]: *Merrill's atlas of radiographic positions and radiologic procedures,* vol 2, 10th ed, St. Louis, 2003, Mosby.)

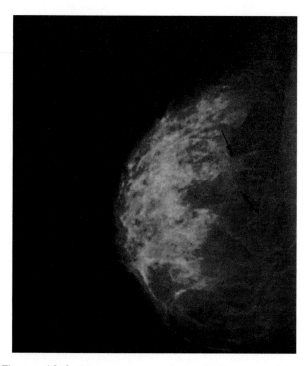

Figure 14-4. Mammogram. *Arrows* indicate suspicious area of increased density that needs further evaluation. (From Prue L: *Atlas of mammographic positioning,* Philadelphia, 1994, Saunders.)

graphic image. To prepare for the examination, the patient must eat a light evening meal and then not eat or drink anything, including water and medications, after midnight the day before the examination. Food and fluid in the GI tract have a degree of density and could cause confusing shadows on the radiograph.

The stomach varies little in density from the structures around it, and in order to make it show up on a radiograph, a contrast medium must be used. The patient drinks a suspension of barium mixed with water and flavoring. The mixture, which has a chalky taste, is known as the barium swallow. As the patient swallows the barium, the radiologist observes its passage down the esophagus and into the stomach and duodenum with fluoroscopy. Radiographs are taken periodically during the examination to allow a detailed study of the upper GI tract and to provide a permanent record. The patient's position is changed at various times so the upper digestive tract can be visualized from different profiles. If the radiologist wants to observe the passage of the barium through the small and large intestines, the patient must return several times for additional radiographs.

The medical assistant should explain to the patient that the barium suspension will appear in the stool the following day and will cause it to have a lighter color. The barium mixture may cause constipation and the

PATIENT TEACHING

Mammography

Answer questions patients may have about mammography.

What is the purpose of mammography?
Mammography is a safe, low-dose radiographic examination used to screen for abnormal changes in the breasts. Mammography allows the physician to detect small lumps in the breast long before they can be felt. Although most breast lumps are not cancerous, breast cancer can be removed at an early stage when detected early, which usually results in treatment that is less deforming and has a much higher survival rate.

Who should have a mammogram?
The American Cancer Society recommends women age 40 years and older have an annual mammogram because the risk of breast cancer increases after this age. Women with a family history of, or other risk factors for, breast cancer should follow the advice of the physician regarding mammography; the age guidelines do not apply because these women undergo examination on a more frequent basis.

What occurs during the mammography procedure?
During mammography, the breast is positioned on a special machine and flattened with a compression paddle. Breast com-

pression may be uncomfortable for some women. The discomfort can be reduced with avoidance of caffeine several days before the procedure and by scheduling the mammography the week following a menstrual period when the breasts are less tender. Each breast is radiographed from above and from the side. The resulting mammogram then is studied by a radiologist to detect any abnormalities. The results are reported to the physician.

Does mammography take the place of breast self-examination?
Mammography is not a substitute for breast self-examination. Women should continue to examine their breasts once a month and also undergo a periodic breast examination by a physician. Most breast lumps are detected by women themselves.

- Encourage the patient to have a mammogram according to the schedule recommended by the American Cancer Society.
- Instruct the patient in the procedure for a breast self-examination.
- Provide the patient with educational materials on breast self-examination and mammography.

need for a laxative. To help prevent constipation, the patient should be instructed to drink water following the procedure.

Lower Gastrointestinal

A lower GI involves filling the colon with a barium sulfate mixture with a tube inserted into the colon. The examination uses both fluoroscopy and radiography to observe and obtain permanent pictures of the colon (Figure 14-5). A lower GI assists in diagnosis of disorders of the lower intestines, such as polyps, tumors, lesions, and diverticulosis. The colon must be thoroughly cleansed in advance to remove gas and fecal material. Gas has a certain degree of density and shows up as confusing shadows on the radiograph. If fecal material appears on the film, the image of the colon is obscured.

The instructions for cleansing the colon may vary somewhat from one medical office to another, but in general the patient is instructed to consume only clear liquids the day before the examination such as water, coffee, tea, clear broth, and strained fruit juice. A laxative should be taken on the day before the scheduled examination, and an enema may also be necessary. The patient should not drink anything (except water) after midnight on the day before the examination. On the morning of the examina-

tion, the patient may be required to perform a warm water cleansing enema until the returns are clear.

The patient should report at the scheduled time and is instructed to relax on one side while the rectal tube is inserted. As the barium enters the colon, the radiologist watches it on the fluoroscopic screen and periodically takes radiographs. The patient will have a sensation of fullness and the urge to defecate as the barium enters the colon. The patient is moved into various positions to allow the barium to fill the colon completely and to obtain better visualization of the colon. The patient then is allowed to evacuate the barium, and another radiograph is taken to finish the radiographic examination.

Cholecystography

Cholecystography is a radiographic examination of the gallbladder used to determine the presence of conditions such as gallstones. The gallbladder is a pear-shaped sac located on the undersurface of the liver that stores bile until it is needed by the body. Bile is produced by the liver and functions to break down fat. When fat enters the small intestine, the gallbladder contracts and releases bile, which enters the small intestine through the common bile duct.

Because the gallbladder does not normally show up on a radiograph, a contrast medium must be used to make it

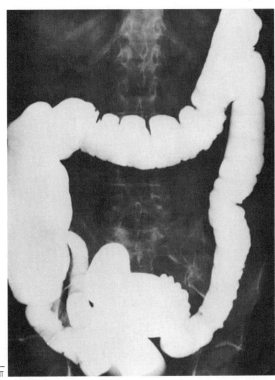

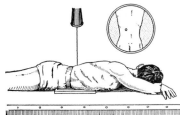

Figure 14-5. Lower GI. Colon is distended with barium: positioning of patient and radiograph. (From Meschan I: *Synopsis of radiologic anatomy with computed tomography,* Philadelphia, 1980, Saunders.)

radiopaque. The patient should eat an evening meal of nonfatty food, such as lean meat, fresh fruit and vegetables, toast or bread, jelly, and tea or coffee. The patient should not consume foods containing fat, such as milk, butter, cheese, cream, eggs, chocolate, or fried or greasy foods. This diet prevents the gallbladder from functioning and contracting and thus emptying the contrast medium before the radiograph is taken.

The patient is given tablets that contain the contrast medium to take at regular intervals (generally 5 to 10 minutes) approximately 2 hours after the evening meal. Specific instructions are included regarding how the tablets should be taken. The contrast medium is absorbed by the gallbladder. Once the tablets have been taken, the patient should have nothing to eat or drink. The patient may also be instructed to cleanse the intestinal tract with a mild laxative and cleansing enemas to prevent gas and fecal material from appearing on the radiograph and obstructing good visualization of the gallbladder.

The patient should report at the scheduled time, and a series of radiographs is taken. The patient then has a meal containing fat to stimulate the gallbladder to empty, and another radiograph is taken for evaluation of the functioning ability of the gallbladder (Figure 14-6).

Intravenous Pyelography

An intravenous pyelogram (IVP) is a radiograph of the kidneys and urinary tract (Figure 14-7). An IVP is used to assist in the diagnosis of kidney stones, blockage or narrowing of the urinary tract, and growths within or near the urinary system.

The patient should eat a light evening meal and not eat or drink anything after 9:00 PM. The patient must remove gas and fecal material from the intestines with a laxative and cleansing enemas. Removal of gas and fecal material permits proper visualization of the urinary tract. Unless the patient is allergic to iodine, a contrast medium consisting of iodine is used and is intravenously administered to the patient. As the iodine enters the bloodstream, the patient may feel warm and flushed and have a metallic or salty taste in the mouth. This reaction is normal and lasts only for a few minutes. If the patient is allergic to iodine, or foods containing iodine such as shellfish, a different type of contrast medium must be used.

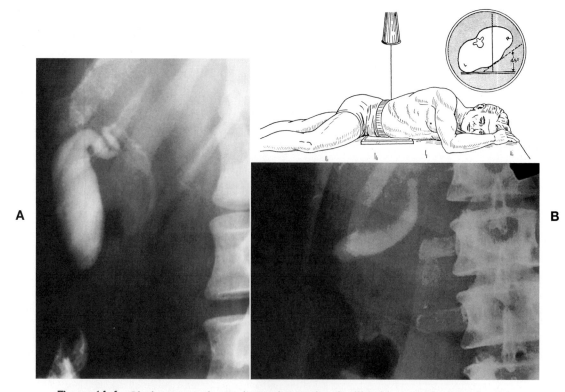

Figure 14-6. Cholecystography. Radiographic study of gallbladder: positioning of patient and radiograph obtained before **(A)** and after **(B)** fatty stimulation. (From Meschan I: *Synopsis of radiologic anatomy with computed tomography,* Philadelphia, 1980, Saunders.)

Other Types of Radiographs

Other types of radiographs that the medical assistant may encounter are in the following list.

Angiocardiogram: A radiograph of the heart in which valves and vessels are examined with radiography and fluoroscopy after the introduction of a radiopaque contrast medium.

Bronchogram: A radiograph of the lungs after introduction of a radiopaque contrast medium.

Cerebral angiogram: A radiograph of the major arteries of the brain after injection of a radiopaque contrast medium.

Cholangiogram: A radiograph of the bile ducts after administration of a radiopaque contrast medium.

Coronary angiogram: A radiograph of the coronary arteries after the injection of a radiopaque contrast medium.

Cystogram: A radiograph of the urinary bladder after injection of a radiopaque contrast medium.

Hysterosalpingogram: A radiograph of the uterus and fallopian tubes after injection of an oily radiopaque contrast medium.

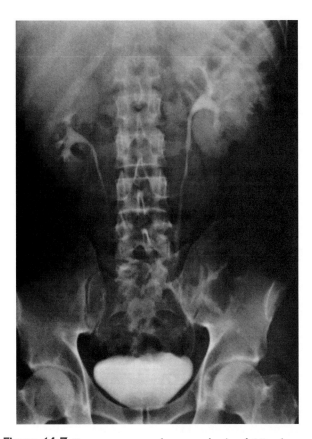

Figure 14-7. Intravenous pyelogram obtained 15 minutes after intravenous injection of suitable contrast agent. (From Meschan I: *Synopsis of radiologic anatomy with computed tomography,* Philadelphia, 1980, Saunders.)

Retrograde pyelogram: A radiograph of the kidneys and urinary tract after injection of radiopaque contrast medium directly into the ureter through a ureteral catheter. The dye flows to the kidneys through the ureters.

Introduction to Diagnostic Imaging

Diagnostic imaging procedures are frequently performed because they allow for the visualization of internal body structures in great detail. The most common procedures are ultrasonography (US), computed tomography (CT), and magnetic resonance imaging (MRI). Diagnostic imaging procedures are almost always performed in a hospital setting; however, information may need to be relayed to a patient scheduled for such a procedure. Therefore, a medical assistant should have a basic knowledge of diagnostic imaging procedures and the preparation necessary for each.

Ultrasonography

Ultrasonography, also called ultrasound, is the oldest of the diagnostic imaging procedures. Ultrasound uses high-frequency sound waves for the study of soft tissue structures. It is frequently used in the diagnosis of conditions of the abdominal and pelvic organs, particularly the liver, gallbladder, spleen, pancreas, kidneys, uterus, and ovaries. An ultrasound examination of the heart is called an **echocardiogram** and is used to determine the size, shape, and position of the heart and the movement of the heart valves and chambers.

Ultrasonography offers a number of advantages as a diagnostic imaging procedure. It shows movement, allows for continuous viewing of a structure, and uses sound waves rather than radiation. Ultrasound does have some minor limitations. Because sound waves are unable to penetrate bone and gas-filled cavities such as the lungs, ultrasound cannot be used in the evaluation of these structures. In addition, ultrasound may be difficult with obese patients because adipose tissue can interfere with sound wave transmission.

During ultrasound, the examiner places a probe containing a transducer firmly on the patient's skin and moves it over the body areas to be examined. The transducer generates sound waves that are directed into the patient's tissues. The sound waves then are reflected back to the transducer, similar to an echo. Deep structures of the body such as the kidneys are visualized by recording the reflections, or echoes, of the sound waves directed into the tissues (Figure 14-8). The image is displayed on an oscilloscope, which is a special type of viewing screen. The image can also be permanently recorded on film and videotape. The recording is called a **sonogram,** and the patient is often permitted to view the sonogram on the oscilloscope as the procedure is performed.

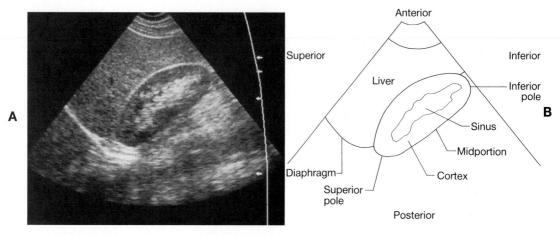

Figure 14-8. Sonogram of right kidney. (From Tempkin BB: *Ultrasound scanning: principles and protocols,* 2nd ed, Philadelphia, 1999, Saunders.)

What Would You DO?
What Would You Not DO?

Case Study 2

Sara-Jayne Monterey has been having heart palpitations. The physician ordered an electrocardiogram, and the results did not show any abnormalities. The physician then ordered a Holter monitor. The results showed the patient was having premature ventricular contractions, especially in the evening. The physician suspects that Sara-Jayne has a prolapsed mitral valve and has scheduled an echocardiogram at the local hospital. Sara-Jayne wants to know whether this procedure involves injecting a dye into her veins. She also wants to know whether the procedure will hurt. Two days before the appointment for the echocardiogram, Sara-Jayne calls the medical office to say that she just found that she is pregnant and wants to know whether the procedure will have to be canceled.

Although ultrasound is commonly used for a wide variety of noninvasive imaging procedures, individuals are most familiar with its use in obstetrics. Obstetric ultrasound is most frequently used to determine gestational age of a fetus and confirm the due date; to detect congenital abnormalities, ectopic pregnancy, and multiple pregnancy; and to determine the baby's position and size late in pregnancy. Because the ultrasound machine is a compact unit, some obstetricians perform this procedure in their medical offices.

Patient Preparation

The medical assistant should tell the patient what to expect during an ultrasound and also instruct the patient in the preparation required for the procedure.

1. Ultrasound is a safe and painless procedure that takes approximately 15 to 45 minutes to complete, depending on the body part examined.
2. The patient may need to prepare for the procedure, depending on the part of the body examined. For example, an ultrasound of the gallbladder and liver ne-

cessitates that the patient fast for 8 to 12 hours. In obstetric ultrasound, the patient needs to have a full bladder. This patient should be instructed to consume approximately 32 oz of fluid about an hour before the procedure.
3. The patient must remain still when requested during the procedure because movement can interfere with accurate results. In addition, the patient may be asked to change positions so the organs can be seen at different angles.

Computed Tomography

Computed (axial) tomography, also known as a CT or CAT scan, is an advanced radiographic examination that uses only a minimal amount of radiation. It produces a series of cross-sectional images of a body part, permitting the imaging of structures that cannot be visualized with conventional radiographic procedures. A CT scan allows the radiologist to view the bones and organs of the head and body in fine detail and has been used most successfully in diagnostic studies of the brain. CT scans are used primarily to detect and evaluate tumors and other abnormalities

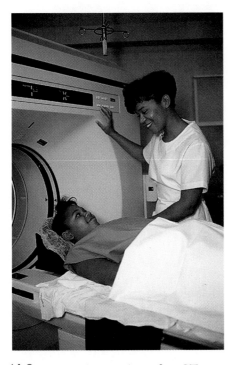

Figure 14-9. Positioning patient for CT scan. (From Kowalczyk N, Donnett K: *Integrated patient care for the imaging professional,* St. Louis, 1996, Mosby.)

During the scan, two examinations are often performed. The first examination is a plain scan, and the second is a repeat scan after a contrast dye has been injected through a vein in the arm. The dye makes a sharper image of internal structures of the body possible. The CT scanner takes multiple radiographic images in a rapid sequence at different angles. The series of radiographs is processed with a computer to produce cross-sectional images, which are displayed on a video monitor and on film (Figure 14-10).

Patient Preparation

The medical assistant should tell the patient what to expect during the CT scan and also instruct the patient in the preparation required for the procedure.

1. If a contrast agent will be used, the patient should fast for 4 hours before the procedure. It is important to ask the patient if he or she is allergic to radiographic contrast media, iodine, or shellfish to avoid an adverse reaction to the contrast medium.
2. Before the procedure, the patient must remove all radiopaque objects such as metal and jewelry because they will interfere with a clear image of the body part examined.
3. The patient should lay motionless and breathe normally during the procedure. When a radiograph is being taken, the patient will be asked to hold his or her breath so the radiograph will not be blurred. The patient will hear mechanical clacking sounds from the scanner as pictures are taken.

Magnetic Resonance Imaging

Magnetic resonance imaging is the newest of the advanced diagnostic imaging procedures. It is used for imaging tissues of high fat and water content that cannot be seen with other radiologic techniques. MRI assists in the diagnosis of intracranial and spinal lesions and cardiovascular and soft tissue abnormalities, such as herniated discs and joint diseases. MRI allows the examiner to see through bone and view fluid-filled soft tissue in great detail.

and to monitor the effects of surgery, radiation therapy, or chemotherapy on tumors.

The scan is conducted by a skilled CT scan technician. The patient is positioned on a special motorized table (Figure 14-9). From an adjoining room, the technician mechanically moves the table into a doughnut-shaped device known as the CT scanner until the part of the body to be examined is inside the tubular opening of the scanner.

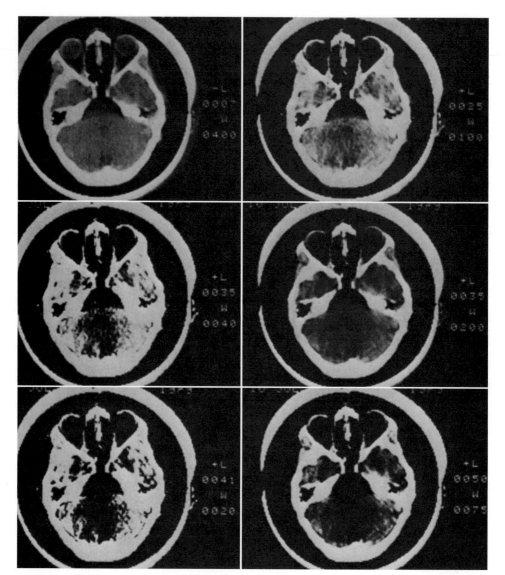

Figure 14-10. Computed tomographic scanner takes multiple cross-sectional radiographic images. The images shown here are cross-sectional pictures of head used to evaluate orbits and sinuses. (From Snopek A: *Fundamentals of special radiographic procedures*, 4th ed, Philadelphia, 1999, Saunders.)

Magnetic resonance imaging is a safe and painless procedure in which a strong magnetic field and ordinary radio waves produce computer-processed images of internal body structures. The patient lays on a table inside the bore of the cylindrical MRI machine while an MRI technician in an adjoining room monitors the procedure (Figure 14-11). Because of the closed space, some patients may have difficulty with claustrophobia. The physician may order a sedative for these patients.

The high-resolution, three-dimensional images that are obtained with MRI are permanently recorded on film or magnetic tape. Because MRI does not involve radiation,

the U.S. Food and Drug Administration has classified the MRI machine as a low-risk device.

Patient Preparation

The medical assistant should tell the patient what to expect during MRI and also instruct the patient in the preparation required for the procedure.

1. Magnetic resonance imaging is a safe and painless procedure with a usual completion time of approximately 1 hour.
2. No special preparation is necessary for the MRI examination. The patient may eat or drink before the examination and take any prescribed medication. The patient

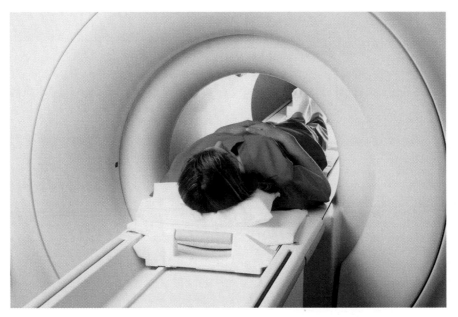

Figure 14-11. Magnetic resonance imaging. Patient lays on table inside bore of cylindrical MRI machine while MRI technicians in adjoining room monitor procedure. (From Ballinger PW, Frank ED [eds]: *Merrill's atlas of radiographic positions and radiologic procedures,* vol 3, 10th ed, St. Louis, 2003, Mosby.)

should wear loose, comfortable clothing, such as a jogging suit, for the procedure.

3. Because the procedure involves a strong magnet, the patient should remove any metal or magnetic-sensitive objects, such as watches, rings, or other metal jewelry and credit cards.

4. The patient must remain completely still for 15- to 20-minute intervals during the procedure. The patient will hear a metallic clacking sound like a muffled drumbeat during the procedure. Earplugs or headphones are available for use if the patient desires.

What Would You DO? What Would You *Not* DO?

Case Study 3

Michael Wendl is an 18-year-old high-school varsity football player. For the past 3 months, he has had pain and swelling in his left knee. The doctor schedules an MRI to assist in determining the cause of the problem. Michael has had several radiographs over the past 2 years and is worried about the radiation exposure to his body. He wants to know how much radiation will be involved with the procedure. Michael has problems with claustrophobia and wants to know whether he can play his Game Boy during the procedure to distract him. He also wants to know whether he is allowed to eat anything before the procedure.

MEDICAL Practice and the LAW

Radiology and diagnostic imaging involve high-technology equipment and procedures that can be frightening and uncomfortable to the patient. Be aware of the patient's reactions, and assist and comfort whenever possible. Be specific in providing the patient with instructions to ensure the best imaging results.

Procedures that involve injectable contrast media or that are invasive usually require written informed consent. Check office policy for procedures that require signed consent forms.

With procedures that use radiation, federal laws regulate usage and exposure testing and record keeping. The acronym ALARA, or As Low As Reasonably Able, reminds workers to minimize exposure to themselves and patients. Be sure to ask female patients if they may be pregnant before starting any radiologic procedure.

Case Study 1
What Did Michelle Do?
❏ Told Mrs. Ramirez that a role-playing game with Jose might help. Suggested that she play the "doctor" and pretend she is taking a radiograph of Jose.

❏ Told Mrs. Ramirez that the barium will have a flavoring in it but that it does taste chalky. Suggested that she explain to Jose why he needs to drink the barium—to help the doctor find what is wrong with him so he will not get sick anymore.

❏ Told Mrs. Ramirez that Jose's truck is made of metal and would interfere with a good radiograph. Suggested that she bring the truck and Jose could have it after the procedure.

❏ Told Mrs. Ramirez that the barium solution should not make Jose sick, but if it does, she should call the office. Explained that the barium might cause constipation and would cause Jose's next bowel movement to be lighter in color. Told her that she should encourage Jose to drink water after the procedure to help prevent constipation.

What Did Michelle Not Do?
❏ Did not tell Mrs. Ramirez that the barium solution would taste good and that she should not have any trouble getting Jose to drink it.

What Would You Do?/What Would You *Not* Do? Review Michelle's response and place a checkmark next to the information you included in your response. List additional information you included in your response below.

_____

_____

_____

_____

Case Study 2
What Did Michelle Do?
❏ Told Sara-Jayne that the procedure uses sound waves to visualize the heart. Explained that the procedure does not use a dye injected into the veins. Gave her an educational brochure on ultrasound imaging.

❏ Reassured Sara-Jayne that no pain is involved with an echocardiogram.

❏ Told Sara-Jayne that an ultrasound is normally safe during pregnancy because radiation is not used. However, the doctor would be informed that she is pregnant and if there is a change in his order, Sara-Jayne would be notified.

What Did Michelle Not Do?
❏ Did not allow Sara-Jayne to go ahead with the procedure without checking with the physician.

What Would You Do?/What Would You *Not* Do? Review Michelle's response and place a checkmark next to the information you included in your response. List additional information you included in your response below.

_____

_____

_____

_____

Case Study 3
What Did Michelle Do?
❏ Explained to Michael that an MRI does not use radiation so he would not be exposed to any radiation during the procedure.

❏ Told Michael that he would not be able to play his Game Boy during the procedure. Explained that the MRI works with a strong magnet that might damage the Game Boy and also interfere with a good image of the knee. Told Michael that he would also need to lay still during the procedure.

❏ Told Michael the physician would be informed of his problem with claustrophobia. Explained that the physician may want to give him something to help him relax during the procedure.

❏ Told Michael that it was fine to eat before the procedure.

What Did Michelle Not Do?
❏ Did not overlook or minimize Michael's concern about claustrophobia.

What Would You Do?/What Would You *Not* Do? Review Michelle's response and place a checkmark next to the information you included in your response. List additional information you included in your response below.

_____

_____

_____

_____

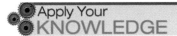
Apply Your
KNOWLEDGE

Choose the best answer for each of the following questions.

1. Joyce Langley, a 45-year-old woman, comes to the office for her gynecologic examination. Dr. Radiolucent asks Michelle Shockey, CMA, to schedule Mrs. Langley for a mammogram at Grant Hospital's radiology department. Michelle provides Mrs. Langley with the following instructions on how to prepare for the examination by telling her to:
   A. Do not wear any lotions, powders, or deodorants to the examination
   B. Fast for 12 hours before the examination
   C. Take a mild sedative before the examination
   D. Cleanse her breasts with isopropyl alcohol the morning of the examination

2. Mrs. Langley returns to the office. Dr. Radiolucent has determined from the results of Mrs. Langley's mammogram that she has fibrocystic breast disease and wants to discuss this condition with her. Mrs. Langley asks Michelle why her breasts were compressed during the mammography procedure. Michelle responds by telling her it was to:
   A. Prevent her from moving during the procedure
   B. Protect her from a radiation burn
   C. Obtain a clear radiograph of her breasts
   D. Make the procedure more comfortable for her

3. James Whitmore, a 62-year-old man, comes to the office with a burning pain that occurs right before he eats. Dr. Radiolucent suspects that James may have a peptic ulcer. He asks Michelle Shockey, CMA, to schedule James for an upper GI radiographic examination at Grant Hospital. Michelle instructs James in the preparation necessary for the radiograph by telling him to:
   A. Perform a cleansing enema on the morning of the examination
   B. Take a laxative the evening before the examination
   C. Not eat or drink anything after midnight on the day before the examination
   D. Take special dye tablets with his evening meal

4. Michelle explains to James that he will be asked to drink a mixture of barium and water before the upper GI examination. Michelle tells James that the barium mixture will be in his stool the next day and will cause his stool to be:
   A. Dark and tarlike
   B. Streaked with mucus
   C. Loose and watery
   D. Lighter in color

5. Susan March comes to the office with cramping in her lower left side. Dr. Radiolucent suspects that Mrs. March may have diverticulitis. He asks Michelle Shockey, CMA, to schedule a lower GI radiographic examination at Grant Hospital. Michelle relays the patient preparation for this examination to Mrs. March. She tells her to do all of the following EXCEPT:
   A. Consume only clear liquids the day before the examination
   B. Eat a breakfast high in fat on the morning of the examination
   C. Take a laxative on the day before the examination
   D. Perform a cleansing enema on the morning of the examination

6. Beth Carroll, a 35-year-old woman, comes to the office with severe pain in her left side, nausea and vomiting, and blood in her urine. Dr. Radiolucent suspects that Beth may have a kidney stone. He asks Michelle Shockey, CMA, to schedule an IVP at Grant Hospital. An important question for Michelle to ask Beth would be:
   A. "Are you allergic to shellfish or iodine?"
   B. "What is the date of your last menstrual period?"
   C. "Is there a history of kidney stones in your family?"
   D. "How much water do you drink every day?"

7. Michelle instructs Beth in how to prepare for the IVP. Michelle tells her to:
   A. Take a laxative the day before the examination
   B. Perform a cleansing enema the morning of the examination
   C. Not eat or drink anything after 9:00 PM the day before the examination
   D. All of the above

8. Megan McCoy, a 35-year-old pregnant woman, comes to the office for an obstetric ultrasound. She is in her fourth month of pregnancy. Megan asks Michelle Shockey, CMA, what kinds of things can be determined from the ultrasound. Michelle responds by saying that it can be used to:
   A. Determine the age of her baby and confirm the due date
   B. Detect certain birth defects
   C. Detect whether or not there is more than one baby
   D. Determine the position of the baby
   E. All of the above

Continued

9. Charles Morrison comes to the office with indigestion and nausea after eating fried foods. Dr. Radiolucent suspects that Charles may be having a problem with his gallbladder. He asks Michelle Shockey, CMA, to schedule an US of the gallbladder at Grant Hospital's diagnostic imaging department. Michelle relays information to Charles regarding this procedure. She includes all of the following EXCEPT:
   A. That Charles must fast for 12 hours before the examination.
   B. That Charles will be required to lay still during the procedure.
   C. That Charles will hear a metallic clacking sound during the procedure.
   D. That it is a safe and painless procedure.

10. Sarah Strong has been diagnosed with colorectal cancer. Dr. Radiolucent asks Michelle Shockey, CMA, to schedule a CT scan at Grant Hospital to determine the extent of the cancer. Michelle explains the preparation required for the examination by telling Sarah to:
   A. Discontinue all medications 2 days before the scan.
   B. Not wear any jewelry.
   C. Consume four glasses of water an hour before the scan.
   D. Perform a cleansing enema on the morning of the scan.
   E. All of the above

CERTIFICATION REVIEW

❏ **X-rays** are used to visualize internal organs and structures and serve as a diagnostic aid in determination of the presence of disease. They are also used therapeutically in the treatment of malignant neoplasms. Radiograph is the term for the permanent record of the picture produced on the radiographic film. Radiology is the branch of medicine that deals with the use of radiant energy in the diagnosis and treatment of disease.

❏ **A structure that permits the passage of X-rays is radiolucent.** A structure that obstructs the passage of x-rays is radiopaque. A contrast medium is used to make a particular structure visible on the radiograph. A fluoroscope is an instrument used to view internal organs and structures of the body directly on a display screen.

❏ **The position of the patient** is determined by the purpose of the examination and the area examined. Different types of radiographic views include AP, PA, lateral, oblique, supine, and prone.

❏ **Mammography** is an radiographic examination of the breasts used to detect breast disease. Mammography can be used to detect a breast tumor when the growth is less than 1 cm in diameter.

❏ **An upper GI** is an examination of the upper digestive tract with both fluoroscopy and radiography. It is used in the diagnosis of disorders of the esophagus, stomach, duodenum, and small intestine.

❏ **A lower GI** involves filling the colon with a barium sulfate mixture with a tube inserted into the colon. The examination is used in the diagnosis of disorders of the lower intestine, such as polyps, tumors, lesions, and diverticulosis.

❏ **Cholecystography** is a radiographic examination of the gallbladder for determination of the presence of conditions such as gallstones.

❏ **An IVP** is a radiograph of the kidneys and urinary tract. It is used to assist in the diagnosis of kidney stones, blockage or narrowing of the urinary tract, and growths within or near the urinary system.

❏ **Ultrasonography** uses high-frequency sound waves to study soft tissue structures. It is frequently used in the diagnosis of conditions of the abdominal and pelvic organs, particularly the liver, gallbladder, spleen, pancreas, kidneys, uterus, and ovaries. An ultrasound examination of the heart is called an echocardiogram. Ultrasound shows movement and allows for continuous viewing of a structure. Obstetric ultrasound is used to determine gestational age of a fetus and confirm date of delivery.

❏ **Computed tomography, CT or CAT scan,** is used to view the bones and organs of the head and body in fine detail. CT scans are used in the detection and evaluation of tumors and other abnormalities and in the monitoring of the effects of surgery, radiation therapy, or chemotherapy on tumors.

❏ **Magnetic resonance imaging** is used to assist in the diagnosis of intracranial and spinal lesions and of cardiovascular and soft tissue abnormalities.

Terminology Review

Contrast medium A substance used to make a particular structure visible on a radiograph.

Echocardiogram An ultrasound examination of the heart.

Enema An injection of fluid into the rectum to aid in the elimination of feces from the colon.

Fluoroscope An instrument used to view internal organs and structures directly.

Fluoroscopy Examination of a patient with a fluoroscope.

Radiograph A permanent record of a picture of an internal body organ or structure produced on radiographic film.

Radiography The taking of permanent records (radiographs) of internal body organs and structures by passing x-rays through the body to act on a specially sensitized film.

Radiologist A medical doctor who specializes in the diagnosis and treatment of disease using radiant energy such as x-rays, radium, and radioactive material.

Radiology The branch of medicine that deals with the use of radiant energy in the diagnosis and treatment of disease.

Radiolucent Describing a structure that permits the passage of x-rays.

Radiopaque Describing a structure that obstructs the passage of x-rays.

Sonogram The record obtained with ultrasonography.

Ultrasonography The use of high-frequency sound waves to produce an image of an organ or tissue.

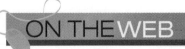

ON THE WEB

For active weblinks to each website visit http://evolve.elsevier.com/Bonewit/.

For Information on Radiography and Diagnostic Imaging

BrighamRAD

Society for Computer Applications in Radiology

Whole Brain Atlas

For Information on Breast Cancer:

American Cancer Society

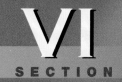

SECTION

Physician's Office Laboratory

15 Introduction to the Clinical Laboratory

16 Urinalysis

17 Phlebotomy

18 Hematology

19 Blood Chemistry and Serology

20 Medical Microbiology

Learning Objectives   ## Procedures

The Clinical Laboratory

1. Explain the general purpose of a laboratory test.
2. List and explain specific uses of laboratory test results.
3. Describe the relationship between the medical office and an outside laboratory.
4. List the information included in a laboratory directory.
5. Identify the purpose of a laboratory request form. List and explain the function of each type of information included on the form.
6. Identify the use of the following profiles and list the tests included in each:
   - Comprehensive metabolic profile
   - Electrolyte profile
   - Hepatic profile
   - Renal profile
   - Lipid profile
   - Thyroid profile
   - Rheumatoid profile
   - Prenatal profile
   - Hepatitis profile
7. Identify the purpose of the laboratory report form and list the information included on it.

Use a laboratory directory.
Complete a laboratory request form.
Read a laboratory report.
Instruct a patient in the preparation necessary for a laboratory test that requires fasting.

Collecting, Transporting, and Handling Specimens

1. Explain the purpose of advance patient preparation for the collection of a laboratory specimen.
2. List examples of specimens.
3. Identify and explain the guidelines that should be followed during specimen collection.
4. Explain why specimens must be handled and stored properly.
5. Identify the proper handling and storage techniques for the following specimens: blood, urine, microbiologic specimen, and stool specimen.

Collect a specimen.
Handle and store a specimen.

The Physician's Office Laboratory

1. Identify and define the eight categories of a laboratory test on the basis of function. List examples of tests included under each category.
2. List the six basic steps involved in testing a specimen.
3. Describe the methods that are used to test a specimen.
4. Explain the purpose of quality control in the laboratory, and list quality control methods that should be used for each of the following: advance patient preparation; specimen collection, handling, and transportation; and laboratory testing.
5. List the laboratory safety guidelines that should be followed in the medical office to prevent accidents.

Use quality control methods.
Practice laboratory safety.

CHAPTER 15

Introduction to the Clinical Laboratory

Chapter Outline

Introduction to the Clinical Laboratory
Laboratory Tests
Purpose of Laboratory Testing
Types of Clinical Laboratories
  Physician's Office Laboratory
  Outside Laboratories
  Laboratory Directory
  Collection and Testing Categories
Laboratory Requests
  Purpose
  Parts of Laboratory Request Form
Laboratory Reports
Patient Preparation and Instructions
  Fasting
  Medication Restrictions
Collecting, Handling, and Transporting Specimens
  Guidelines for Specimen Collection
Clinical Laboratory Improvement Amendments
  Purpose of CLIA 1988
  Categories of Laboratory Testing
  Requirements for Moderate- and High-Complexity Testing
The Physician's Office Laboratory
  Manual Method
  Automated Analyzers
Quality Control
Laboratory Safety

National Competencies

Clinical Competencies
Diagnostic Testing
- Screen and follow-up test results.
- Use methods of quality control.

General Competencies
Patient Instruction
- Instruct individuals according to their needs.
- Instruct and demonstrate the use and care of patient equipment.
- Provide instruction for health care maintenance and disease prevention.
- Identify community resources.

Key Terms

automated method
fasting
homeostasis (hoe-mee-oh-STAY-sis)
in vivo (in-VEE-voe)
laboratory test
manual method
normal range
plasma (PLAZ-ma)
profile
quality control
routine test
serum (SERE-um)
specimen (SPES-i-men)

Introduction to the Clinical Laboratory

Clinical laboratory test results are often used along with a thorough health history and physical examination to provide essential data needed by the physician for accurate diagnosis and management of a patient's condition. Clinical laboratory tests provide objective and quantitative information regarding the status of body conditions and functions. When the body is healthy, its systems will function normally and a state of equilibrium of the internal environment is said to exist; this is termed **homeostasis.** When the body is in a state of homeostasis, the physical and chemical characteristics of the body substances (e.g., fluids, secretions, excretions) will be within a certain acceptable range known as the **normal range** or reference range.

On the other hand, when a pathologic condition exists, biologic changes take place within the body, altering the normal physiology or functioning of the body and resulting in an imbalance. These changes cause the patient to experience the symptoms of that particular pathologic condition. For example, iron deficiency anemia will usually cause the patient to experience weakness, fatigue, pallor, irritability, and, in some cases, shortness of breath on exertion. In addition, these changes in the body's biologic processes may cause an alteration in the characteristics of body substances, such as an alteration of the chemical content of the blood or urine, an alteration in the antibody level, an alteration in cell counts or cellular morphology, and so on.

The physical and chemical alterations of body substances are evidenced through abnormal values or results in laboratory tests—in other words, values outside the accepted normal range or limit for that particular test. Just as certain pathologic conditions cause specific symptoms to occur, certain pathologic conditions cause abnormal values to occur for specific laboratory tests. For example, iron deficiency anemia causes an alteration in normal red blood cell morphology and a decreased hemoglobin level.

An important realization, however, is that an abnormal value for a particular test may be seen with more than one pathologic condition. For example, a decrease in the hemoglobin level also is found with hyperthyroidism and cirrhosis of the liver. In this regard, the physician cannot rely solely on laboratory test results to make a final diagnosis but rather must rely also on the combination of the data obtained from the health history, the physical examination, and diagnostic and laboratory test results.

Laboratory Tests

The number of laboratory tests ordered for a patient varies depending on the physician's clinical findings. A clinical diagnosis of a urinary tract infection, for example, usually necessitates only a urine culture for confirmation. Many diseases, however, have more than one alteration in the physical and chemical characteristics of body substances;

therefore, a series of laboratory tests is often necessary to establish the pattern of abnormalities characteristic of a particular disease.

The medical assistant should realize that not all pathologic conditions necessitate the use of laboratory test results for arrival at a final diagnosis; the information obtained from the patient's clinical signs and symptoms can be sufficient for a final diagnosis of some conditions. In these instances, the physician is so certain of the clinical diagnosis that therapy can be instituted without laboratory confirmation. For example, most physicians diagnose acute purulent otitis media with the information obtained from patient symptoms (earache, fever, feeling of fullness in the ear) and from an otoscopic examination of the tympanic membrane (the tympanic membrane is red and bulging). The information obtained through the clinical signs and symptoms is sufficiently specific to otitis media to allow the physician to make a final diagnosis and to prescribe treatment.

The medical assistant must acquire both knowledge and skill in basic clinical laboratory methods and techniques. It is important that the medical assistant have a knowledge of those laboratory tests that are performed most often, including the purpose of these tests, the normal value or range for each test, any advance patient preparation or special instructions, and any substances that might interfere with accurate test results, such as food or medication.

The medical assistant frequently works with this information when collecting, handling, and storing specimens; performing laboratory tests; typing health histories; and receiving and filing laboratory reports. It is essential that the medical assistant appreciate the value of laboratory tests and alert the physician to any abnormal results as soon as the test is performed or the laboratory report is received.

This chapter is intended to serve as an introduction to the clinical laboratory by providing an overview of methods and general guidelines to follow and by focusing on the relationship between the medical office and an outside laboratory. Specific information for collection, handling, storing, and testing of biologic specimens is presented in the following chapters: Urinalysis, Phlebotomy, Hematology, Blood Chemistry and Serology, and Medical Microbiology.

Purpose of Laboratory Testing

The most frequent use of laboratory test results is to assist in the diagnosis of a patient's condition. However, laboratory test results also have a number of other significant medical uses. A summary of the purpose and function of laboratory testing follows.

1. Laboratory tests are most frequently ordered by the physician *to assist in the diagnosis of pathologic conditions.* Along with the health history and the physical examination, laboratory test results provide the physician with essential data needed to arrive at the final diagnosis and prescription of treatment. After the health history and physical examination, the physician may order laboratory tests for these reasons:

   a. *To confirm a clinical diagnosis.* The patient's signs and symptoms may provide a strong clinical diagnosis of a particular condition, and the physician may order laboratory tests simply to confirm that diagnosis. For example, the patient may have the typical signs and symptoms of diabetes mellitus, which would provide the physician with a fairly certain clinical diagnosis. In this instance, a glucose tolerance test (GTT) would be ordered to confirm the diagnosis and to institute therapy.

   b. *To assist in the differential diagnosis of a patient's condition.* Two or more diseases may have similar signs and symptoms; therefore, the physician will order laboratory tests to assist in the differential diagnosis of the patient's condition. For example, a final diagnosis of streptococcal sore throat must be made with a laboratory test to differentiate it from other pathologic conditions with similar signs and symptoms.

   c. *To obtain information regarding a patient's condition* when not enough concrete evidence exists to support a clinical diagnosis. At times, the patient may have vague signs and symptoms, and laboratory tests are ordered to provide information on what may be causing the patient's problem. For example, the patient may have nonspecific abdominal pain, and the physical examination may not yield enough information to support a clinical diagnosis. In this case, the physician may order a series of tests that may include a number of laboratory tests (usually in the form of profiles) and special diagnostic procedures to assist in pinpointing the cause of the patient's problems.

2. Once the final diagnosis has been made, laboratory testing may be performed *to evaluate the patient's progress and to regulate treatment.* On the basis of the laboratory results, the therapy may need to be adjusted or further treatment prescribed. For example, a patient undergoing iron therapy for iron deficiency anemia should have a complete blood count (CBC) performed every month to assess response to the treatment and to ensure the condition is improving. Another example is a patient with thrombophlebitis who is taking warfarin sodium (Coumadin), an anticoagulant used to inhibit blood clotting. The patient must have a prothrombin time test at regular intervals to assess the clotting ability of the blood. On the basis of the test results, the medication may need to be adjusted to ensure the dosage is at a safe level. The patient with diabetes who measures the blood glucose level each day to regulate insulin dosage provides another example of laboratory tests used to regulate treatment.

3. On the basis of such factors as age, gender, race, and geographic location, individuals will have different normal levels within the established normal range for a particular test. In this respect, laboratory tests can also serve *to establish each patient's baseline or normal level* with which future results can be compared. For example, a patient who is going to undergo warfarin sodium (Coumadin) therapy should have a blood specimen drawn for a prothrombin time test before administration of this anticoagulant. The results serve as a baseline recording for that particular patient with which future prothrombin time test results can be compared.

4. Laboratory tests can also help *to prevent or reduce the severity of disease* by early detection of abnormal findings. Certain conditions, such as high cholesterol, anemia, and diabetes, are relatively common disorders and at times may exist undetected in a patient, especially early in the development of the disease. Laboratory tests known as **routine tests** are performed on a routine basis on apparently healthy patients (usually as part of a general physical examination) to assist in the early detection of disease. These tests are relatively easy to perform and present a minimal hazard to the patient. The most commonly used routine tests include urinalysis, CBC, and routine blood chemistries.

5. Another reason for a laboratory test is its *requirement by state law.* The statutes of most states require a gonorrhea and syphilis test to be performed on pregnant women. The purpose of these tests is to protect the mother and fetus from harm with screening for the presence of these venereal diseases.

Types of Clinical Laboratories

The medical office may use an outside laboratory for testing, or the office may contain its own laboratory, known as a physician's office laboratory (POL), in which the medical assistant performs various tests. Most medical offices use a combination of the two to fulfill the physician's needs for test results.

Physician's Office Laboratory

Generally speaking, laboratory tests that are convenient to perform and commonly required, such as a glucose determination and urinalysis, are performed in the POL. Most physicians consider it too time-consuming and expensive in terms of equipment, supplies, medical laboratory personnel, and quality control to perform in the medical office highly sophisticated and complex tests such as serologic studies and microbiologic studies. Therefore, these tests are usually performed at an outside laboratory. These laboratories use automated equipment to perform the tests, providing the medical offices with fast and reliable test results.

Outside Laboratories

Because the medical assistant usually works closely with an outside laboratory, a basic knowledge of the relationship between the medical office and the laboratory, as described in the following paragraphs, is important. Outside laboratories include hospital and privately owned commercial laboratories, which employ individuals specifically trained in clinical laboratory techniques and methods. The laboratory provides the medical office with the supplies and forms necessary to collect and transport specimens. The medical assistant is responsible for checking these supplies periodically and for reordering them from the laboratory as needed.

Laboratory Directory

The outside laboratory provides the medical office with a laboratory directory that serves as a valuable reference source for the proper collection and handling of specimens. Directories vary in organization, depending on the laboratory. However, the following information is generally included: names of the tests performed by the laboratory, the normal range for each test, instructions on completion of forms, patient preparation necessary for each test, supplies necessary for the collection of each specimen, amount and type of specimen required for each test, techniques to use for the collection of the specimen, proper handling and storage of the specimen, and instructions for transporting specimens.

Table 15-1 is a sample of representative tests taken from a laboratory directory. If the medical assistant has a question regarding any aspect of the collection and handling of the specimen, the laboratory should be called before proceeding.

Collection and Testing Categories

Collection and testing of a specimen can be categorized as follows: (1) the specimen is collected and tested at the medical office; (2) the specimen is collected at the medical office and transferred to an outside medical laboratory for testing; and (3) the patient is given a laboratory request to have the specimen collected and tested at an outside laboratory. The responsibilities of the medical assistant depend on which of these methods is used in the medical office. For example, a specimen collected at the medical office and transferred to an outside laboratory for testing will involve a series of individual steps different from those followed when it is both collected and tested at the medical office.

The following clinical laboratory methods are presented in the remainder of this chapter to provide the student with the information needed to function competently in all three modes just described.

1. Completing laboratory request forms and reviewing laboratory reports.
2. Informing the patient of any necessary advance preparation or special instructions.

TABLE 15-1	Representative Tests from a Laboratory Directory	
Test	**Specimen Requirements**	**Normal Values**
Albumin, Serum	2 ml serum in a SST or transfer tube.	3.5 to 5.5 g/dL
ALT	2 ml serum in a SST or transfer tube.	≤45 U/L
AST	2 ml serum in a SST or transfer tube.	≤40 U/L
Bilirubin, Total	2 ml serum in a SST or transfer tube. Protect from light.	≤1.2-1.3 mg/dL
Blood Group (ABO)	5 ml lavender stoppered tube.	
BUN, Serum	2 ml serum in transfer tube.	7 to 25 mg/dL
Calcium, Serum	2 ml serum in transfer tube.	8.5 to 108 mg/dL
CBC with differential	5 ml lavender stoppered tube. Tube should be inverted 8 to 10 times immediately after drawing. Two blood smears.	Values given with report
Chloride, Serum	2 ml serum in a SST or transfer tube.	96 to 109 mmol/L
CPK	3 ml serum in a SST or transfer tube.	Male: 17 to 148 U/L Female: 10 to 70 U/L
Creatinine, Serum	2 ml serum in a SST or transfer tube.	0.6 to 1.5 to 6 mg/dL
CRP	1 ml serum in a SST or transfer tube. Avoid hemolysis.	<0.8 mg/dL
Glucose, Plasma	5 ml gray stoppered tube. Tube should be inverted 6 to 8 times immediately after drawing.	70 to 110 mg/dL
LD	3 ml serum in a SST or transfer tube. Hemolysis invalidates results.	<240 U/L
Potassium, Serum	2 ml serum in a SST or transfer tube. Hemolysis invalidates results.	3.5 to 5.3 mmol/L
Prothrombin time	1-5 ml blue stoppered tube. Tube should be inverted 8 to 10 times immediately after drawing.	9 to 12 sec
Rapid plasma reagin	2 ml serum in a SST or white topped transfer tube.	Nonreactive
Sedimentation rate	5 ml lavender stoppered tube. Tube should be inverted 6 to 8 times immediately after drawing.	Male: 0 to 15 mm/h Female: 0 to 20 mm/h
Sodium, Serum	2 ml serum in a SST or transfer tube.	135 to 147 mmol/L
Triiodothyronine (T_3)	2 ml serum in a SST or transfer tube.	85 to 205 mg/mL
Thyroxine (T_4)	1 ml serum in a SST or transfer tube.	4.5 to 12 μg/dL
Total protein, Serum	2 ml serum in a SST or transfer tube.	6.0 to 8.5 g/dL
Triglycerides	2 ml serum in a SST or transfer tube. Patient should be fasting 12 to 14 hours.	<150 mg/dL
Uric acid, Serum	2 ml serum in a SST or transfer tube.	Male: 3.9 to 9.0 mg/dL Female: 2.2 to 7.7 mg/dL
Urinalysis, Routine	Random sample. First morning specimen preferred (10 ml).	

ALT, alanine aminotransferase; *AST,* aspartate aminotransferase; *BUN,* blood urea nitrogen; *CPK,* creatine phosphokinase; *CRP,* C-reactive protein; *LD,* lactate dehydrogenase; *RPR,* rapid plasma reagin; *ESR,* erythrocyte sedimentation rate; *SST,* serum separator tube.

3. Collecting, handling, and transporting specimens.
4. Testing the specimens in the medical office.
5. Practicing quality control and laboratory safety.

Laboratory Requests

Purpose

Laboratory requests are printed forms that contain a list of the most frequently ordered laboratory tests (Figure 15-1). A laboratory request is required when the specimen is collected at the medical office and transferred to an outside laboratory for testing or when the specimen will be collected and tested at an outside laboratory, in which case the request is given to the patient at the medical office to take to the laboratory. The request provides the outside laboratory with essential information necessary for accurate testing, reporting of results, and billing. The organizational formats for the request forms vary, depending on the laboratory. In general, most outside laboratories find it more convenient and economic to provide the medical office with one form for designating all tests, with the possible exception of the Pap test, in which case a separate form, known as a cytology request, is provided.

LABORATORY REQUISITION
Biomedical Laboratories, Inc.
100 Main Street
Athens, Georgia 45760

☐ Fax   Send additional copy of report to: ( )
☐ Call   Client Number/Physician's Name   Phone/Fax number
☐ Mail   Physician's Address   City, State, Zip

Patient's Name (Last)	(First)	(MI)	Sex	Date of Birth MO DAY YEAR	Collection Time : AM PM	Fasting YES NO	Collection Date MO DAY YEAR

NPI/UPIN	Physician's ID #	Patient's SS #	Patient's ID #	Urine hrs/vol hrs_____ vol_____

PATIENT / RESP. PARTY

Physician's Name (Last, First) | Physician's Signature
Patient's Address | Phone
Medicare # (Include prefix/suffix) | ☐ Primary ☐ Secondary
City | State | ZIP
Medicaid # | State | Physician's Provider #
Name of Responsible Party (if different from patient)
Diagnosis/Signs/Symptoms in ICD-9 Format (Highest Specificity)
REQUIRED
Address of Responsible Party (if different from patient) | APT #
City | State | ZIP

Patient's Relationship to Responsible Party   ☐ 1–Self   ☐ 2–Spouse   ☐ 3–Child   ☐ 4–Other

Performance Lab ☐	Carrier	Group #	Employee #	Mem

INSURANCE

Insurance Company Name | Plan | Carrier Code
Subscriber/Member # | Location | Group #
Insurance Address | Physician's Provider #
City | State | ZIP
Employer's Name or Number | Insured SS # (If not patient) | Worker's Comp ☐ Yes ☐ No

I hereby authorize the release of medical information related to the service subscribed herein and authorize payment directed to LabCorp.
X _____   Patient's Signature   Date

MEDICARE ADVANCE BENEFICIARY NOTICE
I have read the ABN on the reverse. If Medicare denies payment, I agree to pay for the identified test(s).
X _____   Patient's Signature   Date

NOTE: WHEN ORDERING TESTS FOR WHICH MEDICARE OR MEDICAID REIMBURSEMENT WILL BE SOUGHT, PHYSICIANS SHOULD ONLY ORDER TESTS THAT ARE MEDICALLY NECESSARY FOR THE DIAGNOSIS OR TREATMENT OF THE PATIENT. COMPONENTS OF THE ORGAN OR DISEASE PANELS/COMBINATIONS PRINTED BELOW ARE SHOWN ON THE REVERSE SIDE AND MAY ALSO BE ORDERED INDIVIDUALLY BELOW. COMPONENTS MAY BE BILLED SEPARATELY PER CARRIER POLICY.

PROFILES (See reverse for components)

Code	Test	Tube
80049	Basic Metabolic Profile	SST
80054	Comp Metabolic Profile	SST
80051	Electrolyte Profile	SST
80058	Hepatic Profile	SST
80059	Hepatitis Profile	SST
80061	Lipid Profile	SST
80091	Thyroid Profile	SST
80055	Prenatal Profile	RED LAV
80072	Rheumatoid Profile	SST

HEMATOLOGY

Code	Test	Tube
85025	CBC w Diff	LAV
85027	CBC w/o Diff	LAV
85014	Hematocrit	LAV
85018	Hemoglobin	LAV
85595	Platelet Count	LAV
85041	RBC Count	LAV
85048	WBC Count	LAV
85007	WBC Differential	LAV
89190	Nasal Smear, Eosin	Nasal Smear
85060	Pathologist Consult–Peripheral Smear	LAV

ALPHABETICAL/COMBINATION TESTS

Code	Test	Tube
86900 86901	ABO and Rh	LAV
82040	Albumin	SST
84075	Alkaline Phosphatase	SST
84460	ALT (SGPT)	SST
82150	Amylase, Serum	SST
86038	Antinuclear Antibodies	SST
84450	AST (SGOT)	SST
82607 82746	B12 and Folate	SST
82250	Bilirubin, Total	SST

ALPHABETICAL TESTS CON'T

Code	Test	Tube
84520	BUN	SST
82310	Calcium	SST
80156	Carbamazepine (Tegretol®)	SER
82378	CEA	SST
82465	Cholesterol, Total	SST
82565	Creatinine	SST
80162	Digoxin	SER
82670	Estradiol	SST
82728	Ferritin, Serum	SST
82985	Fructosamine	SST
83001	FSH	SST
83001 83002	FSH and LH	SST
82977	GGT	SST
82947	Glucose, Plasma	GRY
82947	Glucose, Serum	SST
82950	Glucose, 2-hr. PP	SST
83036	Glycohemoglobin, Total	LAV
84703	hCG, Beta Subunit, Qual	SST
84702	hCG, Beta Subunit, Quant	SST
83718	HDL Cholesterol	SST
86677	Helicobacter pylori, IgG	SST
86706	Hep B Surface Antibody	SST
87340	Hep B Surface Antigen	SST
86803	Hep C Antibody	SST
83036	Hemoglobin A1C	LAV
86701	HIV Antibodies	SST
83540	Iron, Total	SST
83540 83550	Iron and IBC	SST
83615	LDH	SST

ALPHABETICAL TESTS CON'T

Code	Test	Tube
83002	LH	SST
83690	Lipase	SER
80178	Lithium (Eskalith®)	SER
83735	Magnesium, Serum	SST
80184	Phenobarbital (Luminal®)	SER
80185	Phenytoin (Dilantin®)	SER
84132	Potassium	SST
84146	Prolactin, Serum	SST
84153	Prostate-Specific Antigen	SST
84066	Prostatic Acid Phos	SST
84155	Protein, Total	SST
85610	Prothrombin Time (PT)	BLU
85610 85730	PT and PTT Activated	BLU
85730	PTT Activated	BLU
86431	Rheumatoid Arthritis Factor	SST
86592	RPR	SST
86762	Rubella Antibodies, IgG	SST
85651	Sed Rate	LAV
84295	Sodium	SST
84403	Testosterone	SST
80198	Theophylline	SER
84436	Thyroxine (T4)	SST
84478	Triglycerides	SST
84480	Triiodothyronine (T3)	SST
84443	TSH, High Sensitivity	SST
84550	Uric Acid	SST
81003	Urinalysis Microscopic on Positives	URN
81001	Urinalysis with Microscopic	URN
80164	Valproic Acid (Depakene®)	SER

MICROBIOLOGY   See Reverse Side

☐ ENDOCERVICAL   ☐ THROAT   ☐ URINE
☐ STOOL   ☐ URETHRAL   INDICATE SOURCE

Code	Test	Transport
87070	Aerobic Bacterial Culture	Bact Trnspt
87490 87590	Chlamydia/GC DNA Probe w/ Confirmation on Positives	Probe Trnspt
87490 87590	Chlamydia/GC DNA Probe Without Confirmation	Probe Trnspt
87490	Chlamydia DNA Probe	Probe Trnspt
87081	Genital, Beta-Hemolytic Strep Cult, Group B	Bact Trnspt
87070	Genital Culture, Routine	Bact Trnspt
87070	Lower Respiratory Culture	Steril Trnspt
87590	N. gonorrhoeae DNA Probe	Probe Trnspt
87015 87211	Ova and Parasites	O & P Kit
87081 X2 87045	Stool Culture	Fecal Trnspt
87081	Throat, Beta-Hemolytic Strep Cult, Group A	Bact Trnspt
87060	Upper Respiratory Culture, Routine	Bact Trnspt
87086	Urine Culture, Routine	Urn Cult Trnspt

Clinical Information/Comments

OTHER TESTS/INDIVIDUAL COMPONENTS
TEST #   TEST NAMES

LAB USE ONLY	STAT ☐ 998074	VENIPUNCTURE ☐ 998085	TRAVEL ☐ 998096	NON LABCORP ☐ 998239	VERBAL ORDER ☐ 998250	CHART ORDER ☐ 998261	HANDWRITTEN ☐ 998272	24 HR TUV ☐ 998283	PST/PSC #

CONTAINERS RECEIVED: SST SPUN | USST UNSPUN | SER SERUM TRNSPT | FRZ FRZ TRNS | RED RED | LAV LAVENDER | SLD SLIDE | BLU LT. BLUE | GRY GREY | GRN GREEN | RYB RYL BLU | YEL ACD | PLS PLASMA | URN URINE | 24U 24 HR URINE | TA-U TART. ACID | FL FLUID | OT OTHER | BACT TRNSP | O & P KIT | PROBE TRNSP | URN CULT TRNSP | STERIL TRNSP | FECAL TRNSP | VIRAL TRNSP

300-0384

Figure 15–1. Laboratory request form.

Case Study 1

Three days ago, Hildy McNicle was given a laboratory requisition at the medical office to have blood drawn and tested at an outside medical laboratory. Hildy calls the medical office and says she is a little confused. She called the laboratory for her test results, and they would not give them to her. They told her to call the medical office. She does not understand this because her blood was collected and tested at the laboratory and it would seem logical to her that they would give her the test results, especially because she is paying the laboratory to perform the tests. The test results have come back with abnormal values, and the physician is at a medical convention and will not return until tomorrow.

Parts of Laboratory Request Form

Specific information that is required on the laboratory request form follows.

1. *Physician's name and address.* The physician's name and address should be clearly indicated on the laboratory request form to facilitate the reporting of test results to the physician. Most laboratories provide request forms with the physician's name and address preprinted on the form. In addition, the forms are usually prenumbered with the physician's account number, which assists in identification, reporting, and billing of laboratory tests.

2. *Patient's name and address.* The patient's name and address should be printed as requested by the laboratory; for example, the laboratory may want the patient's name written with the last name first, middle initial, first name. The patient's address is needed for billing purposes and must include the city, state, and zip code.

3. *Patient's age and gender.* The normal ranges for some tests vary, depending on the patient's age and gender. For example, the normal range for hemoglobin concentration varies according to gender (12 to 16 g/dL for a female; 14 to 18 g/dL for a male).

4. *Date and time of collection of the specimen.* The date of the specimen collection indicates to the laboratory the number of days that have passed since the collection, thus providing the laboratory with information regarding the freshness of the specimen. A time lapse that is too long between collection and testing of a specimen may affect the accuracy of some test results. The time of collection is significant with respect to selected laboratory tests. For example, the normal range for serum cortisol varies depending on whether the specimen is an AM specimen (collected in the morning) or a PM specimen (collected in the afternoon).

5. *Laboratory tests desired.* The tests desired by the physician are usually indicated with checking a box adjacent to those tests (see Figure 15–1). The boxes should be clearly marked to avoid any confusion. A space designated as additional tests or other tests on the laboratory request form provides for writing in a test that is desired but not listed on the request form. As previously indicated, most laboratory request forms include only those tests most frequently ordered. The laboratory directory contains a complete listing of all the tests performed.

   Laboratory tests termed **profiles** contain a number of different tests; the profiles performed by the laboratory and the tests included in each are listed in the directory. A profile may be specific in nature—that is, all the tests included relate to a specific organ of the body or a particular disease state. A specific profile is usually ordered when the physician does not have a definite clinical diagnosis but has a good idea of what organ or organs are involved in the patient's condition. The physician will order a profile of the organ in question. An example of this type of profile is the hepatic profile, which is used to assess liver function and to assist in the diagnosis of a pathologic condition that affects the liver.

   A profile may also be general in nature. A general metabolic profile contains a number of routine laboratory tests and is primarily used in a routine health screen of a patient. General metabolic profiles are used to detect any changes in the body's biologic processes that may be present, although the patient may not have had any symptoms to indicate that these changes have occurred. General metabolic profiles are also used when the patient's symptoms are so vague that the physician does not have enough concrete evidence to support a clinical diagnosis of a specific organ or disease state.

   The medical assistant should have knowledge of the names of common profiles and the tests generally contained in each, which are listed in Table 15-2. The tests contained in each profile may vary slightly from one laboratory to another.

6. *Source of the specimen.* Certain tests require that the source of the specimen (e.g., throat, wound, ear, eye, urine, vagina) be recorded on the laboratory request form. This is for identification of the origin of the specimen for the laboratory because this information is not available from looking at the specimen. In many instances, the source dictates the test method used by the laboratory to evaluate the specimen for the presence of a possible pathogen. For example, the test method used to detect the presence of *Streptococcus* in a specimen obtained from the throat will be different from that used to detect *Candida albicans* in a vaginal specimen.

TABLE 15-2 Laboratory Profiles

Profile	Tests Included	Use
Health screen profile	Glucose	General health screen
	BUN	Assessment of diseases of specific organs
Diabetes assessment	Uric acid	or disease states
Assessment of kidney function	Calcium	
Assessment of infection and nutrition	Phosphorus	
Assessment of liver function	Total protein	
	Albumin	
	Alkaline phosphatase	
Assessment of tissue disease and cardiac function	AST	
	LD	
	Bilirubin	
	Cholesterol	
Liver function profile	Total bilirubin	Detection of pathologic conditions affecting liver
	Total protein	
	Albumin	
	Globulin	
	A/G ratio	
	Alkaline phosphatase	
	AST	
	ALT	
Thyroid function profile	T_4 RIA	Detection of pathologic conditions affecting thyroid gland
	T_3 uptake	
	T_7	
Prenatal profile	Complete blood count	Establishment of baseline recordings and screenings of prenatal patients for disease or potential problems
	ABO blood type	
	Rh factor	
	Serology (VDRL or RPR)	
	Rubella titer	
	Rh antibody titer	
	Antibody screen if Rh−	
Electrolyte profile	Sodium	
	Potassium	
	Chloride	
Rheumatoid profile	ASO titer	Detection of rheumatoid arthritis
	RA test	
	CRP	
	Uric acid	
Lipid profile	Total cholesterol	Detection of coronary heart disease
	Triglycerides	
	HDL cholesterol	
	LDL cholesterol	
	Total cholesterol/HDL ratio	
Hepatitis profile	HBsAg	Detection of viral hepatitis
	HBcAb–IgM	
	HAvAB–IgM	
Renal profile	A/G ratio, albumin globulin ratio	
	ALT, alanine aminotransferase	
	Anti-HBc, IgM, antibody to B core antigen, IgM	
	ASO, antistreptolysin	
	AST, asparate aminotransferase	
	BUN, blood urea nitrogen	
	CRP, C-reactive protein	
	FTI, free thyroxine index	
	HBsAg, B surface antigen	
	HDL, high-density lipoprotien	
	LDL, low-density lipoprotein	
	RA, rheumatoid factor	
	RPR, rapid plasma regain	
	T_3 uptake, thyroid hormone binding ratio	
	T_4, throxine	
	VDRL, Venereal Disease Research Laboratory	

BUN, Blood urea nitrogen; *AST*, aspartate aminotransferase, *ALT*, alanine aminotransferase; *ALP*, alkaline phosphatase; *FTI*, free thyroxine index; *TSH*, thyroid stimulating hormone; *VDRL*, Veneral Disease Research Laboratory; *RPR*, rapid plasma reagin; *ASO*, antistreptolysin O; *RA*, rheumatoid factor; *CRP*, C-reactive protein; *HDL*, high-density lipoprotein; *LDL*, low-density lipoprotein; *VLDL*, very low-density lipoprotein.

7. *Physician's clinical diagnosis.* The clinical diagnosis assists the laboratory in correlating the clinical laboratory data with the needs of the physician. In some instances, further testing is performed by the laboratory if one test method proves inconclusive with respect to providing the physician with the information necessary to confirm or reject the clinical diagnosis. Another function of the clinical diagnosis is to assure laboratory personnel that the test results are within the framework of the diagnosis. When the results of a test disagree with the physician's clinical diagnosis, the laboratory repeats the test on the same or another specimen. The clinical diagnosis also alerts laboratory personnel to the possibility of the presence of a potentially dangerous pathogen, such as the hepatitis virus. In addition, this information is necessary for third-party billing by the laboratory. If the laboratory bills an insurance company for the tests, the clinical diagnosis will be necessary on the insurance form. The processing of insurance forms is facilitated by having the information at hand and not having to contact the medical office to obtain it.

8. *Medications.* Certain medications may interfere with the accuracy and validity of the test results. Therefore, the laboratory should be notified on the request form of any medications taken by the patient.

9. *STAT.* At times, the physician will want the laboratory test results reported as soon as possible. In this case, STAT should be clearly written in bold letters (or the appropriate STAT box checked) on the laboratory request form. Requests that are marked STAT are performed as soon as possible after receipt by the laboratory, and the results are telephoned or faxed to the physician as soon as they are available.

Once the specimen has been collected, the completed request form must be placed with the specimen for transport to the outside laboratory. The medical assistant should realize the significance of this simple but important step. Numerous possible tests can be performed on one particular specimen, and without the request form, the laboratory does not have the information it needs to carry out the physician's orders, causing delays in completing the tests and reporting results.

Laboratory Reports

Laboratory report forms are used to relay the results of the laboratory tests to the physician (Figure 15-2). The report may be in the form of a computer printout, or it may be a preprinted form with the test results written in by the laboratory technologist performing the tests. The report will include the following certain types of information:

1. Name, address, and telephone number of the laboratory.
2. Physician's name and address.
3. Patient's name, age, and gender.
4. Patient accession number.
5. Date the specimen was received by the laboratory.

6. Date the results were reported by the laboratory.
7. Names of the tests performed.
8. Results of the tests.
9. Normal range for each test performed.

A patient accession number or laboratory number is assigned to each specimen received by the laboratory. Its purpose is to provide positive identification of each specimen within the laboratory and to allow easy access to the patient's laboratory records should a test result need to be located again. If the physician desires to have the laboratory test repeated, the accession number listed on the original report form must be included on the laboratory request form.

A normal range, rather than a single value, is necessary for laboratory test results because of individual differences among a general population from factors such as age, gender, race, and geographic location. In addition, no test can be so accurate that a single value is possible. The normal range for each test varies slightly from one laboratory to another, depending on the test method, equipment, and reagents used to perform the test. In this regard, it is essential that the medical assistant compare the test results with the normal range supplied by the laboratory performing the test rather than with a reference source such as a medical laboratory textbook.

Laboratory reports are either hand delivered, faxed, sent electronically, or mailed to the medical office by the laboratory. Abnormal results that pose a threat to the patient's health and laboratory reports marked STAT are telephoned or faxed to the medical office as soon as the tests are

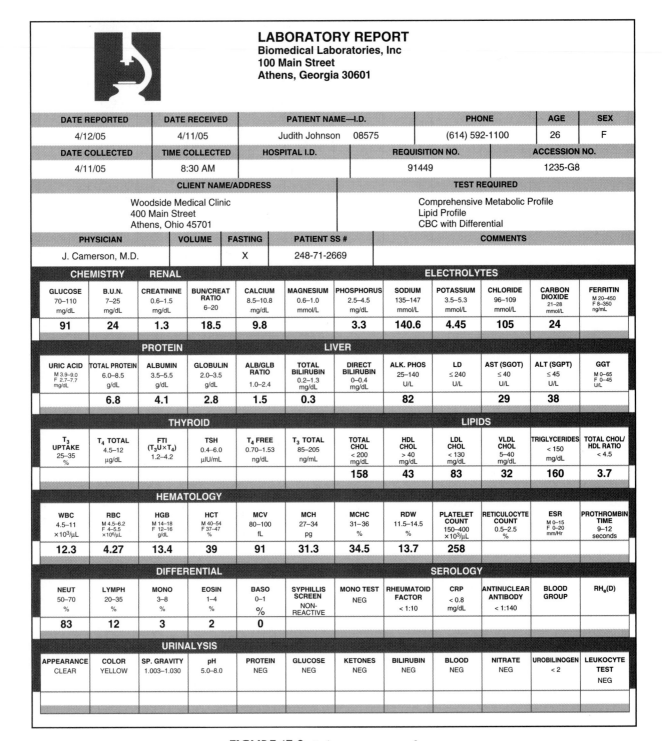

LABORATORY REPORT
Biomedical Laboratories, Inc
100 Main Street
Athens, Georgia 30601

DATE REPORTED	DATE RECEIVED	PATIENT NAME—I.D.		PHONE	AGE	SEX
4/12/05	4/11/05	Judith Johnson 08575		(614) 592-1100	26	F

DATE COLLECTED	TIME COLLECTED	HOSPITAL I.D.	REQUISITION NO.	ACCESSION NO.
4/11/05	8:30 AM		91449	1235-G8

CLIENT NAME/ADDRESS	TEST REQUIRED
Woodside Medical Clinic 400 Main Street Athens, Ohio 45701	Comprehensive Metabolic Profile Lipid Profile CBC with Differential

PHYSICIAN	VOLUME	FASTING	PATIENT SS #	COMMENTS
J. Camerson, M.D.		X	248-71-2669	

CHEMISTRY — RENAL / ELECTROLYTES

GLUCOSE 70–110 mg/dL	B.U.N. 7–25 mg/dL	CREATININE 0.6–1.5 mg/dL	BUN/CREAT RATIO 6–20	CALCIUM 8.5–10.8 mg/dL	MAGNESIUM 0.6–1.0 mmol/L	PHOSPHORUS 2.5–4.5 mg/dL	SODIUM 135–147 mmol/L	POTASSIUM 3.5–5.3 mmol/L	CHLORIDE 96–109 mmol/L	CARBON DIOXIDE 21–28 mmol/L	FERRITIN M 20–450 F 8–350 ng/mL
91	24	1.3	18.5	9.8		3.3	140.6	4.45	105	24	

PROTEIN / LIVER

URIC ACID M 3.9–9.0 F 2.7–7.7 mg/dL	TOTAL PROTEIN 6.0–8.5 g/dL	ALBUMIN 3.5–5.5 g/dL	GLOBULIN 2.0–3.5 g/dL	ALB/GLB RATIO 1.0–2.4	TOTAL BILIRUBIN 0.2–1.3 mg/dL	DIRECT BILIRUBIN 0–0.4 mg/dL	ALK. PHOS 25–140 U/L	LD ≤ 240 U/L	AST (SGOT) ≤ 40 U/L	ALT (SGPT) ≤ 45 U/L	GGT M 0–65 F 0–45 U/L
	6.8	4.1	2.8	1.5	0.3		82		29	38	

THYROID / LIPIDS

T$_3$ UPTAKE 25–35 %	T$_4$ TOTAL 4.5–12 µg/dL	FTI (T$_3$U×T$_4$) 1.2–4.2	TSH 0.4–6.0 µIU/mL	T$_4$ FREE 0.70–1.53 ng/dL	T$_3$ TOTAL 85–205 ng/mL	TOTAL CHOL < 200 mg/dL	HDL CHOL > 40 mg/dL	LDL CHOL < 130 mg/dL	VLDL CHOL 5–40 mg/dL	TRIGLYCERIDES < 150 mg/dL	TOTAL CHOL/ HDL RATIO < 4.5
						158	43	83	32	160	3.7

HEMATOLOGY

WBC 4.5–11 ×10³/µL	RBC M 4.5–6.2 F 4–5.5 ×10⁶/µL	HGB M 14–18 F 12–16 g/dL	HCT M 40–54 F 37–47 %	MCV 80–100 fL	MCH 27–34 pg	MCHC 31–36 %	RDW 11.5–14.5 %	PLATELET COUNT 150–400 ×10³/µL	RETICULOCYTE COUNT 0.5–2.5 %	ESR M 0–15 F 0–20 mm/Hr	PROTHROMBIN TIME 9–12 seconds
12.3	4.27	13.4	39	91	31.3	34.5	13.7	258			

DIFFERENTIAL / SEROLOGY

NEUT 50–70 %	LYMPH 20–35 %	MONO 3–8 %	EOSIN 1–4 %	BASO 0–1 %	SYPHILLIS SCREEN NON-REACTIVE	MONO TEST NEG	RHEUMATOID FACTOR < 1:10	CRP < 0.8 mg/dL	ANTINUCLEAR ANTIBODY < 1:140	BLOOD GROUP	RH$_e$(D)
83	12	3	2	0							

URINALYSIS

APPEARANCE CLEAR	COLOR YELLOW	SP. GRAVITY 1.003–1.030	pH 5.0–8.0	PROTEIN NEG	GLUCOSE NEG	KETONES NEG	BILIRUBIN NEG	BLOOD NEG	NITRATE NEG	UROBILINOGEN < 2	LEUKOCYTE TEST NEG

FIGURE 15-2. Laboratory report form.

completed, and a written report follows immediately thereafter. The laboratory usually supplies the medical office with telephone reporting pads to transcribe the results from the telephone report to reduce errors.

The medical assistant may be responsible for reviewing the laboratory reports as they are received. The medical assistant should compare the patient's test results with the normal ranges supplied by the laboratory and notify the physician of any abnormal test results. Many computer systems automatically identify abnormal results on the laboratory report; if not, the physician may want the medical assistant to identify them by circling them with a red pen. The reports then are reviewed by the physician, and the data obtained are correlated with the information obtained from the health history and physical examination. The physician indicates that he or she is finished with the report usually by placing his or her initials on it. The medical assistant is then responsible for filing the laboratory report in the patient's chart, according to the medical office policy.

Patient Preparation and Instructions

Factors such as food consumption, medication, activity, and time of day affect the laboratory results of certain tests. Therefore, for some laboratory tests, advance patient preparation is necessary to obtain a quality specimen suitable for testing, which leads to accurate results and, in turn, assists the physician in accurate diagnosis and treatment. An important realization is that the quality of the laboratory test results can be only as good as the quality of the specimen obtained from the patient. A specimen obtained from a patient who has not prepared properly may invalidate the test results and necessitate calling the patient back to collect the specimen again.

The medical assistant is usually responsible for instructing the patient in any advance preparation that might be necessary. A complete and thorough explanation of the instructions should be relayed clearly to the patient. The medical assistant should explain the reason for the advance preparation so that the patient will be more likely to comply with the preparation necessary. It should be emphasized to the patient that the preparation is essential to obtain accurate test results and to avoid having to collect the specimen again.

Once the instructions have been explained, it is important that the medical assistant checks that the patient completely understands them and offers to answer any questions. It is also advisable that the patient be provided with a written instruction sheet to serve as a reference, should the patient forget some of the information after leaving the medical office. Some specimen collections may require that the patient remain at the collection site for a specified period of time; an example of this is the GTT, which requires several hours for the collection of multiple, timed specimens. The patient should be told in advance of the time requirement so that any necessary arrangements can be made with an employer or babysitter or such.

At times, the patient will collect the specimen himself or herself, at home. The medical assistant is responsible for explaining detailed instructions to the patient on the proper techniques for collection of the specimen. For example, if a first-voided morning urine specimen is necessary for the laboratory test, the medical assistant will need to provide the patient with the appropriate specimen container and to instruct the patient in the proper collection, handling, and storage of the specimen until it reaches the medical office.

The specific type of preparation necessary for a particular test depends on the test ordered and the method used to run it. If the medical office uses an outside laboratory, the patient preparation necessary for each test will be found in the laboratory directory. If the test is performed in the medical office, the medical assistant should consult the manufacturer's instructions that accompany the testing product to obtain specific information regarding patient preparation. Advance patient preparation is usually in the form of a diet modification (e.g., low-fat diet), fasting, or medication restrictions.

Fasting

Some venous blood specimens require the patient to fast before collection. The composition of blood is altered by the consumption of food because the digested food is absorbed into the circulatory system, thus changing the results of certain laboratory tests. For example, food intake causes the blood glucose and triglyceride laboratory tests to yield falsely high results. Therefore, any individual test (e.g., FBS, GTT) or profile including these tests (e.g., comprehensive metabolic profile, lipid profile), requires the patient to fast before the specimen is collected.

Fasting involves abstaining from food and fluids (except water) for a specified amount of time before the collection of the specimen (usually 12 to 14 hours). Fasting specimens are usually collected in the morning to allow the food from the previous evening meal to be completely digested and absorbed. In addition, collection of the specimen in the morning causes the least amount of inconvenience to the patient in terms of abstaining from food and fluid.

The medical assistant must give detailed instructions to the patient, making certain the patient understands that fasting includes abstaining from both food and fluid. However, the patient should be told that it is permissible—in fact advisable—to drink water because dehydration caused by water abstinence can also alter certain test results.

The medical assistant should indicate a specific time to the patient for initiation of the fast; if the specimen will be collected in the morning, the patient should be instructed to begin fasting at 6:00 PM on the previous evening. The patient must also be told the time to report for collection of the specimen.

Medication Restrictions

Many medications affect the physical and chemical characteristics of body substances; therefore, medications taken by the patient may lead to inaccurate test results. For example, antibiotic therapy administered before collection of a throat specimen for strep testing may cause a falsely negative report. The physician generally will ask the patient to avoid taking medication for a period of time before the collection of the specimen if discontinuing the medication will not cause any health threat or serious discomfort to the patient.

Because medication is more likely to interfere with test results on urine than on blood, the patient is recommended to discontinue medication 48 to 72 hours before the collection of a urine specimen and 4 to 24 hours before the collection of a blood specimen.

If the patient cannot be taken off medication, the information should be recorded on the laboratory request form for those specimens transported to an outside laboratory for testing. This alerts the laboratory personnel to the presence of the medication. If the medication taken by the patient interferes with the method normally used to perform the test, the laboratory may be able to use an alternate method to obtain valid results. If the test is being performed in the medical office, the medical assistant should consult the manufacturer's instructions that accompany the testing materials for the names of the medications that interfere with test results.

The physician determines the need for abstinence from the medication before specimen collection. The medical assistant is responsible for ensuring that the patient understands any instructions regarding restrictions on medication and for recording medications the patient is taking on the laboratory request form.

Collecting, Handling, and Transporting Specimens

Clinical laboratory tests are performed on specimens obtained from the body. A **specimen** is a small sample or part taken from the body to represent the nature of the whole. Most laboratory tests are performed on specimens

that are easily obtained from the body, such as blood, urine, feces, sputum, a cervical and vaginal scraping of cells, or a sample of a secretion or discharge from various parts of the body (eg, nose, throat, wound, ear, eye, vagina, urethra) for microbiologic analysis. Other examples of specimens analyzed in the laboratory but more difficult to obtain from the body include gastric juices, cerebrospinal fluid, pleural fluid, peritoneal fluid, synovial fluid, and tissue biopsy specimens. The source of the specimen may not necessarily be indicative of the pathologic condition in question; for example, T_3 and T_4 tests are performed on blood serum but are used to detect a condition that affects the thyroid gland.

The medical assistant is responsible for the collection of most specimens obtained from patients in the medical office; of these, blood and urine will constitute the largest percentage of specimens collected. Certain specimens, such as a sample of vaginal or urethral discharge, cerebrospinal fluid, or a tissue biopsy, must be collected by the physician; in these cases, the medical assistant assists with the collection.

The most important aspect of specimen collection and handling is to provide the laboratory with a sample that is as biologically representative as possible of the body substance collected. If the specimen is collected or handled improperly, the **in vivo** characteristics of the specimen may be adversely affected, which in turn may cause inaccurate and unreliable test results; this may interfere with the accurate diagnosis and treatment of the patient's condition.

Guidelines for Specimen Collection

Specific guidelines that should be used regarding specimen collection and handling follow:

1. *Review and follow the Occupational Safety and Health Administration (OSHA) Bloodborne Pathogens Standards* during specimen collection (see Chapter 2).

2. *Review the requirements for collection and handling of the specimen,* which include the collection materials necessary, the type of specimen to be collected (e.g., serum, plasma, whole blood, clotted blood, urine), the amount necessary for laboratory analysis, the procedure to follow in collection of the specimen, and its proper handling and storage.

3. *Assemble the equipment and supplies.* Use only the appropriate specimen containers as specified by the medical office or laboratory. Substituting containers may not yield the proper type of specimen required or may affect the test results, as shown by the following examples. If serum is required and a tube containing an anticoagulant is used (instead of a plain tube not containing an anticoagulant), the blood separates into plasma and cells, rather than serum and cells, and the wrong type of blood specimen is obtained, which necessitates another specimen from the patient. Collection of a microbiologic specimen that may contain anaerobic pathogens with supplies meant for aerobic pathogens results in death of the anaerobic pathogen.

    The specimen container should be sterile to prevent contamination of the specimen. Many specimens, especially microbiologic ones, are adversely affected by contaminants, such as extraneous microorganisms, which may affect the accuracy of the test results.

    The medical assistant should check each container before use to ensure it is not broken, chipped, cracked, or otherwise damaged. Damaged containers are unsuitable for specimen collection and should be discarded. The medical assistant should be sure to label each tube and specimen container with the patient's name, the date, the medical assistant's initials, and any other information required by the laboratory, such as the source of the specimen. The information should be printed legibly and the medical assistant should be certain that the information is accurate to avoid a mix-up of specimens.

4. *Identify the patient, and explain the procedure.* It is important for the medical assistant to identify the patient to avoid collection of a specimen from the wrong patient by mistake. An undiscovered problem could lead to invalid test results and could affect the patient's diagnosis and treatment. An explanation of the procedure helps relax and reassure the patient and gains the patient's confidence and cooperation, especially the first time the patient has a specimen collected.

If the patient was required to prepare before the specimen was collected, determine whether this was done properly. Improper preparation may lead to inaccurate test results. For example, if a test that requires fasting, such as FBS, is performed on a nonfasting specimen, the results are altered; in this case, they are falsely high. If the patient has not prepared properly, inform the physician; the physician may want the patient to prepare properly and return, or the physician may tell the medical assistant to go ahead with the collection but to alert the laboratory to the situation by marking the information on the laboratory request. In the example just given, *nonfasting specimen* would be written on the request form.

5. *Collection of the specimen* involves a set of specific techniques for each type of specimen obtained. The information in this section is presented in general terms. The specific procedures for the collection of biologic specimens are included in this text in the following chapters: Urinalysis, Phlebotomy, Hematology, Blood Chemistry and Serology, and Medical Microbiology.

    Specimen collection involves a combination of medical and surgical aseptic techniques. Certain parts of collection materials, such as needles, swabs, and the insides of the specimen containers, must remain sterile. If a culture medium is used to collect a microbiologic specimen, the medical assistant must ensure that the lid of the container is removed only when the specimen is spread on the culture medium. Unnecessary removal of the lid results in contamination of the culture medium with extraneous microorganisms, which interferes with accurate test results. During the collection and handling of the specimen, the medical assistant also must be careful to use medical and surgical asepsis to prevent contamination of the specimen, the patient, or the self.

    The medical assistant must collect the specimen with the proper technique. The procedure should be followed exactly to ensure a high-quality and reliable specimen. The proper type of specimen must be collected as designated either by the outside laboratory or by the instructions that accompany the testing materials. For example, the collection of a random urine specimen when a clean-catch midstream specimen is necessary will affect the accuracy of the test results.

    The medical assistant must be sure to collect the amount necessary for the test, which varies depending on the type of specimen collected and the number of laboratory tests ordered. The medical assistant must refer to the appropriate reference material to determine the amount necessary for each test ordered by the physician. If the specimen is transported to an outside laboratory, the amount necessary is listed next to each test in the laboratory directory (see Table 15–1). The amount necessary for those specimens tested in the medical office is found in the manufacturer's instructions that accompany the testing materials. It is important that the medical assistant strictly observe the stipulated amount requirements, especially for specimens transported to an outside laboratory. If the medical assistant fails to collect the specified amount, the laboratory will be unable to perform the test and the laboratory request will be returned marked *quantity not sufficient* (QNS). This situation warrants calling the patient back for collection of another specimen.

Once the specimen has been collected, the medical assistant records the following information in the patient's chart: the date and time of the collection, the laboratory tests ordered by the physician, the type of specimen, and the source of the specimen. If the specimen is transported to an outside laboratory, this information should be indicated in the patient's chart, including the date the specimen was transported to the laboratory if different from the date of collection.

6. *Properly handle and store the specimen* with care to preserve its in vivo qualities. Some specimens, such as microbiologic specimens, are more sensitive to environmental influences and must be handled with special care. Whenever possible, laboratory tests are best performed on fresh specimens (for most specimens, within 1 hour after collection) because they yield the most reliable test results. When this is not practical, as is usually the case, the specimen must be stored; storage may be required until pickup by an outside laboratory, mailing, or testing at the medical office. Storing of a specimen involves properly preserving so as to maintain its in vivo physical and chemical characteristics until analysis. General guidelines for handling and storing biologic specimens most frequently collected in the medical office are presented in Table 15-3.

TABLE 15-3   Handling and Storage of Biologic Specimens

Specimen	Handling	Storage
Blood	*All Blood Specimens:* Prevent hemolysis. Collect specimen in tube at room temperature. *Serum:* Separate serum from blood within 30 to 45 minutes after collection. *Plasma:* Mix anticoagulant gently but thoroughly with blood specimen immediately after collection.	*For Most Blood Specimens:* Refrigerate at 4°C (39°F) to retard alterations in physical and chemical composition of specimen. Plasma and serum may be frozen; however, whole blood should not be frozen because it will cause hemolysis.
Urine	Avoid contamination of inside of specimen container. Do not leave specimen standing out for more than 1 hour after collection.	If urine specimen cannot be tested within 1 hour after collection, refrigerate it or add appropriate preservative.
Microbiologic specimens	Avoid contamination of swab used to collect specimen. Avoid contamination of inside of microbiologic specimen container. Protect yourself from contamination from microbiologic specimen. Protect anaerobic specimens from exposure to air.	Transport specimen as soon as possible. If not possible, place specimen in transport medium or inoculate it on appropriate culture medium and (for most specimens) place it in refrigerator at 4°C (39°F) to prevent drying and death of specimen or overgrowth of specimen with extraneous microorganisms.
Stool	Collect specimen in clean container. For detection of ova and parasites, keep stool warm.	For most accurate test results, deliver specimen to laboratory immediately. If transportation of specimen will be delayed, mix stool with appropriate preservative or place it in transport medium.

For all specimens: Do not expose to extreme temperature changes.

PROCEDURE 15-1 Collecting a Specimen for Transport to an Outside Laboratory

Outcome Collect a specimen for transport to an outside laboratory. A summary of the series of individual steps required for collecting a specimen in the medical office and transporting it to an outside laboratory is presented in this procedure.

1. Procedural Step. Inform the patient of any advance preparation or special instructions, which may include:
  a. Diet modification.
  b. Fasting.
  c. Medication restriction.
  d. Collection of a specimen at home.
    Explain the instructions thoroughly, and provide the patient with written instructions to take home as a reference. Notify the patient of the time of report to the medical office for the specimen collection.
Principle. The patient must prepare properly to provide a quality specimen that will lead to accurate test results and will avoid a return to have another specimen collected.

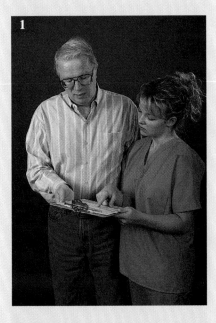

2. Procedural Step. Review the requirements in the laboratory directory for the collection and handling of the specimens ordered by the physician, which include:
  a. Collection materials required.
  b. Type of specimen to be collected.
  c. Amount of the specimen necessary for laboratory analysis.
  d. Procedure to follow to collect the specimen.
  e. Proper handling and storage of the specimen.

Telephone the laboratory with any questions you have regarding any aspect of the collection or handling of the specimen.
Principle. A review of the requirements beforehand prevents errors in collection and handling of the specimen.

3. Procedural Step. Complete the laboratory request form, which must include the following information printed in legible handwriting:
  a. Physician's name and address.
  b. Patient's name (and address if required).
  c. Patient's age and gender.
  d. Date and time of the collection.
  e. Laboratory tests ordered by the physician.
  f. Type of specimen.
  g. Source of specimen.
  h. Physician's clinical diagnosis.
  i. Any medications the patient is taking.
  j. When applicable, third-party billing information (e.g., Blue Cross, Blue Shield, Medicare).
    If the test results are needed by the physician as soon as possible, mark STAT on the request in bold letters.
Principle. The completed form provides the laboratory with the information necessary to perform the tests accurately.

4. Procedural Step. Sanitize your hands.
Principle. Practicing medical asepsis helps protect the specimen from contamination.

5. Procedural Step. Assemble the equipment and supplies. Be sure to use the appropriate specimen container required by the outside laboratory. Ensure the container is sterile, and check to be sure it is not broken, chipped, or cracked.
Principle. The appropriate specimen container must be used to ensure the collection of the proper type of specimen required by the laboratory. Damaged specimen containers are unsuitable for collection and should be discarded.

6. Procedural Step. Clearly label the tubes and containers with the patient's name, the date, your initials, and any other information required by the laboratory, such as the source of the specimen.
Principle. Properly labeled tubes and containers prevent mix-ups of specimens.

Continued

PROCEDURE 15-1

PROCEDURE 15-1 Collecting a Specimen for Transport to an Outside Laboratory—Cont'd

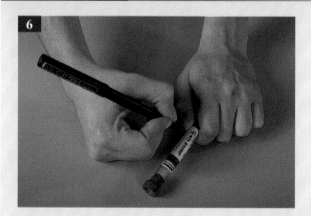

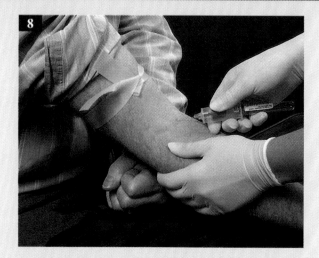

7. **Procedural Step.** Greet and identify the patient. Introduce yourself, and explain the procedure. Be sure you have the correct patient. If patient preparation was required for the test, determine whether the patient prepared properly.
Principle. Identification of the patient prevents collection of a specimen from the wrong person by mistake. Specimen collection is often an anxiety-producing experience for the patient, and reassurance should be offered to help reduce apprehension.

8. **Procedural Step.** Collect the specimen according to the following guidelines:
   a. Follow the OSHA Standard.
   b. Collect the specimen with the proper technique.
   c. Collect the proper type and amount of the specimen required for the test.
   d. Process the specimen further if required by the outside laboratory (e.g., separating serum from whole blood).
   e. Place the lid tightly on the specimen container.
   f. Record information in the patient's chart, including the date and time of the collection, the type and source of the specimen, the laboratory tests ordered by the physician, and information indicating its transport to the outside laboratory, including the date the specimen was sent.
   Principle. Proper collection of a specimen maintains its in vivo qualities and provides the laboratory with a biologically representative sample of the body substance collected.

9. **Procedural Step.** Properly handle and store (if necessary) the specimen, according to the laboratory specifications.
Principle. The specimen must be handled and stored properly to maintain the in vivo characteristics of the specimen.

10. **Procedural Step.** Prepare the specimen for transport to the outside laboratory. Be sure to include the completed laboratory request with the specimen.
Principle. The outside laboratory must have the completed request from to know which laboratory tests have been ordered by the physician.

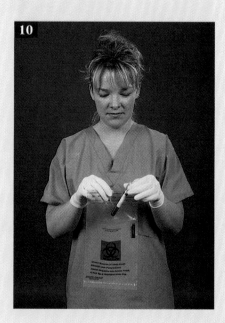

11. **Procedural Step.** Review the laboratory report when it is returned to the medical office. Compare each test result with the normal range provided by the laboratory, and notify the physician of any abnormal results. File the laboratory report in the patient's chart after it has been reviewed by the physician.

CHARTING EXAMPLE	
Date	
3/10/05	8:00 a.m. Venous blood specimen collected from ⓇΓ arm. Tests ordered: total cholesterol, HDL, and triglycerides. Pt was in a fasting state. Courier pick-up by Medical Center Laboratory on 3/10/05. ——— K. McGrew, CMA

PROCEDURE 15-1

Clinical Laboratory Improvement Amendments

Purpose of CLIA 1988

In 1988, Congress passed the Clinical Laboratory Improvement Amendments (CLIA 1988) to improve the quality of laboratory testing in the United States. CLIA 1988 consists of federal regulations that govern all facilities that perform laboratory tests for health assessment or for the diagnosis, prevention, or treatment of disease. CLIA 1988 includes facilities not previously covered under federal legislation, such as POLs and nursing homes. The regulations for implementing CLIA, developed by the Department of Health and Human Services (DHHS), consist of four separate sets of rules: laboratory standards, application and user fees, enforcement procedures, and approval of accreditation programs. The Health Care Financing Administration (HCFA) is a division of DHHS. HCFA is responsible for monitoring compliance with the CLIA regulations.

Categories of Laboratory Testing

The CLIA regulations establish three categories of laboratory testing on the basis of the complexity of the testing methods.

Waived tests. Waived tests are simple procedures and include those that patients can perform at home. Laboratories that perform only waived tests must apply for a certificate of waiver from HCFA, which exempts them from many of the CLIA oversight requirements. Laboratories with certificates of waiver are still expected to adhere to good laboratory practices, which include following the manufacturer's recommended instructions for each product or testing kit. To assist individuals in keeping up with new waived test additions and new methodologies for waived tests, the Centers for Disease Control and Prevention (CDC) maintain the following website: www.cms.hhs.giv/clia. The following tests are examples of waived tests.

Dipstick or tablet reagent urinalysis
Fecal occult blood testing
Ovulation testing with visual color comparisons
Urine pregnancy tests with visual color comparisons
Erythrocyte sedimentation rate, nonautomated
Hemoglobin using a CLIA-waived analyzer
Spun microhematocrit
Blood glucose determination using an FDA-approved blood glucose
Rapid streptococcus testing

Moderate-complexity tests. Moderate-complexity tests account for 75% of the estimated 10,000 laboratory tests performed in the United States every day. Examples of moderate-complexity tests performed in the medical office include hematology and blood chemistry tests performed on automated blood analyzers that are not CLIA-waived, and microscopic analysis of urine sediment.

High-complexity tests. High-complexity tests include all procedures related to cytogenetics, histopathology, histocompatibility, and cytology (includes Pap testing). These tests are not usually performed in medical offices; most of these tests are done in laboratories already subject to federal regulation.

Requirements for Moderate- and High-Complexity Testing

Laboratories that perform moderate- or high-complexity tests or both must meet the CLIA regulations and are subject to unannounced inspections every 2 years by HCFA. The major components of the CLIA 1988 regulations relating to laboratory standards are listed.

Patient test management. A system must be established to maintain the optimal integrity and identification of patient specimens throughout the testing process and to ensure accurate reporting of results.

Quality control. To ensure accurate and reliable test results, each laboratory must establish and follow written quality control procedures that monitor and evaluate the quality of each testing process. These include developing a laboratory procedures manual, following the manufacturer's instructions for each product, performing and documenting calibration procedures at least every 6 months and two levels of controls daily, performing and documenting actions taken when problems or errors are identified, and documenting all quality control activities.

Quality assurance. Each laboratory must establish and follow written policies and procedures to monitor and evaluate the overall quality of the total testing process to ensure the accuracy and reliability of patient test results.

Proficiency testing (PT). PT is a form of external quality control in which laboratory specimens are prepared by an approved PT agency. Three times a year, the physician's laboratory must test a shipment of these unknown specimens with the same procedure as for testing a patient's specimen. The results are then forwarded to the PT agency for evaluation.

Personnel requirements. The CLIA regulations specify qualifications and responsibilities for personnel for laboratory directors, technical consultants, clinical consultants, and testing personnel. The regulations list specific education and training qualifications for the various positions and also define the responsibilities for the persons who fill these positions. Personnel requirements are most stringent for high-complexity testing.

The Physician's Office Laboratory

As previously discussed, a POL consists of an in-house medical office laboratory. The testing of a specimen in a POL involves following a series of steps to measure or identify the presence of a specific substance in the specimen, such as the measurement of a chemical or the identifica-

tion of a microorganism. The medical assistant may be responsible for performing the laboratory tests and recording the results, or the physician may employ a medical laboratory technician or a medical technologist to perform the tests. The decision is based on the number of tests performed in the medical office, the complexity of these tests, and the CLIA regulations. The medical assistant is qualified to perform basic laboratory tests; the more sophisticated tests require the knowledge and skill of the medical laboratory technician.

Laboratory tests can be classified by function into one of the following categories: hematology, clinical chemistry, serology and blood banking, urinalysis, microbiology, parasitology, cytology, and histology. Table 15–4 lists the definitions of each of these categories and provides examples of commonly performed tests in each. Use of these classifications makes it easier to refer to laboratory tests.

Specimens can be analyzed with either the **manual** or **automated methods.** The method the physician uses to test biologic specimens in the medical office is based on the number and type of laboratory tests performed in the office.

Regardless of the method used, a series of basic steps must be followed in testing each specimen.

1. The specific amount of the specimen necessary for the test method is measured from the specimen sample.
2. The necessary chemical reagents necessary for the test are combined with the specimen.
3. The specimen/reagents may require further processing, such as centrifugation, incubation, air drying, or heat fixing.
4. The substance undergoing assessment is manually or automatically measured or identified.
5. The results of the laboratory testing are obtained from a direct readout or with a mathematic calculation.
6. Information is recorded on a laboratory report form or in the patient's chart. The entry includes the patient's name, the date, the time, the name of each laboratory test, the results of the tests, and the name of the individual performing the tests.

These steps are stated in general terms, but a basis is provided for understanding the process of laboratory testing. Textbooks such as this one and the manufacturer's instructions included with testing equipment should be consulted as reference sources to obtain the procedure for performing specific tests. The medical assistant must be sure to follow the procedure exactly to ensure accurate and reliable test results.

Manual Method

The manual method of laboratory testing involves performing the series of steps included in the test method by hand rather than using a self-operating system that performs them automatically. Testing kits, especially in urinalyses, are available to speed up the process, making it more convenient to perform the procedure with the man-

TABLE 15-4 | Categories of Laboratory Tests

Categories of laboratory tests are listed, including definition of each and commonly performed tests or pathologic condition in each category. Those tests that are commonly known by their abbreviations are listed that way.

Category	Definition and Commonly Performed Tests	Category	Definition and Commonly Performed Tests
Hematology	Hematology is science dealing with study of blood and blood-forming tissues. Laboratory analysis in hematology deals with examination of blood for detection of abnormalities and includes areas such as blood cell counts, cellular morphology, clotting ability of blood, and identification of cell types. White Blood Cell Count (WBC) Red Blood Cell count (RBC) Differential white blood cell count (Diff) Hemoglobin (Hgb) Hematocrit (Hct) Platelet count Reticulocyte count Prothrombin time (PT) Erythrocyte sedimentation rate (ESR) Platelet count	Serology and Blood Banking	Laboratory analysis in serology and blood banking deals with studying antigen-antibody reactions to assess presence of substance or to determine presence of disease. Syphilis Tests (VDRL, RPR) C-reactive protein (CRP) ABO Blood Typing Rh Typing Rh Antibody Test Antinuclear Antibody (ANA) Rheumatoid Factor (RA) Latex Mononucleosis Test Hepatitis Tests HIV Tests Antistreptolysin O (ASO) Pregnancy Test
Clinical Chemistry	Laboratory analysis in clinical chemistry determining the amount of chemical substances present in body fluids, excreta, and tissues (e.g., blood, urine, cerebrospinal fluid). The largest area in clinical chemistry is blood chemistry. Glucose Blood urea nitrogen (BUN) Creatinine Total protein Albumin Globulin Calcium Inorganic phosphorus Chloride Sodium Potassium Bilirubin Cholesterol Triglycerides Uric acid Lactate dehydrogenase (LD) Aspartate aminotransferase (AST) Alanine aminotransferase (ALT) Alkaline phosphatase Amylase Carbon dioxide Gamma-glutamyl transpeptidase Thyroxine (T_4) T_3 uptake Creatine phosphokinase (CPK)	Urinalysis	Urinalysis involves physical, chemical, and microscopic analysis of urine. A. Tests included in physical analysis of urine: Color Clarity Specific Gravity B. Tests included in chemical analysis of urine: pH Glucose Protein Ketones Blood Bilirubin Urobilinogen Nitrite Leukocytes C. Tests included in microscopic analysis of urine: Red Blood Cells White Blood Cells Epithelial Cells Casts Crystals

Continued

TABLE 15-4	Categories of Laboratory Tests—cont'd

Categories of laboratory tests are listed, including definition of each and commonly performed tests or pathologic condition in each category. Those tests that are commonly known by their abbreviations are listed that way.

Category	Definition and Commonly Performed Tests	Category	Definition and Commonly Performed Tests
Microbiology	Microbiology is scientific study of microorganisms and their activities. Laboratory analysis in microbiology deals with identification of pathogens present in specimens taken from body (e.g., urine, blood, throat, sputum, wound, urethra, vagina, cerebrospinal fluid). Examples of infectious diseases diagnosed through identification of pathogen present in specimen include: Candidiasis Chlamydia Diphtheria Gonorrhea Meningitis Pertussis Pharyngitis Pneumonia Streptococcal Sore Throat Tetanus Tonsillitis Tuberculosis Urinary Tract Infection	**Parasitology**	Laboratory analysis in parasitology deals with detection of presence of disease-producing human parasites or eggs present in specimens taken from body (e.g., stool, vagina, blood). Examples of human diseases caused by parasites include: Amebiasis Ascariasis Hookworms Malaria Pinworms Scabies Tapeworms Toxoplasmosis Trichinosis Trichomoniasis
		Cytology	Laboratory analysis in cytology deals with detection of presence of abnormal cells. Chromosome Studies Pap Test
		Histology	Histology is microscopic study of form and structure of various tissues that make up living organisms. Laboratory analysis in histology deals with detection of diseased tissues. Tissue Analysis Biopsy Studies

ual method. Because each step in the procedure necessitates a physical manipulation and the application of clinical laboratory theory, the manual method requires a more thorough knowledge and skill in testing procedures than does the automated method. The medical assistant must be especially careful to avoid errors in technique that may lead to inaccurate test results.

Automated Analyzers

Tremendous growth has been seen in the development of automated analyzer systems for performing laboratory tests, especially in the area of blood chemistry. Automated systems are also available for certain tests in the areas of hematology, blood banking, serology, urinalysis, and microbiology. Highly sophisticated automated analyzers are almost always confined to an outside laboratory setting be-

cause the smaller laboratory workload of the medical office does not justify the expense of such systems. However, automated systems have been developed that are more practical and economic for the medical office.

Automated systems designed for use in the medical office permit the processing of a specimen in a short period of time with accurate test results. Automated instruments take less time and provide greater precision than the manual method because the steps in the testing procedure are automated. Such procedures include the measurement of the amount of the specimen necessary, the use of premeasured chemical reagents, measurement of the reaction, and calculation of results. The test results are obtained with a direct (digital display and/or printed) readout.

The ease in operating automated systems, however, should not lead to a false sense of security because these systems have limitations that must be recognized—the most critical one being the mechanical failure of the equipment. Therefore, one of the most important aspects of use of an automated system is the ability to recognize signs that indicate the system is malfunctioning because the malfunctioning may lead to inaccurate test results.

Numerous automated systems are available; they are continually growing in number and are being modified as new technology becomes available. The manufacturer of each automated system provides a detailed operating manual with the instrument that includes the information needed to collect, handle, perform quality control procedures, and test the specimen. In addition, the manufacturer has personnel available for on-site training and service. It is important that the medical assistant become completely familiar with all aspects of any automated system used to perform laboratory tests in the medical office.

Some examples of automated analyzer systems include the QBC hematology analyzer (Becton-Dickinson), the Reflotron blood chemistry analyzer (Roche Diagnostics), and the Clinitek urine analyzer (Bayer Corporation).

Quality Control

The ultimate goal in the clinical laboratory is to ensure the laboratory test accurately measures what it is supposed to measure; this involves practicing and maintaining a quality control program. **Quality control** may be defined as the application of methods and means to ensure that test results are reliable and valid and that errors that may interfere with obtaining accurate test results are detected and eliminated. Quality control is an ongoing process that encompasses every aspect of patient preparation and specimen collection, handling, transport, and testing. The quality control methods that should be used to obtain precision and accuracy in these areas have already been presented in this chapter under their respective headings, with the exception of testing, which is discussed here.

Quality control methods used in testing the specimen include:

1. Using standards and controls to check the precision and accuracy of laboratory equipment and to detect any errors in technique of the individual performing the test.
2. Discarding outdated reagents.
3. Following the procedure exactly to test the specimen.
4. Performing tests in duplicate.
5. Periodically checking the accuracy of the test results with a reference laboratory (PT).
6. Maintaining equipment by having it checked periodically for proper working order.

Practicing quality control methods ensures that the test results represent the true status of the patient's condition and body functions and provides the physician with reliable information with which to make a diagnosis and prescribe treatment.

Laboratory Safety

Laboratory safety is an important aspect of clinical laboratory testing in the medical office. Many of the laboratory tests performed in the medical office involve the use of strong chemical reagents, the handling of specimens that may contain pathogens, and the use of laboratory equipment. Practicing good techniques in testing laboratory specimens and recognizing potential hazards help reduce accidents in the laboratory. Some areas specifically related to laboratory safety in the medical office are described here.

The careful handling and storing of glassware to prevent breakage should be performed as follows:

1. Carefully arrange glassware in storage cabinets to prevent breakage.
2. Carefully remove glassware from storage cabinets.
3. If glassware does break, dispose of it in a puncture-resistant container to protect trash handlers from the shards.

The medical assistant should handle all chemical reagents carefully by adhering to the following instructions:

1. Ensure that all reagent containers are clearly and properly labeled.
2. If a label is loose, reattach it immediately.
3. Recap reagent containers immediately after use to prevent spills.

Laboratory specimens should be handled carefully as follows:

1. Follow the OSHA BBPs Standard in collecting and handling of laboratory specimens.
2. Wash hands immediately if some of the material contained in the specimen is accidentally touched.
3. Avoid hand-to-mouth contact while working with specimens.
4. Immediately clean up any specimen spilled on the work table and cleanse the table with a disinfectant.
5. Properly dispose of all contaminated needles, syringes, specimen containers, and infectious waste.
6. Cover any break in the skin, such as a cut or scratch, with a bandage.
7. Ensure that all specimen containers are tightly capped to prevent leakage.
8. Handle all laboratory equipment and supplies properly and with care as indicated by the manufacturer. For example, wait until the centrifuge comes to a complete stop before opening it.

MEDICAL
Practice and the LAW

Laboratory procedures must be done precisely to obtain accurate results. Pay particular attention to each step in each procedure. Inaccurate laboratory results may cause the physician misdiagnosis and mistreatment, opening both of you to a lawsuit.

Many federal regulations govern laboratory testing, including those from the CLIA, OSHA, and CDC. These regulations help ensure standardization of laboratory tests and safe handling of reagents, blood, and body fluids to prevent contamination of specimens and infection of health care workers. Know and follow all regulations. Failure to do so could result in a legal liability.

Case Study 1
What Did Korey Do?
- ❑ Told Hildy that the laboratory cannot release test results. Explained that they are experts in performing tests but do not have the medical knowledge to know their meanings.
- ❑ Told Hildy that the doctor would need to give her the test results. Explained that the doctor was out of town today but that an appointment could be made for her for tomorrow with the doctor to discuss the results.

What Did Korey Not Do?
- ❑ Did not give Hildy the test results.
- ❑ Did not alarm Hildy that something might be wrong.

What Would You Do?/What Would You *Not* Do? Review Korey's response and place a checkmark next to the information you included in your response. List additional information you included in your response below.

_____

_____

_____

_____

Case Study 2
What Did Korey Do?
- ❑ Told Hanns that the term "clinical diagnosis" means what the physician "thinks" is wrong before the laboratory tests are performed. Explained that when the test results are returned, the doctor will be able to make a final diagnosis and then he will determine what treatment is needed.
- ❑ Told Hanns that a lipid profile includes several tests and one of those tests is a cholesterol test. Explained that the tests in a lipid profile all help to determine whether someone is at risk for heart disease.
- ❑ Told Hanns that, unfortunately, he could not have any coffee until after his blood was drawn because it would affect the test results. Told him that his test could be scheduled first thing in the morning if that would help.

What Did Korey Not Do?
- ❑ Did not tell Hanns he could have a cup of coffee before the laboratory tests.
- ❑ Did not tell Hanns the he should not be eating doughnuts if he was concerned about his heart.

What Would You Do?/What Would You *Not* Do? Review Korey's response and place a checkmark next to the information you included in your response. List additional information you included in your response below.

_____

_____

_____

_____

Case Study 3
What Did Korey Do?
- ❑ Stressed to Kathleen that if the laboratory test results are abnormal, then it is better to know so that the doctor can help make her better.
- ❑ Told Kathleen that many patients feel the same way about having blood drawn so she is not alone. Relayed to her that her fear is normal and she has no reason to be embarrassed.
- ❑ Told Kathleen that she should tell the laboratory about her last experience so they could make it easier for her. Explained that they would probably put her in a reclining position to draw her blood so that she would not get light-headed.
- ❑ Gave Kathleen some suggestions on how to relax during the venipuncture. Told her to turn her head when the blood was drawn.
- ❑ Asked Kathleen if she had any additional symptoms.
- ❑ Checked with the physician to see whether he wanted to keep her appointment for today or have her appointment rescheduled until the laboratory work was completed.

What Did Korey Not Do?
- ❑ Did not ignore or minimize Kathleen's concerns and fears.
- ❑ Did not tell Kathleen that her test results would probably be fine.

What Would You Do?/What Would You *Not* Do? Review Korey's response and place a checkmark next to the information you included in your response. List additional information you included in your response below.

_____

_____

_____

_____

Apply Your KNOWLEDGE

Choose the best answer for each of the following questions.

1. Jennifer Keyes, an 18-year-old woman, comes to the office with a painful sore throat, extreme fatigue, fever, and swollen glands. After taking a health history and performing an examination, Dr. Invivo suspects that Jennifer may have infectious mononucleosis. He asks Korey McGrew, CMA, to run a Monospot test. The purpose of Dr. Invivo ordering this test is to:
   A. Confirm his clinical diagnosis
   B. Ensure Jennifer is not allergic to antibiotics
   C. Regulate Jennifer's treatment
   D. Comply with state regulations

2. Korey performs the Monospot test in the office laboratory. The name given to this type of laboratory is:
   A. CLIA
   B. Reference laboratory
   C. POL
   D. HIPAA

3. Because Jennifer also has paleness and shortness of breath, Dr. Invivo decides to have a CBC performed to rule out iron-deficiency anemia. Korey is getting ready to draw the blood specimen to send to Outside Laboratory for testing. Korey wants to be sure that she uses the correct color stopper blood tube. The best way to obtain this information is to:
   A. Send an e-mail to Outside Laboratory requesting this information
   B. Look at a laboratory report from Outside Laboratory
   C. Look in the *Farmer's Almanac*
   D. Refer to Outside Laboratory's laboratory directory

4. Korey completes the laboratory request form that will accompany the blood specimen to Outside Laboratory. Korey is careful to ensure she includes Jennifer's age on the request form because Korey realizes:
   A. The laboratory needs this information for third-party billing
   B. The normal range for some tests varies based on the age of the patient
   C. The type of test procedure the laboratory uses to analyze the specimen depends on the age of the patient
   D. Outside Laboratory will want to send Jennifer a card on her next birthday

5. Jennifer's test results are returned by Outside Laboratory's courier service the next day. The hemoglobin value on the report is 10 g/dL. To determine whether this value is within normal range, Korey should compare this value with:
   A. Jennifer's social security number
   B. The normal range published in a laboratory reference text
   C. The normal range for hemoglobin on the laboratory report from Outside Laboratory
   D. Jennifer's last hemoglobin test result listed in her medical record

6. After receiving Jennifer's laboratory report and highlighting values outside the normal range, Korey takes the following action:
   A. Files the laboratory report in Jennifer's medical record
   B. Calls Jennifer to inform her of the abnormal test results
   C. Makes a tentative diagnosis of Jennifer's condition
   D. Places the report on Dr. Invivo's desk for his review

7. Keith Thompson comes to the medical office for a complete physical examination. Keith has a history of heart disease in his family. Dr. Invivo wants to have a lipid profile performed. Korey McGrew, CMA, explains to Keith the patient preparation necessary for this test. Keith returns to the office the next morning to have blood drawn. Which of the following statements would indicate that Keith *did not* prepare properly for this test?
   A. "My last meal was at 6 PM last night, but I had a glass of water when I got up this morning"
   B. "I had a cup of black coffee this morning with low-fat milk"
   C. "I ran 5 miles this morning before coming to the office"
   D. "I rinsed out my mouth with mouthwash this morning"

8. Dr. Invivo tells Korey to review the patient preparation instructions again with Keith and have him return the next day. Keith tells Korey that he does not understand why his blood cannot be drawn now. The most appropriate response for Korey to make would be:
   A. "If you would have listened the first time, you would not have to come back"
   B. "The laboratory will refuse to test your blood specimen if you have not prepared properly"
   C. "It is beyond me; Dr. Invivo has a habit of making strange requests"
   D. "If your blood is drawn now, the test results may be inaccurate and you will not receive proper care"

9. Dr. Invivo purchases a blood chemistry analyzer for the office. Korey McGrew, CMA, realizes that the tests run on this analyzer are considered moderate-complexity tests; therefore, the following will need to be performed to comply with CLIA requirements:
   A. Calibration of the analyzer every 6 months
   B. Two levels of controls run each day

C. Documentation of when errors occur and what actions are taken to correct them
D. All of the above

10. Korey is spinning a blood tube in the centrifuge so that she can obtain serum for laboratory tests. Which of the following is an important safety practice to follow with a centrifuge?
    A. Waiting until the centrifuge comes to a complete stop before removing the blood tube
    B. Opening the centrifuge while it is spinning to see whether the blood is separating properly
    C. Using her hand to help the centrifuge come to a complete stop after the timer goes off
    D. Placing the centrifuge on a Mayo stand so that it is easily accessible

CERTIFICATION REVIEW

❏ **The purpose of laboratory testing** is to assist in the diagnosis of pathologic conditions, to evaluate a patient's progress, to regulate treatment, to establish a patient's baseline, to prevent or reduce the severity of disease, and to comply with state law if necessary. A routine test is a laboratory test performed on a routine basis on an apparently healthy patient to assist in the early detection of disease.

❏ **POL** consists of an in-house medical office laboratory. Laboratory tests that are convenient to execute and commonly required are often performed in the POL. Outside laboratories include hospital and privately owned commercial laboratories.

❏ **A laboratory request** is a printed form that contains a list of the most frequently ordered laboratory tests. The laboratory request includes the physician's name and address; the patient's name, age, and gender; the date and time of collection of the specimen; the laboratory tests desired; the source of the specimen; the clinical diagnosis; and medications taken by the patient. A profile consists of a number of laboratory tests that provide related information used to determine the health status of a patient.

❏ **The purpose of the laboratory report** is to relay the results of the laboratory tests to the physician. Information included on a laboratory report is as follows: the name, address, and telephone number of the laboratory; the physician's name and address; the patient's name, age, and gender; the patient accession number; the date the specimen was received by the laboratory; the date the results were reported by the laboratory; the names of the tests performed; the results of the tests; and the normal range for each test performed. The normal range is a certain established and acceptable parameter or reference range within which the laboratory test results of a healthy individual are expected to fall.

❏ **Laboratory safety** is an important aspect of clinical laboratory testing in the medical office. Practicing good techniques in testing laboratory specimens and recognizing potential hazards helps reduce accidents in the laboratory.

❏ **Some laboratory tests** require advance patient preparation to obtain a quality specimen suitable for testing. A specimen obtained from a patient who has not prepared properly may invalidate the test results and necessitate calling the patient back to collect a specimen again. The specific type of preparation necessary for a particular test depends on the test ordered and the method used to perform it. A common patient preparation requirement for laboratory testing is fasting. Fasting means that the patient must abstain from food or fluids (except water) for a specified amount of time (usually 12 to 14 hours) before the collection of a specimen.

❏ **A specimen** is a small sample taken from the body to represent the nature of the whole. Examples of specimens include the following: blood, urine, feces, sputum, a cervical and vaginal scraping of cells, and a sample of a secretion or discharge taken from various parts of the body such as the nose, throat, wound, ear, eye, vagina, or urethra.

❏ **The purpose of the CLIA** is to improve the quality of laboratory testing in the United States. The CLIA consists of federal regulations governing all facilities that perform laboratory tests for health assessment or for the diagnosis, prevention, or treatment of disease.

❏ **The CLIA regulations** establish three categories of laboratory testing that include waived tests, moderate-complexity tests, and high-complexity tests. Laboratories that perform moderate- or high-complexity tests must meet the CLIA regulations. Laboratories that perform only waived tests must apply for a certificate of waiver from HCFA, which exempts them from many of the CLIA requirements.

❏ **Quality control** is the application of methods to ensure that test results are reliable and valid and that errors are detected and eliminated. Quality control is an ongoing process that encompasses every aspect of patient preparation and specimen collection, handling, transport, and testing.

Terminology Review

Automated method *(for testing laboratory specimens)* A method of laboratory testing in which the series of steps in the test method is performed with an automated analyzer.

Fasting Abstaining from food or fluids (except water) for a specified amount of time before the collection of a specimen.

Homeostasis The state in which body systems are functioning normally and the internal environment of the body is in equilibrium; the body is in a healthy state.

In vivo Occurring in the living body or organism.

Laboratory test The clinical analysis and study of materials, fluids, or tissues obtained from patients to assist in diagnosis and treatment of disease.

Manual method A method of laboratory testing in which the series of steps in the test method is performed by hand.

Normal range *(for laboratory tests)* A certain established and acceptable parameter or reference range within which the laboratory test results of a healthy individual are expected to fall.

Plasma The liquid part of the blood, consisting of a clear, yellowish fluid that makes up approximately 55% of the total blood volume.

Profile A number of laboratory tests providing related or complementary information used to determine the health status of a patient.

Quality control The application of methods to ensure that test results are reliable and valid and that errors are detected and eliminated.

Routine test Laboratory test performed routinely on apparently healthy patients to assist in the early detection of disease.

Serum The clear, straw-colored part of the blood (plasma) that remains after the solid elements and the clotting factor fibrinogen have been separated out of it.

Specimen A small sample of something taken to show the nature of the whole.

ON THE WEB

For active weblinks to each website visit http://evolve. elsevier.com/Bonewit/.

For Information on Aging

National Institute on Aging

Administration on Aging

American Association of Retired Persons

Social Security Administration

Centers for Medicare and Medicaid Services

Growth House

Before I Die

Learning Objectives	Procedures

Urinary System

1. Describe the structures that form the urinary system and state the function of each.
2. List conditions that may cause polyuria and oliguria.
3. Define the terms used to describe symptoms of the urinary system.

Instruct a patient in the procedure for collecting a clean-catch midstream urine specimen.
Instruct a patient in the procedure for collecting a 24-hour urine specimen.

Collection of Urine

1. Explain why a first-voided morning specimen is often preferred for urinalysis.
2. Explain the purpose of collecting a clean-catch midstream specimen.
3. Explain the purpose of a 24-hour urine collection.
4. List changes that may occur if urine is allowed to remain standing for more than 1 hour.

Assess the color and appearance of a urine specimen.
Measure the specific gravity of a urine specimen.
Perform a chemical assessment of a urine specimen.

Analysis of Urine

1. List factors that may cause urine to have an unusual color or become cloudy.
2. Identify the various tests that are included in the physical and chemical examination of urine.
3. List the structures that may be found in a microscopic examination of the urine.
4. Explain the purpose of a rapid urine culture test.

Prepare a urine specimen for microscopic analysis and examine the specimen under the microscope.
Perform a rapid urine culture test.

Urine Pregnancy Testing

1. Explain the basis for urine pregnancy tests.
2. List the guidelines that must be followed in a urine pregnancy test to ensure accurate test results.

Perform a urine pregnancy test.

CHAPTER 16

Urinalysis

Chapter Outline

Structure and Function of the Urinary System
Composition of Urine
 Terms Relating to the Urinary System
Collection of Urine
 Guidelines for Urine Collection
 Urine Collection Methods
 The 24-Hour Urine Specimen
Analysis of Urine
 Physical Examination of the Urine
 Chemical Examination of the Urine
 Reagent Strips
 Microscopic Examination of Urine
Rapid Urine Cultures
Urine Pregnancy Testing
 Human Chorionic Gonadotropin
 Testing Methods
 Guidelines for Urine Pregnancy Testing
Serum Pregnancy Test

National Competencies

Clinical Competencies

Specimen Collection
- Instruct patients in the collection of a clean-catch midstream urine specimen.

Diagnostic Testing
- Use methods of quality control.
- Perform urinalysis.
- Screen and follow-up test results.

General Competencies

Patient Instruction
- Instruct individuals according to their needs.
- Instruct and demonstrate the use and care of patient equipment.
- Provide instruction for health care maintenance and disease prevention.

Key Terms

agglutination (ah-gloo-tih-NAY-shun)
bilirubinuria (bill-ih-roo-bin-YUR-ee-ah)
glycosuria (glie-koe-SOO-ree-ah)
ketonuria (kee-toe-NOO-ree-ah)
ketosis (kee-TOE-sis)
micturition (mik-tur-ISH-un)
nephron (NEF-ron)
oliguria (oh-lig-YUR-ee-ah)
pH (PEE-AYCH)
polyuria (pol-ee-YUR-ee-ah)
proteinuria (proe-ten-YUR-ee-ah)
refractive index
refractometer (reh-frak-TOM-ih-tur)
renal threshold (REE-nul-THRESH-hold)
specific gravity
supernatant (soo-per-NAY-tent)
urinalysis (yur-in-AL-ih-sis)
void (VOYD)

Structure and Function of the Urinary System

The function of the urinary system is to regulate the fluid and electrolyte balance of the body and to remove waste products. The structures that comprise the urinary system are the kidneys, the ureters, the urinary bladder, and the urethra (Figure 16-1). The *kidneys* are bean-shaped organs approximately 4.5 inches (11.5 cm) long and 2 to 3 inches (5 to 8 cm) wide; they are located in the lumbar region of the body. Urine drains from the kidneys into the urinary bladder through two tubes known as *ureters*. Each ureter is approximately 10 to 12 inches in length and ½ inch in diameter. The urine produced by the kidneys is propelled into the urinary bladder by the force of gravity and the peristaltic waves of the ureters. The *urinary bladder* is a hollow, muscular sac that can hold approximately 500 ml of urine. Its function is to store and expel urine. The *urethra* is a tube that extends from the urinary bladder to the outside of the body. The *urinary meatus* is the external opening of the urethra. In males, the urethra functions in transporting urine and reproductive secretions. In females, the urethra functions in urination only.

Each kidney is composed of approximately 1 million smaller units known as nephrons (Figure 16-2). The **nephron** is the functional unit of the kidney. It filters waste substances from the blood and dilutes them with water to produce urine. Another function of the nephron is reabsorption. Some substances filtered by the nephron, such as water, glucose, and electrolytes, are needed by the body and are reabsorbed or returned to the body for future use.

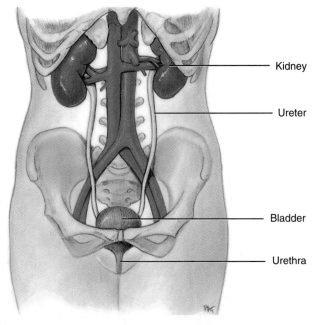

Figure 16-1. Structures that make up the urinary system. (From Applegate EJ: *The anatomy and physiology learning system,* 2nd ed, Philadelphia, 2000, Saunders.)

Composition of Urine

A physiologic change in the body, such as that caused by disease, can create a disturbance in one or more of the functions of the kidney. Detection of such a disturbance can be made with the examination of urine and other body fluids such as blood.

Urine is composed of 95% water and 5% organic and inorganic waste products. Organic waste products consist of urea, uric acid, ammonia, and creatinine. Urea is present in the greatest amounts and is derived from the breakdown of proteins. Inorganic waste products include chloride, sodium, potassium, calcium, magnesium, phosphate, and sulfate.

The normal adult excretes approximately 750 to 2000 ml of urine per day. This amount varies according to the amount of fluid consumed and the amount of fluid lost through other means, such as perspiration, feces, and water vapor from the lungs. An excessive increase in urine output is known as **polyuria,** with the urine volume exceeding 2000 ml in 24 hours. Polyuria may be caused by the excessive intake of fluids or the intake of fluids that contain caffeine (e.g., coffee, tea, cola), which is a mild diuretic. Certain drugs, such as diuretics, and the pathologic conditions of diabetes mellitus, diabetes insipidus, and renal disease in which the kidney is unable to concentrate the urine may also result in polyuria. A decreased or scanty urine output is known as **oliguria.** In the case of oliguria, the urine volume will be less than 400 ml in 24 hours. Oliguria may occur with decreased fluid intake, dehydration, profuse perspiration, vomiting, diarrhea, or kidney disease. The normal act of voiding urine is known as **micturition.**

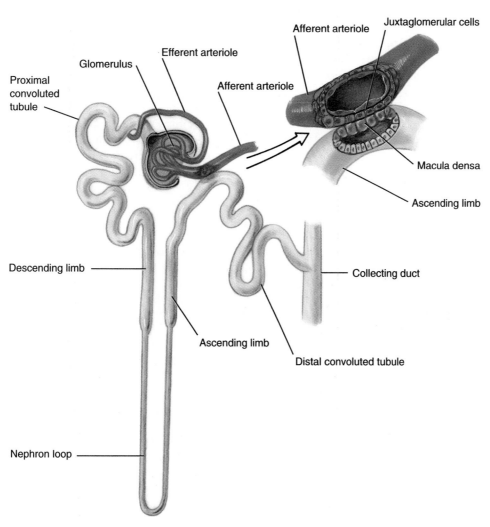

Figure 16-2. Nephron. (From Applegate EJ: *The anatomy and physiology learning system,* 2nd ed, Philadelphia, 2000, Saunders.)

Terms Relating to the Urinary System

The medical assistant should have a thorough knowledge of the following terms used to describe symptoms associated with the urinary system:

Anuria: Failure of the kidneys to produce urine.

Diuresis: Secretion and passage of large amounts of urine.

Dysuria: Difficult or painful urination.

Frequency: The condition of having to urinate often.

Hematuria: Blood present in the urine.

Nocturia: Excessive (voluntary) urination during the night.

Nocturnal enuresis: The inability of the patient to control urination at night during sleep (bedwetting).

Oliguria: Decreased output of urine.

Polyuria: Increased output of urine.

Pyuria: Pus present in the urine.

Retention: The inability to empty the bladder. The urine is being produced normally but is not being voided.

Urgency: The immediate need to urinate.

Urinary incontinence: The inability to retain urine.

Collection of Urine

The advantage of urine testing is that urine is readily available and does not require an invasive procedure or the use of special equipment to obtain. For accurate test results, however, the medical assistant must adhere to proper urine collection procedures and obtain the proper specimen as ordered by the physician.

Guidelines for Urine Collection

The guidelines listed should be followed in collection of a urine specimen.

1. The medical assistant must be sure to obtain an adequate volume of urine as necessary for the type of test (usually between 30 and 50 ml of urine).
2. Each specimen must be properly labeled with the patient's name, the date and time of collection, and the type of specimen (i.e., urine) to avoid any mix-ups in specimens.
3. Any medication the patient is taking should be recorded on the laboratory requisition and in the patient's chart because some medications may interfere with the accuracy of the test results.
4. If possible, the collection of a urine specimen should be avoided in women during menstruation and for several days thereafter because the specimen may become contaminated with blood.
5. The medical assistant should take into consideration that voiding may be difficult for patients under stress and anxiety. In these instances, understanding and patience should be relayed to the patient.
6. A urine specimen may be difficult to obtain from a child, even with the assistance of the parents. In this case, the physician should be informed because another collection method may be used, such as a urine collection bag, suprapubic aspiration, or catheterization of the patient.

What Would You DO? What Would You *Not* DO?

Case Study 1

Yusuke Urameshi is at the office with fever and chills, dysuria, frequency, and difficulty urinating. The physician suspects that Mr. Urameshi has prostatitis and orders a clean-catch urine specimen for a complete urinalysis, including a microscopic examination of the sediment. Mr. Urameshi tries to collect the specimen but is only able to collect 5 ml of urine. He says that he is worried about what is wrong with him and that he thinks his nervousness is making it hard to get a specimen. Mr. Urameshi says that it is probably just as well because he did not quite understand how to cleanse himself and he is not sure that he did it right.

Urine Collection Methods

The type of test to be performed often dictates the method used to collect the urine specimen. For example, a first-voided morning specimen is recommended for pregnancy testing, and a clean-catch midstream specimen is necessary for identification of the presence of a urinary tract infection (UTI).

Most offices use disposable urine specimen containers made of plastic. These containers are available in different sizes and come with lids to reduce bacterial and other types of contamination.

Random Specimen. Urine testing in the medical office is often performed on freshly voided, random specimens. The medical assistant instructs the patient to void into a clean, dry, wide-mouthed container, and the urine is tested immediately at the medical office.

First-Voided Morning Specimen. In many cases, a first-voided morning specimen may be desired for testing because it contains the greatest concentration of dissolved substances. Therefore, a small amount of an abnormal substance that is present would be more easily detected. The patient should be instructed to collect the first specimen of the morning after rising and to preserve the specimen by refrigerating it until it is brought to the medical office. Providing the patient with a specimen container is important to prevent the use of a container that might harbor contaminants.

Clean-Catch Midstream Specimen. The urinary bladder and most of the urethra are normally free of microorganisms, whereas the distal urethra and urinary meatus normally harbor microorganisms. If the urine is being cultured and examined for bacteria, a clean-catch midstream specimen is necessary to prevent contamination of the specimen with these normally present microorganisms. Only those microorganisms that may be causing the patient's condition are desired in the urine specimen. A clean-catch midstream collection may be ordered for both the detection of a UTI and the evaluation of the effectiveness of drug therapy in a patient undergoing treatment for such an infection.

The purpose of the clean-catch midstream collection is the removal of microorganisms from the urinary meatus with thorough cleansing of the area surrounding it and the flushing out of microorganisms in the distal urethra. The urine specimen is collected in a sterile container with medically aseptic conditions. A properly collected specimen reduces the possibility of a bladder catheterization or a suprapubic aspiration of the bladder having to be performed. Bladder catheterization involves the passing of a sterile tube (the catheter) through the urethra and into the bladder to remove urine. Suprapubic aspiration involves the passing of a needle through the abdominal wall into the bladder to remove urine. Both of these procedures must be performed using sterile technique.

Guidelines. The following list contains guidelines that should be followed when collecting a clean-catch midstream specimen.

1. A clean-catch midstream specimen is collected by the patient at the medical office. The medical assistant must provide complete instructions for the collection of this specimen. Failure to adequately instruct the patient may necessitate a return to the medical office for the collection of another specimen because of bacterial contamination. Patient instructions for obtaining a clean-catch midstream specimen are presented in Procedure 16-1.

2. Once the specimen has been collected, the medical assistant should immediately cap and label the container with the patient's name, the date, the time of the collection, and the type of specimen (clean-catch midstream specimen).

3. For reliable test results, the specimen should be tested immediately and not be allowed to stand. If this is not possible, the specimen should be refrigerated or a preservative should be added.

4. If the specimen will be tested at an outside laboratory, completion of a laboratory requisition to accompany it is necessary. An example of a urinalysis laboratory request form is shown in Figure 16-3.

5. The procedure is then completed with sanitizing the hands and recording the procedure in the patient's chart. The information to be charted includes the date and time, type of specimen, and the laboratory tests ordered.

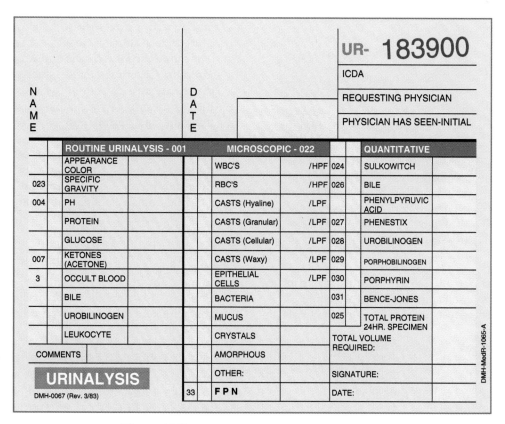

Figure 16-3. Urinalysis laboratory request form.

The 24-Hour Urine Specimen

A 24-hour urine specimen is used for quantitative measurement of specific urinary components. With collection of urine over a 24-hour period, a greater accuracy of measurement exists than with a random specimen. This is because body metabolism, exercise, and hydration can affect the excretion rate of substances in the urine. In addition, at certain times during a 24-hour period, an increased excretion of substances, (e.g., electrolytes, hormones, proteins, and urobilinogen) is seen and, at other times, a decreased excretion is seen.

Examples of substances measured in a 24-hour specimen include calcium, creatinine, lead, potassium, protein, and urea nitrogen. A 24-hour specimen is often used in the diagnosis of the cause of kidney stone formation and in the control and prevention of new stone formation.

A large container (3000 ml) is used to collect the specimen. To prevent changes in the quality of the urine specimen, the specimen must be kept refrigerated or placed in an ice chest. Some containers also contain a preservative to assist in maintaining the quality of the specimen.

The medical assistant should provide the patient with both verbal and written instructions for the collection of the urine specimen (Procedure 16-2). The patient should be advised to moderately limit fluid intake during the collection period and to avoid alcohol intake for 24 hours before and during the collection period.

Certain medications, such as thiazides, phosphorus-binding antacids, allopurinol, or vitamin C, could alter the specimen's testing results. Because of this problem, the physician may want the patient to discontinue these medications for a week before the test.

PROCEDURE 16-1　Clean-Catch Midstream Specimen Collection Instructions

Outcome Instruct a patient in the procedure for collecting a clean-catch midstream urine specimen.

Equipment/Supplies:
- Sterile specimen container and label
- Personal antiseptic towelettes
- Tissues

1. Procedural Step. Sanitize your hands and assemble equipment.

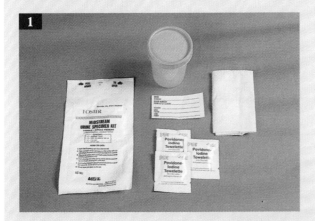

2. Procedural Step. Greet and identify the patient. Introduce yourself and explain the procedure.

Instruct the female patient in the collection of the specimen as follows:

1. Procedural Step. Wash your hands, and remove undergarments.

2. Procedural Step. Expose the urinary meatus by spreading apart the labia with one hand.

3. Procedural Step. Cleanse each side of the urinary meatus with a front-to-back motion (from pubis to anus), with an antiseptic towelette. Use a separate antiseptic towelette for each side of the meatus.
Principle. Cleansing removes microorganisms from the urinary meatus. A front-to-back motion must be used for cleansing to avoid drawing microorganisms from the anal region into the area that is being cleansed.

4. Procedural Step. Cleanse directly across the meatus (front to back) with a third antiseptic towelette.

5. Procedural Step. Continue to hold the labia apart, and void a small amount of urine into the toilet.
Principle. Voiding a small amount flushes microorganisms out of the distal urethra.

6. Procedural Step. Collect the next amount of urine by voiding into the sterile container. Be careful not to touch the inside of the container.
Principle. Touching the inside of the container will contaminate it with microorganisms that normally reside on the skin.

7. Procedural Step. Void the last amount of urine into the toilet. This means that the first and last portion of the urine flow is not included in the specimen.

8. Procedural Step. Wipe the area dry with a tissue, and wash the hands.

9. **Procedural Step.** Provide the patient with instructions about what to do with the specimen once it has been collected (e.g., placing it on a designated shelf or directly handing it to the medical assistant).

Instruct the male patient as follows:

1. **Procedural Step.** Wash the hands and remove undergarments.
2. **Procedural Step.** Retract the foreskin of the penis (if uncircumcised).
3. **Procedural Step.** Cleanse the area around the meatus (glans penis) and the urethral opening (meatal orifice) by wiping each side of the meatus with a separate antiseptic towelette.
4. **Procedural Step.** Cleanse directly across the meatus with a third antiseptic towelette.

5. **Procedural Step.** Void a small amount of urine into the toilet.
6. **Procedural Step.** Collect the next amount of urine by voiding into the sterile container without touching the inside of the container with the hands or penis.
7. **Procedural Step.** Void the last amount of urine into the toilet.
8. **Procedural Step.** Wipe the area dry with a tissue and wash the hands.
9. **Procedural Step.** Provide the patient with instructions about what to do with the specimen once it has been collected

---

PROCEDURE 16-2 Collection of a 24-Hour Urine Specimen

Outcome Collect a 24-hour urine specimen.

Equipment/Supplies:
- Large urine collection container
- Written instructions
- Laboratory requisition

1. Procedural Step. Sanitize your hands, and assemble the equipment.

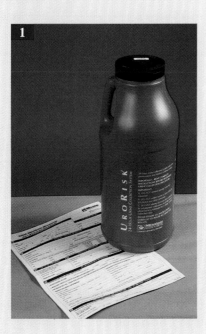

2. Procedural Step. Greet and identify the patient. Introduce yourself to the patient, and explain the procedure.

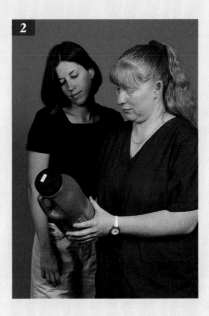

Continued

PROCEDURE 16-2 Collection of a 24-Hour Urine Specimen—Cont'd

Instruct the patient in the collection of the specimen as follows:

3. **Procedural Step.** When you get up in the morning, empty your bladder into the commode just as you normally do. In other words, this urine is not to be saved. Make a note of what time it is, and write this information on a slip of paper.

4. **Procedural Step.** The next time you need to urinate, void the urine directly into the plastic container.

5. **Procedural Step.** Tightly screw the lid onto the container, and put the container into your refrigerator or into an ice chest.

6. **Procedural Step.** Repeat steps 4 and 5 each time you urinate.

7. **Procedural Step.** Emphasize the importance of the following to the patient:
   a. The urine must only be collected in the designated container.
   b. Be sure to collect all the urine during the 24-hour period. The information this test provides will be inaccurate if any urine from the 24-hour period does not go into the container.
   c. The collection must be started again from the beginning if any of the following occur:
      • You forget to urinate into the container at any time.
      • You spill some urine from the container.
      • The child wets the bed (if the specimen is being obtained from a child).

8. **Procedural Step.** On the following morning, get up at the same time (exactly 24 hours after beginning the test). Void into the container for the last time.

9. **Procedural Step.** Put the lid on the container tightly. Return the urine collection container to the office the same morning you complete the urine collection.

10. **Procedural Step.** Provide the patient with the collection container and written instructions. Chart this information in the patient's medical record.

Processing the Specimen

11. **Procedural Step.** When the patient returns the collection container, ask the patient whether he or she encountered any difficulty in following the instructions for the 24-hour collection. If any problems occurred that resulted in undercollection or overcollection of urine, the entire collection process must be repeated.

12. **Procedural Step.** Prepare the specimen for transport to the laboratory. Complete a laboratory request form.

13. **Procedural Step.** Chart the results. Include the date and time, the type of specimen, and information on sending the specimen to the laboratory.

CHARTING EXAMPLE	
Date	
3/26/05	3:30 p.m. Container and verbal/written instructions provided on 24-hour specimen collection. —————— L. Proffitt, CMA
3/28/05	10:00 a.m. 24-hour urine specimen sent to Medical Center Laboratory for kidney stone risk analysis. —————— L. Proffitt, CMA

Analysis of Urine

Urinalysis is the analysis of urine and is the laboratory test most commonly performed in the medical office because a urine specimen is readily obtainable and can be tested easily. Urinalysis consists of a *physical, chemical,* and *microscopic examination.* A deviation from normal in any of the three areas assists the physician in the diagnosis and treatment of pathologic conditions, not only of the urinary system but of other body systems as well. Urinalysis may be performed as a screening measure as part of a general physical examination or to assist in the diagnosis of a pathologic condition. It may also assist in the evaluation of effectiveness of therapy once treatment has been initiated for a pathologic condition.

The urinalysis should be performed on a fresh or preserved specimen. If a specimen cannot be examined within 1 hour of voiding, it should be preserved at once in the refrigerator in a closed container and later returned to room temperature and mixed before testing. Chemical additives, such as toluene and thymol, are also used to preserve urine specimens but are generally used only with specimens that require prolonged storage, such as those that must be shipped a long distance, because the chemical preservative sometimes interferes with the chemicals used to perform the urine test.

If the urine is allowed to stand at room temperature for more than 1 hour, some of the following changes may take place.

1. Bacteria work on the urea present in the urine, converting it to ammonia. Because ammonia is alkaline, an acid urine becomes alkaline, raising the pH measurement. In addition, an alkaline pH may result in a false-positive result on the protein test.
2. Bacteria multiply rapidly in the urine, resulting in a cloudy specimen and a rise in the nitrite.
3. If glucose is present in the specimen, it will decrease in amount because microorganisms use the glucose as a source of food.
4. If any red or white blood cells are present, they may break down.
5. Casts decompose after several hours.

Physical Examination of the Urine

The physical examination of the urine involves determination of the color, appearance, and specific gravity. The color and appearance of the urine specimen may be evaluated during preparation for another testing procedure, such as the chemical testing of the urine, or before centrifugation of the specimen in preparation for microscopic analysis. For an accurate evaluation of the color and appearance, the urine specimen must be in a clear glass or plastic container.

Color. The normal color of urine ranges from almost colorless to dark yellow. Dilute urine tends to be a lighter yellow in color, whereas concentrated urine is a darker yellow. The first-voided morning specimen is usually the most concentrated because consumption of fluids is decreased during the night. The urine becomes more dilute as the day progresses and more fluids are consumed.

The color of the urine is the result of the presence of a yellow pigment known as *urochrome*, produced by the breakdown of hemoglobin. It is not uncommon for the color of urine to vary among different shades of yellow within the course of a day. Classifications that can be used to describe the color of urine include light straw, straw, dark straw, light amber, amber, and dark amber (Figure 16-4).

Abnormal colors may be caused by the presence of hemoglobin or blood (resulting in a red or reddish color), bile pigments (resulting in a yellow-brown or greenish color), and fat droplets or pus (resulting in a milky color). Some drugs and foods may also cause the urine to change to an abnormal color. The color of the specimen assists in determining additional tests that may be necessary.

Appearance. The evaluation of the appearance of urine is usually performed at the same time as the color evaluation. Fresh urine is usually clear, or transparent, but becomes cloudy on standing. Cloudiness in a freshly voided specimen may be the result of the presence of bacteria, pus, blood, fat, yeast, sperm, mucous threads, or fecal contaminants. A microscopic examination of the urine sediment should be performed on all cloudy specimens to de-

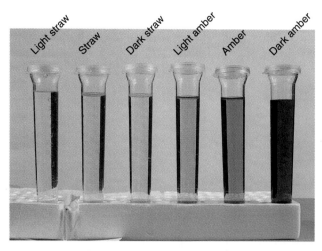

Figure 16-4. Color of urine.

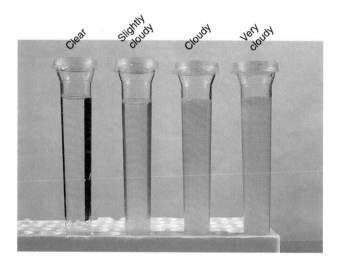

Figure 16-5. Appearance of urine.

termine the cause of the cloudiness. Cloudiness resulting from bacteria may be caused by a UTI.

Terms that may be used to describe the appearance of urine include clear, slightly cloudy, cloudy, and very cloudy (Figure 16-5). The medical assistant should develop skill in recognizing the varying degrees of urine clarity.

Odor. Freshly voided urine normally should have a slightly aromatic odor. Urine that has been standing for a long period of time develops an ammonia odor from the breakdown of urea by bacteria in the specimen. The urine of patients with diabetes mellitus may have a fruity odor from the presence of ketones. The urine of patients with UTIs is usually foul-smelling, and the odor becomes worse on standing. Certain foods, such as asparagus, can cause the urine to have a musty smell. Although the urine may have many characteristic odors, as a rule the odor of the urine is not generally used in the diagnosis of a patient's condition.

Specific Gravity. The **specific gravity** of urine measures the weight of the urine as compared with the weight of an equal volume of distilled water. Specific gravity indicates the amount of dissolved substances present in the urine, thus providing information on the ability of the kidneys to dilute or concentrate the urine. Specific gravity is decreased in conditions in which the kidneys cannot concentrate the urine, such as chronic renal insufficiency, diabetes insipidus, and malignant hypertension. The specific gravity is increased in patients with adrenal insufficiency, congestive heart failure, hepatic disease, diabetes mellitus with glycosuria, and conditions that cause dehydration, such as fever, vomiting, and diarrhea.

Normal specific gravity may range from 1.003 to 1.030 but is usually between 1.010 and 1.025 (the specific gravity of distilled water is 1.000). Specific gravity varies greatly with fluid intake and the state of hydration of an individual. Dilute urine contains fewer dissolved substances and thus has a lower specific gravity. Concentrated urine, on the other hand, will have a higher specific gravity because of the increased amount of dissolved substances. A urine specimen is generally more concentrated in the morning and becomes more dilute after fluid consumption.

Measurement of Specific Gravity. In the medical office, specific gravity is measured with one of the following methods:

Reagent strip method. This method involves a color comparison determination with a reagent strip that contains a reagent area for specific gravity. The reagent strip is dipped into the urine specimen, and the results are compared with a color chart (see Procedure 16-5).

Refractometer method. The amount of dissolved substances in urine can also be measured with a clinical **refractometer,** which is a hand-held optical instrument that consists of a lens and prism system. The refractometer measures the **refractive index** of urine, which is directly correlated with the specific gravity of urine; the results are read directly from a calibrated scale. The advantage of a refractometer is that only one to two drops of urine are necessary to perform the test. The procedure for measuring the specific gravity of urine with a refractometer is presented in Procedure 16-3.

PROCEDURE 16-3 Measuring Specific Gravity of Urine: Refractometer Method

Outcome Measure the specific gravity of a urine specimen.

Equipment/Supplies:
- Disposable gloves
- Refractometer
- Urine specimen
- Disposable pipet
- Antiseptic wipe
- Lint-free tissues

1. Procedural Step. Sanitize your hands, and assemble the equipment. Make sure the surface of the prism is clean.

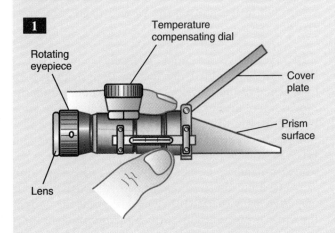

1

Rotating eyepiece

Temperature compensating dial

Cover plate

Prism surface

Lens

2. Procedural Step. Calibrate the refractometer according to the manufacturer's instructions. (Refer to the next procedure for information on calibration.)

3. Procedural Step. Apply gloves. Prepare the urine specimen. The urine specimen must be at room temperature. Mix the urine specimen with the disposable pipet.
Principle. The specimen must be well mixed for accurate test results.

4. Procedural Step. Withdraw a small amount of urine into the disposable pipet. Holding the pipet in a vertical position, place a drop of urine on the surface of the prism.

Depending on the brand of refractometer, this is accomplished in one of two ways as follows:

a. Open the cover plate and place a drop of urine directly on the prism. Tightly close the cover plate.

b. Close the cover plate and place a drop of urine at its notched part. The urine will be drawn across the prism surface (between the over plate and prism) by capillary action.

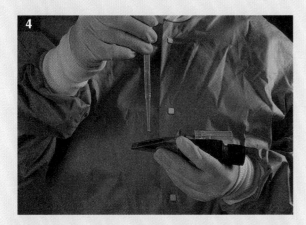

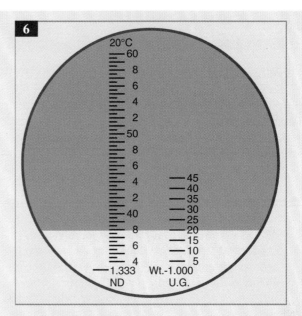

5. **Procedural Step.** Point the instrument toward a light source and rotate the eyepiece to bring the calibrated scale clearly into view. A light area *(bottom)* and a dark area *(top)* will be observed through the eyepiece.

7. **Procedural Step.** Clean the prism surface with a soft lint-free tissue, being careful not to scratch the prism. Disinfect the prism surface with an antiseptic wipe.

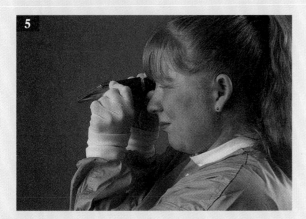

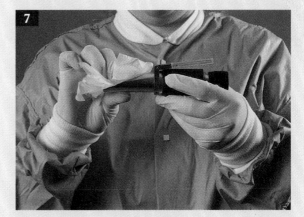

6. **Procedural Step.** Read the value on the scale at the boundary line that shows the distinct division of the light and dark areas. (The specific gravity reading on this scale is 1.020.)

8. **Procedural Step.** Remove the gloves and sanitize your hands.

9. **Procedural Step.** Chart the results. Include the date and time and the specific gravity reading.

CHARTING EXAMPLE

Date	
3/20/05	10:15 a.m. SG: 1.020. ——— L. Proffitt, CMA

PROCEDURE 16-3

PROCEDURE 16-4   Quality Control: Calibration of the Refractometer

Outcome Calibrate the refractometer. If the refractometer does not have a temperature compensating dial, it should be calibrated each day. Calibrating the refractometer compensates for day-to-day temperature variations to ensure accurate test results.

Equipment/Supplies:
- Refractor
- Distilled water
- Small screwdriver

The refractometer is calibrated as follows:

1. **Procedural Step.** Place a drop of distilled water on the surface of the prism with a disposable pipet.
2. **Procedural Step.** Point the instrument toward a light source and rotate the eyepiece to bring the calibrated scale clearly into view. A light area (bottom) and a dark area (top) will be observed through the eyepiece.
3. **Procedural Step.** Read the value on the scale at the boundary line that shows the distinct division of the light and dark areas. If the calibration of the refractometer is correct, the distilled water will have a specific gravity reading of 1.000 and the boundary line will fall exactly on the weight (wt) line.
4. **Procedural Step.** If the calibration of the refractometer is incorrect, the boundary line must be corrected to coincide with the weight line by turning an adjusting screw with a small screwdriver that is supplied by the manufacturer.

5. **Procedural Step.** Clean the prism surface with a soft lint-free tissue, being careful not to scratch the prism.

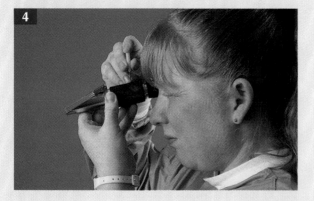
4

Chemical Examination of the Urine

Substances present in excess (abnormal) amounts in the blood are usually removed by the urine. Therefore, the chemical testing of urine is an indirect means of detecting abnormal amounts of chemicals in the body, indicating a pathologic condition. The chemical examination of urine also can be used to detect the presence of substances that, in the absence of disease, do not normally appear in the urine, such as blood and nitrite.

Chemical tests that are routinely performed during a urinalysis include testing for pH, glucose, protein, and ketones. Other chemical tests that may be performed include testing for blood, bilirubin, urobilinogen, nitrite, and leukocytes.

Qualitative tests. The chemical analysis of urine involves the use of both qualitative and quantitative tests. Qualitative tests provide an approximate indication of whether or not a substance is present in abnormal quantities. The interpretation of qualitative tests usually involves the use of a color chart, with results recorded in terms of trace, 1+, 2+, or 3+; trace, small, moderate, or large; or negative or positive. Qualitative tests are useful for screening purposes in the medical office because they are easy to perform and can be used to screen large

numbers of individuals, a procedure that otherwise might be too expensive and time consuming.

Quantitative tests. Quantitative tests indicate the exact amount of a chemical substance that is present; the results are reported in measurable units (e.g., milligrams per deciliter). Quantitative urine tests usually involve the use of more complex equipment and testing procedures than are found in the medical office; they are also more time consuming to run.

Commercial Testing Kits. Commercially prepared diagnostic testing kits are most frequently used in the medical office for the chemical testing of urine. These kits are usually preferred because they contain premeasured reagents, the procedure is easy to follow, and they provide an immediate answer. Most of these tests are qualitative, and a positive result may indicate the need for further testing. Most of the tests are manufactured in the form of reagent strips, and they rely on a color change for interpretation of results. A color chart is provided with the kit for making a visual comparison.

For accurate and reliable test results, the medical assistant should carefully read and follow the instructions that accompany each kit. For example, test strips that contain more than one reagent may require different time intervals for reading results. Certain medications that the patient is taking may also interfere with the test results. These medications will be listed in the manufacturer's instructions accompanying the test.

Before a test is used, its expiration date must be checked. Test material must not be used if a color change has occurred or if the *tested* strip gives off a color that does not match the shades on the color chart. Light, heat, and moisture can alter the effectiveness of the strips; therefore, care must be taken to store the test materials in a cool, dry area. Most test materials are packaged in light-resistant containers to protect them from light. The test materials must never be transferred from their original container to another because the other container may harbor traces of moisture, dirt, or chemicals that could affect the test results.

When results are recorded, the type of test that was used should be specified. A list of commercially available diagnostic kits for chemical tests on urine is presented in Table 16-1.

pH. The **pH** is the unit that indicates the acidity or alkalinity of a solution. The pH scale ranges from 0.0 to 14.0. The lower the number, the greater the acidity; the higher the number, the greater the alkalinity. A pH reading of 7.0 is neutral; a reading below 7.0 indicates acidity; and a reading above 7.0 indicates alkalinity.

The kidneys help regulate the acid-base balance of the body. For an accurate pH reading of the urine, the measurement should be performed on freshly voided urine. If the urine is allowed to remain standing, it becomes more alkaline as urea is converted to ammonia by bacterial action.

Although the pH of the urine can normally range from 4.6 to 8.0, the pH of a freshly voided specimen of a patient on a normal diet is usually acidic and has a pH reading of about 6.0. An abnormally high pH reading on a fresh specimen (that is, an alkaline urine) may indicate a bacterial infection of the urinary tract.

Glucose. Normally no glucose should be detectable in the urine. Glucose in the blood is filtered through the nephrons and is reabsorbed into the body. If the glucose concentration in the blood becomes too high, the kidney is unable to reabsorb all of it back into the blood, the renal threshold is exceeded, and glucose is spilled into the urine—a condition known as **glycosuria.** (The **renal threshold** is the concentration at which a substance in the blood that is not normally excreted by the kidney begins to appear in the urine.) The renal threshold for glucose is generally between 160 and 180 mg/dL (100 ml of blood), but this figure may vary among individuals. Diabetes mellitus is the most common cause of glycosuria. Some individuals have a low renal threshold, and glucose may appear in their urine after the consumption of a large quantity of foods containing sugar. This condition is known as *alimentary glycosuria.*

Protein. An abnormally high amount of protein in the urine is known as **proteinuria.** Protein in the urine usually indicates a pathologic condition if found in several samples over time. A temporary increase in urine protein may be caused by stress or strenuous exercise. Some of the conditions that may cause proteinuria include glomerular filtration problems, renal diseases, and bacterial infections of the urinary tract. If proteinuria occurs, the physician usually requests an examination of the sediment to aid in the determination of the patient's condition.

Ketones. Three types of ketone bodies exist: beta-hydroxybutyric acid, acetoacetic acid, and acetone. *Ketones* are the normal products of fat metabolism and can be used by muscle tissue as a source of energy. When more than normal amounts of fat are used, the muscles cannot handle all of the ketones that result. Large amounts of ketones, therefore, accumulate in the tissues and body fluids; this condition is known as **ketosis. Ketonuria** occurs when excessive amounts of ketones also begin appearing in the urine. Conditions that may lead to ketonuria include uncontrolled diabetes mellitus, starvation, and a diet composed almost entirely of fat.

Bilirubin. The average life span of a red blood cell is 120 days. When a red blood cell breaks down, one of the substances released from the breakdown of hemoglobin is a vivid yellow pigment known as bilirubin. Normally, bilirubin is transported to the liver and excreted into the bile, leaving the body through the intestines. Certain liver conditions such as gallstones, hepatitis, and cirrhosis may result in the presence of bilirubin in the urine, or **bilirubinuria.** The urine becomes yellow-brown or greenish, and a yellow foam appears when the urine is shaken.

Urobilinogen. Normally, bilirubin is excreted by the liver into the intestinal tract. Bacteria present in the intestines convert it to urobilinogen. Approximately 50% of the urobilinogen is then reabsorbed into the body for reexcretion by the liver. Small amounts may appear in the urine, but most of the urobilinogen is excreted in the feces. An increase in the production of bilirubin in turn increases the amount of urobilinogen excreted in the urine. Conditions such as excessive hemolysis of red blood cells, infectious hepatitis, cirrhosis, congestive heart failure, and infectious mononucleosis may increase the level of urobilinogen in the urine.

Blood. Blood is considered an abnormal constituent of urine, unless it is present as a contaminant during menstruation. The condition in which blood is found in the urine is termed *hematuria.* Hematuria may be the result of injury or disorders such as cystitis, tumors of the bladder, urethritis, kidney stones, and certain kidney disorders.

Nitrite. Nitrite in the urine indicates the presence of a pathogen in the (normally sterile) urinary tract, which results in a UTI. The pathogen possesses the ability to

TABLE **16-1**	Diagnostic Kits Used for Chemical Testing of Urine
Brand Name	**Function**

PRODUCTS OF BAYER CORPORATION

Acetest	Reagent tablet to detect ketones
Albustix	Reagent strip to detect protein
Bili-Labstix	Reagent strip to detect pH, protein, glucose, ketones, bilirubin, and blood
Clinistix	Reagent strip to detect glucose
Clinitest	Reagent tablet to detect glucose
Combistix	Reagent strip to detect pH, protein, and glucose
Diastix	Reagent strip to detect glucose
Hema-Combistix	Reagent strip to detect pH, protein, glucose, and blood
Hemastix	Reagent strip to detect blood
Ictotest	Reagent tablet to detect bilirubin
Keto-Diastix	Reagent strip to detect glucose and ketones
Ketostix	Reagent strip to detect ketones
Labstix	Reagent strip to detect pH, protein, glucose, ketones, and blood
Multisix	Reagent strip to detect pH, protein, glucose, ketones, urobilinogen, bilirubin, and blood
Multistix SG	Reagent strip to detect pH, protein, glucose, ketones, urobilinogen, bilirubin, blood, and specific gravity
Multistix 2	Reagent strip to detect leukocytes and nitrite
Multistix 7	Reagent strip to detect pH, protein, glucose, ketones, blood, leukocytes, and nitrite
Multistix 8 SG	Reagent strip to detect pH, protein, glucose, ketones, blood, leukocytes, nitrite, and specific gravity
Multistix 9	Reagent strip to detect pH, protein, glucose, ketones, urobilinogen, bilirubin, blood, leukocytes, and nitrite
Multistix 9 SG	Reagent strip to detect pH, protein, glucose, ketones, bilirubin, blood, leukocytes, nitrite, and specific gravity
Multistix 10 SG	Reagent strip to detect pH, protein, glucose, ketones, urobilinogen, bilirubin, blood, leukocytes, nitrite, and specific gravity
Multistix PRO 10 LS	Reagent strip to detect pH, protein-high, protein-low, glucose, ketones, blood, leukocytes, nitrite, creatinine, and specific gravity
N-Multistix	Reagent strip to detect pH, protein, glucose, ketones, urobilinogen, bilirubin, blood, and nitrite
N-Multistix SG	Reagent strip to detect pH, protein, glucose, ketones, urobilinogen, bilirubin, blood, nitrite, and specific gravity
Uristix	Reagent strip to detect protein and glucose
Uristix 4	Reagent strip to detect protein, glucose, leukocytes, and nitrite

PRODUCTS OF ROCHE LABORATORIES

Chemstrip 6	Reagent strip to detect pH, protein, glucose, ketones, blood, and leukocytes
Chemstrip 7	Reagent strip to detect pH, protein, glucose, ketones, bilirubin, blood, and leukocytes
Chemstrip 8	Reagent strip to detect pH, protein, glucose, ketones, urobilinogen, bilirubin, blood, and nitrite
Chemstrip 10 SG	Reagent strip to detect pH, protein, glucose, ketones, urobilinogen, bilirubin, blood, leukocytes, nitrite, and specific gravity
Chemstrip UG	Reagent strip to detect glucose
Chemstrip 4 OB	Reagent strip to detect glucose, protein, blood, and leukocytes
Chemstrip 2 GP	Reagent strip to detect protein and glucose
Chemstrip 2 LN	Reagent strip to detect leukocytes and nitrite
Chemstrip μGK	Reagent strip to detect glucose and ketones
Chemstrip K	Reagent strip to detect ketones
Chemstrip Micral	Reagent strip to detect protein

Highlight on Drug Testing in the Workplace

Statistics suggest that the problem of drug abuse is growing in the workplace. On any one day, 8.9 to 16 million employees are estimated to be working under the influence of drugs. The effects of on-the-job drug use extend into every segment of the population and touch every business and industry. Occupational Safety and Health Administration (OSHA) estimates that 65% of all work-related accidents can be traced to substance abuse. The Metropolitan Insurance Company states that drug abuse costs industry $85 billion annually because of absenteeism, lowered productivity, and higher health care costs.

Because of these economic and safety factors, businesses across the country are adopting a less permissive attitude toward drug use and are beginning compulsory drug testing in the workplace. Approximately one third of American employers have implemented drug-testing programs in the workplace. Employers include utility companies, transportation operations, sports associations, and governmental agencies. Currently many companies test both blue- and white-collar employees for drug use. Companies with drug-testing programs report a significant reduction in employee accidents, fewer sick days, and healthier employees.

A comprehensive drug-testing program includes the detection of drug use in the workplace, policies to discourage further abuse, and the referral of employees for treatment and rehabilitation. Drug testing may be performed for one or more of the following purposes: (1) preemployment drug screening, (2) testing for probable cause after unexplained behavior or events, and (3) random sample testing of the work force to detect use of controlled substances by employees on the job.

Blood testing is the best means for determining precise information concerning the amount of the drug used and when the drug was taken. However, blood tests are costly and time consuming to perform. Urine drug testing offers the next best alternative; it is noninvasive and technically easier and cheaper to perform. The current urine screening tests target the most common drugs of abuse: amphetamines, barbiturates, benzodiazepines, cocaine, marijuana, opiates, PCP, methaqualone, and methadone.

The usual procedure for urine drug testing involves screening the specimen and then confirming positive results with more specific urine tests. The specimen may be collected at the workplace, at the medical office, or at an outside laboratory. To help ensure reliable and valid drug-testing results, a security system or "chain of custody" must be followed in the collection and handling of the specimen. This typically includes ensuring the identification of the individual undergoing drug testing, taking precautions to avoid faking or tampering with specimens, witnessing the collection of the specimen, properly labeling the urine specimen, sealing the sample in the specimen container after collection, and immediately sending the specimen to the laboratory for analysis or refrigerating it at once for any delay in transporting.

The main disadvantage of urine drug testing is that a positive test result indicates only the presence of a drug in the urine; it does not provide any information regarding when the drug was taken. Drugs that are detected in the urine may or *may not* still be present in the blood where they can affect an individual's behavior and impair performance. Hence, a positive urine test result does not reveal whether an individual is impaired by drugs. In addition the initial urine screening tests are sometimes unreliable; unless positive results are confirmed with a more specific test, an individual may be unjustly accused of drug use. These factors, along with the violation of an individual's right to privacy, are the main areas of dispute for individuals who oppose drug testing in the workplace.

Companies with drug-testing programs have various options when results are positive, such as recommendations for drug treatment programs or disciplinary action. Many companies have established in-house employee assistance programs that include counseling and drug withdrawal therapy for employees who desire help. Most companies prefer to help current employees with rehabilitation instead of discharging them and hiring and training new employees. Studies show a 35% to 60% recovery rate for employees enrolled in drug treatment programs.

---

convert nitrate, which normally occurs in the urine, to nitrite, which is normally absent. The nitrite test must be performed with urine that has been in the bladder for at least 4 to 6 hours to ensure that bacteria have converted nitrate to nitrite. Therefore, use of a first-voided morning specimen is recommended. The test should *not* be performed on specimens that have been left standing out because a false-positive result may occur from bacte-

rial contamination from the atmosphere. Nitrite tests are to be considered only screening tests and must be followed by a quantitative culture and identification of the invading organism.

Leukocytes. The presence of leukocytes in the urine is known as *leukocyturia* and accompanies inflammation of the kidneys and the lower urinary tract. Examples of specific conditions include acute and chronic pyelonephritis, cystitis, and urethritis. Reagent strips are available that contain a reagent area that permits the chemical detection of both intact and lysed leukocytes in the urine. The advantage of detecting lysed leukocytes is that these cells cannot be observed during a microscopic examination of urine sediment and would otherwise remain undetected. The recommended urine specimen, particularly for women, is a clean-catch midstream collection to prevent contamination of the specimen with leukocytes from vaginal secretions leading to false-positive test results.

Reagent Strips

In the medical office, reagent strips are the most commonly used diagnostic urine testing kit. Reagent strips consist of disposable plastic strips on which separate reagent areas are affixed for testing specific chemical constituents that may be present in the urine during pathologic conditions. The results provide the physician with information related to the status of the patient's carbohydrate metabolism, kidney and liver function, acid-base balance, and bacteriuria. Reagent strips are considered qualitative tests, and a positive result necessitates further testing. Table 16-2 (p. 630) presents an outline of reagent strip parameters and the diagnoses in which they assist.

The number and type of reagent areas included on the reagent strip depend on the particular brand of reagent strips. Multistix 10 SG (Bayer Corporation), for example, contains 10 reagent areas for testing pH, protein, glucose, ketones, bilirubin, blood, urobilinogen, nitrite, specific gravity, and leukocytes. Other brands and the tests included for each are listed in Table 16-1.

The reagent strip procedure in this chapter (Procedure 16-5) is specifically for Multistix 10 SG; however, the procedure can be followed for the chemical testing of urine with most reagent strips. In all instances, the medical assistant should read the manufacturer's instructions before performing the test.

Guidelines for Reagent Strip Urine Testing.
Testing urine with reagent strips is a relatively easy procedure to perform. However, specific guidelines must be used to obtain accurate test results.

1. *Type of specimen.* The best results are obtained with a freshly voided urine specimen. Most reagent strips are designed to be used with a random specimen collection; however, clean-catch midstream and first-voided morning specimens are suggested for specific tests. For example, the nitrite test results are optimized with a first-voided morning specimen, whereas a clean-catch midstream collection is recommended for the leukocyte test.
2. *Specimen container.* The specimen container used must be thoroughly clean and free from any detergent or dis-

infectant residue because cleansing agents contain oxidants that react with the chemicals on the reagent strip, leading to inaccurate test results.

3. *Storage of reagent strips.* The reagent strips are sensitive to light, heat, and moisture, and the bottle containing the strips must therefore be stored in a cool, dry area with the cap tightly closed to maintain reactivity of the reagent. The bottle may contain a desiccant that should not be removed because its purpose is to promote dryness by absorbing moisture. The bottle of reagent strips must be stored at a temperature under 30° C (86° F) but should not be stored in the refrigerator or freezer. A tan-to-brown discoloration or darkening on the reagent areas indicates deterioration of the chemical reagent strips, in which case the strips should not be used because the test results would be inaccurate.
4. *Interpretation of results.* Of particular importance is the comparison of the reagent strip with the color chart. The reagent strip must be compared with the color chart in good lighting to obtain a good visual match of the color reactions with the color chart provided with the test kit.

Quality Control.
Quality control should be used in a chemical examination of urine with a reagent strip. Quality control ensures the reliability of test results by (1) determining whether the reagent strips are reacting properly and (2) confirming that the test is being properly performed and accurately interpreted.

To check the reliability of Multistix reagent strips, Chek-Stix (Bayer Corporation) should be used. Each Chek-Stix consists of a firm plastic strip to which are affixed seven synthetic ingredients (Figure 16-6). The strip is reconstituted with immersion in distilled water for 30 minutes, which allows the ingredients on the strip to dissolve in the water.

After reconstitution, the resulting solution is tested in the same manner as a urine specimen. The values to be expected are outlined on a sheet that accompanies the control strips.

TABLE 16-2 Urine Test Strip Parameters and the Diagnoses They Assist*

System/Source	Leukocytes	Nitrite	Urine pH		Protein
Genitourinary	Renal infection/ inflammation • Acute/chronic pyelonephritis • Glomerulo- nephritis • Urolithiasis • Tumors • Lower urinary tract infection (cystitis, urethri- tis, prostatitis)	Bacteriuria • Urinary tract infection (cystitis, urethritis, prostatitis, pyelonephritis)	Up (>pH 6) in • Renal failure • Bacterial infection (e.g., *Proteus* bacteriuria) • Renal tubular acidosis		Renal/glomerular/ tubular disease • Glomerulo- nephritis • Glomerulosclerosis (e.g., in diabetes) • Nephrotic syndrome • Pyelonephritis • Renal tuberculosis
Hepatobiliary					
Gastrointestinal			Up in: • Pyloric obstruction	Down in: • Diarrhea • Malabsorption	
Cardiovascular					Congestive heart failure
Hormonal, Metabolic, and Other Systems			Up in: • Alkalosis (metabolic, respiratory)	Down in: • Acidosis (metabolic, respiratory, diabetic) • Pulmonary emphysema • Dehydration	Gout Hypokalemia Pre-eclampsia Severe febrile infection
Environmental (diet, drugs, stress)	Phenacetin- induced nephritis		Up in: • Diet high in vegetables, citrus fruits • Alkalizing drug use (sodium bicarbonate, acetazolamide)	Down in: • Diet high in meats or other protein, cranberries • Starvation • Acidifying drug use (e.g., ammonium chloride, methenamine mandelate therapy)	Nephrotoxic drugs

Courtesy Boehringer-Mannheim Diagnostics, Indianapolis, Indiana.

Continued

Reagent strip detection of abnormal urine constituent or concentration characteristic of disease (e.g., glycosuria in diabetes mellitus) may provide useful screen or monitor but requires confirmation with other laboratory and clinical evidence.

Modified from: Conn HF, Conn RB (eds): *Current diagnosis 5,* Philadelphia, 1977, Saunders. Davidson I, Henry JB (eds): *Todd-Stanford clinical diagnosis by laboratory methods,* 15th ed, Philadelphia, 1974, Saunders. Raphael SS, et al: *Lynch's medical laboratory technology,* 3rd ed, Philadelphia, 1976, Saunders. Wallach J: *Interpretation of diagnostic tests,* 2nd ed, Boston, 1974, Little, Brown. Widmann FK: *Goodale's clinical interpretation of laboratory tests,* 7th ed, Philadelphia, 1973, F.A. Davis.

Glucose	Ketones	Urobilinogen	Bilirubin	Blood, Erythrocytes (Hematuria)	Hemoglobin
Renal glycosuria (e.g., during pregnancy) Renal tubular disease (e.g., in Fanconi's syndrome) Decreased renal glucose threshold (e.g., in old age)				Renal infection/ inflammation/ injury • Renal tuberculosis • Renal infarction • Calculi (urethral, renal) • Polycystic kidneys • Tumors (bladder, renal pelvis, prostate) • Salpingitis • Cystitis	Renal intravascular Hemolysis Acute glomerulo-nephritis
		Liver cell damage Chronic liver stasis Cirrhosis Dubin-Johnson syndrome *Note:* May be 0 or down in biliary obstruction	Biliary dysfunction • Gallstones Obstructive jaundice Hepatitis (viral toxic) Dubin-Johnson syndrome	Cirrhosis	
	Vomiting Diarrhea	*Note:* May be negative with inhibition of intestinal flora by antimicrobial agents		Colon tumor Diverticulitis	
Myocardial infarction				Bacterial endocarditis	
Diabetes mellitus Hemochromatosis Hyperthyroidism Cushing's syndrome Pheochromocytomas	Diabetic ketosis Glycogen-storage disease Pre-eclampsia Acute fever	Sickle cell anemia Hemolytic disease • Pernicious anemia Leptospirosis	Hemolytic disease Leptospirosis	Blood dyscrasias • Hemophilia • Thrombocytopenia • Sickel cell anemia Disseminated lupus erythemtosus Malignant hypertension	Hemolytic disease Plasmodium (malaria) Clostridia (tetanus) infection
Sudden shock or pain Steroid therapy	Weight-reducing diet Ketogenic diet (e.g., in anti-convulsant therapy) Starvation			Hemorrhagenic drugs (e.g., anticoagulant, salicylates) Nephrotoxic agents Internal injury or foreign body Vitamin C or K deficiency	Overexertion Exposure to cold Incompatible blood transfusion Drug-induced hemolysis

Urine Analyzer. Urine analyzers are used to perform an automatic chemical examination of urine with reagent strips. They offer the advantage of the ability to perform the chemical analysis quickly and to interpret results automatically. These analyzers are used most often in medical offices that perform moderate- to large-volume urine testing.

The Clinitek Analyzer (Bayer Corporation) is an example of a urine analyzer that automatically reads Multistix SG and other (Bayer) urinalysis reagent strips (Figure 16-7). The results are printed out, and abnormal results are highlighted to assist in reviewing results. Different models are available; some can be used to perform a color and appearance analysis and a microscopic examination of the urine.

Text continued on p. 635

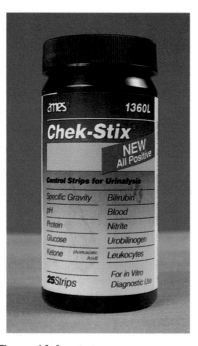

Figure 16-6. Chek-Stix control strips.

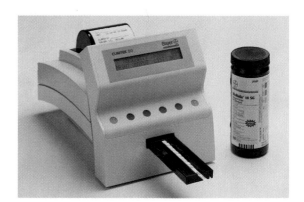

Figure 16-7. Clinitek Urine Analyzer.

What Would You DO?
What Would You Not DO?

Case Study 3

Rita Lavelle is 8½ months pregnant and is at the clinic for a prenatal appointment. She brings in her first-voided urine specimen in a glass jar. She says her dog chewed up the specimen container from the office so she used an empty peanut butter jar. The urine testing results from her specimen show that her glucose level is normal but that her protein level is +4. Until this time, her urine test results have all been normal. Rita is concerned about her baby. She says that she was cleaning her bathroom cabinet yesterday and came across a pregnancy test; just for the fun of it, she decided to run the test. The results were negative, and now she is worried that something is wrong with the baby. Rita says that she has not been sleeping as well at night and that she has noticed more Braxton Hicks contractions but that the baby has been kicking and moving as usual.

PROCEDURE 16-5 Chemical Testing of Urine With the Multistix 10 SG Reagent Strip

Outcome Perform a chemical assessment of a urine specimen.

Equipment/Supplies:
- Disposable gloves
- Multistix 10 SG reagent strips
- Urine container
- Laboratory report form

1. **Procedural Step.** Obtain a freshly voided urine specimen from the patient with a clean container. The specimen should be well mixed, uncentrifuged, and at room temperature.

   Principle. The best results are obtained with a freshly voided specimen. The container should be clean because contaminants could affect the results. Well-mixed, uncentrifuged specimens assure a homogeneous sample.

2. **Procedural Step.** Sanitize your hands.

3. **Procedural Step.** Assemble the equipment. Check the expiration date of the reagent strips.

   Principle. Outdated reagent strips may lead to inaccurate test results.

4. **Procedural Step.** Apply gloves. Remove a reagent strip from the bottle and recap the bottle immediately. Do not touch the test areas with your fingers or lay the strip on the table. However, it is permissible to lay the reagent strip on a clean, dry paper towel.

   Principle. Recapping the bottle is necessary to prevent exposing the strips to environmental moisture, light, and heat, which cause altered reagent reactivity. Contamination of the test areas by the hands or table surface may affect the accuracy of the test results.

5. **Procedural Step.** Completely immerse the reagent strip in the urine specimen, and remove it immediately. While removing, run the edge of the strip against the rim of the urine container to remove excess urine.

   Principle. The strip should be completely immersed to ensure that all test areas are moistened for accurate test results. Prolonged immersion of the reagent strip and failure to remove excess urine may cause the reagents to dissolve and leach onto adjacent test areas, affecting the accuracy of the test results.

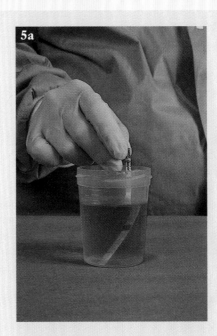

5a

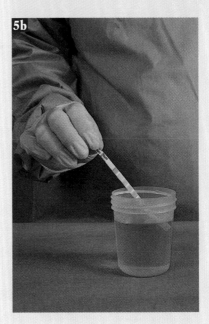

5b

PROCEDURE 16-5

Continued

PROCEDURE 16-5 Chemical Testing of Urine With the Multistix 10 SG Reagent Strip—Cont'd

6. **Procedural Step.** Hold the reagent strip in a horizontal position and place it adjacent to the corresponding color blocks on the color chart. Do not lay the strip directly on the color chart because this will result in the urine soiling the chart. Read the results carefully and at the exact reading times specified on the color chart and as indicated below.
- Glucose, 30 seconds
- Bilirubin, 30 seconds
- Ketones, 40 seconds
- Specific gravity, 45 seconds
- Blood, 60 seconds
- pH, 60 seconds
- Protein, 60 seconds
- Urobilinogen, 60 seconds
- Nitrite, 60 seconds
- Leukocytes, 2 minutes

Principle. Holding the strip in a horizontal position avoids soiling the hands with urine and prevents reagents from running over into the adjacent testing areas, causing inaccurate test results. The strip must be read at the proper time to avoid dissolving out reagents, leading to inaccurate test results.

7. **Procedural Step.** Dispose of the strip in a regular waste container.

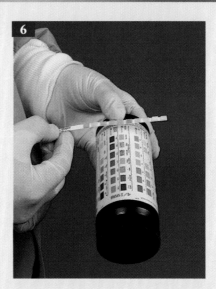

8. **Procedural Step.** Remove gloves and sanitize your hands.

9. **Procedural Step.** Chart the results. The results should be charted following the interpretation guide provided above each color block on the color chart. Be sure to include the date and time, the brand name of the test used (Multistix 10 SG), and the results.

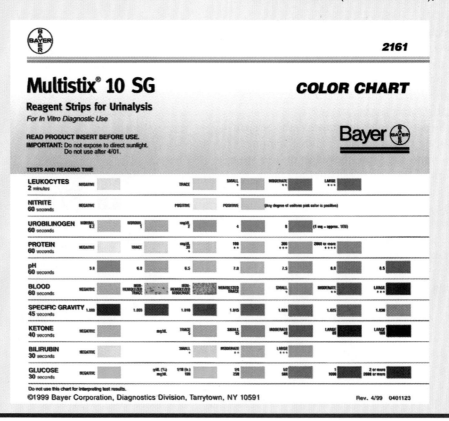

Microscopic Examination of Urine

Urine sediment is the solid material contained in the urine. A microscopic examination of the urine sediment helps clarify results of the physical and chemical examination. A first-voided morning specimen is generally preferred because it is more concentrated and contains more dissolved substances; therefore, small amounts of abnormal substances are more likely to be detected. Use of a fresh specimen is important because changes will take place in a specimen left standing out, as previously discussed. These changes affect the reliability of the test results. The procedures for preparation of a urine specimen for microscopic examination and examination of the sediment under a microscope are presented at the end of this section.

Structures that may be found in a microscopic examination of urine are described next. Tables 16-3 to 16-6 provide an outline of these structures and of the possible causes of their presence.

Red Blood Cells.
Red blood cells appear as round, colorless, biconcave discs that are highly refractile. The presence of 0 to 5 per high-power field is considered normal. More than this amount may indicate bleeding somewhere along the urinary tract. Table 16-3 lists the possible causes of an abnormal number of red blood cells in the urine. Concentrated urine causes the red blood cells to become shrunken or *crenated,* whereas dilute urine causes them to swell and become rounded, which may cause them to hemolyze. If the red blood cells have hemolyzed, they will not be seen under the microscope. The presence of blood in the urine can still be identified, however, with a reagent strip, such as Multistix, designed to detect free hemoglobin.

White Blood Cells.
White blood cells are round and granular and have a nucleus. They are approximately 1.5 times as large as a red blood cell. The presence of 0 to 8 per high-power field is considered normal. More than this amount may indicate inflammation of the genitourinary tract. Table 16-3 lists the possible causes of an abnormal number of white blood cells in the urine.

Epithelial Cells.
Most structures that make up the urinary system are composed of several layers of epithelial cells. The outer layer is constantly sloughed off and replaced by the cells underneath it. *Squamous epithelial cells* are large, clear, flat cells with an irregular shape. They contain a small nucleus and come from the urethra, bladder, and vagina. Squamous epithelial cells are normally present in small amounts in the urine. *Renal epithelial cells* are round and contain a large nucleus. They come from the deeper layers of the urinary tract, and their presence in the urine

is considered abnormal. Table 16-3 lists the types of epithelial cells and possible causes of the presence of abnormal amounts in the urine.

Casts.
Casts are cylindric structures formed in the lumen of the tubules that make up the nephron. Materials in the tubules harden, are flushed out, and appear in the urine in the form of casts. Various types of casts may be present in the urine. Their presence generally indicates a diseased condition.

Casts are named according to what they contain. *Hyaline casts* are pale, colorless cylinders with rounded edges that vary in size. *Granular casts* are hyaline casts that contain granules and are described as "coarsely granular" or "finely granular," depending on the size of the granules. *Fatty casts* are hyaline casts that contain fat droplets. Waxy casts are light yellowish and have serrated edges. Their name is derived from the fact that they appear to be made of wax.

Cellular casts contain organized structures and are named according to what they contain. Examples include red blood cell casts, which are hyaline casts containing red blood cells; white blood cell casts, which are hyaline casts containing white blood cells; epithelial casts, which are hyaline casts containing epithelial cells; and bacterial casts, which are hyaline casts containing bacteria. Table 16-4 lists the types of casts and possible causes of their presence in urine.

Crystals.
A variety of crystals may be found in the urine. The type and number vary with the pH of the urine. Abnormal crystals found include leucine, tyrosine, cystine, and cholesterol. Crystals that commonly appear in acid urine include amorphous urates, uric acid, and calcium oxalate. Those that commonly appear in alkaline urine include amorphous phosphate, triple phosphate, calcium phosphate, and ammonium urate crystals. Table 16-5 lists the types of urine crystals and their significance when found in urine.

Miscellaneous Structures.
Mucous threads are normally present in small amounts in the urine. They appear as long, wavy, threadlike structures with pointed ends.

Bacteria should not normally exist in the urinary tract. The presence of more than a few bacteria may indicate either contamination of the specimen during collection or a UTI. Bacteria are small structures and may be rod shaped or round.

Yeast cells are smooth, refractile bodies with an oval shape. A distinguishing feature of yeast cells is small buds that project from the cells involved with reproduction. Yeast cells in the urine of female patients are usually a vaginal contaminant caused by the yeast *Candida albicans* and produce the vaginal infection known as candidiasis. They may also be present in the urine of patients with diabetes mellitus.

Parasites may be present in the urine sediment as a contaminant from fecal or vaginal material. *Trichomonas vaginalis* is a parasite that causes trichomoniasis vaginitis.

Spermatozoa may be present in the urine of a man or woman after intercourse. The spermatozoa have round heads and long, slender, hairlike tails.

Table 16-6 lists the miscellaneous structures that may be present in the urine and the significance when found.

Text continued on p. 649

▶ PATIENT TEACHING

Urinary Tract Infections

Answer questions patients may have about UTIs.

What is a UTI?

UTI is a general term for the presence of bacteria in any portion of the urinary tract. UTIs, particularly those involving the bladder (cystitis) and urethra (urethritis), are common and treatable. A UTI is usually treated with an antibiotic. Use of all the antibiotic for the full number of days prescribed by the physician is important, even if the symptoms disappear. If the medication is stopped too soon, the infection may recur and be more difficult to treat than the original infection.

What are the symptoms of a UTI?

The symptoms of a simple UTI (cystitis) commonly include the frequent need to urinate, urgency (meaning the immediate need to urinate), a burning sensation during urination, and sometimes blood in the urine. The symptoms of a more complicated UTI involving the kidneys (pyelonephritis) include the preceding symptoms and lower abdominal discomfort, low back pain, fever, cloudy or foul-smelling urine, and blood in the urine.

Why do women have UTIs more frequently than do men?

Women are more prone to the type of UTI called cystitis than are men because the urethra of a woman is much shorter than that of a man, which makes travel up the urethra and into the bladder easier for bacteria. The most common source of infection is bacteria (*Escherichia coli*). This organism is normally found in the large intestine but can travel from the anal area to the urinary bladder, often as the result of poor hygienic practices. Cystitis occurs if *E coli* are able to overcome the body's natural defenses once the bacteria reach the urinary bladder and set up an infection.

What can women do to prevent a UTI?

The prevention measures that a woman prone to development of UTIs should practice are:

Practice good hygienic measures by always cleaning the genital area from front to back after a bowel movement.

Avoid possible irritants, such as bubble baths, perfumed soaps, feminine hygiene sprays, or the use of strong powders and bleaches for washing underclothes.

Avoid clothing that traps moisture and thereby encourages the growth of microorganisms, such as tight, constricting clothing, nylon panties, and panty hose.

Avoid activities that can contribute to irritation of the urinary meatus, such as prolonged bicycling, motorcycling, horseback riding, and traveling involving prolonged sitting.

Urinate as soon as possible when you feel the urge. Holding urine in the bladder gives the bacteria more time to grow, which can cause more infection. The more often you urinate, the quicker the bacteria will be removed from the bladder.

Seek prompt treatment if you experience any of the symptoms of a UTI.

- Encourage the patient with a UTI to drink plenty of water to help flush the bacteria out of the urinary tract.
- Emphasize to the patient the importance of taking all the antibiotic for the duration of time prescribed by the physician.
- Emphasize the importance of practicing preventive measures to prevent the occurrence of UTIs.
- Provide the patient with educational materials on UTIs.

TABLE 16-3	Cells in Urine Sediment		
Type	Presence in Normal Urine	Possible Causes of Abnormal Amounts of Cells in Urine	Microscopic Appearance
Red blood cells	0 to 5 cells per high-power field (depending on preparation of urine sediment)	Inflammatory diseases Acute glomerulonephritis Pyelonephritis Hypertension Renal infarction Trauma Stones Tumor Bleeding diseases Use of anticoagulants	
White blood cells	0 to 8 cells per high-power field (depending on preparation of urine sediment)	Pyelonephritis Cystitis Urethritis Prostatitis Transplant rejection (manifested by lymphocytes in urine) Tissue injury accompanied by severe inflammation (manifested by monocytes in urine) Inflammation, immune mechanisms, and other host defense mechanisms (manifested by histiocytes in urine)	
Squamous epithelial cells	Often present, depending upon collection technique	Vaginal contamination	
Transitional epithelial cells	Moderate number of cells present	Disease of bladder or renal pelvis Catheterization	
Renal tubular epithelial cells	Present in small numbers, higher numbers in infants	Acute tubular necrosis Glomerulonephritis Acute infection Renal toxicity Viral infection	

Text courtesy Boehringer Mannheim Diagnostics, Indianapolis, Indiana.
Photomicrographs courtesy Bayer Corporation, Elkhart, Indiana.

Continued

| TABLE 16-3 | Cells in Urine Sediment—cont'd | | |

Type	Presence in Normal Urine	Possible Causes of Abnormal Amounts of Cells in Urine	Microscopic Appearance
Cytomegalic inclusion bodies	Not normally present in urine	Cytomegalic inclusion disease	
Tumor cells	Not normally present in urine	Tumors of • Renal pelvis • Renal parenchyma • Ureters • Bladder	

Text courtesy Boehringer Mannheim Diagnostics, Indianapolis, Indiana.
Photomicrographs courtesy Bayer Corporation, Elkhart, Indiana.

| TABLE 16-4 | Casts in Urine Sediment | | |

Type	Description	Possible Causes	Microscopic Appearance
Hyaline casts	Colorless, transparent Low refractive index	Normal urine Strenuous exercise Acute glomerulonephritis Acute pyelonephritis Malignant hypertension Chronic renal disease	‡
Red blood cell casts	Red cells in hyaline matrix Yellow-orange color High refractive index	Acute glomerulonephritis Lupus nephritis Severe nephritis Collagen diseases Renal infarction Malignant hypertension	‡
White blood cell casts	Neutrophils in hyaline matrix High refractive index	Acute pyelonephritis Acute glomerulonephritis Chronic renal disease	*

Text courtesy Boehringer Mannheim Diagnostics, Indianapolis, Indiana.
*Photomicrographs courtesy Bayer Corporation, Diagnostics Division, Elkhart, Indiana.
†Photomicrographs from Henry J.B.: *Clinical diagnosis and management by laboratory methods,* ed 20, Philadelphia, W.B. Saunders, 2001.
‡Photomicrographs from Stepp C.A., Woods M.: *Laboratory procedures for medical office personnel.* Philadelphia, W.B. Saunders, 1998.

TABLE 16-4	Casts in Urine Sediment—cont'd		
Type	**Description**	**Possible Causes**	**Microscopic Appearance**
Epithelial cell casts	Renal tubular epithelial cells in hyaline matrix High refractive index	Glomerulonephritis Vascular disease Toxin Virus	†
Granular casts	Opaque granules in matrix	Heavy proteinuria (nephrotic syndrome) Orthostatic proteinuria Congestive heart failure with proteinuria Acute or chronic renal disease	‡
Waxy casts	Sharp, refractile outlines Irregular "broken off" ends Absence of differentiated structures	Severe chronicrenal disease Malignant hypertension Kidney disease resulting from diabetes mellitus Acute renal disease	‡
Fatty casts	Fat globules in transparent matrix	Nephrotic syndrome Diabetes mellitus Mercury poisoning Ethylene glycol poisoning	†
Broad casts	Larger diameter than other casts	Acute tubular necrosis Severe chronic renal disease Urinary tract obstruction	*
Mixed casts	Combination of any of the above	Any of the above, depending on cellular constituents	*

TABLE 16-5   Urine Crystals

Type of Urine	Type of Crystals	Description of Crystals	Significance When Found in Urine	Microscopic Appearance
Normal acid urine	Amorphous urate	Colorless or yellow-brown granules (pink macroscopically)	Nonpathologic	*
	Uric acid	Occur in many shapes; may be colorless, yellow-brown, or red-brown; and square, diamond-shaped, wedge-shaped, or grouped in rosettes	Usually nonpathologic; in large numbers, may indicate gout	*
	Calcium oxalate	Octahedral or dumbbell-shaped; possess double refractive index	Usually nonpathologic; may be associated with stone formation	=
Normal alkaline urine	Amorphous phosphates	Small, colorless granules	Nonpathologic	§

Continued

Triple phosphates	Colorless prisms with three to six sides ("coffin lids") or feathery, shaped like fern leaves	Usually nonpathologic; may be associated with urine stasis or chronic urinary tract infection
Ammonium biurate	Yellow-brown "thorny apple" appearance or yellow-brown spheres	Nonpathologic
Calcium phosphate	Colorless prisms or rosettes	Usually nonpathologic; may be associated with urine stasis or chronic urinary tract infection
Calcium carbonte	Usually appear colorless and amorphous; may be shaped like dumbbells, rhombi, or needles	Usually nonpathologic; may be associated with inorganic calculi formation

Text courtesy Boehringer Mannheim Diagnostics, Indianapolis, Indiana.
*Photomicrographs courtesy Bayer Corporation, Diagnostics Division, Elkhart, Indiana.
†Photomicrograph from Brunzel, N.A: *Fundamentals of Urine and Body Fluid Analysis.* Philadelphia, W.B. Saunders, 1994.
‡Photomicrograph from Lehmann, C.A.: *Saunders Manual of Clinical Laboratory Science.* Philadelphia, W.B. Saunders, 1998.
§Photomicrographs from Henry, J.B.: *Clinical Diagnosis and Management by Laboratory Methods,* ed 20. Philadelphia, W.B. Saunders, 2001.
‖Photomicrographs from Stepp, C.A. Wood, M.: *Laboratory Procedures for Medical Office Personnel.* Philadelphia, W.B. Saunders, 1998.

TABLE 16-5 Urine Crystals—cont'd

Type of Urine	Type of Crystals	Description of Crystals	Significance When Found in Urine	Microscopic Appearance
Abnormal urine	Tyrosine	Thin, dark needles, arranged in sheaves or clumps; usually colorless but may be pale yellow-brown	Liver disease or inherited metabolic disorder	
	Leucine	Yellow-brown spheres with radial striations	Liver disease or inherited metabolic disorder	
	Cystine	Clear, hexagonal plates	Cystinuria	
	Hippuric acid	Star-shaped clusters of needles, rhombic plates, or elongated prisms; may be colorless or yellow-brown	Usually nonpathologic	
	Bilirubin	Delicate needles or rhombic plates; red-brown in color; birefringent	Bilirubinuria	

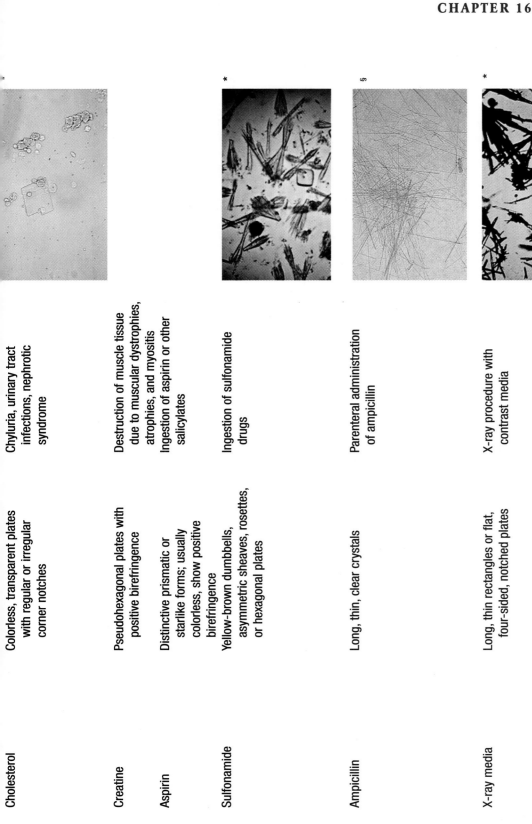

Cholesterol	Colorless, transparent plates with regular or irregular corner notches	Chyluria, urinary tract infections, nephrotic syndrome
Creatine	Pseudohexagonal plates with positive birefringence	Destruction of muscle tissue due to muscular dystrophies, atrophies, and myositis
Aspirin	Distinctive prismatic or starlike forms; usually colorless, show positive birefringence	Ingestion of aspirin or other salicylates
Sulfonamide	Yellow-brown dumbbells, asymmetric sheaves, rosettes, or hexagonal plates	Ingestion of sulfonamide drugs
Ampicillin	Long, thin, clear crystals	Parenteral administration of ampicillin
X-ray media	Long, thin rectangles or flat, four-sided, notched plates	X-ray procedure with contrast media

Text courtesy Boehringer Mannheim Diagnostics, Indianapolis, Indiana.
*Photomicrographs courtesy Bayer Corporation, Diagnostics Division, Elkhart, Indiana.
†Photomicrograph from Brunzel, N.A: *Fundamentals of Urine and Body Fluid Analysis.* Philadelphia, W.B. Saunders, 1994.
‡Photomicrograph from Lehmann, C.A.: *Saunders Manual of Clinical Laboratory Science.* Philadelphia, W.B. Saunders, 1998.
§Photomicrographs from Henry, J.B.: *Clinical Diagnosis and Management by Laboratory Methods,* ed 20. Philadelphia, W.B. Saunders, 2001.
‖Photomicrographs from Stepp, C.A. Wood, M.: *Laboratory Procedures for Medical Office Personnel.* Philadelphia, W.B. Saunders, 1998.

TABLE 16-6 Microorganisms and Artifacts in the Urine

Microorganisms/Artifacts	Significance When Found in the Urine	Microscopic Appearance
Bacteria	More than 100,000 bacteria per ml indicates urinary tract infection 10,000 to 100,000 bacteria per ml indicates that tests should be repeated Less than 10,000 bacteria per ml may signify urine in which any bacteria are due to urethral organisms or contamination Bacterial accompanied by white blood cells and/or white cell or mixed casts may indicate acute pyelonephritis	*
Yeast	May indicate contamination by yeasts from skin or hair May indicate diabetes mellitus or urinary tract infection *Candida albicans* may occur in patients with diabetes mellitus or in the contaminated urine of female patients with candidal vaginitis	*
Parasites and parasitic ova	Usually indicate fecal or vaginal contamination and should be reported *Trichomonas* may be found in patients with urethritis and in the contaminated urine of women with *Trichomonas* vaginitis Pinworm is a common contaminant and should be reported	*
Spermatozoa	Nonpathologic	*

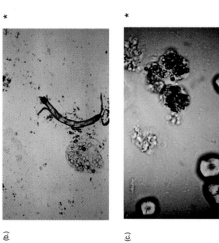

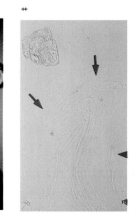

(a.)

(b.)

(c.)

(d.)

Urinary artifacts
Hair (a)
Starch from
  surgical gloves
Pollen grains
Bubbles
Oil droplets
Fibers (b)
Talc (c)
Dust
Mucus threads (d)
Glass particles

Nonpatholgic
May result from improper urine collection,
  improper slide preparation, or
  outside contamination

Text courtesy Boehringer Mannheim Diagnostics, Indianapolis, Indiana.
*Photomicrographs courtesy Bayer Corporation, Diagnostics Division, Elkhart, Indiana.
†Photomicrograph from Lehman C.A.: *Saunders Manual of Clinical Laboratory Science*, Philadelphia. W.B. Saunders, 1998.
‡Photomicrograph from Stepp C.A., Woods M.: *Laboratory Procedures for Medical Office Personnel*. Philadelphia, W.B. Saunders, 1998.

PROCEDURE 16-6 Microscopic Examination of Urine: Kova Method

Outcome Prepare a urine specimen for microscopic analysis and examine the specimen under the microscope.

Equipment/Supplies:
- Disposable gloves
- Urine specimen (first-voided morning specimen)
- Kova urine centrifuge tube
- Kova cap
- Kova pipet
- Kova slide
- Kova stain
- Test tube rack
- Urine centrifuge
- Mechanical stage microscope

Preparing the Specimen:

1. Procedural Step. Sanitize the hands, and assemble the equipment.

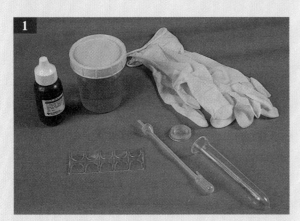

2. Procedural Step. Apply gloves. Mix the urine specimen with the Kova pipet.
Principle. The specimen must be well mixed to ensure accurate test results.

3. Procedural Step. Pour the urine specimen into the urine centrifuge tube. Fill it to the 12-ml graduation mark, and cap the tube.

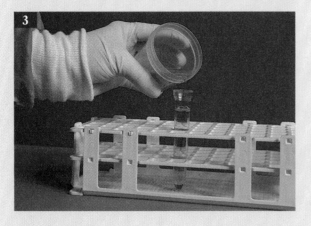

4. Procedural Step. Centrifuge the tube for 5 minutes at approximately 1500 revolutions per minute (rpm).

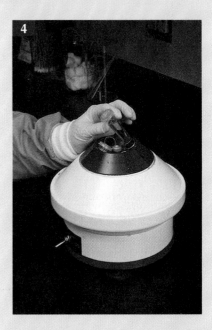

Principle. Centrifuging the specimen causes the solid elements in the urine to settle to the bottom of the tube.

5. Procedural Step. Remove the urine tube from the centrifuge, being careful not to disturb or dislodge the sediment.

6. Procedural Step. Remove the cap. Insert the Kova pipet into the urine tube and push it to the bottom of the tube until it seats firmly. Make sure the clip on the bulb is hooked over the outside edge of the tube.

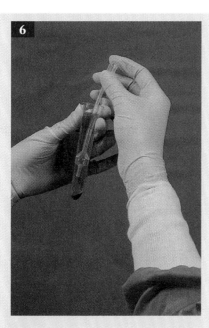

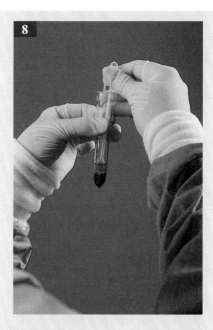

7. **Procedural Step.** Decant the specimen by inverting the tube and pouring off the supernatant fluid. Approximately 1.0 ml of sediment will be retained in the bottom of the tube.

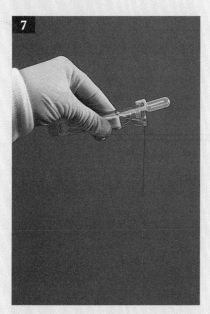

8. **Procedural Step.** Remove the pipet from the tube. Add 1 drop of Kova stain to the tube. Place the pipet back in the tube, and mix the sediment and stain together vigorously with the pipet. Make sure the sediment and stain are well mixed. Place the urine tube in a test tube rack.

Principle. Kova stain improves the detail of the sediment for better visualization of structures under the microscope.

9. **Procedural Step.** Transfer a sample of the sediment to the Kova slide as follows:
a. Place the Kova slide on a flat surface with the open "envelope" areas facing upward.
b. Squeeze the bulb of the pipet to draw a sample of the sediment into the tip of the pipet.
c. Place the tip of the pipet so that it just touches the notched corner edge of the slide.
d. Gently squeeze the bulb to allow the specimen to fill the well. Do not overfill or underfill the well.
e. Place the pipet in the urine tube.

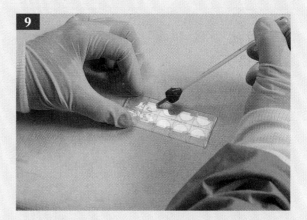

10. **Procedural Step.** Allow the specimen to sit for 1 full minute to permit the sediment to settle in the well.

Principle. Allowing the sediment to settle prevents structures from moving when viewing the slide under the microscope.

Continued

PROCEDURE 16-6 Microscopic Examination of Urine: Kova Method—Cont'd

Examining the Sediment:

11. **Procedural Step.** Focus the specimen under low power as follows:
    (*Note:* Also refer to Chapter 20, Procedure 20-1, for use of a microscope.)
    a. Turn on the light source. Rotate the nosepiece of the microscope to the low-power objective (10 ✕), making sure to click it into place.
    b. Place the slide on the microscope stage, and ensure it is secure.
    c. Look through the ocular. Use the coarse adjustment knob to bring the specimen into coarse focus.
    d. Use the fine adjustment knob to bring the specimen into a sharp clear focus.
    e. Decrease the light intensity with the iris diaphragm as needed to provide maximum focus and contrast.

12. **Procedural Step.** Examine the sediment under low power to scan for the presence of casts.

13. **Procedural Step.** Focus the specimen under high-power as follows:
    a. Rotate the nosepiece to the high-power objective (40✕), making sure it clicks into place.
    b. Use the fine adjustment knob to bring the specimen into a precise focus. Do not use the coarse adjustment to focus the high-power objective to prevent the objective from striking the slide.
    c. Adjust the light intensity with the iris diaphragm as needed to provide maximum focus and contrast.

14. **Procedural Step.** Examine the specimen under high power as follows:
    a. Identify the specific type of casts (if present).
    b. Examine the sediment for the presence of smaller structures, such as red blood cells, white blood cells, bacteria, or crystals. Ten to fifteen high-power fields should be examined, and an average recorded.

15. **Procedural Step.** Turn off the light source, and remove the slide from the stage.

16. **Procedural Step.** Dispose of the plastic slide and pipet in a regular waste container. Rinse the remaining urine down the sink. Cap the empty plastic urine tube and dispose of it in a regular waste container.

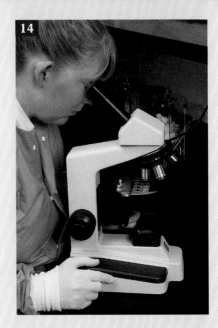

14

17. **Procedural Step.** Remove gloves and sanitize your hands.

18. **Procedural Step.** Chart the results as follows:
    a. Record casts as the average number and type seen per low-power field.
    b. Record red blood cells, white blood cells, and epithelial cells as the average number viewed per high-power field. Record other structures such as crystals, bacteria, yeast, and spermatozoa as occasional, frequent, or many.

LAB REPORT

Date	Time	Name	
3/18/05	10:00 a.m.	Tanya Howe	
		MICROSCOPIC	
	WBC'S		20 /HPF
	RBC'S		3 /HPF
	CASTS (Hyaline)		0 /LPF
	CASTS (Granular)		0 /LPF
	CASTS (Cellular)		0 /LPF
	CASTS (Waxy)		0 /LPF
	EPITHELIAL CELLS		0 /LPF
	BACTERIA		Freq
	MUCUS		Occ
	CRYSTALS		0
			L. Proffitt, CMA

Rapid Urine Cultures

A urine culture is used to assist in diagnosis of a UTI and the assessment of the effectiveness of antibiotic therapy for a patient with a UTI.

Rapid urine culture tests are sometimes used in the medical office to culture a urine specimen; brand names include Uricult and Urichek. They provide more immediate results compared with sending the specimen to an outside laboratory for culture. Rapid urine cultures consist of a slide attached to a screw cap. Each side of the slide is coated with an agar medium suitable for the growth of urinary bacteria. If the surface of the agar medium is dehy-drated or if evidence exists of mold or bacterial growth, the culture test should not be used but discarded in an appropriate receptacle. The slide is suspended in a clean plastic vial, which protects it from contamination during inoculation, storage, or handling.

The type of urine specimen that provides the most accurate results is a clean-catch midstream specimen collected after the urine has been in the bladder at least 4 to 6 hours.

The procedure for performing a rapid urine culture test is presented in Procedure 16-7.

PROCEDURE 16-7   Performing a Rapid Urine Culture Test

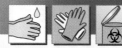

Outcome Perform a rapid urine culture test.

Equipment/Supplies:
- Disposable gloves
- Rapid urine culture kit
- Urine specimen (clean-catch midstream specimen)
- Incubator
- Biohazard waste container

Preparing the Specimen:

1. Procedural Step. Sanitize your hands, and assemble the equipment. Check the expiration date on the rapid culture test. It should not be used if the expiration date has passed. Label the vial with the patient's name and the date and time of inoculation. *Principle.* An expired urine culture test may produce inaccurate test results.

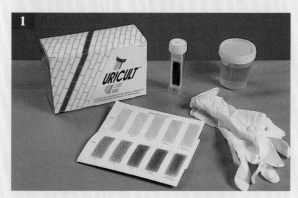

2. Procedural Step. Apply gloves. Remove the slide from its protective vial by unscrewing the cap of the vial, being careful not to touch the culture media.

3. Procedural Step. Dip the agar-coated slide into the urine specimen; it must be completely immersed. If the urine volume is not sufficient to fully immerse the agar slide, the urine may be poured over the agar surfaces.

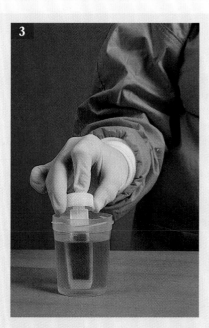

4. Procedural Step. Allow excess urine to drain from the slide.

5. Procedural Step. Immediately replace the inoculated slide in its protective vial. Screw the cap on loosely.

Continued

PROCEDURE 16-7

PROCEDURE 16-7 Performing a Rapid Urine Culture Test—Cont'd

6. Procedural Step. Place the vial upright in an incubator for 18 to 24 hours at 93° to 100° F (35° to 38° C).

Principle. Incubation for more than 24 hours may cause erroneous test results.

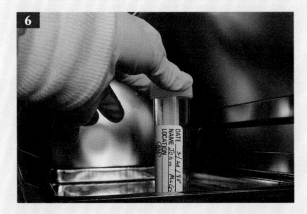

Reading Test Results:

7. Procedural Step. Apply gloves. Remove the vial from the incubator after the incubation period. Remove the slide from its protective vial, and compare the bacterial colony count density on the agar surface with the colony density reference chart provided by the manufacturer. The bacterial colony density on the agar surface should be matched with the printed example it most closely resembles on the colony density chart. (No actual bacterial colony counting is necessary.)

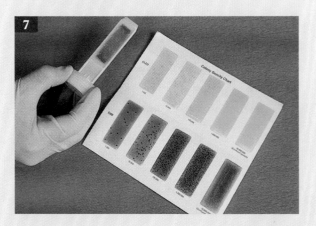

8. Procedural Step. Interpret results. The results of rapid urine tests are interpreted as follows:

Normal: Less than 10,000 bacteria/ml of urine. *Significance:* A normal result indicates the absence of infection.

Borderline: 10,000 to 100,000 bacteria/ml of urine. *Significance:* A borderline result may be caused by chronic and relapsing infections, and it is recommended that the test be repeated.

Positive:

   a. More than 100,000 bacteria/ml of urine.

   b. Confluent growth, or complete coverage of the agar surface with bacterial colonies, which may occasionally occur when a colony count is more than 100,000 bacteria/ml.

   Significance: A positive result indicates that a bacterial infection is present.

9. Procedural Step. Return the slide to the vial and screw on the cap. (*Note:* To aid in the safe disposal of inoculated slides, it is recommended that the slide be immersed in a disinfectant solution, such as 3% phenol solution or Cidex, before placing the slide in the vial.)

10. Procedural Step. Dispose of the rapid culture test in a biohazard waste container. Remove the gloves, and sanitize the hands.

11. Procedural Step. Chart the results. Include the date and time, the name of the test (e.g., Uricult, Urichek), and the results.

CHARTING EXAMPLE	
Date	
3/21/05	10:00 a.m. Uricult: Normal. —— L. Proffitt, CMA

Urine Pregnancy Testing

The determination of pregnacy can be accomplished in a number of ways. By the eighth week after fertilization, pregnancy can be confirmed with the medical history and physical examination. However, the physician may desire an earlier diagnosis with a pregnancy test to initiate early prenatal care. A pregnancy test may also be necessary before certain medications are ordered or procedures are performed that may cause injury to a fetus.

In the medical office, immunologic tests are often used for pregnancy testing. These tests are performed on a concentrated urine specimen and rely on the presence of a hormone known as human chorionic gonadotropin (HCG) for a positive reaction.

Human Chorionic Gonadotropin

Human chorionic gonadotropin is produced by the developing fertilized egg, and small amounts of it are secreted into the urine and blood. Immediately after conception and implantation of the fertilized egg, the plasma level of HCG rises rapidly and can be used to detect pregnancy approximately 1 to 5 days after the first missed menstrual period. The highest plasma levels of HCG occur at about the eighth week after conception. After this time, the production of HCG declines and remains at a lower level for the duration of the pregnancy. Within 72 hours of delivery, HCG disappears entirely from the plasma. As a result, pregnancy tests are more sensitive during the first trimester and may even show a negative reaction once the level of HCG begins to decline during the second and third trimester.

Testing Methods

The two main types of urine pregnancy tests are immunoassay enzyme tests and **agglutination** tests. These tests are used in the medical office because they are convenient to perform and provide immediate test results. Positive and negative reactions are evidenced by a specific visible reaction that is observed and interpreted by the individual performing the test.

Urine pregnancy tests are commercially available in kits that contain all the required reagents and supplies to perform the test. Each kit can be used to perform a specific number of tests, ranging between 10 and 50. The manufacturer's instructions should be carefully followed to prevent inaccurate test results. When used properly, urine pregnancy tests are 95% accurate.

Agglutination Tests. The slide agglutination test is sometimes used to perform pregnancy testing in the medical office. Positive test results are based on the inhibition of latex particle agglutination. The test takes place in two steps and can be performed in only 2 minutes. In the first step, a drop of the urine specimen is placed on a specially provided glass slide that comes with the kit. An HCG antiserum reagent (antibody) is then added to the urine

specimen. If the patient's urine contains HCG, the antiserum combines with the HCG (antigen) in the urine specimen, resulting in an antigen-antibody reaction.

The next step involves the addition of an antigen reagent containing latex particles coated with HCG. If the antigen-antibody reaction has previously occurred in the first step of the procedure, no available HCG antiserum is left in the specimen to react with the latex particles. Therefore, the absence of agglutination on the slide test, known as agglutination inhibition, indicates a positive reaction for pregnancy. On the other hand, if agglutination occurs on the slide, the results are interpreted as negative (Figure 16-8). Coating the HCG with latex permits visible agglutination that can be observed and interpreted as a negative reaction by the individual performing the test. Without the latex, agglutination would not be visible when the HCG antigen and antibody combine.

Immunoassay Tests. Immunoassay tests provide for the rapid, qualitative detection of HCG in a urine specimen; brand names include QuickVue, Clearview, Contrast, and Cards QS. Some brands of tests are able to detect pregnancy as early as 1 week after implantation, or 4 to 5 days before a first missed menstrual period. It is recommended, however, that tests performed this early be repeated later to confirm the results.

Immunoassay tests take approximately 5 minutes to perform and are easier to read than agglutination tests because the results are easily observed as a color change. Specific instructions for the test are included with each commercially available testing kit. The procedure for performing an immunoassay test with QuickVue (Quidel) is outlined in Procedure 16-8.

Guidelines for Urine Pregnancy Testing

Specific guidelines must be followed in a urine pregnancy test to ensure accurate test results.

1. Use clean, preferably disposable, urine containers to collect the specimen. Traces of detergent in the specimen container may cause inaccurate test results.
2. Use a first-voided morning specimen because it contains the highest concentration of HCG. If the urine specimen cannot be tested immediately after voiding, it

Slide agglutination method

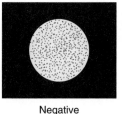
Negative

Positive

Figure 16-8. Urine pregnancy test results: slide agglutination method.

should be preserved in the refrigerator. The patient who collects the specimen at home should be given instructions on preserving the specimen.

3. The specific gravity of the urine specimen should be determined before the test is performed. A specific gravity of less than 1.010 is considered too dilute for pregnancy testing because it may lead to a false-negative test result.

4. The urine specimen should be at room temperature before the procedure is performed.

5. The urine pregnancy testing kit should be stored according to the manufacturer's instructions. Most testing kits can be stored either at room temperature or in the refrigerator. If a kit is stored in the refrigerator, however, the reagents must be brought to room temperature before use to ensure accurate test results.

6. Testing kits past their expiration dates should not be used.

Serum Pregnancy Test

The radioimmunoassay (RIA) for HCG is used to detect HCG in the serum of the blood. This test is more sensitive than a urine test and can detect pregnancy at approximately the eighth day after fertilization; therefore, the pregnancy can be detected even before the time of the missed menstrual period. This test uses a radioisotope technique and is capable of detecting minute amounts of HCG in the blood. This test is generally used to diagnose abnormalities, such as ectopic pregnancy, to follow the course of early pregnancy when abnormalities of embryonic development are suspected, and to provide an early diagnosis of pregnancy in individuals at high risk, such as patients with diabetes.

PROCEDURE 16-8   Performing a Urine Pregnancy Test

Outcome Perform a urine pregnancy test.

Equipment/Supplies:
- Disposable gloves
- Urine pregnancy testing kit (QuickVue by Quidel)
- Urine specimen (first-voided morning specimen)

1. **Procedural Step.** Sanitize the hands, and assemble the equipment. Check the expiration date on the urine pregnancy test. It should not be used if the expiration date has passed.
Principle. An expired pregnancy test may produce inaccurate test results.

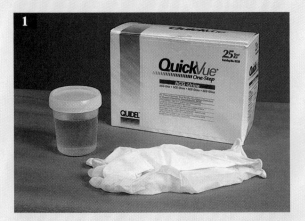

2. **Procedural Step.** Apply gloves. Remove the test cassette from its foil pouch, and place it on a clean, dry, level surface.

3. **Procedural Step.** Add three drops of urine to the round sample well on the test cassette with a disposable pipet supplied with the kit. The test cassette should not be handled again until the test is ready for interpretation. Dispose of the pipet in a regular waste container.

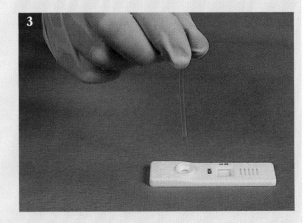

4. **Procedural Step.** Wait 3 minutes, and read the results by observing the result window.
5. **Procedural Step.** Interpret the test results as follows:
Negative: The appearance of the blue procedural control line next to the letter "C" only and no pink-to-purple test line next the letter "T."
Positive: The appearance of any pink-to-purple line next to the letter "T" along with a blue procedural control line next to the letter "C."
No result: If no blue procedural control line appears, the test result is invalid and the specimen must be retested.

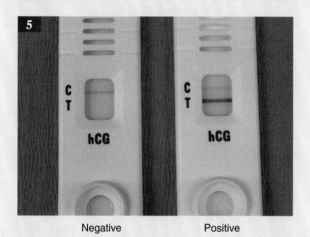

Negative   Positive

6. **Procedural Step.** Dispose of the test cassette in a regular waste container. Remove gloves and sanitize your hands.
7. **Procedural Step.** Chart the results. Include the date and time of the patient's last menstrual period (LMP), the name of the test, and the results recorded as either positive or negative.

CHARTING EXAMPLE

Date	
3/25/05	10:30 a.m. LMP: 2/20/05.
	QuickVue preg test: Positive. ————
	———————— L. Proffitt, CMA

PROCEDURE 16-8

MEDICAL Practice and the LAW

In collection and analysis of patient urine, meticulous attention should be paid to patient instructions such as cleansing and collecting first morning, midstream, or 24-hour specimens.

Patients are often embarrassed to have someone else see their urine, so handle urine specimens in a professional, matter-of-fact manner, with universal precautions to protect yourself.

As with all diagnostic procedures, care must be taken to perform the test correctly and treat results confidentially.

Civil Versus Criminal Law
Civil law involves a conflict with another person, and if found guilty by a preponderance of evidence (>50%), the loser may lose money or property. Malpractice is a type of civil law. Civil law is divided into *torts,* or wrongs, and *contracts,* or promises. Malpractice is a tort, and nonpayment for services is a contract.

Criminal law involves a conflict with society as a whole (local, state, or federal law). If found guilty beyond a reasonable doubt, the loser may lose money, property, freedom (jail), or life (execution). Violation of licensure laws and failure to report child abuse are criminal suits.

What Would You DO?
What Would You *Not* DO? *RESPONSES*

Case Study 1
What Did Linda Do?

❑ Took some time to try to calm and relax Mr. Urameshi. Reassured him that the physician would do everything he could to make him better.

❑ Offered Mr. Urameshi something to drink and told him it might help him obtain a specimen.

❑ Went over the directions again with Mr. Urameshi.

❑ Asked Mr. Urameshi if he would try again to obtain a specimen.

What Did Linda Not Do?

❑ Did not tell Mr. Urameshi that he was not trying hard enough.

What Would You Do?/What Would You *Not* Do? Review Linda's response and place a checkmark next to the information you included in your response. List additional information you included in your response below.

_____
_____
_____
_____

Case Study 2
What Did Linda Do?

❑ Asked Nora if she takes all of the antibiotic she is prescribed when she has a UTI.

❑ Explained to Nora in terms she can understand why women seem to be more prone to development of UTIs.

❑ Explained to Nora what she could do to help prevent UTIs. Gave her a patient education brochure on UTIs to take home.

❑ Told Nora that the physician is not legally or ethically permitted to call in a prescription for her without seeing her. Also explained that it is in the best interests of her health care to be seen by the physician.

What Did Linda Not Do?

❑ Did not tell Nora that she could not test her urine at home.

What Would You Do?/What Would You *Not* Do? Review Linda's response and place a checkmark next to the information you included in your response. List additional information you included in your response below.

_____
_____
_____
_____

Case Study 3
What Did Linda Do?

❑ Told Rita that some peanut butter residue might have been left in the jar she used and might have affected the test results. Asked her to collect another specimen at the office so that the urine could be tested again.

❑ Told Rita if something happens to the specimen container again, she should come to the office and get another one.

❑ Told Rita that several things could have caused her pregnancy test result to be negative. Explained to her that the test could have been outdated or not stored properly. Also explained that as a pregnancy gets further along, less of the hormone that causes the test to be positive is secreted, so negative test results at the end of a pregnancy are not unusual.

❑ Reassured Rita that many women have trouble sleeping during the last month of the pregnancy and that it is normal to have more Braxton-Hicks contractions as she gets closer to delivery.

❑ Told Rita that Linda would inform the physician of her symptoms so that he could discuss them in more detail with her.

What Did Linda Not Do?

❑ Did not criticize Rita for collecting her specimen in a peanut butter jar.

❑ Did not ignore or minimize Rita's concerns.

What Would You Do?/What Would You *Not* Do? Review Linda's response and place a checkmark next to the information you included in your response. List additional information you included in your response below.

_____
_____
_____
_____

Apply Your KNOWLEDGE

Choose the best answer for each of the following questions.

1. Ernie Arnold calls the office and describes symptoms that indicate that he has polyuria. Which of the following *would not* result in polyuria?
   A. Consuming caffeine
   B. Vomiting
   C. Diabetes mellitus
   D. Excessive fluid intake

2. Esther Williams has come to the office with symptoms of dysuria, frequency, and foul-smelling urine. Dr. Frequency asks Linda Proffitt, CMA, to collect a urine specimen that will be evaluated for the presence of bacteria. Linda instructs Esther to obtain a:
   A. Random specimen
   B. First-voided morning specimen
   C. Clean-catch midstream specimen
   D. 24-hour urine specimen

3. Rhonda Gibbs has come to the office for a complete physical. She has brought in a first-voided urine specimen for a urinalysis. Which of the following would indicate that her specimen has been allowed to stand at room temperature for too long?
   A. The urine is cloudy
   B. The pH is acidic
   C. The specific gravity is 1.010
   D. The urine is straw in color

4. Tammy Speakes has *just* obtained a freshly voided urine specimen at the medical office. Linda Proffitt, CMA, is getting ready to test the specimen and notices that the urine is cloudy. This may indicate that:
   A. The specimen has been retained in the bladder for too long
   B. Nitrates are present in the specimen
   C. Tammy used improper technique to collect the specimen
   D. A UTI is present

5. Tom Albert comes to the medical office for a general physical examination. As part of the examination, Linda Proffitt, CMA, needs to perform a complete urinalysis. Dr. Frequency asks Linda to determine whether Mr. Albert's urine is concentrated. Of the following results, which would indicate the concentration of the urine?
   A. pH of 6
   B. RBCs: 3/HPF
   C. Protein: trace
   D. Specific gravity: 1.025

6. Mr. Albert has been on a high protein and low carbohydrate diet for the past week. Mr. Albert's chemical analysis of urine indicates that he has a "small" amount of ketones in his urine. This is an example of a:
   A. Quantitative result
   B. Qualitative result
   C. Microscopic result
   D. Falsely positive result

7. After the chemical analysis of Mr. Albert's urine is performed, Linda is recording the results. In *normal* urine, Linda would expect to find:
   A. Ketones
   B. Urea
   C. Bilirubin
   D. Glucose

8. Jessica Sanders has a UTI. When Linda Profitt, CMA, performs a chemical analysis of Jessica's urine, she would expect all of the following to be positive EXCEPT:
   A. Nitrite
   B. Protein
   C. Bilirubin
   D. Leukocytes

9. Samantha Pidcock, age 18 years, has just given Linda Proffitt, CMA, a freshly voided urine specimen. The specimen is positive for blood. Linda should:
   A. Ask her if she is pregnant
   B. Ask her if she is presently on her menstrual period
   C. Notify the physician that Samantha has a UTI
   D. Tell her she will need to collect another urine specimen

10. Katie Lavelle comes to the medical office. She has missed her menstrual period and hopes she might be pregnant. Linda Proffitt, CMA, performs a urine pregnancy test on Katie. Which of the following would be an ERROR in technique for performing the test?
    A. A random specimen is used to run the test
    B. The specific gravity of the specimen is 1.020
    C. The specimen is at room temperature
    D. The urine pregnancy testing kit is within its expiration date

CERTIFICATIONREVIEW

❑ **The function of the urinary system** is to regulate the fluid and electrolyte balance of the body and to remove waste products. The structures that make up the urinary system are the kidneys, the ureters, the urinary bladder, and the urethra.

❑ **The nephron** is considered the functional unit of the kidney. Each kidney is composed of approximately 1 million nephrons. The nephron filters waste substances from the blood and dilutes them with water to produce urine. Another function of the nephron is reabsorption.

❑ **Urine is composed of** 95% water and 5% organic and inorganic waste products. The normal adult excretes approximately 750 to 2000 ml of urine per day.

❑ **An excessive increase in urine output** is known as polyuria and may be caused by the excessive intake of fluids, certain drugs, diabetes mellitus, and renal disease. A decreased output of urine is known as oliguria and may be caused by decreased fluid intake, dehydration, profuse perspiration, vomiting, diarrhea, or kidney disease.

❑ **The type of test to be performed** often dictates the method used to collect the urine specimen. A first-voided morning specimen contains the greatest concentration of dissolved substances and is recommended for the microscopic examination of urine. A clean-catch midstream specimen is recommended for the detection of a UTI. A 24-hour specimen is used to quantitatively measure specific substances in the urine.

❑ **A complete urinalysis** consists of a physical, chemical, and microscopic examination of urine. A deviation from normal in any of the three areas assists the physician in the diagnosis and treatment of pathologic conditions. A urine specimen should not be left standing out for more than 1 hour because changes take place that affect the test results.

❑ **A physical examination of urine** involves a determination of the color, appearance, and specific gravity of the urine. Dilute urine tends to be a lighter yellow in color, whereas concentrated urine is a darker yellow. Fresh urine is usually clear and transparent.

❑ **The specific gravity of urine** ranges from 1.003 to 1.030 but is usually between 1.010 and 1.025. Dilute urine contains fewer dissolved substances and has a lower specific gravity; concentrated urine has a higher specific gravity from the increased amount of dissolved substances.

❑ **The chemical testing of urine** is a means of detecting abnormal amounts of chemicals in the body, which may indicate a pathologic condition. Chemical tests include pH, glucose, protein, ketones, blood, bilirubin, urobilinogen, nitrite, and leukocytes.

❑ **A microscopic examination** of the urine sediment helps clarify results of the physical and chemical examination. Structures that may be found in microscopic examination of urine include red and white blood cells, epithelial cells, casts, crystals, and miscellaneous structures such as mucous threads, bacteria, yeast cells, parasites, and spermatozoa.

❑ **A urine culture** is used to assist in diagnosis of a UTI and to assess the effectiveness of antibiotic therapy for a patient with a UTI.

❑ **Human chorionic gonadotropin** is produced by the developing fertilized egg, and small amounts of it are secreted into the urine and blood. Urine pregnancy tests are used to detect the presence of HCG and can be used to detect pregnancy approximately 1 to 5 days after the first missed menstrual period.

Terminology Review

Agglutination The aggregation or uniting of separate particles into clumps or masses.

Bilirubinuria The presence of bilirubin in the urine.

Glycosuria The presence of sugar in the urine.

Ketonuria The presence of ketone bodies in the urine.

Ketosis An accumulation of large amounts of ketone bodies in the tissues and body fluids.

Micturition The act of voiding urine.

Nephron The functional unit of the kidney.

Oliguria Decreased or scanty output of urine.

pH The unit that describes the acidity or alkalinity of a solution.

Polyuria Increased output of urine.

Proteinuria The presence of protein in the urine.

Refractive index The ratio of the velocity of light in air to the velocity of light in a solution.

Refractometer *(clinical)* An instrument used to measure the refractive index of urine, which is an indirect measurement of the specific gravity of urine.

Renal threshold The concentration at which a substance in the blood that is not normally excreted by the kidneys begins to appear in the urine.

Specific gravity The weight of a substance as compared with the weight of an equal volume of a substance known as the standard. In urinalysis, the specific gravity refers to the measurement of the amount of dissolved substances present in the urine, as compared with the same amount of distilled water.

Supernatant The clear liquid that remains at the top after a precipitate settles.

Urinalysis The physical, chemical, and microscopic analysis of urine.

Void To empty the bladder.

ON THE WEB

For active weblinks to each website visit http://evolve.elsevier.com/Bonewit/.

For Information on Kidney Disease

National Kidney Foundation

National Institute of Diabetes and Digestive and Kidney Diseases

Renal Net

For Information on Drug Abuse

National Institute on Drug Abuse

American Council for Drug Education

Research Institute on Addictions

Learning Objectives	Procedures

Venipuncture

1. List and describe the patient preparation for venipuncture.
2. Explain how each of the following blood specimens is obtained:
   - Clotted blood
   - Serum
   - Whole blood
   - Plasma
3. List the layers the blood separates into when an anticoagulant is added to the specimen.
4. List the layers the blood separates into when an anticoagulant is *not* added to the specimen.
5. List the OSHA safety precautions that must be followed during venipuncture and separating serum or plasma from whole blood.
6. State the additive content of the following vacuum tubes, and list the type of blood specimens that can be obtained from each: red, lavender, gray, light blue, green, dark blue.
7. Identify and explain the order of draw for the vacuum tube and butterfly methods of venipuncture.
8. List and describe the guidelines for use of evacuated tubes.
9. Identify possible problems during a venipuncture.
10. List four ways to prevent a blood specimen from becoming hemolyzed.
11. Explain how the serum separator tube functions in the collection of a serum specimen.

Collect a venous blood specimen using the vacuum tube venipuncture method.

Collect a venous blood specimen using the butterfly venipuncture method.

Collect a venous blood specimen using the syringe venipuncture method.

Separate serum from a whole blood specimen.

Skin Puncture

1. Explain when a skin puncture would be preferred over a venipuncture.
2. Describe the following skin puncture devices: disposable lancet, disposable semiautomatic lancet, reusable semiautomatic lancet.
3. List and describe the guidelines for performing a finger puncture.

Obtain a capillary blood specimen using a disposable lancet.

Obtain a capillary blood specimen using a disposable semiautomatic lancet.

Obtain a capillary blood specimen using a reusable semiautomatic lancet.

CHAPTER 17

Phlebotomy

Chapter Outline

INTRODUCTION TO PHLEBOTOMY
VENIPUNCTURE
General Guidelines for Venipuncture
  Patient Preparation for Venipuncture
  Patient Position for Venipuncture
  Application of the Tourniquet
  Site Selection for Venipuncture
  Alternative Venipuncture Sites
  Types of Blood Specimen
  OSHA Safety Precautions
Vacuum Tube Method of Venipuncture
  Needle
  Plastic Holder
  Evacuated Tubes
  Order of Draw for Multiple Tubes
  Evacuated Tube Guidelines
Butterfly Method of Venipuncture
  Guidelines for the Butterfly Method
Syringe Method of Venipuncture
Problems Encountered With Venipuncture
  Failure to Obtain Blood
  Inappropriate Puncture Sites
  Scarred and Sclerosed Veins
  Rolling Veins
  Collapsing Veins
  Premature Needle Withdrawal
  Hematoma
  Hemolysis
  Fainting
Obtaining a Serum Specimen
  Serum
  Tube Selection
  Preparation of the Specimen
  Removal of Serum
  Serum Separator Tubes

Obtaining a Plasma Specimen
  Plasma
  Tube Selection
  Preparation and Removal of the Specimen
SKIN PUNCTURE
  Puncture Site
  Skin Puncture Devices
  Microcollection Devices
  Guidelines for a Finger Puncture

National Competencies

Clinical Competencies
Specimen Collection
- Perform venipuncture.
- Perform capillary puncture.

Key Terms

antecubital space (an-tih-KYOO-bih-tul SPAYS)
anticoagulant (an-tih-koe-AG-yoo-lent)
buffy coat
evacuated tube
hematoma (hee-mah-TOE-mah)
hemoconcentration (Hêe-moe-kon-sen-TRAY-shun)
hemolysis (hee-MOL-ih-sis)
osteochondritis (OS-tee-oh-kon-DRY-tis)
osteomyelitis (OS-tee-oh-mie-LIE-tis)
phlebotomist (fleh-BOT-oe-mist)
phlebotomy (fleh-BOT-oe-mee)
plasma
serum
venipuncture (VEN-ih-punk-chur)
venous reflux (VEEN-us-REE-fluks)
venous stasis (VEEN-us-STAE-sis)

Introduction to Phlebotomy

The purpose of phlebotomy is to collect a blood specimen for laboratory analysis. The word *phlebotomy* is derived from the Greek words for vein *(phlebos)* and incision *(tome),* and literally means making an incision into a vein. However, as used in the clinical laboratory sciences, **phlebotomy** is defined generally as the collection of blood. The individual who collects the blood sample is a **phlebotomist.**

Some blood specimens are tested in the medical office, and others are picked up and taken to a laboratory for testing. The latter specimens need to be accompanied by a laboratory request so that the laboratory personnel know what type of test the physician desires. The medical assistant may be responsible for filling out the laboratory request form. It should include the physician's name and address; the patient's name, address, age, and gender; the date and time of collection of the specimen; the physician's clinical diagnosis; and a check mark next to the type of test to be performed.

Phlebotomy encompasses three major areas of blood collection: arterial puncture, venipuncture, and skin puncture. An arterial puncture is typically performed in a hospital to assess the oxygen level, carbon dioxide level, and acid-base balance of arterial blood; hence medical assistants do not perform arterial punctures. In the medical office, medical assistants perform venipunctures and skin punctures; therefore this chapter focuses on these two ways to obtain blood.

VENIPUNCTURE

The term **venipuncture** means the puncturing of a vein for the removal of a venous blood sample. In the medical office a venipuncture is performed when a large blood specimen is needed for testing.

Venipuncture can be performed by the following three methods:
- Vacuum tube method
- Butterfly method
- Syringe method

The vacuum tube method is the fastest and most convenient of the three methods and is used most often. This method relies on the use of an **evacuated tube,** which is a closed glass or plastic tube that contains a vacuum. The butterfly and syringe methods are used for difficult draws such as when a vein is small or sclerosed (hardened). This chapter presents the theory and procedure for each method.

General Guidelines for Venipuncture

General guidelines that are common to all three methods of venipuncture include preparing the patient for the venipuncture, positioning the patient, applying the tourniquet, selecting a site for the venipuncture, obtaining the type of blood specimen required, and following the OSHA safety precautions. These areas are discussed in the following sections.

Patient Preparation for Venipuncture

The patient should be given appropriate instructions on advance preparation, if required. Although most tests require no preparation, some tests require fasting or the avoidance of certain medications. If the medical assistant is unsure whether a laboratory test requires special preparation by the patient, he or she should consult an appropriate reference. Reference sources consist of laboratory directories, instructions included with testing kits, and the laboratory that will test the blood specimen.

When a laboratory test requires advance preparation, before performing the venipuncture, verify that the patient has prepared properly. If the patient has not, do not collect the specimen unless directed otherwise by the physician. If the venipuncture is to be rescheduled, carefully review the preparation requirements with the patient.

Venipuncture is often a frightening experience for the patient. For many patients the anticipation of the procedure is worse than the actual drawing of the blood. The medical assistant should take time to explain the procedure to the patient in an unhurried and confident manner. This should allay the patient's fears, which should help to relax the patient's veins. Relaxed veins make venipuncture easier to perform and result in less pain for the patient.

Instruct the patient to remain still during the procedure. Explain to the patient that a small amount of pain is associated with a venipuncture, but it will be brief. Never tell the patient that the venipuncture will *not* hurt. Just before inserting the needle, tell the patient that he or she will "feel a small stick." This prevents startling the patient, which could cause the patient to move. Movement causes pain for the patient, and it may also damage the venipuncture site.

Patient Position for Venipuncture

The patient position for venipuncture is especially important to the successful collection of a blood specimen. Proper positioning allows easy access to the veins and is more comfortable for the patient. The patient position depends on the vein to be used. The most common site for venipuncture is the **antecubital space,** and the information presented next refers to this site.

The patient should be seated comfortably in a chair. The arm should be extended downward to form a straight line from the shoulder to the wrist with the palm facing up; the arm should not bend at the elbow. The arm should be well supported on the armrest by a rolled towel or by having the patient place the fist of the other hand under the elbow (Figure 17-1).

A venipuncture should never be performed with the patient sitting on a stool or standing. The possibility exists that the patient will faint and injure himself or herself. If the patient appears nervous or has fainted in the past from a venipuncture, it is best to place the patient in a semireclining position on the examining table. A pillow or a cushion should be placed under the patient's arm to support the arm in a straight line from the shoulder to the wrist.

Although unusual, it is possible for blood to flow from the evacuated tube back into the patient's vein during the procedure. This condition is known as **venous reflux.** Venous reflux could cause the patient to have an adverse reaction to a tube additive, particularly if the additive in the tube is EDTA (ethylenediaminetetraacetic acid). Venous reflux can occur only if the contents of the evacuated tube are in contact with the tube stopper while the specimen is being drawn. Venous reflux is prevented by keeping the patient's arm in a downward position so that the evacuated tube remains below the venipuncture site and fills from the bottom up.

Application of the Tourniquet

An important step in the venipuncture procedure is the application of the tourniquet. The tourniquet makes the patient's veins stand out so they are easier to palpate. The tourniquet acts as a "dam," which causes the venous blood to slow down and pool in the veins in front of the tourniquet. This pooling of blood makes the veins more prominent so that they are more visible and can be palpated.

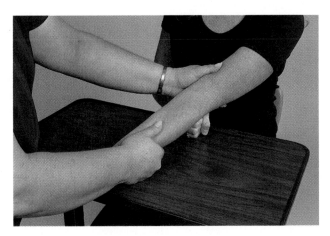

Figure 17-1. Patient position for obtaining blood specimen from the antecubital veins.

MY NAME IS Dori Glover, and I work in a very busy, fast-paced family practice office for two wonderful physicians. I love my job. The physicians are great, with very different styles, the pace is fast, and the time flies by. I am constantly challenged, learning new things, meeting and helping people, and being a part of a team that works well together.

While performing a routine finger stick for a blood glucose determination (a procedure I have performed many, many times), I accidentally stuck myself. I could see the blood inside my glove and I could see the patient's blood clinging to the point—my heart sank. I placed the lancet in the sharps container and tried to keep my cool and not alarm the patient. I mentally assessed the patient. He was an older man from a rural community, but I know you cannot always judge a book by its cover.

I excused myself and immediately proceeded to wash my hands thoroughly with soap and water and rinse, rinse, rinse! I then notified the physician. The physician questioned the patient regarding operations he had had in the previous year. He had undergone bypass surgery, and had received two units of blood. Although blood is effectively screened, I thought about that one-in-a-zillion chance that it could have been contaminated. Thankfully, I had received the hepatitis B immunization series, but there was still concern regarding hepatitis C and, of course, HIV.

The patient was gracious and complied with our request to be tested for hepatitis and HIV. The physician and I discussed the situation and we determined the risk to be low, but he nonetheless offered me the option of getting the HIV post-exposure prophylactic treatment. The window of time for this to be effective is only 1 to 2 hours after the stick. It is very toxic and therefore not something you want to receive needlessly. I declined and proceeded to wait 5 agonizing days for the patient's test results. The word *relief* hardly describes how I felt when the laboratory results came back negative!

This incident confirmed the importance of getting the hepatitis B immunization, as well as paying attention to good technique when performing procedures involving blood.

When applying a tourniquet, it is very important to obtain the correct tourniquet tension. The tourniquet should be applied with enough tension to slow the venous flow without affecting the arterial flow. A tourniquet that is too tight obstructs the arterial blood flow and the venous flow, which may result in a specimen that produces inaccurate test results. On the other hand, a tourniquet that is too loose fails to cause the veins to stand out enough to be palpated. A correctly applied tourniquet should fit snugly and not pinch the patient's skin.

Guidelines for Applying the Tourniquet

The following guidelines help to ensure the successful application of the tourniquet:

1. Do not apply the tourniquet over sores or burned skin.
2. Place the tourniquet 3 to 4 inches above the bend in the elbow. This allows adequate room for cleansing the site and performing the venipuncture without the tourniquet getting in the way.
3. Apply the tourniquet so that it is snug, but not so tight that it pinches the patient's skin or is otherwise painful to the patient.
4. When applying the tourniquet, ask the patient to clench his or her fist. This pushes blood from the lower arm into the veins and makes them easier to palpate. You can ask the patient to clench and unclench the fist a few times; however, vigorous pumping should be avoided because it could lead to hemoconcentration, which could produce inaccurate test results.
5. Never leave the tourniquet on for more than 1 minute because it will be uncomfortable for the patient. In addition, prolonged application of the tourniquet causes the venous blood to stagnate, or stay in one place too long, a condition known as **venous stasis.** When venous stasis occurs, the plasma portion of the blood filters into the tissues, causing **hemoconcentration,** or an increase in the concentration of nonfilterable blood components such as red blood cells, enzymes, iron, and calcium, which can alter test results.
6. Ideally you should remove the tourniquet as soon as a good blood flow is established; however, this may not be practical when first learning the venipuncture procedure. Removing the tourniquet may cause the needle to move so no more blood can be obtained, and the blood has to be redrawn. Therefore when learning the venipuncture procedure, it is better to wait until just before the needle is removed before removing the tourniquet.
7. Always remove the tourniquet before removing the needle from the patient's arm. If the needle is removed first, the pressure of the tourniquet causes blood to be forced out of the puncture site and into the surrounding skin, resulting in a **hematoma.**
8. After use, wipe a tourniquet thoroughly with a disinfectant such as alcohol. Disposable tourniquets are available that are thrown away after one use.

Types of Tourniquet

The most common tourniquets are the *rubber* tourniquet and the *Velcro-closure tourniquet.* The type of tourniquet used is a matter of individual preference.

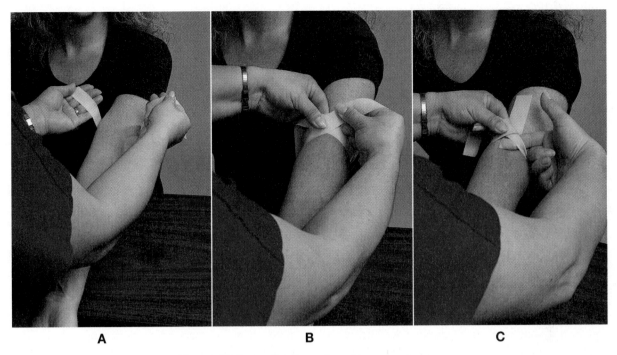

Figure 17-2. Application of a rubber tourniquet.

Rubber Tourniquet. The rubber tourniquet consists of a flat, soft band of rubber approximately 1 inch (2.5 cm) wide and 15 to 18 inches (38 to 45 cm) long. It offers the advantage of being easily removable with one hand. The technique for applying a rubber tourniquet is described next and illustrated in Figure 17-2.

Procedure: Rubber Tourniquet

1. Hold each end of the tourniquet with one hand. Position the tourniquet 3 to 4 inches (7.5 to 10 cm) above the bend in the elbow, making sure that the tourniquet lies flat against the patient's skin. Pull the ends away from each other to create tension (Figure 17-2, *A*).
2. Bring the ends of the tourniquet toward each other and cross one over the other at the point of your grasp with enough tension so that the tourniquet is snug but not pinching the patient's skin (Figure 17-2, *B*).
3. Tuck a portion of the top length into the bottom length, forming a loop. This allows for a one-handed release of the tourniquet when pulled on one end. Make sure the flaps are directed upward so that they do not dangle into the working area (Figure 17-2, *C*).

Velcro-Closure Tourniquet. The Velcro-closure tourniquet consists of a band of rubber or elastic material with Velcro attached at the ends. This type of tourniquet is easier to apply and tends to be more comfortable for the patient than the rubber tourniquet. The disadvantage to the

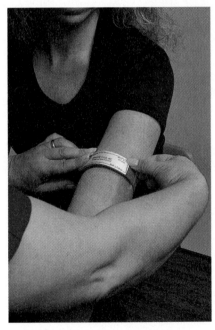

Figure 17-3. Application of a Velcro-closure tourniquet.

Velcro-closure tourniquet is that it is more difficult to remove with one hand than the rubber tourniquet. In addition, this type of tourniquet may not fit around the arms of extremely obese patients. The technique for applying a Velcro-closure tourniquet is described next and illustrated in Figure 17-3.

Procedure: Velcro-Closure Tourniquet

1. Hold each end of the tourniquet with one hand. Position the tourniquet 3 to 4 inches (7.5 to 10 cm) above the bend in the elbow.
2. Wrap the tourniquet around the arm and secure it with the Velcro fastener. The tourniquet should be applied with enough tension so that it is snug but not pinching the patient's skin.

Site Selection for Venipuncture

For most patients, the best site to use is the veins in the antecubital space (Figure 17-4). If the patient has large, accessible antecubital veins, drawing blood is easy. On the other hand, if the patient has small veins or veins that cannot be palpated, obtaining a blood specimen can be quite a challenge, even for the most experienced medical assistant.

The antecubital space is the surface of the arm in front of the elbow. The antecubital veins generally have a wide lumen, are easily accessible, and are close to the surface of the skin. In addition, these veins typically have thick walls, making them less likely to collapse. Using the antecubital space spares the patient unnecessary pain because the skin is less sensitive there than other sites (such as the back of the hand). The medical assistant should not be misled by the presence, in some patients, of many small very blue "spidery" veins that lie very close to the surface of the skin.

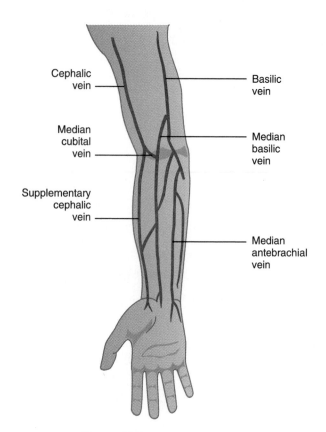

Figure 17-4. Antecubital veins.

These veins are not suitable for performing a venipuncture. The antecubital veins lie beneath these veins.

The best vein to use in the antecubital space is the *median cubital*. The median cubital is a prominent vein in the middle of the antecubital space (see Figure 17-4). At times, however, the median cubital vein cannot be used, for example, when it lies deep in the tissues and cannot be palpated or is scarred from repeated venipunctures.

The *basilic* and *cephalic* veins are located on opposite sides of the antecubital space and are a good alternative when the median cubital vein is not available. The disadvantage of these "side" veins is that they tend to roll or move away from the needle, thereby escaping puncture. To prevent rolling, firm pressure should be applied below the vein to stabilize it as the needle is inserted.

The brachial artery is also located in the antecubital space. Before performing a venipuncture, palpate for the presence of this artery. Unlike a vein, an artery pulsates, is more elastic, and has a thicker wall than a vein. If the brachial artery is inadvertently punctured, the patient feels more than the usual amount of pain and the blood is bright red and comes out in pulsing movements. If this situation occurs, the tourniquet should be removed and then the needle. Pressure with a gauze pad should then be applied for 4 to 5 minutes.

Guidelines for Site Selection

There are specific guidelines that should be followed to facilitate the selection of a good vein. These guidelines are as follows:

1. Ensure that the lighting is adequate. Good lighting facilitates inspection of the veins.
2. Examine the antecubital veins of both arms. The best site to perform a venipuncture varies with each individual. Some patients have larger veins in one arm than in the other. It is advisable to ask the patient if he or she has had a venipuncture before. Most adult patients have had previous venipunctures and know which of their veins are best to use and which should be avoided. Listen to and evaluate information offered by the patient.
3. Ensure that the veins "stand out" as much as possible. Before locating a venipuncture site, always apply the tourniquet and have the patient make a fist. This combination makes the veins more prominent.
4. Always palpate for the median cubital vein first. It is usually bigger and anchored better and bruises less than the other veins. If the median cubital is good in both arms, select the one that appears the fullest. The cephalic vein is the second choice (over the basilic vein) because it does not roll and bruise as easily as the basilic vein.
5. Use inspection and *particularly* palpation to select a vein. A vein does not have to be seen in order to be a good selection. If you cannot see a vein, palpation alone can be used to locate it. A vein feels like an elastic tube that "gives" under the pressure of the fingertips.

6. Thoroughly assess the patient's veins. To assess a vein as a possible site for the venipuncture, place one or two fingertips (index and ring fingers) over it and press lightly, then release pressure. Do not use your thumb to palpate the vein because it is not as sensitive as the index finger. To be suitable for a venipuncture, the vein should feel round, firm, elastic, and engorged. When you depress and release an engorged vein, it should spring back in a rounded, filled state.

7. Determine the size, depth, and direction of the vein. Once a suitable vein has been located, it should be thoroughly and carefully palpated to determine the direction of the vein and to estimate the size and depth of the vein. Palpate and trace the path of the vein several times by rolling your index finger back and forth over the vein to determine its size. Inspect and palpate the vein for problems. Some veins that appear suitable at first sight, feel small, hard, bumpy, or flat when palpated.

8. Map the location of the vein. After locating an acceptable vein, mentally "map" the location of the puncture site on the patient's arm. This technique is particularly helpful if the vein cannot be seen, but only palpated. For example, the puncture site may be located next to a freckle on the patient's arm, a small wrinkle, a pigmented area, and so on.

9. Do not leave the tourniquet on for more than 1 minute. When first learning the venipuncture procedure, you may need to perform a number of assessments of the patient's arms to locate the best vein. After each assessment, remove the tourniquet to prevent patient discomfort and hemoconcentration.

10. If a good vein cannot be found, the following techniques can be employed to make the veins more prominent:
    • Remove the tourniquet and have the patient dangle the arm over the side of the chair for 1 to 2 minutes.
    • Tap at the vein site sharply a few times with your index finger and second finger.
    • Gently massage the arm from the wrist to the elbow.
    • Apply a warm, moist washcloth to the area for 5 minutes.

Alternative Venipuncture Sites

If it is not possible to locate a suitable vein in the antecubital space, alternative sites are available. These include the inner forearm, the wrist area above the thumb, and the back of the hand (Figure 17-5). These alternative veins are smaller and have thinner walls than the antecubital veins and should be used for venipuncture only when all other possibilities for obtaining the blood specimen have been considered. For example, if the medical assistant is able to palpate a small vein in the antecubital space, it may be

possible to obtain blood there using the butterfly method of venipuncture.

The hand veins, in particular, should be used only as a last resort. The veins of the hand have a tendency to roll because they are not supported by much tissue and are close to the surface of the skin. This makes them more difficult to stick. In addition, there is an abundant supply of nerves in the hands, which makes this procedure more uncomfortable for the patient. Hand veins tend to have thin walls, which makes them more susceptible to collapsing as well as bruising and phlebitis. However, in some patients, especially the obese and the elderly, the hand veins may be the only accessible site.

Types of Blood Specimens

The type of blood specimen required depends on the type of test to be performed. For example, serum is required for most blood chemistry studies, whereas whole blood is required for a complete blood count.

The various types of blood specimen that the medical assistant will be required to obtain through the venipuncture procedure are:

1. **Clotted blood.** Clotted blood is obtained from a tube to which an **anticoagulant** has not been added.
2. **Serum.** Serum is obtained from clotted blood by allowing the specimen to stand and then centrifuging it. This causes the specimen to separate into a top layer of serum and a bottom layer of clotted blood cells (Figure 17-6, *A*).
3. **Whole blood.** Whole blood is obtained by using a tube that contains an anticoagulant to prevent clotting. It is important to mix the anticoagulant with the blood by gently inverting the tube eight to ten times.
4. **Plasma.** Plasma is obtained from whole blood that has been centrifuged. This causes the specimen to separate into a top layer of plasma, a middle layer (the **buffy coat**) that contains white blood cells and platelets, and a bottom layer of red blood cells (Figure 17-6, *B*).

What Would You DO? What Would You Not DO?

Case Study 1

Angela Castillo is 21 years old and comes to the office at 9:00 AM to have her blood drawn for a CBC and a thyroid profile. She has brought a friend along with her. Angela seems nervous and her voice is shaking. She says this is the first venipuncture she has ever had. Angela asks if her friend could stay with her to give her moral support while her blood is being drawn. Angela says that the blood has to be taken out of her left arm. She says she is right-handed and has a softball game this evening. When the veins of Angela's left arm are examined, a suitable vein cannot be located; however, she has a very good median cubital vein in her right arm. Angela then wants to know if the blood could be drawn from her left hand like they do on hospital television shows.

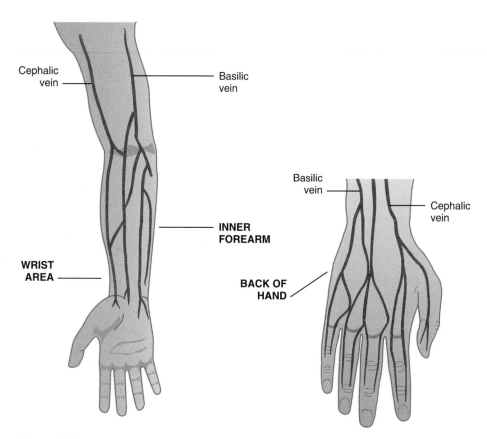

Figure 17-5. Alternative venipuncture sites. These include the inner forearm, the wrist area above the thumb, and the back of the hand.

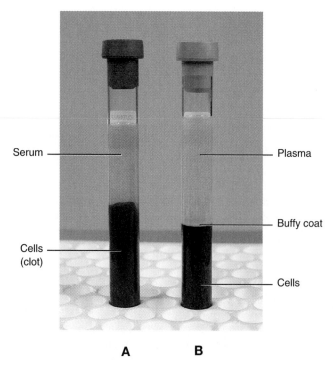

Figure 17-6. Layers the blood separates into **A,** when there is no anticoagulant and, **B,** when an anticoagulant is present.

OSHA Safety Precautions

The OSHA Bloodborne Pathogens Standard presented in Chapter 2 must be carefully followed during a venipuncture procedure to avoid exposure to bloodborne pathogens. The following OSHA requirements apply specifically to the venipuncture procedure, as well as to separation of serum or plasma from whole blood (presented later in this chapter).

1. Wear gloves when it is reasonably anticipated that you will have hand contact with blood.
2. Wear a face shield or mask in combination with an eye protection device whenever splashes, spray, spatter, or droplets of blood may be generated.
3. Perform all procedures involving blood in a manner so as to minimize splashing, spraying, spattering, and generating droplets of blood.
4. Bandage cuts and other lesions on the hands before gloving.
5. Sanitize hands as soon as possible after removing gloves.
6. If your hands or other skin surfaces come in contact with blood, wash the area as soon as possible with soap and water.
7. If your mucous membranes (e.g., eyes, nose, mouth) come in contact with blood, flush them with water as soon as possible.

8. Do not bend, break, or shear contaminated venipuncture needles.
9. Do not recap a contaminated venipuncture needle.
10. Locate the sharps container as close as possible to the area of use. Immediately after use, place the contaminated venipuncture needle (and plastic holder) in the biohazard sharps container.
11. Place blood specimens in containers that prevent leakage during collection, handling, processing, storage, transport, and shipping.
12. If you are exposed to blood, report the incident immediately to your physician-employer.

Vacuum Tube Method of Venipuncture

The vacuum tube method is frequently used to collect venous blood specimens. This method is considered ideal for collecting blood from normal healthy antecubital veins that are adequate in size to withstand the pressure of the vacuum in the evacuated tube. Procedure 17-1 outlines the venipuncture vacuum tube method.

The vacuum tube system consists of a collection needle, a plastic needle holder, and an evacuated tube (Figure 17-7). One such commercially available vacuum tube system is the Vacutainer, manufactured by Becton Dickinson. The components of the vacuum tube system are described next.

Needle

The needle used with the vacuum tube method consists of a double-pointed stainless steel needle with a threaded hub near its center (see Figure 17-8). The needle is coated with silicon, enabling it to penetrate the skin smoothly. The threaded hub of the needle screws into the plastic holder. Vacuum tube needles are packaged in sealed twist-apart containers. The needle gauge and size are printed on the paper label on the container (see Figure 17-8). A needle should not be used if the seal has been broken.

The double-pointed needle consists of an anterior needle and a posterior needle. The *anterior needle* is longer and has a beveled point designed to facilitate entry into the skin and the vein. The *posterior needle* is shorter, and its purpose is to pierce the rubber stopper of the evacuated tube. The posterior needle has a rubber sleeve that functions as a valve. Pushing an evacuated tube into the holder compresses the rubber sleeve and exposes the opening of the needle, allowing blood to enter the tube. When a tube is removed, the sleeve slides back over the needle opening and stops the flow of blood.

Vacuum tube needles are available in sizes 20 to 22 gauge, with 21-gauge needles used most for a routine venipuncture. Vacuum tube needles come in two lengths: 1 inch and 1½ inch. The length used is based on individual preference; medical assistants often prefer the 1-inch needle for routine venipunctures. A 1-inch needle is less intimidating to the patient and tends to offer more control because it allows the medical assistant to rest the fourth and fifth fingers on the patient's arm for stability. On the other hand, a 1½-inch needle allows more room for stabilizing the vein.

Safety Engineered Venipuncture Devices

OSHA stipulates requirements to reduce needlestick and other sharps injuries among health care workers. As discussed in Chapter 2, employers are required to evaluate and implement commercially available safer medical devices that reduce occupational exposure to the lowest extent feasible.

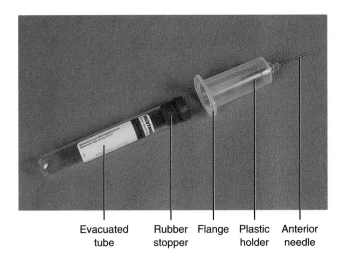

Figure 17-7. Vacuum tube system.

Evacuated tube — Rubber stopper — Flange — Plastic holder — Anterior needle

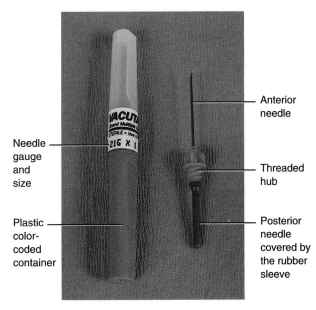

Figure 17-8. Vacuum tube needle in its container showing the size and gauge of the needle.

Needle gauge and size — Plastic color-coded container — Anterior needle — Threaded hub — Posterior needle covered by the rubber sleeve

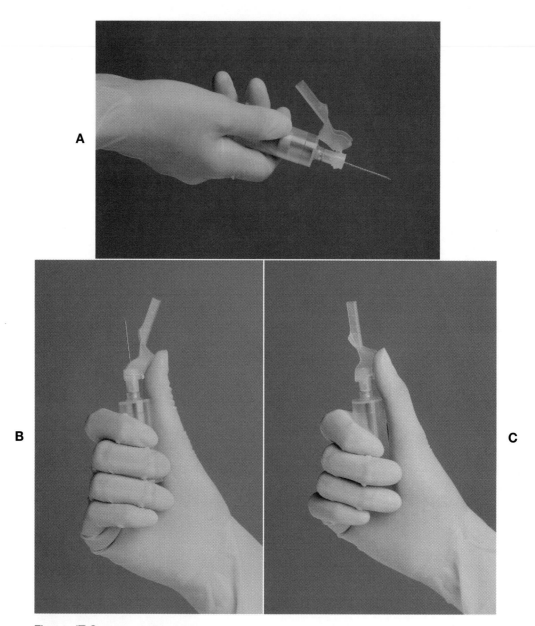

Figure 17-9. Safety engineered venipuncture device. **A,** Perform the venipuncture with the shield in a downward position. **B,** After performing the venipuncture, push the shield forward. **C,** Continue pushing until the needle tip is fully covered by the shield. Discard the needle and holder in a biohazard sharps container.

Safer medical devices include safety engineered venipuncture devices. These devices incorporate a built-in safety feature to reduce risk of a needlestick injury. Figure 17-9 illustrates a safety engineered venipuncture device and method for using it.

Plastic Holder

The plastic holder consists of a plastic cylinder with two openings. The small opening is used to secure the double-pointed needle, and the large opening is used to hold the evacuated tube. The large opening has a plastic extension known as the flange. The flange assists in the insertion and removal of evacuated tubes and prevents the plastic holder from rolling when it is placed on a flat surface.

The plastic holder has an indentation about ½ inch from the hub of the needle. This marks the point at which the posterior needle starts to enter the rubber stopper of the tube. If a tube is inserted past this point before the vein is entered, the tube will fill with air, which will not allow blood to enter.

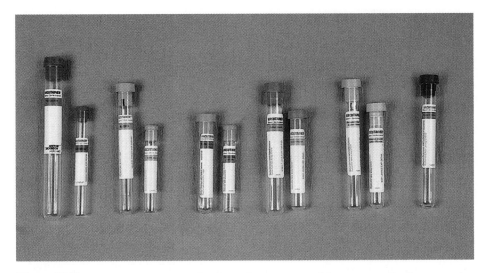

Figure 17-10. Vacutainer evacuated tubes. The stoppers of the evacuated tubes are color coded for ease in identifying the additive content. The lavender, light blue, green, gray, and dark blue tubes contain an anticoagulant and are used to obtain whole blood or plasma. The red-stoppered tubes contain no additive and are used to obtain clotted blood or serum.

Evacuated Tubes

Evacuated tubes consist of a glass tube with a rubber stopper. The tube contains a premeasured vacuum that creates suction to pull the blood specimen into the tube. Evacuated tubes use a color-coded system for ease in identifying the additive content of each type of tube, which is described in the box on p. 670 and illustrated in Figure 17-10. The additive must not alter the blood components or affect the laboratory test to be performed. Additive choice depends on the type of test to be performed. The medical assistant must be sure to use the additive specified by the test ordered. Additives must not be substituted for one another, because inaccurate test results will occur.

Evacuated tubes are available in varying capacities, the most common being the 2-, 3-, 5-, 7-, 10-, and 15-ml sizes (Figure 17-11). The capacity of the tube used depends on the amount of the specimen required for the test. Information regarding additive content, expiration date, and tube capacity is on the label of each box of vacuum tubes. In addition, most tubes have a label affixed to them indicating the additive content and expiration date of the tube.

Hemogard closure tubes, manufactured by Becton Dickinson, are a newer type of evacuated tube (Figure 17-10). A closure tube consists of a special rubber stopper and a plastic closure that overhangs the outside of the tube. Together, these components act as a single unit to reduce the likelihood of coming in contact with the contents of the tube. For example, after collecting a blood specimen, the medical assistant may need to gain access to the blood in the tube for testing it or for further processing such as in separating serum from whole blood. A regular evacuated tube "pops" as the top is removed which may result in splat-

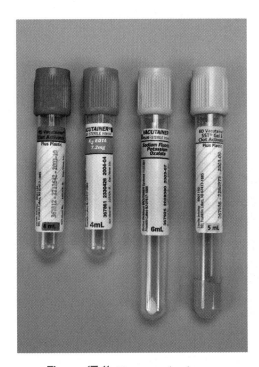

Figure 17-11. Hemogard tubes.

tering of blood. The design of the Hemogard tube works to prevent splattering of blood when the top is removed. In addition, closure tubes are made of plastic which reduces the possibility of tube breakage under normal conditions. It should be noted that the color coding of Hemogard stoppers is similar to that of rubber-stoppered tubes.

Additive Content of Evacuated Tubes

The vacuum tube method uses a color-coded system for ease in identifying the additive content of each type of tube. The most frequently used vacuum tubes are classified here according to the color of the stopper and additive content.

1. **Red.** Red-stoppered tubes do not contain an anticoagulant and are used to obtain clotted blood or serum. Serum is required for serologic tests and most blood chemistries.
2. **Lavender.** Lavender-stoppered tubes contain the anticoagulant ethylenediaminetetraacetic acid (EDTA) and are used to obtain whole blood or plasma. The most common use is to collect a blood specimen for a complete blood count.
3. **Light blue.** Light blue–stoppered tubes contain the anticoagulant sodium citrate and are used to obtain whole blood or plasma; the most common use is for coagulation tests such as the prothrombin time (PT).
4. **Green.** Green-stoppered tubes contain the anticoagulant heparin and are commonly used to collect blood specimens to perform blood gas determinations and pH assays.
5. **Gray.** Gray-stoppered tubes contain the anticoagulant potassium oxalate and are used to obtain whole blood or plasma; the most common use is to collect blood specimens to perform a glucose tolerance test.
6. **Dark blue.** Dark blue–stoppered tubes contain either heparin or no additive at all. These tubes are made of a specially refined glass and rubber stopper and are used for the detection of trace elements, such as lead, zinc, arsenic, and copper, that are contracted through occupational or environmental exposure.

Order of Draw for Multiple Tubes

When using the vacuum tube system and when multiple tubes of blood are to be drawn, the following order of draw is recommended:

1. **Blood culture tubes** (and other tests that require sterile specimens)
   Rationale: To prevent contamination of the specimen by other tubes, which may lead to inaccurate test results.
2. **Red-stoppered tube:** nonadditive tube.
   Rationale: To prevent contamination of nonadditive tubes by additive tubes.
3. **Coagulation tubes** (light blue stopper)
   Rationale: To prevent erroneous test results. When the needle penetrates the patient's skin, thromboplastin, a clotting factor, may be released. Thromboplastin can enter the blood specimen, affecting the test results. (NOTE: If a light blue–stoppered tube is the first or only tube to be drawn, a 5-ml red-stoppered tube should be drawn first and discarded to eliminate contamination from tissue thromboplastin picked up during needle penetration.)

Case Study 2

Buzz Braydon had a heart attack 4 weeks ago and is taking the anticoagulant Coumadin. He is at the office for a checkup and to have his prothrombin time tested. Blood is collected from a vein in Buzz's left arm using the vacuum tube method. After the specimen is collected, Buzz wants to know why a red-topped tube was used to get blood from him and then thrown away. Buzz says that they used something called a butterfly to draw his blood in the hospital and wants to know if a butterfly is ever used in the medical office. Buzz says that he is going on vacation in North Carolina for 2 weeks. He says that they explained to him at the hospital why he should have his blood tested every week, but he's not sure where to go to get his blood tested while he's on vacation. Buzz wants to know if as long as he takes his medication exactly as he should, it would be all right to skip his weekly prothrombin test during that time.

4. **Serum separator tube:** nonadditve tube that contains a gel.
5. **Additive tubes** in this order: green, lavender, gray
   Rationale: To prevent cross-contamination between different types of additive tubes, which may lead to inaccurate test results.

Evacuated Tube Guidelines

Certain guidelines should be followed when using evacuated tubes. They include the following:

1. Select the proper evacuated tubes according to the tests to be performed and amount of specimen required.
2. Check to make sure the tube is not cracked. A cracked tube will no longer have a vacuum.
3. Check the expiration date of each tube. Outdated tubes may no longer contain a vacuum, and, as a result, they may not be able to draw blood into the tube.
4. Label each tube with the patient's name, the date, and your initials. Proper labeling avoids mixing up specimens. Recent advances in specimen identification include the use of computer bar codes to identify specimens (Figure 17-12). The laboratory instruments that do the testing are able to read the bar codes and automatically record results onto the laboratory report.
5. Before using tubes that contain powdered additives, gently tap the tube just below the stopper so that all the additive is dislodged from the stopper. If an additive remains trapped in the stopper, erroneous test results may occur.
6. Take precautions to avoid premature loss of the tube's vacuum. Premature loss of vacuum can occur from dropping the tube or partially pulling the needle out of the arm after penetrating the patient's skin.

7. When multiple tubes are to be drawn, follow the proper *order of draw.* This prevents contamination of nonadditive tubes by additive tubes as well as cross-contamination between different types of additive tubes, which could lead to inaccurate test results.

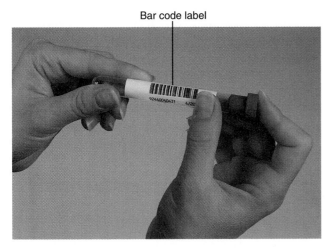

Bar code label

Figure 17-12. Identifying a blood specimen using a computer bar code.

8. Fill evacuated tubes until the vacuum is exhausted, as evidenced by the cessation of the blood flow into the tube. The tube will be almost, but not quite, full when the vacuum is exhausted. If the evacuated tube is removed before the vacuum is exhausted, a rush of air enters the tube, damaging the red blood cells. A tube that contains an additive must be filled completely to ensure the proper ratio of additive to blood.

9. Remove the last tube from the plastic holder before removing the needle. This prevents blood from dripping out of the tip of the needle after it is withdrawn from the patient's skin.

10. Mix tubes that contain an anticoagulant immediately after drawing by gently inverting the tube eight to ten times. This provides adequate mixing without causing **hemolysis,** or breakdown of blood cells. Inadequate mixing may result in clotting, leading to inaccurate test results.

11. After the venipuncture, the top of the stopper may contain residual blood. Be sure to take precautions following the OSHA Standard when handling these tubes.

Text continued on p. 676

PROCEDURE 17-1 Venipuncture—Vacuum Tube Method

Outcome Perform a venipuncture using the vacuum tube method.

Equipment/Supplies:
- Disposable gloves
- Tourniquet
- Antiseptic wipe
- Double-pointed needle
- Plastic holder
- Evacuated tubes with labels
- Sterile 2 × 2 gauze pad
- Adhesive bandage
- Biohazard sharps container

1. **Procedural Step.** Sanitize your hands.
2. **Procedural Step.** Greet and identify the patient, and introduce yourself. If the patient was required to prepare for the test (e.g., fasting, medication restriction), determine whether he or she has prepared properly. If the patient has not followed the patient preparation requirements, notify the physician for instructions on handling this situation.
   Principle. It is important to make sure you have the correct patient. The patient must prepare properly in order to obtain a quality specimen that will lead to accurate test results.
3. **Procedural Step.** Assemble the equipment. Be sure to select the proper evacuated tubes for the tests to be performed. Check the expiration date of the tubes. Label each tube with the patient's name, the date, and your initials. If the specimen will be tested at an outside laboratory, complete a laboratory request form.
   Principle. Outdated tubes may no longer contain a vacuum, and, as a result, they may not be able to draw blood into the tube. Proper labeling of blood specimens avoids a mixup of specimens.

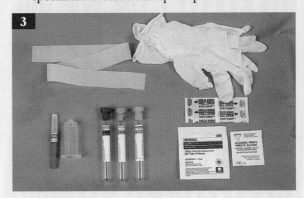

Continued

PROCEDURE 17-1 Venipuncture—Vacuum Tube Method—Cont'd

4. **Procedural Step.** Prepare the vacuum tube system. Insert the posterior needle into the plastic holder. Screw the needle into the plastic holder and tighten it securely.
   Principle. An unsecured needle can fall out of its plastic holder.

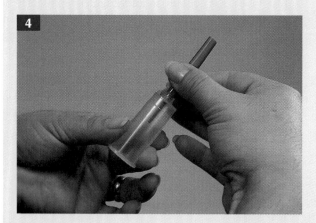

5. **Procedural Step.** Open the sterile gauze packet, and place the gauze pad on the inside of its wrapper. Position the evacuated tubes in the correct order of draw. If the evacuated tube contains a powdered additive, tap the tube just below the stopper to release any additive adhering to the stopper.
   Principle. If an additive remains trapped in the stopper, erroneous test results may occur.

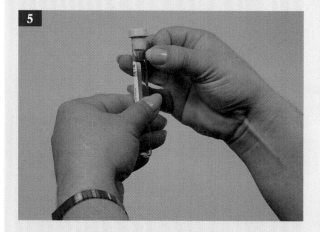

6. **Procedural Step.** Place the first tube loosely in the plastic holder. Place the remaining supplies within comfortable reach of your nondominant hand.

Principle. Items used during the procedure should be positioned so that you do not have to reach over the patient and possibly move the needle.

7. **Procedural Step.** Explain the procedure to the patient, and reassure the patient. Perform a preliminary assessment of both arms to determine the best vein to use. It is also helpful to ask the patient which arm has been used in the past to obtain blood.
   Principle. Venipuncture is often a frightening experience for the patient, and reassurance should be offered to reduce apprehension.

8. **Procedural Step.** Apply the tourniquet. Position the tourniquet 3 to 4 inches above the bend in the elbow. The tourniquet should be snug but not tight. Ask the patient to clench the fist of the arm to which the tourniquet has been applied.
   Principle. The combined effect of the pressure of the tourniquet and the clenched fist should cause the antecubital veins to stand out so that accurate selection of a puncture site can be made.

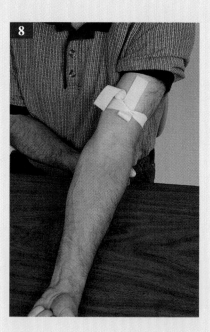

9. **Procedural Step.** With a tourniquet in place, thoroughly assess the veins of first one arm and then the other to determine the best vein to use. Never leave the tourniquet on an arm for more than 1 minute at a time. (NOTE: If you need to perform

several assessments to locate the best vein, the tourniquet can be applied and reapplied as required.)

Principle. Leaving the tourniquet on for more than 1 minute is uncomfortable for the patient and may alter the test results.

10. **Procedural Step.** Position the patient's arm. The arm with the vein selected for the venipuncture should be extended and placed in a straight line from the shoulder to the wrist with the antecubital veins facing anteriorly. The arm should be supported on the armrest by a rolled towel or by having the patient place the fist of the other hand under the elbow.

    Principle. This position allows easy access to the antecubital veins.

11. **Procedural Step.** Thoroughly palpate the selected vein. Gently palpate the vein with the fingertips to determine the direction of the vein and to estimate its size and depth.

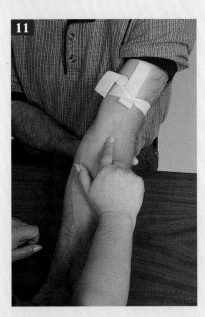

12. **Procedural Step.** Cleanse the site with an antiseptic. Cleansing should be done in a circular motion, starting from the inside and moving away from the puncture site. Allow the site to air dry, and after cleansing do not touch the area or fan the area with your hand.

    Principle. Using a circular motion helps carry foreign particles away from the puncture site. The site must be allowed to dry because alcohol entering the blood specimen contaminates it, leading to inaccurate test results. In addition, the alcohol causes the patient to experience a stinging sensation. Touching or fanning the area causes contamination, and the cleansing process has to be repeated.

13. **Procedural Step.** Apply gloves. Remove the cap from the needle. Hold the vacuum tube system by placing the thumb and index finger of the dominant hand on the plastic holder while supporting the rest of the holder and evacuated tube with the remaining three fingers. The needle should be positioned with the bevel facing up. Position the evacuated tube so that the label is facing down.

    Principle. Gloves provide a barrier against bloodborne pathogens. Positioning the needle with the bevel up allows easier entry into the skin and the vein. With the label facing down, you will be able to observe the blood as it fills the tube, which allows you to know when the tube is full.

14. **Procedural Step.** Anchor the vein. Grasp the patient's arm with the nondominant hand. Your thumb should be placed 1 to 2 inches below and to the side of the puncture site. Using your thumb, draw the skin taut over the vein in the direction of the patient's hand.

    Principle. The thumb helps hold the skin taut for easier entry and helps stabilize the vein to be punctured.

15. **Procedural Step.** Position the needle at a 15-degree angle to the arm. Make sure the needle points in the same direction as the vein to be entered.

    Principle. An angle of less than 15 degrees may cause the needle to enter above the vein, preventing puncture. An angle of more than 15 degrees may cause the needle to go through the vein by puncturing the posterior wall. This could result in a hematoma.

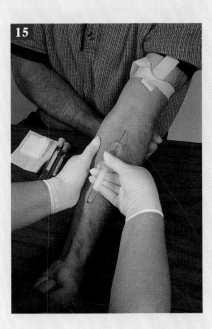

Continued

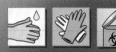

PROCEDURE 17-1   Venipuncture—Vacuum Tube Method —Cont'd

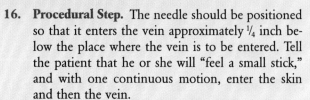

16. **Procedural Step.** The needle should be positioned so that it enters the vein approximately ¼ inch below the place where the vein is to be entered. Tell the patient that he or she will "feel a small stick," and with one continuous motion, enter the skin and then the vein.

    Principle. Using one continuous motion helps to prevent tissue damage.

17. **Procedural Step.** Firmly grasp the holder between the thumb and the underlying fingers to prevent the needle from moving. With the nondominant hand place two fingers on the flange of the plastic holder and with the thumb slowly push the tube forward to the end of the holder. This allows the posterior needle to puncture the rubber stopper. Blood will begin flowing into the tube if the (anterior) needle is in a vein.

    Principle. Firmly grasping the holder prevents the needle from moving deeper into the vein when an evacuated tube is being inserted. Moving the needle is painful for the patient.

18. **Procedural Step.** Allow the evacuated tube to fill to the exhaustion of the vacuum, as indicated by the cessation of the blood flow into the tube. The suction of the evacuated tube automatically draws the blood into the tube.

    Principle. If the evacuated tube is removed before the vacuum is exhausted, a rush of air enters the tube, damaging the red blood cells. Also, a tube containing an additive such as an anticoagulant must be filled completely to ensure accurate test results.

19. **Procedural Step.** Using the flange, remove the tube from the plastic holder, being careful not to change the position of the needle in the vein. If the tube contains an additive, gently rotate the tube eight to ten times before laying it down.

    Principle. The rubber sheath covers the point of the needle, stopping the flow of blood until the next tube is inserted. The tube containing an additive must be inverted immediately to prevent the blood from clotting. Careful mixing of the blood with the additive prevents hemolysis.

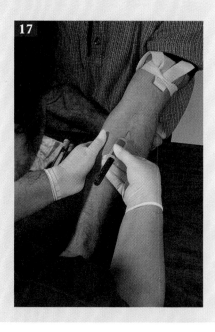

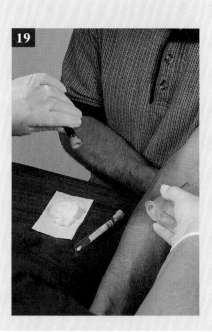

20. **Procedural Step.** Using the flange, carefully insert the next tube into the holder. Continue in this manner until the last tube has been filled.

21. **Procedural Step.** Remove the tension from the tourniquet and ask the patient to unclench the fist. *Principle.* The tourniquet tension must be removed before the needle. Otherwise the pressure on the vein from the tourniquet could cause internal and external bleeding around the puncture site.

22. **Procedural Step.** Remove the last tube from the holder. *Principle.* This prevents blood from dripping out of the tip of the needle.

23. **Procedural Step.** Place a sterile gauze pad over the site and slowly withdraw the needle at the same angle as that for penetration. Do not apply any pressure to the puncture site until the needle is completely removed. *Principle.* Placing the gauze pad over the puncture helps prevent tissue movement as the needle is withdrawn and reduces patient discomfort. Careful withdrawal prevents further tissue damage.

24. **Procedural Step.** Apply pressure with the gauze pad. Ask the patient to apply pressure with the gauze pad for 1 to 2 minutes. The arm can be elevated to facilitate clot formation. Do not allow the patient to bend the arm at the elbow because this increases blood loss from the puncture site. *Principle.* Applying pressure reduces the leakage of blood from the puncture site either externally or internally. Internal leakage of blood into the tissues could result in a hematoma.

25. **Procedural Step.** Properly dispose of the needle and holder in a biohazard sharps container. *Principle.* Proper disposal is required by the OSHA Standard to prevent accidental needlestick injuries.

26. **Procedural Step.** Stay with the patient until the bleeding has stopped. Apply an adhesive bandage to the puncture site. As an alternative, the gauze pad can be folded into quarters and taped on the puncture site to be used as a pressure bandage. Instruct the patient not to pick up anything heavy for about an hour. (NOTE: If swelling or discoloration occurs, apply an ice pack to the site after bandaging it.) *Principle.* Lifting a heavy object causes pressure on the puncture site, which could result in bleeding.

27. **Procedural Step.** Remove the gloves, and sanitize your hands.

28. **Procedural Step.** Chart the procedure. Include the date and time, which arm and vein were used, unusual patient reaction, and your initials.

29. **Procedural Step.** Test, transfer, or store the blood specimen according to the medical office policy. If the specimen is to be transported to an outside laboratory for testing, record this information in the patient's chart, including the date the specimen was transported to the laboratory.

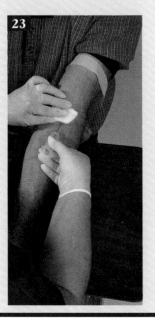

PROCEDURE 17-1

CHARTING EXAMPLE	
Date	
4/5/05	9:00 a.m. Venous blood specimen collected from Ⓛ arm. Picked up by Medical Center Laboratory on 4/5/05. ——— D. Glover, CMA

Butterfly Method of Venipuncture

The butterfly method of venipuncture is also called the *winged infusion method.* This is because a winged infusion set is used to perform the procedure. The term "butterfly" is derived from the plastic "wings" located between the needle and the tubing of the winged infusion set (Figure 17-13).

The butterfly method is used to collect blood from patients who are difficult to stick by conventional methods. This includes adult patients with small antecubital veins and children, who typically have small antecubital veins. The butterfly method is also used when the antecubital veins are not available, and the veins in the forearm, wrist area, or back of the hand are used, as may occur with elderly and obese patients. Procedure 17-2 describes the venipuncture procedure using the butterfly method.

The gauge of the winged infusion needle ranges from 21 to 23, and the length of the needle ranges from ½ to ¾ inch. The needle is short and very sharp, making it easier to stick difficult veins. For extremely small veins, a 23-gauge needle should be used to prevent rupture of the vein by a larger needle. In this case, it is preferable to use smaller volume tubes (e.g., 2-ml evacuated tubes) because large evacuated tubes may put too much vacuum pressure on the vein, causing it to collapse.

The winged infusion needle is attached to a 6- or 12-inch length of tubing and a *Luer adapter,* attached to a (posterior) needle with a rubber sleeve. A plastic evacuated tube holder is screwed onto the Luer adapter (Figure 17-13, *A*). Winged infusion sets are also available with a hub adapter that allows them to be used with a syringe (Figure 17-13, *B*). Safety needles are available that have a shield that covers the contaminated needle after it is withdrawn from the patient's vein (Figure 17-14).

Guidelines for the Butterfly Method

Certain guidelines should be followed when performing the butterfly method of venipuncture. These include the following:

1. Position the patient according to the site selected for the venipuncture as follows:

    Antecubital, wrist and forearm veins. Position the arm in a straight line from the shoulder to the wrist as described in the vacuum tube method of venipuncture.

    Hand veins. Position the patient's hand on the arm rest and ask the patient to make a loose fist or to grasp a rolled towel. This combination causes the hand veins to stand out so that accurate selection of a puncture site can be made. Locate a suitable vein between the knuckles and the wrist bones. Hand veins are usually visible and easy to locate.

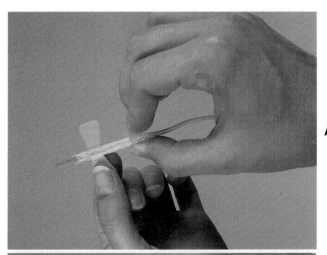

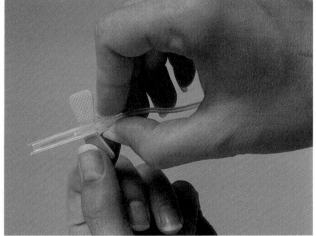

Figure 17-13. Winged infusion set. **A,** Luer adapter with evacuated tube. **B,** Hub adapter with syringe.

Figure 17-14. Butterfly safety needle. The safety needle has a shield that covers the contaminated needle after it is withdrawn from the patient's vein. **A,** The medical assistant has covered half of the needle with the shield. **B,** The needle is completely covered with the shield.

2. Position the tourniquet according to the venipuncture site as follows: If the veins of the forearm or wrist are used, apply the tourniquet to the forearm, approximately 3 inches above the puncture site. For hand veins, position the tourniquet on the arm just above the wrist bone (Figure 17-15).

3. Grasp the needle by compressing the plastic wings together. Insert the needle with the bevel facing up at a 15-degree angle to the skin. Once the vein has been entered, decrease the angle to 5 degrees.

4. After inserting the needle, slowly thread it inside the vein an additional ¼ inch. This anchors the needle in the center of the vein.

5. To prevent venous reflux, keep the evacuated tube and holder in a downward position as in the vacuum tube venipuncture procedure. This technique ensures that the blood fills from the bottom up and not near the rubber stopper.

6. When multiple tubes are to be drawn, follow the proper order of draw. The order of draw for the butterfly method is identical to that for the vacuum tube method (see p. 670). Following this order of draw prevents contamination of nonadditive tubes as well as cross-contamination of additive tubes.

Text continued on p. 682

MEMORIES From EXTERNSHIP

DORI GLOVER: One of the most terrifying things for me as a student was learning venipuncture. Even though I would practice during classroom lab hours and felt comfortable with it, it still scared me to know I would have to draw on a real person one day. When the day arrived to draw on my lab partner, I became sick to my stomach. In the end, we both got through it just fine and walked away without hurting each other. I spent days trying to prepare myself for that first experience, but after it was over, I felt more confident and relaxed that I could do this. At my externship site, I was able to perform several venipunctures a day, which raised my confidence level. Today venipuncture is my favorite responsibility of all. I could sit and draw all day if I could. I know I could draw with my eyes closed, but never would, of course!

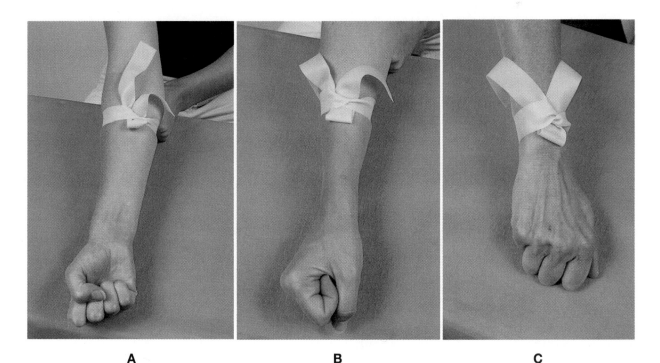

A   **B**   **C**

Figure 17-15. Application of the tourniquet for alternative venipuncture sites: **A,** forearm; **B,** wrist; **C,** hand.

PROCEDURE 17-2 Venipuncture—Butterfly Method

Outcome Perform a venipuncture using the butterfly method.

Equipment/Supplies:
- Disposable gloves
- Tourniquet
- Antiseptic wipe
- Winged infusion set with a Luer adapter

- Plastic holder
- Evacuated tubes with labels
- Sterile 2 × 2 gauze pad
- Adhesive bandage
- Biohazard sharps container

1. **Procedural Step.** Sanitize your hands.
2. **Procedural Step.** Greet and identify the patient, and introduce yourself. If the patient was required to prepare for the test (e.g., fasting, medication restriction), determine whether he or she has prepared properly. If the patient has not followed the patient preparation requirements, notify the physician for instructions on handling this situation.
   Principle. It is important to make sure you have the correct patient. The patient must prepare properly in order to obtain a quality specimen that will lead to accurate test results.
3. **Procedural Step.** Assemble the equipment. Be sure to select the proper evacuated tubes for the tests to be performed. Check the expiration date of the tubes. Label each tube with the patient's name, the date, and your initials. If the specimen will be tested at an outside laboratory, complete a laboratory request form.
   Principle. Outdated tubes may no longer contain a vacuum, and, as a result, they may not be able to draw blood into the tube. Proper labeling of blood specimens avoids mixup of specimens.

4. **Procedural Step.** Prepare the winged infusion set. Remove the winged infusion set from its package. Extend the tubing to its full length and stretch it slightly to prevent it from coiling back up. Insert the Luer adapter and attached needle into the plastic holder. Screw the plastic holder onto the adapter and tighten it securely.
   Principle. Extending the tubing straightens it to permit a free flow of blood in the tubing. An unsecured needle can fall out of its plastic holder.

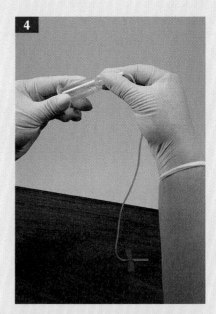

5. **Procedural Step.** Open the sterile gauze packet, and place the gauze pad on the inside of its wrapper. Position the evacuated tubes in the correct order of draw. If the evacuated tube contains a powdered additive, tap the tube just below the stopper to release any additive adhering to the stopper.
   Principle. If an additive remains trapped in the stopper, erroneous test results may occur.

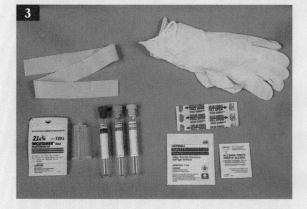

6. **Procedural Step.** Place the first tube loosely in the plastic holder with the label facing down. Place the remaining supplies within comfortable reach.
   Principle. With the label facing down, you will be able to observe the blood as it fills the tube, which allows you to know when the tube is full. Items used during the procedure should be positioned so that you do not have to reach over the patient and possibly move the needle.

7. **Procedural Step.** Explain the procedure to the patient, and reassure the patient. Perform a preliminary assessment of both arms to determine the best vein to use. It is also helpful to ask the patient which arm has been used in the past to obtain blood.
   Principle. Venipuncture is often a frightening experience for the patient, and reassurance should be offered to reduce apprehension.

8. **Procedural Step.** Apply the tourniquet. Position the tourniquet 3 to 4 inches above the bend in the elbow. The tourniquet should be snug but not tight. Ask the patient to clench the fist of the arm to which the tourniquet has been applied.
   Principle. The combined effect of the pressure of the tourniquet and the clenched fist should cause the antecubital veins to stand out so that accurate selection of a puncture site can be made.

9. **Procedural Step.** With a tourniquet in place, thoroughly assess the veins of first one arm and then the other to determine the best vein to use. Never leave the tourniquet on an arm for more than 1 minute at a time. (NOTE: You may need to perform several assessments to locate the best vein by applying and removing the tourniquet several times.)

10. **Procedural Step.** Position the patient's arm. The arm with the vein selected for the venipuncture should be extended and placed in a straight line from the shoulder to the wrist with the antecubital veins facing anteriorly. The arm should be supported on the armrest by a rolled towel or by having the patient place the fist of the other hand under the elbow.
    Principle. This position allows easy access to the antecubital veins.

11. **Procedural Step.** Thoroughly palpate the selected vein. Gently palpate the vein with the fingertips to determine the direction of the vein and to estimate its size and depth.

12. **Procedural Step.** Cleanse the site with an antiseptic. Cleansing should be done in a circular motion, starting from the inside and moving away from the puncture site. Allow the site to air dry, and after cleansing do not touch the area or fan the area with your hand.
    Principle. Using a circular motion helps carry foreign particles away from the puncture site. The site must be allowed to dry because alcohol entering the blood specimen contaminates it, leading to inaccurate test results. In addition, the alcohol causes the patient to experience a stinging sensation. Touching or fanning the area causes contamination, and the cleansing process has to be repeated.

13. **Procedural Step.** Apply gloves. Grasp the winged infusion set by pressing the butterfly tips together. Remove the protective shield from the needle of the infusion set. The needle should be positioned with the bevel facing up.
    Principle. Gloves provide a barrier against bloodborne pathogens. Positioning the needle with the bevel up allows easier entry into the skin and the vein.

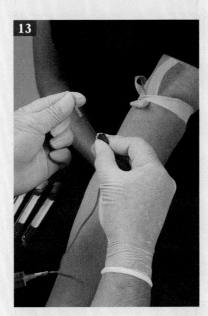

14. **Procedural Step.** Anchor the vein. Grasp the patient's arm with the nondominant hand. The thumb should be placed 1 to 2 inches below and to the side of the puncture site. Using the thumb, draw the skin taut over the vein in the direction of the patient's hand.
    Principle. The thumb helps hold the skin taut for easier entry and helps stabilize the vein to be punctured.

Continued

PROCEDURE 17-2

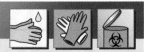

15. Procedural Step. Position the needle at a 15-degree angle to the arm. Make sure the needle points in the same direction as the vein to be entered.

Principle. An angle of less than 15 degrees may cause the needle to enter above the vein, preventing puncture. An angle of more than 15 degrees may cause the needle to go through the vein by puncturing the posterior wall. This could result in a hematoma.

16. Procedural Step. The needle should be positioned so that it enters the vein approximately $1/4$ inch below the place where the vein is to be entered. Tell the patient that he or she will "feel a small stick," and with one continuous motion, enter the skin and then the vein. After penetrating the vein, decrease the angle of the needle to 5 degrees. If the needle is in the vein, a flash of blood will appear in the tubing.

Principle. Using one continuous motion reduces tissue damage.

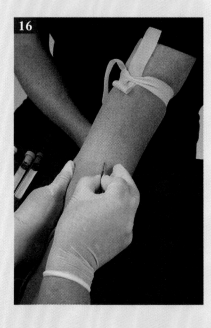

17. Procedural Step. Seat the needle by threading it up the lumen (central area) of the vein slightly so that it will not twist out of the vein, even if you let go of it. Securely rest the needle flat against the skin. Be sure that the needle does not move.

Principle. Seating the needle anchors the needle in the center of the vein. Moving the needle is painful for the patient.

18. Procedural Step. Keep the tube and holder in a downward position so that the tube fills from the bottom up and not near the rubber stopper. Using the flange, slowly push the tube forward to the end of the holder. This allows the needle to puncture the rubber stopper. Blood will begin flowing into the tube. Allow the evacuated tube to fill to the exhaustion of the vacuum, as indicated by the cessation of the blood flow into the tube. The suction of the evacuated tube automatically draws the blood into the tube.

Principle. The tube must fill from the bottom up to prevent venous reflux. If the evacuated tube is removed before the vacuum is exhausted, a rush of air enters the tube, damaging the red blood cells. Also, a tube containing an additive such as an anticoagulant must be filled completely to ensure accurate test results.

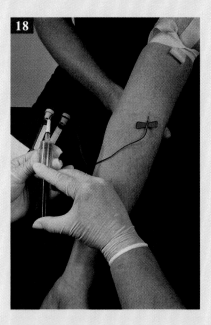

19. **Procedural Step.** Using the flange, remove the tube from the plastic holder, being careful not to change the position of the needle in the vein. If the tube contains an additive, gently rotate the tube eight to ten times before laying it down.

Principle. The rubber sheath covers the point of the needle, stopping the flow of blood until the next tube is inserted. The tube containing an additive must be inverted before laying it down to prevent the blood from clotting. Careful mixing of the blood with the additive prevents hemolysis.

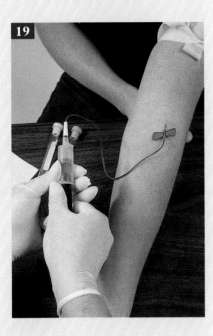

20. **Procedural Step.** Using the flange, carefully insert the next tube into the holder. Continue in this manner until the last tube has been filled.

21. **Procedural Step.** Remove the tension from the tourniquet and ask the patient to unclench the fist.

Principle. The tourniquet tension must be removed before the needle. Otherwise the pressure on the vein from the tourniquet could cause internal and external bleeding around the puncture.

22. **Procedural Step.** Remove the last tube from the holder.

Principle. This prevents blood from dripping out of the tip of the needle.

23. **Procedural Step.** Place a sterile gauze pad over the site. Grasp the wings and slowly withdraw the needle at the same angle as that for penetration. Do not apply pressure to the puncture site until the needle is completely removed.

Principle. Placing the gauze pad over the puncture site helps prevent tissue movement as the needle is withdrawn and reduces patient discomfort. Careful withdrawal prevents further tissue damage.

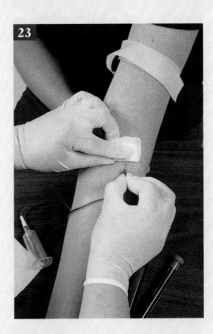

24. **Procedural Step.** Apply pressure with the gauze pad. Ask the patient to apply pressure with the gauze pad for 1 to 2 minutes. The arm can be elevated to facilitate clot formation. Do not allow the patient to bend the arm at the elbow because this increases blood loss from the puncture site.

Principle. Applying pressure reduces the leakage of blood from the puncture site either externally or internally. Internal leakage into the tissues could result in a hematoma.

25. **Procedural Step.** Properly dispose of the winged infusion set. Holding onto the plastic holder, drop the needle and tubing and then the holder into a biohazard sharps container.

Principle. Proper disposal is required by the OSHA Standard to prevent needlestick injuries.

PROCEDURE 17-2

Continued

PROCEDURE 17-2 Venipuncture—Butterfly Method—Cont'd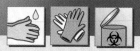

26. Procedural Step. Stay with the patient until the bleeding has stopped. Apply an adhesive bandage to the puncture site. As an alternative, the gauze pad can be folded into quarters and taped on the puncture site to be used as a pressure bandage. Instruct the patient not to pick up anything heavy for about an hour. (NOTE: If swelling or discoloration occurs, apply an ice pack to the site after bandaging it.)
Principle. Lifting a heavy object causes pressure on the puncture site, which could result in bleeding.

27. Procedural Step. Remove the gloves, and sanitize your hands.

28. Procedural Step. Chart the procedure. Include the date and time, which arm and vein were used, unusual patient reaction, and your initials.

29. Procedural Step. Test, transfer, or store the blood specimen according to the medical office policy. If the specimen is to be transported to an outside laboratory for testing, record this information in the patient's chart, including the date the specimen was transported to the laboratory.

CHARTING EXAMPLE	
Date	
4/10/05	10:30 a.m. Venous blood specimen collected from Ⓛ arm. Picked up by Medical Center Laboratory on 4/10/05.———D. Glover, CMA

Syringe Method of Venipuncture

The syringe method is the least used method of venipuncture. This is because once the blood specimen is obtained, it must be transferred from the syringe to an evacuated tube, which presents the risk of an accidental needlestick. Procedure 17-3 describes the venipuncture procedure using a syringe.

The syringe method is used primarily to obtain blood from small veins that are likely to collapse. Because the rate of blood flow into the syringe is not dictated by the premeasured vacuum of an evacuated tube, the syringe method offers more control than other methods of venipuncture. Once the vein has been punctured, the specimen is obtained by pulling back on the plunger of the syringe. Pulling the plunger back slowly minimizes pressure against the vein wall so the vein is less likely to collapse.

The setup for the syringe method includes a disposable needle and syringe. The gauge of the needle ranges from 21 to 23, and the length of the needle ranges from 1 to 1½ inches. For extremely small veins, a 23-gauge needle should be used to prevent rupture of the vein by a larger

needle. The capacity of the syringe depends on the amount of specimen required and ranges from 5 ml (cc) to 20 ml (cc). If more than 20 ml is required, a second venipuncture must be performed; this is another disadvantage of this method.

After the blood specimen is collected, it must be transferred to an evacuated tube. For safety reasons, the tube should always be placed in a test tube rack. The tube should *never* be held in the hand during the transfer because of the danger of a needlestick injury.

If more than one evacuated tube is being filled, a specific "order of fill" is required as follows: blue, lavender, green, gray, and red. It should be noted that this order is the reverse of the vacuum tube and butterfly methods (i.e., the tubes with additives are filled first followed by the tubes without additives). The reason for this is to prevent clotting by combining the blood with the additive as soon as possible after collection. Tubes with additives should be inverted eight to ten times immediately after filling them.

Text continued on p. 686

What Would You DO?
What Would You *Not* DO?

Case Study 3

Maud Gabriel is at the office complaining of persistent headaches over the past 3 months. The physician gives Mrs. Gabriel a laboratory requisition to have her blood drawn and tested at an outside laboratory. Mrs. Gabriel says that her daughter who lives with her works as a phlebotomist at the local hospital. Mrs. Gabriel wants to know if her daughter can draw her blood at home and then drop it off at the laboratory. She says that the last time she had her blood drawn they had to stick her two times and then she got a great big bruise on her arm afterwards She says the lab technician kept digging around in her arm to find the vein and that it was quite painful.

PROCEDURE 17-3 Venipuncture—Syringe Method

Outcome Perform a venipuncture using the syringe method.

Equipment/Supplies:

- Disposable gloves
- Tourniquet
- Antiseptic wipe
- Syringe and needle
- Evacuated tubes with labels
- Test tube rack
- Sterile 2 × 2 gauze pad
- Adhesive bandage
- Biohazard sharps container

1. Procedural Step. Follow steps 1 through 3 of the butterfly method of venipuncture (see Procedure 17-2).

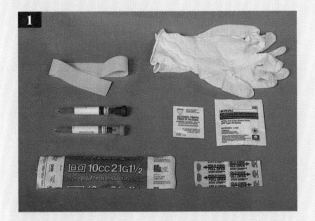

2. Procedural Step. Prepare the needle and syringe, making sure to keep the needle and the inside of the syringe sterile. Break the seal on the syringe by moving the plunger back and forth several times. Loosen the cap on the needle and check to make sure that the hub is screwed tightly into the syringe.

3. Procedural Step. Place the evacuated tubes to be filled in a test tube rack on a work surface. If an evacuated tube contains a powdered additive, tap the tube just below the stopper to release any additive adhering to the stopper. Make sure the tubes are placed in the correct order to be filled. Open the sterile gauze packet and place the gauze pad on the inside of its wrapper.
Principle. If an additive remains trapped in the stopper, erroneous test results may occur.

4. Procedural Step. Follow steps 7 through 12 of the butterfly method of venipuncture.

5. Procedural Step. Apply gloves. Remove the cap from the needle. Hold the syringe by placing the thumb and index finger of the dominant hand near the needle hub while supporting the barrel of the syringe with the three remaining fingers. The needle should be positioned with the bevel facing up.
Principle. Gloves provide a barrier against bloodborne pathogens. Positioning the needle with the bevel up allows easier entry into the skin and the vein.

6. Procedural Step. Anchor the vein. Grasp the patient's arm with the nondominant hand. The thumb should be placed 1 to 2 inches below and to the side of the puncture site. Using the thumb, draw the skin taut over the vein in the direction of the patient's hand.

Continued

PROCEDURE 17-3 Venipuncture—Syringe Method—Cont'd

Principle. The thumb helps hold the skin taut for easier entry and helps stabilize the vein to be punctured.

7. **Procedural Step.** Position the needle at a 15-degree angle to the arm. Make sure the needle points in the same direction as the vein to be entered.

Principle. An angle of less than 15 degrees may cause the needle to enter above the vein, preventing puncture. An angle of more than 15 degrees may cause the needle to go through the vein by puncturing the posterior wall. This could result in a hematoma.

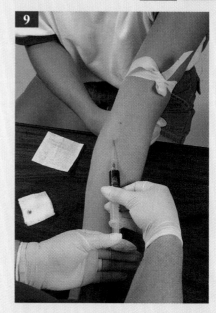

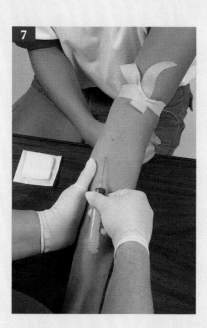

8. **Procedural Step.** Position the needle so that it enters the vein approximately ¼ inch below the place where the vein is to be entered. Tell the patient that he or she will "feel a small stick," and with one continuous motion, enter the skin and then the vein.

Principle. Using one continuous motion helps to prevent tissue damage.

9. **Procedural Step.** Securely grasp the syringe firmly between the thumb and the underlying fingers. Blood may spontaneously enter the top of the syringe. If not, pull back gently on the plunger until blood begins to enter the syringe. Do not move the needle once the venipuncture has been made.

Principle. Moving the needle is painful for the patient.

10. **Procedural Step.** Remove the desired amount of blood by pulling back slowly and gently on the plunger. Care should be taken while pulling back on the plunger to prevent the accidental withdrawal of the needle from the patient's arm.

Principle. Pulling back on the plunger causes a suction effect, which draws the blood into the syringe. The blood should be withdrawn slowly from the vein to prevent hemolysis and to prevent the vein from collapsing.

11. **Procedural Step.** Remove the tension from the tourniquet and ask the patient to unclench the fist.

Principle. The tourniquet tension must be removed before the needle. Otherwise the pressure on the vein from the tourniquet could cause internal and external bleeding around the puncture site.

12. **Procedural Step.** Place a sterile gauze pad over the site and slowly withdraw the needle at the same angle as that for penetration. Do not apply pressure to the puncture site until the needle is completely removed.

Principle. Placing the gauze pad over the puncture site helps prevent tissue movement as the needle is withdrawn and reduces patient discomfort. Careful withdrawal prevents further tissue damage.

13. **Procedural Step.** Apply pressure with the gauze pad. Ask the patient to apply pressure with the gauze pad for 1 to 2 minutes. The arm can be elevated to facilitate clot formation. Do not allow the patient to bend the arm at the elbow because this increases blood loss from the puncture site.
Principle. Applying pressure reduces the leakage of blood from the puncture site either externally or internally. Internal leakage into the tissues could result in a hematoma.

14. **Procedural Step.** Transfer the blood to the labeled evacuated tubes as soon as possible as follows:
Double-check that the tubes are in the correct order of draw in the rack.
Insert the needle through the center of the rubber stopper and allow the vacuum to fill the tube. Do not apply pressure to the plunger of the syringe.
If the blood is added to a tube containing an additive, it must be mixed immediately by gently inverting the tube eight to ten times.
Principle. A delay in transferring the blood to the evacuated tubes causes clotting of the blood in the syringe. To prevent an accidental needlestick, do not hold the tubes in the hand when the needle is inserted through the stopper. The suction action of the vacuum tube will automatically draw the blood into the tube. The tube containing an anticoagulant must be inverted immediately to prevent the blood from clotting. Careful mixing of the blood with the anticoagulant prevents hemolysis.

15. **Procedural Step.** Properly dispose of the needle and syringe in a biohazard sharps container.
Principle. Proper disposal is required by the OSHA Standard to prevent accidental needlestick injuries.

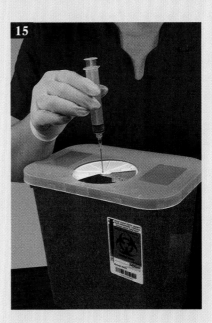

16. **Procedural Step.** Follow steps 26 through 29 of the butterfly method of venipuncture.

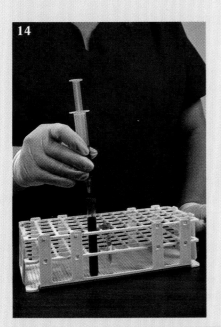

PROCEDURE 17-3

Problems Encountered With Venipuncture

At times the medical assistant will encounter problems when attempting to draw blood from a patient. The appropriate response depends on the type of problem.

Failure to Obtain Blood

Periodically even those highly skilled at performing venipuncture have difficulty obtaining blood. Although large and prominent veins make it easier to collect the blood specimen, conditions often exist that make the procedure more difficult.

It is often difficult to draw blood from obese patients who have small, superficial veins and whose veins suitable for venipuncture are buried in adipose tissue. Elderly patients with arteriosclerosis may have veins that are thick and hard, making them difficult to puncture. Other patients have veins that are small or have a thin wall, making the veins likely to collapse. After two unsuccessful attempts at venipuncture, the medical assistant should notify the physician to get advice or assistance regarding alternative puncture sites.

Factors that result in a failure to obtain blood once the needle has been inserted include not inserting the needle far enough, preventing it from entering the vein (Figure 17-16, *B*); insertion of the needle too far, causing it to go through the vein (Figure 17-16, *C*); and the bevel opening becoming lodged against the wall of the vein. In these instances, most authorities recommend removal of the needle rather than trying to probe the vein. Probing is often uncomfortable for the patient and also can affect the integrity of the blood specimen. Occasionally an evacuated tube loses its vacuum because of a manufacturing defect or through improper handling of the tube. If suspected, this problem can be corrected by removing the defective tube and inserting another vacuum tube.

Inappropriate Puncture Sites

If a patient complains of pain or soreness in a potential venipuncture site, this area should be avoided. In addition, any skin areas that are scarred, bruised, burned, or adjacent to areas of infection should not be used. An arm in a cast or affected by a radical mastectomy should be avoided.

Scarred and Sclerosed Veins

A person who has had many venipunctures over a period of years often develops scar tissue in the wall of the vein. Elderly patients may have veins that have become thickened from arteriosclerosis. In both cases, the veins feel stiff and hard when palpated. A scarred or sclerosed vein is difficult to stick and the blood return may be poor owing to a narrowed lumen; therefore it is recommended that another vein be used for the venipuncture. If this is not possible, the needle should be inserted with careful pressure to avoid going completely through the vein.

Rolling Veins

The median cubital vein, located in the center of the antecubital space, is considered the best vein for a venipuncture. At times, however, it is not possible to use this vein, for example, when it lies deep in the tissues and cannot be palpated or is scarred from repeated venipunctures. The veins on either side of the median cubital can be used; however, they have a tendency to "roll," or move away from the needle, thereby escaping puncture. To prevent rolling, firm pressure should be applied below the vein to stabilize it as the needle is inserted.

Collapsing Veins

Veins are most likely to collapse in people who have small veins or veins with thin walls. This is particularly true when the vacuum tube method is being used. The "sucking action" exerted on the vein when the pressure in the vacuum is released causes the vein to collapse, thereby blocking the flow of blood into the tube (see Figure 17-16, *D*). Because better control is possible, the butterfly or syringe method of venipuncture is recommended to obtain the specimen in patients with small veins.

Premature Needle Withdrawal

Patient movement or improper venipuncture technique can cause the needle to come out of the vein prematurely. Because of the pressure exerted by the tourniquet, blood may be forced out of the puncture site, and immediate action is required to prevent a hematoma. The tourniquet should be removed at once, a gauze pad placed on the puncture site, and pressure applied until the bleeding has stopped.

Hematoma

A hematoma is caused by blood leaking from the vein and into the surrounding tissues, resulting in a bruise. A hematoma is caused by a needle that is inserted too far and that goes through the vein; a bevel opening that is partially in the vein and partially out of the vein (Figure 17-16, *E*); and insufficient pressure at the puncture site after removing the needle. The first sign of a hematoma is a sudden swelling around the puncture site. If this occurs when the needle is in the patient's vein, the tourniquet and needle should be removed immediately, and pressure should be applied to the puncture site until the bleeding stops.

Hemolysis

The blood specimen should be handled carefully at all times. Blood cells are fragile, and rough handling may cause hemolysis, or breakdown of the blood cells. Hemolyzed blood specimens produce inaccurate test results. To prevent hemolysis, these guidelines should be followed:

1. Store the vacuum tubes at room temperature because chilled tubes can result in hemolysis.

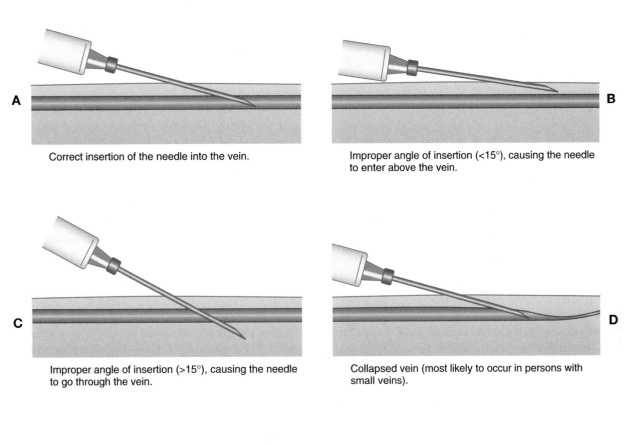

Correct insertion of the needle into the vein.

Improper angle of insertion (<15°), causing the needle to enter above the vein.

Improper angle of insertion (>15°), causing the needle to go through the vein.

Collapsed vein (most likely to occur in persons with small veins).

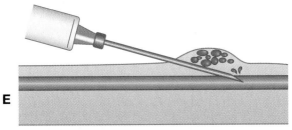

The beveled opening is partially within and partially outside of the vein, causing a hematoma.

Figure 17-16. Problems encountered with venipuncture.

2. Do not use a small-gauge needle to collect the specimen; a needle with a gauge between 20 and 22 should be used.
3. Practice good technique in collecting the specimen; excessive trauma to the blood vessel can result in hemolysis.
4. Always handle the blood specimen carefully; do not shake it or handle it roughly.

Fainting

Occasionally a patient experiences dizziness or fainting during or after a venipuncture. Should this occur, the most immediate concern is to protect the patient from injury, for example, by preventing the patient from falling. The patient should then be placed in a position that promotes blood flow to the brain, and the physician should be notified for further treatment. (See Highlight on Vasovagal Syncope.)

Obtaining a Serum Specimen

Serum

Serum is plasma from which the clotting factor fibrinogen has been removed. A brief discussion of serum is presented here, and a thorough discussion of plasma is presented later in this chapter.

Serum contains numerous dissolved substances such as glucose, cholesterol, lipids, sodium, potassium, chloride, antibodies, hormones, and enzymes. As a result, many laboratory tests require a serum specimen to determine whether these substances are within normal limits and also to detect substances that should not normally be in the serum and that, if present, indicate a pathologic condition. To perform laboratory tests on serum, it must be separated from the blood specimen, which is usually the responsibility of the medical assistant.

Tube Selection

A tube containing no additives (red-stoppered) must be used to collect the blood specimen, to allow the specimen to separate into serum and clotted blood cells. Since the amount of serum recovered is only a portion of the specimen, a blood specimen must be drawn that is 2½ times the amount required for the test. For example, if 2 ml of serum is required, a 5-ml blood specimen must be collected; if 4 ml of serum is required, a 10-ml tube is collected, and if 6 ml of serum is required, a 15-ml tube is needed.

Preparation of the Specimen

Once the blood specimen has been collected, the tube must be allowed to stand upright at room temperature for 30 to 45 minutes before being centrifuged. This allows clot formation, which will yield more serum from the specimen. If the specimen is centrifuged immediately after collection, the clotting factors do not have an opportunity to settle down into the cell layer to form a whole blood clot. The result of this is the formation of a *fibrin clot* in the serum layer. A fibrin clot is a spongy substance that occupies space, interfering with adequate serum collection. However, the blood specimen should not be allowed to stand for longer than 1 hour because changes will take place in the specimen that will lead to inaccurate test results.

Removal of Serum

Once the blood cells have clotted, the specimen is centrifuged, and the serum is then removed from the clot and placed in a separate transfer tube. It is important that proper technique be employed in removing the serum, to avoid disturbing the cell layer of the clot and drawing red blood cells into the serum. If cells do enter the pipet, the entire specimen must be recentrifuged.

When the serum has been removed from the blood specimen, the medical assistant should hold the specimen up to good light to inspect it for the presence of intact red blood cells or hemolyzed blood; in both cases, the specimen has a reddish appearance. A specimen having a reddish appearance must be recentrifuged. If the specimen contains intact red blood cells, they settle to the bottom of the tube and the serum can be removed. If the blood is hemolyzed, recentrifugation will not make the red color disappear because the red blood cells have ruptured and released hemoglobin into the serum. Hemolyzed serum is unsuitable for laboratory tests because the results will be inaccurate; therefore another blood specimen must be collected.

Procedure 17-4 presents the method for separating serum from whole blood using a conventional evacuated tube.

Highlight on Vasovagal Syncope (Fainting)

Most people experience no change in their sense of well-being when they have blood taken. A very small percentage of individuals, however, experience a type of fainting known as vasovagal syncope.

Vasovagal syncope is caused by unpleasant physical or emotional stimuli, such as pain, fright, and the sight of blood. A sudden pooling of blood occurs, which results in a sudden decrease in the blood pressure. This, in turn, momentarily deprives the brain of blood, causing a temporary loss of consciousness, usually lasting only 1 to 2 minutes. Vasovagal syncope usually occurs when an individual is in an upright position, as in standing or sitting. Before fainting, the patient usually experiences some warning signals, such as sudden light-headedness, nausea, weakness, yawning, paleness, blurred vision, a feeling of warmth, and sweating followed by drooping eyelids, weak, rapid pulse, and finally unconsciousness.

A person who is about to faint should be placed in a position that facilitates blood flow to the brain and told to breathe deeply. The preferred position is lying down (supine) with the legs somewhat elevated and the collar and clothing loosened. This position may not always be possible, such as when a patient is seated and the venipuncture needle has already been inserted. In this case, the tourniquet and then the needle should be removed and the patient's head should be lowered between the legs. An individual who has fainted should be protected from injury by falling and then be placed in a position that facilitates blood flow to the brain, as just described.

Fainting during or after venipuncture is more likely in the following individuals: patients having a venipuncture for the first time; young patients; thin patients; patients with a low diastolic or high systolic blood pressure; patients with a history of fainting; nervous and apprehensive patients; and those who are very quiet or very talkative.

Fainting often can be prevented by identifying and closely observing those individuals who are more likely to faint (as described). Talking to the patient often helps relax the patient and divert attention from the venipuncture procedure. If a patient has a history of fainting, he or she should be in a supine position for the venipuncture procedure because people rarely faint in this position. Other factors that contribute to fainting and that should be avoided include fatigue, lack of sleep, hunger, and environmental factors such as a noisy, crowded, or overheated room.

Serum Separator Tubes

A serum separator tube (SST) is an evacuated tube specially designed to facilitate the collection of a serum specimen. The SST glass tube is identified by a red and slate-gray stopper and is used for both collection and separation of blood. The serum separator tube contains a thixotropic gel, which is in a solid state in the bottom of the unused tube (Figure 17-17, *A*).

The blood specimen is collected and processed following the appropriate venipuncture method. The specimen must be allowed to stand in an upright position for proper clot formation and then centrifuged as previously described. During centrifugation, the gel temporarily becomes fluid and moves to the dividing point between the serum and clotted cells, where it re-forms into a solid gel, thus serving as a physical and chemical barrier between the serum and clot (Figure 17-17, *B*).

The serum can be transported or stored in the separator tube; the medical assistant must inspect the tube carefully to ensure that the gel barrier is firmly attached to the glass wall. If a complete barrier has not formed, the serum specimen must be placed in a transfer tube to prevent leaching of substances from the cell layer into the serum, thereby affecting the accuracy of the test results.

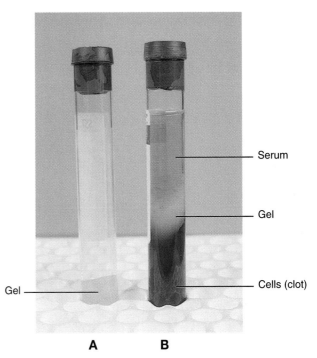

Serum

Gel

Cells (clot)

Gel

A **B**

Figure 17-17. Serum separator tubes. **A,** A tube that contains the thixotropic gel in the bottom of the unused tube. **B,** A tube that has been used to collect a blood specimen. During centrifugation, the gel temporarily becomes fluid and moves to the dividing point between the serum and blood cells in a fibrin clot.

PROCEDURE 17-4

PROCEDURE 17-4 Separating Serum From Whole Blood

Outcome Separate serum from whole blood.

Equipment/Supplies:
- Red-stoppered evacuated tube venipuncture setup
- Test tube rack
- Disposable pipet
- Transfer tube and label
- Disposable gloves
- Face shield or mask and an eye protection device
- Centrifuge
- Biohazard sharps container

1. **Procedural Step.** Collect the blood specimen following the venipuncture procedure. Use a tube containing no additives (red-stoppered) to collect the specimen. The tube selected should have a capacity of 2½ times the amount of serum required. Be sure to label *both* the red-stoppered tube and the transfer tube with the patient's name, the date, and your initials. In addition, the transfer tube should bear the word *serum*. Allow the tube to fill until the vacuum is exhausted.

Principle. To obtain serum, a tube containing no additives must be used. The tube must be allowed to fill completely in order to obtain the proper amount of serum. Several types of specimen such as serum, plasma, and urine are straw colored; therefore the transfer tube containing serum must be labeled as such to avoid confusion and mixup among these specimens.

Continued

PROCEDURE 17-4 Separating Serum From Whole Blood—Cont'd

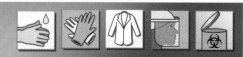

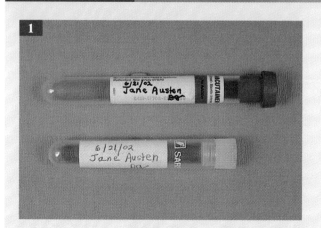

specimen tube. Make sure the tube is stoppered to prevent evaporation of the sample during centrifugation. Centrifuge the specimen for 10 to 15 minutes.
Principle. Centrifuging packs the cells and causes them to settle at the bottom of the tube, thereby yielding more serum. If the centrifuge is not balanced, it may vibrate and move across the table top. An unbalanced centrifuge can also cause specimen tubes to break.

2. Procedural Step. Place the blood specimen tube in an upright position for 30 to 45 minutes at room temperature. To prevent evaporation of the serum sample, do not remove the tube's stopper.
Principle. Specimens must be placed in an upright position and allowed to stand to permit clot formation, which will yield more serum from the specimen. Evaporation of the sample will lead to falsely elevated test results.

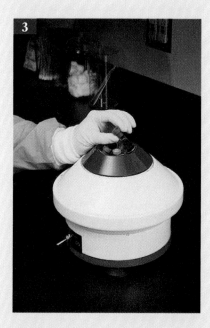

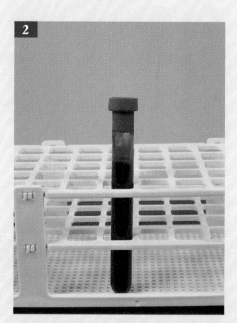

3. Procedural Step. Place the specimen in the centrifuge, stopper end up. Balance the specimen with the same type and weight of tube or another

4. Procedural Step. Put on a face shield or a mask and an eye protection device such as goggles or glasses with solid side-shields. Apply gloves. Carefully remove the tube from the centrifuge without disturbing the contents.
Principle. The OSHA Standard requires the use of personal protective equipment whenever spraying or splashing of blood might be generated. Disturbing the contents may cause the cells to enter the serum, and the specimen will need to be recentrifuged.

5. Procedural Step. Carefully remove the stopper from the tube, pointing the stopper away from you. Squeeze the bulb of the pipet to push the air out, then insert it into the serum. Place the tip of the pipet against the side of the tube approximately ¼ inch above the cell layer. Release the bulb to suction serum into the pipet. Do not allow the tip of the pipet to touch the cell layer.

Principle. Pointing the stopper away prevents accidental spraying or splashing of the specimen onto the medical assistant. The air should be removed from the bulb before inserting the pipet into the serum to prevent disturbance of the cell layer. If the cell layer is disturbed, red blood cells will enter the serum and the specimen will need to be recentrifuged.

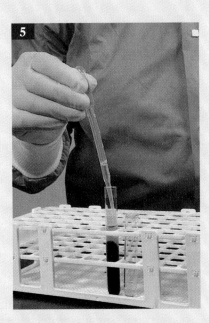

6. **Procedural Step.** Transfer the serum in the pipet to the transfer tube. Continue pipetting until as much serum as possible is removed without disturbing the cell layer. Tightly cap the transfer tube to prevent sample evaporation.

7. **Procedural Step.** Hold the specimen up to the light and examine it for the presence of hemolysis. Make sure the proper amount of serum has been obtained.
Principle. Hemolyzed serum is unsuitable for laboratory testing.

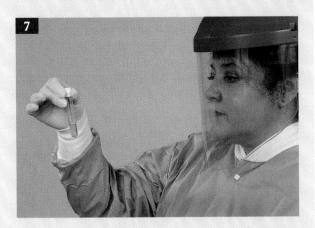

8. **Procedural Step.** Properly dispose of equipment. Following the OSHA Standard, the evacuated tube (containing the blood specimen) and the disposable pipet must be discarded in a biohazard sharps container.
9. **Procedural Step.** Remove the gloves and sanitize your hands.
10. **Procedural Step.** Test, transfer, or store the specimen according to the medical office policy.

PROCEDURE 17-4

Obtaining a Plasma Specimen

Plasma

Plasma is the straw-colored liquid portion of the blood. It serves as a transportation medium in which various substances are dissolved and blood cells are suspended for circulation through the body. Approximately 92% of plasma consists of water; the remaining 8% is dissolved solid substances (solutes) that are carried by the blood to and from the tissues.

The solutes present in greatest amounts are the *plasma proteins,* which include serum albumin, globulins, fibrinogen, and prothrombin. Serum albumin is synthesized in the liver and regulates the volume of plasma in the blood vessels. Globulins play an important role in the immunity

mechanism of the body, and fibrinogen and prothrombin are essential for proper blood clotting.

Various *electrolytes* are carried by the plasma and are needed for normal cell functioning and the maintenance of the normal fluid and acid-base balance of the body. Some of these electrolytes are sodium, chloride, potassium, calcium, phosphate, bicarbonate, and magnesium. *Nutrients* derived from the breakdown of food substances are carried by the plasma to nourish the tissues of the body and include glucose, amino acids, and lipids. *Waste products* formed as the by-products of metabolism are carried by the plasma to be excreted and include urea, uric acid, lactic acid, and creatinine. *Respiratory gases* are dissolved in and carried by the plasma and include carbon dioxide and a small amount of oxygen. Substances in the plasma that help regulate and control body functions include hormones, antibodies, enzymes, and vitamins.

Tube Selection

At times a plasma specimen is required for a laboratory test. The procedure for separating plasma from whole blood is essentially the same as that for separating serum from whole blood with minor variances, which are described here.

A tube containing an anticoagulant must be used to obtain plasma. The medical assistant should check the laboratory directory or the medical office laboratory procedures manual to determine the type of anticoagulant to be used; it is usually specified by the color of the tube stopper. The tube used to collect the specimen *and* the transfer tube should be properly labeled with the patient's name, the date, and the medical assistant's initials. In addition, the transfer tube should bear the word *plasma*.

Preparation and Removal of the Specimen

As with serum, a blood specimen must be collected that is 2½ times the amount required for the test. Before collecting the specimen, evacuated tubes containing a powdered additive should be tapped just below the stopper to release any of the anticoagulant that may have adhered to the stopper. It is important to allow the specimen to fill to the exhaustion of the vacuum to ensure the proper ratio of anticoagulant to blood, which, in turn, will ensure accurate test results.

Immediately after the specimen is drawn, the tube should be gently inverted eight to ten times to mix the anticoagulant with the blood specimen. The specimen is then placed in a centrifuge with the stopper on for 10 to 15 minutes. (The specimen does not need to stand before it is centrifuged.) Centrifuging the specimen packs the blood cells and causes the blood to separate into three layers: a top layer of plasma, a middle layer (the buffy coat), and a bottom layer of red blood cells. The plasma is then separated from the blood specimen using the same procedure as that outlined for the separation of serum from whole blood.

SKIN PUNCTURE

A skin puncture is used to obtain a capillary blood specimen and, therefore, is also called a *capillary puncture*. Laboratory testing of a capillary blood specimen is usually performed at the medical office. Examples of such tests are hemoglobin, hematocrit, and glucose using a glucose monitor.

The reason for performing a skin puncture rather than a venipuncture is as follows. A skin puncture is performed when a test requires only a small blood specimen. Skin puncture is the method preferred for obtaining blood from infants and very young children. Collecting blood in this age-group by venipuncture is difficult and may damage veins and surrounding tissues. In addition, infants and young children have such a small blood volume that removing large quantities of blood may cause anemia. A skin puncture might also be performed as a last resort on an adult when a blood specimen is needed and there are no accessible veins.

Before collecting a capillary blood specimen, the medical assistant must (1) select a puncture site, (2) select the skin puncture device, and (3) obtain the proper microcollection device to collect the specimen. Each of these topics is described next.

Puncture Site

The puncture site varies depending on the age of the patient. The fingertip is the preferred site for a skin puncture on an adult. In the past, the earlobe was also recommended as a skin puncture site for an adult. This is no longer true. Blood obtained by puncturing the earlobe has been found to contain a higher concentration of hemoglobin than fingertip blood. In addition the earlobe produces a slower flow of blood, making it more difficult to obtain a blood specimen.

In an infant (birth to 1 year), the skin puncture should be performed on the plantar surface of the heel. A finger puncture should *never* be performed on infants. The amount of tissue between skin surface and bone is so small that an injury to the bone is very likely. Once a child is walking, the skin puncture should be performed on the finger.

Skin Puncture Devices

A skin puncture can be performed using the following devices: a disposable lancet, a disposable semiautomatic lancet, or a reusable semiautomatic lancet. The device used to perform the skin puncture is a matter of personal preference, and the technique for performing the puncture depends on the equipment. A description of skin puncture devices is presented next, and the procedures for using them are presented at the end of this section.

Regardless of the skin puncture device, the puncture must not penetrate deeper than 3.1 mm on adults and 2.4 mm on infants and children. If the puncture is deeper than this, the bone may be penetrated, which could result in the painful and serious conditions of osteochondritis or osteomyelitis. **Osteochondritis** is the inflammation of bone and cartilage, and **osteomyelitis** is an inflammation of the bone due to bacterial infection. To avoid these complications, a number of companies manufacture special skin puncture devices that control the depth of puncture.

Disposable Lancet

A disposable lancet is a sterile, sharp-pointed device used to pierce the skin (Figure 17-18, *A*). The skin is punctured by pushing the point of the lancet into the skin. A disadvantage of the lancet is that some patients become apprehensive and flinch when they see the point of the lancet coming. Children might even pull their hands out of the medical assistant's grasp. In either case, this could cause the medical assistant to accidentally stick herself or himself. Procedure 17-5 describes the procedure for performing a skin puncture using a disposable lancet.

Disposable Semiautomatic Lancet

A disposable semiautomatic lancet consists of a spring-loaded plastic holder with a metal blade inside the holder. Different sized blades are available to control the depth of the puncture. The plastic holder conceals the blade so the patient cannot see it during the puncture. One such lancet device is the Microtainer Brand Safety Flow Lancet, manufactured by Becton Dickinson (Figure 17-19, *B*). Another example is the Tenderlette, manufactured by International Technidyne Corporation.

To perform the skin puncture, the lancet device is placed on the patient's skin and a plunger is depressed.

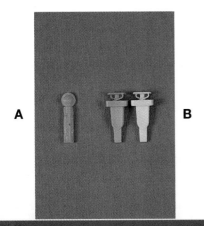

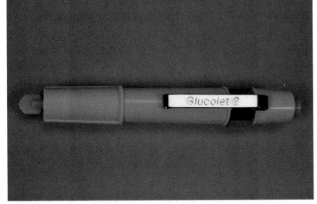

Figure 17-18. Lancet devices. **A,** Disposable lancet. **B,** Microtainer Brand Safety Flow Lancet. **C,** Glucolet II.

The spring forces the blade into the skin and then retracts the blade into the holder. The concealed blade and automatic puncture tend to result in less patient apprehension. After the puncture, the entire lancet device is discarded in a biohazard sharps container. For safety, disposable lancet devices are preferred over other skin puncture devices because not only is the device disposable, but the retractable blade eliminates the possibility of an accidental needlestick. Procedure 17-6 describes the skin puncture procedure using a disposable semiautomatic lancet.

Reusable Semiautomatic Lancet

A wide variety of semiautomatic lancets are commercially available; however, not all are appropriate for use in the medical office. Some of these devices are suitable for use only by an individual patient to perform home blood glucose monitoring. When used by more than one patient in the medical office, they have been associated with the transmission of hepatitis B. The safest reusable device is one in which the part that may become contaminated is disposable. This type of device reduces the risk of needlestick injuries and infection from a contaminated sharp. An example of a reusable lancet that is safe to use in the medical office is the Glucolet II (Bayer Corporation).

The Glucolet II consists of a plastic spring-loaded lancet holder and a lancet/endcap (Figure 17-18, *C*). The lancet holder is reusable while the lancet/endcap is disposable and meant for only one use. To perform the puncture, the lancet/endcap is placed on the patient's skin and a release button is depressed. The spring forces the blade into the skin and then retracts the blade into the endcap. Following the procedure the lancet/endcap is discarded in a biohazard sharps container (see Procedure 17-7).

Microcollection Devices

Once the skin has been punctured, a capillary blood specimen must be collected. The blood specimen can be collected directly onto a reagent strip, such as occurs with blood glucose monitors. It can also be collected in a small container known as a *microcollection* device. The device depends on the laboratory equipment running the test. Common microcollection devices are capillary tubes and microcollection tubes, which are discussed here.

Microcollection Tubes. A microcollection tube consists of a small plastic tube with a removable blood collector tip. The tip is designed to collect capillary blood from a skin puncture and results in a relatively large blood specimen. After the specimen has been collected, the collector tip is removed and discarded and replaced by a plastic plug. Microcollection tubes are available with or without additives. The plugs are color-coded and correspond to the colored-coded evacuated tube system used in venipuncture. One such device is the Microtainer by Becton-Dickinson (Figure 17-19, *A* and *B*).

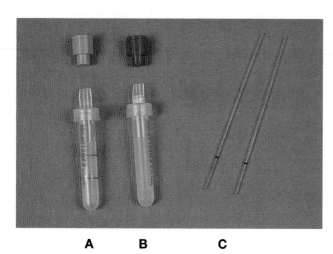

Figure 17-19. Microcollection devices. **A** and **B,** Microcollection tubes. **C,** Capillary tubes.

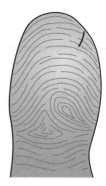

Figure 17-20. Recommended site for a finger puncture.

Capillary Tubes. A capillary tube consists of a disposable glass or plastic tube (Figure 17-19, *C*). Depending on the size of the tube, it can hold between 5 and 75 μl of blood. In the medical office, a capillary tube is used to collect a blood specimen for a hematocrit determination. This procedure is presented in the next chapter.

Guidelines for Performing a Finger Puncture

The following guidelines should be followed when performing a finger puncture:

1. If a laboratory test requires advance preparation, before you perform the finger puncture, verify that the patient has prepared properly. If not, do not collect the specimen unless directed otherwise by the physician. If the finger puncture is to be rescheduled, carefully review the preparation requirements with the patient.
2. The patient should be seated comfortably in a chair. The arm should be firmly supported and extended with the palmar surface of the hand facing up. Never perform a skin puncture with the patient sitting on a stool or standing. The possibility exists that the patient will faint and injure himself or herself.
3. Instruct the patient to remain still during the procedure. Explain to the patient that the procedure should be relatively quick and only slightly uncomfortable. Just before making the puncture, tell the patient that he or she will "feel a small stick." This prevents startling the patient, which could cause the patient to move.
4. Use the lateral part of the tip of the third or fourth fingers (middle and ring fingers) of the nondominant hand for the puncture site. The capillary bed in these fingers is large and the skin is easy to penetrate. The

puncture site should be free of lesions, scars, bruises, and edema. The index finger and the little finger are not recommended as puncture sites. The index finger is more callused and, therefore, harder to penetrate than the other fingers. Also, the patient uses that finger more and will notice the pain longer. The tissue of the little finger is much thinner than that of the others; using this finger as a puncture site could result in an injury to the bone.

5. After selecting the puncture site, warm the site to increase the blood flow to the capillary bed. Warming the site can be accomplished by gently massaging the finger five or six times from base to tip or by placing the hand in warm water for a few minutes (108°F or 42°C). Warming the site promotes bleeding after an effective puncture.
6. Cleanse the site with an antiseptic wipe and allow it to dry thoroughly. The site must be dry to allow a round drop of blood to form. Otherwise the drop will leach out on the patient's skin and be difficult to collect. In addition, alcohol entering the capillary specimen contaminates it, leading to inaccurate test results. Alcohol causes the patient to experience a stinging sensation when the puncture is made.
7. Firmly grasp the finger in front of the most distal knuckle joint. The puncturing area should be hard and red so that adequate penetration and depth of puncture can occur.
8. Make the puncture in the central, fleshy portion of the finger, slightly to the side of center. To prevent injury to the bone, do not puncture the side or very tip of the finger. The puncture should be perpendicular to the lines of the fingerprint rather than parallel to the fingerprint (Figure 17-20). This facilitates the formation of a well-formed drop of blood that is easy to collect. Punctures that are not perpendicular will be difficult to collect because the blood flow will follow the lines of the fingerprint and run down the finger.

9. Perform the puncture. If a good puncture has been made, the blood will flow freely. When learning this procedure, many individuals tend not to press hard enough. If this occurs, a poor blood flow results and the patient has to be punctured again. A deep puncture hurts no more than a superficial one and provides a much better blood flow.
10. Wipe away the first drop of blood with a gauze pad. The first drop of blood is diluted with alcohol and tissue fluid and is not a suitable specimen.
11. Allow a large drop of blood to form by applying continual gentle pressure near the puncture. Collect the

blood specimen using the appropriate microcollection device. If the required amount of blood is not obtained, you can gently massage the tissue surrounding the puncture site. Do not squeeze or massage excessively because doing so causes dilution of the blood specimen with tissue fluids.
12. Check the puncture site to make sure the bleeding has stopped. Apply an adhesive bandage, if needed. A bandage is not recommended for children younger than 2 years of age. The bandage may irritate the skin of a young child, and the child might put the bandage in his or her mouth, aspirate it, and choke.

PROCEDURE 17-5   Skin Puncture—Disposable Lancet

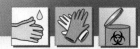

Outcome Obtain a capillary blood specimen.

Equipment/Supplies:
- Disposable gloves
- Antiseptic wipe
- Disposable lancet
- Sterile 2 × 2 gauze pad
- Biohazard sharps container

1. **Procedural Step.** Sanitize your hands.
2. **Procedural Step.** Greet and identify the patient, and introduce yourself. If the patient was required to prepare for the test (e.g., fasting, medication restriction), determine whether he or she has prepared properly. If the patient has not followed the patient preparation requirements, notify the physician for instructions on handling this situation.
3. **Procedural Step.** Assemble the equipment. Open the sterile gauze packet and place the gauze pad on the inside of its wrapper.

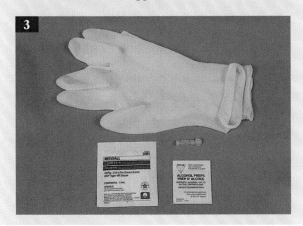

4. **Procedural Step.** Explain the procedure to the patient and reassure the patient.
   Principle. Reassurance should be offered to reduce apprehension.
5. **Procedural Step.** Seat the patient comfortably in a chair. The patient's arm should be firmly supported and extended with the palmar surface of the hand facing up.
6. **Procedural Step.** Using the lateral part of the tip of the third or fourth finger of the nondominant hand, select an appropriate puncture site. If the patient's finger is cold, you can warm it by gently massaging the finger five or six times from base to tip or by placing the hand in warm water for a few minutes.
   Principle. Warming the site increases the blood flow to the area and promotes bleeding from the puncture site.
7. **Procedural Step.** Cleanse the site with an antiseptic wipe. Allow the site to air dry, and after cleansing it do not touch the area or fan the area with your hand.

Continued

PROCEDURE 17-5   Skin Puncture—Disposable Lancet—Cont'd

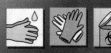

Principle. The site must be dry to prevent a stinging sensation when the puncture is made and to allow a round drop of blood to form. Alcohol in the capillary specimen contaminates it, leading to inaccurate test results. Touching or fanning the site after cleansing contaminates it, and the cleansing process has to be repeated.

8. **Procedural Step.** Apply gloves. Using a twisting motion, remove the plastic cover from the end of the lancet; this exposes its sterile point. If the tip becomes contaminated, a new lancet must be obtained.

   Principle. Gloves provide a barrier against blood-borne pathogens.

9. **Procedural Step.** Without touching the puncture site, firmly grasp the patient's finger and make a puncture with the sterile lancet, using a quick jabbing motion. The puncture should be made perpendicular to the lines of the fingerprint and should be approximately 2 to 3 mm deep for an adult. A well-made puncture results in a free-flowing wound that needs only slight pressure to make it bleed.

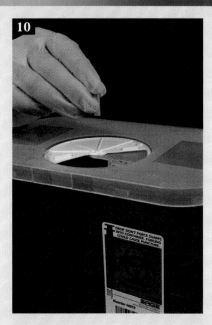

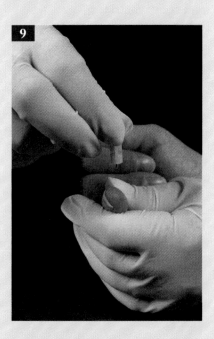

10. **Procedural Step.** Immediately dispose of the lancet in a biohazard sharps container.

    Principle. Proper disposal of contaminated sharps is required by the OSHA Standard to prevent exposure to bloodborne pathogens.

11. **Procedural Step.** Wait a few seconds to allow blood flow to begin. Wipe away the first drop of blood with a gauze pad.

    Principle. The first drop of blood is diluted with alcohol and tissue fluid and is not a suitable specimen.

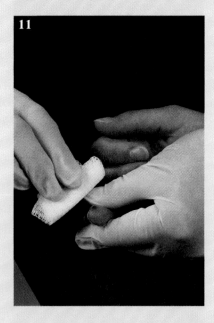

12. Procedural Step. Use the second drop of blood for the test. Allow a large well-rounded drop of blood to form by applying gentle continuous pressure without squeezing the finger. You can massage the tissue surrounding the puncture firmly but gently to encourage blood flow.
Principle. Squeezing or massaging the site excessively causes dilution of the blood sample with tissue fluid; inaccurate test readings result.

13. Procedural Step. Collect the blood specimen in the appropriate microcollection device.

14. Procedural Step. Have the patient hold a gauze pad over the puncture and apply pressure until the bleeding stops. As a safety precaution, remain with the patient until the bleeding stops. If needed, apply an adhesive bandage.

15. Procedural Step. Test the blood specimen as required by the test being performed.

16. Procedural Step. Remove the gloves, and sanitize your hands.

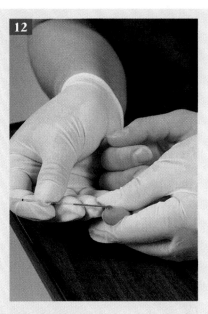

PROCEDURE 17-6 Skin Puncture—Disposable Semiautomatic Lancet Device

Outcome Obtain a capillary blood specimen.

Equipment/Supplies:
- Disposable gloves
- Antiseptic wipe
- Microtainer brand safety flow lancet
- Sterile 2 × 2 gauze pad
- Biohazard sharps container

1. Procedural Step. Follow steps 1 through 7 of the disposable lancet method of skin puncture (see Procedure 17-5).

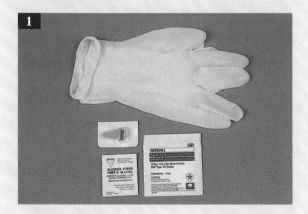

2. Procedural Step. Remove the semiautomatic lancet from its plastic packet. Use the blue (1.9-mm puncture depth) Microtainer lancet for a finger puncture. Apply gloves.
Principle. Gloves provide a barrier precaution against bloodborne pathogens.

3. Procedural Step. Without touching the puncture site, firmly grasp the patient's finger. Place the plastic holder on the patient's finger with moderate pressure. Make the puncture perpendicular to the lines of the fingerprint. Depress the plunger with the index finger. A well-made puncture results in a free-flowing wound that needs only slight pressure to make it bleed.

Continued

PROCEDURE 17-6 Skin Puncture—Disposable Semiautomatic Lancet Device—Cont'd

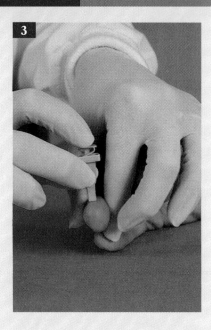

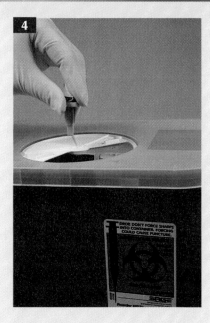

4. Procedural Step. Immediately dispose of the semi-automatic lancet in a biohazard sharps container. *Principle.* Proper disposal of contaminated sharps is required by the OSHA Standard to prevent exposure to bloodborne pathogens.

5. **Procedural Step.** Follow steps 11 through 16 of the disposable lancet method of skin puncture.

PROCEDURE 17-7 Skin Puncture—Reusable Semiautomatic Lancet Device

Outcome Obtain a capillary blood specimen.

Equipment/Supplies:
- Disposable gloves
- Antiseptic wipe
- Glucolet II lancet device
- Disposable lancet/endcap

- Sterile lancet
- Sterile 2 × 2 gauze pad
- Biohazard sharps container

1. **Procedural Step.** Sanitize your hands.

2. **Procedural Step.** Greet and identify the patient, and introduce yourself. If the patient was required to prepare for the test (e.g., fasting, medication restriction), determine whether he or she has prepared properly. If the patient has not followed the patient preparation requirements, notify the physician for instructions on handling this situation.

3. Procedural Step. Assemble the equipment. Push the transparent barrel of the lancet device toward the release button until it clicks into place.

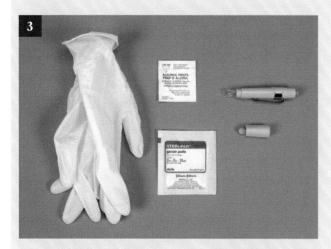

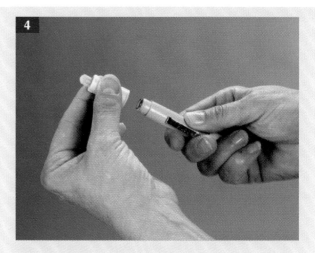

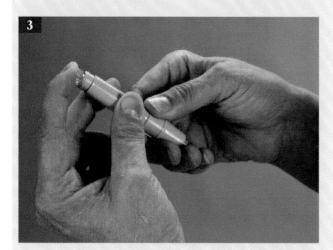

4. Procedural Step. Insert the lancet/endcap onto the lancet device. Open the sterile gauze packet and place the gauze pad on the inside of its wrapper.

5. **Procedural Step.** Explain the procedure to the patient, and reassure the patient.
   Principle. Reassurance should be offered to reduce apprehension.

6. **Procedural Step.** Seat the patient comfortably in a chair. The patient's arm should be firmly supported and extended with the palmar surface of the hand facing up.

7. **Procedural Step.** Using the lateral part of the tip of the third or fourth finger of the nondominant hand, select an appropriate puncture site. If the patient's finger is cold, you can warm it by gently massaging the finger five or six times from base to tip or by placing the hand in warm water for a few minutes.
   Principle. Warming the site increases the blood flow to the area and promotes bleeding from the puncture site.

8. **Procedural Step.** Cleanse the site with an antiseptic wipe. Allow the site to air dry, and after cleansing it do not touch the area or fan the area with your hand.
   Principle. The site must be dry to prevent a stinging sensation when the puncture is made and to allow a round drop of blood to form. Alcohol entering the capillary specimen contaminates it, leading to inaccurate test results. Touching or fanning the site after cleansing contaminates it, and the cleansing process has to be repeated.

9. Procedural Step. Apply gloves. Using a twisting motion, remove the plastic post from the lancet/endcap.
   Principle. Gloves provide a barrier against bloodborne pathogens.

Continued

PROCEDURE 17-7 Skin Puncture—Reusable Semiautomatic Lancet Device—Cont'd

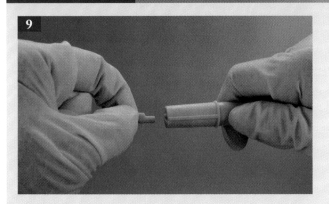

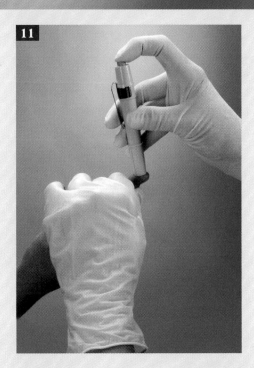

10. **Procedural Step.** Without touching the puncture site, firmly grasp the patient's finger. Place the end-cap firmly against the puncture site.

11. **Procedural Step.** Press the release button without moving the Glucolet or finger. Pressing the release button permits the lancet to puncture the skin. A well-made puncture results in a free-flowing wound that needs only slight pressure to make it bleed.

12. **Procedural Step.** Wait a few seconds to allow blood flow to begin. Wipe away the first drop of blood with a gauze pad.

    Principle. The first drop of blood is diluted with alcohol and tissue fluid and is not a suitable specimen.

13. **Procedural Step.** Use the second drop of blood for the test. Allow a large well-rounded drop of blood to form by applying gentle continuous pressure without squeezing the finger. The tissue surrounding the puncture site can be massaged firmly but gently to encourage blood flow.

    Principle. Squeezing or massaging the site excessively causes dilution of the blood sample with tissue fluid; inaccurate test readings result.

PROCEDURE 17-7

14. **Procedural Step.** Collect the blood specimen in the appropriate microcollection device.

15. **Procedural Step.** Have the patient hold a gauze pad over the puncture site and apply pressure until the bleeding stops. As a safety precaution, remain with the patient until the bleeding stops. If needed, apply an adhesive bandage.

16. **Procedural Step.** Remove the endcap from the lancet device and discard it in a biohazard waste container.

17. **Procedural Step.** Test the blood specimen as required by the test being performed.

18. **Procedural Step** Remove the gloves, and sanitize your hands.

19. **Procedural Step.** Sanitize and disinfect the Glucolet II according to the manufacturer's instructions. Store the Glucolet II in its resting position.

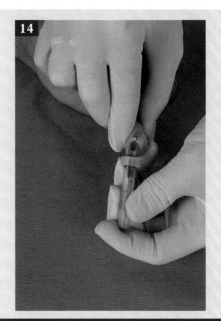

PROCEDURE **17-7**

MEDICAL Practice and the LAW

Phlebotomy is an invasive procedure that can harm the patient if performed incorrectly. Sharps and medical waste contaminated with blood must be disposed of according to federal regulations. Laboratory tests involving blood must be performed correctly for accurate results. Incorrect results can lead to an inaccurate diagnosis and treatment. Currently, performing HIV testing requires the patient's written consent. If the patient has questions regarding HIV, refer him or her to the physician for discussion. Never give out laboratory results without checking with the physician. HIV results should be given only by the physician. Never speculate to the patient or co-workers about the results of any test. All test results must remain confidential.

Use appropriate personal protective equipment to prevent the transmission of bloodborne pathogens to protect yourself, your co-workers, and your patients.

What Would You DO?
What Would You *Not* DO? *RESPONSES*

Case Study 1
What Did Dori Do?

❑ Told Angela that it was fine to have her friends there while she gets her blood drawn.

❑ Told Angela that she could not have the blood drawn out of her left arm because a good vein could not be located in that arm.

❑ Told Angela that using the hand veins are always the last choice when drawing blood. Explained that there are a lot of nerve endings in the hand, which make it hurt more.

❑ Told Angela that most of the time what she sees on TV is someone getting an IV started in the hand, not their blood being drawn.

❑ Explained to Angela that there will just be a small stick and that it would heal quickly, and there should be no reason it would affect her softball game this evening.

❑ Tried to relax and ressure Angela before the venipuncture. Made sure to carefully explain the procedure to her since it was her first one.

❑ Since Angela was nervous, took precautions to prevent her from fainting by placing her in a semi-Fowler's position on the examing table.

❑ Had Angela's friend stand near the head of the table to help calm her down.

What Did Dori Not Do?

❑ Did not try to draw Angela's blood from her left arm or hand.

❑ Did not ignore the fact that Angela was nervous about the venipuncture.

What Would You Do?/What Would You *Not* Do? Review Dori's response and place a checkmark next to the information you included in your response. List additional information you included in your response below.

_____

_____

_____

_____

Case Study 2
What Did Dori Do?

❑ Told Buzz that when the needle enters his skin, the tissues release a substance that could cause inaccurate test results. Explained the red tube is used to get rid of that substance and that's why it is thrown away.

❑ Told Buzz that butterfly setups are also used in the medical office and that the choice of what to use depends on the size of a patient's veins and the policy of the health care facility.

❑ Stressed to Buzz how important it is to have his blood tested every week to make sure there is not too much or too little of the Coumadin in his body. Explained to him again what might occur if his Coumadin was at the wrong level.

❑ Told Buzz that the office would be glad to help him locate a medical laboratory where he will be vacationing so he could have his test done.

❑ Made sure that Buzz had a laboratory requisition so that he could have his test done while he was on vacation.

What Did Dori Not Do?

❑ Did not tell Buzz that it would be all right to skip his pro-thrombin test during his vacation.

What Would You Do?/What Would You *Not* Do? Review Dori's response and place a checkmark next to the information you included in your response. List additional information you included in your response below.

_____

_____

_____

_____

Case Study 3
What Did Dori Do?

❑ Told Mrs. Gabriel that only the laboratory can accept specimens drawn at the lab or the medical office.

❑ Told Mrs. Gabriel that if it would make her feel more comfortable, the lab could drop off the blood-drawing supplies at the office and her blood could be drawn tomorrow at the office.

❑ Informed the physician about Mrs. Gabriel's experience at the laboratory.

What Did Dori Not Do?

❑ Did not tell Mrs. Gabriel that probing a vein could cause the test results to be inaccurate.

What Would You Do?/What Would You *Not* Do? Review Dori's response and place a checkmark next to the information you included in your response. List additional information you included in your response below.

_____

_____

_____

_____

Apply Your
KNOWLEDGE

Choose the best answer to the each of the following questions.

1. Hugh Everett comes to the medical office to have his blood drawn for an FBS and CBC. Of the following, what should Dori Glover, CMA, do *first?*
   A. Cleanse the puncture site thoroughly with an antiseptic wipe
   B. Ask Hugh if he has ever gotten light-headed from having his blood drawn
   C. Label the evacuated tube and complete a laboratory requisition
   D. Ask Hugh when he last ate or drank

2. Dori is getting ready to apply the rubber tourniquet to Hugh's arm. All of the following are correct techniques for Dori to use when applying the tourniquet EXCEPT:
   A. Applying the tourniquet 3 inches above the bend in the elbow
   B. Applying the tourniquet loosely so that it is not uncomfortable for Hugh
   C. Asking Hugh to clench his fist to make the antecubital veins more prominent
   D. Making sure not to leave the tourniquet on for more than 1 minute

3. After applying the tourniquet to Hugh's arm, Dori determines that the median cubital vein on his left arm would be the best vein to use. Dori then proceeds to perform an assessment of the vein by:
   A. Palpating the size and depth of the vein
   B. Tracing the path of the vein
   C. Mentally mapping the location of the vein on Hugh's arm
   D. All of the above

4. Dori is getting ready to draw blood from Hugh using the vacuum tube method of venipuncture. Which of the following would NOT be a correct technique for Dori to use when inserting the needle?
   A. Inserting the needle with the bevel facing up
   B. Pointing the needle in the same direction as the vein to be entered
   C. Inserting the needle at a 30-degree angle to the arm
   D. Positioning the evacuated tube with the label facing downward

5. After filling the lavender-stoppered evacuated tube to the exhaustion of the vacuum and removing it from the plastic holder, Dori proceeds to the next step of the procedure, which is to:
   A. Gently rotate the tube eight times
   B. Remove the needle from the vein
   C. Insert another tube into the plastic holder
   D. Apply pressure to the puncture site with a gauze pad

6. Amy Anderson has come to the medical office to have her blood drawn as part of a college sport's physical requirement. Which of the following would be a good question for Dori Glover, CMA, to ask Amy to facilitate this procedure?
   A. "What kind of sports are you involved in?"
   B. "Who is your next of kin?"
   C. "What vein has been used in the past to draw your blood?"
   D. "Are you allergic to any medications?"

7. Dori examines the veins of both of Amy's arms and cannot palpate a median cubital vein. Dori is able to palpate a large basilic vein on the side of Amy's left arm and decides to draw the blood specimen from that vein. Of the following, what would be an important step to perform when drawing blood from Amy?
   A. Applying the tourniquet as tightly as possible
   B. Applying firm pressure below the vein
   C. Using a small gauge needle to collect the specimen
   D. Using a Hemogard tube to collect the specimen

8. Dori successfully collects a blood specimen from Amy. All of the following are correct techniques for Dori to use when withdrawing the needle EXCEPT:
   A. Removing the tourniquet before withdrawing the needle
   B. Removing the needle at the same angle as that for penetration
   C. Asking Amy to keep her fist clenched as the needle is withdrawn
   D. Applying pressure to the puncture site after withdrawing the needle

9. Dr. Hemolysis asks Dori Glover, CMA, to collect a capillary blood specimen from Ashley Mackenzie, age 6 months, to check her hemoglobin level. An appropriate puncture site for Dori to use would be the:
   A. Plantar surface of the heel
   B. Antecubital veins of the arm
   C. Earlobe
   D. Lateral side of the third finger

10. Dori uses a disposable lancet to collect the blood specimen from Ashley. After making the puncture, Dori should:
    A. Squeeze the puncture site to increase the blood flow
    B. Wipe away the first drop of blood
    C. Collect the blood specimen
    D. Warm the site to increase the blood flow

CERTIFICATION REVIEW

❏ **Phlebotomy** is defined as the collection of blood, and the individual collecting the blood sample is known as a phlebotomist. The term *venipuncture* means the puncturing of a vein for the removal of a venous blood sample. Venipuncture can be performed by the following methods: vacuum tube, butterfly, and syringe.

❏ **The antecubital space** is generally used as the site for drawing blood. The antecubital veins typically have a wide lumen, are easily accessible, and are close to the surface of the skin. The best vein to use in the antecubital space is the median cubital. The basilic and cephalic veins are located on either side of the antecubital space and are considered an alternative when the median cubital vein is not available.

❏ **The various types of blood specimen** that the medical assistant will be required to obtain through the venipuncture procedure include clotted blood, serum, whole blood, and plasma. The blood specimen should be handled carefully at all times. Blood cells are fragile and rough handling may cause hemolysis. Hemolyzed blood specimens produce inaccurate test results.

❏ **The vacuum tube method** is frequently used to collect venous blood specimens. Vacuum tube needles are available in sizes 20 to 22 gauge and come in two lengths: 1 inch and $1\frac{1}{2}$ inch. Evacuated tubes consist of a glass tube with a rubber stopper and a vacuum to pull the blood specimen into the tube. Evacuated tubes use a color-coded system to identify their additive content.

❏ **The butterfly method** of venipuncture is also called the winged infusion method. It is used to collect blood from patients who are difficult to stick by conventional methods, such as adult patients with small antecubital veins and children.

❏ **The syringe method** is the least used method of venipuncture. This is because once the blood specimen is obtained, it must be transferred from the syringe to an evacuated tube, which presents the risk of an accidental needlestick. The syringe method is used primarily to obtain blood from small veins.

❏ **Plasma** is the straw-colored liquid portion of the blood. It serves as a transportation medium in which various substances are dissolved and in which blood cells are suspended for circulation through the body. Approximately 92% of plasma consists of water; the remaining 8% is dissolved solid substances that are carried by the blood to and from the tissues.

❏ **A skin puncture** is used to obtain a capillary blood specimen. A skin puncture is performed when a test requires only a small blood specimen. Also, skin puncture is the method preferred for obtaining blood from infants and very young children. The fingertip is the preferred site for a skin puncture on an adult.

❏ **Once the skin has been punctured,** a capillary blood specimen must be collected. The blood specimen can be collected directly onto a reagent strip or it can be collected in a microcollection device. Examples of microcollection devices are capillary tubes and microcollection tubes.

Terminology Review

Antecubital space The surface of the arm in front of the elbow.

Anticoagulant A substance that inhibits blood clotting.

Buffy coat A thin, light-colored layer of white blood cells and platelets that lays between a top layer of plasma and a bottom layer of red blood cells when an anticoagulant has been added to a blood specimen.

Evacuated tube A closed glass or plastic tube that contains a premeasured vacuum.

Hematoma A swelling or mass of coagulated blood caused by a break in a blood vessel.

Hemoconcentration An increase in the concentration of the nonfilterable blood components, such as red blood cells, enzymes, iron, and calcium, as a result of a decrease in the fluid content of the blood.

Hemolysis The breakdown of blood cells.

Osteochondritis Inflammation of bone and cartilage.

Osteomyelitis Inflammation of the bone due to bacterial infection.

Phlebotomist A health professional trained in the collection of blood specimens.

Phlebotomy Incision of a vein for the removal or withdrawal of blood; the collection of blood.

Plasma The liquid part of the blood consisting of a clear, straw-colored fluid that makes up approximately 55% of the blood volume.

Serum Plasma from which the clotting factor fibrinogen has been removed.

Venipuncture Puncturing of a vein.

Venous reflux The backflow of blood (from an evacuated tube) into the patient's vein.

Venous stasis The temporary cessation or slowing of the venous blood flow.

ON THE WEB

For active weblinks to each website visit http://evolve.elsevier/Bonewit/.

For Information on Phlebotomy:

American Society for Clinical Laboratory Science (ASCLS)

American Society For Clinical Pathology (ASCP)

American Society of Phlebotomy Technicians (ASPT)

Becton Dickinson

National Phlebotomy Association (NPA)

Learning Objectives

Procedures

Hematology Tests

1. List the tests included in a complete blood count (CBC).
2. Describe the shape of an erythrocyte and explain how it acquires this shape.
3. Describe the composition of hemoglobin and explain its function.
4. Describe the normal appearance of leukocytes and explain how they fight infection in the body.
5. State the normal value or range for the following hematologic tests:
   - Hemoglobin
   - Hematocrit
   - Red and white blood cell counts
   - Differential cell count
6. State the purpose of the hematocrit, and list the layers the blood separates into after it has been centrifuged.
7. Explain the purpose of the differential cell count.
8. Describe the appearance of the five types of white blood cells.

Perform a hemoglobin determination using an automated analyzer and the manufacturer's operating manual.

Perform a hematocrit determination.

Perform a white blood cell count using an automated blood cell counter and the manufacturer's operating manual.

Prepare a blood smear.

CHAPTER 18

Hematology

Chapter Outline

INTRODUCTION TO HEMATOLOGY

Components and Function of Blood
  Erythrocytes
  Leukocytes
  Thrombocytes

Hemoglobin Determination

Hematocrit

White Blood Cell Count

Red Blood Cell Count

White Blood Cell Differential Count
  Automated Method
  Manual Method
  Types of White Blood Cells

National Competencies

Clinical Competencies

Diagnostic Testing
- Perform hematology testing.

Patient Care
- Screen and follow up test results.

General Competencies

Patient Instruction
- Provide instruction for health maintenance and disease prevention.

Operational Functions
- Use methods of quality control.

ameboid movement (ah-MEE-boid-MOVE-ment)
anemia (ah-NEE-mee-ah)
bilirubin (bill-ih-ROO-bin)
diapedesis (die-ah-pah-DEE-sis)
hematology (hee-mah-TOL-oe-jee)
hemoglobin (HEE-moe-gloe-bin)
hemolysis (hee-MOL-oe-sis)
leukocytosis (loo-koe-sie-TOE-sis)
leucopenia (loo-koe-PEE-nee-ah)
oxyhemoglobin (ok-see-HEE-moe-gloe-bin)
phagocytosis (fay-goe-sie-TOE-sis)
polycythemia (pol-ee-sie-THEE-mee-ah)

Introduction to Hematology

Hematology is the study of blood, including its morphologic appearance and function, as well as diseases of the blood and blood-forming tissues. Laboratory analysis in hematology is concerned with the examination of blood for the purpose of detecting pathologic conditions. It includes performing blood cell counts, evaluating the clotting ability of the blood, and identifying cell types. These tests are valuable tools that allow the physician to determine whether each blood component falls within its normal value or range.

Examples of hematologic tests include the white blood cell count, red blood cell count, differential white blood cell count, hemoglobin, hematocrit, prothrombin time, erythrocyte sedimentation rate, and platelet count. Table 18-1 summarizes common hematologic tests, including specimen requirements, normal values, and conditions that cause abnormal test results.

Hematologic laboratory tests are often performed in the medical office. Advances in automated blood analyzers designed for use in the medical office have made this possible. Automated blood analyzers perform laboratory tests with accurate test results in a very short time. Each automated analyzer is accompanied by a detailed operating manual that explains its operation, test parameters, care, and maintenance.

The most frequently performed hematologic laboratory test is the *complete blood count (CBC)*. A CBC is routinely performed on new patients and on patients with a pathologic condition. The test results provide valuable information to assist the physician in making a diagnosis, evaluating the patient's progress, and regulating treatment. The tests included in a CBC are as follows:

- White blood cell (WBC) count
- Red blood cell (RBC) count
- Platelet count
- Hemoglobin (Hgb)
- Hematocrit (Hct)
- Differential white blood cell count (diff)
- Red blood cell indices

Components and Function of Blood

Blood consists of two parts: liquid and solid. Plasma, the liquid portion of the blood, consists of a clear yellowish fluid that makes up approximately 55% of the blood volume. The plasma transports nutrients to the tissues of the body to nourish and sustain them. It picks up wastes from the tissues; the wastes are eliminated through the kidneys. The plasma also transports antibodies, enzymes, and hormones to help regulate normal body functioning.

The solid portion of the blood consists of three types of cells: erythrocytes, leukocytes, and thrombocytes, which are described next in detail. The solid portion of the blood accounts for 45% of the total blood volume. The average adult body contains 10 to 12 pints (5 to 6 liters) of blood.

Text continued on p. 712

TABLE 18-1   Common Hematologic Tests

Name of Test	Abbreviation	Purpose	Normal Range	Increased With	Decreased With
White blood cell count	WBC	Assist in diagnosis and prognosis of disease	4,500-11,000/mm³ (or 10⁹ cells/L)	**Leukocytosis** Acute infections (appendicitis, chickenpox, diphtheria, infectious mononucleosis, meningitis, pneumonia, rheumatic fever, smallpox, tonsillitis) Hemorrhaging Trauma Malignant disease Leukemia Polycythemia vera	**Leukopenia** Viral infections Hypersplenism Bone marrow depression Infectious hepatitis Cirrhosis Chemotherapy Radiation therapy
Red blood cell count	RBC	Assist in diagnosis of anemia and poly-cythemia	*Male:* 4.5-6.2 million/mm³, or 10¹² cells/L *Female:* 4-5.5 million/mm³, or 10¹² cells/L MCV 80-100 fL MCH 27-34 pg MCHC 1%-36% RDW 11.5%-14.5%	Polycythemia vera Secondary polycythemia Severe diarrhea Dehydration Acute poisoning Pulmonary fibrosis Severe burns	Iron-deficiency anemia Hodgkin's disease Multiple myeloma Leukemia Hemolytic anemia Pernicious anemia Lupus erythematosus Addison's disease
Hemoglobin	Hgb	To screen for anemia, determine its severity, monitor response to treatment	*Male:* 14-18 g/dL (SI Units: 2.17-2.79 mmol/L) *Female:* 12-16 g/dL (SI Units: 1.86-2.48 mmol/L)	Severe burns Chronic obstructive pulmonary disease Congestive heart failure	Anemia Hyperthyroidism Cirrhosis Severe hemorrhage Hemolytic reactions Hodgkin's disease Leukemia
Hematocrit	Hct	Assist in diagnosis and evaluation of anemia	*Male:* 40%-54% *Female:* 37%-47%	Polycythemia vera Severe dehydration Shock Severe burns	Anemia Leukemia Hyperthyroidism Cirrhosis Acute blood loss Hemolytic reactions

Continued

TABLE 18-1 Common Hematologic Tests—cont'd

Name of Test	Abbreviation	Purpose	Normal Range	Increased With	Decreased With
Differential white blood cell count	diff	Assist in diagnosis and prognosis of disease	Neutrophils 50%-70% Eosinophils 1%-4% Basophils 0%-1% Lymphocytes 20%-35% Monocytes 3%-8%	**Neutrophilia** Acute bacterial infections Parasitic infections Liver disease **Eosinophilia** Allergic conditions Parasitic infections Addison's disease Lung and bone cancer **Basophilia** Leukemia Chronic inflammation Polycythemia vera Hemolytic anemia Hodgkin's disease **Lymphocytosis** Acute and chronic infections Hematopoietic disorders Addison's disease Carcinoma Hyperthyroidism **Monocytosis** Viral infections Bacterial and parasitic infections Collagen diseases Cirrhosis Polycythemia vera	**Neutropenia** Acute viral infections Blood diseases Hormone diseases Chemotherapy **Eosinopenia** Infectious mononucleosis Hypersplenism Congestive heart failure Aplastic and pernicious anemia **Basopenia** Acute allergic reactions Hyperthyroidism Steroid therapy **Lymphopenia** HIV infection Cardiac failure Cushing's disease Hodgkin's disease Leukemia **Monocytopenia** Prednisone treatment Hairy cell leukemia

Prothrombin time	PT	11-16 sec	Screen for coagulation disorders and regulate treatment of patients taking oral anticoagulant therapy with warfarin sodium (Coumadin)	**Thrombocytosis** Prothrombin deficiency Vitamin K deficiency Hemorrhagic disease of the newborn Liver disease Anticoagulant therapy Biliary obstruction Acute leukemia Polycythemia vera	**Thrombocytopenia** Acute thrombophlebitis Diuretics Multiple myeloma Pulmonary embolism Vitamin K therapy
Erythrocyte sedimentation rate	ESR	Westergren's method *Male:* <50 yr, 0-20 mm/hr; ≥50 yr, 0-20 mm/hr *Female:* <50 yr, 0-20 mm/hr; ≥50 yr, 0-30 mm/hr	Nonspecific test for connective tissue diseases, malignancy, and infectious diseases. Also used to evaluate progress of inflammatory diseases. (Elevated test results warrant further testing.)	Collagen diseases Infections Inflammatory diseases Carcinoma Cell or tissue destruction Rheumatoid arthritis	Polycythemia vera Sickle cell anemia Congestive heart failure
Platelet count	Plt	150,000-400,000/mm³ (SI Units: 150-400 × 10⁹/L)	Assist in evaluation of bleeding disorders that occur with liver disease, thrombocytopenia, uremia, and anticoagulant therapy	**Thrombocytosis** Cancer Leukemia Polycythemia vera Splenectomy Acute blood loss Rheumatoid arthritis Trauma (fractures,	**Thrombocytopenia** Pernicious anemia Aplastic anemia Hemolytic anemia Pneumonia Allergic conditions Infection Bone marrow–depressant drugs

Note: SI units — $150\text{-}400 \times 10^9/L$

Erythrocytes

In the adult, erythrocytes, or red blood cells, are formed in the red bone marrow of the ribs, sternum, skull, and pelvic bone and in the ends of the long bones of the limbs. The immature form of an erythrocyte contains a nucleus. As the cell develops and matures, however, it loses its nucleus and acquires the shape of a biconcave disc, thicker at the rim than at the center. This shape provides the erythrocyte with a greater surface area for the exchange of substances. An erythrocyte is approximately 7 to 8 micrometers in diameter. The average number of erythrocytes in the adult female ranges from 4 to 5.5 million per cubic millimeter of blood and in the adult male from 4.5 to 6.2 million per cubic millimeter of blood.

A major portion of the erythrocyte consists of **hemoglobin,** a complex compound that transports oxygen and is responsible for the red color of the erythrocyte. The amount of hemoglobin in the blood averages 12 to 16 g/dL for the adult female and 14 to 18 g/dL for the adult male. A hemoglobin molecule consists of a globin, or protein, and an iron-containing pigment called heme. One hemoglobin molecule loosely combines with four oxygen molecules in the lungs to form a substance called **oxyhemoglobin.** Oxyhemoglobin is transported and distributed to the tissues, where the oxygen is easily released from the hemoglobin. The blood then picks up carbon dioxide, a waste product, and transports it back to the lungs to be expelled. When oxygen combines with hemoglobin, a bright red color results that is characteristic of arterial blood. Venous blood is a darker red, owing to its lower oxygen content.

The average life span of a red blood cell is 120 days. Toward the end of this time, it becomes more and more fragile and eventually ruptures and breaks down; this process is known as **hemolysis.** Hemoglobin, liberated from the red blood cell, also breaks down. The iron is stored and later reused to form new hemoglobin, and the protein is metabolized by the body. **Bilirubin** is formed by metabolism of the heme units and transported to the liver, where it is eventually excreted as a waste product in the bile.

Leukocytes

Leukocytes, or white blood cells, are clear, colorless cells that contain a nucleus. The number of leukocytes in the healthy adult ranges from 4,500 to 11,000 per cubic millimeter of blood. **Leukocytosis** is the condition of having an abnormal increase in the number of leukocytes (above 11,000 per cubic millimeter), and **leukopenia** is having an abnormal decrease in the number of leukocytes (below 4,500 per cubic millimeter).

The function of leukocytes is to defend the body against infection. Pathogens can gain entrance to the body in a variety of ways (review the Infection Process Cycle in Chapter 2). Leukocytes attempt to destroy the invading pathogens and remove them from the body. Unlike erythrocytes, leukocytes do their work in the tissues; they are transported to the site of infection by the circulatory system. During inflammation, the blood vessels in the infected area dilate, resulting in an increased blood supply. More oxygen, nutrients, and white blood cells can then be delivered to the infected area to aid in the healing process. The cells in the capillary walls spread apart, enlarging the pores between the cells. White blood cells squeeze through the pores by **ameboid movement** and move out into the tissues to fight the infection. This movement of the leukocytes through the pores of the capillaries and out into the tissues is known as **diapedesis.**

Leukocytes (especially the granular forms) are phagocytic, and once they arrive at the site of infection they begin the process of **phagocytosis,** the engulfing and destruction of pathogens and damaged cells. In some conditions pus forms in the infected area (suppuration); pus contains dead leukocytes, dead bacteria, and dead tissue cells.

Thrombocytes

Platelets, also known as thrombocytes, are small and clear and shaped like discs. They lack a nucleus and are formed in the red bone marrow from giant cells known as *megakaryocytes.* Platelets function by participating in the blood-clotting mechanism. The number of platelets in the healthy adult ranges from 150,000 to 400,000 per cubic millimeter of blood.

Hemoglobin Determination

Hemoglobin (abbreviated Hgb) is a major component of red blood cells. Hemoglobin transports oxygen to the tissue cells of the body and is responsible for the color of the red blood cell.

The hemoglobin determination is used to measure indirectly the oxygen-carrying capacity of the blood. The normal range for the adult woman is 12 to 16 g/dL, and the normal range for the adult man is 14 to 18 g/dL. A hemoglobin determination is performed as an individual test or as part of the CBC. A hemoglobin determination is often performed as a routine test on individuals, such as children under 2 years of age and pregnant women, who are at risk for developing anemia.

A decreased hemoglobin level occurs with anemia (especially iron-deficiency anemia), hyperthyroidism, cirrhosis of the liver, severe hemorrhaging, hemolytic reactions, and certain systemic diseases such as leukemia and Hodgkin's disease. Increased levels of hemoglobin are present with **polycythemia,** chronic obstructive pulmonary disease (COPD), and congestive heart failure.

The hemoglobin determination can be performed on either capillary or venous blood. The most accurate and reliable method for measuring hemoglobin concentration involves the use of a blood analyzer. An office blood analyzer permits the processing of the specimen in a short time, allowing the physician to evaluate the condition while the patient is still at the medical office.

Hematocrit

The hematocrit (abbreviated Hct) is a simple, reliable, and informative test that is frequently performed in the medical office. The word *hematocrit* means "to separate blood." The solid or cellular elements are separated from the plasma by centrifuging an anticoagulated blood specimen. The heavier red blood cells become packed and settle to the bottom of a tube. The top layer contains the clear, straw-colored plasma. Between the plasma and the packed red blood cells is a small, thin, yellowish-gray layer known as the *buffy coat,* which contains the platelets and white blood cells (Figure 18-1).

The purpose of the hematocrit is to measure the percentage volume of packed red blood cells in whole blood. The normal hematocrit range for the adult female is 37% to 47% and for the adult male is 40% to 54%. A low hematocrit reading may indicate **anemia,** and a high reading may indicate polycythemia. The hematocrit, in conjunction with other hematologic tests, is an aid to the physician in the diagnosis of a patient's condition. The hematocrit is also used as a screening measure for the early detection of anemia and therefore is often included in a general physical examination.

The *microhematocrit method* is used most often in the medical office to perform a hematocrit determination. Through capillary action, blood is drawn directly from a free-flowing skin puncture into a disposable capillary tube lined with an anticoagulant. An anticoagulated blood specimen collected by other means, such as venipuncture, can also be used. The microhematocrit centrifuge spins the blood at an extremely high speed and requires only 3 to 5 minutes to pack the red blood cells. The results are then read at the top of the packed cell column. Procedure 18-1 describes how to perform a hematocrit determination.

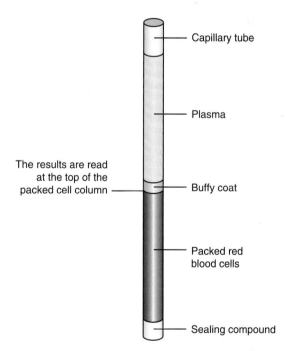

Figure 18-1. Hematocrit test results. The cellular elements are separated from the plasma by centrifuging an anticoagulated blood specimen, and the results are read at the top of the packed cell column.

⫸ PATIENT TEACHING

Iron-Deficiency Anemia

Answer questions patients have about iron-deficiency anemia.

What is anemia?

Anemia is a shortage of red blood cells or hemoglobin. Hemoglobin, the part of the blood that gives red blood cells their color, carries oxygen to all the cells in the body. There are many types of anemia, of which iron-deficiency anemia is by far the most common. Other types of anemia are pernicious anemia, sickle cell anemia, hemolytic anemia, and aplastic anemia.

What causes iron-deficiency anemia?

In general, iron-deficiency anemia is caused by conditions that deplete the iron stored in the body; it can result from an increased need for iron by the body or an increased loss of iron from the body. Iron-deficiency anemia may occur in children under 2 years of age if there is not enough iron in their diet to meet their demands of rapid growth. This is especially true in children whose main source of nutrition during these years is breast milk or bottle milk because milk contains very little iron. Adolescent girls are prone to iron-deficiency anemia because of their growth spurts during puberty and the loss through menstruation. In adults, the most common cause of anemia is chronic blood loss, such as from a bleeding ulcer, bleeding hemorrhoids, and heavy menstrual bleeding. Pregnant women are also at increased risk because of the demands of the growing baby.

What can be done for individuals at risk for iron-deficiency anemia?

Individuals prone to developing iron-deficiency anemia are encouraged to increase foods in their diet that contain iron, such as beef, liver, spinach, eggs, and iron-fortified breads and cereals. As a preventive measure, the physician usually prescribes vitamin supplements for people at an increased risk for developing iron-deficiency anemia, such as pregnant women, infants, and young children. Also, infant formulas and cereals are available that have been supplemented with iron.

What are the symptoms of anemia?

All types of anemia have the same general symptoms. Often these symptoms do not develop right away; when they do develop, feeling tired and run down may be the only sign of anemia. Other symptoms that may occur, particularly as the anemia becomes worse, are paleness of the skin, fingernail beds, and mucous membranes; shortness of breath, especially during physical activity; dizziness; headache; irritability; and inability to concentrate. These symptoms result from the diminished ability of the blood to carry oxygen to the cells of the body. Blood tests are necessary to diagnose anemia and to determine the specific type of anemia present.

How is iron-deficiency anemia treated?

The most important part of treating anemia is to determine its cause, such as not enough iron being consumed in the diet or chronic blood loss, and to correct that condition. The physician usually prescribes an iron supplement to replace the iron that has been depleted from the body. It is generally prescribed in oral form, but it is given through an injection in special situations. An oral iron supplement causes the stool to turn a black tarlike color. This is normal and should not be a cause for concern. Also, an effort should be made to consume foods high in iron content.

- For patients who have had a vitamin supplement prescribed to *prevent* iron-deficiency anemia, such as children under 2 years of age and pregnant women: Emphasize the importance to the patient of taking the vitamin supplement every day to prevent the development of iron-deficiency anemia.
- For patients who have had an iron supplement prescribed to *treat* iron-deficiency anemia: Emphasize to the patient the importance of taking the iron supplement for the period of time prescribed by the physician because replacement of iron takes time.
- Instruct the patient to keep iron supplements out of the reach of children to prevent iron poisoning.
- Provide the patient with written educational materials about anemia.

PROCEDURE 18-1 Hematocrit

Outcome Perform a hematocrit determination.

Equipment/Supplies:

- Microhematocrit centrifuge
- Personal protective equipment, including disposable gloves
- Lancet
- Antiseptic wipe

- Gauze pads
- Capillary tubes
- Sealing compound
- Biohazard sharps container

1. **Procedural Step.** Assemble the equipment. Sanitize your hands, and put on personal protective equipment, including gloves.
2. **Procedural Step.** Greet and identify the patient. Introduce yourself, and explain the procedure.

Perform a finger puncture, then dispose of the lancet in a biohazard sharps container.

Principle. Personal protective equipment and proper disposal of the lancet are required by the OSHA Standard to prevent exposure to bloodborne pathogens.

3. Procedural Step. Wipe away the first drop of blood with a gauze pad. Fill the capillary tube by holding one end of it horizontally, but slightly downward, next to the free-flowing puncture. Keep the tip of the capillary tube in the blood, but do not allow it to press against the patient's skin.

Calibrated tubes are filled to the calibration line; uncalibrated tubes are filled approximately three quarters (within 10 to 20 mm of the end of the tube). The blood will be drawn into the tube through capillary action. Fill a second tube using the method just described.

Principle. Not keeping the tip of the capillary tube in the blood can cause air bubbles in the stem of the tube, which leads to inaccurate test results. Allowing the capillary tube to press against the skin will close the opening of the capillary tubes and not allow blood to enter it.

The type of tube (calibrated or uncalibrated) is based on the method used to read the test results. The hematocrit should be performed in duplicate to ensure accurate and reliable test results.

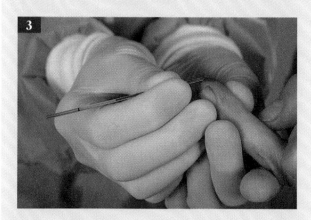

4. Procedural Step. Seal one end of each tube with a small amount of putty or a commercially prepared sealing compound (e.g., Critoseal, Hemato-Seal).
Principle. The capillary tubes must be sealed properly to prevent leakage of the blood specimen during centrifugation.

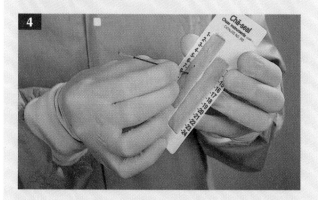

5. Procedural Step. Place the capillary tubes in the microhematocrit centrifuge with the sealed end facing out. Balance one tube with the other capillary tube placed on the opposite side of the centrifuge.
Principle. Placing the sealed end toward the outside prevents the blood specimen from spinning out of the capillary tube when the centrifuge is in operation.

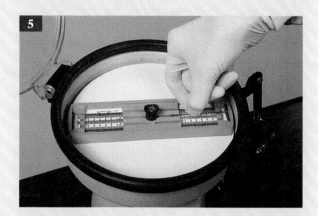

6. Procedural Step. Place the cover on the centrifuge and lock it securely. Centrifuge the blood specimen for 3 to 5 minutes at a speed of 10,000 rpm.
Principle. Centrifuging the blood specimen causes the red blood cells to become packed and to settle on the bottom of the tube.

7. Procedural Step. Allow the centrifuge to come to a complete stop. Read the results, as follows:

Calibrated tube. If a capillary tube with a calibration line was used, read the results using the special graphic reading device that is part of the

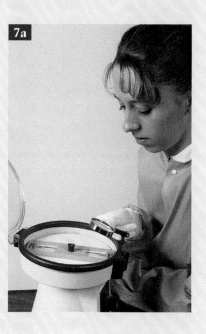

Continued

centrifuge. Adjust the capillary tube so that the bottom of the red blood cell column (just above the sealing compound) is placed on the 0 line. With a magnifying glass, read the results at the top of the packed red blood cell column, and you will see a percentage on the reading device.

Uncalibrated tube. If an uncalibrated tube was used, you must use a microhematocrit reader card to determine the results; place the top of the plasma column on the 100% mark and the bottom of the cell column on the 0 line. Read the results on the scale, which corresponds to the top of the packed cell column.

In both cases, the buffy coat should not be included in the reading. The answer represents the percentage of blood volume occupied by the red blood cells. (The hematocrit determination on this reading device is 38.)

Principle. Stopping the centrifuge with your hands can injure you and can damage the machine.

8. **Procedural Step.** Read the second tube in the manner just described; the results of the tubes should agree within 4 percentage points. If not, the hematocrit procedure must be repeated. If they are within 4 percentage points, the two values are averaged to derive the test results.

9. **Procedural Step.** Properly dispose of the capillary tubes in a biohazard sharps container. Remove personal protective equipment, including gloves, and sanitize your hands. Chart the results. Include the date and time and the hematocrit results.

10. **Procedural Step.** Return the equipment to its proper storage place.

> Normal Range for Hematocrit:
> *Female:* 37% to 47%
> *Male:* 40% to 54%

CHARTING EXAMPLE	
Date	
5/5/05	11:15 a.m. Hct: 38%.———L. Sharpe, CMA

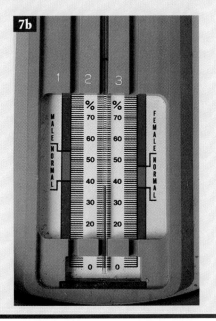

7b

White Blood Cell Count

The white blood cell (WBC) count is used by the physician to assist in the diagnosis and prognosis of disease. The white blood cell count is an approximate measurement of the number of white blood cells in the circulating blood. The normal range for a white blood count is 4,500 to 11,000 white blood cells per cubic millimeter of blood, which is expressed as 4.5 to 11.0 ($\times 10^3/mm^3$) on

laboratory reports. An increase in the white blood count, or leukocytosis, is most commonly seen in acute infection such as appendicitis, chickenpox, diphtheria, infectious mononucleosis, meningitis, and rheumatic fever. A normal elevation of the white blood cell count can occur with pregnancy, strenuous exercise, stress, and treatment with corticosteroids. Conditions that result in **leukopenia,** or a decrease in the white blood cell count,

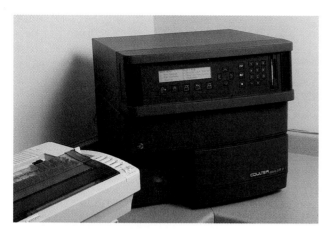

Figure 18-2. Coulter blood cell counter.

include viral infections, chemotherapy, and radiation therapy.

If the white blood cell count is performed in the medical office, a blood cell counter is used. Blood cell counters are also able to perform a red blood count, platelet count, hemoglobin, hematocrit, differential white blood cell count, and calculation of red blood cell indices. Examples of blood cell counters include the QBC Autoread (Beckton-Dickinson), the Cell-Dyn (Abbott), and the Coulter (Coulter Company) (Figure 18-2).

Red Blood Cell Count

The red blood cell (RBC) count is a measurement of the number of red blood cells in whole blood. The range for the red blood count in the healthy adult female is 4 to 5.5 million red blood cells per cubic millimeter of blood, expressed as 4.0-5.5 ($\times 10^6$/mm^3) on laboratory reports. The range for the healthy adult male is 4.5 to 6.2 million red blood cells per cubic millimeter of blood, expressed as 4.5-6.2 ($\times 10^6$/mm^3) on a laboratory report. In the medical office, the red blood count is performed using a blood cell counter.

Conditions that cause a decrease in the red blood cell count include anemia, Hodgkin's disease, and leukemia; conditions that cause an increase of RBCs include polycythemia, dehydration, and pulmonary fibrosis.

White Blood Cell Differential Count

There are five types of white blood cells, or leukocytes, each having a certain size, shape, appearance, and function (Figure 18-3). The purpose of the differential cell count is to identify and count the five types of white blood cell in a representative blood sample. An increase or decrease in one or more types may occur in pathologic conditions, which assists the physician in making a diagnosis.

The differential cell count can be performed automatically or manually. The automatic method is faster and more convenient and, because of this, is growing in popularity. Both methods are described next.

Automatic Method. The automatic method involves the use of a blood cell counter such as the Coulter cell counter (see Figure 18-2). The specimen requirement is an EDTA-anticoagulated blood specimen, which is obtained through venipuncture using a lavender-stoppered tube. The blood cell counter automatically performs the differential cell count, and the results are printed on a laboratory report.

Manual Method. The manual method requires that the medical assistant make two blood smears. The preparation of a blood smear is outlined in Procedure 18-2. Fresh whole blood is preferred for blood smears; however, a satisfactory smear can be made from an EDTA-anticoagulated blood specimen, provided the smear is made within 2 hours after collection. Other anticoagulants should not be used because they could alter the morphology and staining reaction of the white blood cells. After preparing the blood smear, the medical assistant places the slides in a protective container for transportation to an outside laboratory. The blood smear is evaluated at the laboratory by medical laboratory personnel. Because white blood cells are clear and colorless, they must be stained first with an appropriate dye (usually Wright's stain) before a differential count is performed. The nucleus, cytoplasm, and any granules in the cytoplasm take on the characteristic color of their cell type, which aids in proper identification. A minimum of 100 white blood cells is identified on the blood smear, and each is assigned to its appropriate category (neutrophil, eosinophil, basophil, lymphocyte, or monocyte). The number of each type

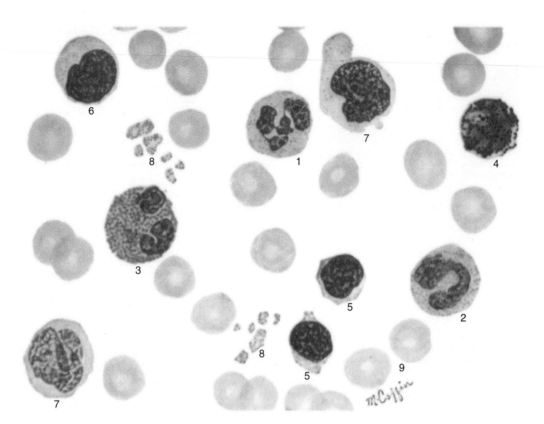

Figure 18-3. Types of human blood cells. *1* to *7,* White cells (leukocytes) stained as they are in the laboratory to show the many types. They play the active role in immune response, or in defense against disease. (*1,* neutrophil; *2,* neutrophilic band; *3,* eosinophil; *4,* basophil; *5,* lymphocyte; *6,* (Large) lymphocyte; and *7,* monocyte). *8,* Platelets (thrombocytes), which are responsible for clotting. *9,* Red blood cells (erythrocytes), which carry oxygen. (From Custer RP: *An Atlas of the Blood and Bone Marrow,* 2nd ed. Philadelphia, 1974, Saunders.)

What Would You DO? What Would You *Not* DO?

Case Study 3

Marjorie Merrick comes to the office for a follow-up visit to discuss her lab results with the physician. Marjorie is in perimenopause and has been having problems with heavy menstrual periods, hot flashes, insomnia, fatigue, and shortness of breath. Marjorie's lab tests indicate that she has iron-deficiency anemia. The physician orders an injection of iron dextran, Z-track technique, and instructs Marjorie to take an iron supplement every day and to return in 3 months for a recheck. Marjorie says she has heard that an iron injection can stain the skin and wants to know if that's true. She says she has a friend that has anemia and he has to go in every week for a vitamin B$_{12}$ shot. Marjorie wants to know if she'll have to do that, too. Marjorie signed up to donate blood this week at her church's Red Cross blood drive. She wants to know if its all right to go ahead and donate.

of leukocyte is recorded as a percentage and reflects the overall distribution of white blood cells in the patient's bloodstream.

Types of White Blood Cells

Leukocytes are classified into two major categories—granular and nongranular. *Granular leukocytes* contain distinct granules in the cytoplasm and include neutrophils, eosinophils, and basophils. Nongranular leukocytes contain few or no granules in the cytoplasm and include lymphocytes and monocytes. The five types of white blood cells are described here, along with their reactions to Wright's stain.

The *neutrophils* are the most numerous of the white blood cells. A neutrophil has a purple, multilobed nucleus that may contain three to five lobes or segments; therefore neutrophils are also known as "segs." The cytoplasm of a neutrophil stains a faint pink and contains many fine granules that stain a violet-pink. Neutrophils exhibit a high degree of ameboid movement and are actively phagocytic. Immature forms of neutrophils known as *bands* can be identified by their curved, non-segmented nuclei. Normally, from zero to five of the neutrophils present will be in the immature band form. When the percentage of band forms increases, this condition is often referred to as a "shift to the left." An increase in the number of neutrophils, including band forms, is generally seen during an acute infection.

An *eosinophil* contains a segmented nucleus, generally of no more than two lobes. Large granules are found in the cytoplasm; they stain a bright reddish-orange. An increase in eosinophils is often seen in allergic conditions and parasitic infestations.

Basophils are the least numerous of the white blood cells. A basophil contains an S-shaped nucleus. The cytoplasm contains large, coarse, dark bluish-black granules that almost completely obscure the details of the nucleus.

Lymphocytes are the smallest white blood cells. A lymphocyte has a round or slightly indented nucleus that almost fills the cell and stains a deep purplish blue. There is a small rim of sky-blue cytoplasm around the nucleus that contains few or no granules. Lymphocytes are involved with the immune system and the production of antibodies. An increase in lymphocytes generally occurs with certain viral diseases, including infectious mononucleosis, mumps, chickenpox, rubella, and viral hepatitis.

MEMORIES From EXTERNSHIP

LATISHA SHARPE: During my externship experience, I had a female patient who drank too much the night before and had been vomiting for 3 hours before coming to the physician's office. Although this incident was self-inflicted, I still found myself feeling deeply sorry for the patient. She was so weak she could not hold her head up, so I stayed with her and held her head up while she was vomiting. I stayed with her throughout this time, and my sympathy for her really made a difference. No matter what the situation is, I always let the patient know that I care.

Monocytes are the largest white blood cells. A monocyte has a large nucleus that is usually kidney- or horseshoe-shaped, but it can be round or oval. Monocytes contain abundant cytoplasm that stains grayish blue.

Normal Range

The healthy adult range for each type of white blood cell making up the total number of leukocytes is listed here:

Neutrophils 50% to 70%
Eosinophils 1% to 4%
Basophils 0% to 1%
Lymphocytes 20% to 35%
Monocytes 3% to 8%

PROCEDURE 18-2   Preparation of a Blood Smear for a Differential Cell Count

Outcome Prepare a blood smear for a differential white blood cell count.

Equipment/Supplies:
- Personal protective equipment, including disposable gloves
- Supplies to perform a finger puncture or venipuncture
- Slides with a frosted edge
- Slide container
- Biohazard sharps container

1. **Procedural Step.** Assemble the equipment. Using a pencil, label two slides on the frosted edge with the patient's name and the date.
   Principle. Laboratories request the preparation of two blood smears as a means of quality control.

2. **Procedural Step.** Sanitize your hands, and put on personal protective equipment, including gloves.

3. **Procedural Step.** Greet and identify the patient. Introduce yourself, and explain the procedure. Obtain a blood sample from the patient, and place a drop of fresh whole blood on each slide as follows:
   From a venipuncture. You can obtain the blood specimen from the fresh whole blood left in the needle immediately after performing a venipuncture as follows: After withdrawing the needle from the patient's arm, deposit the drop of blood remaining in

the needle onto the middle of each slide, approximately ¼ inch from the slide's frosted edge.
   From a skin puncture. Perform a finger puncture and wipe away the first drop of blood. Place a drop of blood from the patient's finger in the middle of each slide, approximately ¼ inch from the slide's frosted edge, by touching the slide to the drop of blood. Do not allow the patient's finger to touch the slide.
   Principle. If the patient's finger touches the slide, it will spread out the blood specimen, producing an uneven smear. In addition, moisture or oil from the patient's finger could interfere with the smear.

4. **Procedural Step.** Hold a second "spreader" slide in front of the drop of blood and at a 30-degree angle to the first slide. Move the spreader slide until it touches the drop of blood. The blood distributes

Continued

PROCEDURE 18-2 Preparation of a Blood Smear for a Differential Cell Count—Cont'd

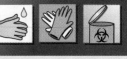

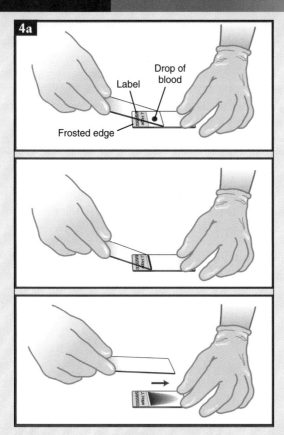

itself along the edge of the spreader by capillary action. Using a smooth, continuous motion, spread the blood thinly and evenly across the surface of the first slide, ending the motion by lifting the spreader slide off the specimen in a smooth, low arc. The smear should be approximately 1½ inches long. The blood smear is thickest at the beginning and gradually thins to a very fine "feathered" edge. If the blood smear has been prepared correctly, it exhibits the following characteristics: (1) it is smooth and even with no ridges, holes, lines, streaks, or clumps; (2) it is not too thick or too thin; (3) there is a feathered edge at the thin end of the smear; and (4) there is a margin on all sides of the smear. Repeat this step with the other slide.

Principle. An angle of more than 30 degrees causes the smear to be too thick; the cells overlap, do not stain well, and are smaller than normal, making them difficult to count. If the angle is smaller than 30 degrees, the smear will be too thin and the cells will be spread out, increasing the time needed to count them.

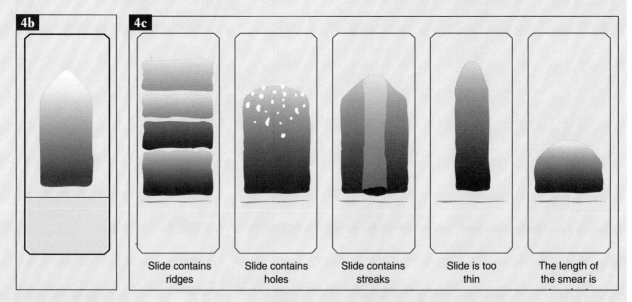

| Slide contains ridges | Slide contains holes | Slide contains streaks | Slide is too thin | The length of the smear is |

Properly prepared blood smear.

Improperly prepared blood smears.

(From Rodak BF: *Hematology: Clinical Principles and Applications.* Philadelphia, 1995, Saunders.)

5. **Procedural Step.** Dispose of the spreader slide in a biohazard sharps container.

6. **Procedural Step.** Lay the blood smears on a flat surface and allow them to dry. Never blow on the slides to dry them.

   Principle. The blood smears must be dried immediately to prevent shrinkage of the blood cells, which makes them difficult to identify. Blowing on the slide might cause exhaled water droplets to make holes in the smears.

7. **Procedural Step.** Prepare the slides for transportation to the laboratory by placing them in a protective slide container.

8. **Procedural Step.** Remove the gloves, and sanitize your hands.

CHARTING EXAMPLE	
Date	
5/05/05	11:15 a.m. Venous blood specimen collected from Ⓡ arm. Specimen to Medical Center Laboratory for CBC c̄ diff on 5/05/05. ———— ———————————— L. Sharpe, CMA

MEDICAL Practice and the LAW

When dealing with blood, remember that any specimen can contain bloodborne pathogens such as hepatitis B and HIV. If spraying or splashing of blood is a possibility, use personal protective equipment, including gloves, mask, and goggles.

Laboratory test results are confidential. Giving out results without the patient's permission can result in an invasion of privacy lawsuit. Usually only the physician gives these results, so he or she can explain their meaning to the patient.

Case Study 1

What Did Latisha Do?

❑ Told Theodore that the doctor was running some routine screening tests on him to make sure he is in good health. Explained that all patients have these tests run as part of a physical examination.

❑ Told Theodore that it was not possible to get the specimen from the earlobe. Explained that the earlobe is not recommended as a good site to obtain blood.

❑ Reassured Theodore that the fingerstick would be made on the least sensitive part of his finger. Told him that it would hurt for just a second, and then it would be all over and it would heal quickly.

❑ Told Theodore that the purpose of the blood test is for the early detection of anemia. Explained that if anemia is present, it can be caught early and treated before symptoms develop.

What Did Latisha Not Do?

❑ Did not collect the specimen from Theodore's earlobe.

❑ Did not tell Theodore that he is healthy and doesn't have anything wrong with him.

What Would You Do?/What Would You *Not* Do? Review Latisha's response and place a checkmark next to the information you included in your response. List additional information you included in your response below.

_____

_____

_____

_____

Case Study 2

What Did Latisha Do?

❑ Commended Mrs. Frasure on eating nutritiously.

❑ Told Mrs. Frasure that breast milk does not contain very much iron. Explained that because of that, it's important to give Travis his liquid vitamins because they have iron in them.

❑ Reassured Mrs. Frasure that breastfeeding does provide very good nutrition for Travis.

❑ Explained to Mrs. Frasure that the iron supplement may cause Travis's stool to be a dark, tarlike color, and she should not be alarmed because this is normal.

What Did Latisha Not Do?

❑ Did not criticize Mrs. Frasure for not giving Travis his vitamins or make her feel that it was her fault that his hemoglobin was low.

What Would You Do?/What Would You *Not* Do? Review Latisha's response and place a checkmark next to the information you included in your response. List additional information you included in your response below.

_____

_____

_____

_____

Case Study 3

What Did Latisha Do?

❑ Told Marjorie that the iron injection can stain the skin, but that it would be given in a special way to prevent that from happening.

❑ Told Marjorie vitamin B_{12} injections are given for pernicious anemia and that her type of anemia is iron-deficiency anemia.

❑ Gave Marjorie a patient education brochure on iron-deficiency anemia to take home with her.

❑ Told Marjorie that the Red Cross requires that a blood donor's hemoglobin level be within normal range. Explained that she could not donate this time, but once her hemoglobin was back to normal she would be able to donate.

❑ Explained to Marjorie that the iron supplement may cause her stool to be a dark, tarlike color, and she should not be alarmed because this is normal.

What Did Latisha Not Do?

❑ Did not tell Marjorie that her friend has pernicious anemia because there is no way of knowing this.

What Would You Do?/What Would You *Not* Do? Review Latisha's response and place a checkmark next to the information you included in your response. List additional information you included in your response below.

_____

_____

_____

_____

Apply Your KNOWLEDGE

Choose the best answer to each of the following questions.

1. Deborah Murray is 6 months pregnant and Dr. Diapedesis wants Latisha Sharpe, CMA, to check her hemoglobin level. Dr. Diapedesis has ordered this test because pregnant women are at increased risk for developing:
A. Osteoporosis
B. Anemia
C. Scurvy
D. Polycythemia

2. Latisha collects a capillary blood specimen from Deborah and runs a hemoglobin test. The hemoglobin value is 14, which is considered:
A. Normal
B. High
C. Low
D. Invalid

3. Richard Wrighter comes in for a general physical examination. As part of his examination, Dr. Diapedesis asks Latisha Sharpe, CMA, to perform a hematocrit. Latisha performs a finger puncture. After inserting the tip of the capillary tube into the drop of blood, Latisha discovers that no blood is entering the tube. The most likely cause of this is:
A. The capillary tubes are outdated
B. Latisha didn't wipe away the first drop of blood
C. Air bubbles have entered the capillary tube
D. The tip of the capillary tube is pressed against Richard's finger

4. Latisha fills two capillary tubes and centrifuges them in the microhematocrit centrifuge. After the centrifuge comes to a complete stop, Latisha reads the results:
A. At the top of the buffy coat
B. At the top of the plasma column
C. At the top of the red blood cell column
D. Next to the black line on the capillary tube

5. Latisha Sharpe, CMA, determines Richard's hematocrit value to be 37. This value is considered:
A. Normal
B. High
C. Low
D. Invalid

6. Anna Lubbers comes to the office with an acute sore throat. Dr. Diapedesis asks Latisha Sharpe, CMA, to perform a rapid strep test on Anna. The test comes out positive. Which of the following test results would Dr. Diapedesis also expect Anna to have?
A. An elevated white blood cell count
B. A low hemoglobin level
C. An increased platelet count
D. An elevated red blood cell count

7. Dr. Diapedesis orders a CBC with differential on Chad Cron. After collecting a lavender tube, Latisha prepares the blood smears. Which of the following techniques would Latisha *not* want to use in preparing the smears?
A. Placing a drop of blood ¼ inch from the frosted edge of the slide
B. Using a 30-degree angle to make the smear
C. Using a smooth continuous motion to make the smear
D. Gently blowing on the slides to dry them

8. Latisha has prepared the blood smears and looks at them to make sure they have been prepared correctly. Which of the following slides would NOT be considered suitable for a blood smear? A slide that has:
A. A margin on all sides of the smear
B. A rounded thick edge at the end of the smear
C. A feathered edge at the end of the smear
D. A smear length of 1½ inches

9. The laboratory report on Chad Cron is sent electronically to the medical office from the laboratory that ran the test. After it prints out at the medical office, Latisha retrieves it and places it on Dr. Diapedesis's desk for review. Which of the following would indicate an abnormal value for Chad's CBC?
A. Hemoglobin: 16 g/dL
B. Hematocrit: 51%
C. White Blood Cell Count: 14.25×10^3 mm³
D. Red Blood Cell Count: 5.85×10^6 mm³

10. The results of the differential cell count are also included on Chad's laboratory report. Which of the following indicates an abnormal value?
A. Neutrophils: 52
B. Eosinophils: 2
C. Basophils: 0
D. Lymphocytes: 41
E. Monocytes: 5

CERTIFICATIONREVIEW

❏ **Hematology** involves the study of blood, including its morphologic appearance and function, and diseases of the blood and blood-forming tissues. The most frequently performed hematologic laboratory test is the complete blood count (CBC). The tests included in a CBC are hemoglobin, hematocrit, white blood cell count, red blood cell count, differential white blood cell count, and red blood cell indices.

❏ **Blood consists of plasma and cells.** The function of plasma is to transport nutrients to the tissues of the body and to pick up wastes from the tissues.

❏ **The three types of cell in the blood** are erythrocytes, leukocytes, and thrombocytes. Erythrocytes are formed in the red bone marrow. The average number of erythrocytes in the adult female ranges from 4 to 5.5 million per cubic millimeter of blood and in the adult male from 4.5 to 6.2 million per cubic millimeter of blood.

❏ **Hemoglobin transports oxygen** and is responsible for the red color of the erythrocyte. The amount of hemoglobin in the blood averages 12 to 16 g/dL for the adult female and 14 to 18 g/dL for the adult male. The average life span of a red blood cell is 120 days.

❏ **Leukocytes are clear, colorless cells** that contain a nucleus. The number of leukocytes in the healthy adult ranges from 4,500 to 11,000 per cubic millimeter of blood. Leukocytosis is an abnormal increase in the number of leukocytes, and leukopenia is an abnormal decrease in the number of leukocytes. The function of leukocytes is to defend the body against infection.

❏ **Thrombocytes,** or platelets, participate in the blood-clotting mechanism. The normal number of platelets in the adult is 150,000 to 400,000 per cubic millimeter.

❏ **The hemoglobin determination** measures indirectly the blood's oxygen-carrying capacity. A hemoglobin determination is often performed as a routine test on individuals at risk for developing anemia, such as children under 2 years of age and pregnant women.

❏ **The purpose of the hematocrit** is to measure the percentage volume of packed red blood cells in whole blood. The normal hematocrit range for the adult female is 37% to 47%, and for the adult male, it is 40% to 54%. A low hematocrit reading may indicate anemia, whereas a high reading may indicate polycythemia.

❏ **The white blood cell count** assists in the diagnosis and prognosis of disease. Leukocytosis is most commonly seen in acute infection. Conditions that result in leukopenia include viral infections, chemotherapy, and radiation therapy.

❏ **The red blood cell count** is a measurement of the number of red blood cells in whole blood. Conditions that cause a decrease in red blood cells include anemia, Hodgkin's disease, and leukemia. Conditions that cause an increase include polycythemia, dehydration, and pulmonary fibrosis.

❏ **The purpose of the differential cell count** is to identify and count the five types of white blood cell in a representative blood sample, which assists the physician in making a diagnosis. An increase or decrease in one or more types can occur in pathologic conditions.

❏ **The five types of white blood cell** are neutrophils, eosinophils, basophils, lymphocytes, and monocytes. Neutrophils are the most numerous of the white blood cells. An increase in the number of neutrophils is generally seen during an acute infection. Basophils are the least numerous of the white blood cells. Lymphocytes are the smallest white blood cells and are involved with the immune system and the production of antibodies. An increase in lymphocytes generally occurs with certain viral diseases. Monocytes are the largest white blood cells.

Terminology Review

Ameboid movement Movement used by leukocytes that permits them to propel themselves from the capillaries into the tissues.

Anemia A condition in which there is a decrease in the erythrocytes or amount of hemoglobin in the blood.

Bilirubin An orange-colored bile pigment produced by the breakdown of heme from the hemoglobin molecule.

Diapedesis The ameboid movement of blood cells (especially leukocytes) through the wall of a capillary and out into the tissues.

Hematology The study of blood and blood-forming tissues.

Hemoglobin The iron-containing pigment of erythrocytes that transports oxygen in the body.

Hemolysis The breakdown of erythrocytes with the release of hemoglobin into the plasma.

Leukocytosis An abnormal increase in the number of white blood cells (above 11,000 per cubic millimeter of blood).

Leukopenia An abnormal decrease in the number of white blood cells (below 4,500 per cubic millimeter of blood).

Oxyhemoglobin Hemoglobin that has combined with oxygen.

Phagocytosis The engulfing and destruction of foreign particles, such as bacteria, by special cells called phagocytes.

Polycythemia A disorder in which there is an increase in the red cell mass.

ON THE WEB

For active weblinks to each website visit http://evolve.elsevier.com/Bonewit/.

For Information on Stress and Stress Management:

The American Institute of Stress

The Medical Basis of Stress, Depression, Anxiety, Sleep Problems, and Drug Use

The Anxiety Panic Internet Resource

Blood Chemistry

1. Explain the purpose of a blood chemistry test.
2. Describe the function of LDL cholesterol and HDL cholesterol in the body.
3. State the desirable ranges for the following tests: total cholesterol, LDL cholesterol, and HDL cholesterol.
4. State the patient preparation for a triglyceride test.
5. Explain the functions of glucose and insulin in the body.
6. State the patient preparation for a fasting blood sugar.
7. Identify the normal range for a fasting blood sugar.
8. State the purpose of the following tests: fasting blood sugar, 2-hour postprandial glucose test, and glucose tolerance test.
9. Describe the procedure for a 2-hour postprandial blood sugar test.
10. Identify the patient preparation for a glucose tolerance test.
11. State the restrictions that must be followed by the patient during the glucose tolerance test.
12. Explain the storage requirements for blood glucose reagent strips.
13. List three advantages of self-monitoring of blood glucose by diabetic patients.

Perform blood chemistry testing, using an automated blood chemistry analyzer and operating manual.

Perform a fasting blood sugar using a glucose monitor.

Instruct a patient how to measure blood glucose using a glucose monitor.

Serology

1. Explain the purpose of the following serologic tests: hepatitis tests, syphilis tests, mono test, rheumatoid factor, antistreptolysin test, C-reactive protein, cold agglutinins, ABO and Rh blood typing, and Rh antibody titer.
2. List the symptoms of infectious mononucleosis.
3. Identify the location of the blood antigens and antibodies.
4. Explain how the blood antigen-antibody reaction is used for blood typing in vitro.
5. List the antigens and antibodies in the following blood types: A, B, AB, and O.
6. Explain the difference between Rh-positive and Rh-negative blood.

Demonstrate the proper care and maintenance of a glucose monitor.

Perform a rapid mononucleosis test.

CHAPTER 19

Blood Chemistry and Serology

Chapter Outline

Introduction to Blood Chemistry and Serology
BLOOD CHEMISTRY
Automated Blood Chemistry Analyzers
Quality Control
Cholesterol
  HDL and LDL Cholesterol
  Cholesterol Testing
  Interpretation of Results
  Patient Preparation
Blood Urea Nitrogen
Blood Glucose
Fasting Blood Sugar
  Two-Hour Postprandial Blood Sugar
  Glucose Tolerance Test
  Glucose Monitors
Self-Monitoring of Blood Glucose
SEROLOGY
Serologic Tests
Rapid Mononucleosis Testing
Blood Typing
  Blood Antigens
  Blood Antibodies
  The Rh Blood Group System
Blood Antigen and Antibody Reactions
Agglutination and Blood Typing

National Competencies

Clinical Competencies
Diagnostic Testing
- Use methods of quality control.
- Perform chemistry testing.
- Perform immunology testing.
- Screen and follow up test results.

General Competencies
Patient Instruction
- Instruct individuals according to their needs.
- Provide instruction for health maintenance and disease prevention.

agglutination (ah-gloo-ti-NAY-shun)
antibody (AN-ti-bod-ee)
antigen (AN-ti-jen)
antiserum (AN-ti-sere-um)
blood antibody
blood antigen
donor
gene (jeen)
glycogen (GLIE-koe-jen))
HDL cholesterol
hyperglycemia (hie-per-glie-SEE-me-ah)
hypoglycemia (hie-poe-glie-SEE-me-ah)
in vitro (in-VEE-troe)
in vivo (in-VEE-voe)
LDL cholesterol
lipoprotein (lie-poe-PROE-teen)
recipient (ree-SIP-ee-ent)

Introduction to Blood Chemistry and Serology

Blood chemistry and serologic laboratory tests are often performed in the medical office. Over the past decade, advances in automated blood analyzers designed for use in the medical office have made this possible. Automated blood analyzers perform laboratory tests in a very short time with accurate test results. Each automated analyzer is accompanied by a detailed operating manual explaining its operation, test parameters, care, and maintenance.

This chapter is divided into two units: The first presents blood chemistry laboratory tests, and the second presents serologic tests.

The material in this chapter about blood testing is intended to serve only as a basic guide for the medical assistant and should be supplemented by much well-supervised practice in a classroom laboratory, the medical office, or both.

BLOOD CHEMISTRY

Blood chemistry testing involves the quantitative measurement of chemical substances in the blood. These chemicals are dissolved in the liquid portion of the blood; therefore most blood chemistry tests require a serum specimen for analysis. There are numerous types of blood chemistry tests; the type of test (or tests) the physician orders depends on the clinical diagnosis. Table 19-1 provides a list of common blood chemistry tests with specimen requirements, normal values, and conditions that cause abnormal test results. The blood chemistry tests that are most frequently performed are described in more detail in this chapter.

Automated Blood Chemistry Analyzers

In the medical office, automated blood chemistry analyzers may be used to perform blood chemistry testing. A blood chemistry analyzer consists of a reflectance photometer that quantitatively measures the amount of chemical substances, or *analytes,* in the blood. Specifically, a reflectance photometer measures light intensity to determine the exact amount of an analyte in a specimen.

Examples of blood chemistry analyzers used in the medical office include the ATAC Lab System (BioMed Laboratories) (Figure 19-1), and the Reflotron Analyzer (Roche Diagnostics).

The manufacturer of each automated analyzer provides a detailed operating manual with the instrument that includes the information necessary to collect, handle, and test the specimen and to perform quality control procedures. In addition, the manufacturer has personnel available for on-site training and service.

Text continued on p. 733

TABLE 19-1	Common Blood Chemistry Tests				
Name of Test	**Abbreviation**	**Purpose**	**Normal Range**	**Increased With**	**Decreased With**
Alanine amino-transferase	ALT	To detect liver disease	≤45 U/L	Hepatocellular disease Active cirrhosis Metastatic liver tumor Obstructive jaundice Pancreatitis	
Alkaline phosphatase	ALP	Assists in diagnosis of liver and bone diseases	25-140 U/L	Liver disease Bone disease Hyperpara-thyroidism Infectious mononucleosis	Hypophosphatasia Malnutrition Hypothyroidism Chronic nephritis
Aspartate amino-transferase	AST	To detect tissue damage	≤40 U/L	Myocardial infarction Liver disease Acute pancreatitis Acute hemolytic anemia	Beriberi Uncontrolled diabetes mellitus with acidosis
Blood urea nitrogen	BUN	Screens for renal disease, especially glomerular functioning	6-20 mg/dL (SI units: 2.5-6.4 mmol/L)	Kidney disease Urinary obstruction Dehydration Gastrointestinal bleeding	Liver failure Malnutrition Impaired absorption
Calcium	Ca	To assess parathyroid functioning and calcium metabolism, and to evaluate malignancies	8.5-10.8 mg/dL (SI units: 2.13-2.76 mmol/L)	**Hypercalcemia** Hyperpara-thyroidism Bone metastases Multiple myeloma Hodgkin's disease Addison's disease Hyperthyroidism	**Hypocalcemia** Hypopara-thyroidism Acute pancreatitis Renal failure
Chloride	Cl	Assists in diagnosing disorders of acid-base and water balance	98-109 mmol/L	Dehydration Cushing's syndrome Hyperventilation Preeclampsia Anemia	Severe vomiting Severe diarrhea Ulcerative colitis Pyloric obstruction Severe burns Heat exhaustion

Continued

TABLE **19-1**	Common Blood Chemistry Tests—cont'd					
Name of Test	**Abbreviation**	**Purpose**	**Normal Range**		**Increased With**	**Decreased With**
Cholesterol	Chol	To screen for athero-sclerosis related to CHD; a secondary aid in study of thyroid and liver functioning	**Total Cholesterol** Below 200 mg/dL 200-239 mg/dL 240 mg/dL or higher (SI units): Below 5.18 mmol/L 5.18-6.19 mmol/L 6.22 mmol/L or higher	Desirable Borderline high High Desirable Borderline high High	Atherosclerosis Cardiovascular disease Obstructive jaundice Hypothyroidism Nephrosis	Malabsorption Liver disease Hyperthyroidism Anemia
			LDL Cholesterol Below 100 mg/dL 100-129 mg/dL 130-159 mg/dL 160-189 mg/dL 190 mg/dL or higher (SI units): Below 2.6 mmol/L 2.6-3.34 mmol/L 3.4-4.12 mmol/L 4.14-4.9 mmol/L 4.92 mmol/L or higher	Optimal Near optimal Borderline high High Very high Optimal Near optimal Borderline high High Very high		
			HDL Cholesterol 60 mg/dL or above 45-59 mg/dL 40-45 mg/dL Below 40 mg/dL (SI units): 1.55 mmol/L or above 1.16-153 mmol/L 1.04-1.17 mmol/L Below 1.04 mmol/L	Optimal Desirable Borderline low Increased risk for CHD Optimal Desirable Borderline low Increased risk for CHD		
Creatinine	Creat	A screening test of renal functioning	0.6-1.5 mg/dL (SI units: 46-115 μmol/L)		Impaired renal function Chronic nephritis Obstruction of the urinary tract Muscle disease	Muscular dystrophy

TABLE 19-1   Common Blood Chemistry Tests—cont'd

Name of Test	Abbreviation	Purpose	Normal Range			Increased With	Decreased With
Globulin	Glob	To identify abnormalities in rate of protein synthesis and removal	2.0-3.5 g/dL (SI units: 20-35 g/L)			Brucellosis Chronic infections Rheumatoid arthritis Dehydration Hepatic carcinoma Hodgkin's disease	Agamma-globulinemia Severe burns
Glucose Fasting blood sugar Two-hour postprandial blood sugar Glucose tolerance test	FBS 2-hr PPBS GTT	To detect disorders of glucose metabolism	**FBS:** 70-110 mg/dL (SI units: 3.9-6.1 mmol/L) **2-hr PPBS:** <140 mg/dL (SI units: <7.8 mmol/L **GTT (mg/dL)**			**Hyperglycemia** Diabetes mellitus Hepatic disease Brain damage Cushing's syndrome	**Hypoglycemia** Excess insulin Addison's disease Bacterial sepsis Carcinoma of the pancreas Hepatic necrosis Hypothyroidism

GTT (mg/dL)

	Normal	Diabetic
FBS	70-110	>120
30 min	150-160	>200
1 hr	160-170	>200
2 hr	120	>140
3 hr	70-110	>140
(SI units: mmol/L)		
FBS	3.9-6.1	>6.7
30 min	8.4-8.9	>11.1
1 hr	8.9-9.5	>11.1
2 hr	6.7	>7.8
3 hr	3.9-6.1	>7.8

≤240 U/L

Name of Test	Abbreviation	Purpose	Normal Range	Increased With	Decreased With
Lactate dehydrogenase, 30° C	LD	Assists in confirming myocardial or pulmonary infarction; also used in differential diagnosis of muscular dystrophy and pernicious anemia		Acute myocardial infarction Acute leukemia Muscular dystrophy Pernicious anemia Hemolytic anemia Hepatic disease Extensive cancer	
Phosphorus	P	Assists in proper evaluation and interpretation of calcium levels; used to detect disorders of endocrine system, bone diseases, and kidney dysfunction	2.5-4.5 mg/dL (SI units: 0.81-1.45 mmol/L)	**Hyperphos-phatemia** Renal insufficiency Severe nephritis Hypopara-thyroidism Hypocalcemia Addison's disease	**Hypophos-phatemia** Hyperpara-thyroidism Rickets and osteomalacia Diabetic coma Hyperinsulinism

Continued

TABLE **19-1**	Common Blood Chemistry Tests—cont'd				
Name of Test	Abbreviation	Purpose	Normal Range	Increased With	Decreased With
Potassium	K	To diagnose disorders of acid-base and water balance in the body	3.5-5.3 mmol/L	**Hyperkalemia** Renal failure Cell damage Acidosis Addison's disease Internal bleeding	**Hypokalemia** Diarrhea Pyloric obstruction Starvation Malabsorption Severe vomiting Severe burns Diuretic administration Chronic stress Liver disease with ascites
Sodium	Na	To detect changes in water and salt balance in the body	135-147 mmol/L	**Hypernatremia** Dehydration Conn's syndrome Primary aldosteronism Coma Cushing's disease Diabetes insipidus	**Hyponatremia** Severe burns Severe diarrhea Vomiting Addison's disease Severe nephritis Pyloric obstruction
Total bilirubin	TB	To evaluate liver functioning and hemolytic anemia	0.2-1.0 mg/dL (SI units: 3.4-22.4 μmol/L)	Liver disease Obstruction of the common bile or hepatic duct Hemolytic anemia	
Total protein	TP	Screens for diseases that alter the protein balance and assesses the state of body hydration	6.0-8.5 g/dL (SI units: 60-85 g/L)	Dehydration (vomiting, diarrhea) Chronic infections Acute liver disease Multiple myeloma Lupus erythematosus	Severe hemorrhaging Hodgkin's disease Severe liver disease Malabsorption
Total thyroxine T_4	Total T_4	To assess thyroid functioning and evaluate thyroid replacement therapy	5-12 μg/dL (SI units: 58-155 nmol/L)	**Hyperthyroidism** Graves' disease Thyrotoxicosis Thyroiditis	**Hypothyroidism** Cretinism Goiter Myxedema Hypoproteinemia

TABLE **19-1**	Common Blood Chemistry Tests—cont'd					
Name of Test	Abbreviation	Purpose	Normal Range		Increased With	Decreased With
Triglycerides	Trig	To evaluate patients with suspected athero-sclerosis	Below 150 mg/dL 150-199 mg/dL 200-499 mg/dL 500 mg/dL or higher	Desirable Borderline high High Very high	Liver disease Nephrotic syndrome Hypothyroidism Poorly controlled diabetes Pancreatitis	Malnutrition Congenital lipoproteinemia
Uric acid	UA	To evaluate renal failure, gout, and leukemia	Male: 3.9-9.0 mg/dL (SI units: 232-596 μmol/L) Female: 2.2-7.7 mg/dL (SI units: 131-458 μmol/L)		Renal failure Gout Leukemia Severe eclampsia Lymphomas	Patients under-going treatment with uricosuric drugs

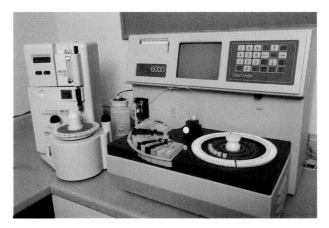

Figure 19-1. A blood chemistry analyzer (ATAC Lab System by BioMed).

Quality Control

Quality control consists of methods and means to ensure that test results are reliable and valid. Two very important quality control measures must be performed routinely when using a blood chemistry analyzer: calibration of the instrument and running controls.

Calibration involves the use of a standard to check the precision of the blood chemistry analyzer. If an analyzer is not properly calibrated, it will be unable to produce accurate test results. If this occurs, the operating manual should be consulted to determine the action that should be taken to correct the problem. Calibration of a blood chemistry analyzer can be compared with placing a scale at zero before weighing a patient. In other words, if the scale is not at zero, the results will not be accurate.

A *control* consists of a sample of a known value. The control is processed in the same manner as a patient specimen, and the results should fall within a specified range as indicated on a reference sheet that accompanies each control. Both normal and abnormal controls are commercially available. Normal controls fall within normal range, whereas abnormal controls fall outside normal range. Low abnormal controls fall below the normal range, and high abnormal controls fall above the normal range. If the control does not fall within its specified range, problems or errors exist, either with the analyzer itself or with the technique used to perform the procedure. The operating manual should be consulted to determine the action to take to correct the situation. A control can be compared with placing an object with a known weight of 5 pounds on a scale. The scale should weigh the object at 5 pounds; otherwise the results are not valid.

The Clinical Laboratory Improvement Amendments of 1988 (CLIA 1988) require the following for moderately complex laboratory tests: the calibration procedure must be performed and documented at least every 6 months and two levels of controls must be performed daily (e.g., running a normal control and a high control). In addition, when problems or errors are identified, the action taken to correct them must be documented.

Cholesterol

Cholesterol is a white, waxy, fatlike substance (lipid) that is essential for normal functioning of the body. It is an important component of cell membranes and is used in the production of hormones and bile. Most of the cholesterol circulating in the blood is manufactured by the liver; however, a portion of it comes from an individual's diet and is

Highlight on Coronary Heart Disease

Coronary heart disease (CHD) affects 6.6 million Americans. The chief forms of CHD are atherosclerosis, high blood pressure, heart attacks, strokes, congestive heart failure, congenital heart disease, and rheumatic heart disease. These various forms of heart disease are interrelated and have elements in common; for example, atherosclerosis can lead to a stroke or heart attack.

Heart disease is the number one killer of adults in the United States today. Because of the national focus on heart disease and cholesterol reduction, since 1985 there has been a decline in heart attacks by 25% and strokes by nearly 40%; however, the death rate from heart disease is likely to remain the number one cause of death until more Americans adopt a more heart-healthy lifestyle.

Not everyone is equal when it comes to coronary heart disease. Some individuals have a much higher risk of developing it than others. The following are risk factors for CHD:

- High total blood cholesterol (above 200 mg/dL confirmed by repeated measurement)
- High blood pressure
- Cigarette smoking (more than 10 cigarettes per day)
- Family history of premature coronary heart disease (definite heart attack or sudden death in a parent or sibling before age 55 years)

- Diabetes mellitus
- History of blood vessel disease
- Obesity (30% or more overweight)
- Low HDL cholesterol (below 40 mg/dL confirmed by repeated measurement)
- Being a man over 45 years of age
- Being a woman over 55 years of age or postmenopausal

Some of these risk factors can be modified; others, such as age, gender, and a family history of CHD, cannot be modified or controlled. The three major risk factors for CHD are high total blood cholesterol, high blood pressure, and cigarette smoking, which fortunately are all modifiable.

Each person's overall risk of coronary heart disease must be assessed individually by the physician, based on the type and number of risk factors present. For example, a 47-year-old man with a cholesterol level of 220 mg/dL who smokes a pack of cigarettes a day and is overweight is at greater risk than a 28-year-old man who is within normal weight, does not smoke, and exercises regularly but has a cholesterol level of 250 mg/dL.

---

known as *dietary cholesterol*. Dietary cholesterol is found only in animal products, such as organ meats, egg yolk, and dairy products.

High blood cholesterol means there is an excessive amount of cholesterol in the blood. An individual's cholesterol level is determined by his or her genetic makeup and by the amount of dietary cholesterol and saturated fat consumed. High blood cholesterol may cause fatty deposits, or plaque, to build up on the walls of the arteries, a condition known as *atherosclerosis*. As the atherosclerosis progresses, the arteries become more occluded, which eventually could lead to a heart attack or stroke. Because of this, high blood cholesterol is considered a major risk for coronary heart disease, and efforts should be made to lower the cholesterol level (see Highlight on Lowering Cholesterol).

HDL and LDL Cholesterol

Cholesterol is transported in the blood as a complex molecule known as **lipoprotein.** Two types of lipoproteins contain cholesterol: low-density lipoprotein (LDL) and high-density lipoprotein (HDL).

LDL picks up cholesterol from ingested fats and from the liver and delivers it to blood vessels and muscles, where it is deposited in the cells. LDL cholesterol is often referred to as "bad" cholesterol because an excess amount of it in the blood can cause plaque to build up on the arterial walls, resulting in atherosclerosis. Refer to Table 19-1 for an interpretation of LDL cholesterol values.

HDL removes excess cholesterol from the cells and carries it to the liver to be excreted. Because HDL removes excess cholesterol from the walls of the blood vessels, it is protective and beneficial to the body and is often called "good" cholesterol. A high HDL cholesterol level has been shown to reduce the risk of heart disease, whereas a low level of HDL cholesterol (less than 40 mg/dL) is a definite risk factor for coronary heart disease.

Cholesterol Testing

All adults over 20 years of age should have a cholesterol test at least once every 5 years. Initial testing includes a *total cholesterol* determination, which is a combined measurement of LDL cholesterol and HDL cholesterol in the blood. To obtain a fuller picture of a patient's cholesterol status, most physicians also order an HDL cholesterol determination, which measures only the HDL cholesterol in the blood. Both these tests are considered screening tests, and elevated results *always* require confirmation through further testing before a diagnosis of high blood cholesterol can be made.

Interpretation of Results

Cholesterol test results are interpreted as follows: Total cholesterol levels under 200 mg/dL are desirable. Levels between 200 and 239 are borderline high, and 240 and above are high. Based on confirmed testing, individuals in the high category are clearly at increased risk for coronary heart disease, and individuals in the

Highlight on Lowering Cholesterol

Research has shown, beyond doubt, that high total blood cholesterol is a major risk factor for coronary heart disease, and the higher the cholesterol, the greater the risk. The National Institutes of Health (NIH) has established guidelines on safe levels of blood cholesterol. The NIH recommends that adults not exceed 200 mg/dL of blood cholesterol.

The National Cholesterol Educational Program (NCEP) was established in 1985 by the federal government to reduce the prevalence of elevated blood cholesterol levels in the United States by educating the public about the health risks associated with high blood cholesterol, and to make recommendations for helping individuals lower their cholesterol levels. It has been shown that for every 1% that an individual lowers his or her total blood cholesterol, the risk of coronary heart disease is lowered by 2%. Taking the following measures can help individuals lower their level of "bad" LDL cholesterol and raise their level of "good" HDL cholesterol.

Diet

Dietary therapy is the first line of treatment of high blood cholesterol. The NCEP recommends that all individuals (over 2 years of age) reduce dietary cholesterol and saturated fats. Many foods high in fat tend to be high in cholesterol. Reading nutrition labels on packaged products helps provide information on the cholesterol and fat content of a food.

Dietary Cholesterol

The body manufactures all the cholesterol it needs for normal functioning, and therefore dietary intake of cholesterol (in foods) serves only to increase the blood cholesterol. According to the NCEP, dietary cholesterol should be limited to 300 mg daily, which is slightly more than the amount of cholesterol in one egg (270 mg). Cholesterol is found only in animal foods and shellfish. Egg yolks, dairy products, and organ meats such as liver and kidneys are especially high in cholesterol.

Saturated Fat

The intake of saturated fat is the single most important dietary factor leading to high blood cholesterol, even more so than consuming dietary cholesterol. In general, the more saturated a fat is, the harder and more solid it is at room temperature. The main source of saturated fat is animal products, including meat fat, poultry skin, and the fat in dairy products (butter, cream, ice cream, cheese, whole milk). Unsaturated fats have little or no effect on the blood cholesterol level; they include olive oil,

canola oil, peanut oil, and sunflower, safflower, and corn oil. The NCEP recommends that no more than 30% of the calories consumed each day come from fat, with no more than 10% of calories coming from saturated fat, and the remaining 20% from unsaturated fat.

Soluble Fiber

Soluble fiber has been shown to lower the cholesterol level by keeping the cholesterol consumed from being absorbed by the body. Examples of foods high in soluble fiber are bran, oats, and beans.

Weight Reduction

It is estimated that one in four Americans is overweight. It is recommended that these individuals follow a sensible eating plan along with an exercise program to reach and maintain desirable weight. Losing weight lowers both total cholesterol and triglyceride levels. Overweight and obese people are at very high risk for CHD because their hearts have to work harder to pump blood through the body.

Exercise

An aerobic exercise program is especially beneficial for weight control because it improves cardiovascular fitness and lowers blood cholesterol level. People who exercise regularly generally have higher HDL cholesterol levels in their blood. Health experts recommend exercising three times a week for 20 to 30 minutes at your target heart rate.

Smoking Cessation

Smoking is one of the three main risk factors for coronary heart disease. By quitting smoking, an individual may be able to strengthen the heart and lower the cholesterol level. Also, non-smokers tend to have higher HDL levels in their blood. A variety of smoking cessation programs are usually offered in the community. Some people have succeeded by using nicotine patches, which help them adjust gradually to lower levels of nicotine.

Generally the cholesterol level begins to drop 2 to 3 weeks after beginning a cholesterol-lowering diet and other cholesterol-lowering measures. Over time it is possible to reduce the total cholesterol level by 30 to 55 mg/dL or even more through these lifestyle changes. If the blood cholesterol level cannot be lowered to an acceptable level, the physician may prescribe cholesterol-lowering medications along with the continuation of the aforementioned measures.

---

borderline high category are at increased risk if they have other risk factors such as being overweight or smoking. An HDL cholesterol level above 60 mg/dL is considered optimal, and a level below 40 mg/dL is a risk factor for coronary heart disease. (45 to 59 mg/dL is considered desirable and 40 to 45 mg/dL is considered borderline low.)

Patient Preparation

Since the total cholesterol and the HDL cholesterol determinations are not affected significantly by food consumption, the patient is usually not required to fast before the collection of the blood specimen. However, some physicians prefer the patient to be in a fasting state.

If the total cholesterol level is 200 mg/dL or higher, the physician usually orders a *lipid profile,* which includes total cholesterol, HDL cholesterol, LDL cholesterol and triglycerides. (The LDL cholesterol level is usually determined as a calculation from the results of the triglyceride and HDL cholesterol levels.) Because triglyceride levels are affected by the consumption of food, the patient must be instructed to fast for at least 12 hours before collection of this blood specimen. An elevated triglyceride level (over 150 mg/dL) places an individual at an increased risk for coronary heart disease, particularly when the LDL cholesterol is high and the HDL cholesterol is low.

Although the primary use of cholesterol testing is to screen for the presence of high blood cholesterol related to coronary heart disease, this test is also used as a secondary aid in the study of thyroid and liver function. See Table 19-1 for a list of specific conditions that cause abnormal cholesterol test results.

Blood Urea Nitrogen

The blood urea nitrogen (BUN) is a kidney function test. Urea is the end product of protein metabolism and is normally present in the blood. However, certain kidney diseases may interfere with the ability of the body to excrete the urea properly, causing an increased level of urea in the blood. See Table 19-1 for a list of specific conditions that cause abnormal BUN test results.

Blood Glucose

Glucose is the end product of carbohydrate metabolism; it is the chief source of energy for the body. Energy is needed to carry out normal functions and to maintain body temperature. The body maintains a constant blood glucose level to ensure a continuous source of energy for the body. Ingested glucose that is not needed for energy can be stored in the form of **glycogen** in muscle and liver tissue for later use. When no more tissue storage is possible, excess glucose is converted to fat and stored as adipose tissue.

Insulin is a hormone secreted by the beta cells of the pancreas and is required for normal use of glucose in the body. Insulin enables glucose to enter the body's cells and be converted to energy. Insulin is also needed for the proper storage of glycogen in liver and muscle cells.

Measuring the amount of glucose in a blood specimen is one of the most common blood chemistry tests. It is used to detect abnormalities in carbohydrate metabolism such as occur in diabetes mellitus, **hypoglycemia,** and liver and adrenocortical dysfunction. Blood glucose is measured by several different testing methods, which include the fasting blood sugar, the 2-hour postprandial blood sugar test, and the glucose tolerance test. Each of these methods serves a specific role in diagnosing and evaluating abnormalities in carbohydrate metabolism and is described in more detail here.

Fasting Blood Sugar

Blood glucose is usually measured when the patient is in a fasting state. This type of test is termed a fasting blood sugar (FBS), which involves collecting a fasting blood sample and measuring the amount of glucose in it. The patient should not have anything to eat or drink, except water, for 12 hours preceding the test. Certain medications, such as oral contraceptives, salicylates, diuretics, and steroids, may affect the test results; therefore the physician may also place the patient on medication restrictions for a specific period of time before the test—usually 3 days. The patient should be scheduled for the test in the morning to minimize the inconvenience of abstaining from food and fluid.

The normal range for a fasting blood sugar varies among laboratories and with the specific type of test, but it usually falls between 70 and 110 mg of glucose per 100 ml of blood (or mg/dL). An FBS is often performed on patients diagnosed with diabetes to evaluate their progress and regulate treatment and as a routine screening procedure to detect diabetes

---

What Would You DO?
What Would You *Not* DO?

Case Study 1

Karen Scrimshaw is at the office. She is 20 years old and is mildly obese. Karen had her cholesterol tested at a health fair and it was 325. The physician orders a CBC, lipid profile, and thyroid profile on Karen and instructs her to return in one week for a follow-up visit to discuss the test results. Karen is very concerned about her cholesterol. She says that she had a candy bar and some potato chips before going to the health fair and wants to know if that could have caused her cholesterol to be so high. She also wants to know how accurate those machines are that are used at health fairs. Karen says that if she has to go on cholesterol medication, it would be hard to decide between Lipitor and Zocor. She says she has seen them advertised on television and they both seem pretty good to her.

PUTTING It All Into PRACTICE

MY NAME IS Michelle Villers, and I work for a physician in an internal medicine medical office. My primary job responsibility includes running the laboratory at the office. I mainly draw blood and perform blood chemistry tests. I also work up patients, run electrocardiograms, apply Holter monitors, and perform pulmonary function tests.

When performing a venipuncture, you need to make sure all the necessary equipment is on hand and ready. Sometimes you may have a tube that has no vacuum in it. In cases like these, it is always better to have a couple of spare tubes on hand. I recently had an experience in which one of my tubes had no vacuum. Luckily I had a few extra tubes within arm's reach so I did not have to interrupt the procedure to get a new one. Basically I have learned that you can never be too prepared.

mellitus. An FBS above 120 mg/dL, considered the dividing point between normal and hyperglycemic values, indicates diabetes mellitus. An elevated test result warrants further testing with the glucose tolerance test.

Two-Hour Postprandial Blood Sugar

The 2-hour postprandial blood sugar (2-hour PPBS) test is used to screen for diabetes mellitus and to monitor the effects of insulin dosage in patients with diabetes. The patient is required to fast, beginning at midnight preceding the test and continuing until breakfast. For breakfast, the patient must consume a prescribed meal that contains 100 grams of carbohydrate, which consists of orange juice, cereal with sugar, toast, and milk. An alternative to this is the consumption of a 100-gram test-load glucose solution. A blood specimen is collected from the patient exactly 2 hours after consumption of the meal or glucose solution.

In the nondiabetic patient, the glucose level returns to the fasting level within 1½ to 2 hours of glucose consumption, whereas the glucose level in the diabetic patient does not return to the fasting level. A postprandial glucose level of 140 g/dL or higher suggests diabetes mellitus and warrants further testing, such as the glucose tolerance test.

Glucose Tolerance Test

The glucose tolerance test (GTT) provides more detailed information about the ability of the body to metabolize glucose by assessing the insulin response to a glucose load. The GTT is used to assist in the diagnosis of diabetes mellitus, hypoglycemia, and liver and adrenocortical dysfunction. It provides a more thorough analysis of glucose utilization than either the FBS or the 2-hour PPBS test.

Testing Requirements

The patient is usually required to consume a high-carbohydrate diet, consisting of 150 grams of carbohydrate per day, for 3 days before the glucose tolerance test. The patient must be in a fasting state when the test begins. On the morning of the test, a blood specimen is drawn from the patient for an FBS and a urine specimen is taken to measure the amount of glucose in each of these samples. If the FBS indicates **hyperglycemia** the physician should be notified because this situation contradicts the administration of a large test load of glucose.

After the FBS has been performed, the patient is instructed to drink a measured amount of a glucose solution (1.75 grams of glucose per kilogram of body weight, or the standard adult dose of 100 grams). Thereafter at regular intervals (generally 30, 60, 120, and 180 minutes), blood and urine samples are taken to determine the patient's ability to handle the increased amount of glucose. Each blood and urine specimen must be labeled carefully with the exact time of collection. The patient is permitted to eat and drink normally after the completion of the test.

It is important that the patient adhere to certain restrictions during the test to ensure accurate results. Since food and fluid affect blood glucose levels, the patient must not eat or drink anything except water during the test. In fact, consumption of water should be encouraged to make it easier for the patient to produce a urine specimen. Smoking is not permitted during the test because tobacco is a stimulant that increases the blood glucose level. The patient should remain at the testing site so that he or she is present when needed for the collection of the blood and urine specimens and to minimize activity. Activity affects the test results by using up glucose; therefore the patient should remain relatively inactive during the test. Sitting and reading, for example, is an activity that would be recommended.

Side Effects

Particularly during the second and third hours of the test, the patient may experience some normal side effects that include weakness, a feeling of faintness, and perspiration. These are considered normal reactions of the body to a fall in the glucose level as insulin is secreted in response to the glucose load. The patient should be reassured that this is a temporary condition. Serious symptoms of severe hypoglycemia should immediately be reported to the physician; they include headache; pale, cold, and clammy skin; irrational speech or behavior; profuse perspiration; and fainting.

Interpretation of Results

The test results are interpreted by evaluating the data obtained for each collection period. If the glucose level is abnormally high compared with established norms for the various blood collection times, a disorder of glucose metabolism, such as diabetes mellitus, may be present. Individuals with diabetes are unable to remove glucose from the bloodstream at the same rate as a nondiabetic individual.

As glucose is absorbed into the bloodstream, the blood glucose level of a nondiabetic rises to a peak level of 160 to 180 mg/dL approximately 30 to 60 minutes after the glucose solution is consumed. The pancreas secretes insulin to compensate for this rise, and the blood glucose returns to the fasting level within 2 to 3 hours of ingestion of the glucose solution. In addition, the urine specimens exhibit negative test results for glucose.

The individual with diabetes does not exhibit the normal use of glucose just described. Rather, the blood glucose peaks at a much higher level, and glucose is present in the urine. In addition, glucose levels are above normal throughout the test because of the lack of insulin. See Table 19-1 for normal and diabetic glucose values.

The glucose tolerance test is generally not used for diagnostic purposes in patients with an FBS above 140 mg/dL or a 2-hour postprandial test result above 180 mg/dL because results greater than these values would qualify for the diagnosis of diabetes mellitus, and the GTT would not be required.

Hypoglycemia

Hypoglycemia is a condition in which the glucose in the blood is abnormally low. During the GTT, patients with this condition exhibit an abnormally low blood glucose level beginning at the 2-hour interval and continuing up to 4 or 5 hours. Hypoglycemia results from glucose removal from the blood at an excessive rate or from a decreased secretion of glucose into the blood, which can be caused by an overdose of insulin, Addison's disease, bacterial sepsis, carcinoma of the pancreas, hepatic necrosis, or hypothyroidism.

Glucose Monitors

In the medical office, a glucose monitor is often used to quantitatively measure the blood glucose level. The test most frequently performed using the glucose monitor is the FBS, although a significant number of offices also perform the GTT and the 2-hour postprandial test. By measuring the blood glucose concentration in the medical office, better patient care can be provided. On-site testing eliminates the time required for an outside laboratory to provide the results, thus allowing the physician to make decisions immediately regarding diagnosis, treatment, and follow-up care. Procedure 19-1 describes how to measure blood glucose using the Accu-Chek Advantage glucose monitor.

Reagent Strips

A reagent strip must be used with the glucose monitor; it consists of a plastic strip with a reaction pad. The pad contains chemicals that react with the glucose in whole blood to determine the blood glucose level in milligrams per deciliter. Through an electronic signal, the glucose results are displayed as a digital readout. The manufacturer's instructions accompanying the glucose monitor must be followed exactly to ensure accurate and reliable test results.

It is important to store the container of reagent strips properly to prevent their deterioration, which affects the test results. The reagents on the strips are sensitive to heat, light, and moisture and must therefore be stored in a cool, dry area at room temperature (cooler than 90°F or

32°C) with the cap tightly closed. Strips that are discolored or that have darkened should be discarded to prevent inaccurate test results. The container of test strips includes a desiccant. Its purpose is to promote dryness by absorbing moisture.

Care and Maintenance

The glucose monitor must be handled carefully. It is a delicate instrument, and a severe physical jar could result in a malfunction. The glucose monitor should not be placed in an area of high humidity, such as a bathroom. In addition, the monitor should not be exposed to severe variations in environmental temperature, such as leaving it in a closed vehicle on a hot or cold day.

Proper cleaning of the glucose monitor is essential for its accurate and reliable operation. On a regular basis, the exterior of the glucose monitor, including the display screen, should be cleaned with a soft, clean cloth slightly dampened with a mild cleaning agent, and it should be dried thoroughly. Do not allow water or detergent to run into the glucose monitor, which could damage the internal components.

Because glucose monitors are battery operated, periodic replacement of the battery is required. The glucose monitor alerts the user to low battery voltage by displaying a special notation on the screen. The type of battery required is specified in the operator's manual, along with directions for installation.

Calibration Procedures

There are usually two calibration procedures required for glucose monitors. Because the Accu-Chek Advantage glucose monitor is presented in Procedure 19-1, the calibration methods discussed here relate specifically to this monitor.

The first calibration procedure ensures that the glucose monitor is functioning properly. It requires the insertion of a plastic check strip into the test strip guide of the monitor (Figure 19-2). Once the plastic strip is inserted, the monitor goes through a series of internal checks to make sure the monitor is functioning properly. The steps presented below should be followed to perform this calibration procedure with the Accu-Chek Advantage glucose monitor.

1. Turn the monitor on.
2. Wait until the strip symbol flashes on the display screen and then insert the check strip into the test strip guide.
3. If the monitor is functioning properly, the word "OK" and a checkmark will appear on the display screen.
4. If the display exhibits the word "error", repeat the calibration procedure. If the error display appears again, the monitor is not working properly and is in need of repair.

The second calibration procedure is performed to ensure accurate and reliable test results. This calibration procedure compensates for variables that occur in the manufacturing process that causes one batch of reagent strips to be a little different from another batch. The calibration procedure programs the electronics of the glucose monitor to match the reactivity of the container of strips that are in current use.

The calibration procedure for the Accu-Chek Advantage is performed using a plastic code key that accompanies each container of Accu-Chek Advantage reagent strips (Figure 19-3). Accu-Chek requires lot-specific calibration, meaning that the calibration procedure needs to be performed only once per container of test strips. This is possible because the Accu-Chek glucose monitor has a built-in memory system that enables it to retain a point of reference, once it has been calibrated. This reference point is retained until the glucose monitor is reprogrammed for a new container of test strips. The calibration procedure delineated next should be followed when a new container of Accu-Chek test strips is opened.

1. Make sure the monitor is turned off.
2. Turn the monitor over so that the back of the monitor is facing you.
3. Remove the old code key if one is installed.
4. Insert a new code key until it snaps into place.
5. Turn the monitor on. A three-digit code number appears on the display screen. This number must match the code number of the vial of reagent strips. If it does not, repeat steps 1 through 3.

Control Procedure

A control check should be run to ensure the test results are reliable and valid and that errors that might interfere with test results are detected and eliminated. A control check is performed on the Accu-Chek Advantage using commercially available glucose control solutions. Two (out of three) levels of controls should be used (high, normal, or low).

A control check should be performed under the following circumstances:

1. Daily, before using the monitor for the first time
2. When a new container of reagent strips is opened

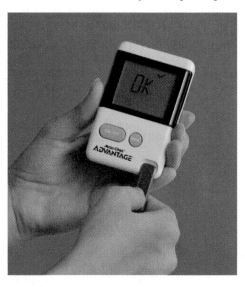

Figure 19-2. Accu-Chek Advantage check strip calibration procedure to ensure the glucose monitor is functioning properly.

❱❱ PATIENT **TEACHING**

Obtaining a Capillary Blood Specimen

The medical assistant may need to instruct the patient in the procedure for obtaining and testing a capillary blood specimen for blood glucose measurement. Properly educating the patient to perform the procedure is the most important factor in obtaining accurate test results.

1. **Obtaining the capillary blood specimen.** Inform the patient of the sites available for obtaining the blood specimen. These include the fingers and the side of the hand where there are no calluses. Most patients prefer to use an automatic lancet to perform the skin puncture. Using such a device makes the puncture less painful, and the preset puncture depth generally ensures a successful stick. For a finger puncture, instruct the patient to obtain the blood specimen from the lateral side of the fingertip because this area contains fewer nerve endings and less pain results. If the patient's hands are cold, tell him or her to rub them together or place them in warm water, which improves the blood flow to the area. Instruct the patient in the proper procedure for obtaining a large drop of blood to ensure accurate test results.

2. **Performing the blood glucose test.** The patient performs the test with a reagent strip using a glucose monitor. Instruct the patient in the proper procedure for performing the test, making sure he or she understands that accurate test results assist in greater glucose control. Patients should also be given detailed instructions on the proper care and maintenance of the glucose monitor.

3. **Recording results.** Instruct the patient to record each test result in a log book to provide a permanent record between office visits. In addition, most glucose monitors are equipped with a memory system that stores test results for later retrieval. The following information should be included with each recording:
   a. Date and time
   b. Number of hours since the patient last ate
   c. Time of the last insulin injection or oral hypoglycemic medication
   d. Any feeling of physical or emotional stress
   e. Amount of exercise the patient has undergone

   Keeping track of these factors helps explain a shift in the blood glucose level and provides the basis for sound self-management decisions.

3. If the cap is left off the vial of reagent strips for any length of time
4. If the monitor is dropped
5. If a test has been repeated and the blood glucose result is still lower or higher than expected

Self-Monitoring of Blood Glucose

Diabetic patients who take insulin must monitor their blood glucose levels to contribute to effective management of diabetes. Based on the results, decisions can be made regarding insulin and dietary adjustments that may be necessary to maintain normal glucose levels and to avoid the extremes of hypoglycemia and hyperglycemia. Satisfactory control of the blood glucose level reduces symptoms of the disease and helps decrease or delay long-term complications that can occur with diabetes mellitus, such as retinopathy and peripheral vascular disease.

Research shows that frequent blood glucose monitoring is the most effective means of maintaining normal blood glucose levels and preventing long-term complications associated with diabetes mellitus. Because of the necessity of performing a finger puncture, however, and the fact that the patient must assume responsibility in self-management decisions, the medical assistant may need to reinforce the advantages of home blood glucose monitoring:

1. **Convenience of testing.** The patient is able to test his or her blood at any time of the day without a physician's order. Before the development of glucose monitors, patients could obtain a blood glucose test only through a laboratory order from the physician. Because of the cost and inconvenience of this process, most patients did not comply with the testing requirements to achieve and maintain satisfactory control. In addition, the patient was unable to obtain the test when the office or laboratory

---

What Would You DO?
What Would You *Not* DO?

Case Study 3
Dave Felden has recently been diagnosed with type 1 diabetes and is taking insulin. He has come to the office for an FBS. A fingerstick will be performed to collect the specimen and a glucose meter will be used to test the specimen. Dave has been performing this test on himself at home now for 2 weeks and wants to know if he can stick his own finger. Dave says that he's been having a few problems giving himself his insulin injections. He says that he has been getting some very large air bubbles in his syringe when he draws up the insulin. He says he's been having trouble getting them out and wants to know how important that is. Dave says he is on a limited income and wants to know if he could use his needle and syringe for more than one injection. He also wants to know if he should throw his used needle and syringes in the regular trash.

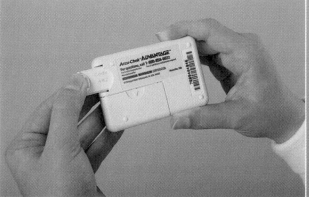
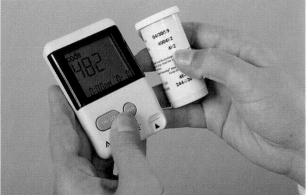

Figure 19-3. Accu-Chek Advantage code key calibration procedure. **A,** The code key is inserted into the monitor. **B,** The code number must match the code number of the vial of reagent strips.

was closed. With some patients, the lowest blood glucose level occurs from 3:00 to 5:00 AM when most laboratory facilities are closed. Testing at home also lets the patient check his or her blood glucose when a side effect common to diabetes mellitus occurs, such as hypoglycemia.

2. **More involvement in self-management decisions.** The patient is able to become more involved in self-management decisions regarding insulin dosage, meal planning, and physical activity. Initially some patients lack confidence in making insulin and dietary adjustments based on the blood glucose test results. The medical assistant should provide encouragement and stress the benefits to be derived in terms of improved regulation of the blood glucose level.

3. **Reliable decisions regarding insulin dosage.** More reliable decisions regarding insulin needs can be made during situations that affect the blood glucose level, such as illness, emotional stress, increased physical activity, or suspected hypoglycemia.

4. **Decrease or delay in long-term complications.** Diabetic patients who maintain good blood glucose control generally experience fewer symptoms and de-

crease or delay long-term complications of the disease; these results can lead to a longer life. Having a record of the patient's daily blood glucose values also assists the physician in making decisions regarding treatment and follow-up care.

The frequency of the blood glucose testing depends on a number of factors, including the severity of the diabetes, special conditions such as pregnancy, and variations in activity level. Ideally, the blood glucose level should be monitored four times a day: in the morning (after an 8-hour fast), before lunch, before dinner, and at bedtime. The FBS test result (obtained in the morning) is the best overall indicator of control, and the other determinations provide guidance for adjusting insulin dosage, diet, and exercise. Some physicians periodically recommend a 2-hour postprandial specimen to further assist in maintaining good control by detecting hyperglycemia that might otherwise be missed.

Overall self-monitoring of the blood glucose level provides an important feedback mechanism to maintain normal blood glucose levels and to assist the diabetic patient in anticipating and treating fluctuations in glucose levels brought on by food, exercise, stress, and infection.

PROCEDURE 19-1 Blood Glucose Measurement Using the Accu-Chek Advantage Glucose Monitor

PROCEDURE 19-1

Outcome Perform a fasting blood sugar.

Equipment/Supplies:
- Personal protective equipment, including disposable gloves
- Accu-Chek Advantage glucose monitor
- Accu-Chek Advantage reagent strips
- Check Strip
- Code Key
- Control solution
- Lancet
- Antiseptic wipe
- Gauze pad
- Biohazard sharps container

1. Procedural Step. Sanitize your hands. Assemble the equipment. Check the expiration date on the container of reagent strips.
Principle. Outdated reagent strips can cause inaccurate test results.

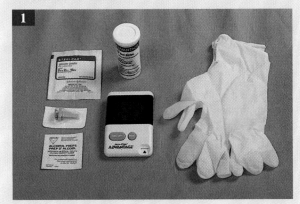

2. Procedural Step. Calibrate the glucose monitor using the Check Strip.
Principle. Calibrating with the Check Strip ensures that the glucose meter is functioning properly.

3. Procedural Step. If necessary, calibrate the glucose monitor using the Code Key that accompanies the container of reagent strips.
Principle. Calibrating with the Code Key compensates for variables that occur in the manufacturing process of the reagent strips.

4. Procedural Step. Run a control check on the glucose meter using control solution.
Principle. Running a control ensures that the test results are reliable and valid.

Continued

PROCEDURE 19-1   Blood Glucose Measurement Using the Accu-Chek Advantage Glucose Monitor—Cont'd

5. **Procedural Step.** Greet and identify the patient. Introduce yourself, and explain the procedure. If a fasting specimen is required, ask the patient if he or she has had anything to eat or drink (besides water) for the past 12 hours.
   Principle. Consumption of food or fluid increases the blood glucose level, leading to inaccurate interpretation of FBS test results.

6. **Procedural Step.** Ask the patient to wash his or her hands in warm water and thoroughly dry them.
   Principle. Washing the hands cleans the fingers and stimulates the flow of blood. The hands must be completely dry to encourage the formation of a hanging drop of blood, which assists in the transfer of the blood to the reagent pad.

7. **Procedural Step.** Turn the monitor on. Check that the code number displayed matches the code number on the vial of test strips that you are using. When the test strip symbol flashes on the display, the monitor is ready to accept a test strip.

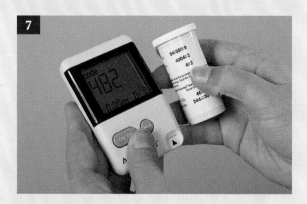

8. **Procedural Step.** Remove a test strip from the container. Promptly replace the lid of the container to prevent the strips from being exposed to moisture.
   Principle. The reagent pads are moisture sensitive and could be affected by environmental moisture, leading to inaccurate test results.

9. **Procedural Step.** Within 30 seconds, gently insert the test strip with the yellow target area facing up into the test strip guide. Once the strip is correctly inserted, a blood drop symbol flashes on the display.

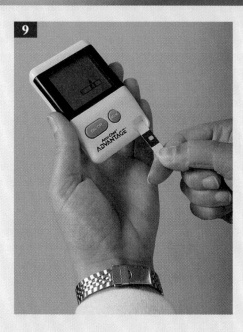

10. **Procedural Step.** Cleanse the puncture site with an antiseptic wipe and allow it to dry. Apply gloves and perform a finger puncture. Dispose of the lancet in a biohazard sharps container.
    Principle. The antiseptic must be allowed to dry to prevent it from reacting with the chemicals on the reagent pad, which would lead to inaccurate test results. Gloves provide a barrier against bloodborne pathogens.

11. **Procedural Step.** Once the puncture has been made, wipe away the first drop of blood with a gauze pad. Place the hand in a dependent position (palm facing down), and gently squeeze the finger around the puncture site until a large drop of blood forms.
    Principle. The first drop of blood contains a large amount of serum, which dilutes the specimen and leads to inaccurate test results. A large drop of blood is needed to completely cover the target area of the reagent strip.

12. **Procedural Step.** Touch the drop of blood to the center of the yellow target area. Do not smear the blood with your finger on the target area. If any yellow mesh is visible after you have applied the initial drop of blood, a second drop of blood may be applied to the target area within 15 seconds of the first drop. If more than 15 seconds has passed, the test result may be erroneous, and you should dis-

card the test strip and repeat the test. When the blood is correctly applied to the strip, a box rotates on the display until the measurement is completed. *Principle.* The entire yellow target area must be completely covered with blood to ensure accurate and reliable test results.

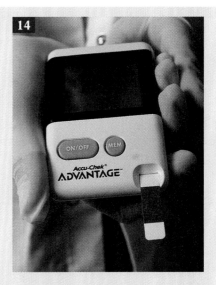

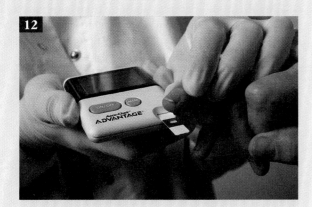

13. **Procedural Step.** Have the patient hold a gauze pad over the puncture site and apply pressure until the bleeding stops.

14. **Procedural Step.** After a short time, the glucose value is displayed in milligrams per deciliter. If the glucose value is higher or lower than expected or if the screen displays something other than the glucose value, see the Troubleshooting Guide section of the operator's manual to obtain instructions for correcting the problem. (The glucose result indicated on this glucose meter is 89 mg/dL.)

15. **Procedural Step.** Remove the reagent strip from the monitor and discard it in a biohazard waste container. Turn the monitor off.

16. **Procedural Step.** Remove gloves and sanitize your hands. Chart the results. Include the date and time, when the patient last ate, the type of test (e.g., FBS, random), the glucose test result, and your initials. If the patient has diabetes mellitus, also record the time of his or her last insulin injection or last consumption of oral hypoglycemic medication.

17. **Procedural Step.** Properly store the glucose meter according the manufacturer's instructions.

CHARTING EXAMPLE	
Date	
5/18/05	8:30 a.m. FBS: 89 mg/dL. Pt last ate on
	5/17 @ 7:00 p.m. —— M. Villers, CMA

SEROLOGY

In the simplest terms, *serology* is defined as the scientific study of the serum of the blood. More specifically, however, serology deals with the study of antigen and antibody reactions.

An **antigen** is a substance that is capable of stimulating the formation of antibodies in an individual. Antigens may consist of protein, glycoprotein, complex polysaccharides, or nucleic acid. Specific examples of antigens include bacteria and viruses, bacterial toxins, allergens, and blood antigens. An **antibody** is a substance that is capable of combining with an antigen, resulting in an antigen-antibody reaction.

Laboratory testing in serology deals with studying antigen-antibody reactions to assess the presence of a substance (e.g., ABO blood typing) or to assist in the diagnosis of disease (e.g., mononucleosis testing). Serologic tests are often used for the early diagnosis of disease and are also used to follow the course of the disease.

Serologic Tests

Some specific examples of serologic tests are listed and described here.

Hepatitis Tests. Hepatitis testing is performed to detect viral hepatitis. There are five types of viral hepatitis: A, B, C, D, and E, which are described in detail in Chapter 2. Hepatitis testing not only detects the presence of viral hepatitis, but it also determines the type of hepatitis present.

Syphilis Test. Syphilis is a sexually transmitted disease (STD) caused by the microorganism *Treponema pallidum.* The most common tests to detect the presence of syphilis are the Venereal Disease Research Laboratories (VDRL) test and the rapid plasma reagin (RPR) test. The test results are reported as nonreactive, weakly reactive, or reactive. Weakly reactive and reactive results are considered positive for the presence of syphilis antibodies. These tests are screening tests, and a positive result warrants more specific testing to arrive at a diagnosis of syphilis.

Mono Test. This test is used to detect the presence of infectious mononucleosis. The theory and procedure for this test are given in detail in this chapter.

Rheumatoid Factor. Rheumatoid arthritis is a chronic inflammatory disease that affects the joints of the body. The blood of individuals with rheumatoid arthritis contains a type of antibody called rheumatoid factor (RF). This test detects the presence of the rheumatoid factor's antibodies and thereby assists in the diagnosis of rheumatoid arthritis.

Antistreptolysin O Test. The antistreptolysin O (ASO) test is used to detect ASO antibodies in the serum. It is the most widely used serologic test for the detection of conditions resulting from streptococcal infections and diseases that occur secondary to a streptococcal infection. This test is useful in assisting in the diagnosis of rheumatic fever, glomerulonephritis, bacterial endocarditis, and scarlet fever.

C-Reactive Protein. During inflammation and tissue destruction, an abnormal protein called C-reactive protein (CRP) appears in the blood. Patients with inflammatory conditions or disorders accompanied by tissue destruction have positive results to this test. Because of this, the CRP test is used to assist in diagnosing or charting the progress of such conditions as rheumatoid arthritis, acute rheumatic fever, widespread malignancy, and bacterial infections.

Cold Agglutinins. This test is used to detect the presence of antibodies called cold agglutinins. The cold agglutinins test is performed by incubating the patient's serum with erythrocytes at cold temperatures. If cold agglutinins are present, this causes **agglutination** of the erythrocytes. Cold agglutinins are found in patients with infectious mononucleosis, mycoplasmal pneumonia, chronic parasitic infections, and lymphoma.

ABO and Rh Blood Typing. Blood typing is performed to determine an individual's ABO and Rh blood type. Knowledge of blood type helps to prevent transfusion and transplant reactions and to identify problems such as hemolytic disease of the newborn. The theory and procedure for ABO and Rh blood typing is presented in this chapter.

Rh Antibody Titer. This test detects the amount of circulating Rh antibodies in the blood. These antibodies can occur in a pregnant woman who is Rh-negative and is carrying an Rh-positive fetus. Therefore this test is most frequently used to detect the presence of an Rh incompatibility problem with a mother and her unborn child.

Rapid Mononucleosis Testing

Infectious mononucleosis is an acute infectious disease caused by the Epstein-Barr virus (EBV). Infectious mononucleosis most frequently affects children and young adults. It is transmitted through saliva by direct oral contact, and because of this, it is often called the "kissing disease." Symptoms of infectious mononucleosis include mental and physical fatigue, fever, sore throat, severe weakness, headache, and swollen lymph nodes.

The rapid mono test is often performed in the medical office and is used to assist in the diagnosis of infectious mononucleosis. Rapid mono tests are easy to perform and provide reliable results in a short time.

Individuals with infectious mononucleosis produce an antibody called heterophile antibody, usually by the sixth to the tenth day of the illness. Rapid mono tests detect this antibody. The presence of the heterophile antibody along with patient symptoms can provide the basis for the diagnosis of infectious mononucleosis. Figure 19-4 outlines the procedure for performing a rapid mono test using the QuickVue+ Mononucleosis Test (Quidel Corporation).

Blood Typing

Blood Antigens

Each individual has a blood type. Blood type depends on the presence of certain factors, or antigens, on the surface of the red blood cells. **Blood antigens** consist of protein and are inherited through **genes,** which program the body to produce a particular antigen. If a blood antigen is present, it appears on the surface of all the red blood cells in the body.

Many types of antigen can appear in the blood. These antigens can be grouped into categories known as blood group systems. The blood group systems that are most likely to cause problems in blood transfusions and in Rh disease of the newborn are the ABO and Rh blood group systems. Therefore, these are the blood group systems most commonly tested for in the medical laboratory.

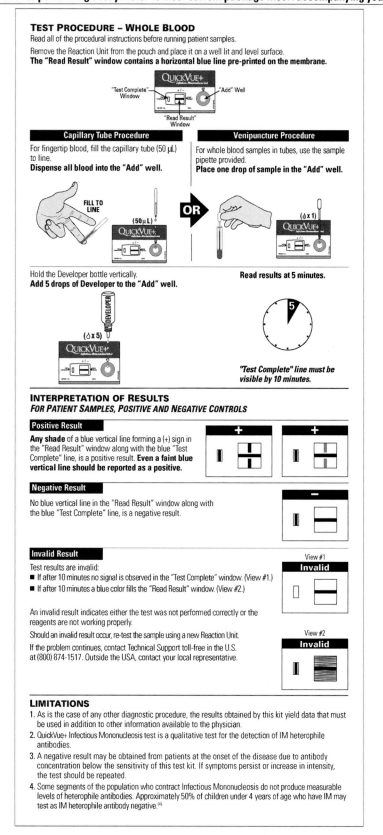

Figure 19-4. Procedure for performing the QuickVue+ Mononucleosis Test (Courtesy Quidel Corporation, San Diego, California.)

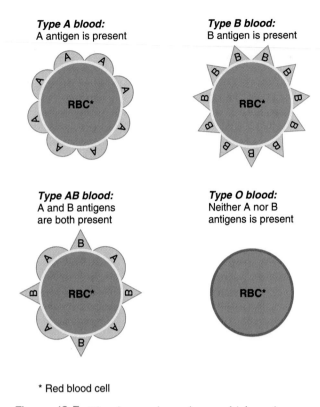

Type A blood:
A antigen is present

Type B blood:
B antigen is present

Type AB blood:
A and B antigens
are both present

Type O blood:
Neither A nor B
antigens is present

* Red blood cell

Figure 19-5. Blood type depends on which antigens are present on the surface of the red blood cells.

Within the ABO blood group system, there are four main blood types: A, B, AB, and O. The blood type depends on which antigens are present on the surface of the red blood cells.
- If the A antigen is present, the blood type is A.
- If the B antigen is present, the blood type is B.
- If both the A and B antigens are present, the blood type is AB.
- If neither the A nor the B antigen is present, the blood type is O. Figure 19-5 helps illustrate this principle.

Blood Antibodies

Blood antibodies are proteins that are naturally present in the plasma of the blood. An antibody is a substance that is capable of combining with an antigen. The body never produces an antibody to combine with its own blood antigen. For example, if the blood type is A, the plasma does not contain the A antibody. However, the B antibody naturally occurs in that plasma. The B antibody cannot combine with the A antigen. If a blood antigen and its corresponding antibody combine (in this case, the A antigen combining with the A antibody), a serious antigen-antibody reaction will take place that could pose a threat to life.
- If the blood type is A, the plasma contains the B antibody.

Highlight on Blood Donor Criteria

Every year approximately 5 million Americans require blood transfusions, resulting in 13.5 million units of blood being transfused. A safe, readily available blood supply is essential for lifesaving medical procedures, such as replacing blood loss from hemorrhages or surgical procedures, replacing plasma in burn and shock victims, and providing platelets to control bleeding. In an average population, 75% of the people are physically and medically eligible to donate blood; unfortunately, only 5% of those eligible decide to donate.

Basic blood donor criteria have been established on a national basis to ensure donor safety and a quality blood donation. All blood collection facilities, such as the American Red Cross, must follow these regulations. In general, blood donors must be in good health and be of a certain age and weight.

Health History

To protect both the donor and recipient, each donor is asked to give a brief health history. The prospective donor is asked to provide information related to diseases that may be transmitted through the blood (such as hepatitis and AIDS) and medications being taken that could affect the quality of the blood donation. Information is also obtained related to medical conditions that might jeopardize the health of the donor if he or she were to donate.

Based on this information, a prospective donor could be *temporarily deferred* from donating blood because of the following: recent immunizations, pregnancy, a human bite, a skin infection, certain medical conditions such as a recent heart attack or tuberculosis, certain prescription medications being taken, recent tattooing, and travel to a malaria-prone area. Temporarily deferred donors will be told how long they must wait and are encouraged to donate blood once the waiting period is over. The waiting period varies based on the condition or situation; for example, there is a one year waiting period following a heart attack, whereas there is only a 2-day wait following the last dose of an antibiotic medication.

A prospective donor is *permanently deferred* from giving blood because of any of the following reasons: a clotting disorder, cancer that was treated with chemotherapy, certain autoimmune disease (e.g., lupus, multiple sclerosis), a history of hepatitis, infection with the AIDS virus (HIV infection), and behavior that is associated with the spread of the AIDS virus. An individual is also permanently deferred if he/she has spent three months or more in the United Kingdom between 1980 and 1996 (a country where "mad cow disease" is found).

Age

An individual must be at least 17 years old to donate blood. With written parental consent, however, some states permit 16-year-old individuals to donate blood. There is no upper age limit for blood donation as long as the individual feels well and has no restrictions or limitations on his or her activities.

- If the blood type is B, the plasma contains the A antibody.
- If the blood type is AB, neither the A nor the B antibodies appear in the plasma.
- If the blood type is O, both the A and B antibodies appear in the plasma. Remember, type O blood has neither the A nor the B antigen on the surface of its red blood cells. The A and B antibodies in the plasma would not have an A or B antigen to combine with them (Table 19-2).

The Rh Blood Group System

In 1940 Landsteiner and Wiener discovered the Rh blood group system while working with rhesus monkeys. Most of the people in the United States have the Rh antigen present on the red blood cells and therefore have type Rh-positive blood. The remaining 15% of the white population and 7% of the African-American population do not have the Rh antigen present on the red blood cells and thus have type Rh-negative blood. Unlike the A and B antibodies, the Rh antibodies do not normally occur in the plasma.

Blood Antigen and Antibody Reactions

When a blood antigen and its corresponding antibody unite, the result is the clumping, or agglutination, of red blood cells. Agglutination of red blood cells can be serious and even fatal if it occurs **in vivo** (in the living body). The clumped red blood cells cannot pass through the small tubules of the kidneys, and this may lead to kidney failure. Also, the clumping of the red blood cells eventually leads to *hemolysis,* or breakdown of the red blood cells.

Blood antigen-antibody reactions can occur if the wrong blood type is administered to an individual during a blood transfusion. If an individual with type A blood is given a transfusion of type B blood, the B antibody of the **recipient** (person receiving the blood) would combine with the B antigen of the **donor** (person donating the blood) and an antigen-antibody reaction would occur, resulting in agglutination of red blood cells. Therefore, we say that type A blood is incompatible with type B blood.

TABLE 19-2	ABO Blood Group System	
Blood Type	**Antigen Present on the Red Blood Cell**	**Antibody Present in the Plasma**
A	A	B
B	B	A
AB	A, B	Neither A nor B
O	Neither A nor B	A, B

Date of Last Donation
At least 56 days (8 weeks) must elapse between donations.

Weight
The donor must weigh at least 110 pounds. (In some states, the minimum weight is 105 pounds.) For the average individual, the total volume of blood is approximately 8% of the body weight. Underweight donors are not accepted because a full donation would result in a proportionately greater reduction in blood volume and might precipitate a reaction. There is no upper weight limit as long as the individual's weight is not higher than the weight limit of the blood donor bed being used.

Temperature
Body temperature of donors may not exceed 99.5° F (37.5° C). The primary purpose of temperature measurement is to eliminate donors who are ill.

Pulse
The acceptable range for the pulse rate is 50 to 110 beats per minute. If the pulse rate appears to be elevated because of physical exertion, the donor may be asked to remain seated for 5 to 10 minutes, with a recheck taken after the resting period.

Blood Pressure
The acceptable limit for blood pressure is a reading no higher than 180 mm Hg for the systolic pressure and a reading no higher than 100 mm Hg for the diastolic pressure.

Hemoglobin
The hemoglobin must be 12.5 g/dL or higher for both men and women.

Blood-Donating Process
It takes approximately 1 hour to donate blood. The process begins with the health history, followed by a mini-physical check of temperature, pulse, blood pressure, and hemoglobin level. Next, a unit (1 pint) of blood is collected using a sterile needle and a sterile plastic bag that contains an additive. A donor should feel no pain during the blood collection procedure, which takes approximately 8 to 10 minutes. It is not possible to contract AIDS or any other infectious disease by donating blood. Following the collection of the unit of blood, the donor is encouraged to have refreshments to begin replenishing the fluids and nutrients temporarily lost during the donation.

Processing the Blood
Each blood donation is tested for AIDS, hepatitis, and syphilis. Any unit of blood that tests positive is rejected for transfusion. The unit of blood is typed and then labeled with its ABO and Rh blood type. It is then available for distribution to hospitals for transfusing.

Agglutination and Blood Typing

Agglutination of red blood cells is the basis for the ABO and Rh blood typing procedure. The antigen-antibody reaction occurs **in vitro,** or "in glass" in the laboratory, so there is no threat to life.

To test for the ABO blood group system, a commercially prepared antiserum is used. An **antiserum** is a serum that contains antibodies. An antiserum containing the A antibody is added to an unknown blood specimen. If the A antigen is present, it combines with the A antibody, resulting in agglutination. An antiserum containing the B antibody is added to another sample of the unknown blood. If the B antigen is present, it will combine with the B antibody, resulting in agglutination. If agglutination occurs in both instances, the sample is type AB. If no agglutination occurs, this indicates the absence of blood antigens, or type O blood. Agglutination that occurs in vitro is visible to the naked eye.

The antigen-antibody reaction that occurs when the unknown blood sample is type A is diagrammed in Figure 19-6.

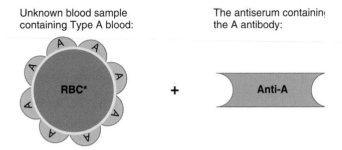

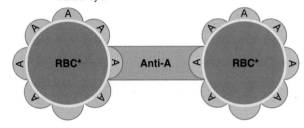

The bridge forming between the antigen and antibody represents the antigen-antibody reaction. This reaction leads to agglutination of red blood cells, which is visible to the naked eye.

Figure 19-6. The antigen-antibody reaction that occurs in vitro when the unknown blood sample is type A.

MEDICAL Practice and the LAW

When running laboratory tests, you must make sure all equipment is functioning properly. This is done by the periodic calibration or running of controls on each piece of equipment. Know how and how often to calibrate or run controls and document appropriately. Without these quality controls, results cannot be trusted to be accurate. Inaccurate results can lead to an inaccurate diagnosis and treatment.

Use personal protective equipment appropriate to each test to avoid transmission of disease and cross-contamination of specimens.

Who can sue?

Anyone can sue for anything. The important thing to know is, can they win? The person filing the lawsuit is called the plaintiff, and the one being sued is called the defendant. In order to win a malpractice lawsuit, four things are necessary:

1. The defendant must have had a duty to the plaintiff, that is, a doctor-patient relationship must exist.

2. Care must have been provided that was not consistent with that of a "reasonably prudent" physician or medical assistant. In other words, a mistake was made and the individual making it should have known better. If you work in a specialty area, you are expected to know more about that specialty than if you worked in a general practice office. Therefore, be very familiar with your office's policy and procedures manual.

3. The plaintiff must prove proximate cause. This means the patient's problem is a direct cause of the physician's or medical assistant's actions.

4. The plaintiff must have been injured by the mistake. Damages may include pain and suffering, loss of income, and medical bills.

To avoid personal lawsuits, practice good care, document everything you do, and maintain good relationships with patients. Few patients who are hurt will sue, but most patients who are hurt and are angry *will* sue.

What Would You DO?
What Would You *Not* DO? *RESPONSES*

Case Study 1
What Did Michelle Do?
- ❏ Tried to calm and reassure Karen.
- ❏ Explained to Karen that the cholesterol results are not affected by food so eating before the health fair should not have affected her results.
- ❏ Told Karen that before a cholesterol analyzer is used, it is usually checked to make sure it is working properly.
- ❏ Explained to Karen that the physician was checking her cholesterol again as well as running some additional tests to determine if she is having any problems.
- ❏ Told Karen that if she must take medication, the physician will determine what drug is best for her.

What Did Michelle Not Do?
- ❏ Did not tell Karen that her cholesterol is extremely high.
- ❏ Did not tell Karen she should be more careful about what she eats since she is overweight.
- ❏ Did not tell Karen that there was no way to know if the cholesterol analyzer used at the health fair was calibrated and had controls run on it.

What Would You Do?/What Would You *Not* Do? Review Michelle's response and place a checkmark next to the information you included in your response. List here additional information you included in your response.

_____
_____
_____
_____

Case Study 2
What Did Michelle Do?
- ❏ Apologized to Crystal for the inconvenience. Explained to her that it takes 3 to 4 hours to run a glucose tolerance test because several specimens must be collected over a period of time to see how her body handles sugar.
- ❏ Explained to Crystal that eating and smoking causes the test results to be inaccurate. Told her that she could eat and smoke as soon as the test was over.
- ❏ Told Crystal that she needs to sit quietly during the test so it would not be possible for her to bring her children.
- ❏ Informed the physician of Crystal's situation to see if he had any suggestions.

What Did Michelle Not Do?
- ❏ Did not get defensive or intimidated by Crystal's behavior.
- ❏ Did not tell Crystal that the staff would watch Crystal's children during the test.

- ❏ Did not tell Crystal that it was not a good idea for her to smoke around her children.

What Would You Do?/What Would You *Not* Do? Review Michelle's response and place a checkmark next to the information you included in your response. List here additional information you included in your response.

_____
_____
_____
_____

Case Study 3
What Did Michelle Do?
- ❏ Told Dave that it would be fine for him to perform his own fingerstick.
- ❏ Made sure that his finger was cleansed with an antiseptic wipe and that he wiped away the first drop of blood.
- ❏ Explained to Dave that the air bubbles take up space that the insulin should occupy and that if he doesn't get rid of them, he will not get his full dose of insulin.
- ❏ Demonstrated how to remove air bubbles and had Dave practice it at the office.
- ❏ Told Dave he must not reuse his needle and syringe. Explained that a used needle could cause him to get an infection. Asked Dave if he had checked to see if his insurance would cover the cost of the needles and syringes.
- ❏ Told Dave that he should put his used needles and syringes in a thick plastic container such as an empty detergent container. After the container is full, he should close it tightly with a screw lid and then it can be thrown out with his regular trash. Explained that this will protect his family and the trash handlers from getting stuck while disposing of the trash.

What Did Michelle Not Do?
- ❏ Did not tell Dave he didn't need to worry about the air bubbles in the syringe.

What Would You Do?/What Would You *Not* Do? Review Michelle's response and place a checkmark next to the information you included in your response. List here additional information you included in your response.

_____
_____
_____
_____

Apply Your KNOWLEDGE

Blood Chemistry

Choose the best answer to each of the following questions.

1. Michelle Villers, CMA, supervises the running of the office laboratory. She is getting ready to run some blood chemistry tests on the automated blood chemistry analyzer. Following the CLIA requirements, Michelle must first perform the following:
   A. Clean the analyzer with a mild detergent
   B. Run two levels of controls on the analyzer
   C. Eat a healthy lunch
   D. Check the warranty on the analyzer

2. Stanley Seaver comes to the office for a general physical examination. Since he has a family history of heart disease, Dr. Donor orders a lipid profile on him. Michelle Villers, CMA, explains the patient preparation for this profile, which includes:
   A. Do not take any medications for 48 hours before the test
   B. Consume a breakfast high in fat
   C. Do not eat or drink anything for 12 hours before the test
   D. Do not consume any foods containing cholesterol for 72 hours before the test

3. Michelle performs a lipid profile on Stanley Seaver. Which of the following test results indicates an abnormal value?
   A. Total Cholesterol: 260
   B. Triglycerides: 175
   C. LDL Cholesterol: 150
   D. HDL Cholesterol: 36
   E. All of the above

4. Michelle is providing patient education to Stanley regarding coronary heart disease. All of the following factors are risk factors for CHD EXCEPT:
   A. Cigarette smoking
   B. Diabetes
   C. Obesity
   D. An elevated HDL cholesterol level

5. Eva Marie is a 56-year-old female who has diabetes. Dr. Donor orders a 2-hour PPBS on Eva. Michelle Villers, CMA, explains the patient preparation to Eva which includes:
   A. Do not eat or drink beginning at midnight
   B. Consume a breakfast of 100 grams of carbohydrate
   C. Drink as much water as you desire
   D. All of the above

6. David Albright has come to the office for a GTT. Michelle Villers, CMA, draws a blood specimen for an FBS and determines the value to be 80 mg/dL. At this point, Michelle should:
   A. Continue with the GTT
   B. Run another FBS
   C. Notify the physician
   D. Discontinue the test

7. Pollyanna Porter is having a GTT. Michelle Villers, CMA, explains to Pollyanna that during the testing period, she is allowed to:
   A. Eat
   B. Smoke
   C. Drink water
   D. Go to her health club and work out

8. During the GTT, Pollyanna experiences some symptoms. Which of the following symptoms should Michelle report to the physician?
   A. Dizziness
   B. Irrational speech
   C. Weakness
   D. Hunger

9. Michelle Villers, CMA, receives an order of reagent strips for the Accu-Chek glucose monitor. Michelle stores the strips in the:
   A. Refrigerator
   B. Cupboard
   C. Freezer
   D. Fireproof safe

10. Michelle gets ready to run a glucose test on the Accu-Chek glucose monitor. She removes a test strip from the container and notices that it is discolored. Michelle should:
    A. Go ahead and run the test
    B. Run the test, but make a notation of the color change in the patient's chart
    C. Obtain a new container of test strips
    D. Ask the physician what should be done

Apply Your KNOWLEDGE—Cont'd

Serology

Choose the best answer to each of the following questions.

1. Stephanie Carter comes to the medical office for a prenatal examination. Dr. Donor has determined that Stephanie's blood type is O-negative and wants to a run a blood test to determine if there is an Rh incompatibility problem. Which of the following tests will Dr. Donor order for Stephanie?
   A. Cold agglutinins
   B. ABO and Rh blood typing
   C. Antistreptolysin O test
   D. Rh Antibody titer

2. Dr. Donor suspects that a patient has syphilis and decides to order a test to screen for this condition. Which of the following is a screening test for syphilis?
   A. RPR
   B. ARP
   C. STD
   D. ELISA

3. The results of the screening test for syphilis come back as weakly reactive. What is Dr. Donor most likely to do?
   A. Perform a TB test on the patient
   B. Make a final diagnosis of syphilis
   C. Order a more specific test to determine if the patient has syphilis
   D. Tell the patient that a weakly reactive test is nothing to worry about

4. Carl Blackburn comes to the office exhibiting the symptoms of infectious mononucleosis. All of the following are symptoms of this condition EXCEPT:
   A. Fatigue
   B. Fever and sore throat
   C. Swollen lymph nodes
   D. Jaundice

5. Dr. Donor asks Michelle Villers, CMA, to run a mono test on Carl. Michelle collects the following specimen to run this test:
   A. Urine specimen
   B. Blood specimen
   C. Throat specimen
   D. Stool specimen

6. Michelle runs a mono test, and the results are positive. Carl wants to know how he contracted mononucleosis. Which of the following would be the most appropriate response to give to Carl?
   A. Through saliva during oral contact such as kissing
   B. Through sexual intercourse
   C. Through contaminated food
   D. Through a spider bite

7. Joan Whitmore is 17 years old. Her high school is having a blood drive and she wants to donate blood. Which of the following is required before Joan can donate blood?
   A. Joan must have a GPA of at least 3.0
   B. Joan must weigh at least 120 pounds
   C. Joan must have a written parental consent
   D. Joan must have a hemoglobin level of at least 12.5 mg/dL

8. Which of the following would temporarily defer Joan from donating blood?
   A. A pulse rate of 82
   B. A recent MMR immunization
   C. Having pierced ears
   D. Being on her menstrual period

9. Joan is getting ready to donate blood and asks a Red Cross volunteer how much blood will be removed. The Red Cross volunteer responds by telling her:
   A. 1 liter
   B. 2 units
   C. 1 pint
   D. 1 gallon

10. Joan asks the Red Cross volunteer how long she must wait before donating blood again. The Red Cross volunteer responds by telling her:
    A. 1 week
    B. 8 weeks
    C. 6 months
    D. 1 year

CERTIFICATION REVIEW

❏ **Blood chemistry testing** involves the quantitative measurement of chemical substances in the blood. These chemicals are dissolved in the liquid portion of the blood; therefore most blood chemistry tests require a serum specimen for analysis. In the medical office, automated blood chemistry analyzers are often used to perform blood chemistry testing.

❏ **Quality control** consists of methods and means to ensure that the test results are reliable and valid.

❏ **Calibration** involves the use of a standard to check the precision of the blood chemistry analyzer. If an analyzer is not properly calibrated, it will be unable to produce accurate test results. A control consists of a sample of a known value. Normal controls fall within normal range, whereas abnormal controls fall outside normal range.

❏ **Cholesterol** is a white, waxy, fatlike substance that is essential for normal functioning of the body. Most of the cholesterol circulating in the blood is manufactured by the liver; a portion of it is dietary. Dietary cholesterol is found only in animal products.

❏ **High blood cholesterol** may cause fatty deposits, or plaque, to build up on the walls of the arteries, a condition known as atherosclerosis. LDL cholesterol is often referred to as "bad" cholesterol because an excess amount of it in the blood can cause atherosclerosis. HDL cholesterol removes excess cholesterol from the walls of the blood vessels and is protective and beneficial to the body.

❏ **Cholesterol test results** are interpreted as follows: Total cholesterol levels under 200 mg/dL are desirable. Levels between 200 and 239 mg/dL are borderline high, and levels of 240 mg/dL and above are high. An HDL cholesterol level above 60 mg/dL is optimal, and a level below 40 mg/dL is a risk factor for coronary heart disease.

❏ **Glucose** is the end product of carbohydrate metabolism; its function is to serve as the chief source of energy for the body. Glucose that is not needed for energy can be stored in the form of glycogen in muscle and liver tissue for later use. Insulin is a hormone secreted by the pancreas and is required for normal use of glucose in the body.

❏ **Measuring the glucose** in a blood specimen is one of the most common blood chemistry tests. It is used to detect abnormalities in carbohydrate metabolism, such as occur in diabetes mellitus, hypoglycemia, and liver and adrenocortical dysfunction.

❏ **Blood glucose** is usually measured when the patient is in a fasting state. This type of test is termed a fasting blood sugar (FBS). The patient should not have anything to eat or drink, except water, for 12 hours preceding the test. The normal range for a fasting blood sugar is 70 to 110 mg/dL. An FBS is often performed on patients with diabetes to evaluate their progress and regulate treatment, and as a routine screening procedure to detect diabetes mellitus.

❏ **The 2-hour postprandial blood sugar** (2-hour PPBS) test is used to screen for diabetes mellitus and to monitor the effects of insulin dosage in diagnosed diabetics. The glucose tolerance test (GTT) provides more detailed information about the ability of the body to metabolize glucose by assessing the insulin response to a glucose load. The GTT is used in the diagnosis of diabetes mellitus, hypoglycemia, and liver and adrenocortical dysfunction.

❏ **Serology** is the scientific study of the serum of the blood. Serologic tests include hepatitis tests, syphilis tests, mono test, rheumatoid factor, antistreptolysin O test, C-reactive protein, cold agglutinins, ABO and Rh blood typing, and Rh antibody titer.

❏ **Infectious mononucleosis** is an acute infectious disease caused by the Epstein-Barr virus (EBV). Symptoms include mental and physical fatigue, fever, sore throat, severe weakness, headache, and swollen lymph nodes.

❏ **Blood antigens** consist of protein and are inherited through genes. Within the ABO blood group system, there are four main blood types: A, B, AB, and O. Blood antibodies are proteins that are naturally present in the plasma of the blood. An antibody is a substance that is capable of combining with an antigen. When a blood antigen and its corresponding antibody unite, the result is the clumping, or agglutination, of red blood cells. Agglutination of red blood cells can be serious and even fatal if it occurs in the living body.

Terminology Review

Agglutination (as it pertains to blood)   Clumping of blood cells.

Antibody A substance that is capable of combining with an antigen, resulting in an antigen-antibody reaction.

Antigen A substance capable of stimulating the formation of antibodies.

Antiserum (pl. antisera) A serum that contains antibodies.

Blood antibody A protein present in the blood plasma that is capable of combining with its corresponding blood antigen to produce an antigen-antibody reaction.

Blood antigen A protein present on the surface of red blood cells that determines a person's blood type.

Donor One who furnishes something, such as blood, tissue, or organs, to be used in another person.

Gene A unit of heredity.

Glycogen The form in which carbohydrate is stored in the body.

HDL cholesterol A lipoprotein, consisting of protein and cholesterol, that removes excess cholesterol from the cells.

Hyperglycemia An abnormally high level of glucose in the blood.

Hypoglycemia An abnormally low level of glucose in the blood.

In vitro Occurring in glass. Refers to tests performed under artificial conditions, as in the laboratory.

In vivo Occurring in the living body or organism.

LDL cholesterol A lipoprotein, consisting of protein and cholesterol, that picks up cholesterol and delivers it to the cells.

Lipoprotein A complex molecule consisting of protein and a lipid fraction such as cholesterol. Lipoproteins function in transporting lipids in the blood.

Recipient One who receives something, such as a blood transfusion, from a donor.

ON THE WEB

For active weblinks to each website visit http://evolve.elsevier.com/Bonewit/.

For Information on Diabetes:

American Diabetes Association

Joslin Diabetes Center

National Diabetes Education Initiative

The National Institute of Diabetes

Microorganisms and Disease
1. List and explain the stages of an infectious disease.
2. List and describe the three classifications of bacteria based on shape.
3. Give examples of infectious diseases caused by the following types of cocci:
   - Staphylococci
   - Streptococci
   - Diplococci
4. State examples of infectious diseases caused by bacilli, spirilla, and viruses.

Microscope
1. Explain the function of the following parts of a compound microscope: base, arm, stage, light source, substage condenser, iris diaphragm, body tube, coarse adjustment, and fine adjustment.
2. Identify the function of the following microscope lenses: low-power, high-power, and oil-immersion.
3. List the guidelines for proper care of the microscope.

Use a microscope.
Properly handle and care for a microscope.

Microbiologic Specimen Collection
1. Explain the purpose of obtaining a specimen, and identify body areas from which a specimen can be taken for microbiologic examination.
2. List ways to prevent contamination of a specimen by extraneous microorganisms.
3. Explain the precautions a medical assistant should take to prevent infection from a pathogenic specimen.
4. Explain the purpose and describe the procedure for culturing a microbiologic specimen.

Collect a specimen for a throat culture.

Microbiologic Tests
1. Explain the importance of the early diagnosis of streptococcal pharyngitis.
2. Explain the purpose and describe the procedure for a sensitivity test.
3. Explain the purpose of microbiologic smear.
4. Explain the purpose of Gram staining.
5. Identify infectious diseases caused by gram-positive bacteria and gram-negative bacteria.
6. Give examples of methods to prevent and control infectious diseases in the community.

Perform a streptococcus test using a rapid strep test.
Perform a streptococcus test using the bacitracin susceptibility test.
Prepare a wet mount.
Prepare a microbiologic smear.

CHAPTER 20

Medical Microbiology

Chapter Outline

INTRODUCTION TO MICROBIOLOGY
The Normal Flora
Infection
  Stages of an Infectious Disease
Microorganisms and Disease
  Bacteria
  Viruses
Microscope
  Support System
  Optical System
  Care of the Microscope
Microbiologic Specimen Collection
  Handling and Transporting Microbiologic Specimens
  Collection and Transport Systems
Cultures
Streptococcus Testing
  Rapid Streptococcus Tests
  Hemolytic Reaction and Bacitracin Susceptibility Test
Sensitivity Testing
Microscopic Examination of Microorganisms
  Wet Mount Method
  Smears
  Gram Stain
Prevention and Control of Infectious Diseases

National Competencies

Clinical Competencies

Specimen Collection
- Obtain specimens for microbiologic testing.

Diagnostic Testing
- Perform microbiology testing.

Patient Care
- Screen and follow up test results.

General Competencies

Patient Instruction
- Provide instruction for health maintenance and disease prevention.

Organizational Functions
- Use methods of quality control.

Key Terms

bacilli (bah-SILL-ie)
cocci (KOK-sie)
colony (KOL-oe-nee)
contagious (kon-TAE-jus)
culture
culture medium
false negative
false positive
fastidious (fas-TID-ee-us)
immunization (im-yoo-ni-ZAY-shun)
incubate (IN-kyoo-bate)
incubation period
infectious disease
inoculate (in-NOK-yoo-late)
inoculum (in-NOK-yoo-lum)
microbiology (mie-kroe-bie-OL-oe-jee)
mucous membrane (MYOO-kus MEM-brain)
normal flora
prodromal period
prodrome (PROE-drome)
resistance
sequela (SEK-kwe-lah)
smear
specimen (SPESS-ih-men)
spirilla (spa-RILL-ah)
streaking
streptolysin (strep-toe-LIE-sin)
susceptible (suh-SEP-tih-bul)

Introduction to Microbiology

Microbiology is the scientific study of microorganisms and their activities. As described in Chapter 2 microorganisms are tiny living plants and animals that cannot be seen by the naked eye but must be viewed under a microscope. Anton van Leeuwenhoek (1632-1723) designed a magnifying glass strong enough for viewing microorganisms. He was the first individual to observe and describe protozoa and bacteria (Figure 20-1). Leeuwenhoek's magnifying glass was the precursor of the modern microscopes used today for studying microorganisms. A microscope allows the observer to see individual microbial cells and thereby to differentiate and identify microorganisms.

For the most part, microbiology deals with unicellular, or one-celled, microscopic organisms. All of the life processes necessary to sustain the microbe are performed by one cell. Among them are the ingestion of food substances and their use for energy, growth, reproduction, and excretion.

Microorganisms are *ubiquitous;* they are found almost everywhere—in the air, in food and water, in the soil, and in association with plants, animals, and human life. Although there are vast numbers of microorganisms, only a relatively small minority are pathogenic and able to cause disease.

When a pathogen infects a host, it often produces a set of symptoms peculiar to that disease. For example, scarlet fever is characterized by a sore throat, swelling of the

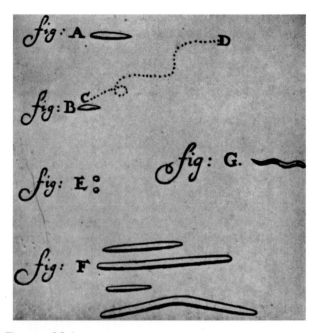

Figure 20-1. Bacteria drawn by van Leeuwenhoek in 1684. (From Fuerst R: *Frobisher and Fuerst's Microbiology in Health and Disease,* ed. 15. Philadelphia, Saunders, 1983.)

lymph nodes in the neck, a red and swollen tongue, and a bright red rash covering the body. These symptoms aid the physician in diagnosing the disease.

Microbiologic laboratory tests are also used to help the physician identify the pathogen causing the disease. Identification of the pathogen leads to the proper treatment of the disease. The medical assistant must be alert to all symptoms the patient describes and relay this information to the physician.

Although most microbiologic tests are performed in the hospital or the medical laboratory, the medical assistant is frequently responsible for the collection of specimens in the medical office. This chapter provides an introduction to the field of microbiology, including a description of techniques that are performed in the medical office. Before undertaking this study, the medical assistant should review Chapter 2, which discusses introductory concepts that are basic to this chapter.

The Normal Flora

Every individual has a *normal flora,* which consists of the harmless microorganisms that normally reside in many parts of the body but do not cause disease. The surface of the skin, the mucous membrane of the gastrointestinal tract, and parts of the respiratory and genitourinary tracts all have an abundant normal flora. Some microorganisms making up the normal flora are beneficial to the body, such as those contained in the intestinal tract that feed on other potentially harmful microscopic organisms. Other examples are those microorganisms found in the intestinal tract that synthesize vitamin K, an essential vitamin needed by the body for proper blood clotting. In rare instances, if the opportunity arises (such as lowered body resistance), certain microorganisms of the normal flora can become pathogenic and cause disease.

Infection

The invasion of the body by pathogenic microorganisms is known as *infection.* Under conditions favorable to the pathogens, they grow and multiply, resulting in an **infectious disease** that produces harmful effects on the host. However, not all pathogens that enter a host are able to cause disease. When a pathogen enters the body, it attempts to invade the tissues so it can grow and multiply. The body, in turn, tries to stop the invasion with its second line of natural defense mechanisms,* which includes inflammation, phagocytosis by white blood cells, and the production of antibodies. These defense mechanisms work to destroy the pathogen and remove it from the body. If the body is successful, the pathogens are destroyed and the individual suffers no adverse effects. If the pathogen is

---

*The first line of natural defense mechanisms, which work to *prevent* the entrance of pathogens into the body (e.g., coughing and sneezing), is described in Chapter 2.

able to overcome the body's natural defense mechanisms, an infectious disease results.

Many infectious diseases are **contagious,** meaning that the pathogen that causes the disease can be spread from one person to another either directly or indirectly. Frequently, *droplet infection* is the mode of transmission of pathogens. This is the inhalation of pathogens from a fine spray emitted by a person infected with the disease. When the infected individual exhales, as during breathing, talking, coughing, or sneezing, the pathogens are dispersed into the air on minute liquid particles. Therefore infected individuals should cover their mouths and noses while coughing or sneezing. See Figure 2-1 for examples of other means of pathogen transmission.

Stages of an Infectious Disease

Once a pathogen becomes established in the host, a series of events generally ensues. The stages of an infectious disease are:

1. The *infection* is the invasion and multiplication of pathogenic microorganisms in the body.
2. The *incubation period* is the interval of time between the invasion by a pathogenic microorganism and the appearance of the first symptoms of the disease. Depending on the type of disease, the incubation period may range from only a few days to several months. During this time, the pathogen is growing and multiplying.
3. The *prodromal period* is a short period in which the first symptoms that indicate an approaching disease occur. Headache and a feeling of illness are common prodromal symptoms.
4. The *acute period* is when the disease is at its peak and symptoms are fully developed. Fever is a common symptom of many infectious diseases.
5. The *decline period* is when the symptoms of the disease begin to subside.
6. The *convalescent period* is the stage in which the patient regains strength and returns to a state of good health.

Microorganisms and Disease

The groups of microorganisms known to contain species capable of causing human disease include bacteria, viruses, protozoa, fungi (including yeasts), and animal parasites. Bacteria and viruses are most frequently responsible for causing human diseases and are discussed next.

Bacteria

Bacteria are microscopic single-celled organisms. Of the 1700 species known to dwell in humans, only approximately 100 produce human disease. The discovery of antibiotics has helped immensely in combating and controlling bacterial infections. It must be remembered, however, that antibiotics are not effective against viral infections.

Bacteria can be classified according to their shape into three basic groups (Figure 20-2). Round bacteria are known as **cocci.** The cocci can be further categorized as diplococci,

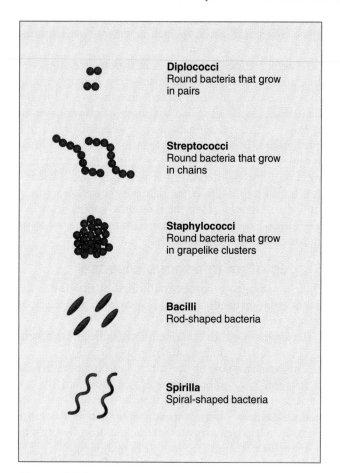

Diplococci
Round bacteria that grow
in pairs

Streptococci
Round bacteria that grow
in chains

Staphylococci
Round bacteria that grow
in grapelike clusters

Bacilli
Rod-shaped bacteria

Spirilla
Spiral-shaped bacteria

Figure 20-2. Classification of bacteria based on shape.

streptococci, or staphylococci, depending on their pattern
of growth. Rod-shaped bacteria are **bacilli.** Spiral and
curve-shaped bacteria are **spirilla,** and they include spiro-
chetes and vibrios.

Cocci

Staphylococci are round bacteria that grow in grapelike clusters (Figure 20-3, *A*). The species *Staphylococcus epidermidis*
is widely distributed and is normally present on the surface
of the skin and the mucous membranes of the mouth,
nose, throat, and intestines. *S. epidermidis* is usually nonpathogenic; however, a cut, abrasion, or other break in the
skin can allow invasion of the tissues by the organism, resulting in a mild infection.

Staphylococcus aureus is the species commonly associated
with pathologic conditions such as boils, carbuncles, pim-
ples, impetigo, abscesses, *Staphylococcus* food poisoning,
and wound infections. Infections caused by staphylococci
usually cause much pus formation (suppuration) and are
termed *pyogenic* infections.

Streptococci are round bacteria that grow in chains
(Figure 20-3, *B*). Before the advent of antibiotics, strep-
tococcal infections were a major cause of human death.
Diseases caused by streptococci include streptococcal

sore throat ("strep throat"), scarlet fever, rheumatic fever,
pneumonia, puerperal sepsis, erysipelas, and skin conditions such as carbuncles and impetigo.

Diplococci are round bacteria that grow in pairs.
Pneumonia, gonorrhea, and meningitis are infectious diseases caused by diplococci.

Bacilli

Bacilli are rod-shaped bacteria that are frequently found
in the soil and air (Figure 20-3, *C*). Some bacilli are able
to form spores, a characteristic that enables them to resist
adverse conditions such as heat and disinfectants.
Diseases caused by bacilli include botulism, tetanus, gas
gangrene, gastroenteritis produced by *Salmonella* food
poisoning, typhoid fever, pertussis (whooping cough),
bacillary dysentery, diphtheria, tuberculosis, leprosy, and
the plague.

Escherichia coli is a species of bacillus that is found
among the normal flora of the intestinal tract in enormous
numbers (Figure 20-3, *D*). It is normally a harmless bacterium; however, if it enters the urinary tract as a result of
lowered resistance or poor hygiene practices, or both, it
may cause a urinary tract infection.

Spirillia

Spirilla are spiral or curve-shaped bacteria. *Treponema pallidum,* a spirochete, is the causative agent of syphilis
(Figure 20-3, *E*). This microorganism cannot be grown in
commonly available culture media; therefore, the diagnosis of syphilis is generally made using serologic tests. A
serologic test is performed on the serum of the blood.
Cholera is caused by another type of spirillum, *Vibrio
cholerae.* Immunization and proper methods of sanitation
and water purification have all but eliminated cholera in
the United States.

Viruses

Viruses are the smallest living organisms. They are so small
that an electron microscope must be used to view them.
Viruses infect plants and animals as well as humans and

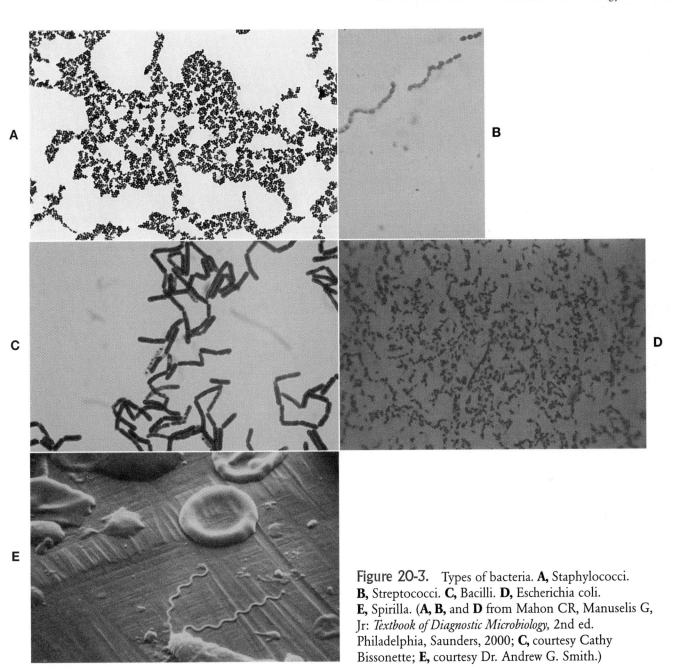

Figure 20-3. Types of bacteria. **A,** Staphylococci. **B,** Streptococci. **C,** Bacilli. **D,** Escherichia coli. **E,** Spirilla. (**A, B,** and **D** from Mahon CR, Manuselis G, Jr: *Textbook of Diagnostic Microbiology,* 2nd ed. Philadelphia, Saunders, 2000; **C,** courtesy Cathy Bissonette; **E,** courtesy Dr. Andrew G. Smith.)

use nutrients inside the host's cells for their metabolic and reproductive needs. Infectious diseases caused by viruses include influenza, chickenpox, rubeola (measles), rubella (German measles), mumps, poliomyelitis, smallpox, rabies, herpes simplex, herpes zoster, yellow fever, hepatitis, and the majority of infectious diseases of the upper respiratory tract, including the common cold.

Microscope

Many kinds of microscope are available, but the type used most often for office laboratory work is the *compound microscope.* The compound microscope consists of a two-lens system, and the magnification of one system is increased by the other. A source of bright light is required for proper illumination of the object to be viewed. This combination of lenses and light permits visualization of structures that cannot be seen with the unaided eye, such as microorganisms and cellular forms. The compound microscope consists of two main components: the support system and the optical system, which are discussed next. The medical assistant should be able to identify the parts of a microscope (Figure 20-4) and be able to properly use and care for it. Procedure 20-1 outlines the correct use and care of a microscope.

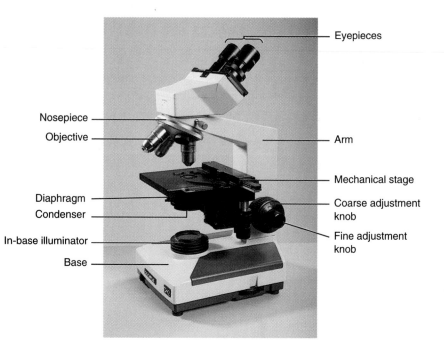

Figure 20-4. Parts of the microscope.

Support System

Frame

The working parts of the microscope are supported by a sturdy frame consisting of a *base* for support and an *arm* for carrying it without damaging the delicate parts. The arm is also needed to support the magnifying and adjusting systems.

Stage

The *stage* of a microscope is the flat, horizontal platform on which the microscope slide is placed. It is located directly over the condenser and beneath the objective lenses. The stage has a small round opening in the center that permits light from below to pass through the object being viewed and up into the lenses above. The slide should be placed on the stage; the object to be viewed is positioned over this opening so that it is satisfactorily illuminated by the light source below. Standard microscope stages have metal clips attached to the stage to hold the glass slide securely in place. With this type of stage, the slide must be moved by hand to examine various areas on it.

Other types of microscope have a *mechanical stage* that allows movement of the slide in a vertical or horizontal position by using adjustment knobs. The mechanical stage provides precise positioning of the slide, which is essential for performing certain procedures, such as differential white blood counts and inspection of Gram-stained smears.

Light Source

The light source is at the base of the microscope and consists of a built-in illuminator, along with a switch for turning it on and off. The light is directed to the condenser above it and then through the object to be viewed.

Condenser

Compound microscopes have a lens system between the light source and object, known as the *substage condenser*. A popular condenser is the *Abbé condenser*, which consists of two lenses used to illuminate objects with transmitted light. The condenser collects and concentrates the light rays and directs them up, bringing them to a focus on the object so that it is well illuminated.

Diaphragm

The amount of light focused on the object can also be controlled by the *iris diaphragm*, located beneath or inside the condenser. The diaphragm consists of a series of horizontally arranged interlocking plates with a central opening, or *aperture*. The iris diaphragm has a lever that is used to increase or decrease the amount of light admitted by increasing or decreasing the aperture.

Appropriate intensity of light is essential for properly viewing the specimens, especially at a higher magnification. A general rule is that as the desired magnification increases, the more intense the light must be. For example, increased light intensity is required for good visualization of a specimen with the oil-immersion objective. On the other hand, with the low-power objective, the light must be somewhat diminished to produce the appropriate contrast for specimen detail and to reduce glare. The degree of illumination is also influenced by the density of the object; therefore stained structures (e.g., a Gram-stained smear of bacteria) usually require more light than do unstained specimens.

Adjustment Knobs

Two adjustment knobs are used to bring the specimen into focus: the coarse adjustment knob and the fine adjustment knob. The *coarse adjustment* is used to obtain an approximate focus quickly. The *fine adjustment* is then used to obtain the precise focusing necessary to produce a sharp, clear image. On some microscope models, the adjustment knobs are mounted as two separate knobs; on others, they are placed together with the smaller fine adjustment knob extending from a larger coarse adjustment wheel.

Optical System

Compound microscopes have a two-lens magnification system. *Magnification* is defined as the ratio of the apparent size of an object viewed through the microscope to the actual size of the object.

The Eyepiece

The first lens system is the eyepiece, or ocular lens, located at the top of the body tube and marked 10×, meaning that it magnifies 10 times. Microscopes that have one eyepiece only are called *monocular* microscopes, and those with two eyepieces are called *binocular*. A binocular microscope is recommended for medical office laboratory work because it causes less eye fatigue than the monocular type. The binocular eyepieces can be adjusted to each individual by moving the eyepieces apart or together as needed.

Objective Lenses

The second lens system consists of three objective lenses located on the revolving *nosepiece,* each with a different degree of magnification. The metal shafts of the objective lenses differ in length and are identified by power of magnification. The short objective is known as the *low-power objective* and has a magnification of 10×. The *high-power objective* is also known as the high-dry objective because it does not require the use of immersion oil; it has a magnification of 40×. The *oil-immersion objective* has the highest power of magnification, which is 100×.

Some microscope manufacturers identify the objective lenses by colored rings. For example, green is used for low power, yellow for high power, and red or black for oil immersion. If the objective is not color coded, it can be identified by the length of the metal shaft; the low-power objective is the shortest, and the oil-immersion objective is the longest.

The objective lens magnifies the specimen, and the ocular lens magnifies the image produced by the objective lens. The *total magnification* of each objective is determined by multiplying the ocular magnification by the objective magnification. The total magnification of the low-power objective is 100 times the actual size of the object being viewed (10 × 10). The total magnification of the high-power objective is 400× (10 × 40), and the oil-immersion magnification is 1000× (10 × 100).

Focus

Depending on the type of microscope, there are two ways to focus on a specimen. Some microscopes are equipped with a *barrel focus*. With this type of microscope, the body tube (or barrel) moves while the stage remains stationary during focusing. Other microscopes focus on the specimen using *stage focus*. With this type of microscope, the stage moves while the body tube remains stationary during focusing.

Low and High Power

The low-power objective is used for the initial focusing and light adjustment of the microscope. The low-power objective is also used for the initial observation and scanning requirements needed for most microscopic work. For example, urine sediment is first examined using the low-power objective to scan the specimen for the presence of casts. The high-power objective is used for a more thorough study, such as observing cells in more detail. The *working distance,* defined as the distance between the tip of the lens and the slide, is short when using this objective. Because of this, care must be taken in focusing the high-power objective to prevent it from striking and breaking the slide or damaging the lens.

Most compound microscopes are *parfocal*. This means that once the specimen is focused with the low-power objective, the nosepiece can be rotated to the high-power objective and focused simply with the fine adjustment knob.

Oil Immersion

The oil-immersion objective provides the highest magnification and is used to view very small structures, such as microorganisms and blood cells. The oil-immersion objective has a very short working distance, and when it is in use, the lens nearly rests on the microscope slide itself. A special grade of oil, known as *immersion oil*, must be used with this lens. Oil has the advantage of not drying out when exposed to air for a long time. A drop of the oil is placed on the slide and resides between the oil-immersion objective and the slide. The oil provides a path for the light to travel on between the slide and the lens, and prevents the scattering of light rays, which, in turn, permits clear viewing of very small structures. The oil also improves the resolution of the objective lens, that is, its ability to provide sharp detail, which is particularly necessary at high magnifications. Procedures that require oil immersion include differential white blood cell counts and examination of Gram-stained smears.

Care of the Microscope

The microscope is a delicate instrument and must be handled carefully. These guidelines should be followed to care for the microscope properly:

1. Always carry the microscope with two hands. Place one hand firmly on the arm, and the other hand under the base for support. Place the microscope down gently to prevent jarring it, which could damage delicate parts.

2. Always handle the microscope in such a way that your fingers do not touch the lenses, to avoid leaving fingerprints on them. When using a microscope, avoid wearing mascara because it is difficult to remove from the ocular lens.

3. When it is not in use, keep the microscope covered with its plastic dust cover and stored in a case or cupboard. Store it with the nosepiece rotated to the low-power objective and as close as possible to the stage.

4. Periodically clean the microscope by washing the enameled surfaces with mild soap and water and drying them thoroughly with a soft cloth. Never use al-cohol on the enameled surfaces because it might remove the finish.

5. After each use, wipe the metal stage clean with gauze or tissue. If immersion oil comes in contact with the stage, remove it with a piece of gauze that is slightly moistened with xylene.

6. The ocular, objectives, and condenser consist of hand-ground optical lenses, which must be kept spotlessly clean by using clean, dry lens paper. Optical glass is softer than ordinary glass; therefore to prevent scratching the lens, do not use tissues or gauze. If the lenses are especially dirty, use a commercial lens cleaner or xylene in the cleaning process. Apply a small amount of cleaner to the lens paper, followed by thorough drying and polishing with a clean piece of lens paper.

7. Keep the light source free of dust, lint, and dirt by periodic polishing with lens paper.

8. A malfunctioning microscope should be repaired only by a qualified service person. Attempting to fix the microscope yourself may result in further damage.

PROCEDURE 20-1 Using the Microscope

Outcome Use a microscope.

Equipment/Supplies:

- Microscope
- Lens paper
- Specimen slide
- Tissue or gauze

- Immersion oil
- Xylene
- Soft cloth

These steps should be followed for proper use of the microscope:

1. Procedural Step. Clean the ocular and objective lenses with lens paper.

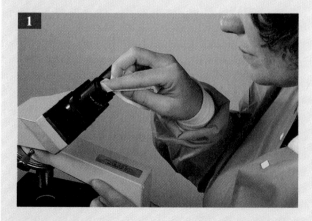

2. Procedural Step. Turn on the light source.

3. Procedural Step. Rotate the nosepiece to the low-power objective (10×), making sure to click it into place. Use the coarse adjustment knob to provide sufficient working space for placing the slide on the stage and to avoid damaging the objective lens as follows:

    a. Barrel focus: Raise the objective all the way up using the coarse adjustment knob.

    b. Stage focus: Lower the stage all the way down using the coarse adjustment knob.

4. Procedural Step. Place the slide on the stage specimen side up and make sure it is secure.

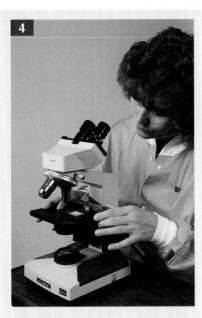

5. **Procedural Step.** Position the low-power objective until it almost touches the slide using the coarse adjustment knob. Be sure to observe this step to prevent the objective from striking the slide.

6. **Procedural Step.** Look through the ocular. If a monocular microscope is being used, keep both eyes open to prevent eyestrain. With a binocular microscope adjust the two oculars to the width between your eyes until a single circular field of vision is obtained.

7. **Procedural Step.** Bring the specimen into coarse focus as follows:

  a. Barrel focus: Slowly raise the objective using the coarse adjustment knob.

  b. Stage focus: Slowly lower the stage using the coarse adjustment knob.

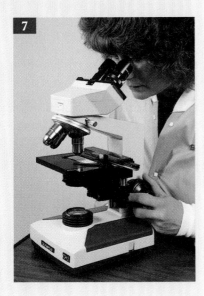

Observe the specimen through the ocular until comes into focus.

8. **Procedural Step.** Use the fine adjustment knob to bring the specimen into a sharp, clear focus.

9. **Procedural Step.** Adjust the light as needed, using the iris diaphragm to provide maximum focus and contrast.

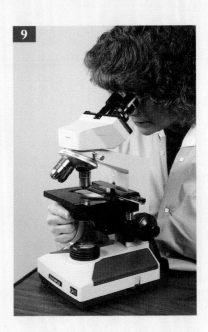

10. **Procedural Step.** Rotate the nosepiece to the high-power objective, making sure it clicks into place. Proper focusing with the low-power objective ensures that the objective does not hit the slide during this operation. Use the fine adjustment knob to bring the specimen into a precise focus. Do not use the coarse adjustment to focus the high-power objective in order to prevent the objective from moving too far and striking the slide.

11. **Procedural Step.** Examine the specimen as required by the test or procedure being performed.

12. **Procedural Step.** Turn off the light after use, and remove the slide from the stage.

13. **Procedural Step.** Clean the stage with a tissue or gauze.

14. **Procedural Step.** Properly care for and store the microscope.

Using the Oil Immersion Objective

Follow these steps for proper use of the oil-immersion objective.

1. **Procedural Step.** Rotate the nosepiece to the oil-immersion objective. Do not click it into place but move it to one side.

PROCEDURE 20-1

Continued

PROCEDURE 20-1 Using the Microscope—Cont'd

2. **Procedural Step.** Place a drop of immersion oil on the slide directly over the center opening in the stage.

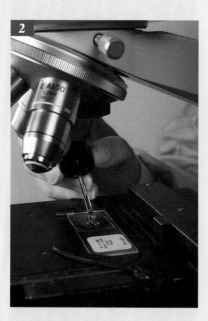

3. **Procedural Step.** Move the oil-immersion objective into place until a click is heard. Make sure that the objective does not touch the stage or slide.

4. **Procedural Step.** Using the coarse adjustment, slowly position the oil-immersion objective until the tip of the lens touches the oil but does not come in contact with the slide. A pop of light will be observed. Be sure to observe carefully this step of the procedure.

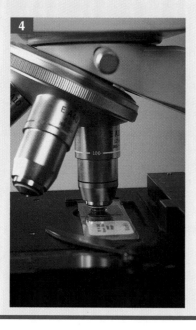

5. **Procedural Step.** Look through the eyepiece, and focus slowly using the coarse adjustment until the object is visible.

6. **Procedural Step.** Use the fine adjustment to bring the object into sharp focus to view fine details.

7. **Procedural Step.** Adjust the light as needed, using the iris diaphragm to provide maximum focus and contrast. Increased light intensity is required for good visualization of the specimen with the oil-immersion objective.

8. **Procedural Step.** Examine the specimen as required by the test or procedure being performed.

9. **Procedural Step.** Turn off the light after use. Remove the slide from the stage, being careful not to get oil on the high-power objective or the stage.

10. **Procedural Step.** Using a piece of clean, dry lens paper, gently clean the oil-immersion objective. The lens must be immediately cleaned after use to prevent oil from drying on the lens surface. In addition, the oil may seep into the lens and perhaps loosen it.

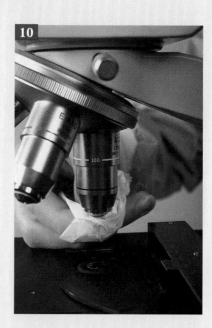

11. **Procedural Step.** Clean the oil from the slide by immersing it in xylene and wiping it off with a soft cloth.

Microbiologic Specimen Collection

If the physician suspects that a particular disease is caused by a pathogen, he or she may want to obtain a specimen for microbiologic examination. This will identify the pathogen causing the disease and aid in the diagnosis. For example, if a urinary tract infection is suspected, a urine specimen is obtained for bacterial examination. In this instance, a clean-catch midstream collection is required to obtain a specimen that excludes the normal flora of the urethra and urinary meatus.

A **specimen** is a small sample or part taken from the body to represent the whole. The medical assistant is often responsible for collecting specimens from certain areas of the body, such as the throat, nose, and wound. He or she may be responsible for assisting the physician in the collection of specimens from other areas, such as the eye, ear, cervix, vagina, urethra, and rectum. In most instances, a swab is used to collect the specimen. A *swab* is a small piece of cotton wrapped around the end of a slender wooden or plastic stick. It is passed across a body surface or opening to obtain a specimen for microbiologic analysis.

To prevent inaccurate test results, good techniques of medical and surgical asepsis must be practiced when a specimen is obtained. The medical assistant must be careful not to contaminate the specimen with *extraneous microorganisms*. These are undesirable microorganisms that can enter the specimen in various ways; they grow and multiply, and possibly obscure and prevent identification of pathogens that might be present. To prevent extraneous organisms from contaminating the specimen, all supplies used to obtain the specimen (e.g., swabs and specimen containers) must be sterile. In addition, the specimen should not contain microorganisms from areas surrounding the collection site. For example, when obtaining a throat specimen, the swab should not be allowed to touch the inside of the mouth.

The OSHA Bloodborne Pathogens Standards presented in Chapter 2 should be carefully followed when performing microbiologic procedures. Specifically, the medical assistant must wear gloves when it is reasonably anticipated that hand contact might occur with blood or other potentially infectious materials. Eating, drinking, smoking, and applying makeup are strictly forbidden when one is working with microorganisms because pathogens can be transmitted to the medical assistant through hand-to-mouth contact. In addition, labels for specimen containers should not be licked, and any break in the skin, such as a cut or scratch, must be covered with a bandage. If the medical assistant accidentally touches some of the material in the specimen, the area of contact should be washed immediately and thoroughly with soap and water. If the specimen comes in contact with the worktable, the table should be

cleaned immediately with soap and water followed by a suitable disinfectant, such as phenol. The worktable should also be cleaned with a disinfectant at the end of every day.

After collection, the specimen must be placed in its proper container with the lid securely fastened. The container must be clearly labeled with the patient's name, the date, the source of the specimen, the medical assistant's initials, and any other required information. Procedure 20-2 outlines the procedure for collecting a specimen for a throat culture.

Handling and Transporting Microbiologic Specimens

Once the specimen has been collected, care should be taken in handling and transporting it. Delay in processing the specimen may cause the death of pathogens or the overgrowth of the specimen by microorganisms that are part of the normal flora usually collected along with the pathogen from the specimen site. If the specimen is to be analyzed in the medical office, it should be examined under the microscope or cultured immediately. Otherwise it should be preserved (if possible) with the method used by the medical office.

Specimens transported to an outside medical laboratory by a courier service are usually placed in a transport medium. The transport medium prevents drying of the specimen and preserves it in its original state until it reaches its destination. An example of a commercially available transport medium is the Starswab II (Starplex Scientific).

Outside laboratories provide the medical office with specific instructions on the care and handling of specimens being transported to them. These specimens must be accompanied by a laboratory request that designates the physician's name and address; the patient's name, age, and gender; the date and time of collection; the type of microbiologic examination requested; the source of the specimen (e.g., throat, wound, urine); and the physician's clinical diagnosis. There is usually a space on the form to indicate whether the patient is receiving antibiotic therapy. Antibiotics may suppress the growth of bacteria, a factor that could produce false-negative results.

Wound Specimens

Wound specimens are collected using many of the techniques described previously. In many cases, two swabs are used to collect the specimen. The specimen is obtained by inserting the swab into the area of the wound that contains the most drainage and gently rotating the swab from side to side to allow it to completely absorb any microorganisms present. The swab is placed in the specimen container, and the process is repeated using a second swab. To obtain accurate and reliable test results it is important to collect a specimen from within the wound, rather than from the surface.

Collection and Transport Systems

Microbiologic collection and transport systems are available to facilitate the collection of a specimen to be transported to an outside laboratory for analysis; examples include Culturette (Beckton Dickinson) and the Starswab II (Starplex Scientific) (Figure 20-5). These systems consist of a sterile swab and a plastic tube that contains a transport medium. The tube comes packaged in a peel-apart envelope and should be stored at room temperature. The procedure for the use of a microbiologic collection and transport system is outlined next.

1. Complete a laboratory request form.
2. Sanitize your hands, and apply gloves.
3. Check the expiration date on the peel-apart envelope.
4. Peel open the envelope and remove the cap/swab unit. The cap is permanently attached to the sterile swab.
5. Using aseptic technique, collect the specimen. Do not allow the swab to touch any area other than the collection site.
6. Remove the cap from the collection tube and insert the swab.
7. Push the cap/swab in as far as it will go to completely immerse the swab in the transport medium. Make sure the cap is tightly in place.
8. Remove gloves and sanitize your hands.
9. Label the tube with the patient's name, the date, the source of the specimen (e.g., throat, wound), and your initials. Place the tube in a biohazard specimen transport bag. Place the laboratory request in the outside pocket of the bag.
10. Chart the procedure.
11. Transport the specimen to the laboratory within 24 hours.

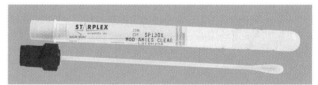

Figure 20-5. Starswab II Collection and Transport System.

PROCEDURE 20-2 Collecting a Specimen for a Throat Culture

Outcome Collect a specimen for a throat culture.

A specimen for a throat culture is obtained by using a sterile swab. It is commonly used to aid in the diagnosis of infections such as streptococcal sore throat, pharyngitis, and tonsillitis. Less frequently, it is used to diagnose whooping cough and diphtheria. These latter diseases are not prevalent today because of the availability of immunizations against them.

The following procedure outlines the steps necessary to obtain a throat specimen that will be used to perform a rapid streptococcus test, which is discussed later in the chapter.

Equipment/Supplies:
- Disposable gloves
- Tongue depressor
- Sterile swab
- Waste container

1. **Procedural Step.** Sanitize your hands and assemble the equipment.
2. **Procedural Step.** Greet and identify the patient. Introduce yourself, and explain the procedure.
3. **Procedural Step.** Position the patient, and adjust the light to provide clear visualization of the throat. *Principle.* The throat must be clearly visible so the medical assistant is able to determine the proper area for obtaining the specimen.
4. **Procedural Step.** Apply gloves. Remove the sterile swab from its peel-apart package, being careful not to contaminate it. *Principle.* Contamination of the swab may lead to inaccurate test results.

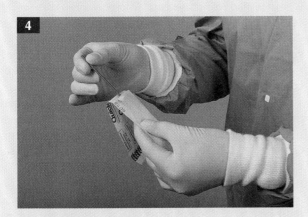

5. **Procedural Step.** Depress the tongue with the tongue depressor. *Principle.* The tongue depressor holds the tongue down and facilitates access to the throat.
6. **Procedural Step.** Place the swab at the back of the throat (posterior pharynx) and firmly rub it over any lesions or white or inflamed areas of the mucous membrane of the tonsillar area and posterior pharyngeal wall. Rotate the swab constantly as you collect the specimen, making sure there is good contact with the tonsillar area. Do not allow the

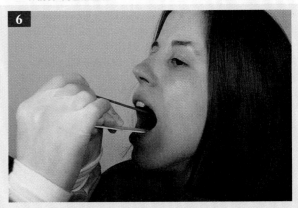

swab to touch any areas other than the throat such as the inside of the mouth. *Principle.* The swab should be rubbed over suspicious-looking areas where pathogens are likely to be found. A rotating motion is used to deposit the maximum amount of material possible on the swab. Touching it to any areas other than the throat contaminates the specimen with extraneous microorganisms.

7. **Procedural Step.** Keeping the patient's tongue depressed, withdraw the swab and remove the tongue depressor from the patient's mouth.
8. **Procedural Step.** Properly dispose of the tongue depressor in a regular waste container to prevent transmission of microorganisms.
9. **Procedural Step.** Process the swab according to the directions accompanying the rapid strep test.
10. **Procedural Step.** Remove gloves, and wash your hands. Chart the test results.

CHARTING EXAMPLE

Date	
7/12/05	10:30 a.m. Throat specimen collected.
	QuickVue Strep Test: Positive.
	N. Moorehead, CMA

PROCEDURE 20-2

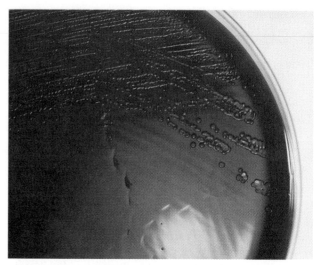

Figure 20-6. Streptococcal colonies growing on a blood agar culture medium contained in a Petri plate. (From Mahon CR, Manuselis G, Jr: *Textbook of Diagnostic Microbiology*, 2nd ed. Philadelphia, Saunders, 2000.)

Cultures

Once a microbiologic specimen is taken, it must be examined to determine the type of microorganisms present. Because most specimens generally contain only a small number of pathogens, it is often desirable to induce any pathogens that are present to grow and multiply.

Most microorganisms, especially bacteria, can be grown on a culture medium. A **culture medium** is a mixture of nutrients on which microorganisms are grown in the laboratory. The culture medium and the environment in which it is placed must contain the requirements to support and encourage the growth of the suspected pathogen. These growth requirements include the presence or the absence of oxygen (depending on the microorganism); proper nutrition, temperature, and pH; and moisture.

The culture medium may be solid or a liquid form. Blood agar is one of the most frequently used solid culture media. It is prepared by adding sheep's blood to a substance known as *agar,* which is transparent and colorless. Blood added to the agar provides nutrients that support the growth of a variety of bacteria. When heated, it melts and becomes a liquid. On cooling, agar solidifies, forming a firm surface on which microorganisms can be grown. A liquid culture medium is often referred to as a broth and is usually contained in a tube; an example is nutrient broth. Culture media must be stored in the refrigerator and then warmed to room temperature before use. A cold culture medium must not be used because the cold temperature results in the death of microorganisms placed on it.

A *Petri plate* is frequently used to hold solid culture medium. The plate consists of a shallow circular dish made of glass or clear plastic with a cover, the diameter of which is greater than that of the base. Microorganisms can be cultured on the surface of the medium in the plate (Figure 20-6). Petri plates allow examination of a culture while preventing microorganisms from entering or escaping. A **culture** is a mass of microorganisms growing in a laboratory culture medium.

Most medical offices use commercially prepared culture media in disposable plastic Petri plates. The plates come packaged in a plastic bag and must be stored in the refrigerator with the medium side facing upward. The plastic bag prevents the medium from drying out; storing the plates medium side upward prevents condensation on the medium surface. The plate has an expiration date that must be checked before using. Plates that are past the expiration date or are dried out or contaminated should not be used.

The solid culture medium in a Petri plate is inoculated by lightly rolling the swab containing the specimen over the surface of the medium; this process is known as **streaking.** The cover of the Petri plate should be removed only when the specimen is being spread on the culture medium. Unnecessary removal of the cover results in contamination of the medium with extraneous microorganisms. The culture is then incubated for 24 to 48 hours in conditions that encourage the growth of the suspected pathogen.

Most specimens taken for analysis contain a mixture of organisms because of the presence of normal flora in most parts of the body. When this is the case, the resulting culture is known as a *mixed culture,* or one that contains two or more types of microorganisms. To analyze most microbiologic specimens, the suspected pathogen must be separated from the mixed culture and permitted to grow alone. This establishes a *pure culture,* or a culture that contains only one type of microorganism. After the culture has grown sufficiently, the appropriate tests are performed to identify the pathogen.

It is not possible to grow viruses by this method; rather, they must be cultured on living tissue or identified using serologic tests.

Streptococcus Testing

The most common streptococcal condition is streptococcal sore throat (streptococcal pharyngitis), which primarily affects children and young adults. The causative agent of streptococcal pharyngitis is a group A beta-hemolytic streptococcus known as *Streptococcus pyogenes.* Streptococcal pharyngitis is a potentially serious condition because some patients develop a poststreptococcal sequela. A **sequela** is a morbid secondary condition that occurs as a result of a less serious primary infection. A small percentage of patients with streptococcal pharyngitis (primary infection) develop rheumatic fever; the rheumatic fever is considered a poststreptococcal sequela. Owing to the risk of sequela, early diagnosis and treatment of streptococcal pharyngitis is important. In the medical office, commercially available tests are often used for identification of group A beta-hemolytic streptococci. The most frequently used testing methods are presented next.

Rapid Streptococcus Tests

Rapid streptococcus tests directly detect group A streptococcus from a throat swab in a very short time. Most tests require only 4 to 10 minutes to process; therefore diagnosis can often be made and antibiotics prescribed, if necessary, before the patient leaves the office.

The most frequently used rapid streptococcus test is the direct antigen identification test, which confirms the presence of group A streptococcus through an antigen-antibody reaction. The test works by combining particles sensitized to the streptococcus antibody with the throat specimen. If group A streptococcal antigen is in the specimen, it combines with the antibody-sensitized particles to produce a color change that can be observed with the unaided eye. Rapid strep tests also include a control that determines if the test results are accurate and reliable.

The advantage of the direct antigen identification test is that it provides the physician with immediate test results rather than requiring an overnight culture. Specific instructions are included with every commercially available antigen identification test; examples of these tests include QTest Strep (Becton Dickinson), Clearview Strep A (Wampole Laboratories), and QuickVue In Line Strep A (Quidel) (Figure 20-7).

Hemolytic Reaction and Bacitracin Susceptibility Test

Streptococci are classified according to their hemolytic properties exhibited on a blood agar medium into three types: **alpha, beta,** and **gamma.** They are further divided according to their antigenic properties into 15 subgroups designated by the letters *A* through *O.* The hemolytic reaction and bacitracin susceptibility test is a biochemical culture test that relies on these hemolytic and antigenic properties of streptococci for the interpretation of the test results.

The testing procedure involves placing a filter paper disc impregnated with 0.04 U of bacitracin on the surface of a sheep-blood sugar agar medium previously inoculated with the throat specimen. The medium is then incubated for 18 to 24 hours to allow growth of the bacteria and to permit diffusion of the bacitracin into the culture medium surrounding the disc.

After the 18- to 24-hour incubation period, the plate is examined for its *hemolytic reaction.* As stated, the causative agent of streptococcal pharyngitis is a (group A) beta-hemolytic streptococcus. Beta-hemolytic streptococci produce and secrete **streptolysin,** an exotoxin that completely hemolyzes red blood cells; therefore, a clear, wide, colorless zone of hemolysis (with no intact red blood cells) around the bacterial colonies indicates their presence. On the other hand, a greenish halo around the colonies indicates the less pathogenic alpha-hemolytic streptococci. The generally nonpathogenic gamma-type streptococci do not cause a reaction on the blood agar medium.

If the hemolytic property exhibited is of the beta type, the area around the bacitracin disc is next inspected for *bacitracin susceptibility.* Group A streptococci are susceptible or sensitive to bacitracin, whereas groups B, C, and G (which are also beta-hemolytic) are resistant to the bacitracin. If group A streptococcus is present, a clear zone of inhibition appears around the disc (Figure 20-8, *A*). Because groups B, C, and G are resistant to the bacitracin, the bacteria grow right up to the edge of the disc; that is, there is no zone of inhibition (Figure 20-8, *B*).

Therefore hemolysis of the blood agar surrounding the bacterial colonies combined with any zone of inhibition around the bacitracin disc is considered presumptive positive for group A beta-hemolytic streptococci. The test is considered presumptive because a small percentage of bacterial strains included in groups B, C, and G are sensitive to bacitracin; therefore a fraction (less than 5%) of the test results will be false positive. A **false positive** is a test result indicating that a condition is present when, in fact, it is not.

The bacitracin disc test is a convenient, reliable, and cost-effective method used in the medical office to determine the presence of streptococcal pharyngitis. However, since the development of the rapid streptococcus tests, it is not used as frequently as it once was.

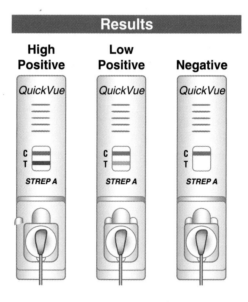

Figure 20-7. Procedure for performing the QuickVue In-Line One-Step Strep A test. (Courtesy Quidel Corporation, San Diego, California.)

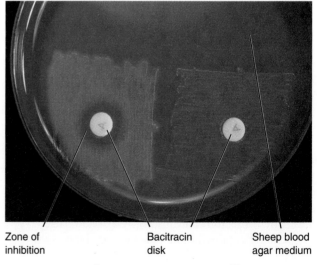

Figure 20-8. Hemolytic reaction and bacitracin susceptibility test. **A,** A positive reaction for Group A beta-hemolytic streptococcus, as evidenced by a clear zone of inhibition present around the bacitracin disc. **B,** A negative reaction as evidenced by the bacteria growing right up to the edge of the disc. (From Mahon CR, Manuselis G, Jr: *Textbook of Diagnostic Microbiology,* 2nd ed. Philadelphia, Saunders, 2000.)

Zone of inhibition

Bacitracin disk

Sheep blood agar medium

A   B

Strep Throat

Answer questions patients have about strep throat.

What is strep throat?

Strep throat is a contagious and acute infection that is medically known as streptococcal pharyngitis. It is caused by a bacterium known as group A streptococcus. Strep throat is transmitted directly from one person to another through droplets of saliva or nasal secretions. It most frequently occurs in children between the ages of 5 and 10 years and during the months of October through April. Strep infections are different from most other infectious diseases because having one strep infection does not prevent the development of another at a future date.

What are the symptoms of strep throat?

The symptoms of strep throat are a sore throat with severe pain on swallowing, a bright red pharynx (called beefy red pharynx), fever, white patches on the tonsils, swollen glands in the neck, muscular aches and pains, and a feeling of tiredness.

How is strep throat diagnosed and treated?

Strep throat is diagnosed by taking a throat specimen and running a laboratory test on it to determine whether group A streptococcus is present. Strep throat is usually treated by antibiotics taken orally for 10 days. It is important to take all the antibiotic prescribed by the physician to prevent complications that can occur from strep throat. The patient with strep throat should also rest in bed and avoid contact with others to prevent spreading it.

What are the complications of strep throat?

Severe complications can result from strep throat if it is not adequately treated. These include rheumatic fever and glomerulonephritis, which is a kidney disorder. Fortunately, these complications do not occur very often since most patients seek early treatment for strep infections.

- Encourage the patient to complete the entire prescribed course of antibiotics.
- Instruct the patient to notify the physician if new symptoms develop.
- Provide the patient with educational materials about strep throat.

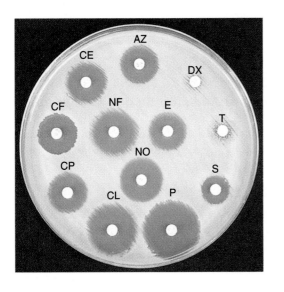

AZ:	Azithromycin
CE:	Cephalothin
CF:	Ciprofloxacin
CP:	Ciprozil
CL:	Clarithromycin
DX:	Doxycycline
E:	Erythromycin
NF:	Nitrofurantoin
NO:	Norfloxacin
P:	Penicillin
S:	Sulfisoxazole
T:	Tetracycline

Figure 20-9.   Sensitivity testing. (From Mahon CR, Manuselis G, Jr: *Textbook of Diagnostic Microbiology,* 2nd ed. Philadelphia, Saunders, 2000.)

Sensitivity Testing

The physician may request not only that the laboratory identify the infecting pathogen but also that a sensitivity test be performed on it to determine the best antibiotic to treat the condition. The test is always performed on a pure rather than a mixed culture. A sensitivity test determines the susceptibility of pathogenic bacteria to various antibiotics; therefore only the growth of the infectious pathogen is desired on the culture.

The most common method for sensitivity testing is the *disc-diffusion method* (Figure 20-9). Commercially prepared discs impregnated with known concentrations of various antibiotics are dropped on the surface of a solid culture medium in a Petri plate inoculated with the pathogen. The culture is then incubated, allowing the antibiotics to diffuse into the culture medium. If the pathogen is susceptible or sensitive to an antibiotic, there is a clear zone without bacterial growth around the disc. This indicates that

Case Study 3

John Seimer calls the medical office. He says that he is not a patient at the office, but would like some assistance. He says that for the past 3 days he has had a headache, fever, chills, and aching muscles. He says that a week ago he pulled a tick off his lower leg, and several days later found a red rash around the tick bite. He says that he went on the Internet and looked up his symptoms and he's sure that he has Lyme disease. The Internet site recommended taking doxycycline for 3 weeks to treat Lyme disease. John says that he doesn't like to go to the doctor and hasn't been to see a doctor for over 10 years. He wants to know if the physician could call in a prescription for doxycycline for him. He says that he has health insurance and the physician could bill him for an appointment, just as long as he doesn't have to come in.

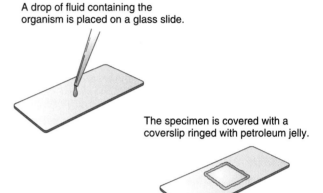

A drop of fluid containing the organism is placed on a glass slide.

The specimen is covered with a coverslip ringed with petroleum jelly.

Figure 20-10. Wet mount method of slide preparation for examining microorganisms in the living state.

the antibiotic was effective in destroying the pathogen. If the pathogen is unaffected by or resistant to the antibiotic, there is not clear zone around the disc, indicating that the antibiotic was unable to kill the pathogen.

Sensitivity testing enables the physician to decide which antibiotics will most likely be effective against the infectious disease in question.

Microscopic Examination of Microorganisms

Microorganisms can be examined under a microscope in the fixed state or in the living state. Examination in the fixed state involves the preparation of a smear through heat fixation, followed by a staining process such as Gram's stain, which is discussed later in this chapter. Most microorganisms are examined in the fixed state because it is easier to examine them when they are stained.

Some microorganisms require examination in the living state, however, owing to special circumstances such as their ability to be readily stained or difficulty in culturing them. The living state also allows visualization of the movement of motile microorganisms. This is espe-

cially helpful in the identification of certain motile microorganisms such as *Trichomonas vaginalis*. To observe the motility of a microorganisms, it must first be suspended in a liquid medium so that it is free to move about.

The most common method of examining microorganisms in the living state is the wet mount method, which is described next.

Wet Mount Method

In the wet mount method, a drop of fluid containing the organism is placed on a glass slide, which is covered with a coverslip (Figure 20-10). The coverslip may be ringed with petroleum jelly to provide a seal between the slide and coverslip. The purpose is to reduce the rate of evaporation through air currents that lead to drying and possible death of the specimen.

The slide is then placed under the microscope for examination, using the high-power objective. For satisfactory visualization, the intensity of the light must be diminished by partially closing the diaphragm of the microscope. The slide and coverslip should then be properly disposed of in a biohazard sharps container.

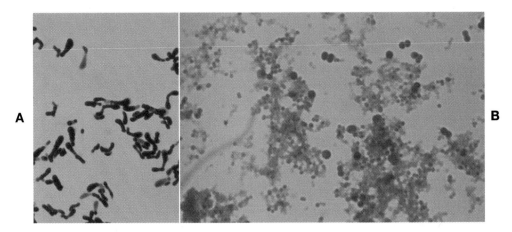

Figure 20-11. Gram-positive and gram-negative bacteria. **A,** Diphtheria is caused by a gram-positive bacillus; **B,** gonorrhea is caused by a gram-negative diplococcus. (**A,** Courtesy Cathy Bissonette; **B,** From Mahon CR, Manuselis G, Jr: *Textbook of Diagnostic Microbiology,* 2nd ed. Philadelphia, Saunders, 2000.)

Smears

A smear consists of material spread on a slide for microscopic examination. It can be prepared directly from the specimen collected on the swab, or the specimen can first be grown on a culture medium and a smear then prepared. Most smears must be stained before they can be viewed under the microscope, using one of a number of staining techniques. Smears are often helpful when time is a factor, because a smear can be prepared immediately from the specimen. This procedure gives the physician a preliminary clue to the causative agent while other, more time-consuming tests are being performed. Procedure 20-3 outlines the method to prepare a microbiologic smear.

The Gram Stain

Gram staining is often used in combination with other tests to help in the diagnosis and treatment of infectious diseases. Bacteria contained in a smear are colorless and usually difficult to identify under the microscope unless some type of staining is used. Staining them allows the observer to view directly the size, shape, and growth patterns of the bacteria.

A very common staining method is the Gram stain. In 1883, Christian Gram, a Danish physician, discovered a way to differentiate bacteria on the basis of their color reactions to various stains. Gram staining is based on the fact that when treated with crystal violet dye, certain bacteria permanently retain this dye after undergoing a decolorization process. These bacteria exhibit a purple color when viewed under the microscope and are known as **gram-positive** bacteria (Figure 20-11, *A*). Other bacteria are unable to retain this dye after being decolorized and become colorless. They must be counterstained with a red dye to become visible under the microscope. These bacteria exhibit a pink or red color and are known as **gram-negative** bacteria (Figure 20-11, *B*). These staining characteristics are due to differences in the chemical composition of the bacterial cell walls.

Gram staining allows for the division of most bacteria into two large groups; gram positive and gram negative. Some of the infectious diseases caused by gram-positive bacteria are streptococcal sore throat, scarlet fever, rheumatic fever, diphtheria, lobar pneumonia, tetanus, and botulism. Infectious diseases caused by gram-negative bacteria include whooping cough, gonorrhea, meningitis, bacillary dysentery, cholera, typhoid fever, and the plague.

Bacteria undergoing Gram staining are also observed for their characteristic shape and fall into one of the following categories: gram-positive rods, gram-negative rods, gram-positive cocci, or gram-negative cocci. For example, the causative agent of gonorrhea is a gram-negative diplococcus.

Prevention and Control of Infectious Diseases

Individuals in the community can help prevent and control infectious diseases by practicing good techniques of medical asepsis, by obtaining proper nutrition and rest, and by using good hygienic measures. In addition, infected individuals should contact their physicians in an effort to ensure early diagnosis and treatment of the disease. Immunizations are available to prevent a wide range of infectious diseases. The medical assistant has a responsibility to help educate community members about practices that reduce the transmission of pathogens and help control and prevent infectious diseases.

PROCEDURE 20-3 Preparing a Smear

Outcome Prepare a microbiology smear.

Equipment/Supplies:
- Disposable gloves
- Bunsen burner
- Clean glass slide
- Microbiologic specimen
- Slide forceps
- Sterile swab
- Biohazard waste container

1. **Procedural Step.** Sanitize your hands.
2. **Procedural Step.** Assemble the equipment. Label the slide with the patient's name and the date.
3. **Procedural Step.** Apply gloves. Hold the edges of the slide between your thumb and index finger. Starting at the right side and using a rolling motion, gently and evenly spread the material from the specimen over the slide. The material should cover approximately one-half to two-thirds of the slide. Do not rub the material vigorously over the slide. Properly dispose of the contaminated swab in a biohazard waste container.

   Principle. The specimen may contain pathogens that are capable of infecting the medical assistant; therefore, it is important to don gloves. A rolling motion is used to deposit the maximum amount of material possible on the slide. Rubbing may disintegrate the cellular structures making up the microorganisms in the specimen.

4. **Procedural Step.** Allow the smear to air dry in a flat position for at least 30 minutes. Heat should not be applied at this time.

   Principle. Air drying allows the bacterial cells to dry slowly. Applying heat at this stage would burst the bacterial cells resulting in an inappropriate smear.

5. **Procedural Step.** Holding the slide with the slide forceps heat fix the smear by quickly passing the slide back and forth (approximately three times) through the flame of a Bunsen burner. The slide has been fixed properly if the back of the slide feels uncomfortable (but not too hot) when touched to the back of your hand. Excessive heat should be avoided. Allow the slide to cool completely. An alternative to heat fixing the slide is to apply ethyl alcohol to the slide and allow it to air dry.

   Principle. Heat fixing the slide kills the microorganisms and attaches them firmly to the slide so they do not wash off during the staining process. An excessive amount of heat could result in distortion of the bacterial cells.

6. **Procedural Step.** Prepare the slide for examination under the microscope. Inform the physician that the slide is ready for examination.

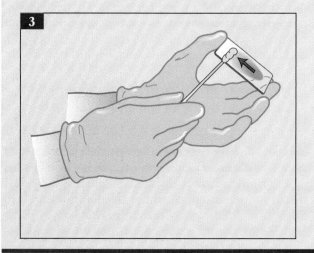

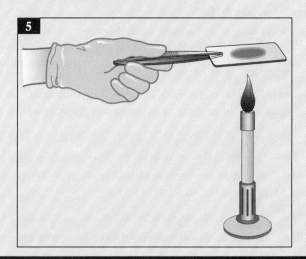

MEDICAL Practice and the LAW

This chapter deals with the collection and identification of microorganisms that cause infections. You must maintain standard precautions whenever handling potentially infectious material to protect yourself, your coworkers, and your patients. Microbiology is an exact science—one stray microorganism can contaminate the entire specimen. Sanitize hands thoroughly, and apply new gloves between handling specimens to avoid cross-contamination. If specimen contamination occurs, immediately discard it and collect a new one. Be precise in your labeling—a mislabeled specimen can cause unnecessary concern and or treatment for the patient.

Maintain confidentiality of information—certain infectious diseases must be reported to the Centers for Disease Control and Prevention (CDC) or local board of health. Otherwise, do not give information to anyone else but the patient or legal guardian.

What Would You DO?
What Would You *Not* DO? *RESPONSES*

Case Study 1
What Did Natalie Do?

❑ Told Paula that it's important that the physician find out whether Caitlin has strep throat because strep can sometimes develop into a more serious infection. Explained that if Caitlin does have strep throat, the physician would want to prescribe the best antibiotic to treat the infection.

❑ Talked with Caitlin about the reason for the test. Explained that it will help the physician find the best way to treat her so that she starts feeling better as soon as possible.

❑ Reassured Caitlin that the procedure would be very quick and it would be over before she knew it.

❑ Told Caitlin that after the specimen was obtained, she could choose a prize from the treasure box.

What Did Natalie Not Do?

❑ Did not force the collection swab into Caitlin's mouth.

What Would You Do?/What Would You *Not* Do? Review Natalie's response and place a checkmark next to the information you included in your response. List additional information you included in your response below.

_____
_____
_____
_____

Case Study 2
What Did Natalie Do?

❑ Told Hollie that mononucleosis is usually transmitted by kissing, but it can sometimes be transmitted by coughs and sneezes from an infected person.

❑ Sympathized with Hollie and told her that it probably *feels* like she is going to die, but she should start to feel better as her body starts to fight off the disease.

❑ Explained to Hollie that mononucleosis is caused by a virus and that antibiotics don't work against viruses.

❑ Told Hollie to try drinking cold fluids or sucking on a Popsicle until she feels more like eating.

What Did Natalie Not Do?

❑ Did not ignore or minimize Hollie's concerns.

What Would You Do?/What Would You *Not* Do? Review Natalie's response and place a checkmark next to the information you included in your response. List additional information you included in your response below.

_____
_____
_____
_____

Case Study 3
What Did Natalie Do?

❑ Empathized with John and told him that a lot of people don't like coming to see the doctor. Told him that the physician could not legally or ethically prescribe medication for him without seeing him.

❑ Told John that the office could not bill him for an appointment that he did not have.

❑ Asked John if he wanted to make an appointment to see the doctor.

What Did Natalie Not Do?

❑ Did not tell John he shouldn't be diagnosing himself with information he found on the Internet.

What Would You Do?/What Would You *Not* Do? Review Natalie's response and place a checkmark next to the information you included in your response. List additional information you included in your response below.

_____
_____
_____
_____

Apply Your KNOWLEDGE

Choose the best answer for each of the following questions.

1. Martha Keplar brings her daughter Megan, age 6, to the office. Megan has had a fever and sore throat for the past 24 hours. Dr. Petri suspects that Megan has strep throat. The type of pathogen that causes strep throat is a:
   A. Bacteria
   B. Virus
   C. Parasite
   D. Fungus

2. Dr. Petri asks Natalie Moorehead, CMA, to collect a throat specimen from Megan and run a rapid strep test. Natalie removes the sterile swab from its peel-apart package. All of the following would result in contamination of the swab with extraneous microorganisms EXCEPT:
   A. Allowing the swab to touch Megan's tongue
   B. Letting the tip of the swab touch the outside of the peel-apart package
   C. Rubbing the swab over Megan's tonsils
   D. Allowing the swab to touch Natalie's clean gloves

3. Natalie collects the throat specimen from Megan by:
   A. Adjusting the light so that the throat is clearly visible.
   B. Firmly rubbing the swab over any inflamed areas
   C. Rubbing the swab over any lesions
   D. Rotating the swab constantly while collecting the specimen
   E. All of the above

4. After collecting the specimen, Natalie properly discards her gloves in:
   A. The regular waste container
   B. A biohazard sharps container
   C. A biohazard waste container
   D. A recycling bin

5. Emily Bresser comes to the office complaining of pain and burning when she urinates. Dr. Petri suspects that Emily has a urinary tract infection. He asks Natalie Moorehead, CMA, to set up for a microscopic examination of Emily's urine sediment. Natalie prepares the microscope by:
   A. Cleaning the ocular and objective lenses with lens paper
   B. Rotating the nosepiece to the high-power objective
   C. Applying oil to the low-power objective
   D. Wiping off the surface of the microscope with xylene

6. Natalie places the urine sediment slide on the microscope. The next step that should be taken is to:
   A. Call the physician in to focus the slide
   B. Position the low-power objective until it almost touches the slide
   C. Focus the slide under the high-power objective
   D. Apply a drop of oil to the slide

7. Natalie begins focusing the slide under the microscope. While looking through the ocular of the monocular microscope, Natalie should:
   A. Keep both eyes open
   B. Close the eye that is not being used to view the specimen
   C. Blink frequently to keep her eyes moist
   D. Squint as much as possible to improve her vision

8. Natalie brings the slide into an initial focus using the coarse adjustment. To bring the slide into a sharp clear focus, Natalie uses the:
   A. Diaphragm adjustment know
   B. Mechanical stage adjustment knobs
   C. Revolving nosepiece
   D. Fine adjustment knob

9. Natalie next focuses the urine sediment under the high-power objective. This objective has a total magnification of:
   A. 100×
   B. 200×
   C. 400×
   D. 1000×

10. Dr. Petri examines Emily's urine sediment under the microscope. After he is finished, Natalie properly cares for the microscope. All of the following are correct techniques to use EXCEPT:
    A. Carrying the microscope with two hands
    B. Storing the microscope with the nosepiece rotated to the high-power objective
    C. Cleaning the enameled surfaces of the microscope with soap and water
    D. Cleaning the lenses of the microscope with lens paper

CERTIFICATION REVIEW

- ❑ **Microbiology** is the scientific study of microorganisms and their activities. Each individual has a normal flora, which consists of the harmless, nonpathogenic microorganisms that normally reside in many parts of the body but do not cause disease.

- ❑ **The invasion of the body** by pathogenic microorganisms is known as infection. Many infectious diseases are contagious, meaning that the pathogen causing the disease can be spread from one person to another either directly or indirectly. Frequently, droplet infection is the mode of transmission of pathogens.

- ❑ **The incubation period** is the interval of time between the invasion by a pathogenic microorganism and the appearance of the first symptoms of the disease. The prodromal period is when the first symptoms of a disease occur. The acute period is when the disease is at its peak and the symptoms are fully developed. The decline period is when the symptoms of the disease begin to subside. The convalescent period is the stage in which the patient regains strength and returns to health.

- ❑ **Bacteria** can be classified into three basic groups, according to their shape. Staphylococci are round bacteria that grow in grapelike clusters. Streptococci are round bacteria that grow in chains. Diplococci are round bacteria that grow in pairs. Bacilli are rod-shaped bacteria that are frequently found in the soil and air. Spirilla are spiral and curve-shaped bacteria. Viruses are the smallest living organisms, and an electron microscope must be used to view them.

- ❑ **A compound microscope** is used for office laboratory work. It contains three objective lenses. The low-power objective has a magnification of 10× and is used for the initial observation and scanning requirements needed for most microscopic work. The high-power objective has a magnification of 40× and is used for a more thorough study. The oil-immersion objective has the highest power of magnification, which is 100×.

- ❑ **A specimen** is a small sample taken from the body to represent the nature of the whole. Throat specimens are frequently collected in the medical office to aid in the diagnosis of streptococcal sore throat. Specimens can also be collected from wounds, the eye, ear, cervix, vagina, urethra, and rectum.

- ❑ **A culture medium** is a mixture of nutrients on which microorganisms are grown in the laboratory. A culture is a mass of microorganisms growing in a laboratory culture medium. A mixed culture contains two or more different types of microorganisms. A pure culture contains only one type of microorganism.

- ❑ **The most common streptococcal condition** is streptococcal sore throat. A sequela is a morbid secondary condition that occurs as a result of a less serious primary infection. A small percentage of patients with streptococcal pharyngitis develop rheumatic fever; rheumatic fever is considered a poststreptococcal sequela.

- ❑ **A sensitivity test** determines the best antibiotic to treat a condition caused by a pathogenic bacterium. A sensitivity test must be performed on a pure culture.

- ❑ **Microorganisms** can be examined under a microscope in the fixed state or in the living state. Examination in the fixed state involves the preparation of a smear followed by a staining process such as Gram's stain. A smear consists of material spread on a slide for microscopic examination. The wet mount method is used to examine microorganisms in the living state.

- ❑ **Gram staining** is used to differentiate bacteria on the basis of their color reactions to various stains. Bacteria exhibiting a purple color when they are viewed under the microscope are known as gram-positive bacteria. Bacteria exhibiting a pink or red color are known as gram-negative bacteria.

Terminology Review

bacilli (singular, bacillus) Bacteria that have a rod shape

cocci (singular, coccus) Bacteria that have a round shape

colony A mass of bacteria growing on a solid culture medium that have arisen from the multiplication of a single bacterium.

contagious Capable of being transmitted directly or indirectly from one person to another.

culture The propagation of a mass of microorganisms in a laboratory culture medium.

culture medium A mixture of nutrients on which microorganisms are grown in the laboratory.

false negative A test result denoting that a condition is absent when, in actuality, it is present.

false positive A test result denoting that a condition is present when, in actuality, it is absent.

fastidious Extremely delicate, difficult to culture, therefore involving specialized growth requirements.

immunization The process of becoming protected from a disease through vaccination.

incubate In microbiology, the act of placing a culture in a chamber (incubator), which provides optimal growth requirements for the multiplication of the organisms, such as the proper temperature, humidity, and darkness.

incubation period The interval of time between the invasion by a pathogenic microorganism and the appearance of first symptoms of the disease.

infectious disease A disease caused by a pathogen that produces harmful effects on its host.

inoculate To introduce microorganisms into a culture medium for growth and multiplication.

microbiology The scientific study of microorganisms and their activities.

mucous membrane A membrane lining body passages or cavities that open to the outside.

normal flora Harmless, nonpathogenic microorganisms that normally reside in many parts of the body but do not cause disease.

resistance The natural ability of an organism to remain unaffected by harmful substances in its environment.

sequela A morbid (secondary) condition occurring as a result of a less serious primary infection.

smear Material spread on a slide for microscope examination.

specimen A small sample or part taken from the body to show the nature of the whole.

spirilla (singular, spirillum) Bacteria that have a spiral or curved shape.

streaking In microbiology, the process of inoculating a culture to provide for the growth of colonies on the surface of a solid medium. Streaking is accomplished by skimming a wire inoculating loop that contains the specimen across the surface of the medium, using a back and forth motion.

streptolysin An exotoxin produced by beta-hemolytic streptococci, which completely hemolyzes red blood cells.

susceptible Easily affected, lacking resistance

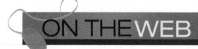

For active weblinks to each website visit http://evolve. elsevier.com/Bonewit/.

For Information on Disease and Infection Control:

American Society for Microbiology

Association for Professionals in Infection Control and Epidemiology

Centers for Disease Control and Prevention

World Health Organization (WHO)

Outbreak

Infection Control Today

Infectious Diseases Society of America (IDSA)

National Multiple Sclerosis Society

Cystic Fibrosis Foundation (CFF)

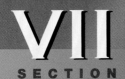

Emergency Medical Procedures

21 Emergency Medical Procedures

Learning Objectives	Procedures

First Aid

1. State the purpose of first aid.
2. Explain the purpose of the emergency medical services (EMS) system.
3. List the OSHA Standards for administering first aid.
4. List the guidelines that should be followed when providing emergency care.

Respond to common emergency situations.

Common Emergency Situations

1. List and describe conditions that cause respiratory distress.
2. List the symptoms of a heart attack and a stroke.
3. Explain the causes the following types of shock: cardiogenic, neurogenic, anaphylactic, and psychogenic.
4. Identify and describe the three classifications of external bleeding.
5. Explain the difference between an open wound and a closed wound.
6. Describe the characteristics of the following fractures: impacted, greenstick, transverse, oblique, comminuted, and spiral.
7. Identify the characteristics of the following burns: superficial, partial thickness, and full thickness.
8. Explain the difference between a partial seizure and a generalized seizure.
9. List examples of the following types of poisoning: ingested, inhaled, absorbed, and injected.
10. Identify factors that place an individual at higher risk for developing heat- and cold-related injuries.
11. Describe the difference between type 1 and type 2 diabetes mellitus.
12. Explain the causes of insulin shock and diabetic coma.
13. Identify the symptoms and describe the emergency care for the following conditions: respiratory distress, heart attack, stroke, shock, bleeding, wounds, musculoskeletal injuries, burns, seizures, poisoning, heat and cold exposure, and diabetic emergencies.

CHAPTER 21

Emergency Medical Procedures

Chapter Outline

INTRODUCTION TO EMERGENCY MEDICAL PROCEDURES
The Office Crash Cart
Emergency Medical Services System
First Aid Kit
OSHA Safety Precautions
Guidelines for Providing Emergency Care
Respiratory Distress
Heart Attack
Stroke
Shock
Bleeding
Wounds
Musculoskeletal Injuries
Burns
Seizures
Poisoning
Heat and Cold Exposure
Diabetic Emergencies

National Competencies

General Competencies
Communication
- Recognize and respond to verbal communications.
- Recognize and respond to nonverbal communications.

Introduction to Emergency Medical Procedures

Medical emergencies often arise both in and outside of the workplace that can result in the sudden loss of life or permanent disability. If an emergency situation occurs in the medical office, the physician provides immediate medical care for the patient. Some medical offices maintain a crash cart for this purpose, which is discussed next. In these situations, the medical assistant may be required to assist the physician in providing the emergency medical care.

The medical assistant may need to administer first aid for medical emergencies that occur outside of the medical office environment. **First aid** is defined as the immediate care administered to an individual who is injured or suddenly becomes ill before complete medical care can be obtained. The medical assistant is most likely to administer first aid to a family member or friend. The purpose of first aid is to save a life, reduce pain and suffering, prevent further injury, reduce the incidence of permanent disability, and increase the opportunity for an early recovery.

This chapter focuses on common emergency situations that the medical assistant may encounter and the first aid required for each. It is not intended, however, as a substitute for thorough first aid instruction through the American Red Cross, National Safety Council, or the American Heart Association.

The Office Crash Cart

A **crash cart** is a specially equipped cart for holding and transporting medications, equipment, and supplies needed to perform life-saving procedures in an emergency. A growing number of physicians are incorporating crash carts into their medical offices. Patients who are injured or suddenly become ill might be brought to the medical office for emergency medical care. In addition, a patient might develop a sudden illness at the medical office that requires emergency medical care. Examples of these situations include life-threatening cardiac arrhythmias, shock, cardiac arrest, poisoning, and traumatic injury.

The items on an office crash cart vary widely among medical offices depending on the extent of the emergency medical care that is likely to be administered. This, in turn, is directly related to the time it takes for emergency medical personnel to arrive and the location of the nearest hospital. Table 21-1 provides a general list of the medications, equipment, and supplies that may be included on an office crash cart. The medical assistant may be responsible for regularly checking the crash cart to replenish supplies and to check the expiration dates on medications.

Text continued on p. 788

TABLE 21-1	The Office Crash Cart	
Name	**Drug Category**	**Emergency Use**
MEDICATIONS USED IN CARDIOVASCULAR EMERGENCIES		
Epinephrine (Adrenalin)	Sympathomimetic*	Helps restore cardiac rhythm in cardiac arrest
Sodium bicarbonate	Alkalinizing agent	To correct metabolic acidosis after a cardiac arrest
Lidocaine (Xylocaine)	Antiarrhythmic	For rapid control of acute ventricular arrhythmias following a myocardial infarction
Bretylium tosylate	Antiarrhythmic	For treatment of ventricular fibrillation or ventricular tachycardia that fails to respond to lidocaine
Procainamide (Pronestyl)	Antiarrhythmic	An alternative drug when lidocaine fails to suppress ventricular arrhythmias
Atropine	Parasympatholytic**	For treating bradycardia associated with hypotension
Isoproterenol (Isuprel)	Sympathomimetic	To increase the heart rate in bradycardia that fails to respond to atropine
Dopamine (Intropin)	Sympathomimetic	One of the most common agents for treatment of hypotension associated with cardiogenic shock
Dobutamine (Dobutrex)	Sympathomimetic	To manage congestive heart failure when an increase in heart rate is not desired
Nitroprusside (Nitropress)	Antihypertensive-vasodilator	For immediate reduction of blood pressure in hypertensive crisis and cardiogenic shock
Norepinephrine (Levophed)	Sympathomimetic	To increase blood pressure in cardiogenic shock and other hypotensive emergencies
Adenosine (Adenocard)	Antiarrhythmic	To manage complex paroxysmal supraventricular tachycardia
Verapamil (Calan, Isoptin)	Antiarrhythmic	For treatment of supraventricular tachycardia that fails to respond to adenosine
Furosemide (Lasix)	Diuretic	For treatment of congestive heart failure and acute pulmonary edema
Nitroglycerin (Nitrostat)	Coronary vasodilator	For treatment of chest pain associated with both angina pectoris and acute myocardial infarction
IV SOLUTIONS		
Dextrose, 5% (D5W)	Glucose	A solution of 5% glucose in water used to replace fluid and nutrients
Isotonic saline	Electrolyte	A solution of sodium chloride in purified water used to replace lost fluid, sodium, and chloride
Lactated Ringer's solution	Electrolyte	A sterile solution of sodium chloride, potassium chloride, and calcium chloride in purified waters, used to replace fluids and electrolytes
MEDICATIONS USED IN BREATHING EMERGENCIES		
Epinephrine (Adrenalin)	Sympathomimetic	For symptomatic relief in acute attacks of bronchial asthma or bronchospasm associated with chronic bronchitis and emphysema
Terbutaline (Brethine)	Sympathomimetic	For symptomatic relief of bronchial asthma and reversible bronchospasm associated with bronchitis and emphysema
Aminophylline	Bronchodilator	For symptomatic relief in acute attacks of bronchial asthma or reversible bronchospasm associated with chronic bronchitis and emphysema
Albuterol (Proventil, Ventolin)	Sympathomimetic	For symptomatic relief of bronchial asthma and reversible bronchospasm associated with chronic bronchitis and emphysem

* A drug that stimulates the sympathetic nervous system; also called an adrenergic.
** A drug that inhibits the action of the parasympathetic nervous system; also called an anticholinergic.

Continued

TABLE 21-1	The Office Crash Cart—cont'd	
Name	**Drug Category**	**Emergency Use**

MEDICATIONS USED IN ANAPHYLACTIC REACTIONS

Epinephrine (Adrenalin)	Sympathomimetic	For treatment of hypersensitivity reactions caused by medications, allergens, or insect stings
Diphenhydramine (Benadryl)	Antihistamine	To counteract histamine in the treatment of hypersensitivity reactions
Methylprednisolone (Solu-Medrol)	Glucocorticoid	For severe anaphylactic reactions when epinephrine does not effect a satisfactory response

MEDICATIONS USED FOR POISONING

Ipecac syrup	Emetic	To induce vomiting of ingested poisons
Activated charcoal	Antidote, adsorbent	Used as a general purpose antidote to adsorb swallowed poisons; to decrease the absorption of the poison or drug by binding with any unabsorbed drug from the digestive tract
Naloxone (Narcan)	Narcotic antagonist	For the treatment of overdoses caused by narcotics or synthetic narcotic agents

MEDICATIONS USED IN NEUROLOGIC EMERGENCIES

Diazepam (Valium)	Anticonvulsant, antianxiety	For the treatment of convulsions in major motor seizures, status epilepticus, and acute anxiety states
Phenytoin (Dilantin)	Anticonvulsant	For controlling status epilepticus; for management of generalized tonic-clonic seizures, complex partial seizures, and critical focal seizures
Phenobarbital	Anticonvulsant, sedative/hypnotic	For management of generalized tonic-clonic seizures and partial seizures, and in the control of acute convulsive episodes (status epilepticus, febrile seizures)

MEDICATIONS USED IN METABOLIC EMERGENCIES

Glucose (e.g., orange juice)	Glucose	To provide glucose for conscious patients with hypoglycemia
Dextrose, 50%	Glucose	To provide glucose for unconscious patients with hypoglycemia

EQUIPMENT AND SUPPLIES

Cardiac Equipment
Defibrillator
Defibrillator pads

IV Equipment
Tourniquet
Surgical tape
IV catheters
IV cannulas
IV tubing and needles
Armboard
IV cut-down tray
Scalpel

---

* A drug that stimulates the sympathetic nervous system; also called an adrenergic.
** A drug that inhibits the action of the parasympathetic nervous system; also called an anticholinergic.

TABLE 21-1	The Office Crash Cart—cont'd	
Name	**Drug Category**	**Emergency Use**
Curved and straight hemostats		
Needle holder		
Tissue forceps		
Small scissors		
Local anesthetic		
Gauze squares		
Airway Equipment		
Suction equipment		
Suction pumps		
Suction tubing		
Suction catheters		
Oral and nasal airways		
Oxygen equipment		
Oxygen		
Oxygen face mask		
Nasal cannula		
Oxygen tubing		
Laryngoscope handle and blades		
Endotracheal tubes		
Lubricant		
Miscellaneous Supplies		
Sterile gloves		
Clean gloves		
Biohazard containers		
Syringes (assorted sizes)		
Needles (assorted sizes)		
Filter needles		
Tubex syringe		
Alcohol swabs		
Betadine swabs		
Sterile dressings		
Roller gauze (various widths)		
Adhesive tape		
Band-Aids		
Bandage scissors		
Local anesthetic (Xylocaine)		
Lidocaine ointment		
Lidocaine spray		
Lubricant		
Tongue blades		
Flashlight		
Cold packs		
Sphygmomanometer		
Stethoscope		

Emergency Medical Services System

The **emergency medical services (EMS) system** is a network of community resources, equipment, and medical personnel that provides emergency care to victims of injury or sudden illness. An *emergency medical technician-basic (EMT-B)* is a professional provider of prehospital emergency care, which includes care both at the scene and during transportation to the hospital. An EMT-B has received formal training and is certified to provide basic life support measures. An *EMT-Paramedic (EMT-P)* is qualified to provide advanced life support care, including advanced airway maintenance, starting intravenous drips, administration of medication, cardiac monitoring and interpretation, and cardiac defibrillation.

Activating the emergency medical services is often the most important step in an emergency. The rapid arrival of emergency medical technicians increases the patient's chances of surviving a life-threatening emergency. In the majority of urban and in some rural areas in the United States, the medical assistant can activate the local emergency medical services by dialing 911 on the telephone. Other areas have a local seven-digit number, in which case it is important to keep the number at hand.

When calling local emergency medical services, the medical assistant will speak with an *emergency medical dispatcher (EMD)*. An EMD has had formal training in handling emergency situations over the phone. The responsibility of the EMD is to answer the emergency call, listen to the caller, obtain critical information, determine what help is needed, and send the appropriate personnel and equipment. The EMD is also responsible for relaying instructions to the caller about providing emergency care until the emergency medical technicians arrive.

These guidelines should be followed when calling the emergency medical services:

- Speak clearly and calmly to the EMD. Identify the problem as accurately and concisely as possible so that proper equipment and personnel will be sent. The EMD needs to know the number of victims, the condition of the victim or victims, and the emergency care that has already been administered.
- The EMD will ask you for your phone number and address. In responding, be sure to relay the exact location of the victim to the dispatcher, including the correct street name and house number, and (if applicable) the building name, the floor, and the room number. With the 911 enhanced emergency system, the address automatically appears on a monitor; however, there is a chance that the address will not show up on the monitor. In addition, the emergency may not be in the same location as the caller. If possible, have someone meet the ambulance personnel and direct them to the scene.
- Do not hang up until the EMD gives you permission to do so. The dispatcher may need additional information

or may give you instructions on treating the patient until emergency medical technicians arrive.

First Aid Kit

It is important that the medical assistant acquire and maintain a first aid kit. A first aid kit contains basic supplies to provide emergency care to individuals who have been injured or become suddenly ill (Figure 21-1). It is recommended that a first aid kit be kept both at home and in the car.

First aid kits are available at most drug stores. It is also possible to make your own. Along with the items shown in Figure 21-1, the first aid kit should include the phone numbers of the local emergency medical service, the poison control center, and the police and fire departments. It is important to check the first aid kit regularly and replace supplies as needed.

OSHA Safety Precautions

To avoid exposure to bloodborne pathogens and other potentially infectious materials, the OSHA Bloodborne Pathogens Standards presented in Chapter 2 should be followed when performing first aid. The following guidelines help reduce or eliminate the risk of infection:

1. Make sure that your first aid kit contains personal protective equipment such as gloves, a face shield and mask, and a pocket mask.
2. Wear gloves when it is reasonably anticipated that your hand will come into contact with the following: blood and other potentially infectious materials, mucous membranes, nonintact skin, and contaminated articles or surfaces.
3. Perform all first aid procedures involving blood or other potentially infectious materials in a manner that minimizes splashing, spraying, spattering, and generation of droplets of these substances.
4. Wear protective clothing and gloves to cover cuts or other lesions of the skin.
5. Sanitize your hands as soon as possible after removing gloves.
6. Avoid touching objects that may be contaminated with blood or other potentially infectious materials.
7. If your hands or other skin surfaces come in contact with blood or other potentially infectious materials, wash the area as soon as possible with soap and water.
8. If your mucous membranes (in eyes, nose, and mouth) come in contact with blood or other potentially infectious materials, flush them with water as soon as possible.
9. Avoid eating, drinking, and touching your mouth, eyes, and nose while providing emergency care or before you sanitize your hands.
10. If you are exposed to blood or other potentially infectious materials, report the incident as soon as possible to your physician so that postexposure procedures can be instituted.

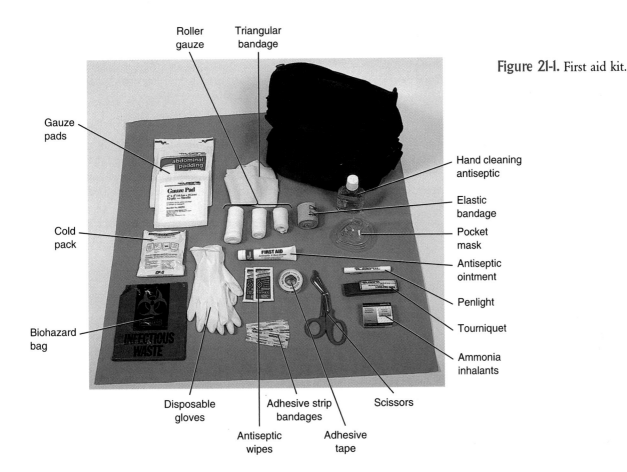

Roller gauze

Triangular bandage

Gauze pads

Cold pack

Biohazard bag

Disposable gloves

Antiseptic wipes

Adhesive strip bandages

Adhesive tape

Scissors

Hand cleaning antiseptic

Elastic bandage

Pocket mask

Antiseptic ointment

Penlight

Tourniquet

Ammonia inhalants

Figure 21-1. First aid kit.

Guidelines for Providing Emergency Care

The remainder of this chapter presents specific emergency situations that may be encountered by the medical assistant and the emergency care for each. The following guidelines should be followed when providing emergency care:

1. Remain calm, and speak in a normal tone of voice. These measures help calm and reassure the patient.

2. Make sure that the scene is safe before approaching the patient. It is important that you protect yourself from harm in an emergency situation.

3. Before administering emergency care to a conscious patient, you must first have permission or consent. To obtain consent, you must inform the patient who you are, your level of training, and what you are going to do to help. *Never* administer care to a conscious patient who refuses it. When a life-threatening condition exists and the patient is unconscious or otherwise unable to give consent, consent is assumed or implied. Under law, it is implied that if the patient could give consent to care, he or she would.

4. Follow the OSHA Standards when providing emergency care to reduce or eliminate exposure to bloodborne pathogens or other potentially infectious materials.

Highlight on Good Samaritan Laws

In most states, Good Samaritan laws have been enacted to provide immunity to individuals, such as the medical assistant, who administer first aid at the scene of an emergency. These laws were enacted to encourage individuals to help others in an emergency. They assume that an individual would do her or his best to save a life or prevent further injury.

The legal immunity provided by Good Samaritan laws protects an individual from being sued and found financially responsible for a patient's injury. The individual is immune from liability (except for "gross negligence") if he or she acts in good faith and uses a reasonable level of skill that does not exceed the scope of the individual's training.

Good Samaritan laws do not mean that an individual *cannot* be sued for administering first aid. An individual is *not* protected from liability if he or she is grossly careless or reckless in handling the situation. Because the components of Good Samaritan laws vary from state to state, the medical assistant must become familiar with the laws that govern his or her state.

5. Know how to activate your local emergency medical services (EMS) system. Activating the EMS is often the most important step you can take to help a patient who has experienced an injury or sudden illness.

6. Do not move the patient unnecessarily. Unnecessary movement can result in further injury or even be life-threatening to a patient with a serious condition.
7. Obtain information as to what happened from the patient, family members, coworkers, bystanders, and so on.
8. Look for a medical alert tag on the patient's wrist or neck. A medical alert tag provides information on a medical condition the patient may have.
9. Continue caring for the patient until more highly trained personnel arrive. On the arrival of emergency medical personnel or a physician, relay the condition in which you found the patient and the emergency care that has been administered.

Respiratory Distress

Respiratory distress indicates that the patient is breathing but is having great difficulty in doing so. Respiratory distress may sometimes lead to respiratory arrest. It is therefore important that the medical assistant be alert for the signs and symptoms of respiratory distress. These signs and symptoms may include noisy breathing, such as gasping for air, or rasping, gurgling, or whistling sounds; breathing that is unusually fast or slow; and breathing that is painful. The general care for respiratory distress is to place the patient in a comfortable position that facilitates breathing. Most patients prefer a sitting or semi-reclining position. Remain calm, and reassure the patient to help reduce anxiety. Calming the patient may help the patient breathe easier. If the patient's condition worsens or does not resolve within a few minutes, activate the local emergency medical services.

Examples of conditions frequently causing respiratory distress are described next.

Asthma

Asthma is a condition characterized by wheezing, coughing, and dyspnea. During an asthmatic attack, the bronchioles constrict and become clogged with mucus, which accounts for many of the symptoms of asthma.

Asthma may occur at any age, but it is more common in children and young adults. If the condition is not treated, it can lead to serious complications such as permanent lung damage. It is frequently, but not always, associated with a family history of allergies. Any of the common allergens, such as house dust, pollens, molds, or animal danders, may trigger an asthmatic attack. Asthmatic attacks also may be caused by nonspecific factors such as air pollutants, tobacco smoke, chemical fumes, vigorous exercise, respiratory infections, exposure to cold, and emotional stress. Normally, an individual with asthma easily controls attacks with medications. These medications stop the muscle spasms and open the airway, making breathing easier.

Some patients may develop a severe prolonged asthma attack that is life-threatening, which is known as **status asthmaticus.** These patients can move only a small amount of air. Because so little air is being moved, the typical breathing sounds associated with asthma may not be audible. The patient may have a bluish discoloration of the skin and extremely labored breathing. Status asthmaticus is a true emergency and requires immediate transportation of the patient to an emergency care facility by the fastest way possible.

Emphysema

Emphysema is a progressive lung disorder in which the terminal bronchioles that lead into the alveoli become plugged with mucus. Because of this problem, the alveoli become damaged, resulting in less surface area to diffuse oxygen into the blood. Eventually, this condition results in a loss of elasticity of the alveoli, causing inhaled air to become trapped in the lungs. This makes breathing difficult, particularly during exhalation.

Emphysema usually develops over many years and is found most frequently in heavy smokers. It also occurs in patients with chronic bronchitis and in elderly patients whose lungs have lost their natural elasticity.

Chronic emphysema is one of the major causes of death in the United States. As the lungs progressively become less efficient, breathing becomes more and more difficult. Patients with advanced cases may go into respiratory or cardiac arrest.

Hyperventilation

Hyperventilation literally means "overbreathing." Hyperventilation is a manner of breathing in which the respirations become rapid and deep, causing an individual to exhale too much carbon dioxide. In fact, the low carbon dioxide levels in the body account for many of the symptoms of hyperventilation.

Hyperventilation is often the result of fear or anxiety and is more likely to occur in people who are tense and nervous. It is also caused by serious organic conditions such as diabetic coma, pneumonia, pulmonary edema, pulmonary embolism, head injuries, high fever, and aspirin poisoning.

In addition to rapid and deep respirations, the signs and symptoms of hyperventilation include dizziness, faintness, light-headedness, visual disturbances, chest pain, tachycardia, palpitations, fullness in the throat, and numbness and tingling of the fingers, toes, and the area around the mouth. Despite their rapid breathing efforts, patients complain that they cannot get enough air. They often think they are having a heart attack.

Treatment for hyperventilation caused by emotional factors is as follows: Calm and reassure the patient, and encourage him or her to slow the respirations, thereby allowing the carbon dioxide level to return to normal. In the past, breathing into a paper bag was advocated as a remedy for hyperventilation. Recent studies no longer recommend this practice because it could be harmful if an underlying medical condition exists or if the patient is not actually hyperventilating. If the medical assistant suspects that hyperventilation has been caused by an organic problem, the emergency medical services should be activated immediately.

Heart Attack

A heart attack, also known as a myocardial infarction (MI), is caused by partial or complete obstruction of one or both of the coronary arteries or their branches. In most cases, the severity of the attack depends on the size of the obstructed artery and the amount of myocardial tissue nourished by that artery. For example, if a small branch of a coronary artery is obstructed, the myocardial damage and symptoms may be mild, whereas the damage is usually extensive and the symptoms intense if a coronary artery is completely blocked.

The principal symptom of a heart attack is chest pain or discomfort. The chest pain is described by patients as squeezing or crushing pressure, severe indigestion or burning, heaviness, or aching. The chest discomfort can range in severity from feeling only mildly uncomfortable to being intense and accompanied by a feeling of suffocation and doom. The pain is usually felt behind the sternum and may radiate to the neck, throat, jaw, both shoulders, and arms. The pain associated with a heart attack is prolonged and is usually not relieved by resting or taking nitroglycerin. Other signs and symptoms of a heart attack include shortness of breath, profuse perspiration, nausea, and fainting.

If the medical assistant suspects that the patient is having a heart attack, EMS should be activated immediately. Meanwhile, loosen tight clothing and have the patient rest in a comfortable position that facilitates breathing. If cardiac arrest occurs, the medical assistant should begin CPR immediately.

Stroke

A stroke, also called a cerebrovascular accident (CVA), results when an artery to the brain is blocked or ruptures, causing an interruption of the blood flow to the brain.

The signs and symptoms of a stroke include sudden weakness or numbness of the face, arm, or leg on one side of the body; difficulty in speaking; dimmed vision or loss of vision in one eye; double vision; dizziness; confusion; severe headache; and loss of consciousness.

If the medical assistant suspects that the patient is having a stroke, EMS should be activated immediately. Meanwhile, loosen tight clothing and have the patient rest in a comfortable position. If respiratory arrest or cardiac arrest or both occur, begin rescue breathing or CPR, or both, as required.

Shock

For the body to function properly, adequate blood flow must be maintained to all the vital organs. This is accomplished by the three important cardiovascular functions:
- Adequate pumping action of the heart,
- Sufficient blood circulating in the blood vessels, and
- Blood vessels being able to respond to blood flow.

When an individual suffers a severe injury or illness, one or more of these cardiovascular functions may be affected, which can lead to shock.

Shock is defined as the failure of the cardiovascular system to deliver enough blood to all the body's vital organs. Shock accompanies different types of emergency situation such as: hemorrhaging, a myocardial infarction, and severe allergic reaction.

The five major types of shock are categorized according to cause: hypovolemic, cardiogenic, neurogenic, anaphylactic, and psychogenic. Each type of shock is described in this section. If not treated, most types of shock become life threatening. This is because shock is progressive; once it reaches a certain point, it becomes irreversible and the patient's life cannot be saved.

The signs and symptoms of shock are caused by the failure of the vital organs to receive enough oxygen and nutrients. The organs most affected are the heart, brain, and lungs, which can be irreparably damaged in just 4 to 6 minutes. The general signs and symptoms of shock are weakness, restlessness, anxiety, disorientation, pallor, cold and clammy skin, rapid breathing, and rapid pulse.

If not treated, these symptoms can rapidly progress to a significant drop in the blood pressure, cyanosis, loss of consciousness, and death. It is important to know that the signs and symptoms of shock may be subtle or pronounced. In addition, no single sign or symptom will determine accurately the presence or severity of the shock. Because of this, it is extremely important to consider the nature of the illness or injury in determining whether the patient is a possible victim of shock. For example, if a patient suffers a traumatic injury to the abdomen, shock should be considered a possibility, even if the patient's signs and symptoms do not suggest shock.

Shock (with the exception of psychogenic shock) requires immediate medical care. The medical assistant should activate the emergency medical services without delay so that proper medical care can be obtained as soon as possible.

Hypovolemic Shock

Hypovolemic shock is caused by a loss of blood or other body fluids. Conditions that result in this type of shock include external and internal hemorrhaging, plasma loss from severe burns, and severe dehydration from vomiting, diarrhea, or profuse perspiration. The first priority of hypovolemic shock is to control bleeding. The patient in hypovolemic shock must have the volume of fluid that was lost replaced and therefore must be transported to an emergency care facility immediately.

Cardiogenic Shock

Cardiogenic shock is caused by the failure of the heart to pump blood adequately to all the body's vital organs. This type of shock occurs when the heart has been injured or damaged. Cardiogenic shock is most frequently seen with myocardial infarction. Other causes include arrhythmias, severe congestive heart failure, acute valvular damage, and pulmonary embolism. Once a patient develops cardiogenic shock, it is very difficult to reverse and, therefore, has a high fatality rate (80% to 90%).

Neurogenic Shock

Neurogenic shock occurs when the nervous system is unable to control the diameter of the blood vessels. In normal situations, the nervous system instructs the blood vessels to constrict or dilate, which controls blood pressure. In neurogenic shock, that control is lost and the blood vessels dilate, causing the blood to pool in peripheral areas of the body away from vital organs.

This type of shock is most often seen with brain and spinal injuries. The blood vessels become dilated, and there is not enough blood in the circulatory system to fill the dilated vessels, causing the blood pressure to drop significantly.

Anaphylactic Shock

Anaphylactic shock is a life-threatening reaction of the body to a substance to which an individual is highly allergic. Allergens that are most apt to result in anaphylaxis are drugs (e.g., penicillin), insect venoms, foods, and allergen extracts used in hyposensitization injections.

An anaphylactic reaction causes the release of large amounts of histamine, resulting in dilation of the blood vessels throughout the entire body and a drop in the blood pressure. The symptoms of anaphylactic shock begin with sneezing, hives, itching, angioedema, erythema, and disorientation and progress to difficulty in breathing, dizziness, faintness, and loss of consciousness. Medical care should be obtained immediately because most fatalities occur within the first 2 hours.

The emergency care for anaphylactic shock is the administration of epinephrine. Because time is a factor, individuals known to have a severe allergy carry an anaphylactic emergency treatment kit that contains injectable epinephrine (Figure 21-2) and oral antihistamines. With the kit, treatment for a severe allergic reaction can be started immediately.

Psychogenic Shock

Psychogenic shock is the least serious type of shock. It is caused by unpleasant physical or emotional stimuli, such as pain, fright, and the sight of blood.

With psychogenic shock, a sudden dilation of the blood vessels causes the blood to pool in the abdomen and extremities. This, in turn, temporarily deprives the brain of blood, causing a temporary loss of consciousness (fainting), usually lasting only 1 to 2 minutes. Fainting generally occurs when an individual is in an upright position. Before fainting, the patient usually experiences some warning signals such as sudden light-headedness, pallor, nausea, weakness, yawning, blurred vision, a feeling of warmth, and sweating.

An individual who is about to faint should be placed in a position that facilitates blood flow to the brain and told to breathe deeply. The preferred position is to move the patient into a supine position with the legs elevated approximately 12 inches and the collar and clothing loosened (Figure 21-3). This position is not always be possible, such as when a patient is seated; in this case, the patient's head should be lowered between the legs (Figure 21-4). A patient who has fainted should be placed in the supine position with the legs elevated. It is recommended that a patient who has fainted contact her or his physician for further evaluation.

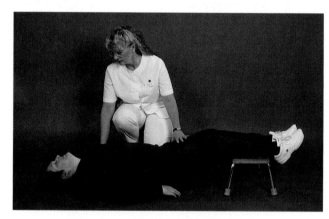

Figure 21-3. Prevention and treatment of fainting.

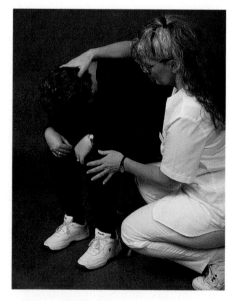

Figure 21-4. Prevention of fainting.

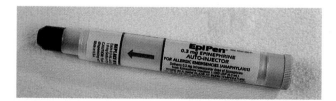

Figure 21-2. Anaphylactic emergency epinephrine injector.

Bleeding

Bleeding, or hemorrhaging, is the escape of blood from a severed blood vessel. Bleeding can range from very minor to very serious, which could lead to shock and death. The amount of blood that can be lost before bleeding becomes life threatening varies according to each individual. In general, a loss of 25% to 40% of an individual's total blood volume can be fatal. This equates to approximately 2 to 4 pints of blood for the average adult.

External Bleeding

External bleeding is bleeding that can be seen coming from a wound. Common examples of external bleeding include bleeding from open fractures, lacerations, and the nose.

Individuals with serious external bleeding exhibit the following symptoms: obvious bleeding, restlessness, cold and clammy skin, thirst, increased and thready pulse, rapid and shallow respirations, a drop in the blood pressure (a late symptom), and decreasing levels of consciousness.

There are three types of external bleeding, classified according to the type of blood vessel that has been injured: capillary, venous, and arterial.

Capillary Bleeding.
Capillary bleeding is the most common type of external bleeding and consists of a slow oozing of bright red blood. This type of bleeding occurs with minor cuts, scratches, and abrasions.

Venous Bleeding.
Venous bleeding occurs when a vein has been punctured or severed. This type of bleeding is characterized by a slow and steady flow of dark red blood.

Arterial Bleeding.
Arterial bleeding is the most serious type of external bleeding and occurs when an artery is punctured or severed. Fortunately, it is the least common type of bleeding because arteries are situated deeper in the body and are protected by bone. Arterial bleeding is characterized by bright red blood that spurts. The arteries most frequently involved in accidents are the carotid, brachial, radial, and femoral.

Emergency Care for External Bleeding

The most effective way to control bleeding is by applying direct pressure to the bleeding site. The pressure functions by either slowing down or stopping the flow of blood. The amount of pressure required depends on the type of bleeding. A small amount of pressure is usually sufficient to control capillary bleeding, whereas significant pressure is often required to control arterial bleeding.

If bleeding cannot be controlled with direct pressure, a pressure point can be used. A **pressure point** is a site on the body where an artery lies close to the surface of the skin and can be compressed against an underlying bone. See Figure 21-5 for an illustration of pressure points. Using a pressure point helps slow or stop the flow of blood from the wound. The pressure points used most often are on the brachial and femoral arteries. The brachial artery is located on the inside of the upper arm midway between the elbow and shoulder. Squeezing the brachial artery helps control severe bleeding in the arm. The femoral artery is located in the groin and helps control severe bleeding in the leg.

The specific steps for controlling bleeding are:

1. Apply direct pressure to the wound with a clean covering such as a large, thick gauze dressing (Figure 21-6, *A*). If gauze is not available, a clean material such as a sanitary napkin, washcloth, handkerchief, or sock can be used. If the wound is located on an extremity, elevate the limb while continuing to apply direct pressure.
2. Apply additional dressings if needed. If the dressing soaks through, apply another dressing over the first one and continue to apply pressure (Figure 21-6, *B*). (Never remove a dressing once it has been applied because this could result in more bleeding.) If the bleeding cannot be controlled with direct pressure, apply pressure to the appropriate pressure point while continuing to apply direct local pressure.
3. Apply a pressure bandage. When bleeding has been controlled, apply a bandage snugly over the dressing to maintain pressure on the wound (Figure 21-6, *C*).
4. Transport the patient to an emergency care facility, or, if the case is serious enough, activate the local emergency medical services.

Nosebleeds

A nosebleed, or epistaxis, is a common form of external bleeding and is usually not serious but is more of a nuisance. Nosebleeds are usually caused by an upper respiratory infection but can also result from a direct blow from a blunt object, hypertension, strenuous activity, and exposure to high altitudes.

PUTTING It All Into **PRACTICE**

MY NAME IS Judy Markins. I work at a large clinic in the family medicine department with 12 physicians. We also have 6 to 10 physicians that do their internships and residency programs with us.

One day as I was performing my usual morning duties of getting the office ready for that day's patients, the office door opened. There stood a mother with her very ill child. I immediately took the patients back to a room. When I took the boy's temperature, it was 104°F. I asked the mother if she had been giving him any type of fever reducer. She said she had but that it was not helping. Under the direction of our physician I immediately started trying to reduce the fever. The fever started to come down and the look of relief on the mother's face was beyond words. That was one of the many days that reinforced how satisfied I am with my career choice.

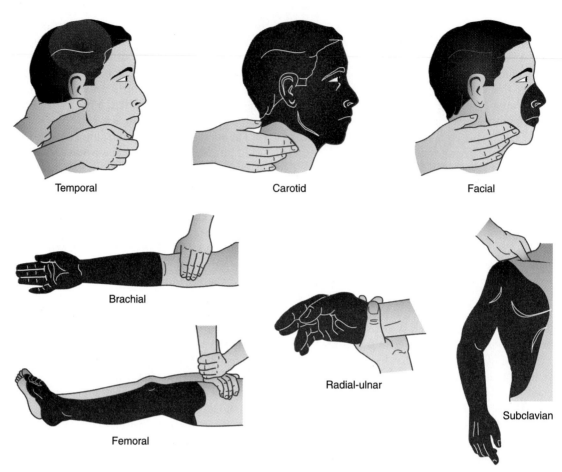

Temporal

Carotid

Facial

Brachial

Radial-ulnar

Femoral

Subclavian

Figure 21-5. Location of pressure points. Shaded areas show the regions in which bleeding may be controlled by pressure at the points indicated. (From Miller BF, Keane CB: *Encyclopedia and dictionary of medicine, nursing, and allied health*, 7th ed., Philadelphia, 2003, Saunders.)

Emergency Care for a Nosebleed

1. Position the patient in a sitting position with the head tilted forward. This prevents the blood from running down the back of the throat, which may result in nausea.
2. Apply direct pressure by pinching the nostrils together (Figure 21-7, *A*). Do not release the pressure too soon, because the bleeding may resume. It usually takes about 15 minutes for adequate clot formation. An ice pack can also be applied to the bridge of the nose to help control the bleeding (Figure 21-7, *B*). If these measures do not control the bleeding, apply pressure on the upper lip, just below the nose.
3. After the bleeding has stopped, tell the patient not to blow the nose for several hours because it could loosen the clot, causing the bleeding to start again.
4. If bleeding cannot be controlled, transport the patient to an emergency care facility for further treatment.

Internal Bleeding

Internal bleeding is bleeding that flows into a body cavity, an organ, or between tissues. It may be minor, as in the case of a contusion, or it may be very serious, such as a severe, blunt blow to the abdomen.

Severe internal bleeding is a life-threatening emergency. Because there is no obvious blood flow, the nature of the injury and the signs and symptoms of bleeding must be used to recognize internal bleeding. Signs and symptoms include bruises, pain, tenderness, or swelling at the site of the injury; rapid weak pulse; cold and clammy skin; nausea and vomiting; excessive thirst; a drop in the blood pressure; and decreased levels of consciousness.

If a patient is suspected of having internal bleeding, the local emergency medical services should be activated immediately. Until emergency medical personnel arrive, the patient should be kept quiet and treated for shock.

Wounds

A **wound** is a break in the continuity of an external or internal surface, caused by physical means. Wounds are either open or closed.

Open Wounds

An open wound is a break in the skin surface or mucous membrane that exposes the underlying tissues. Because the skin is broken, hemorrhaging and wound contamination

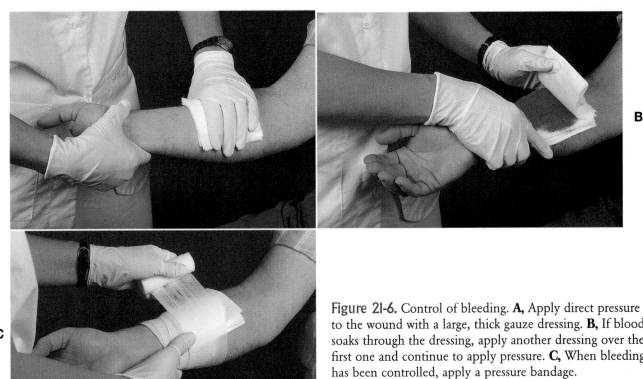

Figure 21-6. Control of bleeding. **A,** Apply direct pressure to the wound with a large, thick gauze dressing. **B,** If blood soaks through the dressing, apply another dressing over the first one and continue to apply pressure. **C,** When bleeding has been controlled, apply a pressure bandage.

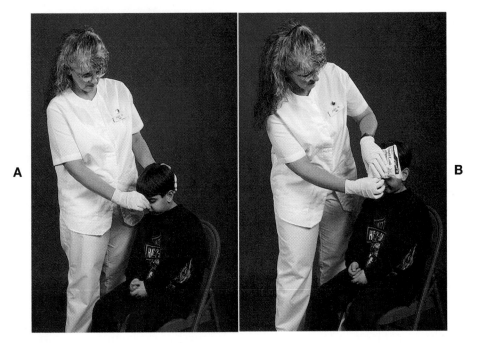

Figure 21-7. Care of a nosebleed. **A,** Apply direct pressure by pinching the nostrils together. **B,** An ice pack can be applied to the bridge of the nose to help control the bleeding.

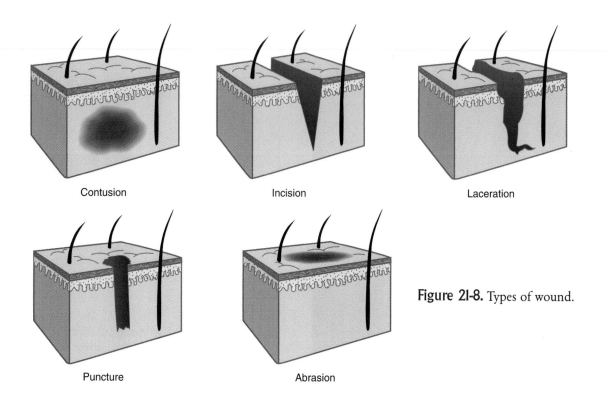

Contusion

Incision

Laceration

Puncture

Abrasion

Figure 21-8. Types of wound.

are primary concerns with open wounds. Open wounds include incisions, lacerations, punctures, and abrasions (Figure 21-8). An individual with an open wound should receive prompt medical attention by a physician if any of the following occur: spurting blood; bleeding that cannot be controlled; a break in the skin that is deeper than just the outer skin layers; embedded debris or an embedded object in the wound; involvement of nerves, muscles, or tendons; and occurrence on the mouth, tongue, face, genitals, or other area where scarring would be apparent.

Incisions and Lacerations

An incision is a clean, smooth cut caused by a sharp cutting instrument such as a knife, razor, or a piece of glass. Deep incisions are accompanied by profuse bleeding; in addition, damage to muscles, tendons, and nerves may occur. Because the edges of the wound are smooth and straight, incisions usually heal better than lacerations.

A laceration is a wound in which the tissues are torn apart, rather than cut, leaving ragged and irregular edges. Lacerations are caused by dull knives, large objects that have been driven into the skin, and heavy machinery. Deep lacerations result in profuse bleeding, and a scar often results from the jagged tearing of the tissues.

Emergency Care for Incisions and Lacerations

Minor Incisions and Lacerations

1. Assess the length, depth, and location of the wound.
2. Control bleeding by covering the wound with a dressing and applying firm pressure.

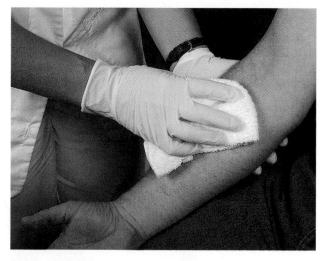

Figure 21-9. Minor incisions and lacerations should be cleaned with soap and water to remove dirt and other debris.

3. Clean the wound with soap and water to remove dirt and other debris (Figure 21-9).
4. Cover the wound with a dry, sterile dressing. Instruct the patient to check the wound for redness, swelling, discharge, or increase in pain and to contact a physician if any of these problems occur.

Serious Incisions and Lacerations

1. Control bleeding by covering the wound with a large, thick gauze dressing and applying firm pressure. Do not clean or probe the wound because this may result in more bleeding.

2. Transport the individual to a physician or, if the wound is serious enough, activate the local EMS.

Punctures

A puncture is a wound made by a sharp, pointed object piercing the skin layers and sometimes the underlying structures. Objects that cause a puncture wound include a nail, splinter, needle, wire, knife, bullet, and animal bite. A puncture wound has a very small external skin opening, and for this reason bleeding is usually minor. A tetanus booster may be administered because the tetanus bacteria grow best in a warm, anaerobic environment, as would be found in a puncture wound.

Emergency Care for Puncture Wounds

1. Allow the wound to bleed freely for a few minutes to help wash out bacteria.
2. Clean the wound with soap and water.
3. Apply a dry, sterile dressing to prevent contamination.
4. Transport the individual to a physician so that medical care can be provided to prevent infection and to ensure that the patient's tetanus toxoid immunization is up to date.

Abrasions

An abrasion, or scrape, is a wound in which the outer layers of the skin are scraped or rubbed off. Blood may ooze from ruptured capillaries; however, the bleeding is not usually severe. Abrasions are caused by falls, resulting in floor burns and skinned knees and elbows. Dirt and other debris are frequently rubbed into the wound; therefore it is important to clean scrapes thoroughly to prevent infection.

Emergency Care for Abrasions

1. Rinse the wound with cold running water.
2. Wash the wound gently with soap and water to remove dirt and other debris. Embedded debris should be removed by a physician.
3. Cover large abrasions with a dry, sterile dressing. Small minor abrasions do not require a dressing.
4. Instruct the patient to check the wound for signs of inflammation, including redness, swelling, discharge, or increase in pain and to contact a physician if they occur.

Closed Wounds

A closed wound involves an injury to the underlying tissues of the body without a break in the skin surface or mucous membrane; an example is a contusion or bruise.

A contusion results when the tissues under the skin are injured (see Figure 21-8) and is often caused by a sudden blow or force from a blunt object. Blood vessels rupture, allowing blood to seep into the tissues, resulting in a bluish discoloration of the skin and swelling. Most contusions heal without special treatment, but cold compresses may reduce bleeding and thus reduce swelling and discoloration and relieve pain. After several days, the color of the contusion turns greenish or yellow, owing to oxidation of blood pigments. Contusions commonly occur with injuries such as fractures, sprains, strains, and black eyes. These injuries, along with the corresponding emergency care, are discussed next.

Musculoskeletal Injuries

The musculoskeletal system is made up of all the bones, muscles, tendons, and ligaments of the body. Injuries that affect the musculoskeletal system include fractures, dislocations, sprains, and strains.

Fracture

A **fracture** is any break in a bone. The break may range in severity from a simple chip or a crack to a complete break or shattering of the bone. Fractures can occur anywhere on the surface of the bone, including across the surface of a joint such as the wrist or ankle. Fractures are caused by a direct blow, a fall, bone disease, or a twisting force as may occur in a sports injury. Although fractures often cause severe pain, they are seldom life-threatening.

The two basic types of fracture are closed fractures and open fractures (Figure 21-10). A *closed fracture* is the most common type and occurs when there is a break in a bone but no break in the skin over the fracture site. An *open fracture* involves a break in the bone along with a penetration of the overlying skin surface. Open fractures are more serious due to the risk of blood loss and contamination leading to infection.

The signs and symptoms of a fracture include pain and tenderness, deformity, swelling and discoloration, loss of function of the body part, and numbness or tingling. The patient usually guards the injured part and may relay to you that he or she heard the bone break or snap or felt a grating sensation. This grating sensation, known as **crepitus,** is caused by the bone fragments rubbing against each other.

Fractures can also be classified according to the nature of the break: impacted, greenstick, transverse, oblique, comminuted, and spiral. Figure 21-11 illustrates and describes these types of fracture.

Dislocation

A **dislocation** is an injury in which one end of a bone making up a joint is separated or displaced from its normal position. A dislocation is caused by a violent pulling or pushing force that tears the ligaments. Dislocations usually result from falls, sports injuries, and motor vehicle accidents. The signs and symptoms of a dislocation include significant deformity of the joint, pain and swelling, and loss of function.

Sprain

A **sprain** is a tearing of ligaments at a joint. Sprains may result from a fall, a sports injury, or a motor vehicle accident. The joints most often sprained are the ankle, knee, wrist, and fingers. The signs and symptoms of a sprain

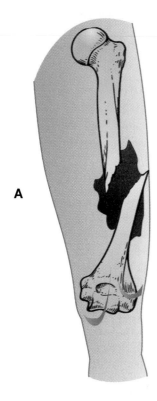

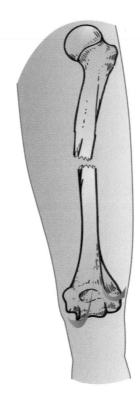

A

B

Figure 21-10. Fractures. **A,** Open fracture. **B,** Closed fracture. (From Connolly JF: *DePalma's the Management of fractures and dislocations: An atlas.* Philadelphia, 1981, Saunders.)

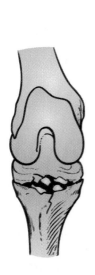

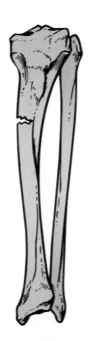

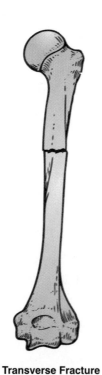

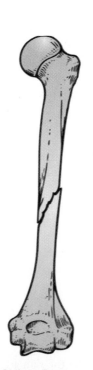

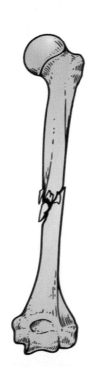

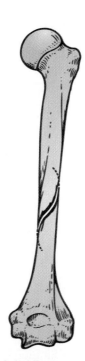

Impacted Fracture
The broken ends of the bones are forcefully jammed together.

Greenstick Fracture
The bone remains intact on one side, but broken on the other, in much the same way a that a "green stick" bends; common in children, whose bones are more flexible than those of adults.

Transverse Fracture
The break occurs perpendicular to the long axis of the bone.

Oblique Fracture
The break occurs diagonally across the bone; generally the result of a twisting force.

Comminuted Fracture
The bone is splintered or shattered into three or more fragments; usually caused by an extremely traumatic direct force.

Spiral Fracture
The bone is broken into a spiral or S-shape; caused by a twisting force.

Figure 21-11. Types of fractures.

include pain, swelling, and discoloration. Sprains can vary in seriousness from mild to severe, depending on the amount of damage to the ligaments.

Strain

A **strain** is a stretching and tearing of muscles or tendons. Strains are most likely to occur when an individual lifts a heavy object or overworks a muscle, as during exercise. The muscles most commonly strained are those of the neck, back, thigh, and calf. The signs and symptoms of a strain are pain and swelling. Strains do not usually cause the intense symptoms associated with fractures, dislocations, and sprains.

Emergency Care for a Fracture

It is often difficult to determine whether a patient has a fracture, dislocation, or sprain because the symptoms of these injuries are similar. Because of this, any serious musculoskeletal injury to an extremity should be treated as if it were a fracture.

The primary goal of emergency care for a fracture is to immobilize the body part. Immobilization reduces pain and prevents further damage. A **splint** is any item that will immobilize a body part. In an emergency situation, a length of wood, cardboard, or rolled newspapers or magazines are items that can be used for splinting. The splint should be padded with a soft material such as a rolled-up towel.

The body part should be splinted in the position in which you found it. However, severely angulated fractures may have to be straightened before splinting. If you attempt to straighten an angulated fracture, be careful not to force the affected part. A dislocated bone end can become "locked" and will have to be realigned at the hospital. If you straighten an angulated bone and encounter pain, stop and splint it in the position in which you found it. The splint should also immobilize the area above and below the injury. For example, when splinting an injury to the wrist, the hand and forearm also should be immobilized (Figure 21-12, *A*). When splinting an injury to the shaft of the bone, the joints both above and below the injury should be immobilized. For example, when splinting the forearm, both the elbow joint and the wrist joint should be immobilized.

The splint should be held in place with a roller gauze bandage or other suitable material such as neckties, scarves, or strips of cloth (Figure 21-12, *B*). The splint should be applied snugly but not so tightly that it interferes with proper circulation. After applying the splint,

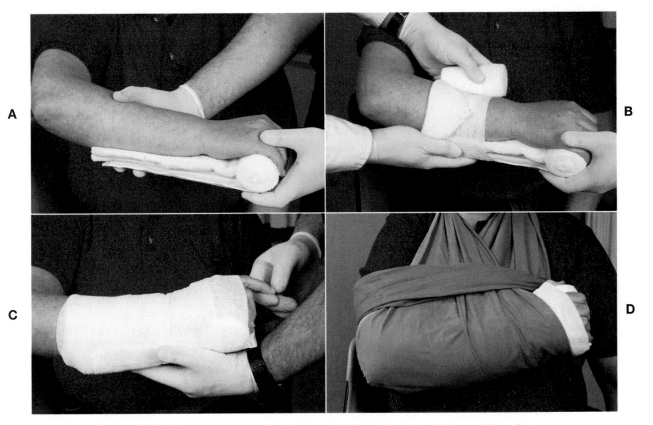

Figure 21-12. Emergency care of a fracture. **A,** The splint should immobilize the area above and below the injury. **B,** The splint is held in place with a gauze roller bandage. **C,** After the splint is applied, the pulse below the splint should be checked to make sure the splint has not been applied too tightly. **D,** A sling can be used to elevate the extremity to reduce swelling. (From Henry M, Stapleton E: *EMT prehospital care,* 2nd ed. Philadelphia, Saunders, 1997.)

check the pulse below the splint to make sure the splint has not been applied too tightly. If you cannot detect a pulse, immediately loosen the splint until you can feel the pulse (Figure 21-12, *C*).

Whenever possible, elevate an injured extremity after it has been immobilized to reduce swelling (Figure 21-12, *D*). An ice pack can also be applied to the injured part. The cold limits the accumulation of fluid in the body tissues by constricting blood vessels and reducing leakage of fluid into the tissues. In addition, cold temporarily relieves pain because of its anesthetic or numbing effect, which reduces stimulation of nerve receptors.

Once you have properly immobilized the injury, transport the patient to an emergency care facility, or if the injury is serious enough, activate the local emergency medical services. In any situation in which an injury to the spine is suspected, activate the local EMS system.

Burns

A **burn** is an injury to the tissues caused by exposure to thermal, chemical, electrical, or radioactive agents. The severity of a burn depends on the depth of the burn, the percentage of the body involved, the type of agent causing the burn, the duration and intensity of the agent, and the part of the body.

Burns are classified according to the depth of tissue injury, as illustrated in Figure 21-13, and are described as follows:

Superficial (First-Degree) Burn. A superficial burn is the most common type of burn. It involves only the top layer of skin, the epidermis. With this type of burn, the skin appears red, is warm and dry to the touch, and is usually painful. Sunburn is a common example of a superficial burn. A superficial burn heals in 2 to 5 days of its own accord and does not cause scarring.

Partial-Thickness (Second-Degree) Burn. A partial-thickness burn involves the epidermis and extends into the dermis but does not pass through the dermis to the underlying tissues. The burned area usually appears red, mottled, and blistered. In most cases, the blisters should not be broken because they provide a protective barrier against infection. Partial-thickness burns are usually very painful, and the area often swells. This type of burn usually heals within 3 to 4 weeks and may result in some scarring.

Full-Thickness (Third-Degree) Burn. A full-thickness burn completely destroys both the epidermis and the dermis and extends into the underlying tissues such as fat, muscle,

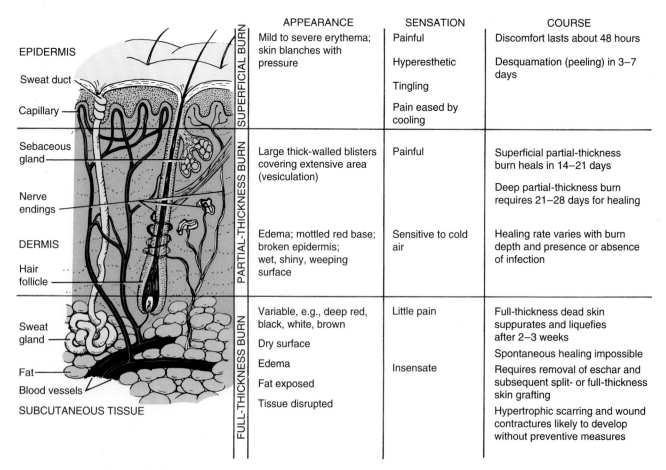

Figure 21-13. Types of burns. (From Polaski AL, Tatro SE: *Luckmann's core principles and practice of medical-surgical nursing.* Philadelphia, 1996, Saunders.)

bone, and nerves. The affected area appears charred black, brown, and cherry red, with the damaged tissues underneath often pearly white. The patient may experience intense pain; however, if there has been substantial damage to the nerve endings, the patient may feel no pain at all. During the healing process, dense scars typically result. Infection is a major concern, and the patient must be carefully monitored.

Thermal Burns

Thermal burns usually occur in the home, often as a result of fire, scalding water, or coming into contact with a hot object such as a stove or curling iron.

Emergency Care for Major Thermal Burns

1. Stop the burning process to prevent further injury. If the individual is on fire, wrap him or her in a blanket, rug, or heavy coat and push him or her to the ground to help smother the flames. If a covering is not available, shout at the individual to drop to the ground and roll around to smother the flames.
2. Cool the burn, using large amounts of cool water from a faucet or garden hose. Do not use ice or ice water because this may result in further tissue damage; it also causes heat loss from the body. If the burn covers a large surface area (greater than 20%), do not use water. The loss of a large amount of skin surface places the patient at risk for hypothermia (generalized body cooling). With large surface area burns you may cool the most painful areas but not an area greater than 20% of the body (i.e., two arms, one leg, and so on).
3. Activate your local EMS.
4. Cover the patient with a clean, nonfuzzy material such as a tablecloth or sheet. The cover serves to maintain warmth, reduce pain, and reduce the risk of contamination. Do not apply any type of ointment, antiseptic, or other substance to the burned area.

Emergency Care for Minor Thermal Burns

1. Immerse the affected area in cold water for 2 to 5 minutes. Be careful not to break any blisters because they provide a protective barrier against infection.
2. Cover the burn with a dry sterile dressing.

Chemical Burns

Chemical burns occur both in the workplace and at home. The severity of the burn depends on the type and strength of the chemical and the duration of exposure to the chemical. The main difference between a chemical burn and a thermal burn is that the chemical continues to burn the patient's tissues as long as it is on the skin. Because of this factor, it is important to remove the chemical from the skin as quickly as possible and then to activate the local emergency medical services.

Liquid chemical burns should be treated by flooding the area with large amounts of cool running water until emergency personnel arrive. If a solid substance such as lime has been spilled on the patient, it should be brushed off before flooding the area with water. This is because a dry chemical may be activated by contact with water.

Seizures

A **seizure** is a sudden episode of involuntary muscular contractions and relaxation, often accompanied by a change in sensation, behavior, and level of consciousness. A seizure results when the normal electrical activity of the brain is disturbed, causing the brain cells to become irritated and overactive. Specific conditions that trigger a seizure include epilepsy, encephalitis, a recent or old head injury, high fever in infants and young children, drug and alcohol abuse or withdrawal, eclampsia associated with toxemia of pregnancy, diabetic conditions, and heat stroke.

Seizures are classified as partial or generalized according to the location of the abnormal electrical activity in the brain.

Partial seizures are the most common type, occurring in approximately 80% of individuals who have seizures. With a partial seizure, the abnormal electrical activity is localized into very specific areas of the brain; therefore only the brain functions in those areas are affected.

Partial seizures are further classified as simple or complex, depending on whether the patient's level of consciousness is affected. The symptoms of a *simple partial seizure* include twitching or jerking in just one part of the body. This type of seizure lasts less than a minute, and the patient remains awake and alert during the seizure. With a *complex partial seizure*, the patient's level of consciousness is affected, and the patient has little or no memory of the seizure afterward.

The symptoms of this type of seizure include abnormal behavior such as confusion, a glassy stare, aimless wandering, lip smacking or chewing, or fidgeting with clothing, which lasts from a few seconds up to a minute or two. Both a simple and a complex partial seizure can progress to a generalized seizure.

With a *generalized seizure,* the abnormal electrical activity spreads through the entire brain. The best-known type of generalized seizure is a *tonic-clonic seizure* (formerly known as a grand mal seizure). With this type of seizure, the patient exhibits tonic-clonic activity followed by a postictal state. During the tonic phase, the patient suddenly loses consciousness and exhibits rigid muscular contractions, which result in odd posturing of the body. Respirations are inhibited, which may cause cyanosis around the mouth and lips. The patient may lose control of the bladder or bowels, resulting in involuntary urination and defecation. The tonic phase lasts up to 30 seconds, followed by the clonic phase. During the clonic phase, the patient's body jerks about violently. The patient's jaw muscles contract, which may cause the patient to bite the tongue or lips. The final phase of the seizure is the postictal state, lasting between 10 and 30 minutes, in which the patient exhibits a depressed level of consciousness, is disoriented, and often has a headache. The patient generally has little or no

What Would You DO?
What Would You *Not* DO?

Case Study 1

Beth Eaton calls the office. She says that she thinks her 3-year-old daughter, Olivia, has eaten some chewable vitamins. Beth was taking a shower and when she came out, Olivia was holding an empty vitamin bottle and saying "Good candy." Beth says she doesn't know how Olivia got the child-proof top off. She thinks the bottle was about a third of the way full. Beth says that Olivia is complaining that her tummy hurts. Beth says she has syrup of ipecac and wants to know if she should give some to Olivia.

memory of the seizure and feels confused and exhausted for several hours after the seizure.

In some instances of seizures, particularly in patients with epilepsy, an aura precedes the seizure. An *aura* is a sensation perceived by the patient that something is about to happen: examples include a strange taste, smell, or sound, a twitch, or a feeling of dizziness or anxiety. An aura provides the patient with a warning signal that a seizure is about to begin.

Although seizures are frightening to observe, they are usually not as bad as they look. Most patients fully recover within a few minutes after the seizure begins. An exception to this is *status epilepticus,* in which the seizures are prolonged or come in rapid succession without full recovery of consciousness between them. Status epilepticus is a potentially life-threatening situation that requires immediate medical care.

Emergency Care for Seizures

The most important criterion in caring for a patient in a seizure is to protect the patient from harm. Remove hazards from the immediate area to prevent the patient from injury by striking a surrounding object. Do not restrain the patient. Loosen restrictive clothing that may interfere with breathing, such as collars, neckties, scarves, and jewelry. It is important to realize that the seizure will occur no matter what you do; restraining the patient could seriously injure the patient's muscles, bones, or joints. Do not insert anything into the patient's mouth during the seizure because this could damage the teeth or mouth or interfere with breathing. In addition, it could trigger the gag reflex, causing the patient to vomit and possibly aspirate the vomitus into the lungs. If the patient vomits, roll him or her onto one side so that the vomitus can drain from the mouth.

If you are uncertain as to the cause of the seizure or suspect that the patient is having status epilepticus, activate your local emergency medical services immediately.

Otherwise transport the patient to an emergency medical care facility for further evaluation and treatment once the seizure is over.

Poisoning

A **poison** is any substance that causes illness, injury, or death if it enters the body. Most poisoning episodes take place in the home, are accidental, and occur in children under the age of 5 years. Poisoning usually involves common substances such as cleaning agents, medications, and pesticides. For most poisonous substances, the reaction is more serious in children and the elderly than in adults.

Poison control centers are valuable resources that are easily accessible to medical personnel and the community. There are more than 500 regional poison control centers across the United States; most are located in the emergency departments of large hospitals. These centers are staffed by personnel who have access to information about almost all poisonous substances. Most of the centers are staffed 24 hours a day, and calls are toll free. There is also a National Poison Control Hotline number (1-800-222-1222), which can be called 24 hours a day.

A poison can enter the body in four ways: ingestion, inhalation, absorption, or injection. Each of these is described here along with the corresponding emergency care.

Ingested Poisons

Poisons that are ingested enter the body by being swallowed. Ingestion is the most common route of entry for poisons. Examples of poisons that are often ingested include cleaning products, pesticides, contaminated food, petroleum products (e.g., gasoline, kerosene), and poisonous plants. The abuse of drugs or alcohol or both also can result in poisoning from an accidental or intentional overdose.

The signs and symptoms of poisoning by ingestion are based on the specific substance that has been consumed but often include strange odors, burns or stains around the mouth, nausea, vomiting, abdominal pain, diarrhea, difficulty in breathing, profuse perspiration, excessive salivation, dilated or constricted pupils, unconsciousness, and convulsions.

Emergency Care for Poisoning by Ingestion

1. Acquire as much information as possible about the type of poison, the amount ingested, and when it was ingested.
2. Call your poison control center or local emergency medical services. *Never* induce vomiting unless directed to do so by a medical authority. Vomiting is often contraindicated, for example, when an individual is unconscious, has swallowed a petroleum product, or has swallowed a corrosive poison such as a strong acid or base. Corrosive poisons may cause more injury to the esophagus, throat, and mouth if they are vomited back up. If it is available, you may be directed by the poison control center to administer activated charcoal. Activated charcoal is used to absorb the poison that remains in the stomach and prevents absorption by the intestine.
3. If the individual vomits, collect some of the vomitus for transport with the patient to the hospital for analysis by a toxicologist, if necessary. In addition, bring along containers of any substances ingested, such as empty medication bottles and household cleaner containers because the label of the container often lists the ingredients in the product.

Inhaled Poisons

A poison that is inhaled is breathed into the body in the form of gas, vapor, or spray. The most commonly inhaled poison is carbon monoxide, such as from car exhausts, malfunctioning furnaces, and fires. Other inhaled poisons include carbon dioxide from wells and sewers and fumes from household products such as glues, paints, insect sprays, and cleaners (e.g., ammonia, chlorine).

The signs and symptoms of inhaled poisoning often include severe headache; nausea and vomiting; coughing or wheezing; shortness of breath; chest pain or tightness; facial burns; burning of the mouth, nose, eyes, throat or chest; cyanosis; confusion; dizziness; and unconsciousness.

Emergency Care for Inhaled Poisons

1. Determine whether it is safe to approach the patient. Toxic gases and fumes can also be dangerous to individuals helping the patient.
2. Remove the individual from the source of the poison and into fresh air as quickly as possible.
3. Call your poison control center or local emergency medical services.
4. If oxygen is available, you may be directed to administer it under the supervision of a physician. Oxygen is the primary antidote for carbon monoxide poisoning.

Absorbed Poisons

A poison that is absorbed enters the body through the skin. Examples of absorbed poisons include fertilizers and pesticides used for lawn and garden care. The signs and symptoms of absorbed poisoning are irritation, burning and itching, burning of the skin or eyes, headache, and abnormal pulse or respiration or both.

What Would You DO?
What Would You *Not* DO?

Case Study 2

Anita Alland calls the office and says that her son, Garon, was stung by a yellow jacket about an hour ago while mowing the grass. She says that his entire arm and back are red and swollen and that he also has a lot of redness and swelling around his eyes. Garon is itching all over and seems fuzzy-headed. Anita says she has never seen anyone do this after being stung. She says she had Garon take a cold shower to see if it would help. After the shower he started feeling faint and dizzy and now he's having a little trouble breathing. Anita wants to know if she can bring him to the office so he can be seen by the physician.

Emergency Care for Absorbed Poisons

1. Remove the patient from the source of the poison. Be sure to avoid contact with the toxic substance.
2. Call your poison control center or local emergency medical services. In most cases, you will be instructed to flood the area that has been exposed to the poison with water. Dry chemicals should be brushed from the skin before flooding with water.

Injected Poisons

An injected poison enters the body through bites, through stings, or by a needle. Examples of injected poisons include the venom of insects, spiders, snakes, and marine creatures such as jellyfish, and the bite of rabid animals. The poison may also be a drug that is self-administered with a hypodermic needle, such as heroin.

The general signs and symptoms of injected poisoning include an altered state of awareness; evidence of stings, bites, or puncture marks on the skin; mottled skin; localized pain or itching; burning, swelling, or blistering at the site; difficulty in breathing; abnormal pulse rate; nausea and vomiting; and anaphylactic shock.

The emergency care for specific types of injected poison is described in more detail in the following paragraphs.

Insect Stings

It is estimated that 1 of every 125 Americans is allergic to insect stings. Approximately 40 people in the United States die every year from a severe allergic reaction to insect stings. The incidence of deaths is low because most people know they need to obtain medical attention immediately if an allergic reaction begins.

Almost all the insects whose venom can cause allergic reactions belong to a group called *Hymenoptera*, which includes honeybees and bumblebees, wasps, yellow jackets, and hornets. When a honeybee stings, its stinger remains embedded in the victim's skin, causing the bee to die as it tries to tear itself away. Wasps, yellow jackets, and hornets are more aggressive than bees and can sting repeatedly. Hornets are the most aggressive of the group and may sting even when not provoked. Yellow jackets are close behind in aggressiveness, and wasps usually sting only if someone interferes with them near their nest.

If an insect sting does not cause an allergic reaction within 30 minutes, chances are excellent that no problem will occur. A normal reaction to an insect sting includes localized pain, redness, swelling, and itching lasting 1 to 2 days. Any generalized reaction not arising directly from the area of the sting is almost certain to be an allergic reaction, which begins with such symptoms as sneezing, hives, itching, angioedema, erythema, and disorientation and progresses to difficulty in breathing, dizziness, faintness, and loss of consciousness.

Medical care should be sought immediately because these are the symptoms of an anaphylactic reaction, and most fatalities occur within 2 hours of the sting. Because time is a factor, individuals known to have a severe allergy to insect stings carry an anaphylactic emergency treatment kit containing injectable epinephrine and oral antihistamines (see Figure 21-2). With this kit, treatment for a severe allergic reaction can be started immediately.

Emergency Care for Insect Stings

1. Remove the stinger and attached venom sac. Scrape the stinger off the patient's skin with your fingernail or a plastic card such as a credit card (Figure 21-14). Do not use tweezers or forceps as squeezing the venom sac may cause more venom to be injected into the patient's tissues.
2. Wash the site with soap and water.
3. Apply a cold pack to the affected area to reduce pain and swelling.
4. Observe the patient for the signs of an anaphylactic reaction.

Spider Bites

Although spiders are numerous throughout the United States, most do not cause injuries or serious complications. Only two spiders have bites that cause serious or even life-threatening reactions: the black widow spider and the brown recluse spider. Both these spiders prefer dark, out-of-the-way places such as woodpiles, brush piles, under rocks, and in dark garages and attics. Because of this, bites usually occur on the hands and arms of individuals reaching into places where the spiders are hiding. Often the individual does not know that she or he has been bitten until she or he begins to feel ill or notices swelling and a bite mark on the skin.

The black widow spider is approximately 1 inch long and is black with a distinctive bright red hourglass shape on its abdomen. The venom injected when this spider bites an individual is toxic to the central nervous system. The signs and symptoms of a black widow bite are swelling and a dull pain at the injection site; nausea and vomiting; a rigid, boardlike abdomen; fever; rash; and difficulty in breathing or swallowing. Although the symptoms are severe, they are not usually fatal. An antivenin is available; however, because of its undesirable and frequent side effects, it is generally administered only

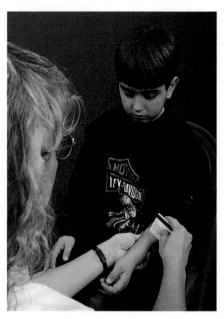

Figure 21-14. Removing a honeybee stinger and venom sac using the edge of a credit card.

to individuals with severe bites and to individuals who may have a heightened reaction, such as elderly people and children younger than 5 years old.

The brown recluse spider is light brown with a dark brown violin-shaped mark on its back. The bite of a brown recluse causes severe local effects including tenderness, redness, and swelling at the injection site. On the other hand, systemic effects, such as difficulty in breathing or swallowing, seldom occur.

Emergency Care for Spider Bites

1. Wash the wound.
2. Apply a cold pack to the affected area to reduce pain and swelling.
3. Obtain medical help immediately if you suspect the individual has been bitten by a black widow spider or a brown recluse spider or if a severe reaction begins to occur.

Snakebites

Snakebites kill very few people in the United States. Every year approximately 45,000 persons are bitten by a snake; however only 7,000 of these bites involve a poisonous snake, and fewer than 15 of the individuals die.

The species of snakes that are poisonous in the United States include rattlesnakes, copperheads, cottonmouths (water moccasins), and coral snakes. However, other poisonous species may be privately owned by individuals, zoos, or labs. Rattlesnakes account for most snakebites and nearly all fatalities from snakebites. Most snakebites occur near the home, as opposed to in the wild. Because it is often difficult to identify a snake, any unidentified snake should be considered poisonous.

The general signs and symptoms of a bite from a poisonous snake include puncture marks on the skin, pain and swelling at the puncture site, rapid pulse, nausea, vomiting, unconsciousness, and convulsions.

Emergency Care for Snakebites

1. Wash the bite area gently with soap and water.
2. Immobilize the injured part and position it below the level of the heart.
3. Call emergency personnel. Do not apply ice to a snakebite. Do not apply a tourniquet, and do not cut or suction the wound.
4. If the snake is dead, inform emergency personnel of its location so that it can be transported to the hospital for identification.

Animal Bites

Bites and other injuries from animals range in severity from minor to serious and even fatal. Most people who are bitten by animals do not report the bite to a physician. Because of this factor, the incidence of animal bites in the United States each year is not known but has been estimated at approximately 1 to 2 million for dog bites and 400,000 for cat bites.

The most serious type of bite is one from an animal with rabies. Rabies is a viral infection transmitted through the saliva of an infected animal. If the condition is not treated, rabies is generally fatal.

Certain animals tend to have a higher incidence of rabies than others. These include skunks, bats, raccoons, cats, dogs, cattle, and foxes. On the other hand, hamsters, gerbils, guinea pigs, chipmunks, rats, mice, gophers, and rabbits are rarely infected with the rabies virus.

An individual who has been bitten by an animal that has rabies or is suspected of having rabies must obtain medical care. To prevent rabies, a rabies vaccine, which produces antibodies to fight the rabies virus, is administered to the individual.

Emergency Care for Animal Bites

Minor Animal Bites. Wash the wound with soap and water. Apply an antibiotic ointment and a dry sterile dressing. Transport the individual to a physician so that medical care can be provided to prevent infection and to ensure that the patient's tetanus toxoid immunization is up to date.

Serious Bites. If the wound is bleeding heavily, first control the bleeding with direct pressure. Do not clean the wound because this may result in more bleeding. Transport the patient to a physician, or if the bite is serious enough, call the local emergency medical service.

All Animal Bites. If you suspect that the animal has rabies, relay this information to the appropriate authorities, such as medical personnel, the police, or animal control personnel. If possible, try to remember what the animal looked like and the area in which you last saw it.

Heat and Cold Exposure

Exposure to excessive environmental heat or cold can result in injury to the body ranging in severity from minor to life-threatening.

Heat-related injuries are most apt to occur on very hot days that are accompanied by high humidity with little or no air movement. The three conditions caused by overexposure to heat are heat cramps, heat exhaustion, and heat stroke.

The two major types of cold-related injury are frostbite and hypothermia. Although cold-related injuries are most apt to occur in the winter months, they can also occur at other times of the year, such as when an individual is exposed to cold water in a near-drowning incident.

Certain individuals are at higher risk for developing heat- and cold-related injuries:

- Elderly people
- Young children, particularly infants
- Individuals who work or exercise outdoors
- Individuals with medical conditions that cause poor blood circulation, such as diabetes mellitus and cardiovascular disease
- Individuals who have had heat- or cold-related injuries in the past
- Individuals under the influence of drugs or alcohol

Heat Cramps

Heat cramps are the least serious of the three types of heat-related injury. Heat cramps are most apt to occur when an individual is exercising or working in a hot environment and fails to replace lost fluids and electrolytes. Lost electrolytes can be replaced with a commercial sports drink (e.g., Gatorade).

The signs and symptoms of heat cramps include painful muscle spasms, particularly of the legs, calves, and abdomen; hot, sweaty skin; weakness; and a rapid pulse. These symptoms are a warning that an individual is having a problem with the heat. If the problem is ignored, heat cramps may progress to a more serious condition, such as heat exhaustion or heat stroke.

Treatment of heat cramps consists of removal of the patient to a cool environment, rest, and replacement of fluids and electrolytes. If the patient's condition does not improve, she or he should be transported to an emergency care facility for further treatment.

Heat Exhaustion

Heat exhaustion is the most common heat-related injury. It occurs most often in individuals involved in vigorous physical activity on a hot and humid day, such as athletes and construction workers. It can also occur in people who are wearing too much clothing on a hot and humid day.

The signs and symptoms of heat exhaustion are very similar to those of influenza: cold and clammy skin that is pale or gray, profuse sweating, headache, nausea, dizziness, weakness, and diarrhea.

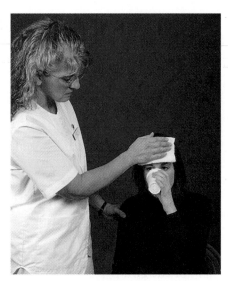

Figure 21-15. Treatment of heat exhaustion consists of removing the patient to a cool environment, replacing fluids and electrolytes, and applying a cold compress to the forehead; the patient should then rest.

Treatment of heat exhaustion consists of removal of the patient to a cool environment, replacement of fluids and electrolytes, application of a cold compress to the forehead, and rest (Figure 21-15). Tight clothing should be loosened and excessive layers of clothing should be removed. In most cases, these measures will improve the patient's condition in approximately 30 minutes. If the patient's condition does not improve, however, he or she should be transported to an emergency care facility.

Heat Stroke

Heat stroke is the least common, but most serious, of the three heat-related injuries. Heat stroke is most apt to occur in elderly people during a heat wave and in athletes who overexert in a hot and humid environment. Heat stroke can occur in a very short time, as when a child has been left to wait in a closed car on a hot day.

During heat stroke, the body becomes so overheated that the heat-regulating mechanism breaks down and is unable to cool the body. The body temperature rises to a dangerous level, causing the destruction of tissues. The signs and symptoms of heat stroke include a body temperature of 105°F (40°C) or higher; red, hot dry skin; a rapid weak pulse; dizziness and weakness; rapid, shallow breathing; decreased levels of consciousness; and seizures.

Heat stroke is a life-threatening emergency and requires immediate transport of the patient to an emergency care facility by the fastest way possible. If not treated, heat stroke is always fatal. During transport, every attempt should be made to lower the body temperature, such as setting the air conditioner to its maximum capacity, covering the victim with cool, wet sheets, or fanning the victim.

Frostbite

Frostbite is the localized freezing of body tissue as a result of exposure to cold. The severity of the frostbite depends on the environmental temperature, the duration of exposure, and the wind-chill factor. Frostbite most commonly affects the hands, fingers, feet, toes, ears, nose, and cheeks. Although frostbite is not life-threatening, it can cause severe tissue damage that may require amputation of the affected body part. The signs and symptoms of frostbite include loss of feeling in the affected area, cold and waxy skin, and white, yellow, or blue discoloration of the skin.

Treatment of frostbite requires rewarming of the affected body part to prevent permanent damage. This is best accomplished in an emergency care facility since improper rewarming can result in further tissue damage. To transport the patient, loosely wrap warm clothing or blankets around the affected body part. The frozen area can also be placed in contact with another body part that is warm. It is very important to handle the affected area gently. Do not rub or massage the affected area because this can further damage frozen tissue.

Hypothermia

Hypothermia is a life-threatening emergency in which the temperature of the entire body falls to a dangerously low level. Hypothermia can occur rapidly, such as when an individual falls through the ice on a frozen lake. It can also occur slowly when an individual is exposed to a cold environment for a long time, such as a hiker lost in the woods.

When the core body temperature falls too low, the body loses its ability to regulate its temperature and to generate body heat. The signs and symptoms of hypothermia are shivering, numbness, drowsiness, apathy, a glassy stare, and decreased levels of consciousness.

Treatment of hypothermia should focus on preventing further heat loss. Remove the patient from the cold, or if this is not possible, wrap him or her in blankets. Do not attempt to rewarm the patient such as through immersion in warm water. Rapid rewarming can result in serious respiratory and cardiac problems. The patient should be transported immediately to an emergency care facility.

Diabetic Emergencies

Glucose is the end product of carbohydrate metabolism. Its serves as the chief source of energy to carry out normal body functions and to assist in maintaining body temperature. The body maintains a constant blood glucose level to ensure a continuous source of energy for the body. Glucose that is not needed for energy can be stored in the form of glycogen in muscle and liver tissue for later use. When no more tissue storage is possible, excess glucose is converted to fat and stored as adipose tissue.

Insulin is a hormone secreted by the beta cells of the pancreas and is required for normal use of glucose in the body. Insulin enables glucose to enter the body's cells and be converted to energy. Insulin is also needed for the proper storage of glycogen in liver and muscle cells.

Diabetes mellitus is a disease in which the body is unable to use glucose for energy due to a lack of insulin in the body. There are two types of diabetes: a severe form, usually appearing in childhood, known as type 1 diabetes, and a mild form, usually appearing in adulthood, known as type 2 diabetes. Most individuals with diabetes (90%) have type 2 diabetes. There is no cure for diabetes mellitus, but significant advances have been made in controlling the disease through a combination of drug therapy, diet therapy, and activity. The goal for the diabetic patient is to balance food intake and level of activity with the body's insulin.

Two types of emergency can be experienced by a diabetic patient: *hypoglycemia,* commonly referred to as insulin shock, and *diabetic ketoacidosis,* commonly known as diabetic coma.

Insulin shock (hypoglycemia) occurs when there is too much insulin in the body and not enough glucose. Insulin shock can be caused by administration of too much insulin, skipping meals, and unexpected or unusual exercise. The symptoms of insulin shock are normal or rapid respirations; pale, cold, and clammy skin; sweating; dizziness and headache; full rapid pulse; normal or high blood pressure; extreme hunger; aggressive or unusual behavior; fainting; and seizure or coma. The onset of insulin shock occurs rapidly, usually over a period of 5 to 20 minutes, after the blood glucose level begins to fall. Because the brain requires a constant supply of glucose for proper functioning, permanent brain damage or even death can result from severe hypoglycemia.

Diabetic coma (diabetic ketoacidosis) occurs when there is not enough insulin in the body. This causes the blood glucose level to rise, resulting in hyperglycemia. When glucose cannot be used for energy, fat is broken down. This results in a buildup of acid waste products in the blood, known as ketoacidosis. The combined effect of the hyperglycemia and ketoacidosis causes the following symptoms: polyuria, excessive thirst and hunger, vomiting, abdominal pain, dry, warm skin, rapid and deep sighing respirations, a sweet or fruity (acetone) odor to the breath, and a rapid, weak pulse.

If the condition is not treated, diabetic coma can progress to dehydration, hypotension, coma, and death. Unlike insulin shock, however, the onset of diabetic coma is gradual, usually developing over a period of 12 to 48 hours. Diabetic coma can be caused by illness and

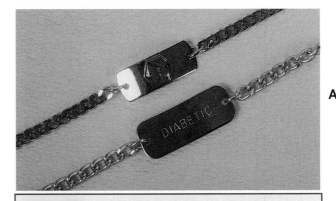

Figure 21-16. Diabetic medical identification. **A,** Diabetic medical alert bracelet. **B,** Diabetic wallet card.

infection, overeating, forgetting to administer an insulin injection, or administering an insufficient amount of insulin.

Most individuals with diabetes have a thorough knowledge of their disease and manage it effectively. Because of this, diabetic emergencies are most apt to occur when there is an unusual upset in the insulin/glucose balance in the body, such as might be caused by illness or infection. An emergency situation may also arise in an individual who has diabetes but in whom the condition has not yet been diagnosed.

It may be difficult to tell the difference between insulin shock and diabetic coma because the symptoms are similar. Often a patient suffering from either of these conditions appears to be intoxicated. If he or she is conscious, the diabetic patient usually knows what the trouble is; therefore, you should listen carefully to the patient to determine what may have caused the problem (e.g., not eating, forgetting to administer an insulin injection). If the patient is unconscious, and therefore unable to communicate, you should observe the patient's respirations. A patient in insulin shock has normal or rapid respirations, whereas a patient in diabetic coma has deep, labored respirations.

Most diabetic patients carry an emergency medical identification to alert others to their condition when they cannot; examples include a medical alert bracelet or necklace, and a wallet card (Figure 21-16).

Emergency Care in Diabetes
Insulin Shock (Hypoglycemia)

A patient in insulin shock needs sugar immediately. For the conscious patient, glucose should be administered by mouth in the form of fruit juice (e.g., orange juice), nondiet soft drinks, candy, honey, or table sugar dissolved in water (Figure 21-17). Improvement is usually fairly rapid after the glucose has been consumed. If the patient is unconscious, do not give anything by mouth because it may be aspirated into the lungs. Instead, provide the fastest possible transportation of the patient to an emergency care facility.

Diabetic Coma (Diabetic Ketoacidosis)

The patient in diabetic coma needs insulin and therefore must be transported as soon as possible to an emergency care facility.

Doubtful Situations

If you are ever in doubt as to whether a patient is developing insulin shock or diabetic coma, give sugar, even though the final diagnosis actually may be diabetic coma. This is because insulin shock develops much more rapidly than diabetic coma and can quickly cause permanent brain damage or death. If you give sugar to a patient in diabetic coma, there is very little risk of making the condition worse because a patient can withstand a high blood glucose level longer than he or she can tolerate a low blood glucose level.

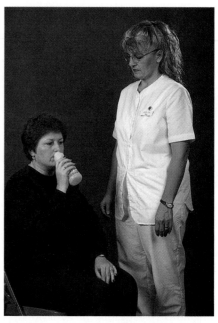

Figure 21-17. Orange juice is administered to a diabetic patient showing signs and symptoms of insulin shock.

MEDICAL Practice and the LAW

Emergency medicine is one of the most litigious (lawsuit-prone) areas of health care. Owing to the nature of emergencies, there is little time to plan your actions, and one misstep could cause damage. Keep in mind that your actions will be compared in court to those of a "reasonably prudent medical assistant with similar education and experience." Do not perform procedures you are not comfortable performing.

Whenever possible, obtain written consent for all procedures. In a life or death situation, this is not usually possible. In this case, you are held accountable to try to save the life of the patient, even without consent.

Many times, patients or families become hysterical during emergencies. As a health care professional, you are expected to keep a cool head and calm the patient and family while attending to the emergency situation.

If you are out of the office and encounter an emergency situation, many states have a "Good Samaritan" law that protects you from legal action if you perform only procedures with which you are familiar, such as emergency first aid or CPR.

What Would You DO?
What Would You Not DO? RESPONSES

Case Study 1

What Did Judy Do?

❑ Gave Beth the National Poison Control hotline number (1-800-222-1222) and told her to call them immediately. Explained that was the fastest way to obtain information on what to do.

❑ Told Beth not to give the syrup of ipecac to Olivia unless she was told to do so by poison control.

❑ Told Beth to have the vitamin bottle in her hand when she calls. Told her that poison control would want to know information from the label and would especially want to know if the vitamins contained iron.

❑ Told Beth to call the office back if she needs any more help after talking with poison control.

What Did Judy Not Do?

❑ Did not tell Beth she should give Olivia syrup of ipecac, because some poisons can cause additional problems if they are brought back up.

What Would You Do?/What Would You Not Do? Review Judy's response and place a checkmark next to the information you included in your response. List additional information you included in your response below.

_____

_____

_____

_____

What Would You DO?
What Would You *Not* DO? *RESPONSES*—Cont'd

Case Study 2

What Did Judy Do?

❑ Told Anita that Garon needs to get to the hospital as soon as possible. Explained that he is having a *very* serious allergic reaction that could be life-threatening.

❑ Told her to stay calm and call 911 immediately.

❑ Notified the physician of the situation.

What Did Judy Not Do?

❑ Told her to bring Garon to the office because he may need special life-support equipment available at the hospital.

What Would You Do?/What Would You *Not* Do? Review Judy's response and place a checkmark next to the information you included in your response. List additional information you included in your response below.

_____

_____

_____

_____

Case Study 3

What Did Judy Do?

❑ Took David to an examining room that was cool and gave him a glass of water.

❑ Told David we needed to get his costume off as soon as possible. Explained that if his condition gets worse, it could become life-threatening.

❑ Helped David out of the costume and gave him another glass of water.

What Did Judy Not Do?

❑ Did not let David keep the costume on.

What Would You Do?/What Would You *Not* Do? Review Judy's response and place a checkmark next to the information you included in your response. List additional information you included in your response below.

_____

_____

_____

_____

Apply Your
KNOWLEDGE

Choose the best answer to each of the following questions.

1. John Adams is a 56-year-old male with a history of an MI. While at the office for a health examination, Mr. Adams starts complaining of chest pain. Dr. Cardio directs Judy Markins, CMA to call 911 for an ambulance. Judy does all of the following when speaking to the EMS dispatcher EXCEPT:
   A. Speaks clearly and calmly
   B. Relays the condition of the patient
   C. Gives the dispatcher the suite number of the office
   D. Hangs up as soon as possible

2. Judy Markins, CMA is assembling a first aid kit for the medical office. Which of the following would she include in the kit?
   A. Cold packs
   B. Pocket mask
   C. Tourniquet
   D. Roller gauze
   E. All of the above

3. Teresa Marquez is seated in the venipuncture chair. Judy Markins, CMA is about to perform a venipuncture on Teresa. Teresa indicates that she feels warm and light-headed. Which of the following is the best step for Judy to take?
   A. Have Teresa put her head between her knees
   B. Offer Teresa a Popsicle
   C. Continue with the venipuncture
   D. Have Teresa stand up and walk around slowly

4. Timmy Tompkins is brought to the office for a recheck after recently being discharged from the hospital. He developed anaphylactic shock after being stung by a yellow jacket. Dr. Cardio explains to Timmy and his parents that anytime Timmy is stung by a yellow jacket, he will develop an anaphylactic reaction. The quickest method of treating anaphylactic shock is to:
   A. Call the EMS immediately
   B. Place a belt around the area where Timmy is stung to prevent the spread of the venom
   C. Use an emergency treatment kit with injectable epinephrine and an oral antihistamine, and then call EMS
   D. Timmy's parents should drive him to the ER after the sting because an anaphylactic reaction usually doesn't occur for several hours

Continued

5. Sherry Walters, a 10-year-old girl, is brought to the office by her mother. Sherry fell while she was inline skating and has a deep laceration on the inner aspect of her right forearm. Sherry's mother had wrapped a clean dishtowel around the wound, but the towel was saturated with blood and the bleeding continued. Judy Markins, CMA, should:
   A. Apply a dressing over the towel, elevate the arm, and apply direct pressure over the site
   B. Tie a tight bandage above the site to decrease the circulation and slow the bleeding
   C. Remove the saturated towel and rinse the wound with warm water
   D. Scream for help and have Sherry keep her arm below the level of her heart

6. John Collins is a 38-year-old who stepped on a nail. He calls the office to ask what to do. It would be most important for Judy Markins, CMA, to ask:
   A. How Mr. Collins cleaned his wound
   B. If Mr. Collins knows the signs and symptoms of infection
   C. If the nail Mr. Collins stepped on was rusty
   D. When Mr. Collins last had a tetanus toxoid immunization

7. Beatrice Ellis is a 25-year-old woman who comes to the office because she has a sore throat and fever. She also has a history of epilepsy. While taking her chief complaint and checking vital signs, she tells Judy Markins, CMA, she is having an aura. The most appropriate response for Judy would be to:
   A. Continue taking vital signs and reassure Beatrice that everything is okay
   B. Have Beatrice lie down on the floor, remove all objects around her, loosen restrictive clothing, and stay with her
   C. Run and get Dr. Cardio and make sure there is a tongue depressor in position in Beatrice's mouth
   D. Finish taking vitals and tell Beatrice she will be back to check on her in 10 minutes

8. Jane White calls the office and states that the 3-year-old she is babysitting has been chewing on leaves from her jade plant. She asks Judy Markins, CMA, if jade plants are poisonous. Judy should:
   A. Recommend that Mrs. White watch the toddler closely for symptoms of poisoning
   B. Have Mrs. White take the child to the local ER immediately
   C. Tell Mrs. White to call the Poison Control Center for information about the toxicity of jade plants
   D. Call Children's Services and report Mrs. White for child endangerment

9. Jeremy Jenkins is 6 years old and is brought to the office because he was bitten on the leg by a dog in his neighborhood. The bite is small and superficial. Appropriate actions for Judy Markins, CMA, to take would include all of the following EXCEPT:
   A. Ask for the name and address of the owner of the dog to determine if the animal's rabies vaccination is current
   B. Call the local dog warden to have the animal removed and exterminated
   C. Wash the area with soap and water, apply antibiotic ointment, and bandage
   D. Ask Jeremy's mother if his immunizations are up to date

10. Judy Markins, CMA, receives a frantic phone call from her next-door neighbor's niece. She states she came to visit her aunt and found her unconscious on the floor. When Judy goes to the house, she finds Mrs. Oxford to be very warm and dry to the touch, and her pulse is rapid and weak. Her breath has a "fruity" odor, and her respirations are rapid and deep. Mrs. Oxford has been an insulin-dependent diabetic for many years. Judy should:
   A. Call Mrs. Oxford's doctor and let him know about her condition
   B. Give Mrs. Oxford some orange juice because she is in insulin shock
   C. Administer 40 U of Regular Insulin because Mrs. Oxford is in a diabetic coma
   D. Call the EMS to take Mrs. Oxford to the hospital because her symptoms are suggestive of ketoacidosis

CERTIFICATIONREVIEW

❏ **First aid** is the immediate care that is administered to an individual who is injured or suddenly becomes ill before complete medical care can be obtained. The emergency medical services (EMS) system is a network of community resources, equipment, and medical personnel that provides emergency care to victims of injury or sudden illness.

❏ **Respiratory distress** indicates that the patient is breathing, but is having great difficulty in doing so. Asthma is a condition characterized by wheezing, coughing, and dyspnea. Emphysema is a progressive lung disorder in which the terminal bronchioles that lead into the alveoli become plugged with mucus. Hyperventilation is a manner of breathing, in which the respirations become rapid and deep, causing an individual to exhale too much carbon dioxide.

❏ **A heart attack,** also known as a myocardial infarction (MI), is caused by partial or complete obstruction of one or both of the coronary arteries or their branches. The principal symptom of a heart attack is chest pain or discomfort. The pain is usually felt behind the sternum and may radiate to the neck, throat, jaw, both shoulders, and arms.

❏ **A stroke** results when an artery to the brain is blocked or ruptures, interrupting the blood flow to the brain. The signs and symptoms of a stroke are sudden weakness or numbness of the face, arm, or leg on one side of the body; difficulty in speaking; dimmed vision or loss of vision in one eye; double vision; dizziness; confusion; severe headache; and loss of consciousness.

❏ **Shock** is the failure of the cardiovascular system to deliver enough blood to all the body's vital organs. Shock accompanies many types of emergency: hemorrhaging, a myocardial infarction, a severe allergic reaction. There are five major types of shock: hypovolemic, cardiogenic, neurogenic, anaphylactic, and psychogenic. The general signs and symptoms of shock are weakness, restlessness, anxiety, disorientation, pallor, cold, clammy skin, rapid breathing, and rapid pulse.

❏ **Hypovolemic shock** is caused by a loss of blood or other body fluids. Cardiogenic shock is caused by the failure of the heart to pump blood adequately to all the vital organs of the body. Neurogenic shock occurs when the nervous system is unable to control the diameter of the blood vessels. Anaphylactic shock is a life-threatening reaction of the body to an allergen. Psychogenic shock is caused by an unpleasant experience or emotional stimuli, such as pain, fright, or the sight of blood.

❏ **Bleeding or hemorrhaging** is the escape of blood from a severed blood vessel. External bleeding is bleeding that can be seen coming from a wound. The most effective way to control bleeding is through the application of direct pressure to the bleeding site. If bleeding cannot be controlled with di-rect pressure, a pressure point can be used. A pressure point is a site on the body where an artery lies close to the surface of the skin and can be compressed against an underlying bone. Internal bleeding is bleeding that flows into a body cavity, an organ, or between tissues.

❏ **A wound** is a break in the continuity of an external or internal surface caused by physical means. An open wound is a break in the skin surface or mucous membrane that exposes the underlying tissues; examples include incisions, lacerations, punctures, and abrasions.

❏ **An incision** is a clean, smooth cut caused by a sharp cutting instrument such as a knife, a razor, or a piece of glass. A laceration is a wound in which the tissues are torn apart, rather than cut, leaving ragged and irregular edges. A puncture is a wound made by a sharp, pointed object piercing the skin layers and sometimes the underlying structures. An abrasion is a wound in which the outer layers of the skin are scraped or rubbed off.

❏ **A closed wound** involves an injury to the underlying tissues of the body without a break in the skin or mucous membrane; an example is a contusion or bruise.

❏ **A fracture** is any break of a bone. A closed fracture occurs when there is a broken bone but no break in the skin over the fracture site. An open fracture involves a break in the bone along with a penetration of the overlying skin surface. The signs and symptoms of a fracture include pain and tenderness, deformity, swelling and discoloration, loss of function of the body part, and numbness or tingling.

❏ **A dislocation** is an injury in which one end of a bone making up a joint is separated or displaced from its normal position. A sprain is a tearing of ligaments at a joint. A strain is a stretching and tearing of muscles or tendons. A splint is any item that will immobilize a body part.

❏ **A burn** is an injury to the tissues caused by exposure to thermal, chemical, electrical, or radioactive agents. A superficial (first-degree) burn involves only the epidermis; an example is sunburn. A partial-thickness (second-degree) burn involves the epidermis and extends into the dermis. A full-thickness (third-degree) burn completely destroys both the epidermis and the dermis and extends into the underlying tissues such as fat, muscle, bone, and nerves.

❏ **A seizure** is a sudden episode of involuntary muscle contractions and relaxation often accompanied by a change in sensation, behavior, and level of consciousness. Seizures are classified as partial and generalized. In a partial seizure, the abnormal electrical activity is localized into very specific areas of the brain; only the brain functions in those areas are affected. With a generalized seizure, the abnormal electrical activity spreads through the entire brain.

Continued

CERTIFICATION REVIEW—Cont'd

❑ **A poison** is any substance that causes illness, injury, or death if it enters the body. Poisons that are ingested enter the body by being swallowed. A poison that is inhaled is breathed into the body in the form of gas, vapor, or spray. A poison that is absorbed enters the body through the skin. An injected poison enters the body through bites, through stings, or by a needle.

❑ **Heat cramps** are most apt to occur when an individual is exercising or working in a hot environment and fails to replace lost fluids and electrolytes. The symptoms are painful muscle spasms, particularly of the legs, calves, and abdomen; hot, sweaty skin; weakness; and a rapid pulse.

❑ **Heat exhaustion** occurs most often in individuals involved in vigorous physical activity on a hot and humid day. The symptoms of heat exhaustion are cold and clammy skin, profuse sweating, headache, nausea, dizziness, weakness, and diarrhea.

❑ **Heat stroke** is the most serious heat-related injury and is most apt to occur in elderly people during a heat wave and in athletes who overexert in a hot and humid environment. The symptoms of heat stroke are a body temperature of 105°F or higher; red, hot, dry skin; a rapid, weak pulse; dizziness and weakness; rapid, shallow breathing; decreased levels of consciousness; and seizures.

❑ **Frostbite** is the localized freezing of body tissue as a result of exposure to cold. Frostbite commonly affects the hands, fingers, feet, toes, ears, nose, and cheeks. Hypothermia is a life-threatening emergency in which the temperature of the entire body falls to a dangerously low level.

❑ **Diabetes mellitus** is a disease in which the body is unable to use glucose for energy because the body lacks enough insulin. Insulin shock (hypoglycemia) occurs when there is too much insulin in the body and not enough glucose. Diabetic coma occurs when there is not enough insulin in the body. This causes the blood glucose level to rise in the body, resulting in hyperglycemia.

Terminology Review

Burn An injury to the tissues caused by exposure to thermal, chemical, electrical, or radioactive agents.

Crash cart A specially equipped cart for holding and transporting medications, equipment, and supplies needed for life-saving procedures in an emergency.

Crepitus A grating sensation caused by fractured bone fragments rubbing against each other.

Dislocation An injury in which one end of a bone making up a joint is separated or displaced from its normal anatomic position.

Emergency medical services (EMS) system A network of community resources, equipment, and personnel that provides care to victims of injury or sudden illness.

First aid The immediate care administered to an individual who is injured or suddenly becomes ill before complete medical care can be obtained.

Fracture Any break in a bone.

Hypothermia A life-threatening condition in which the temperature of the entire body falls to a dangerously low level.

Poison Any substance that causes illness, injury, or death if it enters the body.

Pressure point A site on the body where an artery lies close to the surface of the skin and can be compressed against an underlying bone to control bleeding.

Seizure A sudden episode of involuntary muscular contractions and relaxation, often accompanied by a change in sensation, behavior, and level of consciousness.

Shock The failure of the cardiovascular system to deliver enough blood to all the vital organs of the body.

Splint Any device that will immobilize a body part.

Sprain Trauma to a joint, which causes tearing of ligaments.

Strain A stretching or tearing of muscles or tendons caused by trauma.

Wound A break in the continuity of an external or internal surface, caused by physical means.

ON THE WEB

For active weblinks to each website visit http://evolve.elsevier.com/Bonewit/.

For Information on Emergency Medicine:

American Red Cross

Federal Emergency Management Agency

Appendices

A Medical Abbreviations

B The Human Body Highlights
of Structure and Function

Medical Abbreviations

a̅a̅	of each
AA	affected area; Alcoholics Anonymous
AAA	abdominal aortic aneurysm
AAL	anterior axillary line
AAMA	American Association of Medical Assistants
Ab	abortion; antibody
ABC	airway, breathing, circulation
abd	abdomen
ABE	acute bacterial endocarditis
ABG	arterial blood gases
ABN	abnormal
ABO	a blood group system
ABP	arterial blood pressure
Abs	absent
ac	before meals (Latin: *ante cibum*)
ACLS	advanced cardiac life support
ACOA	adult child of an alcoholic
ACTH	adrenocorticotropic hormone
AD	right ear (Latin: *auris dextra*)
ADA	American Diabetic Association; American Dental Association
ADH	antidiuretic hormone
ADL	activities of daily living
ad lib	as desired
adm	admission, admit
admin	administer
AFB	acid-fast bacillus
A Fib	atrial fibrillation
AFL	atrial flutter
AFP	alpha-fetoprotein
A/G	albumin-to-globulin ratio
AGA	appropriate for gestational age
AGN	acute glomerular nephritis
AHA	American Heart Association
AI	aortic insufficiency
AICD	automatic implantable cardioverter-defibrillator
AIDS	acquired immunodeficiency syndrome
AJ	ankle jerk
AKA	above the knee amputation
AL	acute leukemia
alb	albumin
ALL	acute lymphoblastic leukemia
ALP	alkaline phosphatase
ALS	amyotrophic lateral sclerosis
ALT	alanine aminotransferase
AM or a.m.	before noon, morning (Latin: *ante meridiem*)
AMA	against medical advice; American Medical Association
amb	ambulatory
AMI	acute myocardial infarction
amnio	amniocentesis
amt	amount
anes	anesthesia, anesthetist
ant.	anterior
A/O	alert and oriented
AOM	acute otitis media
AP	apical pulse; angina pectoris
APC	atrial premature complex
approx	approximately
appt	appointment
aq	water
ARC	American Red Cross; AIDS-related complex
ARD	acute respiratory distress
ARDS	acute respiratory distress syndrome
AS	left ear (Latin: *auris sinistra*)
ASA	acetylsalicylic acid (aspirin)
ASAP	as soon as possible
ASCVD	arteriosclerotic cardiovascular disease
ASD	atrial septal defect
ASHD	arteriosclerotic heart disease
ASO	antistreptolysin-O; arteriosclerosis obliterans
AST	aspartate aminotransferase
ATR	Achilles tendon reflex
AU	both ears (Latin: *aurus unitas*); in each ear (Latin: *auris uterque*)
aud	auditory
AVR	aortic valve replacement
A & W	alive and well
ax	axillary
BA	backache
Ba	barium
Bab	Babinski (reflex)

bas	basophil		cc	cubic centimeter
BBB	bundle branch block; blood-brain barrier		CCU	coronary care unit; critical care unit
BBT	basal body temperature		CD	chemical dependence
b/c	because		C & D	cystoscopy and dilation
BC	birth control; bone conduction		CDC	Centers for Disease Control and Prevention
BCP	birth control pills		cerv	cervical, cervix
BE	barium enema		CF	cystic fibrosis
BEA	below elbow amputation		CFS	chronic fatigue syndrome
BG	blood glucose		CGL	chronic granulocytic leukemia
bid	twice a day (Latin: *bis in die*)		CH	crown-heel (length of baby)
bili	bilirubin		CHB	complete heart block
BJ	biceps jerk		CHD	congenital heart disease; coronary heart disease
BJM	bones, joints, and muscles		chemo	chemotherapy
BK	below knee		CHF	congestive heart failure
BKA	below knee amputation		CHL	conductive hearing loss
BLS	basic life support		Chol	cholesterol
BM	bowel movement		CIS	carcinoma in situ
BMR	basal metabolic rate		CK	creatine kinase
BOM	bilateral otitis media		cl	chloride, chlorine
BP	blood pressure		CLD	chronic lung disease
BPAD	bipolar affective disorder		cldy	cloudy
BPH	benign prostatic hypertrophy		cm	centimeter
BPM	beats per minute		cm^3	cubic centimeter
BR	bathroom		CMA	Certified Medical Assistant
BRB	bright red blood		CMV	cytomegalovirus
BrBx	breast biopsy		CNS	central nervous system
BS	blood sugar; breath sounds		CO	cardiac output
BSA	body surface area		c/o	complains of
BSE	breast self-examination		CO_2	carbon dioxide
BSN	bowel sounds normal		COPD	chronic obstructive pulmonary disease
BTL	bilateral tubal ligation		CP	cerebral palsy
BUN	blood urea nitrogen		CPK	creatine phosphokinase
BW	birth weight		CPN	chronic pyelonephritis
Bx	biopsy		CPR	cardiopulmonary resuscitation
			CR	crown-rump (length of baby)
$\bar{c}$	with		CRC	colorectal cancer
C	Celsius		CRD	chronic respiratory disease
C1	first cervical vertebra		CS	cesarean section
C2	second cervical vertebra		C & S	culture and sensitivity
Ca	calcium		CSF	cerebrospinal fluid
CA	cancer; cardiac arrest		CST	contraction stress test
CAD	coronary artery disease		CT	computed tomography
CAHD	coronary atherosclerotic heart disease		CTS	carpal tunnel syndrome
cal	calorie(s)		CV	cardiovascular
CAPD	continuous ambulatory peritoneal dialysis		CVA	cerebrovascular accident
			CVP	central venous pressure
caps	capsules		CVS	chorionic villus sampling; cardiovascular system
CAT	computerized axial tomography			
cath	catheter, catheterize		Cx	cervix
CB	cesarean birth		CXR	chest x-ray
CBC	complete blood count		Cysto	cystoscopy
CBD	common bile duct			
CBF	cerebral blood flow		d	day
CBR	complete bed rest		/day	per day
CC	chief complaint			

db	decibel	D/W	dextrose in water
DBE	deep breathing exercise	Dx	diagnosis
DBM	diabetic management	Dz	disease
DBP	diastolic blood pressure		
d/c	discontinue	ea	each
D & C	dilation and curettage	EAB	elective abortion
DD	discharge diagnosis	EAC	external auditory canal
DDD	degenerative disc disease	EAM	external auditory meatus
D/DW	dextrose, distilled water	EBL	estimated blood loss
DDx	differential diagnosis	EBV	Epstein-Barr virus
D & E	dilation and evacuation	EC	enteric-coated
DEA	Drug Enforcement Administration	ECD	esophago-gastroduodenoscopy
del	delivery	ECF	extended care facility
DES	diethylstilbestrol	ECG	electrocardiogram
DI	diabetes insipidus	Echo	echocardiogram
D & I	dry and intact	E. coli	Escherichia coli
diab	diabetic	ECT	electroconvulsive therapy
diff	differential white blood cell count	ED	emergency department
dil	dilute	EDD	expected date of delivery
disch	discharge	EEG	electroencephalogram
disp	dispense	EENT	eye, ear, nose, and throat
DIU	death in utero	EGA	estimated gestational age
DJD	degenerative joint disease	elect stim	electrical stimulation
DKA	diabetic ketoacidosis	ELISA	enzyme-linked immunosorbent assay
dL	deciliter		
DM	diabetes mellitus	elix	elixir
DNA	deoxyribonucleic acid	EmBx	endometrial biopsy
DNKA	did not keep appointment	EMG	electromyogram
DNR	do not resuscitate	EMS	emergency medical service
d/o	disorder	ENT	ear, nose, and throat
DOA	dead on arrival	EOM	extraocular movement
DOB	date of birth	eos	eosinophil
DOE	dyspnea on exertion	ER	emergency room
DOI	date of injury	ESR	erythrocyte sedimentation rate
DP	diastolic pressure	est	estimated
DPT	diphtheria, pertussis, and tetanus (vaccine)	ESWL	extracorporeal shock-wave lithotripsy
		ETT	endotracheal tube
DR	delivery room	EVAL	evaluation
dr	dram	ex	exercise
DRE	digital rectal exam	ext	extract
DRG	diagnosis-related group	Ez	eczema
drsg	dressing		
DS	double strength	F	Fahrenheit
D/S	discharge summary	FA	fluorescent antibody
DSD	dry sterile dressing	FB	foreign body
DT	diphtheria and tetanus toxoid	FBP	femoral blood pressure
DTaP	diphtheria and tetanus toxoids and acellular pertussis vaccine	FBS	fasting blood sugar
		FD	fully dilated
DTR	deep tendon reflex	FDA	Food and Drug Administration
DU	duodenal ulcer	Fe	iron
DUB	dysfunctional uterine bleeding	Fe def	iron deficiency
DUI	driving under the influence (of alcohol)	FEF	forced expiratory flow
D & V	diarrhea and vomiting	FEKG	fetal electrocardiogram
DVA	distance visual acuity	FEV	forced expiratory volume
DVT	deep venous thrombosis	FFP	fresh frozen plasma
DW	distilled water	FH	family history

FHR	fetal heart rate	Hct	hematocrit
FHT	fetal heart tones	HCVD	hypertensive cardiovascular disease
fl	fluid	HD	Hodgkin's disease
flex sig	flexible sigmoidoscopy	HDL	high-density lipoprotein
FMP	first menstrual period	HDN	hemolytic disease of the newborn
FOB	fetal occult blood	HEENT	head, eye, ear, nose, and throat
FOBT	fecal occult blood test	Hep	heparin
FP	family practice	Hep B	hepatitis B vaccine
freq	frequent	Hg	mercury
FS	finger stick	Hgb	hemoglobin
FSH	follicle-stimulating hormone	HGM	home glucose monitoring
ft	foot	HH	home health
FT	full term	H & H	hemoglobin and hematocrit
FTND	full-term normal delivery	Hib	Haemophilus influenzae type b
FTT	failure to thrive		conjugate vaccine
F/U	follow-up	HIV	human immunodeficiency virus
FUO	fever of undetermined origin	H & L	heart and lungs
FVC	forced vital capacity	HMO	health maintenance organization
FWB	full weight bearing	H/O	history of
Fx	fracture	H_2O	water
		H & P	history and physical
g	gram	HPF	high-power field
G	gravida	HPI	history of present illness
GA	general anesthesia; gestational age	*H. pylori*	*Helicobacter pylori*
GB	gallbladder	HR	heart rate
GC	gonorrhea; gas chromatography	HRT	hormone replacement therapy
GCT	glucose challenge test	hs	at bedtime (Latin: *hora somni*)
GDM	gestational diabetes mellitus	HSV	herpes simplex virus
gen	general	ht	height
GFR	glomerular filtration rate	HTN	hypertension
GH	growth hormone	HVD	hypertensive vascular disease
GI	gastrointestinal	Hx	history
glu	glucose	Hz	hertz
Gm−	gram negative		
Gm+	gram positive	IA	intraarterial
GM	gross motor	IABP	intraaortic balloon pump
GP	general practitioner	IBS	irritable bowel syndrome
gr	grain	IBW	ideal body weight
GSW	gunshot wound	ICCU	intensive coronary care unit
gtt(s)	drop (drops)	ICD	International Classification of Diseases
GTT	glucose tolerance test		(of the World Health Organization)
GU	genitourinary	ICDA	International Classification of Diseases,
G/W	glucose in water		Adapted
GYN	gynecology	ICF	intracellular fluid
		ICP	intracranial pressure
h	hour	ICS	intercostals space
H/A	headache	ICU	intensive care unit
HAL	hyperalimentation	ID	intradermal
HAV	hepatitis A virus	I & D	incision and drainage
HBIG	hepatitis B immunoglobulin	IDDM	insulin-dependent diabetes mellitus
HBP	high blood pressure	IM	intramuscular
HBsAg	hepatitis B surface antigen	Immuniz	immunizations
HBV	hepatitis B virus	imp	impression
HC	head circumference	in	inch
HCG	human chorionic gonadotropin	I & O	intake and output
HCl	hydrochloric acid	IOP	intraocular pressure

IPPB	intermittent positive pressure breathing
IPV	inactivated polio vaccine
IQ	intelligence quotient
IU	international unit
IUD	intrauterine device
IUFD	intrauterine fetal death
IUGR	intrauterine growth rate
IV	intravenous
IVP	intravenous pyelogram
JAMA	*Journal of the American Medical Association*
jaund	jaundice
JODM	juvenile onset diabetes mellitus
JP	Jackson Pratt (drain)
JRA	juvenile rheumatoid arthritis
JVD	jugular venous distention
JVP	jugular venous pressure
K	potassium
KCl	potassium chloride
kg	kilogram
KOH	potassium hydroxide
KUB	kidney, ureter, and bladder
L	liter
l	length
LA	left atrium
lab	laboratory
lac	laceration
lap	laparotomy
lat	lateral
LAVH	laparoscopic assisted vaginal hysterectomy
lax	laxative
LB	lower back
lb	pound
LBBB	left bundle branch block
LBP	low back pain
LBW	low birth weight
LD	lactate dehydrogenase
L & D	labor and delivery
LDL	low-density lipoprotein
LE	lupus erythematosus
LFD	low forceps delivery
LFT	liver function test
lg	large
LGA	large for gestational age
LH	luteinizing hormone
liq	liquid
LLC	long leg cast
LLE	left lower extremity
LLL	left lower leg
LLQ	left lower quadrant
LMP	last menstrual period
LNMP	last normal menstrual period

LOC	loss of consciousness
LOM	loss of motion
LP	lumbar puncture
LPF	low-power field
LR	labor room
LRQ	lower right quadrant
LS	lumbosacral
lt	left
LTC	long-term care
LTM	long-term memory
LUE	left upper extremity
LUQ	left upper quadrant
LV	left ventricle
L & W	living and well
lymphs	lymphocytes
m	meter
mcg	microgram
MCH	mean corpuscular hemoglobin
MCHC	mean corpuscular hemoglobin concentration
MCL	midclavicular line
MCV	mean corpuscular volume
MD	muscular dystrophy; medical doctor
MDE	major depressive episode
MDI	metered dose inhaler
MDR	minimum daily requirement
med(s)	medication(s)
mEq/L	milliequivalents per liter
mg	milligram
MG	myasthenia gravis
MGF	maternal grandfather
MGM	maternal grandmother
MH	marital history
MHx	medical history
MI	myocardial infarction
min	minute
ml	milliliter
mm	millimeter
mm^3	cubic millimeter
mm Hg	millimeters of mercury
mmol	millimole
MMR	measles, mumps, and rubella (vaccine)
MO	month old
mod	moderate
MODM	mature-onset diabetes mellitus
mono	mononucleosis
MP	menstrual period
MR	mitral regurgitation; mental retardation
MRI	magnetic resonance imaging
MRM	modified radical mastectomy
MS	multiple sclerosis
MSL	midsternal line
MSU	midstream urine specimen
MT	medical technologist
multip	multipara

MV	mitral valve		O	oral
MVA	motor vehicle accident		O$_2$	oxygen
MVP	mitral valve prolapse		OA	osteoarthritis
MVR	mitral valve replacement		OB	obstetrics
			OB/GYN	obstetrics and gynecology
Na	sodium		obs	observed
N/A	not applicable		occ	occasionally
NaCl	sodium chloride		OCD	obsessive-compulsive disorder
NAD	nothing abnormal detected; no appreciable disease		OCT	oxytocin challenge test
			OD	right eye
narc	narcotic		O & E	observation and examination
NB	newborn		O/E	on examination
NBS	normal bowel sounds: normal breath sounds		OH	occupational history
			oint	ointment
NBW	normal birth weight		OM	otitis media
NC	no change		OOB	out of bed
N/C	no complaints		op	operation
NED	no evidence of disease		OP	outpatient
neg	negative		O & P	ova and parasites
NG	nasogastric		OPV	oral polio vaccine
NGT	nasogastric tube		OR	operating room
NGU	nongonococcal urethritis		ortho	orthopedics
NH	nursing home		OS	left eye
NHL	non-Hodgkin's lymphoma		OT	occupational therapy
NI	not improved		OTC	over the counter (nonprescription medication)
NICU	newborn intensive care unit			
NIDDM	non–insulin-dependent diabetes mellitus		OU	in each eye (Latin: *oculus uterque*); both eyes
NKA	no known allergies			
NKDA	no known drug allergies		OV	office visit
NL	normal limits		oz	ounce
NMP	normal menstrual period			
NMR	nuclear magnetic resonance		P	pulse
noct	nocturnal		PA	posteroanterior; physician assistant
non rep	do not repeat		PAC	premature atrial contraction
nor.	normal		Pap	Pap test
NPO	nothing by mouth (Latin: *nil per os*)		PAT	paroxysmal atrial tachycardia
NR	no refill		path	pathology
N/R	not responsible		Pb	lead
NS	normal saline		PBI	protein-bound iodine
NSAID	nonsteroidal antiinflammatory drug		pc	after meals (Latin: *post cibum*)
			PC	platelet count
NSR	normal sinus rhythm		PCC	Poison Control Center
NSS	normal saline solution		PCV	packed cell volume
NST	nonstress test		PD	Parkinson's disease
NSU	nonspecific urethritis		*PDR*	*Physician's Desk Reference*
NSVD	normal spontaneous vaginal delivery		PE	physical examination
			peds	pediatrics
NT	nontender		PEG	pneumoencephalogram; pneumoencephalography
N & T	nose and throat			
nullip	nullipara (never gave birth)		PEN	penicillin; pharmacy equivalent name
N & V	nausea and vomiting		per	by, through
NVA	near visual acuity		peri	perineal
NVD	nausea, vomiting, and diarrhea		PERRLA	pupils equal, round, regular, react to light, and accommodation (normal)
N & W	normal and well			
NWB	non-weight-bearing		PET	positron emission tomography
NYD	not yet diagnosed		PFS	pulmonary function studies

PFT	pulmonary function test	q	each; every (Latin: *quaque*)
PGF	paternal grandfather	q AM	every morning
PGH	pituitary growth hormone	qd	every day (Latin: *quaque die*)
PGM	paternal grandmother	qh	every hour (Latin: *quaque hora*)
pH	hydrogen ion concentration	q2h (q3h, q4h)	every 2 (3, 4) hours
PH	past history	qid	four times a day (Latin: *quater in die*)
pharm	pharmacy	qn	every night (Latin: *quaque nocturnus*)
PI	present illness	QNS	quantity not sufficient
PID	pelvic inflammatory disease	qod	every other day (Latin: *quater in die*)
PIH	pregnancy induced hypertension	QS	quantity sufficient
PKU	phenylketonuria	qt	quart
PM or p.m.	afternoon, evening (Latin: *post meridiem*)	quad	quadriplegic
PMB	postmenopausal bleeding		
PMH	past medical history	R	respiration
PMN	polymorphonuclear neutrophils	RA	rheumatoid arthritis
PMP	past menstrual period	RAF	rheumatoid arthritis factor
PMS	premenstrual syndrome	RAST	radioallergosorbent test
PMT	premenstrual tension	RBC/HPF	red blood cells per high power field
PN	progress notes		
PND	paroxysmal nocturnal dyspnea	RBC	red blood cell; red blood (cell) count
PNX	pneumothorax		
po	by mouth (Latin: *per os*)	RBCV	red blood cell volume
PO	by mouth (Latin: *per os*)	RBS	random blood sugar
POL	physician's office laboratory	RCV	red cell volume
POR	problem-oriented medical record	RD	respiratory distress
pos	positive	RDA	recommended daily allowance
postop	postoperative (after surgery)	RDS	respiratory distress syndrome
PP	postpartum	RE	rectal examination
PPB	positive pressure breathing	reg	regular
PPBS	postprandial blood sugar	rehab	rehabilitation
PPD	purified protein derivative	REM	rapid eye movement
PPH	postpartum hemorrhage	REP	retrograde pyelogram
PPT	partial prothrombin time	resp	respiration
preop	preoperative (before surgery)	RF	rheumatic fever
prep	preparation	RG	random glucose
primip	woman bearing first child	Rh	rhesus blood factor
prn	as the occasion arises, as necessary (Latin: *pro re nata*)	RHD	rheumatic heart disease
		RHF	right heart failure
procto	proctoscopy	RI	respiratory illness
prog	prognosis	RLQ	right lower quadrant
PROM	premature rupture of membranes	RMA	Registered Medical Assistant
prox	proximal	RMSF	Rocky Mountain spotted fever
PSA	prostate-specific antigen	RNA	ribonucleic acid
pt	patient; pint	R/O	rule out
Pt	patient	ROM	rupture of membranes; range of motion
PT	physical therapy; prothrombin time		
PTA	prior to admission	ROS	review of systems
PTB	prior to birth	RP	retrograde pyelogram
PTD	prior to discharge	RQ	respiratory quotient
PTH	parathyroid hormone	RRR	regular rate and rhythm
PTT	partial thromboplastin time	RSV	respiratory syncytial virus
PUD	peptic ulcer disease	rt	right
PVC	premature ventricular contraction	RT	room temperature; radiation therapy
PVD	peripheral vascular disease	R/T	related to
PWB	partial weight-bearing	RTW	return to work
Px	physical examination	RUE	right upper extremity

RUQ	right upper quadrant		std	standard
RV	right ventricle		STM	short-term memory
RVH	right ventricular hypertrophy		*Strep*	*Streptococcus*
Rx	prescription		subcut	subcutaneous
			sup	superior
s̄	without		supp	suppository
SA	sinoatrial		surg	surgery
SAB	spontaneous abortion		SV	stroke volume
SARS	severe acute respiratory syndrome		Sx	symptoms
SB	stillborn; sinus bradycardia		Sz	seizure
SBE	subacute bacterial endocarditis			
SBO	small bowel obstruction		T	temperature
SBP	systolic blood pressure		T_3	triiodothyronine
SC	subcutaneous		T_4	thyroxine
SCD	sudden cardiac death		T & A	tonsils and adenoids
schiz	schizophrenia		tab(s)	tablet(s)
SCI	spinal cord injury		TAB	therapeutic abortion
SD	spontaneous delivery; standard deviation		TAH	total abdominal hysterectomy
			TB	tuberculosis
SDH	subdural hematoma		TBF	total body fat
S/E	side effects		TBLC	term birth, living child
sec	second		tbsp	tablespoon
sed rate	sedimentation rate		TBW	total body water
segs	segmented neutrophils		TC	total capacity
seq	sequela		T & C	type and crossmatch
SF	scarlet fever; spinal fluid		temp	temperature
SG	specific gravity		TENS	transcutaneous electrical nerve stimulation
SGA	small for gestational age			
SH	social history; serum hepatitis		TF	tube feeding; transfer factor
sid	once a day (Latin: *semel in die*)		ther	therapy
SIDS	sudden infant death syndrome		THR	total hip replacement
sig	write on label		TIA	transient ischemic attack
sigmoid	sigmoidoscopy		tid	three times a day (Latin: *ter in die*)
sl	slight		tinct	tincture
SLC	short leg cast		TKR	total knee replacement
SLE	systemic lupus erythematosus		TLC	total lung capacity; tender loving care
SM	simple mastectomy		TM	tympanic membrane
sm	small		TMJ	temporomandibular joint
SNF	skilled nursing facility		TND	term normal delivery
SOAP	subjective data, objective data, assessment, and plan		TO	telephone order
			tol	tolerate, tolerated
SOB	shortness of breath		TOP	termination of pregnancy
sol	solution		TOPV	trivalent oral poliovirus vaccine
SOM	serous otitis media		TP	total protein
sp gr	specific gravity		TPM	temporary pacemaker
SP	systolic pressure		TPN	total parenteral nutrition
SPA	suprapubic aspiration		TPR	temperature, pulse, and respiration
spec	specimen		Tq	tourniquet
spont ab	spontaneous abortion		tr	trace
SQ	subcutaneous		trig	triglycerides
SR	sustained release		TRUS	transrectal ultrasound
SROM	spontaneous rupture of membranes		TSE	testicular self-examination
ss	one-half		TSH	thyroid-stimulating hormone
Staph	*Staphylococcus*		tsp	teaspoon
STAT	immediately		TSP	total serum protein
STD	sexually transmitted disease		TSS	toxic shock syndrome

TVH	total vaginal hysterectomy	VHDL	very-high-density lipoprotein
Tx	treatment	vit	vitamin
		VLDL	very-low-density lipoprotein
U	unit	VO	verbal order
UA	urinalysis	VP	venipuncture
UC	ulcerative colitis	VS	vital signs
U/C	urine culture	VSD	ventricular septal defect
UCG	urinary chorionic gonadotropin	VSS	vital signs stable
UCHD	usual childhood diseases	VT	ventricular tachycardia
UE	upper extremity	VV	varicose veins
UGI	upper gastrointestinal		
ULQ	upper left quadrant	WB	weight bearing
UOQ	upper outer quadrant	WBAT	weight bearing as tolerated
UR	upper respiratory	WBC	white blood cell; white blood (cell) count
URI	upper respiratory infection		
Urol	urology	WC	white cell
URQ	upper right quadrant	W/C	wheelchair
US	ultrasound	WDWN	well developed, well nourished
USI	urinary stress incontinence	wk	week
USP	*United States Pharmacopoeia*	WN	well nourished
UT	urinary tract	WNF	well-nourished female
UTI	urinary tract infection	WNL	within normal limits
UV	ultraviolet	WNM	well-nourished male
		WO	written order
VA	visual acuity	w/o	without
VAD	vascular access device	WR	weakly reactive
vag	vagina; vaginal	wt	weight
VAP	vascular access port	W/U	workup
VC	vital capacity		
VD	venereal disease	X	magnification
VDRL	Venereal Disease Research Laboratory (test)	XM	crossmatch
		XR	x-ray
VE	vaginal examination		
VFib	ventricular fibrillation	y	year(s)
VH	vaginal hysterectomy	yd	yard(s)
VHD	valvular heart disease	YOB	year of birth

The Human Body Highlights of Structure and Function

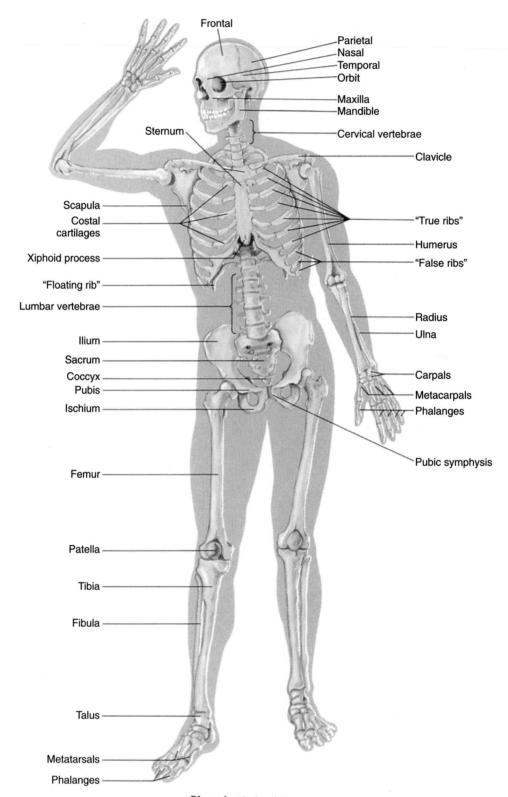

Plate 1. Skeletal System

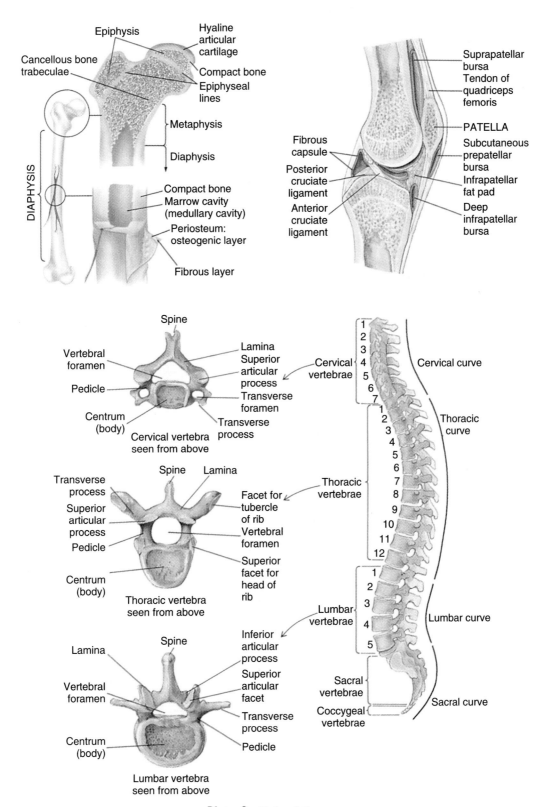

Epiphysis

Hyaline articular cartilage

Cancellous bone trabeculae

Compact bone

Epiphyseal lines

Metaphysis

Diaphysis

DIAPHYSIS

Compact bone

Marrow cavity (medullary cavity)

Periosteum: osteogenic layer

Fibrous layer

Suprapatellar bursa

Tendon of quadriceps femoris

Fibrous capsule

PATELLA

Posterior cruciate ligament

Subcutaneous prepatellar bursa

Infrapatellar fat pad

Anterior cruciate ligament

Deep infrapatellar bursa

Spine

Vertebral foramen

Lamina

Superior articular process

Pedicle

Transverse foramen

Centrum (body)

Transverse process

Cervical vertebra seen from above

Cervical vertebrae

1 2 3 4 5 6 7

Cervical curve

Transverse process

Spine

Lamina

Superior articular process

Facet for tubercle of rib

Pedicle

Vertebral foramen

Centrum (body)

Superior facet for head of rib

Thoracic vertebra seen from above

Thoracic vertebrae

1 2 3 4 5 6 7 8 9 10 11 12

Thoracic curve

Lamina

Spine

Inferior articular process

Vertebral foramen

Superior articular facet

Centrum (body)

Transverse process

Pedicle

Lumbar vertebra seen from above

Lumbar vertebrae

1 2 3 4 5

Lumbar curve

Sacral vertebrae

Coccygeal vertebrae

Sacral curve

Plate 2. Skeletal System.

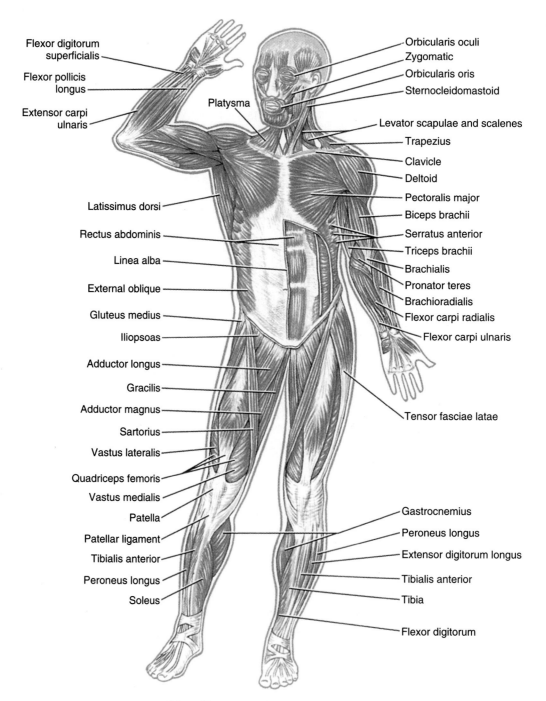

Flexor digitorum superficialis

Flexor pollicis longus

Extensor carpi ulnaris

Platysma

Latissimus dorsi

Rectus abdominis

Linea alba

External oblique

Gluteus medius

Iliopsoas

Adductor longus

Gracilis

Adductor magnus

Sartorius

Vastus lateralis

Quadriceps femoris

Vastus medialis

Patella

Patellar ligament

Tibialis anterior

Peroneus longus

Soleus

Orbicularis oculi

Zygomatic

Orbicularis oris

Sternocleidomastoid

Levator scapulae and scalenes

Trapezius

Clavicle

Deltoid

Pectoralis major

Biceps brachii

Serratus anterior

Triceps brachii

Brachialis

Pronator teres

Brachioradialis

Flexor carpi radialis

Flexor carpi ulnaris

Tensor fasciae latae

Gastrocnemius

Peroneus longus

Extensor digitorum longus

Tibialis anterior

Tibia

Flexor digitorum

Plate 3. Anterior Superficial Muscles

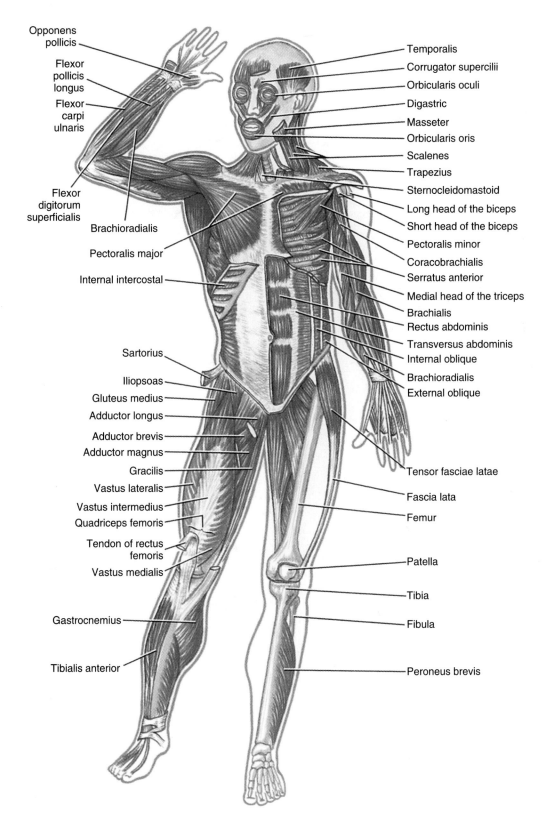

Opponens pollicis
Flexor pollicis longus
Flexor carpi ulnaris
Flexor digitorum superficialis
Brachioradialis
Pectoralis major
Internal intercostal
Sartorius
Iliopsoas
Gluteus medius
Adductor longus
Adductor brevis
Adductor magnus
Gracilis
Vastus lateralis
Vastus intermedius
Quadriceps femoris
Tendon of rectus femoris
Vastus medialis
Gastrocnemius
Tibialis anterior

Temporalis
Corrugator supercilii
Orbicularis oculi
Digastric
Masseter
Orbicularis oris
Scalenes
Trapezius
Sternocleidomastoid
Long head of the biceps
Short head of the biceps
Pectoralis minor
Coracobrachialis
Serratus anterior
Medial head of the triceps
Brachialis
Rectus abdominis
Transversus abdominis
Internal oblique
Brachioradialis
External oblique
Tensor fasciae latae
Fascia lata
Femur
Patella
Tibia
Fibula
Peroneus brevis

Plate 4. Anterior Deep Muscles

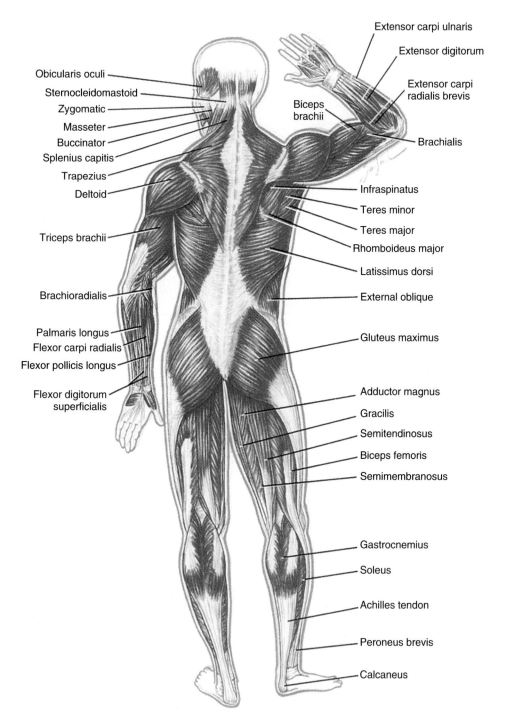

Obicularis oculi

Sternocleidomastoid

Zygomatic

Masseter

Buccinator

Splenius capitis

Trapezius

Deltoid

Triceps brachii

Brachioradialis

Palmaris longus

Flexor carpi radialis

Flexor pollicis longus

Flexor digitorum
superficialis

Extensor carpi ulnaris

Extensor digitorum

Extensor carpi
radialis brevis

Biceps
brachii

Brachialis

Infraspinatus

Teres minor

Teres major

Rhomboideus major

Latissimus dorsi

External oblique

Gluteus maximus

Adductor magnus

Gracilis

Semitendinosus

Biceps femoris

Semimembranosus

Gastrocnemius

Soleus

Achilles tendon

Peroneus brevis

Calcaneus

Plate 5. Posterior Superficial Muscles

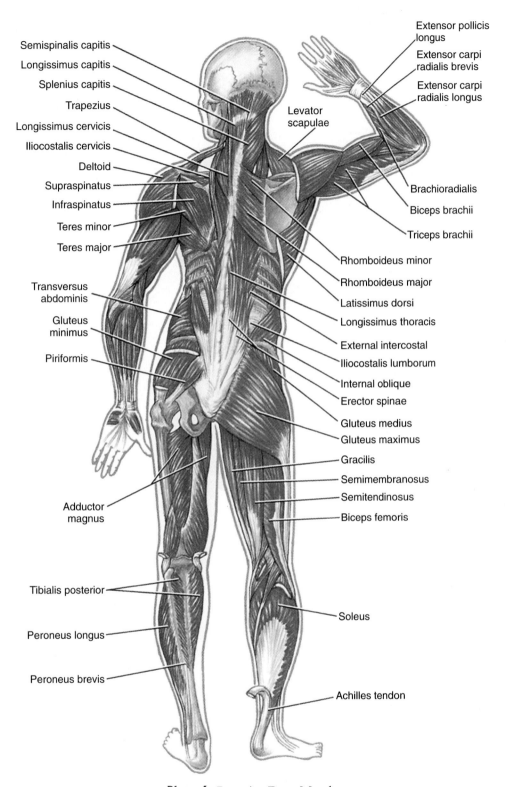

Semispinalis capitis

Longissimus capitis

Splenius capitis

Trapezius

Longissimus cervicis

Iliocostalis cervicis

Deltoid

Supraspinatus

Infraspinatus

Teres minor

Teres major

Transversus abdominis

Gluteus minimus

Piriformis

Adductor magnus

Tibialis posterior

Peroneus longus

Peroneus brevis

Extensor pollicis longus

Extensor carpi radialis brevis

Extensor carpi radialis longus

Levator scapulae

Brachioradialis

Biceps brachii

Triceps brachii

Rhomboideus minor

Rhomboideus major

Latissimus dorsi

Longissimus thoracis

External intercostal

Iliocostalis lumborum

Internal oblique

Erector spinae

Gluteus medius

Gluteus maximus

Gracilis

Semimembranosus

Semitendinosus

Biceps femoris

Soleus

Achilles tendon

Plate 6. Posterior Deep Muscles

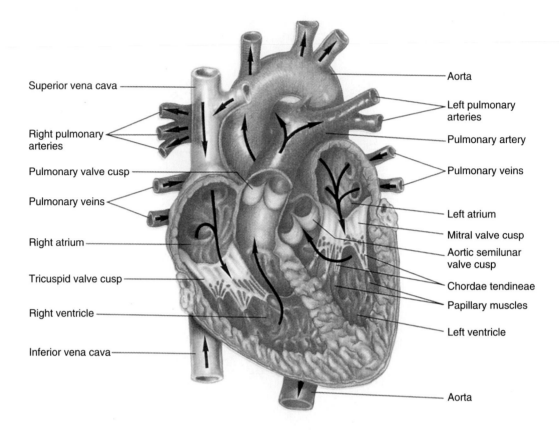

Superior vena cava

Right pulmonary arteries

Pulmonary valve cusp

Pulmonary veins

Right atrium

Tricuspid valve cusp

Right ventricle

Inferior vena cava

Aorta

Left pulmonary arteries

Pulmonary artery

Pulmonary veins

Left atrium

Mitral valve cusp

Aortic semilunar valve cusp

Chordae tendineae

Papillary muscles

Left ventricle

Aorta

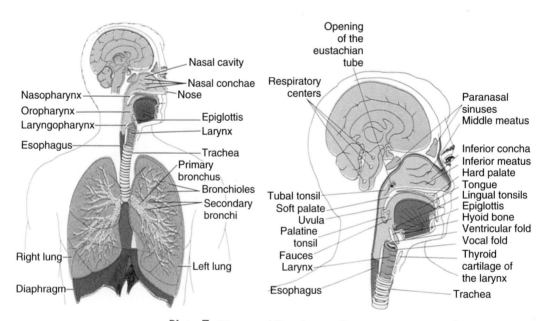

Nasal cavity

Nasal conchae

Nose

Nasopharynx

Oropharynx

Laryngopharynx

Esophagus

Epiglottis

Larynx

Trachea

Primary bronchus

Bronchioles

Secondary bronchi

Right lung

Left lung

Diaphragm

Opening of the eustachian tube

Respiratory centers

Paranasal sinuses

Middle meatus

Inferior concha

Inferior meatus

Hard palate

Tongue

Lingual tonsils

Epiglottis

Hyoid bone

Ventricular fold

Vocal fold

Thyroid cartilage of the larynx

Trachea

Tubal tonsil

Soft palate

Uvula

Palatine tonsil

Fauces

Larynx

Esophagus

Plate 7. Heart and Respiratory System

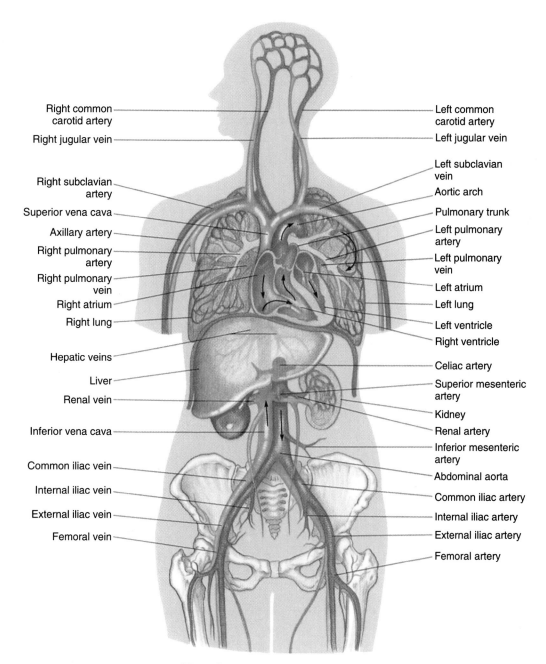

Right common carotid artery
Right jugular vein
Right subclavian artery
Superior vena cava
Axillary artery
Right pulmonary artery
Right pulmonary vein
Right atrium
Right lung
Hepatic veins
Liver
Renal vein
Inferior vena cava
Common iliac vein
Internal iliac vein
External iliac vein
Femoral vein

Left common carotid artery
Left jugular vein
Left subclavian vein
Aortic arch
Pulmonary trunk
Left pulmonary artery
Left pulmonary vein
Left atrium
Left lung
Left ventricle
Right ventricle
Celiac artery
Superior mesenteric artery
Kidney
Renal artery
Inferior mesenteric artery
Abdominal aorta
Common iliac artery
Internal iliac artery
External iliac artery
Femoral artery

Plate 8. Circulatory System—Blood

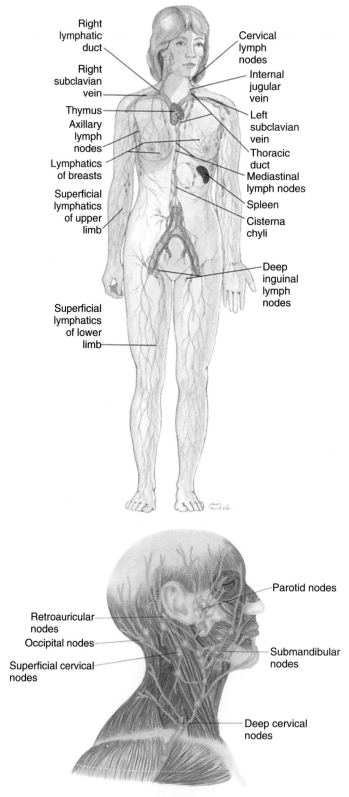

Right lymphatic duct

Right subclavian vein

Thymus

Axillary lymph nodes

Lymphatics of breasts

Superficial lymphatics of upper limb

Superficial lymphatics of lower limb

Cervical lymph nodes

Internal jugular vein

Left subclavian vein

Thoracic duct

Mediastinal lymph nodes

Spleen

Cisterna chyli

Deep inguinal lymph nodes

Parotid nodes

Retroauricular nodes

Occipital nodes

Superficial cervical nodes

Submandibular nodes

Deep cervical nodes

Plate 9. Circulatory System–Lymph

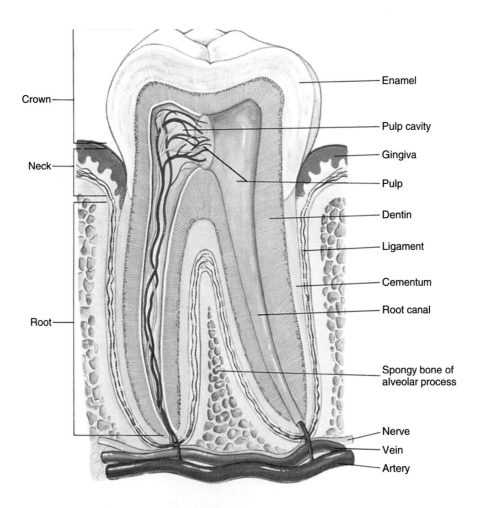

Crown

Neck

Root

Enamel

Pulp cavity

Gingiva

Pulp

Dentin

Ligament

Cementum

Root canal

Spongy bone of alveolar process

Nerve

Vein

Artery

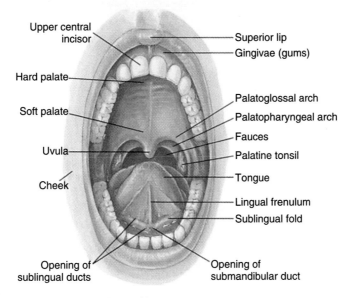

Upper central incisor

Hard palate

Soft palate

Uvula

Cheek

Opening of sublingual ducts

Superior lip

Gingivae (gums)

Palatoglossal arch

Palatopharyngeal arch

Fauces

Palatine tonsil

Tongue

Lingual frenulum

Sublingual fold

Opening of submandibular duct

Plate 10. Digestive System

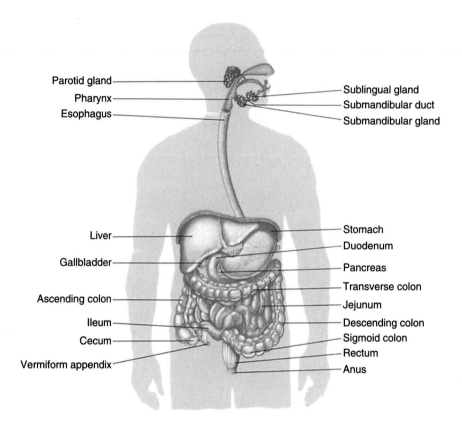

Parotid gland
Pharynx
Esophagus
Sublingual gland
Submandibular duct
Submandibular gland

Liver
Gallbladder
Ascending colon
Ileum
Cecum
Vermiform appendix

Stomach
Duodenum
Pancreas
Transverse colon
Jejunum
Descending colon
Sigmoid colon
Rectum
Anus

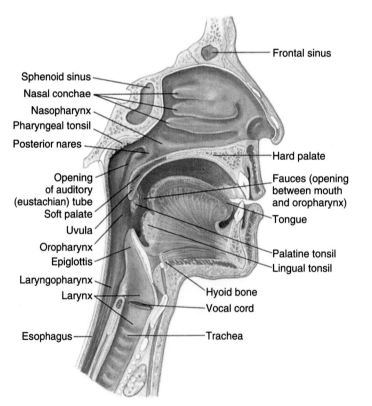

Frontal sinus

Sphenoid sinus
Nasal conchae
Nasopharynx
Pharyngeal tonsil
Posterior nares

Opening
of auditory
(eustachian) tube
Soft palate
Uvula
Oropharynx
Epiglottis
Laryngopharynx
Larynx
Esophagus

Hard palate
Fauces (opening
between mouth
and oropharynx)
Tongue
Palatine tonsil
Lingual tonsil
Hyoid bone
Vocal cord
Trachea

Plate 11. Digestive System.

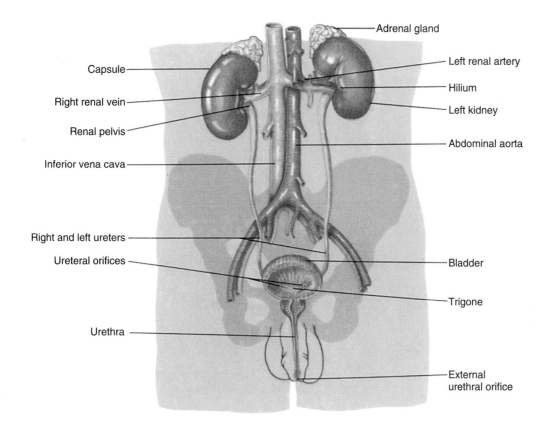

Adrenal gland

Capsule

Right renal vein

Renal pelvis

Inferior vena cava

Left renal artery

Hilium

Left kidney

Abdominal aorta

Right and left ureters

Ureteral orifices

Urethra

Bladder

Trigone

External urethral orifice

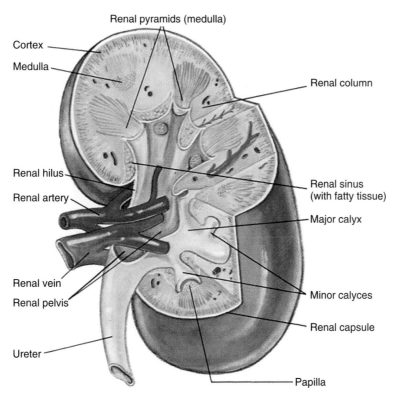

Renal pyramids (medulla)

Cortex

Medulla

Renal hilus

Renal artery

Renal vein

Renal pelvis

Ureter

Renal column

Renal sinus (with fatty tissue)

Major calyx

Minor calyces

Renal capsule

Papilla

Plate 12. Genitourinary System

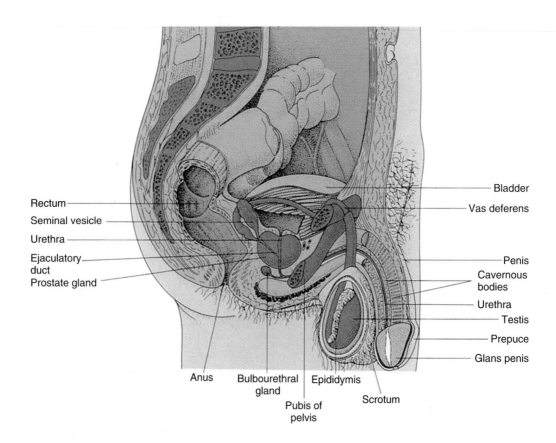

Rectum

Seminal vesicle

Urethra

Ejaculatory
duct

Prostate gland

Bladder

Vas deferens

Penis

Cavernous
bodies

Urethra

Testis

Prepuce

Glans penis

Anus   Bulbourethral   Epididymis
            gland

                              Scrotum

Pubis of
pelvis

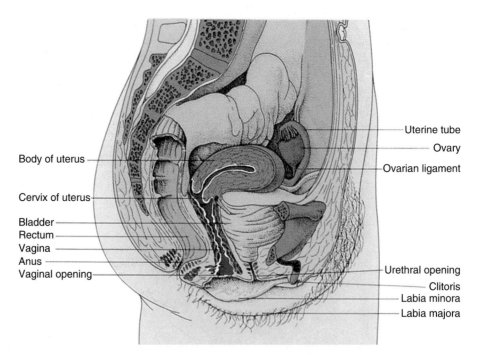

Body of uterus

Cervix of uterus

Bladder
Rectum
Vagina
Anus
Vaginal opening

Uterine tube

Ovary

Ovarian ligament

Urethral opening

Clitoris

Labia minora

Labia majora

Plate 13. Genitourinary System.

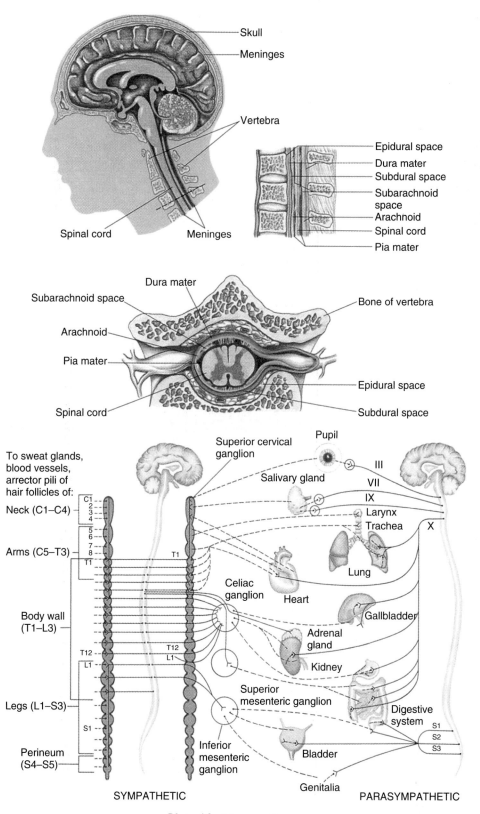

Plate 14. Nervous System

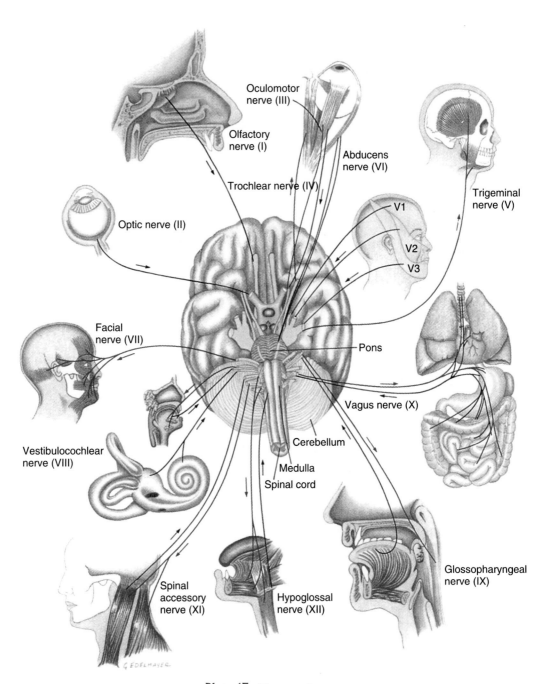

Plate 15. Nervous System.

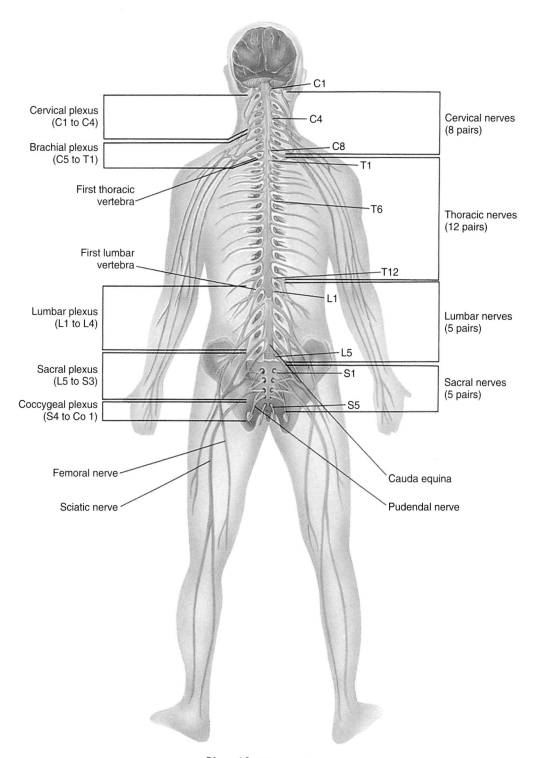

Plate 16. Nervous System.

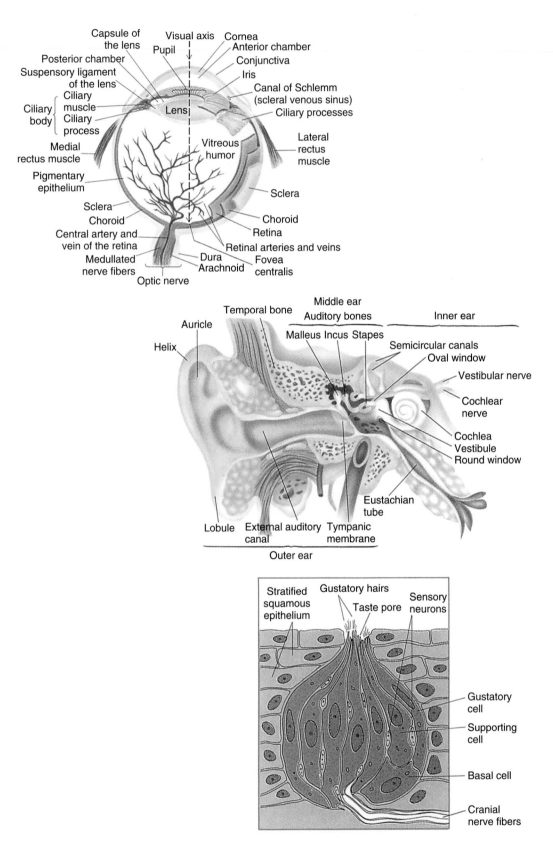

Plate 17. Organs of Special Sense

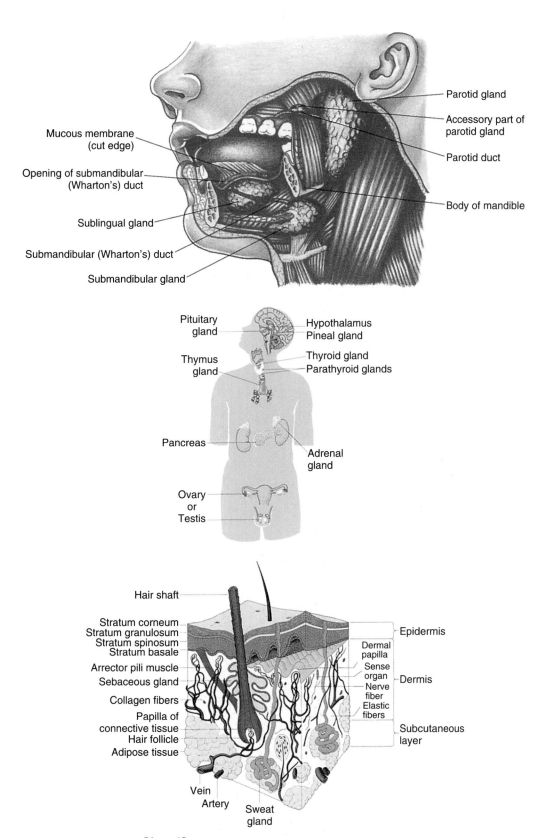

Parotid gland

Accessory part of
parotid gland

Parotid duct

Mucous membrane
(cut edge)

Opening of submandibular
(Wharton's) duct

Body of mandible

Sublingual gland

Submandibular (Wharton's) duct

Submandibular gland

Pituitary
gland

Hypothalamus
Pineal gland

Thymus
gland

Thyroid gland
Parathyroid glands

Pancreas

Adrenal
gland

Ovary
or
Testis

Hair shaft

Stratum corneum
Stratum granulosum
Stratum spinosum
Stratum basale

Epidermis

Dermal
papilla

Arrector pili muscle

Sense
organ

Sebaceous gland

Dermis

Nerve
fiber
Elastic
fibers

Collagen fibers

Papilla of
connective tissue
Hair follicle

Subcutaneous
layer

Adipose tissue

Vein
Artery

Sweat
gland

Plate 18. Salivary and Endocrine Glands and Skin

Glossary

Abortion The termination of a pregnancy before the fetus reached the stage of viability.

Abrasion A wound in which the outer layers of the skin are damaged; a scrape.

Abscess A collection of pus in a cavity surrounded by inflamed tissue.

Absorbable suture Suture material that is gradually digested by tissue enzymes and absorbed by the body.

Adolescent An individual from 12- to 18-years of age.

Adnexal Adjacent.

Adventitious sounds Abnormal breath sounds.

Adverse reaction An unintended and undesirable effect produced by a drug.

Aerobe A microorganism that needs oxygen in order to live and grow.

Afebrile Without fever; the body temperature is normal.

Agglutination The aggregation or uniting of separate particles into clumps or masses; the clumping of blood cells.

Allergen A substance that is capable of causing an allergic reaction.

Allergy An abnormal hypersensitivity of the body to substances that are ordinarily harmless.

Alveolus (pl. **alveoli**) A thin-walled air sac of the lungs in which the exchange of oxygen and carbon dioxide takes place.

Ambulation Walking or moving from one place to another.

Ambulatory Able to walk, as opposed to being confined to bed.

Ameboid movement Movement used by leukocytes that permits them to propel themselves from the capillaries out into the tissues.

Amenorrhea The absence or cessation of menstrual period. Amenorrhea occurs normally before puberty, during pregnancy, and after menopause.

Amplitude Refers to amount, extent, size, abundance, or fullness.

Ampule A small sealed glass container that holds a single dose of medication.

Anaerobe A microorganism that grows best in the absence of oxygen.

Anaphylactic reaction A serious allergic reaction that requires immediate treatment.

Anemia A condition in which there is a decrease in the number of erythrocytes or in the amount of hemoglobin in the blood.

Antecubital space The surface of the arm in front of the elbow.

Antibody A substance capable of combining with an antigen, resulting in an antigen-antibody reaction.

Anticoagulant A substance that inhibits blood clotting.

Antigen A substance capable of stimulating the formation of antibodies.

Antipyretic An agent that reduces fever.

Antiseptic An agent that kills disease-producing microorganisms but not their spores. An antiseptic is usually applied to living tissue.

Antiserum (pl. **antisera**) A serum that contains antibodies.

Aorta The major trunk of the arterial system of the body. The aorta arises from the upper surface of the left ventricle.

Apnea The temporary cessation of breathing.

Approximation The process of bringing two parts, such as tissue, together, through the use of sutures or other means.

Arrhythmia An irregular heart rhythm; also termed dysrhythmia.

Artifact Additional electrical activity picked up by the electrocardiograph that interferes with the normal appearance of the ECG cycles.

Asepsis Free from infection or pathogens; the actions practiced to make and maintain an object free from infection or pathogens.

Atherosclerosis Build-up of fibrous plaques of fatty deposits and cholesterol on the inner walls of the coronary arteries.

Attending physician The physician responsible for the care of a hospitalized patient.

Atypical Deviation from the normal.

Audiometer An instrument used to measure hearing acuity quantitatively for the various frequencies of sound waves.

Auscultation The process of listening to the sounds produced within the body to detect signs of disease.

Autoclave An apparatus for the sterilization of materials, using steam under pressure.

Automated method (for testing laboratory specimens) A method of laboratory testing in which the series of steps in the test is performed by an automated analyzer.

Axilla The armpit.

Bacilli (sing. **bacillus**) Bacteria that have a rod shape.

Bandage A strip of woven material used to wrap or cover a part of the body.

Bariatrics The branch of medicine that deals with the treatment and control of obesity including diseases associated with obesity.

Baseline The flat horizontal line that separates the various waves of the ECG cycle.

Bilirubin An orange-colored bile pigment produced by the breakdown of heme from the hemoglobin molecule.

Bilirubinuria The presence of bilirubin in the urine.

Biopsy The surgical removal and examination of tissue from the living body. Biopsies are generally performed to determine whether a tumor is benign or malignant.

Blood antibody A protein in blood plasma that is capable of combining with its corresponding blood antigen to produce an antigen-antibody reaction.

Blood antigen A protein present on the surface of red blood cells that determines a person's blood type.

Bounding pulse A pulse with an increased volume that feels very strong and full.

Brace An orthopedic device used to support and hold a part of the body in the correct position to allow functioning and healing.

Bradycardia An abnormally slow heart rate (fewer than 60 beats per minute).

Bradypnea An abnormal decrease in the respiratory rate of fewer than 10 respirations per minute.

Braxton Hicks contractions Intermittent and irregular painless uterine contractions that occur throughout pregnancy. They occur more frequently toward the end of pregnancy and are sometimes mistaken for true labor pains.

Buffy coat A thin, light-colored layer of white blood cells and platelets that lays between a top layer of plasma and a bottom layer of red blood cells when an anticoagulant has been added to a blood specimen.

Burn An injury to the tissues caused by exposure to thermal, chemical, electrical, or radioactive agents.

Canthus The junction of the eyelids at either corner of the eye.

Capillary action The action that causes liquid to rise along a wick, a tube, or a gauze dressing.

Cardiac arrest A condition in which the heart has stopped beating or beats too irregularly to circulate blood effectively through the body.

Cardiac cycle One complete heartbeat.

Celsius scale A temperature scale on which the freezing point of water is 0° and the boiling point of water is 100°; also called the centigrade scale.

Cerumen Ear wax.

Cervix The lower narrow end of the uterus that opens into the vagina.

Charting The process of making written entries about a patient in the medical record.

Cilia Slender, hairlike projections.

Clinical diagnosis A tentative diagnosis of a patient's condition obtained through the evaluation of the health history and the physical examination, without the benefit of laboratory or diagnostic tests.

Cocci (sing. **coccus**) Bacteria that have a round shape.

Colonoscopy The visualization of the entire colon using a colonoscope.

Colony A mass of bacteria growing in a solid culture medium that have arisen from the multiplication of a single bacterium.

Colposcope A lighted instrument with a binocular magnifying lens used to examine the vagina and cervix.

Colposcopy The visual examination of the vagina and cervix using a colposcope.

Compress A soft, moist, absorbent cloth that is folded in several layers and applied to a part of the body in the local application of heat or cold.

Conduction The transfer of energy, such as heat, from one object to another.

Consultation report A narrative report of an opinion about a patient's condition by a practitioner other than the attending physician.

Contagious Capable of being transmitted directly or indirectly from one person to another.

Contaminate To soil or to make impure.

Contrast medium A substance that is used to make a particular structure visible on a radiograph.

Controlled drug A drug that has restrictions placed on it by the federal government because of its potential for abuse.

Contusion An injury to the tissues under the skin causing blood vessels to rupture, allowing blood to seep into the tissues; a bruise.

Convection The transfer of energy, such as heat, through air currents.

Conversion Changing from one system of measurement to another.

Crash cart A specially equipped cart for holding and transporting medications, equipment, and supplies needed for performing life-saving procedures in an emergency.

Crepitus A grating sensation caused by fractured bone fragments rubbing against each other.

Crisis (pertaining to fever) A sudden falling of an elevated body temperature to normal.

Critical item An item that comes in contact with sterile tissue or the vascular system.

Cryosurgery The therapeutic use of freezing temperatures to destroy abnormal tissue.

Cubic centimeter The amount of space occupied by 1 milliliter (1 ml = 1 cc).

Culture The propagation of a mass of microorganisms in a laboratory culture medium.

Culture medium A mixture of nutrients in which microorganisms are grown in the laboratory.

Cyanosis A bluish discoloration of the skin and mucous membranes.

Cytology The science that deals with the study of cells, including their origin, structure, function, and pathology.

DEA number A registration number assigned to physicians by the Drug Enforcement Administration for prescribing or dispensing controlled drugs.

Decontamination The use of physical or chemical means to remove, inactivate, or destroy bloodborne pathogens on a surface or item to the point where they are no longer capable of transmitting infectious particles, and the surface or item is rendered safe for handling, use, or disposal.

Detergent An agent that cleanses by emulsifying dirt and oil.

Diagnosis The scientific method of determining and identifying a patient's condition.

Diagnostic procedure A procedure performed to assist in the diagnosis, management, and treatment of a patient's condition.

Diapedesis The ameboid movement of blood cells (especially leukocytes) through the wall of a capillary and out into the tissues.

Diastole The phase in the cardiac cycle in which the heart relaxes between contractions.

Diastolic pressure The point of lesser pressure on the arterial wall, which is recorded during diastole.

Differential diagnosis A determination of which of two or more diseases with similar symptoms is producing the patient's symptoms.

Dilation (of the cervix) The stretching of the external os from an opening a few millimeters wide to an opening large enough to allow the passage of an infant (approximately 10 cm).

Discharge summary report A brief statement of the significant events of a patient's hospitalization.

Disinfectant An agent used to destroy pathogenic microorganisms but not necessarily their spores. Disinfectants are usually applied to inanimate objects.

Dislocation An injury in which one end of a bone making up a joint is separated or displaced from its normal anatomic position.

Donor One who furnishes something such as blood, tissue, or organs to be used in another person.

Dose The quantity of a drug to be administered at one time.

Drug A chemical used for the treatment, prevention, or diagnosis of disease.

Dysmenorrhea Pain associated with the menstrual period.

Dyspareunia Pain in the vagina or pelvis experienced by a woman during sexual intercourse.

Dysplasia The growth of abnormal cells. Dysplasia is a precancerous condition that may or may not develop into cancer.

Dyspnea Shortness of breath or difficulty in breathing.

Dysrhythmia An irregular heart rhythm; also termed arrhythmia.

ECG cycle The graphic representation of a heartbeat.

Echocardiogram An ultrasound examination of the heart.

EDD Expected date of delivery, or due date.

Edema The retention of fluid in the tissues, resulting in swelling.

Effacement The thinning and shortening of the cervical canal from its normal length of 1 to 2 cm to a structure with paper-thin edges in which there is no canal at all. Effacement occurs late in pregnancy or during labor, or both. The purpose of effacement along with dilation is to permit the passage of the infant into the birth canal.

Electrocardiogram (ECG) The graphic representation of the electrical activity of the heart.

Electrocardiograph The instrument used to record the electrical activity of the heart.

Electrode A conductor of electricity, which is used to promote contact between the body and the electrocardiograph.

Electrolyte A chemical substance that promotes conduction of an electrical current.

Electronic medical record (EMR) A medical record that is stored on a computer.

Embryo The child in utero from the time of conception to the beginning of the first trimester.

Emergency medical services (EMS) system A network of community resources, equipment, and personnel that provides care to victims of injury or sudden illness.

Endocervix The mucous membrane lining the cervical canal.

Endoscope An instrument that consists of a tube and an optical system that is used for direct visual inspection of organs or cavities.

Enema An injection of fluid into the rectum to aid in the elimination of feces from the colon.

Engagement The entrance of the fetal head or the presenting part into the pelvic inlet.

Erythema Reddening of the skin caused by dilation of superficial blood vessels in the skin.

Eupnea Normal respiration. The rate is 16 to 20 respirations per minute, the rhythm is even and regular, and the depth is normal.

Evacuated tube A closed glass or plastic tube that contains a premeasured vacuum.

Exhalation The act of breathing out.

External os The opening of the cervical canal of the uterus into the vagina.

Exudate A discharge produced by the body's tissues.

Fahrenheit scale A temperature scale on which the freezing point of water is 32° and the boiling point of water is 212°.

False negative A test result indicating that a condition is absent when, in actuality, it is present.

False positive A test result indicating that a condition is present when, in actuality, it is absent.

Familial Occurring or affecting members of a family more frequently than would be expected by chance.

Fastidious Extremely delicate, difficult to culture, therefore involving specialized growth requirements.

Fasting Abstaining from food or fluids (except water) for a specified amount of time before the collection of a specimen.

Febrile Pertaining to fever.

Fetal heart rate The number of times the fetal heart beats per minute.

Fetal heart tones The sounds of the heartbeat of the fetus heard through the mother's abdominal wall.

Fetus The child in utero, from the third month after conception to birth; during the first 2 months of development, it is called an embryo.

Fever A body temperature that is above normal. Synonym for pyrexia.

Fibroblast An immature cell from which connective tissue can develop.

First aid The immediate care that is administered to an individual who is injured or suddenly becomes ill before complete medical care can be obtained.

Fluoroscope An instrument used to view internal organs and structures directly.

Fluoroscopy Examination of a patient with a fluoroscope.

Forceps A two-pronged instrument for grasping and squeezing.

Fracture Any break in a bone.

Frenulum linguae The midline fold that connects the undersurface of the tongue with the floor of the mouth.

Fundus The dome-shaped upper portion of the uterus between the fallopian tubes.

Furuncle A localized staphylococcal infection that originates deep within a hair follicle; also known as a boil.

Gauge The diameter of the lumen of a needle used to administer medication.

Gene A unit of heredity.

Gestation The period of intrauterine development from conception to birth; the period of pregnancy. The average pregnancy lasts about 280 days, or 40 weeks, from the date of conception to childbirth.

Gestational age The age of the fetus between conception and birth.

Glycogen The form in which carbohydrate is stored in the body.

Glycosuria The presence of sugar in the urine.

Gravidity The total number of pregnancies a woman has had regardless of duration, including a current pregnancy.

Gynecology The branch of medicine that deals with the diseases of the reproductive organs of women.

Hand hygiene The process of cleansing or sanitizing the hands.

HDL cholesterol A lipoprotein consisting of protein and cholesterol that removes excess cholesterol from the cells.

Health history report A collection of subjective data about a patient.

Hematology The study of blood and blood-forming tissues.

Hematoma A swelling or mass of coagulated blood caused by a break in a blood vessel.

Hemoconcentration An increase in the concentration of the nonfilterable blood components such as red blood cells, enzymes, iron, and calcium as a result of a decrease in the fluid content of the blood.

Hemoglobin The iron-containing pigment of erythrocytes that transports oxygen in the body.

Hemolysis The breakdown of erythrocytes with the release of hemoglobin into the plasma; the breakdown of blood cells.

Hemostasis The arrest of bleeding by natural or artificial means.

Home health care The provision of medical and nonmedical care in a patient's home or place of residence.

Homeostasis The state in which body systems are functioning normally and the internal environment of the body is in equilibrium; the body is in a healthy state.

Hyperglycemia An abnormally high level of glucose in the blood.

Hyperopia Farsightedness.

Hyperpnea An abnormal increase in the rate and depth of respiration.

Hyperpyrexia An extremely high fever.

Hypertension High blood pressure.

Hyperventilation An abnormally fast and deep type of breathing usually associated with acute anxiety conditions.

Hypoglycemia An abnormally low level of glucose in the blood.

Hypopnea An abnormal decrease in the rate and depth of respiration.

Hypotension Low blood pressure.

Hypothermia A body temperature that is below normal.

Hypoxia A reduction in the oxygen supply to the tissues of the body.

Immunity The resistance of the body to the effects of a harmful agent such as a pathogenic microorganism or its toxins.

Immunization (active, artificial) The process of becoming immune or of rendering an individual immune through the use of a vaccine or toxoid.

Impacted Wedged firmly together so as to be immovable.

Incision A clean cut caused by a cutting instrument.

Incubate To provide proper conditions for growth and development. In microbiology, the act of placing a culture in a chamber (incubator), which provides optimal growth requirements for the multiplication of the organisms, such as the proper temperature, humidity, and darkness.

Incubation period The interval of time between the invasion by a pathogenic microorganism and the appearance of first symptoms of the disease.

Induration An area of hardened tissue.

Infant A child from birth to 12 months of age.

Infection The condition in which the body, or part of it, is invaded by a pathogen.

Infectious disease A disease caused by a pathogen that produces harmful effects on its host.

Infiltration The process by which a substance passes into and is deposited within the substance of a cell, tissue, or organ.

Inflammation A protective response of the body in trauma and the entrance of foreign matter. The purpose of inflammation is to destroy invading microorganisms and to repair injured tissue. Symptoms at the site of the inflammation include pain, swelling, redness, and warmth.

Informed consent Consent given by a patient for a medical procedure after being informed of the nature of his or her condition, the purpose of the procedure, the risks involved with the procedure, alternative treatments or procedure available, the likely outcome of the procedure, and the risks involved with declining or delaying the procedure.

Inhalation The act of breathing in.

Inhalation administration The administration of medication by way of air or other vapor being drawn into the lungs.

Inoculate To introduce microorganisms into a culture medium for growth and multiplication.

Inoculum The specimen used to inoculate a medium.

Inpatient A patient who has been admitted to a hospital for at least one overnight stay.

Inspection The process of observing a patient to detect signs of disease.

Instillation The dropping of a liquid into a body cavity.

Insufflate To blow a powder, vapor, or gas (such as air) into a body cavity.

Intercostal Between the ribs.

Internal os The internal opening of the cervical canal into the uterus.

Interval The length of a wave or the length of a wave with a segment.

Intradermal injection Introduction of medication into the dermal layer of the skin.

Intramuscular injection Introduction of medication into the muscular layer of the body.

Intravenous injection Introduction of medication directly into the bloodstream through a vein.

In vitro Occurring in glass. Refers to tests performed under artificial conditions, as in the laboratory.

In vivo Occurring in the living body or organism.

Irrigation The washing of a body canal with a flowing solution.

Ischemia Deficiency of blood in a body part.

Ketonuria The presence of ketone bodies in the urine.

Ketosis An accumulation of large amounts of ketone bodies in the tissues and body fluids.

Korotkoff sounds Sounds heard during the measurement of blood pressure that are used to determine the systolic and diastolic blood pressures readings.

Laboratory test The clinical analysis and study of materials, fluids, or tissues obtained from patients to assist in diagnosing and treating disease.

Laceration A wound in which the tissues are torn apart, leaving ragged and irregular edges.

LDL cholesterol A lipoprotein, consisting of protein and cholesterol, that picks up cholesterol and delivers it to the cells.

Length (recumbent) The measurement from the vertex of the head to the heel of the foot in a supine position.

Leukocytosis An abnormally high number of white blood cells (more than 11,000 per cubic millimeter of blood).

Leukopenia An abnormal decrease in the number of white blood cells (below 4,500 per cubic millimeter of blood).

Ligate To tie off and close a structure such as a severed blood vessel.

Lipoprotein A complex molecule consisting of protein and a lipid fraction such as cholesterol. Lipoproteins transport lipids in the blood.

Load Articles that are being sterilized.

Local anesthetic A drug that produces a loss of feeling and an inability to perceive pain in only a specific part of the body.

Lochia A discharge from the uterus after delivery, consisting of blood, tissue, white blood cells, and some bacteria.

Long arm cast A cast that extends from the axilla to the fingers, usually with a bend in the elbow.

Long leg cast A cast that extends from the midthigh to the toes.

Maceration The softening and breaking down of the skin as a result of prolonged exposure to moisture.

Malaise A vague sense of body discomfort, weakness, and fatigue that often marks the onset of a disease and continues through the course of the illness.

Manometer An instrument for measuring pressure.

Manual method A method of laboratory testing in which the series of steps in the test is performed by hand.

Material safety data sheet (MSDS) A sheet that provides information regarding a chemical, its hazards, and measures to take to prevent injury and illness when handling the chemical.

Mayo tray A broad, flat metal tray placed on a stand and used to hold sterile instruments and supplies once it has been covered with a sterile towel.

Medical asepsis Practices that are employed to reduce the number and hinder the transmission of pathogens.

Medical impressions Conclusions drawn by the physician from an interpretation of data. Other terms for impressions include *provisional diagnosis* and *tentative diagnosis*.

Medical record A written record of the important information regarding a patient, including the care of that individual and the progress of the patient's condition.

Medical record format The way a medical record is organized. The two main types of medical record format are the source-oriented record and the problem-oriented record.

Melena The darkening of the stool caused by the presence of blood in an amount of 50 ml or greater.

Meniscus The curved upper surface of liquid in a tube or container. The surface is convex if the liquid does not wet the container and concave if it does.

Menopause The permanent cessation of menstruation, which usually occurs between the ages of 35 and 58.

Menorrhagia Excessive bleeding during a menstrual period, either in the number of days or the amount of blood or both; also called dysfunctional uterine bleeding (DUB).

Mensuration The process of measuring the patient.

Metrorrhagia Bleeding between menstrual periods.

Microbiology The scientific study of microorganisms and their activities.

Microorganism A microscopic plant or animal.

Micturition The act of voiding urine.

Mucous membrane A membrane lining body passages or cavities that open to the outside.

Multigravida A woman who has been pregnant more than once.

Multipara A woman who has completed two or more pregnancies to the age of fetal viability regardless of whether they ended in live infants or stillbirths.

Myopia Nearsightedness.

Needle biopsy A type of biopsy in which tissue from deep within the body is obtained by the insertion of a biopsy needle through the skin.

Nephron The functional unit of the kidney.

Nonabsorbable suture Suture material that is not absorbed by the body and either remains permanently in the body tissue and becomes encapsulated by fibrous tissue or is removed.

Noncritical item An item that comes into contact with intact skin but not mucous membranes.

Nonintact skin Skin that has a break in the surface. It includes, but is not limited to, abrasions, cuts, hangnails, paper cuts, and burns.

Nonpathogen A microorganism that does not normally produce disease.

Normal flora Harmless, nonpathogenic microorganisms that normally reside in many parts of the body.

Normal range (for laboratory tests) A certain established and acceptable parameter or reference range within which the laboratory test results of a healthy individual are expected to fall.

Normal sinus rhythm Refers to an electrocardiogram that is within normal limits.

Nullipara A woman who has not carried a pregnancy to the point of fetal viability (20 weeks of gestation).

Objective symptom A symptom that can be observed by an examiner.

Obstetrics The branch of medicine concerned with the care of the woman during pregnancy, childbirth, and the postpartal period.

Occult blood Blood in such a small amount that it is not detectable by the unaided eye.

Oliguria Decreased or scanty output of urine.

Ophthalmoscope An instrument for examining the interior of the eye.

Opportunistic infection An infection that results from a defective immune system that cannot defend the body from pathogens normally found in the environment.

Optimum growth temperature The temperature at which an organism grows best.

Oral administration Administration of medication by mouth.

Orthopedist A physician who specializes in the diagnosis and treatment of disorders of the musculoskeletal system, which includes the bones, joints, ligaments, tendons, muscles, and nerves.

Orthopnea The condition in which breathing is easier when an individual is standing or sitting.

Osteochondritis Inflammation of bone and cartilage.

Osteomyelitis Inflammation of the bone due to bacterial infection.

Otoscope An instrument for examining the external ear canal and tympanic membrane.

Oxyhemoglobin Hemoglobin that has combined with oxygen.

Palpation The process of feeling with the hands to detect signs of disease.

Paper-based patient record (PPR) A medical record in paper form.

Parenteral Taken into the body through the piercing of the skin barrier or mucous membranes, such as through needlesticks, human bites, cuts, abrasions, and so on. Administration of medication by injection.

Parity The condition of having borne offspring regardless of the outcome.

Pathogen A disease-producing microorganism.

Pediatrician A medical doctor who specializes in the care and development of children and the diagnosis and treatment of children's diseases.

Pediatrics The branch of medicine that deals with the care and development of children and the diagnosis and treatment of children's diseases.

Pelvimetry Measurement of the capacity and diameter of the maternal pelvis, which helps determine whether it will be possible to deliver the infant via the vaginal route.

Percussion The process of tapping the body to detect signs of disease.

Percussion hammer An instrument with a rubber head, used for testing reflexes.

Perimenopause Before the onset of menopause, the phase during which the woman with regular periods changes to irregular cycles and increased periods of amenorrhea.

Perinatal Relating to the period shortly before and after birth.

Perineum The external region between the vaginal orifice and the anus in a female and between the scrotum and the anus in a male.

Peroxidase (as it pertains to the guaiac slide test) A substance that is able to transfer oxygen from hydrogen peroxide to oxidize guaiac, causing the guaiac to turn blue.

pH The unit that describes the acidity or alkalinity of a solution.

Phagocytosis The engulfing and destruction of foreign particles, such as bacteria, by special cells called phagocytes.

Pharmacology The study of drugs.

Phlebotomist A health professional trained in the collection of blood specimens.

Phlebotomy Incision of a vein for the removal or withdrawal of blood; the collection of blood.

Physical examination An assessment of each part of the patient's body to obtain objective data about the patient that assists in determining the patient's state of health.

Physical examination report A report of the objective findings from the physician's assessment of each body system.

Plasma The liquid part of the blood, consisting of a clear, straw-colored fluid that makes up approximately 55% of the total blood volume.

Poison Any substance that causes illness, injury, or death if it enters the body.

Polycythemia A disorder in which there is an increase in the red cell mass.

Polyuria Increased output of urine.

Position The relation of the presenting part of the fetus to the maternal pelvis.

Post-exposure prophylaxis (PEP) Treatment administered to an individual after exposure to an infectious disease to prevent the disease.

Postoperative After a surgical operation.

Postpartum Occurring after childbirth.

Preeclampsia A major complication of pregnancy, the cause of which is unknown, characterized by increasing hypertension, albuminuria, and edema. If this condition is neglected or not treated properly, it may develop into eclampsia, which could cause maternal convulsions and coma. Preeclampsia generally occurs between the twentieth week of pregnancy and the end of the first week postpartum.

Prenatal Before birth.

Preoperative Preceding a surgical operation.

Presbyopia A decrease in the elasticity of the lens that occurs with aging, resulting in a decreased ability to focus on close objects.

Preschooler A child from 3 to 6 years of age.

Prescription A physician's order authorizing the dispensing of a drug by a pharmacist.

Presentation Indication of the part of the fetus that is closest to the cervix and will be delivered first. A cephalic presentation is a delivery in which the fetal head is presenting against the cervix. A breech presentation is a delivery in which the buttocks or feet are presented instead of the head.

Pressure point A site on the body where an artery lies close to the surface of the skin and can be compressed against an underlying bone to control bleeding.

Preterm birth Delivery occurring between 20 and 37 weeks regardless of whether the child was born alive or stillborn.

Primigravida A woman who is pregnant for the first time.

Primipara A woman who has carried a pregnancy to viability (20 weeks of gestation) for the first time, regardless of whether the infant was stillborn or alive at birth.

Problem Any patient condition that requires further observation, diagnosis, management, or patient education.

Prodrome A symptom that indicates an approaching disease.

Profile A number of laboratory tests providing related or complementary information used to determine the health status of a patient.

Prognosis The probable course and outcome of a patient's condition and the patient's prospects for a recovery.

Proteinuria The presence of protein in the urine.

Puerperium The period of time, usually 4 to 6 weeks after delivery, in which the uterus and the body systems are returning to normal.

Pulse pressure The difference between the systolic and diastolic pressures.

Pulse rhythm The time interval between heartbeats.

Pulse volume The strength of the heartbeat.

Puncture A wound made by a sharp pointed object piercing the skin.

Quality control The application of methods to ensure that test results are reliable and valid and that errors are detected and eliminated.

Quickening The first movements of the fetus in utero as felt by the mother, which usually occurs between the sixteenth and twentieth weeks of gestation and is felt consistently thereafter.

Radiation The transfer of energy, such as heat, in the form of waves.

Radiograph A permanent record of a picture of an internal body organ or structure produced on radiographic film.

Radiography The taking of permanent records (radiographs) of internal body organs and structures by passing x-rays through the body to act on a specially sensitized film.

Radiologist A medical doctor who specializes in the diagnosis and treatment of disease using radiant energy such as x-rays, radium, and radioactive material.

Radiology The branch of medicine that deals with the use of radiant energy in the diagnosis and treatment of disease.

Radiolucent Describing a structure that permits the passage of x-rays.

Radiopaque Describing a structure that obstructs the passage of x-rays.

Recipient One who receives something, such as a blood transfusion, from a donor.

Refraction The deflection or bending of light rays by a lens.

Refractive index The ratio of the velocity of light in air to the velocity of light in a solution.

Refractometer (clinical) An instrument used to measure the refractive index of urine, which is an indirect measurement of the specific gravity of urine.

Regulated medical waste Medical waste that poses a threat to health and safety.

Renal threshold The concentration at which a substance in the blood that is not normally excreted by the kidneys begins to appear in the urine.

Reservoir host The organism that becomes infected by a pathogen and also serves as a source of transfer of the pathogen to others.

Resident flora Harmless, nonpathogenic microorganisms that normally reside on the skin and usually do not cause disease; also known as normal flora.

Resistance The natural ability of an organism to remain unaffected by harmful substances in its environment.

Reverse chronological order Arrangement of documents with the most recent document on top or in the front, which means that oldest document is on the bottom or at the back of a section or file.

Risk factor Anything that increases an individual's chance of developing a disease. Some risk factors (e.g., smoking) can be avoided, but others cannot (e.g., age and family history).

Routine test Laboratory test performed routinely on apparently healthy patients to assist in the early detection of disease.

Sanitization A process to remove organic matter from an article and to lower the number of microorganisms to a safe level as determined by public health requirements.

Scalpel A surgical knife used to divide tissues.

School-age child A child from 6 to 12 years of age.

Scissors A cutting instrument.

Sebaceous cyst A thin, closed sac or capsule that contains fatty secretions from a sebaceous gland.

Segment The portion of the ECG between two waves.

Seizure A sudden episode of involuntary muscular contractions and relaxation, often accompanied by a change in sensation, behavior, and level of consciousness.

Semicritical item An item that comes into contact with nonintact skin intact mucous membranes.

Sequela (pl. **sequelae**) A morbid (secondary) condition occurring as a result of a less serious primary infection.

Serum The clear, straw-colored part of the blood (plasma) that remains after the solid elements and the clotting factor fibrinogen have been removed.

Shock The failure of the cardiovascular system to deliver enough blood to all the vital organs of the body.

Short arm cast A cast that extends from below the elbow to the fingers.

Short leg cast A cast that begins just below the knee and extends to the toes.

Sigmoidoscope An endoscope that is specially designed for passage through the anus to permit visualization of the rectum and sigmoid colon.

Sigmoidoscopy The visual examination of the rectum and sigmoid colon using a sigmoidoscope.

Signatura The part of a prescription that indicates the information to print on the medication label.

Smear Material spread on a slide for microscope examination.

Soak The direct immersion of a body part in water or a medicated solution.

SOAP format A method of organization for recording progress notes. The SOAP format includes the following categories: subjective data, objective data, assessment, and plan.

Sonogram The record obtained with ultrasonography.

Specific gravity The weight of a substance compared with the weight of an equal volume of a substance known as the standard. In urinalysis, the specific gravity refers to the measurement of the amount of dissolved substances in the urine, compared with the same amount of distilled water.

Specimen A small sample of something taken to show the nature of the whole.

Speculum An instrument for opening a body orifice or cavity for viewing.

Sphygmomanometer An instrument for measuring arterial blood pressure.

Spirilla (sing. **spirillum**) Bacteria that have a spiral or curved shape.

Spirometer An instrument for measuring air taken into and expelled from the lungs.

Spirometry Measurement of an individual's breathing capacity by means of a spirometer.

Splint An orthopedic device used to immobilize, restrain, or support a part of the body.

Sponge A porous, absorbent pad, such as a 4-inch gauze pad or cotton surrounded by gauze, used to absorb fluids, to apply medication, or to cleanse an area.

Spore A hard, thick-walled capsule formed by some bacteria that contains only the essential parts of the protoplasm of the bacterial cell.

Sprain Trauma to a joint that causes injury to the ligaments.

Stature The height of the body in a standing position.

Sterile Free of all living microorganisms and bacterial spores.

Sterilization The process of destroying all forms of microbial life, including bacterial spores.

Stethoscope An instrument for amplifying and hearing sounds produced by the body.

Strain An overstretching of a muscle caused by trauma.

Streaking In microbiology, the process of inoculating a culture to provide for the growth of colonies on the surface of a solid medium. Streaking is accomplished by skimming a wire inoculating loop that contains the specimen across the surface of the medium, using a back and forth motion.

Streptolysin An exotoxin produced by beta-hemolytic streptococci, which completely hemolyzes red blood cells.

Subcutaneous injection Introduction of medication beneath the skin, into the subcutaneous or fatty layer of the body.

Subjective symptom A symptom that is felt by the patient but is not observable by an examiner.

Sublingual administration Administration of medication by placing it under the tongue, where it dissolves and is absorbed through the mucous membrane.

Subscription The part of the prescription that gives directions to the pharmacist and usually designates the number of doses to be dispensed.

Supernatant The clear liquid that remains at the top after a precipitate settles.

Superscription The part of a prescription consisting of the symbol Rx (from the Latin word *recipe*, meaning "take").

Suppuration The process of pus formation.

Surgical asepsis Practices that keep objects and areas sterile or free from microorganisms.

Susceptible Easily affected; lacking resistance.

Sutures Material used to approximate tissues with surgical stitches.

Swaged needle A needle with suturing material permanently attached to its end.

Symptom Any change in the body or its functioning that indicates that a disease might be present.

Systole The phase in the cardiac cycle in which the ventricles contract, sending blood out of the heart and into the aorta and pulmonary aorta.

Systolic pressure The point of maximum pressure on the arterial walls, which is recorded during systole.

Tachycardia An abnormally fast heart rate (more than 100 beats per minute).

Tachypnea An abnormal increase in the respiratory rate of more than 20 respirations per minute.

Termbirth Delivery occurring after 37 weeks, regardless of whether the child was born alive or stillborn.

Thermolabile Easily affected or changed by heat.

Thready pulse A pulse with a decreased volume that feels weak and thin.

Toddler A child from 1 to 3 years of age.

Topical administration Application of a drug to a particular spot, usually for a local action.

Toxemia A pathologic condition occurring in pregnant women that includes preeclampsia and eclampsia. If preeclampsia goes undiagnosed or is not satisfactorily controlled, it could develop into eclampsia, characterized by convulsions and coma.

Toxin A poisonous or noxious substance.

Toxoid A toxin (poisonous substance produced by a bacterium) that has been treated by heat or chemicals to destroy its harmful properties. It is administered to an individual to prevent an infectious disease by stimulating the production of antibodies in that individual.

Transient flora Microorganisms that reside on the superficial skin layers and are picked up in the course of daily activities. They are often pathogenic but can be removed easily from the skin by good handwashing techniques.

Trimester Three months, or one third, of the gestational period of pregnancy.

Tympanic membrane A thin, semitransparent membrane located between the external ear canal and the middle ear that receives and transmits sound waves; also known as the eardrum.

Ultrasonography The use of high-frequency sound waves (ultrasound) to produce an image of an organ or tissue.

Urinalysis The physical, chemical, and microscopic analysis of urine.

Vaccine A suspension of attenuated (weakened) or killed microorganisms administered to an individual to prevent an infectious disease by stimulating the production of antibodies in that individual.

Venipuncture Puncturing of a vein.

Venous reflux The backflow of blood (from an evacuated tube) into the patient's vein.

Venous stasis The temporary cessation or slowing of the venous blood flow.

Vertex The summit, or top, especially the top of the head.

Vial A closed glass container with a rubber stopper that holds medication.

Void To empty the bladder.

Vulva The region of the external female genital organs.

Wheal A small raised area of the skin.

Wound A break in the continuity of an external or internal surface caused by physical means.

Index

A

Abbé condenser, 760
Abbreviations
  medical, 815-823
  in medical record, 37-39
  in medication documentation, 462t
Abdominal aorta, 833f, 837f
Abdominal examination, 193t
  prenatal, 302t
Abducens nerve, 840f
Abnormal breath sounds, 147t
ABO blood type, 744-747, 745f, 748f
  in blood donation, 747t
  in prenatal examination, 304
Abortion, 298, 323
  minor and, 317
Abrasion, 392, 392f, 433, 795f, 796
Abscess, 416-417, 417f, 433
Absorbable suture, 397, 398f, 433
Absorbed poison, 803
Access to medical record, 5
Accolate. See Zafirlukast.
Accu-Chek glucose monitor, 739, 741-743
Accupril. See Quinapril.
Acel-Imune. See Diphtheria, tetanus toxoids
  and acellular pertussis vaccine.
Acetaminophen, 442t
Acetest, 627t
Acetoacetic acid, 626
Acetone, 626
Achilles tendon, 830f, 831f
Achromycin. See Tetracycline.
Acoustical stethoscope, 151
Acquired defects of color vision, 212
Acquired immune deficiency syndrome, 73-79,
  77-78t
  antiretrovirals for, 449t
  website information on, 83
Acquired immune deficiency syndrome–
  defining conditions, 77-78t
ActHIB. See Haemophilus b conjugate vaccine.
Activase. See Alteplase.
Activated charcoal, 786t
Active immunizing agent, 71
Activella. See Estradiol-norethindrone.
Activity diary for Holter monitor, 528, 528f
Actonel. See Risedronate.
Actos. See Pioglitazone.
Acute illness, 169
Acute otitis media, 222
Acute viral hepatitis B, 72, 73
Acyclovir, 450t
Adalat. See Nifedipine.
Adderall. See Dextroamphetamine-saccinarate
  and sulfate.
Additive tube, 670
Additives in evacuated tubes, 670
Adductor brevis, 829t
Adductor longus, 828f, 829f
Adductor magnus, 828-831f
Adenocard. See Adenosine.
Adenosine, 785t
Adhesive skin closures, 401, 401f, 404-407
Adipose tissue, 843f
Adjustment knobs of microscope, 761
Administration of medication, 435-508
  allergy testing in, 493-496, 494t, 495t, 495-
    496f
  application of knowledge in, 504-505
  certification review in, 505-506
  charting of, 42
  controlled drugs and, 459-462, 460-461t
  converting units of measurement, 458-459,
    458-459t
  drug nomenclature and, 440
  drugs classified on action, 441, 442-455t
  drugs classified on preparation, 440-441
  factors affecting drug action, 467-468
  Food and Drug Administration and, 440
  guidelines for, 468
  legal issues in, 503
  medication record and, 465f, 465-466
  oral, 468-470
  parenteral, 470-489
    intradermal injections in, 489, 489f, 497-
      499
    intramuscular injections in, 475-479, 479t,
      486-488
    parts of needle and syringe for, 471-472,
      471-472f
    prefilled syringes and cartridges for, 475,
      475f, 476f

Administration of medication (Continued)
    preparation from ampule, 472-473, 474f,
      480-483
    preparation from vial, 472, 474f, 480-483
    reconstitution of powdered drugs for, 475,
      477f, 483-484
    safety engineered syringes for, 472, 473f,
      474f
    storage for drugs for, 475
    subcutaneous injections in, 475, 477f, 484-
      487
    Z-track injection technique in, 479, 479f,
      488-489
  patient teaching in prescription
    medications, 466
  Physician's Desk Reference and, 437-439f
  prescription for, 462t, 462-465, 463f
  systems of measurement for, 455-458, 458t
  terminology review in, 507
  tuberculin testing in, 489-492, 500-502
  website information on, 508
Administration on Aging, 611
Administrative documents, 4-6
Adnexal, term, 323
Adnexal region, 282
Adolescent
  pulse rate of, 141t
  respiratory rates of, 145t
  safety guidelines for, 339t
  techniques for interaction with, 341t
Adrenal gland, 837f, 843f
Adrenalin. See Epinephrine.
Adson dressing forceps, 382f
Adventitious sounds, 147, 164
Adverse reaction, 467, 507
Advil. See Ibuprofen.
Aerobes, 52, 83
Aerobic exercise, 143
  for high blood cholesterol, 735
Aerosol, 441
Afebrile, term, 127, 164
Afferent arteriole, 615f
Afrin. See Oxymetazoline.
Agar, 768, 768f
Age
  application of heat or cold and, 239
  blood donation and, 746
  blood pressure and, 150
  body temperature variations and, 126,
    127t
  effect on drug action, 467
  hypertension and, 156
  pulse rate and, 141
  respiratory rate and, 145, 145t
  risk of breast cancer and, 274
Agglutination, 651, 651f, 657, 744, 747, 748f,
  753
Aggression, preschool child and, 334t
Aging, website information on, 611
AIDS. See Acquired immune deficiency
  syndrome.
Airborne Express, 48
Al-Anon, 508
Alanine aminotransferase, 589t, 729t
ALARA acronym, 577
Albumin, 589t
Albustix, 627t
Albuterol, 450t, 785t
Alcohol
  as disinfectant, 98t, 98-99
  hypertension and, 156
Alcohol abuse, 508
Alcohol-based hand rubs, 55, 55f, 58-59
Alcoholics Anonymous, 508
Aldactone. See Triamterene.
Alendronate, 450t
Alesse. See Ethinyl estradiol-levonorgestrel.
Aleve. See Naproxen.
Alimentary glycosuria, 626
Alka-Seltzer. See Sodium bicarbonate.
Alkaline phosphatase, 729t
Allegra. See Fexofenadine.
Allergen, 492, 493, 507
  direct skin testing for, 493-494, 495t
  intradermal skin testing for, 496, 496f
  patch testing for, 494-495, 495f, 495t
  radioallergosorbent test for, 496
  skin-prick testing for, 495f, 495t,
    495-496
Allergic drug reaction, 467-468
Allergic reaction, 493, 494t
Allergic rhinitis, 451t, 494t

Allergy, 507
  antihistamines for, 445t
  corticosteroids for, 451t
  vasopressors for, 455t
  website information on, 508
Allergy testing, 493-496, 494-495t, 495-496f,
  498
Allis tissue forceps, 382f
Allopurinol, 445t
ALP. See Alkaline phosphatase.
Alphafetoprotein, 309
Alprazolam, 443t
ALT. See Alanine aminotransferase.
Altace. See Ramipril.
Alteplase, 454t
Alternating current artifact, 522f, 523
Aluminum hydroxide-magnesium hydroxide,
  442t
Alveolar process, 835f
Alveolus, 144, 145f, 164
Amaryl. See Glimepiride.
Ambien. See Zolpidem.
Ambulation, 257, 269
Ambulatory, 269
Ambulatory aids, 257-264
  canes in, 259, 259f, 264
  crutches in, 257-259, 258f, 259f, 260-263
  walkers in, 259f, 259-260, 264
Ameboid movement, 712, 725
Amenorrhea, 273, 323
American Academy of Allergy, Asthma, and
  Immunology, 508
American Academy of Audiology, 235
American Academy of Ophthalmology, 235
American Academy of Orthopedic Surgeons,
  269
American Academy of Otolaryngology, 235
American Academy of Pediatrics, 374
American Association of Retired Persons, 611
American Cancer Society, 563, 582
American Chiropractic Association, 269
American College of Cardiology, 545
American College of Surgeons, 433
American Council for Drug Education, 657
American Dietic Association, 202
American Heart Association, 165, 545
American Institute of Stress, 725
American Lung Association, 165, 545
American Occupational Therapy Association,
  269
American Optometric Association, 235
American Physical Therapy Association, 269
American Red Cross, 433, 812
American Social Health Organization, 325
American Society for Clinical Laboratory
  Science, 705
American Society of Clinical Pathologists, 705
American Society of Hypertension, 545
American Society of Phlebotomy Technicians,
  705
American Thoracic Society, 508
Aminoglycosides, 447t
Aminophylline, 785t
Amitriptyline, 444t
Amlodipine
  for angina, 443t
  for hypertension, 446t
Amlopidine-benazepril, 446t
Ammonium biurate, 635t
Amniocentesis, 311t, 312, 312f
Amorphous phosphates, 640t
Amorphous urate, 640t
Amoxicillin, 447t
Amoxicillin-clavulanate, 447t
Amoxil. See Amoxicillin.
Amphotericin B, 445t
Ampicillin, 643t
Amplifier of electrocardiograph, 517, 517f
Amplitude, term, 545
Ampule, 507
  drug preparation from, 472-473, 474f, 480-
    483
Anabolic steroids, 460t
Anaerobes, 52, 83
Analgesics, 442t
  controlled, 460t, 461t
  otic, 454t
Analgesics-antipyretics, 442t
Analytes, 728
Anaphylactic reaction, 467-468, 507
  in insect sting, 492, 804
Anaphylactic shock, 792

Anaprox. See Naproxen.
Anemia, 709t, 713, 725
  antianemics for, 442-443t
  iron-deficiency, 713-714
Aneroid sphygmomanometer, 152, 152f, 153f
Anesthetics, local, 433, 442t
  for minor office surgery, 408-410, 410f
  before suturing, 397
Angina pectoris, 531, 532
  antianginals for, 443t
Angioedema, 467
Angiotensin-converting enzyme inhibitors,
  446t
Angiotensin II receptor antagonists, 446t
Animal bite, 805
Anistreplase, 454t
Anorexia, 40
Antacids, 442t
Antecubital space, 164, 661, 664, 705
Antecubital veins, 664f
Anterior cavity, 207f
Anterior chamber, 207, 842f
Anterior cruciate ligament, 827f
Anteroposterior view, 568
Anthelmintics, 445t
Anti-impotence agents, 447t
Antianemics, 442-443t
Antianginals, 443t
Antianxiety agents, 443t, 461t
Antibiotics, 536
Antibody, 743, 753
  blood, 744-746, 747t
  Rh, 304-305, 744
  rubella, 304
Anticholinergics, 443t
Anticipatory guidance, 328, 329-339t
  for infant, 329-331t
  for preschooler, 334-335t
  for school-age child, 335-337t
  for toddler, 331-333t
Anticoagulants, 443t, 705
  in blood specimen, 665, 692
Anticonvulsants, 444t, 461t
Antidepressants, 444t
Antidiabetics, 444t
Antidiarrheals, 445t
Antidysrhythmics, 445t
Antiflatulents, 445t
Antifungals, 445t
Antigen, 743, 753
Antigen-antibody reaction, 747, 748f
Antigout agents, 445t
Antihistamines, 445t
Antihypertensives, 446t
Antiinfectives, 447t
  ophthalmic, 453t
  otic, 454t
Antiinflammatory agents, 448t
Antimanics, 448t
Antimicrobial soap, 54, 55, 55f
Antimigraines, 448t
Antineoplastics, 448t
Antiparkinson agents, 448t
Antiprotozoals, 449t
Antipsychotics, 449t
Antipyretic, 127, 164
Antiretrovirals, 449t
Antiseptic hand washing, 55, 55f
Antiseptic wipe, 170t
Antiseptics, 55, 83, 120, 408
Antiserum, 747, 753
Antispasmodics, 449t
Antistreptolysin O test, 743-744
Antithyroid agents, 455t
Antituberculars, 449t
Antitussives, 449t
Antiulcers, 449t
Antivirals, 449t
Anuria, 616
Anus, 836f, 838f
Anxiety
  antianxiety agents for, 443t
  toddlers and, 332t
Aorta, 141, 164, 513, 513f, 832f
Aortic arch, 833f
Aortic semilunar valve, 513f, 832f
Apical pulse, 141-142, 142f, 149
Apnea, 146, 164
Apothecary system, 456-457, 458-459t
Appearance of urine, 621, 621f
Appendix, 836f
Appetite suppressants, 455t

Applicator head of ultrasound machine, 247
Approximate, term, 397
Approximation, 433
Apresoline. See Hydralazine.
Aqueous humor, 207, 207f
Arachnoid, 839f
Aristocort. See Triamcinolone.
Arm
  lymphatics of, 834f
  physical examination of, 190t
Arm splint, 256t
Arrector pili muscle, 843f
Arrhythmia, 143
Arterial bleeding, 792-793
Arterial blood, 712
Arterial puncture, 660
Arthritis Foundation, 269
Artifact, 545
  in electrocardiography, 521-523, 522f
  in urine, 644-645t, 635
Artifact filter, 521
Ascending colon, 836f
Ascending limb, 615f
Asepsis, 51-83, 83
  application of knowledge in, 81
  bloodborne diseases and, 71-79
    acquired immunodeficiency syndrome in, 73-79, 77-78t
    hepatitis B in, 71-72, 74-75t
    hepatitis C in, 72, 73, 74-75t
  microorganisms and, 52-60
    alcohol-based hand rubs and, 58-59
    gloves and, 55, 59-60
    growth requirements for, 52-53
    hand hygiene and, 53-55, 54t
    handwashing in, 56-58
    infection control and, 55
    infection process cycle and, 53, 53f
    protective mechanisms of body and, 53
  OSHA Bloodborne Pathogens Standard and, 61-69
    communicating hazards to employees in, 63
    engineering controls in, 64
    exposure control plan in, 61-63, 62f
    hepatitis B vaccination and, 68, 69f
    housekeeping in, 67f, 67-68, 68f
    labeling requirements in, 63, 64f
    Needlestick Safety and Prevention Act and, 61
    personal protective equipment and, 65-67, 66f, 67f
    record keeping in, 64
    safer medical devices and, 63, 63f
    terminology in, 61
    universal precautions and, 68-69
    work practice controls in, 64-65
  in parenteral administration of medication, 471
  regulated medical waste and, 69-71, 70t, 71f
  surgical, 378-380
Aspartate aminotransferase, 589t, 729t
Aspiration, suprapubic, 617
Aspirin
  for fever, 442t
  for inflammation, 448t
  in urine, 643t
Association for Advancement of Medical Instrumentation, 83
AST. See Aspartate aminotransferase.
Asthma, 494t
  chronic, 536
  corticosteroids for, 451t
ATAC Lab System, 728, 733f
Atacand. See Candesartan.
Atarax. See Hydroxyzine.
Atenolol
  for angina, 443t
  for hypertension, 446t
Atherosclerosis, 531, 545, 734
Ativan. See Lorazepam.
Atorvastatin, 453t
Atrial depolarization, 525
Atrial fibrillation, 534
Atrial flutter, 533
Atrial premature contractions, 532
Atrial septum, 513f
Atrioventricular node, 514, 514f
Atro-Pen. See Atropine.
Atropine, 443t, 785t
AT&T Toll-Free Directory, 48
Attending physician, 12, 48
Atypical, term, 323
Atypical cell, 276
Audiogram, 224
Audiometer, 202, 206, 224, 235
Audiometry, 224-226, 226f
Auditory meatus, 221f
Augmented leads in electrocardiography, 517, 518f
Augmentin. See Amoxicillin-clavulanate.
Aura, 801
Aural temperature, 129, 131, 138-140
Auralgan. See Benzocaine.
Auricle, 221f, 842f
Auscultation, 196, 202

Autoclave, 102, 120
  maintenance of, 112-113
  operating of, 110f, 110-112, 111f
  wrapping articles for, 105-109, 106f
Autoclave cycle, 110, 110f
Autoclave log, 103, 103f
Autoclave tape, 104, 105f
AutoCyte Pap Test, 278
Autolet II, 693
Automated analyzer, 604-605
Automated blood chemistry analyzer, 728, 733f
Automated method, 611
Autotrophs, 52
Avandia. See Rosiglitazone.
Avapro. See Irbesartan.
Avoirdupois, 457
Axilla, 164
Axillary artery, 833f
Axillary crutch measurement, 257-258, 258f, 260
Axillary lymph nodes, 834f
Axillary temperature, 128, 135-136
Azithromycin, 292, 447t

B
Bacilli, 758, 758f, 759f, 780
Bacitracin susceptibility test, 769, 770f
Back pain, 246
Backhaus towel clamp, 384f
Bacteria, 757-758, 758f-759f
  gram staining of, 773
  in urine, 620, 644t, 635
Bactrim. See Trimethoprim-sulfamethoxazole.
Bactroban. See Mupirocin.
Bandage, 422, 433
Bandage scissors, 380, 381f
Bandaging, 422-472, 423-425f, 425t
Bands, 719
Bariatrics, 177, 202
Barium enema, 566, 571, 571f
Barium sulfate, 567
Barium swallow, 570
Barrel focus, 761
Barrel of syringe, 471f, 471-472
Baseline in electrocardiography, 515, 545
Basilic vein, 664f, 666f
Basin, 170t
Basopenia, 710t
Basophil, 718f, 719
Basophilia, 710t
Beclomethasone, 451t
Becton Dickinson, 705
Bedtime struggles, 332-333t
Bee sting, 492, 803-804, 804f
Benadryl. See Diphenhydramine.
Benazepril, 446t
Beneficence, 560
Bentyl. See Dicyclomine.
Benzathine penicillin, 447t
Benzocaine, 454t
Benzonatate, 449t
Bepridil, 443t
Beta blockers
  for angina, 443t
  for hypertension, 446t
Beta-hydroxybutyric acid, 626
Bethesda system, 280-282, 281f, 282t
Bevel of needle, 471, 471f
Bextra. See Valdecoxib.
Biaxin. See Clarithromycin.
Biceps brachii, 828f, 830f, 831f
Biceps femoris, 830f, 831f
Bicillin. See Benzathine penicillin.
Bicuspid valve, 513f
Big E chart, 208
Bili-Labstix, 627t
Bilirubin, 712, 725
  total, 589t
  in urine, 626, 632t, 643t
Bilirubinuria, 626, 643t, 657
Billing information, 6
Bimanual pelvic examination, 282, 283f
Binocular microscope, 761
Biohazard bag waste container, 64f, 70, 70t, 71f, 170t
Biohazard sharps container, 68, 68f, 70, 70t
Biohazard warning label, 63, 64f
Biologic indicators, 104-105, 105f
Biopsy, 417, 433, 563
  breast, 274
  cervical, 420-421, 421f
  needle, 417-418, 418f
  rectal, 555
Biopsy needle, 417, 418f
Biopsy requisition, 410, 411f
Bipolar disorder, 525
Bipolar leads, 517, 518f
Bisacodyl, 453t
Bismuth subsalicylate, 445t
Bisoprolol-hydrochlorothiazide, 446t
Bite
  animal, 805
  snake, 804-805
Black widow spider, 804
Bladder, 614, 614f, 837f, 838f

Bladder catheterization, 617
Bladecon. See Guaifenesin.
Bleach, 99
Bleeding, 792-793, 794-795f
  in animal bite, 805
  hypovolemic shock in, 791
Blood
  components and function of, 708
  donation of, 746-747
  handling and storage of, 598t
  separate layers in sample of, 666f
  in urine, 626, 632t
Blood agar, 768, 768f
Blood antibody, 744-746, 747t, 753
Blood antigen, 744, 753
Blood banking, 603t
Blood chemistry, 728-743
  Accu-Chek glucose monitor and, 741-743
  application of knowledge in, 750
  automated blood chemistry analyzers in, 728, 733f
  blood glucose in, 736
  blood urea nitrogen in, 736
  certification review in, 752
  cholesterol testing in, 734-736
  common tests in, 729-733t
  fasting blood sugar in, 736-737
  glucose monitors and, 738-739
  quality control in, 733-734
  self-monitoring of blood glucose and, 739-740
  terminology review in, 753
Blood cholesterol, 734, 735
Blood culture tube, 670
Blood donation, 746-747
Blood glucose, 731t, 736-743
  Accu-Chek glucose monitor and, 741-743
  fasting blood sugar and, 736-737
  glucose monitors and, 738-739
  recommended frequency for testing, 169
  self-monitoring of, 739-740
Blood group, 589t
Blood loss, 793-794
Blood pressure, 150-160
  blood donation and, 747
  cuff sizes for, 153, 153f, 154t
  in initial prenatal examination, 301t
  Korotkoff sounds and, 153, 155t
  measurement of, 157-159
  mechanism of, 150-151, 151t
  palpation for determining systolic pressure and, 160
  patient teaching in, 156
  pediatric, 354t, 354-355, 354-355f
  postpartal, 316t
  prevention of errors in measurement of, 154
  recommended frequency for, 169
  sphygmomanometer for, 151-153, 152f, 153f
  stethoscope for, 151, 151f, 152
Blood pressure cuff, 153, 153f, 154t
  for child, 354, 354f, 354t
Blood smear, 719-721
Blood specimens, 659-705
  application of knowledge in, 703
  for blood glucose, 739
  certification review in, 704
  legal issues in, 701
  safety engineered device for, 63f
  skin puncture in, 692-701
    disposable lancet for, 695-697
    disposable semiautomatic lancet device for, 697-698
    guidelines for finger puncture in, 694f, 694-695
    microcollection devices for, 693-694, 694f
    puncture devices for, 692-693, 693f
    puncture site for, 692
    reusable semiautomatic lancet device for, 698-701
  terminology review in, 705
  venipuncture in, 660-692
    application of tourniquet in, 661-664, 663f
    butterfly method of, 676-677f, 676-682
    evacuated tubes for, 669f, 669-670
    guidelines for evacuated tube method of, 670-675, 671f
    needle for, 667, 667f, 668f
    obtaining plasma specimen in, 691-692
    obtaining serum specimen in, 687-691, 689f
    order of draw for multiple tubes, 670
    OSHA safety precautions in, 666-668
    patient positioning for, 661, 662f
    patient preparation for, 661
    plastic holder for, 668
    problems encountered in, 686-687, 687f
    site selection for, 664f, 664-665, 666f
    syringe method of, 682-685
    types of blood specimens in, 665, 666f
  website information on, 705
Blood tests, 707-725, 709-711t
  application of knowledge in, 723
  certification review in, 724
  components and function of blood and, 708
  erythrocytes and, 712

Blood tests (Continued)
  hematocrit and, 713f, 713-716
  hemoglobin determination in, 712-713
  iron deficiency anemia and, 714
  legal issues in, 721
  leukocytes and, 712
  in prenatal examination, 304
  red blood cell count in, 717
  terminology review in, 725
  thrombocytes and, 712
  white blood cell count in, 716-717, 717f
  white blood cell differential count in, 717-721, 718f
Blood typing, 744-747, 745f, 748f
  in prenatal examination, 304
Blood urea nitrogen, 589t, 729t, 736
Blood vessels, 833f
Bloodborne diseases, 71-79
  acquired immunodeficiency syndrome in, 73-79, 77-78t
  hepatitis B in, 71-72, 74-75t
  hepatitis C in, 72, 73, 74-75t
Bloodborne Pathogens Standard, 61-69
  communicating hazards to employees in, 63
  in emergency medical procedures, 788
  engineering controls in, 64
  exposure control plan in, 61-63, 62f
  hepatitis B vaccination and, 68, 69f
  housekeeping and, 67f, 67-68, 68f
  labeling requirements in, 63, 64f
  in microbiologic procedures, 765
  Needlestick Safety and Prevention Act and, 61
  personal protective equipment and, 65-67, 66f, 67f
  record keeping in, 64
  safer medical devices and, 63, 63f
  terminology in, 61
  universal precautions and, 68-69
  in venipuncture, 666-667
  work practice controls in, 64-65
Body mass index, 177
Body mechanics, 247
Body of uterus, 273f, 838f
Body position, blood pressure and, 151
Body structure and function, 825-844
  circulatory system in, 833-834f
  digestive system in, 835-836f
  genitourinary system in, 837-838f
  heart and respiratory system in, 832f
  muscles in, 828-831f
  nervous system in, 839-841f
  salivary and endocrine glands in, 843f
  sense organs in, 842f
  skeletal system in, 826-827f
  skin in, 843f
Body temperature, 124-140
  alterations in, 126, 126f
  assessment sites for, 128
  aural, 129, 131, 138-140
  axillary, 128, 135-136
  blood donation and, 747
  fever and, 127-128, 128t
  growth of microorganisms and, 52
  in initial prenatal examination, 301t
  oral, 128, 133-135
  postpartal, 316t
  rectal, 128, 137-138
  regulation of, 124-125, 125f
  thermometers for, 129-130f, 129-132
  variations in, 126-127, 127t
Boil, 416
Bone resorption inhibitors, 450t
Bones, 221f, 826-827f
Bonine. See Meclizine.
Botulism, 758
Bounding pulse, 143, 164
Brace, 256, 256f, 257f, 269
Brachial artery, 664
Brachial plexus, 841f
Brachial pressure point, 794f
Brachial pulse, 141t, 142
Brachialis, 828-830f
Brachioradialis, 828-831f
Bradycardia, 40, 143, 164, 531
Bradypnea, 145, 164
Brain, control of respiration by, 144-145
Brand name of drug, 440
Braxton-Hicks contractions, 294, 323
Breast
  biopsy of, 274
  cancer of, 274, 582
  examination of, 192t, 274-275, 283-285
    in initial prenatal examination, 302t
    postpartal, 316t
    recommended frequency for, 169
  lymphatics of, 834f
  mammography in, 569, 569f, 570f
  self-examination of, 275, 283-285
Breast cancer gene, 274
Breast sounds, 147, 147t
Breathing emergency, 785-786t
Breathing exercises, 536
Brethine. See Terbutaline.
Bretylium tosylate, 785t
Broad casts, 639t

Broad ligament, 273*f*
Brompheniramine, 445*t*
Bronchiole, 832*f*
Bronchitis, chronic, 536
Bronchodilators, 450*t*, 536
Bronchogram, 573
Bronkodyl. See Theophylline.
Broom for Pap specimen, 278, 278*f*, 287
Brown recluse spider, 804
Buccinator, 830*f*
Buffy coat, 665, 666*f*, 705, 713, 713*f*
Bulbourethral gland, 838*f*
Bumetanide, 451*t*
Bumex. See Bumetanide.
BUN. See Blood urea nitrogen.
Bundle branches, 514, 514*f*
Bundle of His, 514, 514*f*
Bupropion, 444*t*
Burns, 812
adolescent and, 339*t*
emergency care of, 799*f*, 799-800
infant and, 337*t*
preschool child and, 338*t*
toddler and, 338*t*
BuSpar. See Buspirone.
Buspirone, 443*t*
Butterfly method of venipuncture, 676-677*f*, 676-682

C
C-reactive protein, 589*t*, 744
CAD. See Coronary artery disease.
Calan. See Verapamil.
Calcaneus, 830*f*
Calcium, 589*t*, 729*t*
Calcium carbonate, 442*t*, 641*t*
Calcium channel blockers
for angina, 443*t*
for hypertension, 446*t*
Calcium oxalate, 640*t*
Calcium phosphate, 641*t*
Calibration
of blood chemistry analyzer, 733-734
of glucose monitor, 739
of refractometer, 624
of spirometer, 538
Calibration bar, 174, 175*f*
Calorie Control Council, 202
Canal of Schlemm, 842*f*
Cancellous bone, 827*f*
Cancer
in acquired immune deficiency syndrome, 77*t*
antineoplastics for, 448*t*
breast, 274
prostate, 558-559, 559*f*
website information on, 563
Candesartan, 446*t*
Candida albicans, 291, 291*f*
in acquired immune deficiency syndrome, 78*t*
prenatal testing for, 303
in urine, 644*t*
Cane, 259, 259*f*, 264
Canthus, 218, 235
Capillary action, 380, 433
Capillary bleeding, 793
Capillary puncture, 692-701
for blood glucose, 739
disposable lancet for, 695-697
disposable semiautomatic lancet device for, 697-698
guidelines for finger puncture in, 694*f*, 694-695
microcollection devices for, 693-694, 694*f*
puncture devices for, 692-693, 693*f*
puncture site for, 692
reusable semiautomatic lancet device for, 698-701
Capillary tube, 694, 694*f*
Caplet, 441
Capoten. See Captopril.
Capsule, 441
Captopril, 446*t*
Carbamazepine, 444*t*
Carbamide peroxide, 454*t*
Carbidopa-levodopa, 448*t*
Carbon dioxide, respiration and, 144, 145*f*
Cardiac arrest, 784, 791, 812
Cardiac arteriogram, 573
Cardiac cycle, 514*f*, 514-515, 545
Cardiac dysrhythmias, 531-535
antidysrhythmics for, 445*t*
atrial fibrillation in, 534
atrial flutter in, 533
paroxysmal atrial tachycardia in, 533
premature ventricular contractions in, 534
ventricular fibrillation in, 535
ventricular tachycardia in, 535
Cardiac glycosides, 450*t*
Cardiogenic shock, 791-792
Cardiology Channel, 545
Cardiopulmonary procedures, 511-545
application of knowledge in, 542
certification review in, 544
electrocardiography in, 512-535
artifacts in, 521-523, 522*f*
for atrial fibrillation, 534
Cardiopulmonary procedures *(Continued)*
for atrial flutter, 533
for atrial premature contractions, 532
augmented leads in, 517, 518*f*
baseline, segments, and intervals in, 515
bipolar leads in, 517, 518*f*
chest leads in, 518-519, 519*f*
conduction of heart and, 514, 514*f*
electrocardiograph capabilities and, 519
electrocardiograph in, 512*f*, 512-513
electrocardiograph leads for, 516-517, 517*f*
electrocardiograph paper for, 515, 515*f*
fro ventricular fibrillation, 535
Holter monitor in, 526-531, 527*f*, 538*f*
interpretative electrocardiographs in, 520, 521*f*
maintenance of electrocardiograph in, 519
for paroxysmal atrial tachycardia, 533
for premature ventricular contractions, 534
standardization of, 516, 516*f*
structure of heart and, 513, 513*f*
telephone transmission of, 520
three-channel recording capability of, 519, 520*f*
twelve-lead, three-channel electrocardiogram in, 524-526
for ventricular tachycardia, 535
waves in, 514*f*, 514-515
legal issues in, 540
pulmonary function tests in, 536-540, 538*f*
terminology review in, 545
website information on, 545
Cardiovascular emergency, 785*t*, 791
Cardiovascular system, 832*f*
conduction of heart and, 514, 514*f*
dysrhythmias and, 531-535
atrial fibrillation in, 534
atrial flutter in, 533
paroxysmal atrial tachycardia in, 533
premature ventricular contractions in, 534
ventricular fibrillation in, 535
ventricular tachycardia in, 535
electrocardiography and, 512-535
artifacts in, 521-523, 522*f*
for atrial fibrillation, 534
for atrial flutter, 533
for atrial premature contractions, 532
augmented leads in, 517, 518*f*
baseline, segments, and intervals in, 515
bipolar leads in, 517, 518*f*
chest leads in, 518-519, 519*f*
electrocardiograph capabilities and, 519
electrocardiograph in, 512*f*, 512-513
electrocardiograph leads for, 516-517, 517*f*
electrocardiograph paper for, 515, 515*f*
fro ventricular fibrillation, 535
Holter monitor in, 526-531, 527*f*, 538*f*
interpretative electrocardiographs in, 520, 521*f*
maintenance of electrocardiograph in, 519
for paroxysmal atrial tachycardia, 533
for premature ventricular contractions, 534
standardization of, 516, 516*f*
structure of heart and, 513, 513*f*
telephone transmission of, 520
three-channel recording capability of, 519, 520*f*
twelve-lead, three-channel electrocardiogram in, 524-526
for ventricular tachycardia, 535
waves in, 514*f*, 514-515
physical examination of, 192*t*
pulmonary function tests and, 536-540, 538*f*
structures of, 513, 513*f*
urine test strip parameters and, 630*t*
website information on, 545
Cardizem. See Diltiazem.
Cards O.S. Mono test, 745*f*
Cardura. See Doxazosin.
Carisoprodol, 453*t*
Carotid artery, 833*f*
Carotid pressure point, 794*f*
Carotid pulse, 141*t*, 142
Carpals, 826*f*
Cartilage, 221*f*
Cartridge for parenteral medication administration, 475, 475*f*, 476*f*
Cast care, 254-255
Cast padding, 253, 253*f*
Casting of fracture, 251-254*f*, 251-255, 256*f*
Casts, urinary, 635, 638-639*t*,
Cat bite, 805
Catapres. See Clonidine.
Cauda equina, 841*f*
Cavernous bodies, 838*f*
CBC. See Complete blood count.
Ceclor. See Cefaclor.
Cecum, 836*f*
Cefaclor, 447*t*
Cefprozil, 447*t*
Ceftriaxone, 292, 447*t*
Cefzil. See Cefprozil.
Celebrex. See Celecoxib.
Celecoxib, 448*t*
Celexa. See Citalopram.
Celiac artery, 833*f*
Cell metabolism, heat production and, 125
Cells in urine, 630-631*t*,
Cellular casts, 635
Celsius temperature, 126, 126*t*, 164
Cementum, 835*f*
Centers for Disease Control and Prevention, 83, 374, 508, 780
guidelines for hand hygiene, 54*t*
Centers for Medicare and Medicaid Services, 611
Centimeters to inches, 175
Central nervous system stimulants, 450*t*, 460*t*, 461*t*
Central retinal artery, 842*f*
Centrum, 827*f*
Cephalexin, 447*t*
Cephalic vein, 664*f*, 666*f*
Cephalosporins, 447*t*
Cerebellum, 840*f*
Cerebral angiogram, 573
Cerebral palsy, 374
Cerebrovascular accident, 791
Certification review
in blood chemistry and serology, 752
in cardiopulmonary procedures, 544
in clinical laboratory, 610
in colon procedures, 563
in disinfection and sterilization, 119
in emergency medical procedures, 810-811
in eye and ear assessment, 234
in hematology, 724
in measurement of vital signs, 163
in medical asepsis, 82
in medication administration, 505-506
in microbiology, 779
in minor office surgery, 431-432
in phlebotomy, 704
in physical agents for tissue healing, 268
in physical examination, 201
in radiology and diagnostic imaging, 581
in urinalysis, 656
Cerumen, 221, 235
Cerumenolytics, 454*t*
Cervical canal, 273*f*
Cervical curve, 827*f*
Cervical lymph nodes, 834*f*
Cervical plexus, 841*f*
Cervical vertebrae, 826*f*, 827*f*
Cervix, 273, 273*f*, 323, 838*f*
biopsy of, 420-421, 421*f*
cryosurgery of, 421*f*, 421-422
inspection of, 276, 276*f*
specimen for Pap test, 277, 277*f*
Cetirizine, 445*t*
Chart dividers, 29, 30
Charting, 34-43, 48
abbreviations used in, 37-39
of Accu-Chek glucose monitor use, 743
of adhesive skin closure application, 406
of administration of medication, 42
of allergy skin test, 498
of apical pulse, 148
of aural temperature, 140
of axillary temperature, 136
of blood pressure, 159
of breast self-examination instructions, 285
of butterfly venipuncture, 682
of chest circumference, 346
of child growth percentiles, 347
of cold compress, 245
of diagnostic procedures and laboratory tests, 43
of diagnostic tests, 43
of differential cell count, 721
of dressing change, 397
of ear instillation, 230
of ear irrigation, 228
of electrocardiogram, 526
of eye instillation, 220
of eye irrigation, 219
of fasting blood sugar, 743
of flexible sigmoidoscopy, 558
guidelines for, 34-36, 36*f*
of head circumference, 346
of heating pad, 241
of hematocrit, 716
of Hemoccult, 555
of Holter monitor application, 531
of hot compress, 243
of hot soak, 242
of ice bag, 244
of infant length and weight, 345
of intramuscular injection, 488
of Ishihara test, 216
of laboratory tests, 43
of Mantoux test, 499
of minor office surgery, 415
of newborn screening test, 368
of oral medication administration, 470
of oral temperature, 135
of Pap test, 289
of patient instructions, 43, 44*t*
of patient symptoms, 36, 40, 43
of pediatric urine specimen, 357
of pregnancy test, 653
of procedures, 41
of progress notes, 36
Charting *(Continued)*
of pulse respiration, 148
of rapid urine culture test, 650
of rectal temperature, 138
of removal of adhesive skin closure, 407
of Snellen test, 215
of specimen collection, 42, 43, 601
of spirometry, 540
of subcutaneous injection, 486
of suture removal, 403
of throat culture, 767
of tine test, 501, 502
of tubular gauze bandage, 427
of twenty-four hour urine specimen, 620
of ultrasound therapy, 250
of urine specific gravity, 624
of vacuum tube venipuncture, 675
of weight and height, 179
of Z-track injection, 489
Chek-Stix control strips, 632*f*
Chemical burn, 800
Chemical cold pack, 246
Chemical disinfection, 97-101, 98*f*, 98*t*
Chemical examination of urine, 625-629, 627*t*
Chemical hot pack, 246
Chemical indicators, 104
Chemical name of drug, 440
Chemical sterilization methods, 102
Chemical thermometer, 130
Chemstrip, 627*t*
Chest
physical examination of, 192*t*
radiography of, 567, 567*f*
Chest circumference, 343, 346
Chest leads, 518-519, 519*f*
Chest pain, 531, 532, 791
Chestpiece of stethoscope, 151
Chewable tablet, 441
Chickenpox vaccine, 362*t*
Chief complaint, 30
Child abuse, 374
Child health, 327-374
anticipatory guidance and, 329-339*t*
for infant, 329-331*t*
for preschooler, 334-335*t*
for school-age child, 335-337*t*
for toddler, 331-333*t*
application of knowledge in, 371-372
blood pressure measurement and, 354*t*, 354-355, 354-355*f*
carrying of infant, 342, 342*f*
certification review in, 372
development of rapport during examination, 340*f*, 340-341, 341*t*
growth measurements and, 342-353
growth charts in, 344, 347-355
head and chest circumferences in, 343, 346
length and height and, 342, 343*f*, 344-345
weight and, 342, 344-345
hearing impairment and, 224
immunizations and, 359-360, 361*f*, 362*t*
injections and, 358-359, 358-359*f*
legal issues in, 369
milestones of gross and fine motor development in infancy, 329*t*
newborn screening test, 362, 367-368, 369*f*
safety guidelines in, 337-339*t*
terminology review in, 373
urine specimen collection in, 355-357
variations in body temperature, 127*t*
visual acuity and, 209
website information on, 374
Childbearing, risk of breast cancer and, 274
Childbirth, 325
Chills, 40, 127
Chlamydial infection, 292-293, 303
Chlor-Trimetron. See Chlorpheniramine.
Chloramphenicol, 447*t*
Chlordiazepoxide, 443*t*
Chloride, 589*t*, 729*t*
Chlorine, 99
Chlorine compounds, 99
Chloromycetin. See Chloramphenicol.
Chlorpheniramine, 445*t*
Chlorpheniramine-hydrocodone, 449*t*
Chlorthalidone, 451*t*
Choking
adolescent and, 339*t*
infant and, 338*t*
preschool child and, 338*t*
school-age child and, 339*t*
toddler and, 338*t*
Cholangiogram, 573
Cholecystography, 571-572, 572*f*
Cholera, 758
Cholesterol, 734-736
recommended frequency for testing, 169
serum, 730*t*
in urine, 643*t*
Chordae tendineae, 832*f*
Choroid, 206, 207*f*, 842*f*
Chromic surgical gut, 397
Chronic asthma, 536
Chronic bronchitis, 536
Chronic illness, 169
Chronic obstructive pulmonary disease, 146, 536

Chronic viral hepatitis B, 72
Chyluria, 643*t*
Cilia, 53, 83
Ciliary body, 206, 207*f*, 842*t*
Ciliary process, 842*f*
Cimetidine, 449*t*
Ciprofloxacin, 447*t*
Circular turn in bandaging, 423, 423*f*
Circulatory system
  application of heat or cold and, 239
  common symptoms of, 40
  structure and function of, 833-834*f*
Cisterna chyli, 834*f*
Citalopram, 444*t*
Civil law, 653
Clarithromycin, 447*t*
Claritin. See Loratadine.
Clavicle, 826*f*, 828*f*
Clean-catch midstream specimen, 616-617, 618*f*, 618-619
Cleaning of surgical site, 408, 408*f*
Cleansing solutions, 408, 408*f*
Clinical chemistry, 11, 603*t*
Clinical diagnosis, 168, 202, 587
Clinical laboratory, 585-611
  application of knowledge in, 608-609
  automated analyzers in, 604-605
  blood chemistry in, 728-743
    Accu-Chek glucose monitor and, 741-743
    automated blood chemistry analyzers in, 728, 733*f*
    blood glucose in, 736
    blood urea nitrogen in, 736
    cholesterol testing in, 734-736
    common tests in, 729-733*t*
    fasting blood sugar in, 736-737
    glucose monitors and, 738-739
    quality control in, 733-734
    self-monitoring of blood glucose and, 739-740
  certification review in, 610
  Clinical Laboratory Improvement Amendments of 1988, 601-602
  collecting, handling, and transporting specimens, 596-601, 598*t*
  hematologic tests in, 707-725, 709-711*t*
    application of knowledge in, 723
    certification review in, 724
    components and function of blood and, 708
    erythrocytes and, 712
    hematocrit and, 713*f*, 713-716
    hemoglobin determination in, 712-713
    iron deficiency anemia and, 714
    legal issues in, 721
    leukocytes and, 712
    red blood cell count in, 717
    terminology review in, 725
    thrombocytes and, 712
    white blood cell count in, 716-717, 717*f*
    white blood cell differential count in, 717-721, 718*f*
  laboratory reports and, 593-595, 594*f*
  laboratory requests and, 589-593, 590*f*, 592*t*
  laboratory tests and, 586-587
  legal issues in, 606
  manual method of laboratory testing, 602-604
  microbiology and, 755-780
    application of knowledge in, 778
    certification review in, 779
    cultures and, 768*f*, 768-769
    disease and, 757-759, 758*f*, 759*f*
    Gram stain and, 773, 773*f*
    hanging drop slide in, 774
    infection and, 757
    laboratory tests in, 604*t*
    legal issues in, 776
    microscope and, 759-764, 760*f*
    normal flora and, 757
    in prevention and control of infectious diseases, 773
    sensitivity testing and, 771*f*, 771-772
    smears and, 772, 775
    specimen collection in, 765-766, 766*f*
    streptococcus testing and, 769, 770*f*
    terminology review in, 780
    throat culture and, 767
    website information on, 780
    wet mount method and, 772, 772*f*
  patient preparation and instructions for testing, 595-596
  purpose of laboratory testing and, 587-588
  quality control in, 605
  safety in, 605
  serology in, 11, 743-747
    application of knowledge in, 751
    blood typing in, 744-747, 745*f*, 748*f*
    certification review in, 752
    rapid mononucleosis testing in, 744, 745*f*
    for syphilis, 304
    terminology review in, 753
  skin puncture in, 692-701
    disposable lancet for, 695-697
    disposable semiautomatic lancet device for, 697-698
    guidelines for finger puncture in, 694*f*, 694-695
Clinical laboratory *(Continued)*
    microcollection devices for, 693-694, 694*f*
    puncture devices for, 692-693, 693*f*
    puncture site for, 692
    reusable semiautomatic lancet device for, 698-701
  terminology review in, 611
  types of, 588-589, 589*t*
  urinalysis and, 11, 613-657
    application of knowledge in, 655
    calibration of refractometer for, 624
    casts in urine sediment, 635, 638-639*t*, 635
    cells in urine sediment, 637-638*t*, 639-640
    certification review in, 656
    chemical examination of urine in, 625-629, 627*t*
    collection of urine for, 616-621, 618*f*
    composition of urine and, 615
    Kova method of, 646-648
    legal issues in, 653
    measurement of urine specific gravity, 622-623
    microorganisms and artifacts in urine, 636, 644-645*t*,
    physical examination of urine in, 621, 621*f*, 623*f*
    rapid urine cultures in, 649-650
    reagent strips for, 627, 629-635*t*, 632*f*, 644-645
    structure and function of urinary system and, 614, 614*f*, 615*f*
    terminology review in, 657
    urine crystals, 635, 640-643*t*,
    urine pregnancy testing and, 651*f*, 651-653
    website information on, 657
  venipuncture in, 660-692
    application of tourniquet in, 661-664, 663*f*
    butterfly method of, 676-677*f*, 676-682
    evacuated tubes for, 669*f*, 669-670
    guidelines for evacuated tube method of, 670-675, 671*f*
    needle for, 667, 667*f*, 668*f*
    obtaining plasma specimen in, 691-692
    obtaining serum specimen in, 687-691, 689*f*
    order of draw for multiple tubes, 670
    OSHA safety precautions in, 666-668
    patient positioning for, 661, 662*f*
    patient preparation for, 661
    plastic holder for, 668
    problems encountered in, 686-687, 687*f*
    site selection for, 664*f*, 664-665, 666*f*
    syringe method of, 682-685
    types of blood specimens in, 665, 666*f*
  website information on, 611
Clinical Laboratory Improvement Amendments of 1988, 601-602, 733
Clinistix, 627*t*
Clinitek Analyzer, 629, 632
Clinitest, 627*t*
Clitoris, 838*f*
Clonazepam, 444*t*
Clonidine, 446*t*
Clopidogrel, 454*t*
Closed fracture, 796, 797*f*
Closed wound, 392, 796
Clotrimazole, 291, 445*t*
Clotted blood specimen, 665
Coagulation tube, 670
Coarse adjustment, 761
Cobex. See Cyanocobalamin.
Cocci, 757, 758, 780
Coccygeal plexus, 841*f*
Coccygeal vertebrae, 827*f*
Coccyx, 826*f*
Cochlea, 221, 221*f*, 842*f*
Cochlear nerve, 842*f*
Codeine, 442*t*
Colace. See Docusate.
Colchicine, 445*t*
Cold agglutinins, 744
Cold compress, 245
Cold exposure, 806
Cold pack, 246
Cold sterilization, 113
Cold therapy, 238-246
  chemical cold pack in, 246
  cold compress in, 245
  factors affecting, 238-239, 240*f*
  ice bag in, 244
Colic, 331*t*
Collagen, wound healing and, 393
Collapsing veins, 686, 687*f*
Collecting duct, 615*f*
Colon Cancer Alliance, 563
Colon procedures, 547-558
  application of knowledge in, 562-563
  certification review in, 563
  fecal occult blood testing in, 548-555
    colorectal cancer and, 551
    guaiac slide test in, 548*f*, 548-549, 554-555
    patient preparation for, 549
    quality control in, 550
  flexible sigmoidoscopy in, 555-558, 556*f*
  legal issues in, 560
  terminology review in, 563
  website information on, 563
Colonoscopy, 549, 563
Colonoscopy report, 11
Colony, 780
Color
  respiration and, 146
  of urine, 621, 621*f*
Color vision assessment, 212*f*, 212-213, 215-216
Color vision defect, 209
Colorectal cancer, 551
  fecal occult blood testing for, 548-555
  website information on, 563
ColoScreen, 548-549, 549*f*
Colposcope, 419, 419*f*, 433
Colposcopy, 273, 323, 419*f*, 419-420, 433
Coma, diabetic, 807, 808
Commercial urine testing kits, 625-626
Commercially prepared sterile package, 386, 387*f*
Comminuted fracture, 797
Commit Lozenges, 454*t*
Common carotid artery, 833*f*
Common iliac artery, 833*f*
Common iliac vein, 833*f*
Communication
  with patient, 35
  website information on, 48
Compact bone, 827*f*
Compazine. See Prochlorperazine.
Complete blood count, 708
  with differential, 589*t*
  in prenatal examination, 304
Complex partial seizure, 800-801
Compliance to exposure control plan, 62
Compound microscope, 759
Compress, 239, 269
  cold, 245
  hot, 243
Computed tomography, 574-575, 575-576*f*
Computerized patient record, 24, 48
Concerta. See Methylphenidate.
Condenser of microscope, 760
Conduction, 164
  of heart, 514, 514*f*
  heat loss and, 125, 125*f*
Conductive hearing loss, 222
Congenital defects of color vision, 212
Congestive heart failure
  application of heat or cold and, 239
  diuretics for, 451*t*
Conjugated estrogens, 452*t*
Conjugated estrogens-progesterone, 452*t*
Conjunctiva, 207, 207*f*, 842*f*
Conjunctivitis, 217
Consent by minor, 317
Consent documents, 19-24
  consent to treatment form in, 19-21, 21*f*, 379*f*
  release of medical information form in, 21-24, 22*f*
Constipation, 40
Consultation report, 8-10, 9*f*, 48
Contact dermatitis, 494*t*
Contagious, term, 780
Contagious disease, 757
Container label requirements, 87-88
Contaminate, term, 83, 120, 433
Contaminated sharps, 65
Contamination, 61
Continuous fever, 128*t*
Contraceptives, 325, 451*t*
Contraction stress test, 312
Contrast medium, 566-567, 567*f*, 582
  for cholecystography, 572
  for intravenous pyelogram, 572
  for lower gastrointestinal series, 571, 571*f*
  for upper gastrointestinal series, 570
  in urine, 643*t*
Controlled drugs, 459-462, 460-461*t*, 503, 507
Contusion, 392, 392*f*, 433, 795*f*, 796
Convection, 125, 125*f*, 164
Conversion, 458-459, 458-459*t*, 507
Converting units of measurement, 458-459, 458-459*t*
Convulsion, 40
COPD. See Chronic obstructive pulmonary disease.
Copperhead snake, 804-805
Copy capability of electrocardiogram, 519
Coracobrachialis, 829*f*
Coral snake, 804-805
Cornea, 206, 207*f*, 842*f*
Coronary artery disease, 734
Correspondence, 6
Corrosive poison, 802
Corrugator supercilii, 829*f*
Cortef. See Hydrocortisone.
Corticosteroids, 451*t*
Cortisone, 451*t*
Cortisporin Otic. See Neomycin-polymyxin-hydrocortisone.
Cortone. See Cortisone.
Corzide. See Nadolol-bendroflumethiazide.
Costal cartilage, 826*f*
Cotton-tipped applicator, 170*t*
Cottonmouth snake, 804-805
Coughing, 40
  antitussives for, 449*t*
  as defense mechanism, 53
  expectorants for, 452*t*
Coulter blood cell counter, 717, 717*f*
Coumadin. See Warfarin.
Coupling agents, 247-248
Cozaar. See Losartan.
Crackles, 147*t*
Cradle position, 342, 342*f*
Cranial nerves, 840*f*
Crash cart, 784, 785-787*t*, 812
Cream, 441
Creatine, 643*t*
Creatine phosphokinase, 589*t*
Creatinine, 589*t*, 730*t*
Crepitus, 796, 812
Crile-Wood needle holder, 383*f*
Criminal law, 653
Crisis, 164
Critical item, 102, 120
Crown, 835*f*
Crutch gaits, 259, 261-263
Crutch palsy, 258
Crutches, 257-259, 258*f*, 259*f*, 260-263
Crying, infant and, 331*t*
Cryosurgery, 421*f*, 421-422, 433
Cryptococcosis, 78*t*
Cryptosporidiosis, 78*t*
Crystals in urine, 635
Crystodigin. See Digitoxin.
CT. See Computed tomography.
Cubic centimeter, 456, 507
Cultural awareness, 35
Cultural competence, 35
Cultural diversity, 35, 48
Cultural sensitivity, 35
Culture, 768*f*, 768-769, 780
  collection and transport system for, 766, 766*f*
  rapid urine, 649-650
  throat, 767
Culture medium, 768, 780
Cup, 458, 458*t*
Curette, 385*f*, 386
Curved needles, 398, 399*f*
Cushing's syndrome, 632*t*
Cutting needle, 398, 399*f*
CVA. See Cerebrovascular accident.
Cyanocobalamin, 443*t*
Cyanoject. See Cyanocobalamin.
Cyanosis, 40, 146, 164
Cyber Diet, 202
Cyclobenzaprine, 453*t*
Cyclophosphamide, 448*t*
Cyclosporine, 453*t*
Cyst, sebaceous, 415-416, 416*f*
Cystic fibrosis, 374, 780
Cystine crystals, 642*t*
Cystitis, 636
Cystogram, 573
Cytology, 11, 276, 323, 604*t*
Cytology report, 280-282, 281*f*, 282*t*
Cytology request for Pap test, 279
Cytomegalic inclusion bodies, 638*t*
Cytomegalovirus, 77*t*
Cytopathologist, 279
Cytotechnologist, 279
Cytoxan. See Cyclophosphamide.

D

Dalmane. See Flurazepam.
Daptacel. See Diphtheria, tetanus toxoids and acellular pertussis vaccine.
Darvocet. See Propoxyphene.
Darvon. See Propoxyphene.
Database, 25
Daycare, 334*t*
DEA number, 462, 464, 507
Debrox. See Carbamide peroxide.
Decibels, 224
Decongestants, 451*t*
Decontamination, 61, 83, 86, 120
Deep cervical lymph nodes, 834*f*
Deep infrapatellar bursa, 827*f*
Deep inguinal lymph nodes, 834*f*
Deep palpation, 195
Deep respirations, 146
Defense mechanisms of body, 53
Dehydration, 40
Deltasone. See Prednisone.
Deltoid intramuscular injection site, 359, 359*f*, 477-478, 478*f*
Deltoid muscle, 828*f*, 830*f*, 831*f*
Demerol. See Meperidine.
Demographic information in patient registration record, 6
Dental caries, 336*t*
Dental health, 374
Dental problems, 336*t*
Dentin, 835*f*
Depakene. See Valproic acid.
Depakote. See Divalproex.
Department of Health and Human Services, 601
Depo-Medrol. See Methylprednisolone.
Depo-Provera. See Medroxyprogesterone.
Depolarization, 525
Depression, 444*t*
Dermis, 843*f*
Descending colon, 836*f*
Descending limb, 615*f*

Detergent, 86, 92-93, 120
  for hand washing, 54
Dex-Ferrum. See Iron dextran.
Dexamethasone-tobramycin, 453t
Dexedrine. See Dextroamphetamine.
Dextroamphetamine, 450t
Dextroamphetamine-saccinarate and sulfate, 450t
Dextromethorphan, 449t
Dextrose in water, 785t
DiaBeta. See Glyburide.
Diabetes mellitus
  antidiabetics for, 444t
  application of heat or cold and, 239
  assessment of, 592t
  emergency care in, 807-808, 807f, 808f
  gestational, 304, 305
  glycosuria in, 626
  urine test strip parameters and, 632t
  website information on, 374, 753
Diabetic coma, 807, 808
Diabetic ketoacidosis, 808
Diagnosis, 6, 48, 168, 202
Diagnostic imaging, 565-582
  application of knowledge in, 579-580
  certification review in, 581
  cholecystography and, 571-572, 572f
  computed tomography and, 574-575, 575-576f
  contrast media in, 566-567, 567f
  fluoroscopy and, 568
  gastrointestinal series and, 569-571, 571f
  intravenous pyelography and, 572, 573f
  legal issues in, 577
  magnetic resonance imaging and, 575-577, 577f
  mammography and, 569, 569f, 570f
  patient positioning in, 568
  radiography and, 566
  terminology review in, 582
  ultrasonography and, 573-574, 574f
  website information on, 582
Diagnostic imaging report, 11-12, 13f
Diagnostic procedure, 48, 169
Diagnostic procedure documents, 11-12
Diagnostic testing, 168, 509-582
  charting of, 43
  colon procedures in, 547-558
    application of knowledge in, 562-563
    certification review in, 563
    fecal occult blood testing in, 548f, 548-555
    flexible sigmoidoscopy in, 555-558, 556f
    legal issues in, 560
    terminology review in, 563
    website information on, 563
  electrocardiography in, 512-535
    artifacts in, 521-523, 522f
    for atrial fibrillation, 534
    for atrial flutter, 533
    for atrial premature contractions, 532
    augmented leads in, 517, 518f
    baseline, segments, and intervals in, 515
    bipolar leads in, 517, 518f
    chest leads in, 518-519, 519f
    conduction of heart and, 514, 514f
    electrocardiograph capabilities and, 519
    electrocardiograph in, 512f, 512-513
    electrocardiograph leads for, 516-517, 517f
    electrocardiograph paper for, 515, 515f
    Holter monitor in, 526-531, 527f, 538f
    interpretative electrocardiographs in, 520, 521f
    maintenance of electrocardiograph in, 519
    for paroxysmal atrial tachycardia, 533
    for premature ventricular contractions, 534
    standardization of, 516, 516f
    structure of heart and, 513, 513f
    telephone transmission of, 520
    three-channel recording capability of, 519, 520f
    twelve-lead, three-channel electrocardiogram in, 524-526
    for ventricular fibrillation, 535
    for ventricular tachycardia, 535
    waves in, 514f, 514-515
  prostate cancer screening in, 558-559, 559f
  pulmonary function tests in, 536-540, 538f
  radiology in, 565-582
    application of knowledge in, 579-580
    certification review in, 581
    cholecystography and, 571-572, 572f
    computed tomography and, 574-575, 575-576f
    contrast media in, 566-567, 567f
    fluoroscopy and, 568
    gastrointestinal series and, 569-571, 571f
    intravenous pyelography and, 572, 573f
    legal issues in, 577
    magnetic resonance imaging and, 575-577, 577f
    mammography and, 569, 569f, 570f
    patient positioning in, 568
    radiography and, 566
    terminology review in, 582
    ultrasonography and, 573-574, 574f
    website information on, 582
  testicular self-examination in, 559-560, 560f
Diapedesis, 712, 725
Diaphoresis, 40, 127
Diaphragm, 832f
  of microscope, 760-761
  respiration and, 144, 144f
Diaphragm chestpiece, 151
Diaphysis, 827f
Diarrhea, 40, 445t
Diastix, 627t
Diastole, 150, 164
Diastolic pressure, 150, 155t, 164
Diazepam, 443t, 786t
Dibucaine, 442t
Dicyclomine, 449t
Dietary cholesterol, 734, 735
Diethylpropion, 455t
Differential diagnosis, 168-169, 202, 587
Differential white blood cell count, 709-710t
Diflucan. See Fluconazole.
Digastric muscle, 829f
Digestive system, 835-836f
Digital rectal examination
  for colorectal cancer, 555
  for prostate cancer, 558, 559f
Digitoxin, 450t
Digoxin, 450t
Dilantin. See Phenytoin.
Dilation, 308, 308f
  of cervix, 294, 323
Diltiazem
  for angina, 443t
  for hypertension, 446t
Diluent, 475
Dimetane. See Brompheniramine.
Diovan. See Valsartan.
Diphenhydramine, 445t, 786t
Diphenoxylate-atropine, 445t
Diphtheria, tetanus toxoids and acellular pertussis vaccine, 362t, 364-365f, 452t
Diplococci, 758, 758f
Direct antigen identification test, 769
Direct pressure to wound, 794f, 793-794
Direct skin testing, 493-494, 495t
Direct smear for Pap test, 278, 287
Disability, 269
Disc-plate method for sensitivity testing, 771f, 771-772
Discharge summary report, 16, 17f, 48
Disease
  microorganisms and, 757-759, 758f, 759f
  patient teaching in prevention of, 173
  website information on, 780
Disinfectants, 86, 98t, 98-99, 120
Disinfection, 97-101, 98f, 98t
  after completing procedures involving blood, 67, 67f
  application of knowledge in, 118
  certification review in, 119
  definition of terms in, 86-87
  sterilization and, 116
  terminology review in, 120
  website information in, 120
Dislocation, 798, 812
Dispensed medication, 436
Disposable chemical single-use thermometer, 132, 132f
Disposable gloves, 170t
Disposable lancet for skin puncture, 693, 693f, 695-697
Disposable semiautomatic lancet device, 683, 693f, 697-698
Dissecting scissors, 380, 382f
Distal convoluted tubule, 615f
Distance visual acuity, 208-210, 208-210f, 213-215
Diuresis, 616
Diuretics, 451t
Diurnal variations
  in blood pressure, 150
  in body temperature, 126
Divalproex, 444t
Division of Healthcare Quality Promotion, 83
Dobutamine, 785t
Dobutrex. See Dobutamine.
Documentation, 3-50
  application of knowledge in, 45-46
  certification review in, 47
  charting in, 34-43
    abbreviations used in, 37-39
    administration of medication and, 42
    diagnostic procedures and laboratory tests and, 43
    guidelines for, 34-36, 36f
    patient instruction and, 43, 44t
    patient symptoms and, 36, 40
    procedures and, 41
    progress notes and, 36
    specimen collection and, 42
  components of, 4
  consent documents in, 19-24
    consent to treatment form in, 19-21, 21f
    release of medical information form in, 21-24, 22f
  correspondence in, 6
  diagnostic procedure documents in, 11-12
  formats for, 24-26f, 24-27
  hospital documents in, 12-19
    discharge summary report in, 16, 17f
Documentation *(Continued)*
    emergency room report in, 17-19, 19f
    history and physical report in, 13-15, 15f
    operative report in, 15-16, 16f
    pathology report in, 17, 17f
  laboratory documents in, 10-11
  legal issues in, 44
  medical office administrative documents in, 4-6
  medical office clinical documents in, 6-10
    consultation report in, 8-10, 9f
    health history report in, 6-7
    home health care report in, 10, 10f
    medication record in, 8, 8f
    physical examination report in, 7
    progress notes in, 8
  patient registration record in, 6, 7f
  preparation of medical record in, 27-29
  taking health history, 29-34, 41-42
    chief complaint in, 30
    family history in, 34
    introductory data in, 29, 31-33f
    past history in, 34
    present illness in, 30-34
    review of systems in, 34
    social history in, 34
  terminology review in, 48
  therapeutic service documents in, 12, 14f
  website information on, 48
Docusate, 453t
Dog bite, 805
Donation of blood, 746-747
Donor, 747, 753
Dopamine, 785t
Doppler fetal pulse detector, 307f, 307-308
Dorsal recumbent position, 184
Dorsalis pedis pulse, 141t, 142
Dorsogluteal intramuscular injection site, 358, 358f, 477, 478f
Doryx. See Doxycycline.
Dosage range, 468
Dose, 468, 507
Down syndrome
  amniocentesis for, 312
  triple screen test for, 309
  website information on, 374
Doxazosin, 446t
Doxycycline, 292, 447t
Dram, 457
Drape, 170t
Draping, 180-189
  in dorsal recumbent position, 184
  in Fowler's position, 189
  in knee-chest position, 187-188
  in lithotomy position, 185-186
  in prone position, 183
  in Sims position, 186-187
  in sitting position, 180-181
  in supine position, 181-182
Dressing
  for external bleeding, 794f, 793-794
  sterile, 394-397
Dressing forceps, 381, 382f
Dristan. See Oxymetazoline.
Driving, body mechanics and, 247
Dronabinol, 445t
Drop, 458, 458t
Droplet infection, 757
Drowning
  adolescent and, 339t
  infant and, 337t
  school-age child and, 339t
  toddler and, 338t
Drug, defined, 507
Drug abuse, 508, 657
Drug Enforcement Agency, 508
Drug interactions, 467
Drug overdose, 452t
Drug-testing programs in workplace, 628
Drugs. See also Medication administration.
  blood pressure and, 151
  for breathing emergencies, 785-786t
  for cardiovascular emergencies, 785t
  classified on action, 441, 442-455t
  classified on preparation, 440-441
  controlled, 459-462, 460-461t
  factors affecting action of, 467-468
  Food and Drug Administration and, 440
  for metabolic emergency, 786t
  for neurologic emergencies, 786t
  nomenclature of, 440
  patient teaching in, 466
  Physician's Desk Reference and, 436, 437-439f
  for poison reversal, 786t
  powdered, 475, 477f, 483-484
  preparation from ampule, 472-473, 474f, 480-483
  preparation from vial, 472, 474f, 480-483
  prescription for, 462t, 462-465, 463f
  pulse rate and, 141
  respiratory rate and, 146
  storage of, 475
  systems of measurement for, 455-458, 458t
  website information on, 508
Dry cold, 238
Dry heat, 238
Dry heat oven, 113
Dry sterile dressing, 394-397
Dulcolax. See Bisacodyl.
Duodenum, 836f
Duplay uterine tenaculum, 385f
DuPont Analyst, 728
Dura mater, 839f
Dust mite, 492
Dyrenium. See Triamterene.
Dysmenorrhea, 273, 323
Dyspareunia, 273, 323
Dysplasia, 273, 323
Dyspnea, 40, 146-147, 164
Dysrhythmias, 143, 164, 531-535, 545
  antidysrhythmics for, 445t
  atrial fibrillation in, 534
  atrial flutter in, 533
  paroxysmal atrial tachycardia in, 533
  premature ventricular contractions in, 534
  ventricular fibrillation in, 535
  ventricular tachycardia in, 535
Dysuria, 616

E
Ear, 221-230
  acute otitis media and, 222
  application of knowledge of, 232-233
  certification review in, 234
  hearing acuity tests, 223-226, 225f, 226f
  hearing loss and, 222, 224
  instillations in, 227, 229-230
  irrigation of, 226-228
  legal issues in assessment of, 230
  otic preparations for, 454t
  physical examination of, 191t
  structure of, 221, 221f, 842f
  terminology review in, 235
  website information on, 235
Ear wax, 221
Echocardiogram, 573, 582
Eclampsia, 295
Ecotrin. See Aspirin.
Eczema, 494t
EDD. See Expected date of delivery.
Edema, 40, 269
  angioedema, 467
  application of heat for, 239
Effacement, 294, 308, 308f, 323
Efferent arteriole, 615f
Effexor XR. See Venlafaxine.
Ejaculatory duct, 838f
Elastic bandage, 423, 425f
Elavil. See Amitriptyline.
Elderly
  pulse rate of, 141t
  variations in body temperature, 127t
Electrocardiogram report, 11
Electrocardiograph leads, 516-517, 517f
Electrocardiograph paper, 515, 515f
Electrocardiography, 512f, 512-535, 545
  artifacts in, 521-523, 522f
  for atrial fibrillation, 534
  for atrial flutter, 533
  for atrial premature contractions, 532
  augmented leads in, 517, 518f
  baseline, segments, and intervals in, 515
  bipolar leads in, 517, 518f
  chest leads in, 518-519, 519f
  components of, 516-517, 517f
  conduction of heart and, 514, 514f
  Holter monitor in, 526-531
    activity diary for, 528, 528f
    application of, 529-531
    electrode placement in, 526-528, 527f
    event marker of, 528
    patient guidelines for, 527
  interpretative, 520, 521f
  maintenance of equipment in, 519
  paper for, 515, 515f
  for paroxysmal atrial tachycardia, 533
  for premature ventricular contractions, 534
  recommended frequency for, 169
  standardization of, 516, 516f
  structure of heart and, 513, 513f
  telephone transmission of, 520
  twelve-lead, three-channel, 519, 520f, 524-526
  for ventricular fibrillation, 535
  for ventricular tachycardia, 535
  waves in, 514f, 514-515
Electrode, 545
  for electrocardiogram, 516-517, 517f
  for Holter monitor, 526-528, 527f
Electrolyte profile, 592t
Electrolyte replacements, 452t
Electrolytes, 545
  electrical impulse of heart and, 517
  in plasma, 691
Electronic thermometer, 129, 129f
  for axillary body temperature, 135-136
  for oral body temperature, 133-135
  for rectal body temperature, 137-138
Elixir, 440
Embryo, 294, 323
Emergency medical dispatcher, 788
Emergency medical procedures, 783-812
  application of knowledge in, 808-809
  in bleeding, 793-794, 794-795f
  in burns, 799f, 799-800
  certification review in, 810-811

Emergency medical procedures *(Continued)*
  in diabetic emergencies, 807-808, 807f, 808f
  Emergency Medical Services system, 788
  first aid kit for, 788, 789f
  in heart attack, 791
  in musculoskeletal injuries, 796-799, 797f, 798f
  office crash cart for, 784, 785-787t
  OSHA safety precautions and, 788
  in poisoning, 801-804, 804f
  in seizures, 800-801
  in shock, 791-792, 792f
  in stroke, 791-792
  terminology review in, 812
  website information on, 812
  in wounds, 794-796, 795f, 796f
Emergency Medical Services system, 788, 812
Emergency medical technician, 788
Emergency medicine, 433
Emergency room report, 17-19, 19f
Emetics, 452t
Eminase. See Anistreplase.
Emotional states
  blood pressure and, 150-151
  body temperature variations and, 126-127
  pulse rate and, 141
  respiratory rate and, 145
Emphysema, 536
Employee information and training in
    hazardous chemicals, 91
EMS. See Emergency Medical Services system.
Emulsion, 440
Enalapril, 446t
Enamel, 835f
Endocardium, 513f
Endocervical specimen, 277, 277f
Endocervix, 323
Endocrine system
  structure and function of, 843f
  urine test strip parameters and, 632t
Endometrium, 273f
Endoscope, 555, 563
Endovaginal ultrasound scan, 310, 311t
Enema, 582
  barium, 566, 571, 571f
Engagement, 294, 323
Engerix-B. See Hepatitis B vaccine.
Engineering controls, 64
Enteric-coated tablet, 441
Environment, body temperature variations
    and, 127
Environmental Protection Agency, 83, 120
Enzyme-linked immunosorbent assay test, 76
Eosinopenia, 709t
Eosinophil, 718f, 719
Eosinophilia, 709t
Epicardium, 513f
Epidemiology Program Office, 83
Epidermis, 843f
Epididymis, 838f
Epidural space, 839f
Epiglottis, 832f, 836f
Epinephrine, 455t
  for anaphylactic shock, 468, 791, 791f
  for cardiovascular emergency, 785t
  in local anesthetic, 409
EpiPen. See Epinephrine.
Epiphyseal lines, 827f
Epiphysis, 827f
Epistaxis, 40, 794
Epithelial cell, 639-640
Epithelial cell casts, 639t
Epstein-Barr virus, 744
Equipment
  on crash cart, 786-787t
  in electrocardiography, 519
  for physical examination, 170t
Erector spinae, 831f
Error in patient medical record, 36, 36f
Errors of refraction, 207f, 207-208
Ery-Tab. See Erythromycin.
Erythema, 239, 269, 467
Erythrocyte, 718f
Erythrocyte sedimentation rate, 589t, 711t
Erythromycin, 447t
Escherichia coli, 758, 759f
Esidrix. See Hydrochlorothiazide.
Eskalith. See Lithium.
Esomeprazole, 449t
Esophagus, 832f, 836f
ESR. See Erythrocyte sedimentation rate.
Essential hypertension, 156
Estradiol-norethindrone, 452t
Ethicon Incorporated, 433
Ethics, 79
Ethinyl estradiol-etonogestrel, 451t
Ethinyl estradiol-levonorgestrel, 451t
Ethinyl estradiol-norelgestromin, 451t
Ethinyl estradiol-norethindrone, 451t
Ethinyl estradiol-norgestimate, 451t
Ethyl alcohol, 98t, 98-99
Ethylene oxide gas sterilization, 113
Etodolac, 448t
Eupnea, 146, 164
Eustachian tube, 221, 221f, 832f, 842f
Evacuated tube, 660, 669, 669f, 705
  serum separator, 689, 689f

Evacuated tube method of venipuncture,
    667-675
  guidelines for, 670-675, 671f
  needle for, 667, 667f, 668f
  order of draw for multiple tubes, 670
  plastic holder for, 668
  site selection for, 664f, 664-665, 666f
  tubes for, 669f, 669-670
  types of blood specimens in, 665,
    666f
Event marker of Holter monitor, 528
Event-related sterility, 112
Evista. See Raloxifene.
Examining room preparation, 170t, 170-171,
    171f
Exercise
  aerobic, 143
  blood pressure and, 151
  body temperature variations and, 126
  for high blood cholesterol, 735
Exercise tolerance testing, 516
Exhalation, 144, 144f, 164
Expected date of delivery, 300, 323
Expectorants, 452t, 536
Expiration, 144, 144f
Exposure control plan, 61-63, 62f
Exposure incident, 61, 64
Extensor carpi radialis brevis, 831f
Extensor carpi radialis longus, 831f
Extensor carpi ulnaris, 828f, 830f
Extensor digitorum longus, 828f, 830f
Extensor pollicis longus, 831f
External auditory canal, 221, 221f, 842f
External auditory meatus, 221
External bleeding, 793-794
External ear, 221
External female genitalia, 276, 276f
External iliac artery, 833f
External iliac vein, 833f
External intercostal muscle, 831f
External oblique, 828f, 829f, 830f
External os, 273f, 277, 323
External respiration, 144, 145f
External urethral orifice, 837f
Extraneous microorganisms, 765
Exudate, 239, 269, 394, 433
Eye, 206-220
  antiinfectives for, 453t
  application of knowledge of, 232-233
  certification review in, 234
  color vision assessment, 212f, 212-213,
    215-216
  conjunctivitis and, 217
  instillations in, 216, 219-220
  irrigation of, 216, 217-219
  legal issues in assessment of, 230
  physical examination of, 191t
  structure of, 206-207, 207f, 842f
  terminology review in, 235
  visual acuity assessment, 207-212
    distance, 208-210, 208-210f, 213-215
    near, 210-212, 211f
    in preschooler, 210, 210f
  website information on, 235
Eye contact, 35
Eye ointment, 216, 220
Eye-protection devices, 66, 67f
Eyedrops, 220
Eyepiece of microscope, 761

F
Face shield, 65, 66f, 67f
Facial nerve, 840f
Facial pressure point, 794f
Fahrenheit scale, 126, 126t, 164
Fainting, 781f, 791
  venipuncture-related, 687, 688
Fallopian tube, 273f
Falls
  adolescent and, 339t
  infant and, 337t
  preschooler and, 338t
  school-age child and, 339t
  toddler and, 338t
False negative, 780
False positive, 769, 780
False rib, 826f
Familial, term, 48
Familial disease, 34
Family Doctor, 202
Family history, 34, 274
  in hypertension, 156
Famotidine, 449t
Farsighted, 208
Fascia lata, 829f
Fastidious, 761
Fastin. See Phentermine.
Fasting, 595, 611
Fasting blood sugar, 731t, 736-737
Fatty casts, 639t, 640
Fauces, 832f, 835f, 836f
FDA. See Food and Drug Administration.
Fear
  preschooler and, 334t
  toddler and, 332t
Febrile, term, 127, 164

Fecal occult blood test, 548-555
  for colorectal cancer, 551
  guaiac slide test in, 548f, 548-549, 554-555
  patient preparation for, 549
  quality control in, 550
  recommended frequency of, 169
Federal Emergency Management Agency, 433,
    812
Federal Express, 48
Felodipine, 446t
Female
  genitalia of, 193t
  growth charts for
    head circumference-for-age and weight-
      for-length percentiles, 349
    length-for-age and weight-for-age
      percentiles, 348
    stature-for-age and weight-for age
      percentiles, 352
  reproductive system of, 273f
Femoral artery, 833f
Femoral nerve, 841f
Femoral pressure point, 794f
Femoral pulse, 141t, 142
Femoral vein, 833f
Femur, 826f, 829f
Fenestrated drape, 408, 408f
Feosol. See Ferrous sulfate.
Ferrous sulfate, 442t
Fetal heart rate, 312, 323
Fetal heart tones, 307f, 307-308, 323
Fetus, 294, 323
  problems of, 303
Fever, 40, 126, 126f, 127-128, 128t, 164
  pulse rate and, 141
  respiratory rate and, 146
Fexofenadine, 445t
Fibrillation
  atrial, 534
  ventricular, 535
Fibrin clot, 688
Fibrinogen, 691
Fibroblast, 393, 393f, 433
Fibrous capsule, 827f
Fibula, 826f, 829f
Figure-eight turn in bandaging, 424-425, 425f
File folder, 27-29
Fimbriae, 273f
Final diagnosis, 168
Fine adjustment, 761
Fine motor development, 329t
Finger puncture, 694f, 694-695
Firearm injury
  adolescent and, 339t
  school-age child and, 339t
First aid, 784, 812
First aid kit, 788, 789f
First-degree burn, 799f, 799-800
First-voided morning specimen, 616
Flagyl. See Metronidazole.
Flange of syringe, 471f, 471-472
Flatulence, 40
Flexeril. See Cyclobenzaprine.
Flexible sigmoidoscope, 555-558, 556f
Flexor carpi radialis, 828f, 830f
Flexor carpi ulnaris, 828f, 829f
Flexor digitorum, 828f
Flexor digitorum superficialis, 828-830f
Flexor pollicis longus, 828f, 829f
Floating rib, 826f
Flogen. See Influenza virus vaccine.
Flonase. See Fluticasone.
Flovent. See Fluticasone.
Floxin. See Ofloxacin.
Fluconazole, 291, 445t
Fluidounce, 457
Fluidram, 457
Fluoroquinolones, 447t
Fluoroscopy, 568, 582
Fluoxetine, 444t
Flurazepam, 454t
Fluticasone, 451t
Flutter, atrial, 533
Fluvastatin, 453t
Fluzone. See Influenza virus vaccine.
Focus of microscope, 761
Foerster sponge forceps, 383f
Folder labels, 29
Folex. See Methotrexate.
Food and Drug Administration, 83, 440, 508
Food poisoning, 758
Foot, linear measurement term, 457
Forced expiratory volume in 1 second, 537,
    538f
Forced expiratory volume in 1 second-forced
    vital capacity ratio, 537, 538f
Forced vital capacity, 537, 538f
Forceps, 380-381, 381f, 383f, 433
Forearm crutch, 257, 258f
Forearm veins, 666f
Fornix of vagina, 273f
Fosamax. See Alendronate.
Four-point gait, 261
Fovea centralis, 207f, 842f
Fowler's position, 189

Fracture, 796, 797f, 812
  casts for, 251-254f, 251-255, 256f
  emergency care of, 798f, 798-799
Frenulum linguae, 128, 164
Frequency, 616
Frontal bone, 826f
Frontal sinus, 836f
Frostbite, 806
Full-thickness burn, 799f, 800
Fulminant hepatitis, 72
Fundal height measurement, 306-307, 307-307f
Fundus of uterus, 273f, 294, 323
Fungal infection
  in acquired immune deficiency syndrome,
    78t
  antifungals for, 445t
Fungizone. See Amphotericin B.
Furosemide, 451t, 785t
Furuncle, 416, 433

G
Gabapentin, 444t
Gallbladder, 836f
  cholecystography of, 571-572, 572f
Gallon, 457
Galvanometer of electrocardiograph, 517, 517f
Gantanol. See Sulfamethoxazole.
Garamycin. See Gentamicin.
Gastric pump inhibitors, 449t
Gastrocnemius, 828f, 829f
Gastroesophageal reflux disease
  antacids for, 442t
  antiulcers for, 449t
Gastrointestinal series, 569-571, 571f
Gastrointestinal system
  common symptoms of, 40
  urine test strip parameters and, 630t
Gauge, 471, 507
Gauze pads, 394
Gender
  blood pressure and, 150
  pulse rate and, 141
Gene, 744, 753
General appearance, 190t
Generalized seizure, 801
Generator of ultrasound machine, 247
Generic name of drug, 440
Generic prescribing, 465
Genitalia examination, 193t
Genitourinary system
  anatomy of, 837-838f
  urine test strip parameters and, 630t
Gentamicin, 447t
Gestation, 294, 323
Gestation calculator, 300, 300f
Gestational age, 294, 323
Gestational diabetes mellitus, 304, 305
Gingiva, 835f
Glans penis, 838f
Glimepiride, 444t
Glipizide, 444t
Global Emergency Medical Services, 433, 812
Globulins, 691, 730t
Glomerulus, 615f
Glossopharyngeal nerve, 840f
Gloves, 55, 65
  application and removal of, 59-60
  for rectal body temperature, 137-138
  sanitization process and, 92
  sterile, 387-389
Glucolet 2, 693f
Glucophage. See Metformin.
Glucose, 807-808
  blood, 731t
    for hypoglycemia, 786t
  plasma, 589t
  in urine, 626, 632t
Glucose challenge test, 304
Glucose monitor, 738-739
Glucose tolerance test, 731t, 737-738
Glucotrol XL. See Glipizide.
Glutaraldehyde, 98, 98f, 98t
Gluteus maximus, 830f, 831f
Gluteus medius, 828f, 829f, 831f
Gluteus minimus, 831f
Glyburide, 444t
Glycogen, 736, 753
Glycosuria, 626, 657
Goniometer, 260
Gonorrhea, 292-293
  prenatal testing for, 303
Good Samaritan laws, 789
Gooseneck lamp, 170t
Gout, 445t
Gracilis, 828-831f
Grain, 456-457
Gram, 456
Gram-negative bacteria, 773, 773f
Gram-positive bacteria, 773, 773f
Gram stain, 773, 773f
Granular casts, 639t, 640
Granular leukocyte, 718
Granulation phase of wound healing, 393,
    393f
Graves vaginal speculum, 385f
Gravidity, 297-298, 323

- Greenstick fracture, 797
- Gross hearing test, 223
- Gross motor development, 329t
- Group A streptococci, 769
- Group B streptococci, 303
- Growth charts, 344, 347-353
  - female
    - head circumference-for-age and weight-for-length percentiles, 349
    - length-for-age and weight-for-age percentiles, 348
    - stature-for-age and weight-for age percentiles, 352
  - male
    - head circumference-for-age and weight-for-length percentiles, 351
    - length-for-age and weight-for-age percentiles, 350
    - stature-for-age and weight-for age percentiles, 353
- Growth measurements, 342-353
  - growth charts in, 344, 347-353
    - female, 348-349, 352
    - male, 350-351, 353
  - head and chest circumferences in, 343, 346
  - length and height in, 342, 343f, 344-345
  - weight in, 342, 344-345
- GTT. See Glucose tolerance test.
- Guaiac slide test, 548f, 548-549, 549f, 551-555
- Guaifenesin, 452t
- Guaifenesin-codeine, 449t
- Gums, 835f
- Gustatory hairs, 842f
- Gyne-Lotrimin. See Clotrimazole.
- Gynecologic examination, 272-293
  - assisting with, 286-289
  - breast examination and, 274-275, 283-285
  - pelvic examination and, 275-289
    - bimanual, 282, 283f
    - inspection of external genitalia, vagina, and cervix in, 276, 276f
    - Pap test and, 276-282, 277-278f, 280-281f, 282t
    - rectal-vaginal examination in, 282
  - terms related to, 272-273, 273f
  - vaginal infections and, 289-293
    - candidiasis in, 291, 291f
    - chlamydia in, 292, 293
    - gonorrhea in, 292-293
    - trichomoniasis in, 290, 291f
- Gynecologic instruments, 384-386, 385f
- Gynecology, 272, 323

H

- *Haemophilus* b conjugate vaccine, 362t, 452t
- Hair, 843f
- Hair follicle, 843f
- Haldol. See Haloperidol.
- Haloperidol, 449t
- Halsted mosquito hemostatic forceps, 383f
- Hand
  - physical examination of, 190t
  - veins for venipuncture, 665, 666f
- Hand hygiene, 53-55, 54t, 83
- Hand washing, 56-58
- Handgrip positioning for crutches, 260
- Handling of specimen, 596-601, 598t
- Hanging drop slide, 774
- Hard palate, 832f, 835f, 836f
- Havrix. See Hepatitis A vaccine.
- Hay fever, 494t
- Hazard communication program, 87
- Hazard Communication Standard, 87-91, 88-90f
- Hazardous chemical, 87
- HDL cholesterol, 753
- Head, physical examination of, 190t
- Head circumference, 343, 346
- Head circumference-for-age and weight-for-length percentiles
  - female, 349
  - male, 351
- Headache, 40, 448t
- Healing, 237-269
  - ambulatory aids in, 257-264
    - canes in, 259, 259f, 264
    - crutches in, 257-259, 258f, 259f, 260-263
    - walkers in, 259f, 259-260, 264
  - application of knowledge in, 267
  - certification review in, 268
  - fracture casting and, 251-254f, 251-255, 256f
  - legal issues in, 265
  - local application of heat and cold for, 238-246
    - cold, 240-241, 244-246
    - factors affecting, 238-239
    - heat, 239, 240f, 241-243
  - splints and braces in, 256, 256f, 257f
  - terminology review in, 269
  - therapeutic ultrasound in, 247-250, 248f
  - website information on, 269
- Health Care Financing Administration, 601
- Health Finder, 202
- Health history, 29-34, 41-42, 168
  - of blood donor, 746
  - chief complaint in, 30
- Health history *(Continued)*
  - family history in, 34
  - introductory data in, 29, 31-33f
  - past history in, 34
  - present illness in, 30-34
  - review of systems in, 34
  - social history in, 34
- Health history form, 31-33f
- Health history report, 6-7, 48
- Health Insurance Portability and Accountability Act, 5
- Health promotion, 173
- Health screen profile, 592t
- Hearing acuity, 221-226
  - audiometry and, 224-226, 226f
  - gross screening test of, 223
  - tuning fork tests of, 223-224, 225f
  - tympanometry and, 226, 226f
  - types of hearing loss and, 222
- Hearing loss, 222, 224
- Heart, 832f
  - conduction of, 514, 514f
  - dysrhythmias of, 531-535
    - atrial fibrillation in, 534
    - atrial flutter in, 533
    - paroxysmal atrial tachycardia in, 533
    - premature ventricular contractions in, 534
    - ventricular fibrillation in, 535
    - ventricular tachycardia in, 535
  - electrocardiography and, 512-535
    - artifacts in, 521-523, 522f
    - for atrial fibrillation, 534
    - for atrial flutter, 533
    - for atrial premature contractions, 532
    - augmented leads in, 517, 518f
    - baseline, segments, and intervals in, 515
    - bipolar leads in, 517, 518f
    - chest leads in, 518-519, 519f
    - electrocardiograph capabilities and, 519
    - electrocardiograph in, 512f, 512-513
    - electrocardiograph leads for, 516-517, 517f
    - electrocardiograph paper for, 515, 515f
    - Holter monitor in, 526-531, 527f, 538f
    - interpretative electrocardiographs in, 520, 521f
    - maintenance of electrocardiograph in, 519
    - for paroxysmal atrial tachycardia, 533
    - for premature ventricular contractions, 534
    - standardization of, 516, 516f
    - telephone transmission of, 520
    - three-channel recording capability in, 519, 520f
    - twelve-lead, three-channel electrocardiogram in, 524-526
    - for ventricular fibrillation, 535
    - for ventricular tachycardia, 535
    - waves in, 514f, 514-515
  - physical examination of, 192t
  - pulmonary function tests and, 536-540, 538f
  - structure of, 513, 513f
  - urine test strip parameters and, 630t
  - website information on, 545
- Heart attack, 784, 791
- Heart Center Online, 545
- Heart disease, 734
- Heart rate, 143
- Heartburn
  - antacids for, 442t
  - antiulcers for, 449t
- Heat cramps, 805
- Heat exhaustion, 805-806, 806f
- Heat exposure, 805-806, 806f
- Heat loss, 125
- Heat production, 125
- Heat stroke, 806
- Heat therapy, 238-246
  - chemical hot pack in, 246
  - factors affecting, 238-239, 240f
  - heating pad in, 241
  - hot compress in, 243
  - hot soak in, 242
- Heating pad, 241
- Height
  - length-for-age and weight-for-age percentiles, 348, 350
  - measurement in child, 342, 343f, 344-345
  - measurement of, 173-179, 174-176t
  - stature-for-age and weight-for age percentiles, 352, 353
- Height conversion, 175
- Helix, 842f
- Hema-Combistix, 627t
- Hemastix, 627t
- Hematocrit, 710t, 713f, 713-716
  - in prenatal examination, 304
- Hematology, 10, 707-725
  - application of knowledge in, 723
  - certification review in, 724
  - common tests in, 603t, 709-711t
  - components and function of blood, 708
  - erythrocytes and, 712
  - hematocrit and, 713f, 713-716
  - hemoglobin determination and, 712-713
  - iron deficiency anemia and, 714
- Hematology *(Continued)*
  - legal issues in, 721
  - leukocytes and, 712
  - in prenatal examination, 304
  - red blood cell count in, 717
  - terminology review in, 725
  - thrombocytes and, 712
  - white blood cell count in, 716-717, 717f
  - white blood cell differential count in, 717-721, 718f
- Hematoma, 662, 705
  - venipuncture-related, 686, 687f
- Hematuria, 616, 626
- Hemoccult, 548-549, 549f
- Hemochromatosis, 632t
- Hemoconcentration, 662, 705
- Hemogard closure tube, 669, 669f
- Hemoglobin, 710t
  - blood donation and, 747
  - determination of, 712-713
  - in prenatal examination, 304
- Hemolysis, 671, 686-687, 705, 712, 725
  - in blood antigen and antibody reactions, 746-747
- Hemolytic reaction, 769, 770f
- Hemorrhage, 793-794, 794-795f
- Hemostasis, 381, 433
- Hemostatic forceps, 381, 383f
- Heparin, 443t
- Hepatic vein, 833f
- Hepatitis
  - prenatal testing for, 305
  - testing for, 743
  - website information on, 83
- Hepatitis A, 73, 74-75t
- Hepatitis A vaccine, 452t
- Hepatitis B, 71-72, 74-75t, 305
- Hepatitis B vaccine, 71f, 71-72, 362t, 452t
- Hepatitis B vaccine waiver form, 68, 69f
- Hepatitis C, 72, 73, 74-75t
- Hepatitis D, 74-75t
- Hepatitis E, 74-75t
- Hepatitis profile, 592t
- Hepatobiliary system, 630t
- Heredity, hypertension and, 156
- Herpes simplex, 77t
- Heterotrophs, 52
- HibTITER. See *Haemophilus* b conjugate vaccine.
- High-complexity test, 601-602
- High-density lipoprotein cholesterol, 730t, 734-735
- High-level disinfection, 97
- High-power objective, 761
- Hilum, renal, 837f
- HIPAA privacy rule, 5
- Hippuric acid crystals, 642t
- Histamine$_2$-receptor antagonists, 449t
- Histology, 11, 604t
- History, 29-34, 41-42
  - chief complaint in, 30
  - family history in, 34
  - introductory data in, 29, 31-33f
  - past history in, 34
  - present illness in, 30-34
  - review of systems in, 34
  - social history in, 34
- History and physical report, 13-15, 15f
- HIV. See Human immunodeficiency virus.
- Hives, 467, 494t
- Holter monitor, 526-531, 527f, 538f
  - activity diary for, 528, 528f
  - application of, 529-531
  - electrode placement in, 526-528, 527f
  - event marker of, 528
  - patient guidelines for, 527
- Holter monitor report, 11, 528
- Home health care, 10, 48
- Home health care report, 10, 10f
- Homeostasis, 586, 611
- Hookworm infection, 445t
- Hormonal contraceptives, 451t
- Hormone replacement therapy, 274, 452t
- Hornet sting, 492, 803-804, 804f
- Hospital documents, 12-19
  - discharge summary report in, 16, 17f
  - emergency room report in, 17-19, 19f
  - history and physical report in, 13-15, 15f
  - operative report in, 15-16, 16f
  - pathology report in, 17, 17f
- Hot compress, 243
- Hot pack, 246
- Hot soak, 242
- House dust, 492
- Household bleach, 99
- Household system, 457-458, 458-459t
- Housekeeping, 67-68, 67-68f
- Hub adapter with syringe, 676, 676f
- Humalog, 444t
- Human body, 825-844
  - circulatory system of, 833-834f
  - digestive system of, 835-836f
  - genitourinary system of, 837-838f
  - heart and respiratory system of, 832f
  - muscles of, 828-831f
  - nervous system of, 839-841f
- Human body *(Continued)*
  - salivary and endocrine glands of, 843f
  - sense organs of, 842f
  - skeletal system of, 826-827f
  - skin of, 843f
- Human chorionic gonadotropin, 309, 651
- Human immunodeficiency virus, 73-79, 77-78t
  - antiretrovirals for, 449t
  - prenatal testing for, 305
- Humerus, 826f
- Humulin, 444t
- Hyaline articular cartilage, 827f
- Hyaline casts, 632t, 64038
- Hydralazine, 446t
- Hydrochloric acid, 53
- Hydrochlorothiazide, 451t
- Hydrocodone, 442t
- Hydrocortisone, 451t
- Hydroxyzine, 445t
- Hygroton. See Chlorthalidone.
- Hyoid bone, 832f, 836f
- Hyoscyamine, 449t
- Hyperacidity
  - antacids for, 442t
  - antiulcers for, 449t
- Hypercalcemia, 729t
- Hyperglycemia, 731t, 737, 753
- Hyperkalemia, 732t
- Hypernatremia, 732t
- Hyperopia, 207f, 208, 235
- Hyperphosphatemia, 731t
- Hyperpnea, 146, 164
- Hyperpyrexia, 126, 126f, 164
- Hypertension, 150, 164
  - antihypertensives for, 446t
  - diuretics for, 451t
  - website information on, 165
- Hyperthyroidism, 732t
  - antithyroid agents for, 455t
  - urine test strip parameters and, 632t
- Hyperventilation, 146, 164
- Hypnotics and sedatives, 454t, 460t, 461t
- Hypocalcemia, 729t
- Hypodermic syringe, 472, 472f
- Hypoglossal nerve, 840f
- Hypoglycemia, 731t, 736, 736-737, 753, 807-808
  - emergency medications for, 786t
- Hypokalemia, 732t
- Hyponatremia, 732t
- Hypophosphatemia, 731t
- Hypopnea, 146, 164
- Hypotension, 150, 164
- Hypothalamus, 124, 843f
- Hypothermia, 126, 126f, 164, 806, 812
- Hypothyroidism, 732t
- Hypovolemic shock, 791
- Hypoxia, 146, 164
- Hysterosalpingogram, 573
- Hyzaar. See Losartan-hydrochlorothiazide.

I

- Ibuprofen
  - for fever, 442t
  - for inflammation, 448t
- Ice bag, 244
- Ice pack
  - for musculoskeletal injury, 799
  - for nosebleed, 794f
- Ictotest, 627t
- Idiosyncratic reaction, 468
- Ileum, 836f
- Iliocostalis cervicis, 831f
- Iliocostalis lumborum, 831f
- Iliopsoas, 828f, 829f
- Ilium, 826f
- Imaginative play, 333t
- Imaging studies, 565-582
  - application of knowledge in, 579-580
  - certification review in, 581
  - cholecystography and, 571-572, 572f
  - computed tomography and, 574-575, 575-576f
  - contrast media in, 566-567, 567f
  - fluoroscopy and, 568
  - gastrointestinal series and, 569-571, 571f
  - intravenous pyelography and, 572, 573f
  - legal issues in, 577
  - magnetic resonance imaging and, 575-577, 577f
  - mammography and, 569, 569f, 570f
  - patient positioning in, 568
  - radiography and, 566
  - terminology review in, 582
  - ultrasonography and, 573-574, 574f
  - website information on, 582
- Imdur. See Isosorbide mononitrate.
- Imitrex. See Sumatriptan.
- Immersion oil, 761-762
- Immobilization of fracture, 798f, 798-799
- Immunity, 359, 373
- Immunization, 359-360, 373, 780
  - diphtheria, tetanus and pertussis vaccine information, 364-365f
  - National Childhood Vaccine Injury Act and, 359

Immunization, 359-360, 373, 780
patient teaching in, 360
recommended schedule for, 361*f*
record card for, 363*f*
vaccine administration record for, 366*f*
vaccines for, 362*t*, 452-453*t*
website information on, 374
Immunoassay test for pregnancy, 651
Immunosuppressants, 453*t*
Imodium. See Loperamide.
Impacted, term, 235
Impacted fracture, 797
Impotence, 447*t*
In vitro, 753
In vivo, 611, 753
Inactivated polio vaccine, 362*t*, 452*t*
Inch, 457
Inches to centimeters, 175
Incision, 392, 392*f*, 433, 795, 795*f*
Incision and drainage, 416-417, 417*f*
Incisor, 835*f*
Incubate, term, 120, 780
Incubation period, 757, 780
Incus, 221, 221*f*, 842*f*
Inderal. See Propranolol.
Indigestion
antacids for, 442*t*
antiulcers for, 449*t*
Indocin. See Indomethacin.
Indomethacin, 448*t*
Induration, 490, 491, 507
Infanrix. See Diphtheria, tetanus toxoids and acellular pertussis vaccine.
Infant, 294, 323, 373
anticipatory guidance for, 329-331*t*
blood pressure cuff for, 354*t*
carrying of, 342, 342*f*
gross and fine motor development, 329*t*
head circumference of, 343
length of, 342, 343*f*, 344-345
measuring head and chest circumference of, 346
measuring weight and length of, 344-345
safety guidelines for, 337-338*t*
skin puncture in, 692
techniques for interaction with, 341*t*
Infection, 83, 433, 757
antiinfectives for, 447*t*
chlamydial, 292-293
fever in, 127
of middle ear, 222
during pregnancy, 303
sexually transmitted, 290, 325
in strep throat, 771
in tuberculosis, 489-490
acquired immune deficiency syndrome and, 78*t*
antituberculars for, 449*t*
website information on, 508
in viral hepatitis, 72, 73
Infection control, 51-120
bloodborne diseases and, 71-79
acquired immunodeficiency syndrome in, 73-79, 77-78*t*
hepatitis B in, 71-72, 74-75*t*
hepatitis C in, 72, 73, 74-75*t*
disinfection and, 97-101, 98*f*, 98*t*
Hazard Communication Standard and, 87-91, 88-90*f*
microorganisms and, 52-60
alcohol-based hand rubs and, 58-59
gloves and, 55, 59-60
growth requirements for, 52-53
hand hygiene and, 53-55, 54*t*
handwashing and, 56-58
infection process cycle and, 53, 53*f*
protective mechanisms of body and, 53
OSHA Bloodborne Pathogens Standard and, 61-69
communicating hazards to employees in, 63
engineering controls in, 64
exposure control plan in, 61-63, 62*f*
hepatitis B vaccination and, 68, 69*f*
housekeeping and, 67*f*, 67-68, 68*f*
labeling requirements in, 63, 64*f*
Needlestick Safety and Prevention Act and, 61
personal protective equipment and, 65-67, 66*f*, 67*f*
record keeping in, 64
safer medical devices and, 63, 63*f*
terminology in, 61
universal precautions and, 68-69
work practice controls in, 64-65
regulated medical waste and, 69-71, 70*t*, 71*f*
sanitization and, 91-97
manual method of, 91-92, 94-95
rinsing in, 96-97
ultrasound method of, 92, 92*f*, 95
sterilization and, 102-116
autoclave in, 102, 110*f*, 110-112, 111*f*, 114-116
cold techniques in, 113
dry heat oven in, 113
ethylene oxide gas for, 113
handling and storing sterilized packs, 112
legal issues in, 116
Infection control *(Continued)*
maintenance of autoclave, 112-113
monitoring program in, 102-103, 103*f*, 104*f*
radiation for, 113
sterilization indicators in, 103-105, 105*f*
wrapping articles for, 105-109, 106*f*
website information on, 120, 780
Infection process cycle, 53, 53*f*
Infectious disease, 780
prevention and control of, 773
stages of, 757
Infectious Diseases Society of America, 780
Infectious mononucleosis, 744
InFeD. See Iron dextran.
Inferior articular process, 827*f*
Inferior concha, 832*f*
Inferior meatus, 832*f*
Inferior mesenteric artery, 833*f*
Inferior vena cava, 513*f*, 832-833*f*, 837*f*
Infiltration, 409, 433
Inflammation, 433
antiinflammatory agents for, 448*t*
corticosteroids for, 451*t*
leukocytes and, 712
wound healing and, 393
Inflammatory phase of wound healing, 393, 393*f*
Influenza virus vaccine, 452*t*
Informed consent, 19, 48
Infrapatellar fat pad, 827*f*
Infraspinatus, 830*f*, 831*f*
Ingested poison, 802
Ingrown toenail removal, 418-419, 419*f*
Inguinal lymph node, 834*f*
INH. See Isoniazid.
Inhalation, 144, 144*f*, 164
Inhalation administration, 507
Inhaled poison, 803
Injectable contraceptives, 451*t*
Injected poison, 803
Injection
intradermal, 489, 489*f*, 497-499
intramuscular, 475-479, 479*t*, 486-488
parts of needle and syringe for, 471-472, 471-472*f*
pediatric, 358-359, 358-359*f*
prefilled syringes and cartridges for, 475, 475*f*, 476*f*
preparation from ampule, 472-473, 474*f*, 480-483
preparation from vial, 472, 474*f*, 480-483
reconstitution of powdered drugs for, 475, 477*f*, 483-484
safety engineered syringes for, 472, 473*f*, 474*f*
storage for drugs for, 475
subcutaneous, 475, 477*f*, 484-487
Z-track technique in, 479, 479*f*, 488-489
Injury prevention
infant and, 331*t*
toddler and, 333*t*
Inner canthus, 218
Inner ear, 221, 842*f*
Inoculate, 780
Inoculum, 780
Inorganic iodine compounds, 567
Inorganic waste products, 615
Inpatient, term, 13, 48
Inscription, 463, 507
Insect sting, 492, 803-804, 804*f*
Insomnia, 454*t*
Inspection, 195, 202
Inspiration, 144, 144*f*
Instillation, 206, 235
ear, 227, 229-230
eye, 216, 219-220
Instruments, 380-386, 381-385*f*
for cervical punch biopsy, 420
for colposcopy, 419, 419*f*
for cryosurgery, 422
gynecologic, 384-386, 385*f*
for incision and drainage, 417
for ingrown toenail removal, 418
for needle biopsy, 418
for physical examination, 171, 171*f*
sanitization of, 91-97, 92*f*, 93-97
for sebaceous cyst removal, 416
Insufflate, 556, 563
Insulin, 444*t*, 807-808
blood glucose and, 736
Insulin glargine, 444*t*
Insulin lispro, 444*t*
Insulin shock, 807, 808, 808*f*
Insulin syringe, 472, 472*f*
Integumentary system symptoms, 40
InteliHealth, 202
Intensity control of ultrasound machine, 247
Intercostal, term, 164
Intermediate-level disinfection, 97-98
Intermittent fever, 128*t*
Internal bleeding, 794
Internal iliac artery, 833*f*
Internal iliac vein, 833*f*
Internal intercostal muscle, 829*t*
Internal jugular vein, 834*f*
Internal oblique muscle, 829*f*, 831*f*
Internal os, 273*f*, 323
Internal respiration, 144
International Stress Management Association, 725
Interpretative electrocardiograph, 520, 521*f*
Interrupted baseline artifact, 522*f*, 523
Interval in electrocardiogram, 515, 545
Interval prenatal history, 300
Intradermal injection, 489, 489*f*, 497-499, 507
Intradermal skin testing, 496, 496*f*
Intramuscular injection, 475-479, 479*t*, 507
administration of, 486-488
pediatric, 358-359, 358-359*f*
sites for, 477, 478*f*
Intravenous injection, 470, 507
Intravenous pyelography, 572, 573*f*
Intravenous solutions, 785*t*
Introductory data in health history, 29, 31-33*f*
Intropin. See Dopamine.
Inventory of hazardous chemicals, 87
Iodine-sensitivity test, 567
Ipecac syrup, 452*t*, 786*t*
IPOL. See Inactivated polio vaccine.
Irbesartan, 446*t*
Iris, 207, 207*f*, 842*f*
Iris diaphragm, 760
Iron-deficiency anemia, 713-714
Iron dextran, 442*t*
Iron supplements, 442*t*
Irrigation, 206, 235
of ear, 226-228
of eye, 216, 217-219
Irritable bowel syndrome, 449*t*
Ischemia, 545
Ischemic heart disease, 516
Ischium, 826*f*
Ishihara test, 212*f*, 213, 215-216
Isoniazid, 449*t*
Isopropyl alcohol, 98*t*, 98-99
Isoproterenol, 785*t*
Isoptin. See Verapamil.
Isosorbide dinitrate, 443*t*
Isosorbide mononitrate, 443*t*
Isotamine. See Isoniazid.
Isotonic saline, 785*t*
Isuprel. See Isoproterenol.

J
Jaundice, 40
Jejunum, 836*f*
Joslin Diabetes Center, 753
Jugular vein, 833*f*
Juxtaglomerular cell, 615*f*

K
Kanamycin, 447*t*
Kantrex. See Kanamycin.
Kaolin pectin, 445*t*
Kaopectate. See Kaolin pectin.
Kaposi's sarcoma, 77, 77*t*
Keflex. See Cephalexin.
Kelly hemostatic forceps, 383*f*
Keto-Diastix, 62*t*
Ketoconazole, 445*t*
Ketones, 626, 632*t*
Ketonuria, 626, 657
Ketosis, 626, 657
Ketostix, 627*t*
Kevorkian punch tip, 421*f*
Kidney, 614, 614*f*, 615*f*, 833*f*, 837*f*
intravenous pyelography and, 572, 573*f*
sonogram of, 574*f*
website information on, 657
Kilogram, 456
Kilograms to pounds, 175
Kling gauze, 423
Klonopin. See Clonazepam.
Knee, 827*f*
Knee-chest position, 187-188
Korotkoff sounds, 153, 155*t*, 164
Kova method, 646-648

L
Labeling of hazardous chemicals, 63, 64*f*, 87-88, 88*f*
Labia majora, 838*f*
Labia minora, 838*f*
Laboratory directory, 588, 589*t*
Laboratory documents, 10-11
Laboratory profiles, 591, 592*t*
Laboratory report, 593-595, 594*f*
Laboratory request, 589-593, 590*f*, 592*t*
Laboratory safety, 605
Laboratory tests, 169, 586-587, 611
blood chemistry in, 728-743
Accu-Chek glucose monitor and, 741-743
automated blood chemistry analyzers in, 728, 733*f*
blood glucose in, 736
blood urea nitrogen in, 736
cholesterol testing in, 734-736
common tests in, 729-733*t*
fasting blood sugar in, 736-737
glucose monitors and, 738-739
quality control in, 733-734
self-monitoring of blood glucose and, 739-740
charting of, 43
hematologic, 707-725, 709-711*t*
application of knowledge in, 723
Laboratory tests *(Continued)*
certification review in, 724
components and function of blood and, 708
erythrocytes and, 712
hematocrit and, 713*f*, 713-716
hemoglobin determination in, 712-713
iron-deficiency anemia and, 714
legal issues in, 721
leukocytes and, 712
red blood cell count in, 717
terminology review in, 725
thrombocytes and, 712
white blood cell count in, 716-717, 717*f*
white blood cell differential count in, 717-721, 718*f*
in initial prenatal examination, 302-305
microbiologic, 604*t*, 755-780
application of knowledge in, 778
certification review in, 779
cultures and, 768*f*, 768-769
disease and, 757-759, 758*f*, 759*f*
Gram stain and, 773, 773*f*
hanging drop slide in, 774
infection and, 757
legal issues in, 776
microscope and, 759-764, 760*f*
normal flora and, 757
in prevention and control of infectious diseases, 773
sensitivity testing and, 771*f*, 771-772
smears and, 772, 775
specimen collection in, 765-766, 766*f*
streptococcus testing and, 769, 770*f*
terminology review in, 780
throat culture and, 767
website information on, 780
wet mount method and, 772, 772*f*
patient preparation and instructions for, 595-596
purpose of, 587-588
reporting of, 593-595, 594*f*
requests for, 589-593, 590*f*, 592*t*
in serology, 11, 743-747
application of knowledge in, 751
blood typing in, 744-747, 745*f*, 748*f*
certification review in, 752
rapid mononucleosis testing in, 744, 745*f*
for syphilis, 304
terminology review in, 753
skin puncture and, 692-701
disposable lancet for, 695-697
disposable semiautomatic lancet device for, 697-698
guidelines for finger puncture in, 694*f*, 694-695
microcollection devices for, 693-694, 694*f*
puncture devices for, 692-693, 693*f*
puncture site for, 692
reusable semiautomatic lancet device for, 698-701
urinalysis in, 11, 613-657
application of knowledge in, 655
calibration of refractometer for, 624
casts in urine sediment, 635, 638-639*t*, 640-641
cells in urine sediment, 637-638*t*, 639-640
certification review in, 656
chemical examination of urine in, 625-629, 627*t*
collection of urine for, 616-621, 618*f*
composition of urine and, 615
Kova method of, 646-648
legal issues in, 653
measurement of urine specific gravity, 622-623
microorganisms and artifacts in urine, 644-645*t*, 641
physical examination of urine in, 621, 621*f*, 623*f*
rapid urine cultures in, 649-650
reagent strips for, 629-635, 630-631*t*, 632*f*, 644-645
structure and function of urinary system and, 614, 614*f*, 615*f*
terminology review in, 657
urine crystals, 635, 640-643*t*,
urine pregnancy testing and, 651*f*, 651-653
website information on, 657
venipuncture and, 660-692
application of tourniquet in, 661-664, 663*f*
butterfly method of, 676-677*f*, 676-682
evacuated tubes for, 669*f*, 669-670
guidelines for evacuated tube method of, 670-675, 671*f*
needle for, 667, 667*f*, 668*f*
obtaining plasma specimen in, 691-692
obtaining serum specimen in, 687-691, 689*f*
order of draw for multiple tubes, 670
OSHA safety precautions in, 666-668
patient positioning for, 661, 662*f*
patient preparation for, 661
plastic holder for, 668
problems encountered in, 686-687, 687*f*
site selection for, 664*f*, 664-665, 666*f*
syringe method of, 682-685
types of blood specimens in, 665, 666*f*

Labstix, 627*t*
Laceration, 392, 392*f*, 433, 795, 795*f*
Lactate dehydrogenase, 589*t*, 731*t*
Lactated Ringer's solution, 785*t*
LaLeche League, 325
Lamaze Method of Childbirth, 325
Lamina, 827*f*
Lancet devices, 693, 693*f*
Lanoxicaps. See Digoxin.
Lanoxin. See Digoxin.
Lansoprazole, 449*t*
Lantus. See Insulin glargine.
Laryngopharynx, 832*f*, 836*f*
Larynx, 832*f*, 836*f*
Lasix. See Furosemide.
Last menstrual period, 300
Latent tuberculosis infection, 489
Lateral position, 186-187
Lateral rectus muscle, 842*f*
Lateral view, 568
Latissimus dorsi, 828*f*, 830*f*, 831*f*
Law, 79
Laxatives, 453*t*
LDL cholesterol, 753
Leads in electrocardiograph, 516-517, 517*f*
Left atrium, 513, 513*f*, 832*f*, 833*f*
Left common carotid artery, 833*f*
Left jugular vein, 833*f*
Left lateral position, 186-187
Left lateral view, 568
Left pulmonary artery, 832*f*, 833*f*
Left pulmonary vein, 833*f*
Left renal artery, 837*f*
Left subclavian vein, 833*f*, 834*f*
Left ventricle, 513, 513*f*, 832*f*, 833*f*
Legal blindness, 209
Legal guardian, 369
Legal issues
  in cardiopulmonary procedures, 540
  in colon procedures, 560
  in consent by minors, 317
  in documentation, 44
  in emergency medicine, 807
  in eye and ear assessment, 230
  in hematologic tests, 721
  in laboratory procedures, 606
  in laboratory testing, 748
  in measurement of vital signs, 160
  in medical asepsis, 79
  in medication administration, 503
  in microbiology, 776
  in minor office surgery, 428
  in pediatrics, 369
  in phlebotomy, 701
  in physical agents for tissue healing, 265
  in physical examination, 198
  in radiology and diagnostic imaging, 577
  in sterilization and disinfection, 116
  in surgical procedures, 428
  in urinalysis, 653
Length, 373
  of infant, 342, 343*f*, 344-345
Length-for-age and weight-for-age percentiles
  female, 348
  male, 350
Lens, 207, 207*f*, 842*f*
Lescol. See Fluvastatin.
Leucine crystals, 642*t*
Leukocyte, 712, 718*f*
  in urine, 628, 630*t*
Leukocytosis, 709*t*, 712, 725
Leukocyturia, 628-629
Leukopenia, 709*t*, 712, 716-717, 725
Levaquin. See Levofloxacin.
Levator scapulae, 828*f*
Levofloxacin, 447*t*
Levophed. See Norepinephrine.
Levothyroxine, 454*t*
Levoxyl. See Levothyroxine.
Levsin. See Hyoscyamine.
Librium. See Chlordiazepoxide.
Lidocaine, 442*t*, 785*t*
Lifestyle, risk of breast cancer and, 274
Lifting, body mechanics and, 247
Ligament
  ovarian, 838*f*
  patellar, 828*f*
  periodontal, 835*f*
Ligate, 397, 433
Light palpation, 195
Light source of microscope, 760
Limit setting for infant, 330*t*
Linea alba, 828*f*
Lingual frenulum, 835*f*
Lingual tonsil, 832*f*, 836*f*
Liniment, 440
Lipase inhibitors, 455*t*
Lipid-lowering agents, 453*t*
Lipid profile, 592*t*, 736
Lipitor. See Atorvastatin.
Lipoprotein, 734, 753
Liquid-based preparation for Pap test, 278*f*, 278-279, 286-287
Liquid chemical burn, 800
Liquid nitrogen, 422
Liquid preparations of medication, 440-441, 469-470
Lisinopril, 446*t*
Lister bandage scissors, 381*f*
Liter, 456
Lithium, 448*t*
Lithotomy position, 185-186, 275
Littauer suture scissors, 381*f*
Liver, 833*f*, 836*f*
Liver function profile, 592*t*
Living children, 298
Load, 120
Lobule of ear, 842*f*
Local anesthetics, 433, 442*t*
  for minor office surgery, 408-410, 410*f*
  before suturing, 397
Lochia, 315, 323
Lodine. See Etodolac.
Lofstrand crutch, 257
Lomotil. See Diphenoxylate-atropine.
Long arm cast, 252, 253, 269
Long head of biceps, 829*f*
Long leg cast, 252, 269
Longissimus capitis, 831*f*
Longissimus cervicis, 831*f*
Loop diuretics, 451*t*
Loperamide, 445*t*
Lopressor. See Metoprolol.
Loratadine, 445*t*
Lorazepam, 443*t*
Lortab. See Hydrocodone.
Losartan, 446*t*
Losartan-hydrochlorothiazide, 446*t*
Lotensin. See Benazepril.
Lotion, 441
Lotrel. See Amlopidine-benazepril.
Lovastatin, 453*t*
Low-density lipoprotein cholesterol, 730*t*, 734
Low-grade fever, 126, 126*f*
Low-level disinfection, 98
Low-power objective, 761
Lower extremities
  lymphatics of, 834*f*
  physical examination of, 193*t*
Lower gastrointestinal series, 571, 571*f*
Lozenge, 441
Lubricant, 170*t*
Lubrication of hinged instruments, 93, 97
Luer adapter, 676, 676*f*
Lumbar curve, 827*f*
Lumbar plexus, 841*f*
Lumbar vertebrae, 826*f*, 827*f*
Lumen of needle, 471, 471*f*
Luminal. See Phenobarbital.
Lung, 832*f*, 833*f*
  physical examination of, 192*t*
  transplantation for chronic obstructive pulmonary disease, 536
  website information on diseases of, 165, 545
Lymphatics, 834*f*
Lymphocyte, 718*f*, 719
Lymphocytosis, 710*t*
Lymphopenia, 710*t*

M
Maalox. See Aluminum hydroxide-magnesium hydroxide.
Maceration, 255, 269
Macrobid. See Nitrofurantoin.
Macrodantin. See Nitrofurantoin.
Macrolides, 447*t*
Macula densa, 615*f*
Magnetic resonance imaging, 575-577, 577*f*
Magnification, 761
Major calyx, 837*f*
Malaise, 40, 128, 164
Male
  genitalia of, 193*t*
  growth charts for
    head circumference-for-age and weight-for-length percentiles, 351
    length-for-age and weight-for-age percentiles, 350
    stature-for-age and weight-for age percentiles, 353
  reproductive health of, 558-560, 559*f*
Malignant neoplasm, 77*t*
Malleus, 221, 221*f*, 842*f*
Malpractice, 560, 653
Mammography, 169, 569, 569*f*, 570*f*
Mandible, 826*f*
Manometer, 152, 164
Mantoux test, 490, 491, 498-499
Manual cleaning, 91-92, 94-95
Manual method, 611
  of laboratory testing, 602-604
  in white blood cell differential count, 717-718
Marinol. See Dronabinol.
Marrow cavity, 827*f*
Masseter, 829*f*, 830*f*
Material safety data sheet, 88-91, 89-90*f*, 120
Maturation index, 279-280
Maturation phase of wound healing, 393*f*, 394
Mature minor, 317
Maxilla, 826*f*
Maximum heart rate, 143
Mayo Clinic, 202
Mayo dissecting scissors, 382*f*
Mayo tray, 407, 433
McDonald's rule, 307
Measles, mumps, and rubella vaccine, 362*t*, 453*t*
Measured values in spirometry, 537, 538*f*
Mebendazole, 445*t*
Meclizine, 445*t*
Medial head of triceps, 829*f*
Medial rectus muscle, 842*f*
Median antebrachial vein, 664*f*
Median basilic vein, 664*f*
Median cubital vein, 664*f*
Mediastinal lymph node, 834*f*
Medical abbreviations, 815-823
Medical asepsis, 51-83, 83
  application of knowledge in, 81
  bloodborne diseases and, 71-79
    acquired immunodeficiency syndrome in, 73-79, 77-78*t*
    hepatitis B in, 71-72, 74-75*t*
    hepatitis C in, 72, 73, 74-75*t*
  microorganisms and, 52-60
    alcohol-based hand rubs and, 58-59
    gloves and, 55, 59-60
    growth requirements for, 52-53
    hand hygiene and, 53-55, 54*t*
    hand washing and, 56-58
    infection control and, 55
    infection process cycle and, 53, 53*f*
    protective mechanisms of body and, 53
  OSHA Bloodborne Pathogens Standard and, 61-69
    communicating hazards to employees in, 63
    engineering controls in, 64
    exposure control plan in, 61-63, 62*f*
    hepatitis B vaccination and, 68, 69*f*
    housekeeping and, 67*f*, 67-68, 68*f*
    labeling requirements in, 63, 64*f*
    Needlestick Safety and Prevention Act and, 61
    personal protective equipment and, 65-67, 66*f*, 67*f*
    record keeping in, 64
    safer medical devices and, 63, 63*f*
    terminology in, 61
    universal precautions and, 68-69
    work practice controls in, 64-65
  in parenteral administration of medication, 471
  regulated medical waste and, 69-71, 70*t*, 71*f*
Medical impressions, 13, 48
Medical office administrative documents, 4-6
Medical office clinical documents, 6-10
  consultation report in, 8-10, 9*f*
  health history report in, 6-7
  home health care report in, 10, 10*f*
  medication record in, 8, 8*f*
  physical examination report in, 7
  progress notes in, 8
Medical record, 3-50
  application of knowledge in, 45-46
  certification review in, 47
  charting in, 34-43
    abbreviations used in, 37-39
    administration of medication and, 42
    diagnostic procedures and laboratory tests and, 43
    guidelines for, 34-36, 36*f*
    patient instruction and, 43, 44*t*
    patient symptoms and, 36, 40
    procedures and, 41
    progress notes and, 36
    specimen collection and, 42
  components of, 4
  consent documents in, 19-24
    consent to treatment form in, 19-21, 21*f*
    release of medical information form in, 21-24, 22*f*
  correspondence in, 6
  diagnostic procedure documents in, 11-12
  formats for, 24-26*f*, 24-27
  hospital documents in, 12-19
    discharge summary report in, 16, 17*f*
    emergency room report in, 17-19, 19*f*
    history and physical report in, 13-15, 15*f*
    operative report in, 15-16, 16*f*
    pathology report in, 17, 17*f*
  laboratory documents in, 10-11
  legal issues in, 44
  medical office administrative documents in, 4-6
  medical office clinical documents in, 6-10
    consultation report in, 8-10, 9*f*
    health history report in, 6-7
    home health care report in, 10, 10*f*
    medication record in, 8, 8*f*
    physical examination report in, 7
    progress notes in, 8
  patient registration record in, 6, 7*f*
  preparation of, 27-29
  taking health history for, 29-34, 41-42
    chief complaint in, 30
    family history in, 34
    introductory data in, 29, 31-33*f*
    past history in, 34
    present illness in, 30-34
    review of systems in, 34
    social history in, 34
  terminology review in, 48
  therapeutic service documents in, 12, 14*f*
  website information on, 48
Medical record format, 48
Medical waste, 69-71, 70*t*
Medication administration, 435-508
  allergy testing in, 493-496, 494*t*, 495*t*, 495-496*f*
  application of knowledge in, 504-505
  certification review in, 505-506
  controlled drugs and, 459-462, 460-461*t*
  converting units of measurement, 458-459, 458-459*t*
  drug nomenclature and, 440
  drugs classified on action, 441, 442-455*t*
  drugs classified on preparation, 440-441
  factors affecting drug action, 467-468
  Food and Drug Administration and, 440
  guidelines for, 468
  legal issues in, 503
  medication record and, 465*f*, 465-466
  oral, 468-470
  parenteral, 470-489
    intradermal injections in, 489, 489*f*, 497-499
    intramuscular injections in, 475-479, 479*t*, 486-488
    parts of needle and syringe for, 471-472, 471-472*f*
    prefilled syringes and cartridges for, 475, 475*f*, 476*f*
    preparation from ampule, 472-473, 474*f*, 480-483
    preparation from vial, 472, 474*f*, 480-483
    reconstitution of powdered drugs for, 475, 477*f*, 483-484
    safety engineered syringes for, 472, 473*f*, 474*f*
    storage for drugs for, 475
    subcutaneous injections in, 475, 477*f*, 484-487
    Z-track injection technique in, 479, 479*f*, 488-489
  patient teaching in prescription medications, 466
  Physician's Desk Reference and, 437-439*f*
  prescription for, 462*t*, 462-465, 463*f*
  systems of measurement for, 455-458, 458*t*
  terminology review in, 507
  tuberculin testing in, 489-492, 500-502
  website information on, 508
Medication record, 8, 8*f*, 465*f*, 465-466
Medication restrictions, 596
Medrol. See Methylprednisolone.
Medroxyprogesterone, 451*t*
Medulla, 840*f*
Medulla oblongata, 144-145
Medullary cavity, 827*f*
Megakaryocyte, 712
Melena, 548, 563
Meninges, 839*f*
Meniscus, 164, 657
  of mercury sphygmomanometer, 153
Menopause, 273, 323
  hormone replacements for, 452*t*
  website information on, 325
Menorrhagia, 273, 323
Menstrual history in prenatal record, 296-297
Mensuration, 173, 202
Meperidine, 442*t*
Mercury glass thermometer, 129
Mercury sphygmomanometer, 152-153, 153*f*
Meridia. See Sibutramine.
Metabolic emergency, 786*t*
Metabolic system
  pulse rate and, 141
  urine test strip parameters and, 630*t*
Metacarpals, 826*f*
Metamucil. See Psyllium.
Metaphysis, 827*f*
Metatarsals, 826*f*
Metaxalone, 453*t*
Meter, 456
Metformin, 444*t*
Methimazole, 455*t*
Methocarbamol, 453*t*
Methotrexate, 448*t*, 453*t*
Methylphenidate, 450*t*
Methylprednisolone, 451*t*, 786*t*
Metoprolol, 446*t*
Metric system, 455-456, 458-459*t*
Metronidazole, 290, 449*t*
Metrorrhagia, 273, 323
Mevacor. See Lovastatin.
Mexate. See Methotrexate.
Miconazole, 291, 445*t*
Microbiologic specimens
  collection and transport systems for, 766, 766*f*
  handling and storage of, 598*t*, 765-766
Microbiology, 11, 755-780
  application of knowledge in, 778
  certification review in, 779
  cultures and, 768*f*, 768-769
  disease and, 757-759, 758*f*, 759*f*
  Gram stain and, 773, 773*f*
  hanging drop slide in, 774
  infection and, 757
  laboratory tests in, 604*t*
  legal issues in, 776
  microscope and, 759-764, 760*f*

Microbiology (Continued)
normal flora and, 757
in prevention and control of infectious diseases, 773
sensitivity testing and, 771f, 771-772
smears and, 772, 775
specimen collection in, 765-766, 766f
streptococcus testing and, 769, 770f
terminology review in, 780
throat culture and, 767
website information on, 780
wet mount method and, 772, 772f
Microcollection devices, 693-694, 694f
Microhematocrit method, 713
Micronase. See Glyburide.
Microorganisms, 52-60, 83, 756
alcohol-based hand rubs and, 58-59
Bloodborne Pathogens Standard and, 61-69
communicating hazards to employees in, 63
engineering controls in, 64
exposure control plan in, 61-63, 62f
hepatitis B vaccination and, 68, 69f
housekeeping and, 67f, 67-68, 68f
labeling requirements in, 63, 64f
Needlestick Safety and Prevention Act and, 61
personal protective equipment and, 65-67, 66f, 67f
record keeping in, 64
safer medical devices and, 63, 63f
terminology in, 61
universal precautions and, 68-69
work practice controls in, 64-65
culture of, 768f, 768-769
disease and, 757-759, 758f, 759f
gloves and, 55, 59-60
growth requirements for, 52-53
hand hygiene and, 53-55, 54t
hand washing and, 56-58
infection control and, 55
infection process cycle and, 53, 53f
microscopic examination of, 772-773, 773f
normal flora, 757
protective mechanisms of body and, 53
in urine, 635, 644t,
Microscope, 759-764, 760f
care of, 762
optical system of, 761
support system of, 760-761
Microscopic examination of urine, 635-649
calibration of refractometer for, 624
casts in urine sediment, 635, 638-639t, 640-641
cells in urine sediment, 637-638t, 639-640
Kova method of, 646-648
measurement of urine specific gravity, 622-623
microorganisms and artifacts in urine, 635, 644-645t,
urine crystals and, 635, 640-643t,
Microtainer Brand Safety Flow Lancet, 693, 693f
Micturition, 615, 657
Middle ear, 221, 842f
infection of, 222
Middle meatus, 832f
Migraine, 448t
Milligram, 456
Milliliter, 456
Minim, 457
Minipress. See Prazosin.
Minor, 317
Minor calyx, 837f
Minor office surgery, 377-433
application of knowledge in, 430-431
assisting physician in, 410-411f, 410-415
bandaging in, 422-472, 423-425f, 425t
certification review in, 431-432
cervical punch biopsy in, 420-421, 421f
colposcopy in, 419f, 419-420
commercially prepared sterile packages for, 386, 387f
cryosurgery in, 421f, 421-422
incision and drainage of abscess in, 416-417, 417f
ingrown toenail removal in, 418-419, 419f
instruments used in, 380-386, 381-385f
legal issues in, 428
local anesthetics for, 408-410, 410f
needle biopsy in, 417-418, 418f
opening of sterile packages in, 390-391
pouring of sterile solution in, 391
sebaceous cyst removal in, 415-416, 416f
sterile dressing change in, 394-397
sterile gloves for, 387-389
surgical asepsis for, 378-380
sutures in, 397-407
adhesive skin closures and, 401, 401f, 404-407
insertion of, 398-400, 399f
needles for, 398, 399f
surgical skin staples and, 400f, 400-401
suture size and packaging, 397
types of, 397, 398f
terminology review in, 433
tray setup for, 407-408, 411
website information on, 433
wounds and, 392-393f, 392-394
Mircette. See Ethinyl estradiol-norethindrone.
Mitral valve, 513f, 832f
Mixed casts, 639t
Mixed culture, 769
Mixed hearing loss, 222
Moderate-complexity tests, 601-602
Moist cold, 238
Moist heat, 238
Mometasone, 451t
Monistat. See Miconazole.
Monitoring
of fetal heart rate, 312
self-monitoring of blood glucose, 739-740
of sterilization process, 102-103, 103f, 104f
Mono test, 743, 745f
Monocular microscope, 761
Monocyte, 718f, 719
Monocytopenia, 710t
Monocytosis, 710t
Montelukast, 450t
Mothers Against Drunk Drivers, 508
Motor vehicle crash
adolescent and, 339t
infant and, 337t
preschool child and, 338t
school-age child and, 339t
toddler and, 338t
Motrin. See Ibuprofen.
Mouth, 191-192t
MRI. See Magnetic resonance imaging.
MSNBC Health, 202
Mucous membrane, 53, 780, 843f
Mucous threads in urine, 635
Mucus, 53
Multigravida, 294, 323
Multipara, 294, 323
Multistix reagent strip, 627t, 633-634
Mupirocin, 447t
Muscle artifact, 521-523, 522f
Muscle contraction, heat production and, 125
Muscle relaxants, 453t
Muscles, 828-831f
Musculoskeletal injuries, 796-799, 797-798f
Muslin for wrapping instruments, 106
Mycobacterial infection, 78t
Mycobacterium avium complex, 78t
Mycobacterium tuberculosis, 78t, 489
Mycostatin. See Nystatin.
Mylanta. See Aluminum hydroxide-magnesium hydroxide.
Mylanta-Gas. See Simethicone.
Myocardial infarction, 791
cardiogenic shock in, 791-792
urine test strip parameters and, 632t
Myocardium, 513f
Myometrium, 273f
Myopia, 207f, 208, 235

N
Nabumetone, 448t
Nadolol-bendroflumethiazide, 446t
Nägele's rule, 300
Naloxone, 786t
Naprosyn. See Naproxen.
Naproxen
for analgesia, 442t
for inflammation, 448t
Narcan. See Naloxone.
Nasacort. See Triamcinolone.
Nasal bone, 826f
Nasal cavity, 832f
Nasal conchae, 832f, 836f
Nasal congestion, 451t
Nasal corticosteroids, 451t
Nasal inflammation, 451t
Nasonex. See Mometasone.
Nasopharynx, 832f, 836f
National Center for Tobacco-free Kids, 545
National Childhood Vaccine Injury Act, 359
National Cholesterol Educational Program, 735
National Diabetes Education Initiative, 753
National Down Syndrome Society, 374
National Eye Institute, 235
National Geographic Society, 48
National Heart, Lung, and Blood Institute, 165, 545
National Institute of Allergy and Infectious Disease, 325, 508
National Institute of Arthritis and Musculoskeletal and Skin Diseases, 269
National Institute of Diabetes, 753
National Institute of Diabetes and Digestive and Kidney Diseases, 657
National Institute of Environmental Health Services, 120
National Institute of Health, 508
National Institute of Occupational Safety and Health, 83
National Institute on Aging, 611
National Institute on Alcohol Abuse and Alcoholism, 508
National Institute on Drug Abuse, 657
National Kidney foundation, 657
National Library of Medicine, 508
National Multiple Sclerosis Society, 780
National Phlebotomy Association, 705
National Rehabilitation Information Center, 269
National Stroke Association, 269
National Women's Health Information Center, 325
Nausea, 40, 445t
Near visual acuity, 210-212, 211f
Nearsighted, 208
Neck examination, 190t
Neck of tooth, 835f
Needle
angle for injection, 477f
biopsy, 417, 418f
for intradermal injection, 489
for parenteral injection, 471-472, 471-472f
for pediatric injection, 358
recapping of, 65
for suturing, 398, 399f
for venipuncture, 667, 667f, 668f
Needle biopsy, 417-418, 418f, 433
Needle holder, 382
Needleless system, 63
Needlestick injury, 66
Needlestick Safety and Prevention Act, 61
Nefazodone, 444t
Neisseria gonorrhoeae, 292-293
prenatal testing for, 303
Neo-Synephrine. See Phenylephrine.
Neobiotic. See Neomycin.
Neomycin, 447t
Neomycin-polymyxin-hydrocortisone, 454t
Neoral. See Cyclosporine.
Neosporin. See Polymyxin-neomycin.
Nephron, 614, 615f, 657
Nervous system
common symptoms of, 40
structure and function of, 839-841f
Neurogenic shock, 791
Neurologic emergency, 786t
Neurologic examination, 193t
Neurontin. See Gabapentin.
Neutropenia, 709t
Neutrophil, 718, 718f
Neutrophilia, 709t
Neutrophilic band, 718f
Newborn
blood pressure cuff for, 354t
head circumference of, 343
pulse rate of, 141t
respiratory rates of, 145t
screening test for, 362, 367-368, 369f
variations in body temperature, 127t
visual acuity in, 209
Nexium. See Esomeprazole.
Nicoderm patch, 454t
Nicorette gum, 454t
Nicotine, 454t
Nicotrol inhaler, 454t
Nifedipine, 443t
Night terrors, 335t
Nightmares, 335t
Nitrates, 443t
Nitrite in urine, 626, 628, 630t
Nitro-Bid. See Nitroglycerin.
Nitro-Dur. See Nitroglycerin.
Nitrofurantoin, 447t
Nitroglycerin, 443t
for cardiovascular emergency, 785t
for chest pain, 532
Nitropress. See Nitroprusside.
Nitroprusside, 785t
Nitrostat. See Nitroglycerin.
Nizoral. See Ketoconazole.
Nocturia, 616
Nocturnal enuresis, 616
Noise-induced hearing loss, 224
Nonabsorbable suture, 397, 398f, 433
Nonadherent pads, 394
Noncritical item, 97-98, 120
Noncutting needle, 398, 399f
Nonintact skin, 61, 83
Nonpathogens, 52, 83
Nonsteroidal antiinflammatory drugs, 442t
Nonstress test, 312
Norepinephrine, 785t
Normal acid urine, 640t
Normal alkaline urine, 640-641t
Normal flora, 54, 757, 780
Normal range, 586, 611
Normal sinus rhythm, 531, 545
North American Menopause Society, 325
Norvasc. See Amlodipine.
Nose, 191t, 832f
Nosebleed, 794
Notice of Privacy Practices, 5
Novolin, 444t
NPH insulin, 444t
Nullipara, 294, 323
Nupercainal ointment. See Dibucaine.
Nutrients in plasma, 691
Nutrition website, 202
NuvaRing. See Ethinyl estradiol-etonogestrel.
Nystatin, 291, 445t

O
Obesity
body mass index and, 177
in child, 343
Objective data, 27
Objective lenses of microscope, 761
Objective symptom, 36, 48
Oblique fracture, 797
Oblique view, 568
Obstetric history, 297-299
Obstetric US, 574
Obstetrics, 294-295, 323
Occipital node, 834f
Occult blood, 548, 563
Occupational exposure, 61
engineering controls for, 64
exposure control plan and, 61-63, 62f
hepatitis B vaccination after, 68
recording of, 64
work practice controls and, 64-65
Occupational Safety and Health Administration, 83
Bloodborne Pathogens Standard of, 61-69
communicating hazards to employees in, 63
in emergency medical procedures, 788
engineering controls in, 64
exposure control plan in, 61-63, 62f
hepatitis B vaccination and, 68, 69f
housekeeping and, 67f, 67-68, 68f
labeling requirements in, 63, 64f
in microbiologic procedures, 765
Needlestick Safety and Prevention Act and, 61
personal protective equipment and, 65-67, 66f, 67f
record keeping in, 64
safer medical devices and, 63, 63f
terminology in, 61
universal precautions and, 68-69
in venipuncture, 666-667
work practice controls in, 64-65
Occupational therapy, 12
Ochsner-Kocher hemostatic forceps, 383f
Ocular lens of microscope, 761
Oculomotor nerve, 840f
Odor of urine, 621
Office crash cart, 784, 785-787t
Office laboratory, 585-611
application of knowledge in, 608-609
automated analyzers in, 604-605
blood chemistry in, 728-743
Accu-Chek glucose monitor and, 741-743
automated blood chemistry analyzers in, 728, 733f
blood glucose in, 736
blood urea nitrogen in, 736
cholesterol testing in, 734-736
common tests in, 729-733t
fasting blood sugar in, 736-737
glucose monitors and, 738-739
quality control in, 733-734
self-monitoring of blood glucose and, 739-740
certification review in, 610
Clinical Laboratory Improvement Amendments of 1988, 601-602
collecting, handling, and transporting specimens, 596-601, 598t
hematologic tests in, 707-725, 709-711t
application of knowledge in, 723
certification review in, 724
components and function of blood, 708
erythrocytes and, 712
hematocrit and, 713f, 713-716
hemoglobin determination in, 712-713
iron deficiency anemia and, 714
legal issues in, 721
leukocytes and, 712
red blood cell count in, 717
terminology review in, 725
thrombocytes and, 712
white blood cell count in, 716-717, 717f
white blood cell differential count in, 717-721, 718f
laboratory reports and, 593-595, 594f
laboratory requests and, 589-593, 590f, 592t
laboratory tests and, 586-587
legal issues in, 606
manual method of laboratory testing, 602-604
microbiology and, 755-780
application of knowledge in, 778
certification review in, 779
cultures and, 768f, 768-769
disease and, 757-759, 758f, 759f
Gram stain and, 773, 773f
hanging drop slide in, 774
infection and, 757
laboratory tests in, 604t
legal issues in, 776
microscope and, 759-764, 760f
normal flora and, 757
in prevention and control of infectious diseases, 773
sensitivity testing and, 771f, 771-772
smears and, 772, 775
specimen collection in, 765-766, 766f
streptococcus testing and, 769, 770f
terminology review in, 780
throat culture and, 767
website information on, 780
wet mount method and, 772, 772f

Office laboratory *(Continued)*
patient preparation and instructions for testing, 595-596
purpose of laboratory testing and, 587-588
quality control in, 605
safety in, 605
serology in, 11, 743-747
application of knowledge in, 751
blood typing in, 744-747, 745*f*, 748*f*
certification review in, 752
laboratory tests in, 603*t*
rapid mononucleosis testing in, 744, 745*f*
for syphilis, 304
terminology review in, 753
skin puncture in, 692-701
disposable lancet for, 695-697
disposable semiautomatic lancet device for, 697-698
guidelines for finger puncture in, 694*f*, 694-695
microcollection devices for, 693-694, 694*f*
puncture devices for, 692-693, 693*f*
puncture site for, 692
reusable semiautomatic lancet device for, 698-701
terminology review in, 611
types of, 588-589, 589*t*
urinalysis and, 11, 613-657
application of knowledge in, 655
calibration of refractometer for, 624
casts in urine sediment, 635, 638-639*t*,
cells in urine sediment, 637-638*t*, 639-640
certification review in, 656
chemical examination of urine in, 625-629, 627*t*
collection of urine for, 616-621, 618*f*
composition of urine and, 615
Kova method of, 646-648
legal issues in, 653
measurement of urine specific gravity, 622-623
microorganisms and artifacts in urine, 635-636, 644-645*t*,
physical examination of urine in, 621-623, 621*f*, 623*f*
rapid urine cultures in, 649-650
reagent strips for, 629-635, 630-631*t*, 632*f*, 644-645
structure and function of urinary system and, 614, 614*f*, 615*f*
terminology review in, 657
urine crystals, 635, 640-643*t*,
urine pregnancy testing and, 651*f*, 651-653
website information on, 657
venipuncture in, 660-692
application of tourniquet in, 661-664, 663*f*
butterfly method of, 676-677*f*, 676-682
evacuated tubes for, 669*f*, 669-670
guidelines for evacuated tube method of, 670-675, 671*f*
needle for, 667, 667*f*, 668*f*
obtaining plasma specimen in, 691-692
obtaining serum specimen in, 687-691, 689*f*
order of draw for multiple tubes, 670
OSHA safety precautions in, 666-668
patient positioning for, 661, 662*f*
patient preparation for, 661
plastic holder for, 668
problems encountered in, 686-687, 687*f*
site selection for, 664*f*, 664-665, 666*f*
syringe method of, 682-685
types of blood specimens in, 665, 666*f*
website information on, 611
Office surgery, 377-433
application of knowledge in, 430-431
assisting physician in, 410-411*f*, 410-415
bandaging in, 422-472, 423-425*f*, 425*t*
certification review in, 431-432
cervical punch biopsy in, 420-421, 421*f*
colposcopy in, 419*f*, 419-420
commercially prepared sterile packages for, 386, 387*f*
cryosurgery in, 421*f*, 421-422
incision and drainage of abscess in, 416-417, 417*f*
ingrown toenail removal in, 418-419, 419*f*
instruments used in, 380-386, 381-385*f*
legal issues in, 428
local anesthetics for, 408-410, 410*f*
needle biopsy in, 417-418, 418*f*
opening of sterile packages in, 390-391
pouring of sterile solution in, 391
sebaceous cyst removal in, 415-416, 416*f*
sterile dressing change in, 394-397
sterile gloves for, 387-389
surgical asepsis for, 378-380
sutures in, 397-407
adhesive skin closures and, 401, 401*f*, 404-407
insertion of, 398-400, 399*f*
needles for, 398, 399*f*
surgical skin staples and, 400*f*, 400-401
suture size and packaging, 397
types of, 397, 398*f*
Office surgery *(Continued)*
terminology review in, 433
tray setup for, 407-408, 411
website information on, 433
wounds and, 392-393*f*, 392-394
Official name of drug, 440
Ofloxacin, 447*t*, 454*t*
Oil immersion objective, 761-764
Ointment, 441
Olanzapine, 449*t*
Olfactory nerve, 840*f*
Oliguria, 615, 616, 657
Omeprazole, 449*t*
Oncology Channel, 563
Ondansetron, 445*t*
One-handed recapping technique, 65
Open fracture, 796, 797*f*
Open wound, 392, 795
Opening of sterile package, 390-391
Operating scissors, 380, 381*f*
Operative report, 15-16, 16*f*
Ophthalmia neonatorum, 303
Ophthalmic antiinfectives, 453*t*
Ophthalmologist, 208
Ophthalmoscope, 170*t*, 202
Opponens pollicis, 829*f*
Opportunistic infection, 76, 77*t*, 83
Optic disk, 207*f*
Optic nerve, 207*f*, 840*f*, 842*f*
Optical system of microscope, 761
Optician, 208
Optimum growth temperature, 52, 83
Optometrist, 208
Oral administration, 468-470, 507
Oral contraceptives, 451*t*
Oral hypoglycemics, 444*t*
Oral temperature, 128, 133-135
Orbicularis oculi, 828-830*f*
Orbicularis oris, 828-829*f*
Orbit, 826*f*
Order of draw in venipuncture, 670
Organic waste products, 615
Orlistat, 455*t*
Oropharynx, 832*f*, 836*f*
Ortho Evra. See Ethinyl estradiol-norelgestromin.
Ortho-Novum. See Ethinyl estradiol-norethindrone.
Ortho Tri-Cyclen. See Ethinyl estradiol-norgestimate.
Orthopedist, 251, 269
Orthopnea, 147, 164
OSHA. See Occupational Safety and Health Administration.
Ossicle, 221
Osteochondritis, 692m705
Osteomyelitis, 692, 705
Other potentially infectious materials, 61
Otic preparations, 454*t*
Otitis media, 222
Otoscope, 170*t*, 202, 235
Ounce, 457, 458, 458*t*
Outer canthus, 218
Outer ear, 842*f*
Outside laboratories, 588
Oval window, 221*f*, 842*f*
Ovarian ligament, 838*f*
Ovary, 273*f*, 838*f*, 843*f*
Over-the-counter drugs, 466
use during pregnancy, 300
Oxycodone, 442*t*
OxyContin. See Oxycodone.
Oxygen
growth of microorganisms and, 52
respiration and, 144, 145*f*
Oxygen therapy, 536
Oxyhemoglobin, 712, 725
Oxymetazoline, 451*t*

P

P-R interval, 514*f*, 514-515
P-R segment, 514*f*, 514-515
P wave, 514*f*, 514-515
Pain, 40
analgesics for, 442*t*
back, 246
chest, 531, 532, 791
in fracture, 796
muscle relaxants for, 453*t*
Palate, 832*f*
Palatine tonsil, 832*f*, 835*f*, 836*f*
Palatoglossal arch, 835*f*
Palatopharyngeal arch, 835*f*
Palmaris longus, 830*f*
Palpation, 195, 195*f*, 202
of systolic pressure, 160
of vein for venipuncture, 664-665
Pancreas, 836*f*, 843*f*
Pap test, 276-282
cytology report in, 280-282, 281*f*, 282*t*
cytology request in, 279, 280*f*
evaluation of, 279
in initial prenatal examination, 303
maturation index and, 279-280
patient history and, 279
patient instructions for, 276
preparation of specimen in, 278*f*, 278-279, 286-287
Pap test *(Continued)*
previous treatment and, 279
recommended frequency for, 169
specimen collection for, 277, 277*f*
Paper-based patient record, 24, 48
Papilla, renal, 837*f*
Papillary muscles, 832*f*
Paramedic, 788
Paranasal sinuses, 832*f*
Parasitology, 11
laboratory tests in, 604*t*
microorganisms in urine, 635-636, 644*t*,
Parasympathetic nervous system, 839*f*
Parathyroid gland, 843*f*
Parenteral, term, 83, 436, 507
Parenteral contact, 61
Parenteral medication administration, 470-489
intradermal injections in, 489, 489*f*, 497-499
intramuscular injections in, 475-479, 479*t*, 486-488
parts of needle and syringe for, 471-472, 471-472*f*
prefilled syringes and cartridges for, 475, 475*f*, 476*f*
preparation from ampule, 472-473, 474*f*, 480-483
preparation from vial, 472, 474*f*, 480-483
reconstitution of powdered drugs for, 475, 477*f*, 483-484
safety engineered syringes for, 472, 473*f*, 474*f*
storage for drugs for, 475
subcutaneous injections in, 475, 477*f*, 484-487
Z-track injection technique in, 479, 479*f*, 488-489
Parietal bone, 826*f*
Parity, 298, 323
Parker-Mott retractor, 384*f*
Parkinson's disease, 448*t*
Parotid duct, 843*f*
Parotid gland, 836*f*, 843*f*
Parotid node, 834*f*
Paroxetine, 444*t*
Paroxysmal atrial tachycardia, 533
Partial seizure, 800
Partial-thickness burn, 799*f*, 800
Past medical history, 34
in prenatal record, 295
Patch testing, 494-495, 495*f*, 495*t*
Patella, 826*f*, 828*f*, 829*f*
Patellar ligament, 828*f*
Pathogen, 52, 83, 757
Pathology report, 17, 18*f*
Patient, 48
access to medical record, 5
assessment during physical examination, 190-193*t*, 190-195, 194*f*
Patient examination gown, 170*t*
Patient history, 29-34, 41-42
chief complaint in, 30
family history in, 34
introductory data in, 29, 31-33*f*
in Pap test, 279
past history in, 34
present illness in, 30-34
review of systems in, 34
social history in, 34
Patient instructions
for breast self-examination, 283-285
charting of, 43, 44*f*
for Holter monitor, 527
for laboratory tests, 595-596
for Pap test, 276
Patient positioning, 180-189
for computed tomography, 575, 575*f*
dorsal recumbent position in, 184
Fowler's position in, 189
knee-chest position in, 187-188
lithotomy position in, 185-186
for magnetic resonance imaging, 576, 577*f*
for pelvic examination, 275
prone position in, 183
in radiology and diagnostic imaging, 568
for rectal body temperature, 137-138
Sims position in, 186-187
sitting position in, 180-181
supine position in, 181-182
for venipuncture, 661, 662*f*
Patient preparation
for cholesterol testing, 736
for Hemoccult, 549
for initial prenatal examination, 301-302*t*
for laboratory tests, 595-596
for physical examination, 172-173
for pulmonary function tests, 538
for sigmoidoscopy, 555
for venipuncture, 661
Patient record, 3-50
application of knowledge in, 45-46
certification review in, 47
charting in, 34-43
abbreviations used in, 37-39
administration of medication and, 42
diagnostic procedures and laboratory tests and, 43
guidelines for, 34-36, 36*f*
patient instruction and, 43, 44*t*
patient symptoms and, 36, 40
Patient record *(Continued)*
procedures and, 41
progress notes and, 36
specimen collection and, 42
components of, 4
consent documents in, 19-24
consent to treatment form in, 19-21, 21*f*
release of medical information form in, 21-24, 22*f*
correspondence in, 6
diagnostic procedure documents in, 11-12
formats for, 24-26*f*, 24-27
hospital documents in, 12-19
discharge summary report in, 16, 17*f*
emergency room report in, 17-19, 19*f*
history and physical report in, 13-15, 15*f*
operative report in, 15-16, 16*f*
pathology report in, 17, 17*f*
laboratory documents in, 10-11
legal issues in, 44
medical office administrative documents in, 4-6
medical office clinical documents in, 6-10
consultation report in, 8-10, 9*f*
health history report in, 6-7
home health care report in, 10, 10*f*
medication record in, 8, 8*f*
physical examination report in, 7
progress notes in, 8
patient registration record in, 6, 7*f*
preparation of, 27-29
taking health history for, 29-34, 41-42
chief complaint in, 30
family history in, 34
introductory data in, 29, 31-33*f*
past history in, 34
present illness in, 30-34
review of systems in, 34
social history in, 34
terminology review in, 48
therapeutic service documents in, 12, 14*f*
website information on, 48
Patient registration record, 6, 7*f*
Patient rights, 230
Patient teaching, 171-172
in acquired immune deficiency syndrome, 79
in aerobic exercise, 143
in angina pectoris, 531, 532
in body mechanics, 247
in breast self-examination, 275
in cast care, 255
in childhood immunizations, 360
in chronic obstructive pulmonary disease, 146
in conjunctivitis, 217
in crutches, 258
in health promotion and disease prevention, 173
in hypertension, 156
in initial prenatal examination, 302
in iron deficiency anemia, 713-714
in low back pain, 246
in mammography, 570
in obstetric ultrasound scan, 309
in otitis media, 222
in prescription medications, 466
in strep throat, 771
in taking capillary blood specimen, 739
in urinary tract infection, 636
in wound care, 393
Paxil. See Paroxetine.
Pectoralis major, 828*f*, 829*f*
Pectoralis minor, 829*f*
Pediatric examination, 327-374
anticipatory guidance and, 329-339*t*
for infant, 329-331*t*
for preschooler, 334-335*t*
for school-age child, 335-337*t*
for toddler, 331-333*t*
application of knowledge in, 371-372
blood pressure measurement in, 354*t*, 354-355, 354-355*f*
carrying infant in, 342, 342*f*
certification review in, 372
child safety guidelines and, 337-339*t*
development of rapport during, 340*f*, 340-341, 341*t*
growth measurements in, 342-353
growth charts in, 344, 347-355
head and chest circumferences in, 343, 346
length and height and, 342, 343*f*, 344-345
weight and, 342, 344-345
immunizations in, 359-360, 361*f*, 362*t*
injections in, 358-359, 358-359*f*
legal issues in, 369
milestones of gross and fine motor development in infancy, 329*t*
newborn screening test in, 362, 367-368, 369*f*
terminology review in, 373
urine specimen collection in, 355-357
website information on child health, 374
Pediatric vaccine administration record, 366
Pediatrician, 328, 373
Pediatrics, 328, 373
Pediazole. See Erythromycin.

- Pedicle, 827*f*
- Peel-pack, 386, 387*f*
- Pelvic examination, 275-289
  - bimanual, 282, 283*f*
  - in initial prenatal examination, 302*t*
  - inspection of external genitalia, vagina, and cervix in, 276, 276*f*
  - Pap test and, 276-282, 277-278*f*, 280-281*f*, 282*t*
  - postpartal, 316*t*
  - recommended frequency for, 169
  - rectal-vaginal examination in, 282
- Pelvic inflammatory disease, 292
- Pelvic measurements in prenatal examination, 302*t*
- Penicillin, 447*t*
  - allergy to, 492
- Penis, 838*f*
- Pepcid AC. See Famotidine.
- Pepto-Bismol. See Bismuth subsalicylate.
- Percocet. See Oxycodone.
- Percodan. See Oxycodone.
- Percussion, 195*f*, 195-196, 202
- Percussion hammer, 170*t*, 202
- Perimenopause, 273, 323
- Perinatal, 83
- Perineum, 273, 323
- Periodic health screening, 169
- Periosteum, 827*f*
- Peripherally acting adrenergic blocking agents, 446*t*
- Peroneus brevis, 829-831*f*
- Peroneus longus, 828*f*, 831*t*
- Peroxidase, 563
- Personal protective equipment, 65, 66*f*, 67, 67*f*
- Personnel requirements in laboratory procedures, 602
- Perspiration
  - during fever, 127
  - heat loss and, 125
- Petri plate, 768, 768*f*
- PFTs. See Pulmonary function tests.
- pH, 83, 657
  - growth of microorganisms and, 53
  - of urine, 626, 630*t*
- Phagocytosis, 712, 725
- Phalanges, 826*f*
- Pharmacology, 435-508
  - allergy testing and, 493-496, 494*t*, 495*t*, 495-496*f*
  - application of knowledge in, 504-505
  - certification review in, 505-506
  - controlled drugs and, 459-462, 460-461*t*
  - converting units of measurement, 458-459, 458-459*t*
  - drug nomenclature and, 440
  - drugs classified on action, 441, 442-455*t*
  - drugs classified on preparation, 440-441
  - factors affecting drug action, 467-468
  - Food and Drug Administration and, 440
  - guidelines for medication administration, 468
  - legal issues in, 503
  - medication record and, 465*f*, 465-466
  - oral administration and, 468-470
  - parenteral administration and, 470-489
    - intradermal injections in, 489, 489*f*, 497-499
    - intramuscular injections in, 475-479, 479*t*, 486-488
    - parts of needle and syringe for, 471-472, 471-472*f*
    - prefilled syringes and cartridges for, 475, 475*f*, 476*f*
    - preparation from ampule, 472-473, 474*f*, 480-483
    - preparation from vial, 472, 474*f*, 480-483
    - reconstitution of powdered drugs for, 475, 477*f*, 483-484
    - safety engineered syringes for, 472, 473*f*, 474*f*
    - storage for drugs for, 475
    - subcutaneous injections in, 475, 477*f*, 484-487
    - Z-track injection technique in, 479, 479*f*, 488-489
  - patient teaching in prescription medications, 466
  - *Physician's Desk Reference* and, 437-439*f*
  - prescription for medication and, 462*t*, 462-465, 463*f*
  - systems of measurement for, 455-458, 458*t*
  - terminology review in, 507
  - tuberculin testing and, 489-492, 500-502
  - website information on, 508
- Pharyngeal tonsil, 836*f*
- Pharynx, 191-192*t*, 836*f*
- Phenergan. See Promethazine.
- Phenobarbital, 454*t*, 786*t*
- Phenolax. See Phenolphthalein.
- Phenolics, 99
- Phenolphthalein, 453*t*
- Phentermine, 455*t*
- Phenylalanine hydroxylase, 362
- Phenylephrine, 451*t*
- Phenylketonuria, 362
- Phenytoin, 444*t*, 786*t*
- Pheochromocytoma, 632*t*
- Phlebotomist, 660, 705
- Phlebotomy, 659-705
  - application of knowledge in, 703
  - certification review in, 704
  - legal issues in, 701
  - skin puncture in, 692-701
    - disposable lancet for, 695-697
    - disposable semiautomatic lancet device for, 697-698
    - guidelines for finger puncture in, 694*f*, 694-695
    - microcollection devices for, 693-694, 694*f*
    - puncture devices for, 692-693, 693*f*
    - puncture site for, 692
    - reusable semiautomatic lancet device for, 698-701
  - terminology review in, 705
  - venipuncture in, 660-692
    - application of tourniquet in, 661-664, 663*f*
    - butterfly method of, 676-677*f*, 676-682
    - evacuated tubes for, 669*f*, 669-670
    - guidelines for evacuated tube method of, 670-675, 671*f*
    - needle for, 667, 667*f*, 668*f*
    - obtaining plasma specimen in, 691-692
    - obtaining serum specimen in, 687-691, 689*f*
    - order of draw for multiple tubes, 670
    - OSHA safety precautions in, 666-668
    - patient positioning for, 661, 662*f*
    - patient preparation for, 661
    - plastic holder for, 668
    - problems encountered in, 686-687, 687*f*
    - site selection for, 664*f*, 664-665, 666*f*
    - syringe method of, 682-685
    - types of blood specimens in, 665, 666*f*
  - website information on, 705
- Phobia, 335*t*
- Phosphorus, 731*t*
- Physical activity
  - blood pressure and, 151
  - pulse rate and, 141
  - respiratory rate and, 145
- Physical agents for tissue healing, 237-269
  - ambulatory aids in, 257-264
    - canes in, 259, 259*f*, 264
    - crutches in, 257-259, 258*f*, 259*f*, 260-263
    - walkers in, 259*f*, 259-260, 264
  - application of knowledge in, 267
  - certification review in, 268
  - fracture casting in, 251-254*f*, 251-255, 256*f*
  - legal issues in, 265
  - local application of heat and cold, 238-246
    - cold, 240-241, 244-246
    - factors affecting, 238-239
    - heat, 239, 240*f*, 241-243
  - splints and braces in, 256, 256*f*, 257*f*
  - terminology review in, 269
  - therapeutic ultrasound in, 247-250, 248*f*
  - website information on, 269
- Physical examination, 7, 48, 167-202
  - application of knowledge in, 200
  - assisting with, 196-198
  - auscultation in, 196
  - certification review in, 201
  - definition of terms in, 168-169
  - in initial prenatal visit, 301*t*
  - inspection in, 195
  - legal issues in, 198
  - measuring weight and height in, 173-179, 174-176*t*
  - palpation in, 195, 195*f*
  - patient assessment during, 190-193*t*, 190-195, 194*f*
  - patient preparation for, 172-173
  - percussion in, 195*f*, 195-196
  - positioning and draping for, 180-189
    - dorsal recumbent position in, 184
    - Fowler's position in, 189
    - knee-chest position in, 187-188
    - lithotomy position in, 185-186
    - prone position in, 183
    - Sims position in, 186-187
    - sitting position in, 180-181
    - supine position in, 181-182
  - postpartum, 316, 316*t*
  - preparation of examining room for, 170*t*, 170-171, 171*f*
  - terminology review in, 202
  - of urine, 621, 621*f*, 623*f*
  - website information on, 202
- Physical examination report, 7, 48, 194*f*
- Physical fitness, 202
- Physical therapy, 12, 14*f*
- *Physician's Desk Reference*, 436, 437-439*f*
- Physician's office laboratory, 585-611, 588
  - application of knowledge in, 608-609
  - automated analyzers in, 604-605
  - blood chemistry in, 728-743
    - Accu-Chek glucose monitor and, 741-743
    - automated blood chemistry analyzers in, 728, 733*f*
    - blood glucose in, 736
    - blood urea nitrogen in, 736
    - cholesterol testing in, 734-736
    - common tests in, 729-733*t*
    - fasting blood sugar in, 737-738
- Physician's office laboratory *(Continued)*
    - glucose monitors and, 738-739
    - quality control in, 733-734
    - self-monitoring of blood glucose and, 739-740
  - certification review in, 610
  - Clinical Laboratory Improvement Amendments of 1988, 601-602
  - collecting, handling, and transporting specimens, 596-601, 598*t*
  - hematologic tests in, 707-725, 709-711*t*
    - application of knowledge in, 723
    - certification review in, 724
    - components and function of blood, 708
    - erythrocytes and, 712
    - hematocrit and, 713*f*, 713-716
    - hemoglobin determination in, 712-713
    - iron deficiency anemia and, 714
    - legal issues in, 721
    - leukocytes and, 712
    - red blood cell count in, 717
    - terminology review in, 725
    - thrombocytes and, 712
    - white blood cell count in, 716-717, 717*f*
    - white blood cell differential count in, 717-721, 718*f*
  - laboratory reports and, 593-595, 594*f*
  - laboratory requests and, 589-593, 590*f*, 592*t*
  - laboratory tests and, 586-587
  - legal issues in, 606
  - manual method of laboratory testing, 602-604
  - microbiology and, 755-780
    - application of knowledge in, 778
    - certification review in, 779
    - cultures and, 768*f*, 768-769
    - disease and, 757-759, 758*f*, 759*f*
    - Gram stain and, 773, 773*f*
    - hanging drop slide in, 774
    - infection and, 757
    - laboratory tests in, 604*t*
    - legal issues in, 776
    - microscope and, 759-764, 760*f*
    - normal flora and, 757
    - in prevention and control of infectious diseases, 773
    - sensitivity testing and, 771*f*, 771-772
    - smears and, 772, 775
    - specimen collection in, 765-766, 766*f*
    - streptococcus testing and, 769, 770*f*
    - terminology review in, 780
    - throat culture and, 767
    - website information on, 780
    - wet mount method and, 772, 772*f*
  - patient preparation and instructions for testing, 595-596
  - purpose of laboratory testing and, 587-588
  - quality control in, 605
  - safety in, 605
  - serology in, 11, 743-747
    - application of knowledge in, 751
    - blood typing in, 744-747, 745*f*, 748*f*
    - certification review in, 752
    - laboratory tests in, 603*t*
    - rapid mononucleosis testing in, 744, 745*f*
    - for syphilis, 304
    - terminology review in, 753
  - skin puncture in, 692-701
    - disposable lancet for, 695-697
    - disposable semiautomatic lancet device for, 697-698
    - guidelines for finger puncture in, 694*f*, 694-695
    - microcollection devices for, 693-694, 694*f*
    - puncture devices for, 692-693, 693*f*
    - puncture site for, 692
    - reusable semiautomatic lancet device for, 698-701
  - terminology review in, 611
  - types of, 588-589, 589*t*
  - urinalysis and, 11, 613-657
    - application of knowledge in, 655
    - calibration of refractometer for, 624
    - casts in urine sediment, 635, 638-639*t*,
    - cells in urine sediment, 635, 637-638*t*, 639-640
    - certification review in, 656
    - chemical examination of urine in, 625-629, 627*t*
    - collection of urine for, 616-621, 618*f*
    - composition of urine and, 615
    - Kova method of, 646-648
    - legal issues in, 653
    - measurement of urine specific gravity, 622-623
    - microorganisms and artifacts in urine, 635-636, 644-645*t*,
    - physical examination of urine in, 621-623, 621*f*, 623*f*
    - rapid urine cultures in, 649-650
    - reagent strips for, 629-635, 630-631*t*, 632*f*, 644-645
    - structure and function of urinary system and, 614, 614*f*, 615*f*
    - terminology review in, 657
    - urine crystals, 635, 640-643*t*,
    - urine pregnancy testing and, 651*f*, 651-653
    - website information on, 657
- Physician's office laboratory *(Continued)*
  - venipuncture in, 660-692
    - application of tourniquet in, 661-664, 663*f*
    - butterfly method of, 676-677*f*, 676-682
    - evacuated tubes for, 669*f*, 669-670
    - guidelines for evacuated tube method of, 670-675, 671*f*
    - needle for, 667, 667*f*, 668*f*
    - obtaining plasma specimen in, 691-692
    - obtaining serum specimen in, 687-691, 689*f*
    - order of draw for multiple tubes, 670
    - OSHA safety precautions in, 666-668
    - patient positioning for, 661, 662*f*
    - patient preparation for, 661
    - plastic holder for, 668
    - problems encountered in, 686-687, 687*f*
    - site selection for, 664*f*, 664-665, 666*f*
    - syringe method of, 682-685
    - types of blood specimens in, 665, 666*f*
  - website information on, 611
- Pia mater, 839*f*
- Pigmentary epithelium of eye, 842*f*
- Pineal gland, 843*f*
- Pink eye, 217
- Pint, 457
- Pinworms, 445*t*, 644*t*
- Pioglitazone, 444*t*
- Piriformis, 831*f*
- Pituitary gland, 843*f*
- Placental problems, 303
- Plain surgical gut, 397
- Planned Parenthood, 325
- Plasma, 611, 705, 708
- Plasma proteins, 691
- Plasma specimen, 665, 691-692
- Plaster cast, 251, 253-254
- Plastic holder for venipuncture, 668
- Platelet, 712, 718*f*
- Platelet count, 711*t*
- Platelet inhibitors, 454*t*
- Plavix. See Clopidogrel.
- Play, toddler and, 333*t*
- Plendil. See Felodipine.
- Pleural friction rub, 147*t*
- Plunger of syringe, 471*f*, 471-472
- Pneumococcal vaccine, 362*t*, 453*t*
- *Pneumocystis carinii* pneumonia, 77*t*
- Point of needle, 471, 471*f*
- Poison, 801, 812
- Poison control center, 801
- Poisoning, 801-804, 803*f*
  - adolescent and, 339*t*
  - emetics for, 452*t*
  - infant and, 338*t*
  - medications for, 786*t*
  - preschool child and, 338*t*
  - school-age child and, 339*t*
  - toddler and, 338*t*
- Polycythemia, 709*t*, 713, 725
- Polymyxin-bacitracin, 453*t*
- Polymyxin-neomycin, 453*t*
- Polymyxin-trimethoprim, 453*t*
- Polysporin. See Polymyxin-bacitracin.
- Polytrim. See Polymyxin-trimethoprim.
- Polyuria, 615, 616, 657
- Pons, 840*f*
- Popliteal pulse, 141*t*, 142
- Position, 323
- Position of fetus, 294
- Positioning, 180-189
  - for computed tomography, 575, 575*f*
  - dorsal recumbent position in, 184
  - Fowler's position in, 189
  - knee-chest position in, 187-188
  - lithotomy position in, 185-186
  - for magnetic resonance imaging, 576, 577*f*
  - for pelvic examination, 275
  - prone position in, 183
  - in radiology and diagnostic imaging, 568
  - for rectal body temperature, 137-138
  - Sims position in, 186-187
  - sitting position in, 180-181
  - supine position in, 181-182
  - for venipuncture, 661, 662*f*
- Post-bronchodilator spirometry, 538-539
- Post-exposure evaluation, 62
- Post-exposure prophylaxis, 71*f*, 71-72, 83
- Posterior chamber, 207, 842*f*
- Posterior cruciate ligament, 827*f*
- Posterior nares, 836*f*
- Posterior tibial pulse, 141*t*, 142
- Posteroanterior view, 568
- Postoperative, 433
- Postpartum, 294, 323
- Postpartum physical examination, 316, 316*t*
- Postural bronchial drainage, 536
- Posture, 247
- Potassium, 589*t*, 732*t*
- Potassium chloride, 452*t*
- Potassium hydroxide preparation, 291
- Potassium-sparing diuretics, 451*t*
- Potassium supplements, 452*t*
- Pound, 457
- Pounds to kilograms, 175
- Pouring of sterile solution, 391

Powdered drug, reconstitution of, 475, 477f, 483-484
Pravachol. See Pravastatin.
Pravastatin, 453t
Prazosin, 446t
Predicted values in spirometry, 537, 538f
Prednisone, 451t
Preeclampsia, 294, 303, 323
Prefilled disposable syringe, 475, 475f, 476f
Pregnancy
  body temperature variations and, 127
  prenatal care in, 294-325
    amniocentesis in, 311t, 312, 312f
    fetal heart rate monitoring in, 312
    fetal heart tones and, 307f, 307-308
    fundal height measurement and, 306-307, 306-307f
    gestational diabetes and, 305
    laboratory tests in, 302-305
    medical assisting responsibilities in, 312-315
    obstetric terminology in, 294-295
    obstetric ultrasound scan in, 309-310, 310f, 310-311f
    patient education in, 302
    patient preparation in prenatal visit, 301-302t
    prenatal record and, 295-300, 296-299f
    sex weeks-postpartum examination and, 316, 316t
    triple screen test in, 309
    vaginal examination in, 308, 308f
  testing for, 651f, 651-653
  warning signs during, 303
  website information on, 325
Pregnancy test, 651f, 651-653
Prehypertension, 150
Premarin. See Conjugated estrogens.
Premature contractions
  atrial, 534
  ventricular, 534
Premature needle withdrawal in venipuncture, 686
Prempro. See Conjugated estrogens-progesterone.
Prenatal, term, 323
Prenatal care, 294-325
  amniocentesis in, 311t, 312, 312f
  fetal heart rate monitoring in, 312
  fetal heart tones and, 307f, 307-308
  fundal height measurement and, 306-307, 306-307f
  gestational diabetes and, 305
  laboratory tests in, 302-305
  medical assisting responsibilities in, 312-315
  obstetric terminology in, 294-295
  obstetric ultrasound scan in, 309-310, 310f, 310-311f
  patient education in, 302
  patient preparation in prenatal visit, 301-302t
  prenatal record and, 295-300, 296-299f
  sex weeks-postpartum examination and, 316, 316t
  triple screen test in, 309
  vaginal examination in, 308, 308f
Prenatal profile, 592t
Prenatal record, 295-300, 296-299f
Preoperative, term, 433
Preparation of examining room, 170t, 170-171, 171f
Prepuce, 838f
Presbyopia, 208, 235
Preschooler, 373
  anticipatory guidance for, 334-335t
  distance visual acuity in, 210, 210f
  pulse rate of, 141t
  respiratory rates of, 145t
  safety guidelines for, 338t
  techniques for interaction with, 341t
  visual acuity in, 209
Prescription, 462t, 462-465, 463f, 507
Prescription and over-the-counter medication record form, 8
Present illness, 30-34
Present pregnancy history, 299-300, 300f
Presentation, 323
Presentation of fetus, 294
Pressure area, 251
Pressure bandage, 794
Pressure points, 793, 794f, 812
Pressure ulcer, 251
Pretending, 333t
Preterm birth, 298, 323
Preterm labor, 303
Prevacid. See Lansoprazole.
Prevnar. See Pneumococcal vaccine.
Prilosec. See Omeprazole.
Primary bronchus, 832f
Primary hypertension, 156
Primigravida, 295, 324
Primipara, 295, 324
Prinivil. See Lisinopril.
Probe, 382, 384f
Problem, defined, 25, 48
Problem list, 25f, 25-27
Problem-oriented record, 24-27, 25-26f
Procainamide, 445t, 785t

Procaine penicillin, 447t
Procardia-XL. See Nifedipine.
Prochlorperazine, 445t
Prodromal period, 757, 780
Prodrome, 780
Proficiency testing in laboratory procedures, 602
Profile, 591, 592t, 611, 736
Prognosis, 48, 169, 202
Progress note sheets, 36
Progress notes, 8, 26f, 27
Promethazine, 445t
Pronator teres, 828f
Prone position, 183, 568
Pronestyl. See Procainamide.
Propoxyphene, 442t
Propranolol
  for angina, 443t
  for dysrhythmias, 445t
  for hypertension, 446t
Prostate, 838f
Prostate cancer
  screening for, 169, 558-559, 559f
  website information on, 563
Prostate-specific antigen test, 558-559
Protected health information, 5, 21
Protective clothing, 65, 66
Proteinuria, 626, 657
Prothrombin, 691
Prothrombin time, 711t
Protozoal infection, 449t
Proventil. See Albuterol.
Provisional diagnosis, 15
Proxi-Strip, 401
Proximal convoluted tubule, 615f
Prozac. See Fluoxetine.
Pruritus, 40
Pseudoephedrine, 451t
Psychogenic shock, 791
Psychosis, 449t
Psyllium, 453t
PT. See Prothrombin time.
Pubic symphysis, 826f
Pubis, 826f, 838f
Public Health Service, 120
Pudendal nerve, 841f
Puerperium, 295, 315, 324
Pulmonary artery, 513, 513f, 832f, 833f
Pulmonary Channel, 545
Pulmonary function tests, 536-540, 538f
Pulmonary semilunar valve, 513f
Pulmonary trunk, 833f
Pulmonary tuberculosis, 490
Pulmonary valve cusp, 832f
Pulmonary vein, 832f, 833f
Pulp, 835f
Pulp cavity, 835f
Pulse, 141t, 141-142f, 141-143
  blood donation and, 747
  in initial prenatal examination, 301t
  measurement of, 147-148
  postpartal, 316t
Pulse pressure, 150, 164
Pulse rate, 141t, 142-143
Pulse rhythm, 143, 164
Pulse sites, 141-142, 141-142f
Pulse volume, 143, 164
Puncture, 433, 795f, 796
Puncture devices, 692-693, 693f
Puncture wound, 392, 392f
Pupil, 207, 207f, 842f
Pure culture, 769
Purkinje fiber, 514, 514f
Purosanguineous exudate, 394
Purulent exudate, 394
Pus, 394
Pyrazinamide, 449t
Pyrexia, 40, 126, 126f
Pyrogen, 127

Q
Q-T interval, 514f, 514-515
Q wave, 514f, 514-515
QRS complex, 514f, 514-515
Quad cane, 259, 259f
Quadriceps femoris, 828f, 829f
Qualitative tests, 625
Quality assurance, 602
Quality control, 611
  in blood chemistry, 783-784
  in clinical laboratory, 605
  in glucose testing, 739
  in guaiac slide testing, 550
  in laboratory procedures, 602
  reagent strip and, 629
Quantitative tests, 625
Quart, 457
Quaternary ammonium compounds, 99
Quickening, 295, 324
QuickVue In-Line One-Step A test, 770f
Quinapril, 446t

R
R wave, 514f, 514-515
Rabies, 805
Radial pulse, 141
Radial-ulnar pressure point, 794f

Radiation, 164
  heat loss and, 125, 125f
  to sterilize articles, 113
Radiation treatment, risk of breast cancer and, 274
Radioallergosorbent test, 496
Radiography, 566, 582
Radioimmunoassay for human chorionic gonadotropin, 653
Radiologist, 566, 582
Radiology, 565-582
  application of knowledge in, 579-580
  certification review in, 581
  cholecystography and, 571-572, 572f
  computed tomography and, 574-575, 575-576f
  contrast media in, 566-567, 567f
  fluoroscopy and, 568
  gastrointestinal series and, 569-571, 571f
  intravenous pyelography and, 572, 573f
  legal issues in, 577
  magnetic resonance imaging and, 575-577, 577f
  mammography and, 569, 569f, 570f
  patient positioning in, 568
  radiography and, 566
  terminology review in, 582
  ultrasonography and, 573-574, 574f
  website information on, 582
Radiology report, 11, 12f
Radiolucent, term, 567, 582
Radiopaque, term, 567, 582
Radius, 826f
Rales, 147t
Raloxifene, 450t
Ramipril, 446t
Random specimen, 616
Ranitidine, 449t
Rapid mononucleosis testing, 744, 745f
Rapid plasma reagin, 589t, 743
Rapid streptococcus test, 769, 770f
Rapid urine culture, 649-650
Rash, 40, 494t
RAST. See Radioallergosorbent test.
Rattlesnake, 804-805
Reagent strip, 629-632, 627, 630-631t, 632f, 644-645, 738
Recapping of needle, 65
Recipient, 747, 753
Recombivax HB. See Hepatitis B vaccine.
Reconstitution of powdered drugs, 475, 477f, 483-484
Record keeping, OSHA Bloodborne Pathogens Standard and, 64
Rectal biopsy, 555
Rectal temperature, 128, 137-138
Rectal-vaginal examination, 282
  in initial prenatal examination, 302t
  postpartal, 316t
Rectum, 191t, 836f, 838f
Rectus abdominis, 828-829f
Recurrent turn in bandaging, 425, 425f
Red blood cell, 712, 718f
  in urine, 643t, 639
Red blood cell casts, 638t
Red blood cell count, 709t
Reference range, 586
Reflotron Analyzer, 728
Refraction, 207, 235
Refractive index, 622, 657
Refractometer, 622-624, 622-623, 657
Regular insulin, 444t
Regulated medical waste, 69-71, 70t, 71f
Rehabilitation, 259
Relafen. See Nabumetone.
Release of medical information, 24
Release of medical information form, 21
Remittent fever, 128t
Removal of cast, 255, 256f
Renal artery, 833f
Renal capsule, 837f
Renal column, 837f
Renal cortex, 837f
Renal disease
  diuretics for, 451t
  urine test strip parameters and, 632t
  website information on, 657
Renal epithelial cell in urine, 640
Renal hilum, 837f
Renal medulla, 837f
Renal pelvis, 837f
Renal pyramid, 837f
Renal sinus, 837f
Renal threshold, 625, 657
Renal tubular epithelial cell in urine, 643t
Renal vein, 833f, 837f
Repolarization, 525
Reproductive history, risk of breast cancer and, 274
Research Institute on Addictions, 657
Reservoir host, 83
Resident flora, 54, 83
Resistance, 780
Respiration, 144-149
  abnormalities in, 146-147
  breath sounds and, 147, 147t
  in initial prenatal examination, 301t
  measurement of, 147-148

Respiration (Continued)
  mechanism of, 144-145, 144-145f
  patient color and, 146
  postpartal, 316t
  respiratory rate and, 145t, 145-146
  rhythm and depth of, 146
Respiratory depth, 146
Respiratory gases, 691
Respiratory system
  anatomy of, 832f
  common symptoms of, 40
Restoril. See Temazepam.
Retavase. See Reteplase.
Retention, 616
Reteplase, 454t
Retina, 207, 207f, 842f
Retinal artery, 842f
Retinal vein, 842f
Retractable needle, 474
Retractable venipuncture holder, 668f
Retractor, 382, 384f
Retroauricular node, 834f
Retrograde pyelogram, 573
Retrograde pyelogram angiocardiogram, 573
Retrovir. See Zidovudine.
Reusable semiautomatic lancet device, 693, 698-701
Reuse life, 100
Reverse chronological order, 24, 48
Review of systems, 34
Rh antibody titer, 304-305, 744
Rh blood group system, 746
Rh factor, 304
Rh immune globulin, 305
Rh-negative blood specimen, 304-305
Rheumatoid factor, 743
Rheumatoid profile, 592t
Rheumatrex. See Methotrexate.
Rhinorrhea, 445t
Rhomboideus major, 830-831f
Rhomboideus minor, 831f
Rhonchi, 147t
Rhythm strip, 517, 520f, 521f
Rifadin. See Rifampin.
Rifampin, 449t
Right atrium, 513, 513f, 832-833f
Right common carotid artery, 833f
Right jugular vein, 833f
Right lateral view, 568
Right lymphatic duct, 834f
Right pulmonary artery, 832f, 833f
Right pulmonary vein, 833f
Right renal vein, 837f
Right subclavian artery, 833f
Right subclavian vein, 833f
Right ventricle, 513, 513f, 832-833f
Rinne test, 223-224, 225f
Risedronate, 450t
Risk factor, 169, 273, 324
Risperdal. See Risperidone.
Risperidone, 449t
Robaxin. See Methocarbamol.
Robitussin. See Guaifenesin.
Robitussin A-C. See Guaifenesin-codeine.
Robitussin DM. See Dextromethorphan.
Rocephin. See Ceftriaxone.
Rochester-Pean hemostatic forceps, 383f
Rofecoxib, 448t
Roller bandage, 423, 423f
Rolling veins, 686
Root canal, 835f
Root of tooth, 835f
Rosiglitazone, 444t
Round window, 221f, 842f
Roundworm infection, 445t
Route of administration
  effect on drug action, 467
  oral, 468-470, 507
  parenteral, 470-489
    intradermal injections in, 489, 489f, 497-499
    intramuscular injections in, 475-479, 479t, 486-488
    parts of needle and syringe for, 471-472, 471-472f
    prefilled syringes and cartridges for, 475, 475f, 476f
    preparation from ampule, 472-473, 474f, 480-483
    preparation from vial, 472, 474f, 480-483
    reconstitution of powdered drugs for, 475, 477f, 483-484
    safety engineered syringes for, 472, 473f, 474f
    storage for drugs for, 475
    subcutaneous injections in, 475, 477f, 484-487
    Z-track injection technique in, 479, 479f, 488-489
Routine test, 588, 611
Rubber tourniquet, 663, 663f
Rubella, pregnancy and, 296
Rubella antibody titer, 304
Rubella vaccine, 453t

S
S-T segment, 514f, 514-515
S wave, 514f, 514-515

Sacral curve, 827*f*
Sacral plexus, 841*f*
Sacral vertebrae, 827*f*
Sacrum, 826*f*
Safer medical devices, 63, 63*f*
Safety engineered phlebotomy device, 63*f*
Safety engineered syringe, 63*f*, 472, 473-474*f*
Safety engineered venipuncture device, 668*f*
Safety precautions
  Bloodborne Pathogens Standard and, 61-69
    communicating hazards to employees in, 63
    in emergency medical procedures, 788
    engineering controls in, 64
    exposure control plan in, 61-63, 62*f*
    hepatitis B vaccination and, 68, 69*f*
    housekeeping and, 67*f*, 67-68, 68*f*
    labeling requirements in, 63, 64*f*
    in microbiologic procedures, 765
    Needlestick Safety and Prevention Act and, 61
    personal protective equipment and, 65-67, 66*f*, 67*f*
    record keeping in, 64
    safer medical devices and, 63, 63*f*
    terminology in, 61
    universal precautions and, 68-69
    in venipuncture, 666-667
    work practice controls in, 64-65
  for child, 337-339*t*
  in clinical laboratory, 605
  in disinfection, 99
  in using autoclave, 113
Salicylates, 454*t*
Salivary gland, 843*f*
Salmeterol, 450*t*
Salmonella, 758
Sandimmune. See Cyclosporine.
Sanguineous exudate, 394
Sanitary sewer, 70*t*
Sanitization, 86, 91-97, 120
  before disinfection, 99
  manual method of, 91-92, 94-95
  rinsing in, 96-97
  ultrasound method of, 92, 92*f*, 95
Sartorius, 828*f*, 829*t*
Saturated fat, 735
Scab, 393
Scalds, 337*t*, 338*t*
Scalenes, 828*f*, 829*f*
Scalpel, 380, 381*f*, 433
Scapula, 826*f*
School-age child, 373
  anticipatory guidance for, 335-337*t*
  pulse rate of, 141*t*
  respiratory rates of, 145*t*
  safety guidelines for, 339*t*
  techniques for interaction with, 341*t*
  visual acuity in, 209
School anxiety, 335*t*
Schroeder uterine tenaculum, 385*f*
Sciatic nerve, 841*f*
Scissors, 380, 381*f*, 382*f*, 433
Sclera, 206, 207*f*, 842*f*
Scleral venous sinus, 842*f*
Scrape, 392, 795*f*, 796
Screening
  hearing, 223
  newborn, 362, 367-368, 369*f*
  prostate cancer, 558-559, 559*f*
  triple screen test, 309
Scrotum, 838*f*
Scruple, 457
Sebaceous cyst, 415-416, 416*f*, 433
Second-degree burn, 799*f*, 800
Secondary bronchus, 832*f*
Sedatives and hypnotics, 454*t*, 460-461*t*
Segment in electrocardiogram, 515, 545
Seizure, 812
  anticonvulsants for, 444*t*
  emergency care of, 800-801
Selective serotonin reuptake inhibitors, 444*t*
Self-monitoring of blood glucose, 739-740
Semicircular canal, 221, 221*f*, 842*f*
Semicritical item, 97, 120
Semimembranosus, 831*f*
Seminal vesicle, 838*f*
Semispinalis capitis, 831*f*
Semitendinosus, 830*f*, 831*f*
Senn-Mueller retractor, 384*f*
Sensation, application of heat or cold and, 239
Sense organs, 842*f*
Sensitivity testing, 771*f*, 771-772
Sensorineural hearing loss, 222
Separation fear, 330*t*
Sequela, 769, 780
Serevent. See Salmeterol.
Serology, 11, 743-747
  application of knowledge in, 751
  blood typing in, 744-747, 745*f*, 748*f*
  certification review in, 752
  laboratory tests in, 603*t*
  rapid mononucleosis testing in, 744, 745*f*
  for syphilis, 304
  terminology review in, 753
Serosanguineous exudate, 394
Serous exudate, 394
Serratus anterior, 828-829*f*
Sertraline, 444*t*
Serum, 394, 433, 611, 687-688, 705
Serum albumin, 589*t*, 691
Serum calcium, 729*t*
Serum chloride, 729*t*
Serum cholesterol, 730*t*
Serum creatinine, 730*t*
Serum globulin, 730*t*
Serum glucose tolerance test, 731*t*
Serum lactate dehydrogenase, 731*t*
Serum phosphorus, 731*t*
Serum potassium, 732*t*
Serum pregnancy test, 653
Serum separator evacuated tubes, 689, 689*f*
Serum sodium, 732*t*
Serum specimen, 665, 687-691, 689*f*
Serum triglycerides, 733*t*
Serum uric acid, 733*t*
Serzone. See Nefazodone.
Seton Resource Center, 120
Sex education, 337*t*
Sexually transmitted diseases, 290, 325
Shape Up America, 202
Sharps injury log, 64
Shaving of surgical site, 408
Shelf life, 100
Shock, 791-792, 792*f*, 812
  insulin, 807, 808, 808*f*
  urine test strip parameters and, 632*t*
Short arm cast, 252, 253, 269
Short head of biceps, 829*f*
Short leg cast, 252, 269
Short leg walker, 256, 257*f*
Sibutramine, 455*t*
Sick child visit, 328
Sick role, 35
Side effects, 467
Sight and Hearing Association, 235
Sigmoid colon, 836*f*
Sigmoidoscope, 555, 563
Sigmoidoscopy, 169, 549, 563
Sigmoidoscopy report, 11
Signatura, 464, 507
Sildenafil, 447*t*
Simethicone, 445*t*
Simple partial seizure, 800
Sims position, 186-187
Sims uterine curette, 385*f*
Simvastatin, 453*t*
Sinemet. See Carbidopa-levodopa.
Singulair. See Montelukast.
Sinoatrial node, 514, 514*f*
Sinus bradycardia, 531
Sinus tachycardia, 531
Sitting, body mechanics and, 247
Sitting position, 180-181
Skelaxin. See Metaxalone.
Skeletal relaxants, 453*t*
Skeletal system, 826-827*f*
Skin, 843*f*
  application of heat or cold and, 239, 240*f*
  applying of cast and, 253
  cryosurgery for lesions of, 422
  as defense mechanism, 53
  intradermal injections and, 489, 489*f*, 497-499
  physical examination of, 190*t*
  Z-track injection method and, 479*f*
Skin-prick testing, 495*f*, 495*t*, 495-496
Skin puncture, 692-701
  disposable lancet for, 695-697
  disposable semiautomatic lancet device for, 697-698
  guidelines for finger puncture in, 694*f*, 694-695
  microcollection devices for, 693-694, 694*f*
  puncture devices for, 692-693, 693*f*
  puncture site for, 692
  reusable semiautomatic lancet device for, 698-701
Skin staples, 400*f*, 400-401
Skin testing
  direct, 493-494, 495*t*
  intradermal, 496, 496*f*
  patch, 494-495, 495*f*, 495*t*
  skin-prick testing in, 495*f*, 495*t*, 495-496
Skull, 221*f*, 839*f*
Sleep
  body mechanics and, 247
  body temperature during, 126
  disorders of, 335*t*
Sleep apnea, 146
Sleeptalking, 336*t*
Sleepwalking, 336*t*
Slide agglutination test, 651, 651*f*
Slide table, 408
Sliding shield syringe, 473
Sling, 798*f*
Smear, 772, 780
  preparation of, 775
  for white blood cell differential count, 719-721
Smoking
  chronic obstructive pulmonary disease and, 146, 536
  deterrent medications for, 454*t*
  high blood cholesterol and, 735
Smoking *(Continued)*
  hypertension and, 156
  website information on, 545
Snakebite, 804-805
Sneezing, 53
Snellen big E eye chart, 209*f*
Snellen eye chart, 208, 208*f*, 213-215
Snellen test, 208-210
Soak, 269
Soap, 54
SOAP format, 27, 48
Social history, 34
Social Security Administration, 611
Sodium, 589*t*
  hypertension and, 156
  normal values of, 732*t*
Sodium bicarbonate, 442*t*, 785*t*
Sodium hypochlorite, 99
Soft palate, 832*f*, 835*f*, 836*f*
Soleus, 828*f*, 830*f*, 831*f*
Solid preparations of medications, 441, 469
Solu-Medrol. See Methylprednisolone.
Soluble fiber, 735
Solution, 441
Soma. See Carisoprodol.
Sonogram, 310, 573, 582
Sorbitrate. See Isosorbide dinitrate.
Sound vibration, 195*f*, 195-196
Source individual, 62
Source-oriented record, 24, 24*f*
Spanking, 334*t*
Specific gravity, 622-623, 657
Specimen, 611, 765, 780
Specimen collection, 596-601, 598*t*
  charting of, 42
  for chlamydia and gonorrhea, 293
  microbiologic, 765-766, 766*f*
  in Pap test, 277, 277*f*
  skin puncture for, 692-701
    disposable lancet for, 695-697
    disposable semiautomatic lancet device for, 697-698
    guidelines for finger puncture in, 694*f*, 694-695
    microcollection devices for, 693-694, 694*f*
    puncture devices for, 692-693, 693*f*
    puncture site for, 692
    reusable semiautomatic lancet device for, 698-701
  testing categories and, 588-589
  urine, 616-617, 618*f*
    clean-catch midstream, 617, 618*f*, 618-619
    first-voided morning, 616
    pediatric, 355-357
    random, 616
    twenty-four hour, 618, 619-620
  vaginal, 289
  venipuncture for, 660-692
    application of tourniquet in, 661-664, 663*f*
    butterfly method of, 676-677*f*, 676-682
    evacuated tubes for, 669*f*, 669-670
    guidelines for evacuated tube method of, 670-675, 671*f*
    needle for, 667, 667*f*, 668*f*
    obtaining plasma specimen in, 691-692
    obtaining serum specimen in, 687-691, 689*f*
    order of draw for multiple tubes, 670
    OSHA safety precautions in, 666-668
    patient positioning for, 661, 662*f*
    patient preparation for, 661
    plastic holder for, 668
    problems encountered in, 686-687, 687*f*
    site selection for, 664*f*, 664-665, 666*f*
    syringe method of, 682-685
    types of blood specimens in, 665, 666*f*
Specimen container, 170*t*
Speculum, 202, 384, 385*f*
  for physical examination, 170*t*
  vaginal, 276, 276*f*
Speech therapy, 12
Spermatozoa, 636, 644*t*,
Sphenoid sinus, 836*f*
Sphygmomanometer, 164, 170*t*
Spider bite, 804
Spina bifida, 374
Spinal accessory nerve, 840*f*
Spinal cord, 839*f*, 840*f*
Spine, 827*f*
Spiral fracture, 797
Spiral-reverse turn in bandaging, 424, 424*f*
Spiral turn in bandaging, 424, 424*f*
Spirilla, 758-759*f*, 780
Spirit, 441
Spirometer, 536-538, 545
Spirometry, 536-540, 538*f*, 545
Spirometry report, 11
Spironolactone, 451*t*
Spleen, 834*f*
Splenius capitis, 830*f*, 831*f*
Splint, 256-257*f*, 269, 798*f*, 798-799, 812
Splinter forceps, 381, 382*f*
Spoiling of infant, 330*t*
Sponge forceps, 381, 383*f*
Spontaneous abortion, 303
Spore, 86-87, 120
Sprain, 240, 269, 798, 812
Spray, 441
Squamous epithelial cell in urine, 637*t*
Stabs, 719
Stage focus, 761
Stain
  Gram, 773, 773*f*
  of Pap specimen, 279
Stain remover, 93
Standard cane, 259, 259*f*
Standardization mark, 516, 516*f*
Standardization of electrocardiograph, 516, 516*f*
Standing, body mechanics and, 247
Stapes, 221, 221*f*, 842*f*
Staphylococci, 758-759*f*
Staples, 400*f*, 400-403
Stature-for-age and weight-for age percentiles
  female, 352
  male, 353
Status epilepticus, 801
Stereotyping, 35
Steri-Strip, 401
Sterile, 433
Sterile dressing, 394-397
Sterile field, 380
  adding sutures to, 398, 399*f*
  items included on, 400
  transferring articles to, 411-412
Sterile gloves, 55, 387-389
Sterile package
  commercially prepared, 386, 387*f*
  opening of, 390-391
Sterile solution, 391
Sterile technique, 378-380
Sterile tray setup, 407-408, 411
Sterilization, 87, 102-116, 120
  application of knowledge in, 118
  autoclave in, 102, 110-111*f*, 110-112, 114-116
  certification review in, 119
  cold techniques in, 113
  definition of terms in, 86-87
  dry heat oven in, 113
  ethylene oxide gas for, 113
  handling and storing sterilized packs, 112
  legal issues in, 116
  maintenance of autoclave, 112-113
  monitoring program in, 102-103, 103-104*f*
  radiation for, 113
  sterilization indicators in, 103-105, 105*f*
  terminology review in, 120
  website information in, 120
  wrapping articles for, 105-109, 106*f*
Sterilization indicators, 103-105, 105*f*
Sterilization paper wrap, 106, 106*f*
Sterilization pouch, 106, 106*f*
Sterilization strip, 104, 105*f*
Sterilized pack, 112
Sternocleidomastoid, 828-830*f*
Sternum, 826*f*
Stethoscope, 151, 164, 170*t*
Sting, 803-804, 804*f*
Stockinette, 253, 253*f*
Stomach, 836*f*
Stool, handling and storage of, 598*t*
Storage
  of biologic specimens, 598*t*
  of disinfectants, 100
  of medications, 475
  of sterilized packs, 112
Straight needle, 398, 399*f*
Strain, 240, 269, 798, 812
Stranger fear, 330*t*
Stratum basale, 843*f*
Stratum corneum, 843*f*
Stratum granulosum, 843*f*
Stratum spinosum, 843*f*
Streaking, 768, 780
Strep throat, 771
Streptase. See Streptokinase.
Streptococcal pharyngitis, 769
Streptococci, 758, 758*f*, 759*f*
  testing for, 769, 770*f*
Streptococcus pyogenes, 769
Streptokinase, 454*t*
Streptolysin, 769, 780
Stress
  hypertension and, 156
  toddler and, 332*t*
  website information on, 725
Stress management, 725
Stress testing, 516
Stroke, 791-792
Subarachnoid space, 839*f*
Subclavian artery, 833*f*
Subclavian pressure point, 794*f*
Subcutaneous injection, 475, 477*f*, 484-487, 507
Subcutaneous layer, 843*f*
Subcutaneous prepatellar bursa, 827*f*
Subdural space, 839*f*
Subjective data, 27
Subjective symptom, 36, 48
Sublingual administration, 507
Sublingual fold, 835*f*
Sublingual gland, 836*f*, 843*f*
Sublingual tablet, 441
Submandibular duct, 836*f*, 843*f*
Submandibular gland, 836*f*, 843*f*

Submandibular node, 834f
Subscription, 463-464, 507
Substage condenser, 760
Substance abuse
  drug testing in workplace and, 628
  website information on, 508
Sudafed. See Pseudoephedrine.
Sudden infant death syndrome, 374
Suffocation
  infant and, 338t
  school-age child and, 339t
Sulfamethoxazole, 447t
Sulfonamides, 447t, 643t
Sumatriptan, 448t
Sumycin. See Tetracycline.
Superficial burn, 799f, 799-800
Superficial cervical node, 834f
Superior articular facet, 827f
Superior articular process, 827f
Superior mesenteric artery, 833f
Superior vena cava, 513f, 832-833f
Supernatant, 657
Superscription, 463, 507
Supine position, 181-182, 568
Supplementary cephalic vein, 664f
Supplies on crash cart, 786-787t
Suppository, 441
Suppuration, 239, 269, 394
Suprapatellar bursa, 827f
Suprapubic aspiration, 617
Supraspinatus, 831f
Surgical asepsis, 378-380, 433
Surgical gut, 397
Surgical instrument cleaners, 92f, 92-93
Surgical instruments, 380-386, 381-385f
Surgical procedures, 377-433
  application of knowledge in, 430-431
  assisting physician in, 410-411f, 410-415
  bandaging in, 422-472, 423-425f, 425t
  certification review in, 431-432
  cervical punch biopsy in, 420-421, 421f
  colposcopy in, 419f, 419-420
  commercially prepared sterile packages for, 386, 387f
  cryosurgery in, 421f, 421-422
  incision and drainage of abscess in, 416-417, 417f
  ingrown toenail removal in, 418-419, 419f
  instruments used in, 380-386, 381-385f
  legal issues in, 428
  local anesthetics for, 408-410, 410f
  needle biopsy in, 417-418, 418f
  opening of sterile packages in, 390-391
  pouring of sterile solution in, 391
  sebaceous cyst removal in, 415-416, 416f
  sterile dressing change in, 394-397
  sterile gloves for, 387-389
  surgical asepsis for, 378-380
  sutures in, 397-407
    adhesive skin closures and, 401, 401f, 404-407
    insertion of, 398-400, 399f
    needles for, 398, 399f
    surgical skin staples and, 400f, 400-401
    suture size and packaging, 397
    types of, 397, 398f
  terminology review in, 433
  tray setup for, 407-408, 411
  website information on, 433
  wounds and, 392-393f, 392-394
Surgical skin staples, 400f, 400-401
Susceptible, term, 83, 780
Suspension, 441
Suspensory ligament of lens, 206, 207f, 842f
Sustained-release capsule, 441
Suture, 397-407, 433
  adhesive skin closures and, 401, 401f, 404-407
  insertion of, 398-400, 399f
  needles for, 398, 399f
  size and packaging for, 397
  surgical skin staples and, 400f, 400-401
  types of, 397, 398f
Suture scissors, 380, 381f
Swab, 765
Swaged needle, 398, 399f, 433
Sweat, 53
Sweat gland, 843f
Swing gaits, 263
Symbols used in medication documentation, 462t
Sympathetic nervous system, 839f
Symptom, 36, 48, 202
Synthetic cast, 251-252, 252f
Synthroid. See Levothyroxine.
Syphilis, 304, 743, 758
Syringe
  for parenteral injection, 471-472, 471-472f
  prefilled, 475, 475f, 476f
  safety engineered, 63f, 472, 473f, 474f
Syringe method of venipuncture, 682-685
Syrup, 441
Syrup of ipecac, 452t, 786t
Systemic corticosteroids, 451t
Systole, 150, 164
Systolic pressure, 150, 155t, 160, 164

T
T wave, 514f, 514-515
Tablespoon, 458, 458t
Tablet, 441
Tachycardia, 40, 143, 164
  paroxysmal atrial, 533
  sinus, 531
  ventricular, 535
Tachypnea, 145, 164
Tagamet. See Cimetidine.
Talus, 826f
Tapazole. See Methimazole.
Tape measure, 170t
Target heart rate, 143
Teaspoon, 458, 458t
Teething, 330t
Tegretol. See Carbamazepine.
Teldrin. See Chlorpheniramine.
Telephone transmission of electrocardiogram, 520
Temazepam, 454t
Temper tantrum, 332t
Temperature, 124-140
  alterations in, 126, 126f
  assessment sites for, 128
  aural, 129, 131, 138-140
  axillary, 128, 135-136
  blood donation and, 747
  fever and, 127-128, 128t
  growth of microorganisms and, 52
  in initial prenatal examination, 301t
  oral, 128, 133-135
  postpartal, 316t
  rectal, 128, 137-138
  regulation of, 124-125, 125f
  thermometers for, 129-130f, 129-132
  variations in, 126-127, 127t
Temperature conversion table, 126t
Temperature-sensitive strip, 132, 132f
Temporal bone, 826f, 842f
Temporal pressure point, 794f
Temporal pulse, 141f, 142
Temporalis, 829f
Tenaculum, 384, 385f
Tendon
  Achilles, 830-831f
  quadriceps, 827f
  rectus femoris, 829f
Tenormin. See Atenolol.
Tensor fasciae latae, 828f, 829f
Tentative diagnosis, 15
Tenuate. See Diethylpropion.
Terazol. See Terconazole.
Terbutaline, 785t
Terconazole, 445t
Teres major, 830f, 831f
Teres minor, 830f, 831f
Term birth, 298, 324
Terminology review
  in blood chemistry and serology, 753
  in cardiopulmonary procedures, 545
  in clinical laboratory, 611
  in colon procedures, 583
  in disinfection and sterilization, 120
  in emergency medical procedures, 812
  in eye and ear assessment, 235
  in hematology, 725
  in medical asepsis, 83
  in medication administration, 507
  in microbiology, 780
  in minor office surgery, 433
  in phlebotomy, 705
  in physical agents for tissue healing, 269
  in physical examination, 202
  in radiology and diagnostic imaging, 582
  in urinalysis, 657
  in vital signs, 164
Tessalon. See Benzonatate.
Test cable of Holter monitor, 526
Testicular cancer, 559-560
Testicular examination
  recommended frequency of, 169
  self-examination, 559-560, 560f
Testis, 838f, 843f
Tetracycline, 447t
Theophylline, 450t
Therapeutic effect, 467
Therapeutic procedure, 169
Therapeutic service documents, 12, 14f
Therapeutic ultrasound, 247-250, 248f
Thermal burn, 800
Thermolabile dye, 104, 120
Thermometer, 129-132, 130f, 132f, 170t
Thiazide diuretics, 451t
ThinPrep Pap Test, 278
Third-degree burn, 799f, 800
Thoracic curve, 827f
Thoracic duct, 834f
Thoracic nerves, 841f
Thoracic vertebrae, 827f
Thready pulse, 143, 164
Three-channel electrocardiograph, 512f, 519, 520f
Three-point gait, 262
Throat culture, 767
Thrombocyte, 712, 718t
Thrombocytopenia, 711t

Thrombocytosis, 711t
Thrombolytic agents, 454t
Thumb forceps, 380, 382f
Thumb sucking, 329t
Thymus, 834f, 843f
Thyroid, 843f
Thyroid cartilage, 832f
Thyroid function profile, 592t
Thyroid hormones, 454t
Thyroid preparations, 454-455t
Thyroxine, 589t
Tibia, 826f, 829f
Tibialis anterior, 828f, 829f
Tibialis posterior, 831f
Timing control of ultrasound machine, 247
Tincture, 441
Tine test, 491, 492, 500-502
Tine test, 489-492, 500-502
Tissue forceps, 380-381, 382f
Tissue healing, 237-269
  ambulatory aids in, 257-264
    canes in, 259, 259f, 264
    crutches in, 257-259, 258f, 259f, 260-263
    walkers in, 259f, 259-260, 264
  application of knowledge in, 267
  certification review in, 268
  fracture casting and, 251-254f, 251-255, 256f
  legal issues in, 265
  local application of heat and cold for, 238-246
    cold, 240-241, 244-246
    factors affecting, 238-239
    heat, 239, 240f, 241-243
  splints and braces in, 256, 256f, 257f
  terminology review in, 269
  therapeutic ultrasound in, 247-250, 248f
  website information on, 269
TobraDex. See Dexamethasone-tobramycin.
Tobramycin, 447t, 453t
Tobrex. See Tobramycin.
Toddler, 373
  anticipatory guidance for, 331-333t
  pulse rate of, 141t
  respiratory rates of, 145t
  safety guidelines for, 338t
  techniques for interaction with, 341t
  visual acuity in, 209
Toenail, ingrown, 418-419, 419f
Toilet training, 331-332t
Tolerance
  to change in temperature, 239
  drug, 467
Tongue, 832f, 835f, 836f
Tongue depressor, 170t
Tonic-clonic seizure, 801
Tonsil, 832f
Tooth, 835f
  evulsion of, 336t
Topical administration, 507
Toprol XL. See Metoprolol.
Total bilirubin, 732t
Total cholesterol, 730t, 734-735, 736
Total magnification, 761
Total protein, 589t, 732t
Total thyroxine, 589t
Tourniquet in venipuncture, 661-664, 663f, 677f
Towel clamp, 382, 384f
Toxemia, 295, 324
Toxoid, 373
Toxoplasmosis, 78t
Trabeculae, 827f
Trachea, 832f, 836f
Tramadol, 442t
Transabdominal ultrasound scan, 310
Transcutaneous electrical nerve stimulation. See TENS.
Transdermal contraceptives, 451t
Transdermal patch, 441
Transducer, 247
Transient flora, 54, 83
Transitional epithelial cell in urine, 637t
Transporting of specimen, 596-601, 598f
Transverse abdominis, 829f, 831f
Transverse colon, 836f
Transverse foramen, 827f
Transverse fracture, 797
Transverse process, 827f
Trapezius, 828-831f
Tray setup for surgical procedure, 407-408, 411
Treponema pallidum, 304, 758
Triamcinolone, 451t
Triamterene, 451t
Triceps brachii, 828f, 830f, 831f
Trichomonas vaginalis, 290, 291f
  prenatal testing for, 303
  in urine, 636, 644t
Tricuspid valve, 513f, 832f
Trigeminal nerve, 840f
Triglycerides, 589t, 733t
Trigone, 837f
Triiodothyronine, 589t
Trimester, 295, 324
Trimethoprim-sulfamethoxazole, 447t
Trimox. See Amoxicillin.
Tripedia. See Diphtheria, tetanus toxoids and acellular pertussis vaccine.
Triple phosphates, 641f
Triple screen test, 309
Tripod cane, 259
Tripod position in crutch stance, 261

Trochlear nerve, 840f
True ribs, 826f
Tubal tonsil, 832f
Tuberculin syringe, 472, 472f
Tuberculin test, 489-492, 500-502
Tuberculosis, 489-490
  in acquired immune deficiency syndrome, 78t
  antituberculars for, 449t
  website information on, 508
Tubex Injector, 476f
Tubular aluminum crutches, 260
Tubular gauze bandage, 425t, 425-427
Tumor cell in urine, 638t
Tumor in acquired immune deficiency syndrome, 77t
Tums. See Calcium carbonate.
Tuning fork, 170t, 223-224, 225f
Tussionex. See Chlorpheniramine-hydrocodone.
Twelve-lead, three-channel electrocardiogram, 524-526
Twenty-four-hour urine specimen, 618, 619-620
Two-hour postprandial blood sugar, 731t, 737
Two-point gait, 262
Tylenol. See Acetaminophen.
Tympanic membrane, 221, 221f, 235, 842f
Tympanic membrane thermometer, 129-130, 130f, 131, 138-140
Tympanogram, 226
Tympanometer, 226
Tympanometry, 226, 226f
Tyrosine crystals, 642t

U
U wave, 514f, 514-515
Ulna, 826f
Ulnar pulse, 141t, 142
Ultram. See Tramadol.
Ultrasonic cleaner, 92, 92f, 95
Ultrasonography, 573-574, 574f, 582
Ultrasound therapy, 247-250, 248f
Unconjugated estriol, 309
Unintentional injury
  infant and, 331t
  preschool child and, 335t
  toddler and, 333t
United Parcel Service, 48
United States Department of Health and Human Services, 202
United States Information Agency Gateway to Information on Substance Abuse, 657
United States Postal Service Zip Code Access, 48
Universal precautions, 68-69
Unsaturated fat, 735
Upper gastrointestinal series, 569-570
Upright balance scale, 170t, 175f, 175-176
Upright position, 342, 342f
Urea, 615
Ureter, 614, 614f, 837f
Ureteral orifice, 837f
Urethra, 614, 614f, 837-838f
Urgency, 616
Uric acid, 589t, 640t, 733t
Uricult, 649
Urinalysis, 11, 613-657
  application of knowledge in, 655
  certification review in, 656
  chemical examination of urine in, 625-629, 627t
  collection of urine for, 616-621, 618f
  composition of urine and, 615
  in initial prenatal examination, 303
  laboratory tests in, 603t
  legal issues in, 653
  microscopic examination of urine in, 635-649
    calibration of refractometer for, 624
    casts in urine sediment, 635, 638-639t, 640-641
    cells in urine sediment, 637-638t, 639-640
    Kova method of, 646-648
    measurement of urine specific gravity, 622-623
    microorganisms and artifacts in urine, 635-636, 644-645t
    urine crystals, 640-643t, 641
  normal values in, 589t
  physical examination of urine in, 621-623, 621f, 623f
  rapid urine cultures in, 649-650
  reagent strips for, 629-635, 630-631f, 632f, 644-645
  structure and function of urinary system and, 614, 614f, 615f
  terminology review in, 657
  urine pregnancy testing and, 651f, 651-653
  website information on, 657
Urinalysis laboratory request form, 617
Urinary bladder, 614, 614f, 837-838f
Urinary incontinence, 616
Urinary meatus, 614, 614f
Urinary system
  intravenous pyelography and, 572, 573f
  structure and function of, 614, 614f, 615f, 837-838f
  terms relating to, 616
  urine test strip parameters and, 630t

Urinary tract infection, 641
Urine
  chemical examination of, 625-629, 627*t*
  collection of, 616-621, 618*f*
  composition of, 615
  as defense mechanism, 53
  handling and storage of, 598*t*
  microscopic examination of, 635-649
    calibration of refractometer for, 624
    casts in urine sediment, 635, 638-639*t*,
      640-641
    cells in urine sediment, 637-638*t*, 639-640
    Kova method of, 646-648
    measurement of urine specific gravity,
      622-623
    microorganisms and artifacts in urine,
      635-636, 644-645*t*,
    urine crystals, 635, 640-643*t*,
  physical examination of, 621-623, 621*f*, 623*f*
Urine analyzer, 632*f*
Urine crystals, 635, 640-643*t*,
Urine drug testing, 628
Urine pregnancy testing, 651*f*, 651-653
Urine sediment, 632, 637-638*t*
Urine sediment casts, 638-639*t*
Urine specific gravity, 622-623
Urine specimen, 616-621
  clean-catch midstream, 616-617, 618*f*, 618-
    619
  first-voided morning, 616
  pediatric, 355-357
  for pregnancy test, 652
  random, 616
  twenty-four hour, 618, 619-620
Uristix, 627*t*
Urobilinogen, 626, 632*t*
Urochrome, 621
Urticaria, 467, 494*t*
US. See Ultrasonography.
Use life, 100
Uterine body cavity, 273*f*
Uterine curette, 385*f*
Uterine dressing forceps, 385*f*
Uterine sound, 385*f*, 386
Uterine tube, 838*f*
Uvula, 832*f*, 835-836*f*

V
Vaccine, 359, 373, 452-453*t*
Vaccine administration record, 366*f*
Vaccine Education Center, 374
Vacutainer-evacuated tube, 669*f*
Vacuum tube method of venipuncture, 667-
  675
  evacuated tubes for, 669*f*, 669-670
  guidelines for, 670-675, 671*f*
  needle for, 667, 667*f*, 668*f*
  order of draw for multiple tubes, 670
  plastic holder for, 668
  site selection for, 664*f*, 664-665, 666*f*
  types of blood specimens in, 665, 666*f*
Vagina, 273*f*, 838*f*
  discharge in gonorrhea, 292-293
  examination during pregnancy, 308, 308*f*
  infection of, 289-293
    candidiasis in, 291, 291*f*
    chlamydia in, 292, 293
    gonorrhea in, 292-293
    trichomoniasis in, 290, 291*f*
  inspection of, 276, 276*f*
  secretions as defense mechanism, 53
  specimen in Pap test, 277, 277*f*
Vaginal ring contraceptives, 451*t*
Vaginal speculum, 276, 276*f*
Vaginitis, 289
Vagus nerve, 840*f*
Valacyclovir, 450*t*
Valdecoxib, 448*t*
Valium. See Diazepam.
Valproic acid, 444*t*
Valsartan, 446*t*
Valtrex. See Valacyclovir.
Vancenase. See Beclomethasone.
Vancocin. See Vancomycin.
Vancomycin, 447*t*
Vaqta. See Hepatitis A vaccine.
Varicella vaccine, 453*t*
Varivax. See Varicella vaccine.
Vas deferens, 838*f*
Vascor. See Bepridil.
Vasodilators, 446*t*
Vasopressors, 455*t*
Vasotec. See Enalapril.
Vasovagal syncope, 688
Vastus intermedius, 829*t*
Vastus lateralis, 828*f*, 829*f*

Vastus lateralis intramuscular injection site,
  358, 358*f*, 478*f*, 478-479
Vastus medialis, 828*f*, 829*f*
Veetids. See Penicillin V.
Velcro-closure tourniquet, 663*f*, 663-664
Venereal Disease Research Laboratories, 743
Venipuncture, 660-692
  application of tourniquet in, 661-664, 663*f*
  butterfly method of, 676-677*f*, 676-682
  evacuated tubes for, 669*f*, 669-670
  guidelines for evacuated tube method of,
    670-675, 671*f*
  needle for, 667, 667*f*, 668*f*
  obtaining plasma specimen in, 691-692
  obtaining serum specimen in, 687-691, 689*f*
  order of draw for multiple tubes, 670
  OSHA safety precautions in, 666-668
  patient positioning for, 661, 662*f*
  patient preparation for, 661
  plastic holder for, 668
  problems encountered in, 686-687, 687*f*
  safety engineered devices, 667
  site selection for, 664*f*, 664-665, 666*f*
  syringe method of, 682-685
  types of blood specimens in, 665, 666*f*
Venous bleeding, 792
Venous blood, 712
Venous reflux, 661, 705
Venous stasis, 662, 705
Ventolin. See Albuterol.
Ventricular depolarization, 525
Ventricular fibrillation, 535
Ventricular fold, 832*f*
Ventricular repolarization, 525
Ventricular septum, 513*f*
Ventricular tachycardia, 535
Ventrogluteal site, 478*f*, 479
Venlafaxine, 444*t*
Verapamil, 443*t*, 785*t*
Verelan. See Verapamil.
Vermiform appendix, 836*f*
Vermox. See Mebendazole.
Vertebra, 839*f*
Vertebral foramen, 827*f*
Vertex, 373
Vertigo, 40
Vesication in Mantoux test, 491, 502
Vestibular nerve, 842*f*
Vestibule of ear, 221*f*, 842*f*
Vestibulocochlear nerve, 221*f*, 840*f*
Viagra. See Sildenafil.
Vial, 507
  drug preparation from, 472, 474*f*, 480-483
Vibramycin. See Doxycycline.
Vibrio cholera, 758
Vicodin. See Hydrocodone.
Vioxx. See Rofecoxib.
Viral hepatitis, 72, 73
Virtual Hospital, 202
Viruses, 450*t*, 758-759
Vistaril. See Hydroxyzine.
Visual acuity, 207-212
  distance, 208-210, 208-210*f*, 213-215
  near, 210-212, 211*f*
  in preschooler, 210, 210*f*
Visual acuity charts, 208
Visual axis, 842*f*
Vital signs, 123-165
  application of knowledge in, 162
  blood pressure in, 150-160
    cuff sizes for, 153, 153*f*, 154*t*
    Korotkoff sounds and, 153, 155*t*
    measurement of, 157-159
    mechanism of, 150-151, 151*t*
    palpation for determining systolic
      pressure, 160
    patient teaching in, 156
    pediatric, 354*t*, 354-355, 354-355*f*
    prevention of errors in measurement of,
      154
    sphygmomanometer for, 151-153, 152*f*,
      153*f*
    stethoscope for, 151, 151*t*, 152
  body temperature in, 124-140
    alterations in, 126, 126*f*
    assessment sites for, 128
    aural, 129, 131, 138-140
    axillary, 128, 135-136
    fever and, 127-128, 128*t*
    oral, 128, 133-135
    rectal, 128, 137-138
    regulation of, 124-125, 125*f*
    thermometers for, 129-130*f*, 129-132
    variations in, 126-127, 127*f*
  case studies in, 161
  certification review in, 163

Vital signs (*Continued*)
  in initial prenatal examination, 301*t*
  legal issues in, 160
  postpartal, 316*t*
  pulse in, 141*f*, 141-142*f*, 141-143
  respiration in, 144-149
    abnormalities in, 146-147
    breath sounds and, 147, 147*t*
    measurement of, 147-148
    mechanism of, 144-145, 144-145*f*
    patient color and, 146
    respiratory rate and, 145*t*, 145-146
    rhythm and depth of, 146
  terminology review in, 164
  website information on, 165
Vitreous humor, 207, 207*f*, 842*f*
Vocal cord, 836*f*
Vocal fold, 832*f*
Void, 657
Volkmann rake retractor, 384*f*
Volume, conversion charts for, 458-459*t*
Voluntary respiration, 145
Vomiting, 40, 445*t*
Vulva, 324

W
Waived tests, 601
Walker, 259*f*, 259-260, 264
Walking, body mechanics and, 247
Wandering baseline artifact, 522*f*, 523
Warfarin, 443*t*
Warning label, 63
Wart, 422
Wasp sting, 492, 803-804, 804*f*
Waste container, 70*t*
Waste disposal, 69-71, 70*t*, 71*f*
Waste products in plasma, 691
Waste receptacle, 170*t*
Water moccasin, 804-805
Water reservoir of autoclave, 111
Waves in electrocardiography, 514*f*, 514-515
Waxy casts, 639*t*, 640
WBC. See White blood cell count.
Web MD, 202
Weber test, 223, 225*f*
Website information
  on cardiopulmonary procedures, 545
  on colon procedures, 563
  on disinfection and sterilization, 120
  on emergency medicine, 812
  on medical asepsis, 83
  on medications, 508
  on microbiology, 780
  on minor office surgery, 433
  on phlebotomy, 705
  on physical agents for tissue healing, 269
  on physical examination, 202
  on radiology and diagnostic imaging,
    582
  on urinalysis, 657
  on vital signs, 165
Weight, 173-179, 174-176*t*
  blood donation and, 747
  conversion charts for, 458-459*t*
  female
    head circumference-for-age and weight-
      for-length percentiles, 349
    length-for-age and weight-for-age
      percentiles, 348
    stature-for-age and weight-for age
      percentiles, 352
  hypertension and, 156
  in initial prenatal examination, 301*t*
  male
    head circumference-for-age and weight-
      for-length percentiles, 351
    length-for-age and weight-for-age
      percentiles, 350
    stature-for-age and weight-for-age
      percentiles, 353
  measurement in child, 342, 344-345
  postpartal, 316*t*
Weight control
  for high blood cholesterol, 735
  website information on, 202
Weight control agents, 455*t*, 461*t*
Weight conversion, 175
Weight Watchers, 202
Well-child visit, 328
Wellbutrin-SR. See Bupropion.
Westergren's method, 711*t*
Wet mount method, 772, 772*f*
Wet preparation, 291*f*
Wharton's duct, 843*f*
Wheal, 489, 507
Wheezing, 147*t*

White blood cell, 718*f*
  in urine, 637*t*, 639
White blood cell casts, 632*t*
White blood cell count, 709*t*
Whole blood
  separating serum from, 689-691
  specimen of, 665
Winged infusion method of venipuncture,
  676-677*f*, 676-682
Witnessing of signature, 20
Wittner punch tip, 421*f*
Women's health, 272-325
  application of knowledge in, 319-320
  assisting with gynecologic examination, 286-
    289
  breast examination and, 274-275, 283-285
  certification review in, 321-322
  legal issues in, 317
  pelvic examination and, 275-289
    bimanual, 282, 283*f*
    inspection of external genitalia, vagina,
      and cervix in, 276, 276*f*
    Pap test and, 276-282, 277-278*f*, 280-281*f*,
      282*t*
    rectal-vaginal examination in, 282
  prenatal care and, 294-325
    amniocentesis in, 311*t*, 312, 312*f*
    fetal heart rate monitoring in, 312
    fetal heart tones and, 307*f*, 307-308
    fundal height measurement and, 306-307,
      306-307*f*
    gestational diabetes and, 305
    laboratory tests in, 302-305
    medical assisting responsibilities in, 312-315
    obstetric terminology in, 294-295
    obstetric ultrasound scan in, 309-310,
      310*f*, 310-311*f*
    patient education in, 302
    patient preparation in prenatal visit,
      301-302*t*
    prenatal record and, 295-300, 296-299*f*
    sex weeks-postpartum examination and,
      316, 316*t*
    triple screen test in, 309
    vaginal examination in, 308, 308*f*
  terminology review in, 323-324
  terms related to, 272-273, 273*f*
  vaginal infections and, 289-293
    candidiasis in, 291, 291*f*
    chlamydia in, 292, 293
    gonorrhea in, 292-293
    trichomoniasis in, 290, 291*f*
  website information on, 325
Wooden crutches, 260
Work practice controls, 64-65
World Health Organization, 780
Worm infection, 445*t*
Wound, 392-393*f*, 392-394, 433, 812
  direct pressure to, 794*f*, 793-794
  emergency care of, 794-796, 795*f*, 796*f*
Wound care, 393
Wound drainage, 394
Wound healing, 393
Wound specimen, 766
Wrapping articles, 105-109, 106*f*
Wrist veins, 666*f*

X
Xanax. See Alprazolam.
Xenical. See Orlistat.
Xiphoid process, 826*f*
Xylocaine. See Lidocaine.

Y
Yard, 457
Yeast, urinary, 635-636, 644*t*,
Yeast infection, 78*t*, 291, 291*f*
Yellow jacket sting, 492, 803-804, 804*f*

Z
Z-track injection method, 479, 479*f*, 488-489
Zafirlukast, 450*t*
Zantac. See Ranitidine.
Zestril. See Lisinopril.
Ziac. See Bisoprolol-hydrochlorothiazide.
Zidovudine, 449*t*
Zithromax. See Azithromycin.
Zocor. See Simvastatin.
Zofran. See Ondansetron.
Zoloft. See Sertraline.
Zolpidem, 454*t*
Zovirax. See Acyclovir.
Zygomatic, 828*f*, 830*f*
Zyloprim. See Allopurinol.
Zyprexa. See Olanzapine.
Zyrtec. See Cetirizine.